MOSBY'S TEXTBOOK FOR

Nursing Assistants

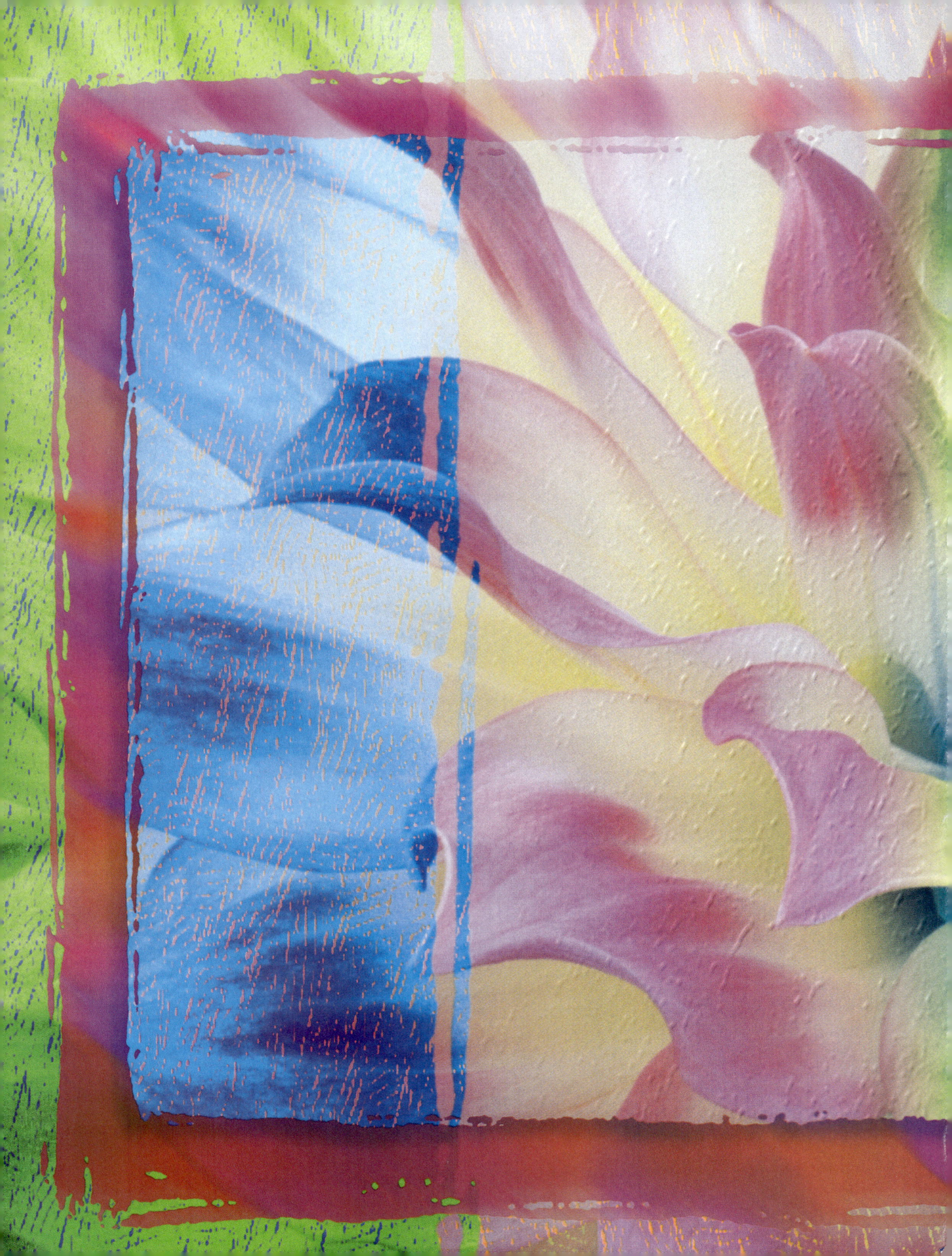

MOSBY'S TEXTBOOK FOR

Nursing Assistants

SHEILA A. SORRENTINO, R.N., PH.D.

Consultant and former Dean of Human Services and Career Education at Heartland Community College, Bloomington, IL

Mosby Lifeline

St. Louis Baltimore Boston Carlsbad Chicago Naples New York Philadelphia Portland
London Madrid Mexico City Singapore Sydney Tokyo Toronto Wiesbaden

Mosby Lifeline
Dedicated to Publishing Excellence

A Times Mirror Company

Publisher: David Dusthimer
Managing Editor: Doris Smith
Developmental Editor: Mary Beth Ryan Warthen
Assistant Editor: Elaine Wilburt
Project Manager: Chris Baumle
Production Editor: David Orzechowski
Book Design: Studio Montage
Artwork: Rick Brady, Vincent Knaus, Donald O'Connor

Fourth Edition

Printed in the United States of America

Mosby–Year Book, Inc.
11830 Westline Industrial Drive
St. Louis, MO 63146

Sorrentino, Sheila A.
Mosby's Textbook for Nursing Assistants / Sheila A. Sorrentino.--
4th ed.
p. cm.
Includes bibliographical references and index
ISBN 0-8151-8026-8
1. Nurses' Aides. 2. Care of the Sick. I. Title
[DNLM: 1. Nurses' Aides. 2. Nursing Care. WY 193 S714m 1995]
RT84.S67 1995
610.73′06′98--dc20
DNLM/DLC
for Library of Congress 95-43198
CIP

Dedication

To my sister, Sandra,
my best friend

Acknowledgments

Many individuals have contributed to the quality and comprehensiveness of the fourth edition of *Mosby's Textbook for Nursing Assistants.* Their insights, suggestions, and contributions are sincerely appreciated. I want specifically and publicly to acknowledge the following people at Heartland Community College in Bloomington, Illinois:

Katie Williams, reading specialist, for offering design and manuscript preparation ideas that make the book more readable, usable, and comfortable for students and instructors. She also provided information for the student preface.

Linda Hamilton, Director of Nursing, for being a consultant and for providing additional resources and insights.

Tammy Taylor, nursing assistant instructor, for reviewing parts of the manuscript and for being a consultant during manuscript preparation.

Johnna Darragh, Chair of the Division of Human Services and head of the college's Early Childhood Care and Education program, for reviewing Chapter 6 (Growth and Development) for currency and relevancy in today's society.

Jan Rampey, Academic Advisor/Special Needs and expert in signing. Jan provided resources and was a resource herself for Chapter 27 (Persons with Hearing and Vision Problems).

Dee Armsworth, my secretary while at Heartland Community College, for her patience, support, and assistance while I tried to do numerous things at one time.

My sincere appreciation is also extended to: Carol Miller, Employee Recruiter and Nursing Recruiter, St. Joseph's Medical Center, Bloomington, Illinois, for providing information on finding a job (job application and common interview questions). Carol also provided a sample job description and other documents used in manuscript development. Her contributions to Chapter 2 (The Nursing Assistant) will be most helpful to students in job searches.

Mark Burgess, D.M.D., for providing resources and advice on oral hygiene practices.

Steve Breinen, Sheriff of McLean County, Illinois, for providing information on personal safety in Chapter 35 (The Home Health Care Assistant).

W. Michael Shinkle, attorney and beloved friend, for providing resources and insights into the legal content included in this book.

The instructors and employers who wrote to us about the successes of their students and employees. Those success stories are featured in "Spotlight on..." boxes throughout the text.

The nursing assistants featured in "Spotlight on..." boxes. The work you do is important, and you now serve as role models to future nursing assistants across the country and throughout the world.

Debbie Fedor, my former secretary who returned to college to become a professional nurse, for serving as my research and secretarial assistant. She allowed me to use my time efficiently.

The manuscript reviewers for their candor and the many hours spent reading the manuscript. They have contributed to the thoroughness and accuracy of this book.

Relda Kelly for again writing the accompanying workbook and Eleanor Kirouff for doing the Instructor's Resource Kit and the Instructor's Guide.

Studio Montage for a vibrant and unique book design.

Connie Leinicke, colleague and trusted friend from the first edition, for returning to the project as copy editor.

Mary Beth Ryan Warthen and Elaine Wilburt, Mosby Lifeline, for their contributions to the development of the book, and Chris Baumle and Dave Orzechowski, Mosby–Year Book in Philadelphia for their production efforts.

David Dusthimer, Publisher, Mosby Lifeline, for his special interest in this book.

And finally, special thanks to Doris Smith, Managing Editor, Mosby Lifeline, for her friendship and dedication to this book. Her personal interest and ties to this book help to ensure its success. And to Richard Weimer, Editor-in-Chief, Mosby Lifeline; David Culverwell, Senior Vice-President, Mosby Lifeline; and Virgil Mette, President, Mosby Lifeline, for their remarkable vision.

Sheila A. Sorrentino

Preface to the Instructor

The fourth edition of *Mosby's Textbook for Nursing Assistants* is an exciting and comprehensive textbook and resource for nursing assistants and unlicensed assistive personnel in today's health care industry. Whether the outcome is employment in a hospital, long-term care facility, or home setting, this textbook serves the needs of students, instructors, and employees in clinical and home settings.

While retaining the features and organization of previous editions, considerable effort was made to make the fourth edition more inviting, appealing, readable, and usable for students and instructors. Attention was given to increasing the student's sensitivity to patients and residents being persons and to the importance of the nursing assistant's role in today's health care delivery systems. New standards and guidelines, scope of practice issues, and cross-training trends were major factors in content decisions. The following provide insight into this fourth edition of *Mosby's Textbook for Nursing Assistants.*

The Cover

The unique and inviting cover is intended to convey and appeal to a variety of emotions. The bright colors communicate excitement and stimulation; being a nursing assistant can be very exciting and stimulating. The shades of pink and red also convey warmth, for warmth along with caring and sensitivity are the very essence of the nursing assistant's role. The blues and greens symbolize calm. To bring calm to the bedside and to patient, resident, and family is also central to the nursing assistant's purpose. Come into this book, come into this world—that is what the cover invites.

Readability

Considerable attention was given to the readability of the fourth edition. On the advice of a reading specialist, the design features the following.

- Key terms with definitions remain at the beginning of each chapter and appear in bold print in the text where they are again defined.
- Procedure boxes are divided into preprocedure, procedure, and postprocedure steps. Besides labeling the sections, color gradients differentiate the sections.
- The review question and answer format was modified. Answers appear at the back of the book while the review questions remain at the end of each chapter.
- Boxes are used for the listing of principles, rules, signs and symptoms, and other information. The boxes present an efficient way for instructors to highlight content and provide useful study guides for students.
- Content and illustrations from Chapter 5 (Body Structure and Function) are repeated in appropriate chapters throughout the text. For example, Chapter 10 (Body Mechanics) begins with a review of the musculoskeletal system.
- Bullets are used for each item in a list rather than numbering.

Scope of Practice

Besides new standards and guidelines, content selected for inclusion in the fourth edition was based on state curricula, a survey of randomly selected instructors across the United States, comments made to sales representatives, and reviewer comments. Careful attention was given to the scope of nursing assistant practice and nursing and health care delivery trends. Safe nursing assistant practice, while acknowledging that scope of practice may be expanded in some areas, remains an emphasis of this and previous editions of *Mosby's Textbook for Nursing Assistants.*

Valuing the Person

This edition also emphasizes the desirable qualities of a nursing assistant. The importance of caring and treating the patient or resident as a person are important messages throughout this book. The words "person" or "persons" are used whenever possible in reference to the individual to instill the value that the recipient of care is more than a "patient" or a "resident." When necessary in relation to specific content, "patient" and/or "resident" are used.

Spotlight on…

The nursing assistant's role and self-esteem were also important considerations in the development of the fourth edition. While the author and instructors can say that the role is important and the nursing assistant is valued, more effective avenues are role modeling, supervisor appreciation, and nursing team attitude. Therefore instructors and facility staff were asked to share the success stories of exemplary nursing assistants. Those success stories are featured throughout the book in "Spotlight on..." boxes to support the role and enhance the self-esteem of nursing assistants.

Culture

Nursing assistants come from various cultural groups and care for persons of different cultures. Because nursing assistants need to appreciate the significance of cultural diversity and how culture influences health and illness practices, the importance of culture is integrated throughout this book. The following cultural practices of the top 10 countries of origin of immigrants to the United States (based on information from the U.S. Department of Immigration and Naturalization Services) appear in box format.

- Health care belief
- Sick care practices
- Touch practices
- Eye contact practices
- Family roles in hospital care
- Food practices
- Pain reactions
- Death rites

New Content and Chapters

The fourth edition of *Mosby's Textbook for Nursing Assistants* contains new chapters, new content, and expanded information. Like scope of practice, content selected for inclusion was based on new standards and guidelines, instructor surveys and comments, state curricula, and trends in nursing practice and health care delivery. The new chapters are:

- Personal Care and Grooming
- Comfort, Rest, and Sleep
- Persons with Vision and Hearing Problems
- Mental Health Problems

Expanded and new content include the following:

- Case management, health care system, managed care
- Becoming employed (finding a job, what employers look for, sample job application, interview questions, completing a job application, and grooming and dressing for the interview)
- Cross-training (introduced in Chapter 2 and integrated throughout the text)
- International time (introduced in Chapter 3 and integrated throughout the text with 12: hour time in parentheses)
- Nursing process (introduced in Chapter 3 and integrated throughout the text)
- Techniques for effective communication (listening, paraphrasing, direct questions, open-ended questions, clarifying, focusing, and silence)
- Extensive revised coverage of restraints
- Restraint alternatives
- Nosocomial infection
- Bloodborne pathogen standard (introduced in Chapter 9 and integrated throughout text)
- OBRA Requirements for Resident Rooms
- Expanded content on urinary incontinence
- Expanded content on fecal impaction
- Testing stools for blood
- Food Guide Pyramid
- OBRA dietary requirements
- High-sodium foods
- Tympanic thermometer
- Recreational activities
- Expanded coverage of IV therapy
- Binders and bandages
- Expanded coverage on the person having surgery (wound healing, early ambulation, nutrition and fluids, elimination, comfort and rest, personal hygiene)
- OBRA requirements for rehabilitation
- Signing
- Total joint replacement under arthritis
- Aphasia
- Tuberculosis
- Risk factors for hypertension
- Disorders of the urinary system (urinary tract infection, renal calculi, renal failure)
- Type I and type II diabetes
- Expanded AIDS content
- Expanded content on Alzheimer's disease
- Legal aspects of dying (Patient Self-Determination Act, living wills, durable power of attorney, "Do not resuscitate" orders)
- Food labels
- Personal safety for home health care assistants

Nursing Process

Because of its importance to nursing practice and its role in communicating the person's needs and care to the nursing team, the nursing process was included in the fourth edition. The purpose and components of the nursing process are presented in Chapter 3 (Communicating in the Health Care Facility). Thereafter, the nursing process is integrated throughout the text. Students using this text will be better able to understand and use the nursing process if they choose to access career ladder nursing programs for upward career mobility.

Cross-Training

Patient-focused care and the cross-training of personnel are trends in today's health care industry. The student is introduced to the purpose of cross-training to the person as a recipient of health care, the health care facility, and to the potential or current employee. Throughout the text the student is acquainted with cross-training opportunities that may be interesting or beneficial to his or her employment status.

Intended for use in community colleges, technical colleges, high schools, vocational-career centers, hospitals, long-term care facilities, home care agencies, and other agencies educating nursing assistants and unlicensed assistive personnel, the book focuses on safe and effective functioning when giving nursing care to persons in a variety of settings. It also incorporates the Omnibus Budget Reconciliation Act (OBRA) of 1987 guidelines for nursing assistant education. A resource for students in preparing for competency evaluations, the book also is a reference for the expansion of skills and knowledge.

With instruction being a primary purpose, *Mosby's Textbook for Nursing Assistants* is organized to accommodate variability in program length among curricula and instructor choice in the order of content presentation. The instructor can select which chapters or parts of chapters to include based on state requirements and the order of presentation. For example, an instructor may begin a course with infection control, body mechanics, bedmaking, and giving a bed bath. The appropriate chapters and sections of this book can be assigned for reading in the above order without jeopardizing content or learning. Or the instructor may choose to present the structure and function of a body system when students study a particular content area. For example, the instructor may want to introduce the cardiovascular and respiratory systems when students study vital signs. The instructor can assign reading from Chapter 5 (Body Structure and Function) or assign the body structure and function section in Chapter 18 (Measurement of Vital Signs). The fourth edition of *Mosby's Textbook for Nursing Assistants* retains values and principles that were integral to the organization and success of previous editions. They include:

- Safe functioning within the scope of practice of nursing assistants while recognizing that the scope of practice may vary among states.
- Respect for the person and recognition that each person is a physical, psychological, and spiritual human being with basic needs.
- The importance of personal choice and dignity of the person.
- The need for nursing assistants to be aware of and understand their work environment and the individuals in that environment.
- That understanding body structure and function and normal growth and development are helpful for developing desirable attitudes toward individuals and for performing nursing skills safely and competently.
- Learning proceeds from the simple to the complex. Those concepts and procedures integral to other activities and functions (safety, body mechanics, and medical asepsis) are presented early. Those skills that are easy to learn and basic to the role of nursing assistants are then presented (bedmaking, personal care, certain urinary and bowel elimination procedures, measuring intake and output, serving food trays, and feeding persons). More complex content is then presented. Measuring vital signs, the application of heat and cold, and care of surgical patients are more complex in regard to learning and safe practice and may not be nursing assistant functions in all facilities.

The following instructional supplements are available for use by you and/or your students:

- Instructor's Resource kit
- Instructor's Guide
- Student Workbook to accompany the text
- Student Education Evaluation Disk (SEED)

The editors at Mosby Lifeline and I believe that this fourth edition will serve you and your students well. We hope that safe care, respect for the person, and enhanced nursing assistant self-esteem will be outcomes of the learning experience.

Sheila A. Sorrentino

Preface for the Student

This book was designed for you. It was designed to help you learn. After completing your education program, you can use the book to study for the competency evaluation. Also, the book is a useful resource as you gain experience and expand your knowledge.

This preface gives some study guidelines and helps you use the book. When given a reading assignment, do you read from the first page to the last page without stopping? How much do you remember? You will learn more if you use a study system. A useful study system has these steps:

- Preview (or survey)
- Question
- Read and record
- Recite and review

Preview

Before you start a reading assignment, preview or survey the assignment. This will give you an idea of what the assignment covers. It also helps you recall what you already know about the subject. Carefully look over the assignment. Preview the chapter title, headings, subheadings, and terms or ideas in bold print or italics. Also survey the objectives, key terms, first paragraph, boxes, summary, and review questions at the end of the chapter. Previewing only takes a few minutes. Remember, previewing helps you become familiar with the material.

Question

After previewing, you need to form questions to answer while you read. Questions should relate to what might be asked on a test or how the information applies to giving care. Use the title, headings, and subheadings to form questions. Avoid questions that have one-word answers. Questions that begin with what, how, or why are helpful. While reading, you may find that a question does not help you study. If so, just change the question. Remember, questioning sets a purpose for reading. So changing a question only makes this step more useful.

Read and Record

Reading is the next step. Reading is more productive after determining what you already know and what you need to learn. Read to find answers to your questions. The purpose of reading is to:

- Gain new information
- Connect the new information to what you know already

Break the assignment into smaller parts. Then answer your questions as you read each part. Also, mark important information. The information can be marked by underlining, highlighting, or making notes. Underlining and highlighting remind you what you need to learn. You need to go back and review the marked parts later. Making notes results in more immediate learning. When making notes, you write down important information in the margins or in a notebook. Use words and summary statements that will jog your memory about the material.

After reading the assignment, you need to remember the information. To remember the material, you must work with the information. This step involves organizing information into a study guide. Study guides have many forms. Diagrams or charts help show relationships or steps in a process. Much of the information in this text is organized in this manner to help you learn. Note taking in outline format is also very useful. The following is a sample outline.

I. Main heading
  A. Second level
  B. Second level
    1. Third level
    2. Third level

Recite and Review

Finally, recite and review. Use your notes and the study guides. Answer the questions you formed earlier. Also answer any other questions that came up during the reading and the review questions at the end of the chapter. Answer all questions out loud (recite).

Reviewing is more about when to study rather than what to study. You already determined what to study during the preview, question, and reading steps. The best times to review the material are right after the first study session, 1 week later, and regularly before a test, midterm, or final exam.

The editors at Mosby Lifeline and I want you to enjoy learning. We also want you to enjoy your work as a nursing assistant. You and your work are important. You and the care you give may be

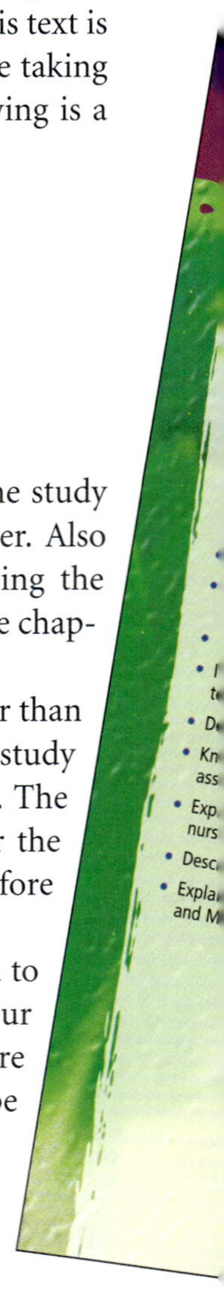

bright spots in a person's day. The book's cover was designed to convey and appeal to many emotions. The bright colors communicate excitement and stimulation; being a nursing assistant can be very exciting and stimulating. The shades of pink and red also convey warmth, for warmth along with caring and sensitivity are the very essence of your role. The blues and greens symbolize calm. To bring calm to the person and family is also central to your purpose as a nursing assistant. Come into this book, come into this world—this is our invitation to you.

This book was also designed to help you study. Special design features are described on the next pages. Objectives tell you what will be presented and what you need to learn.

Bold type is used to highlight the key terms in the text. You again see the key term and read its definition. This helps reinforce your learning.

Key terms are the important words and phrases in the chapter. Definitions are given for each term. The key terms introduce you to the chapter content. They are also useful study guides.

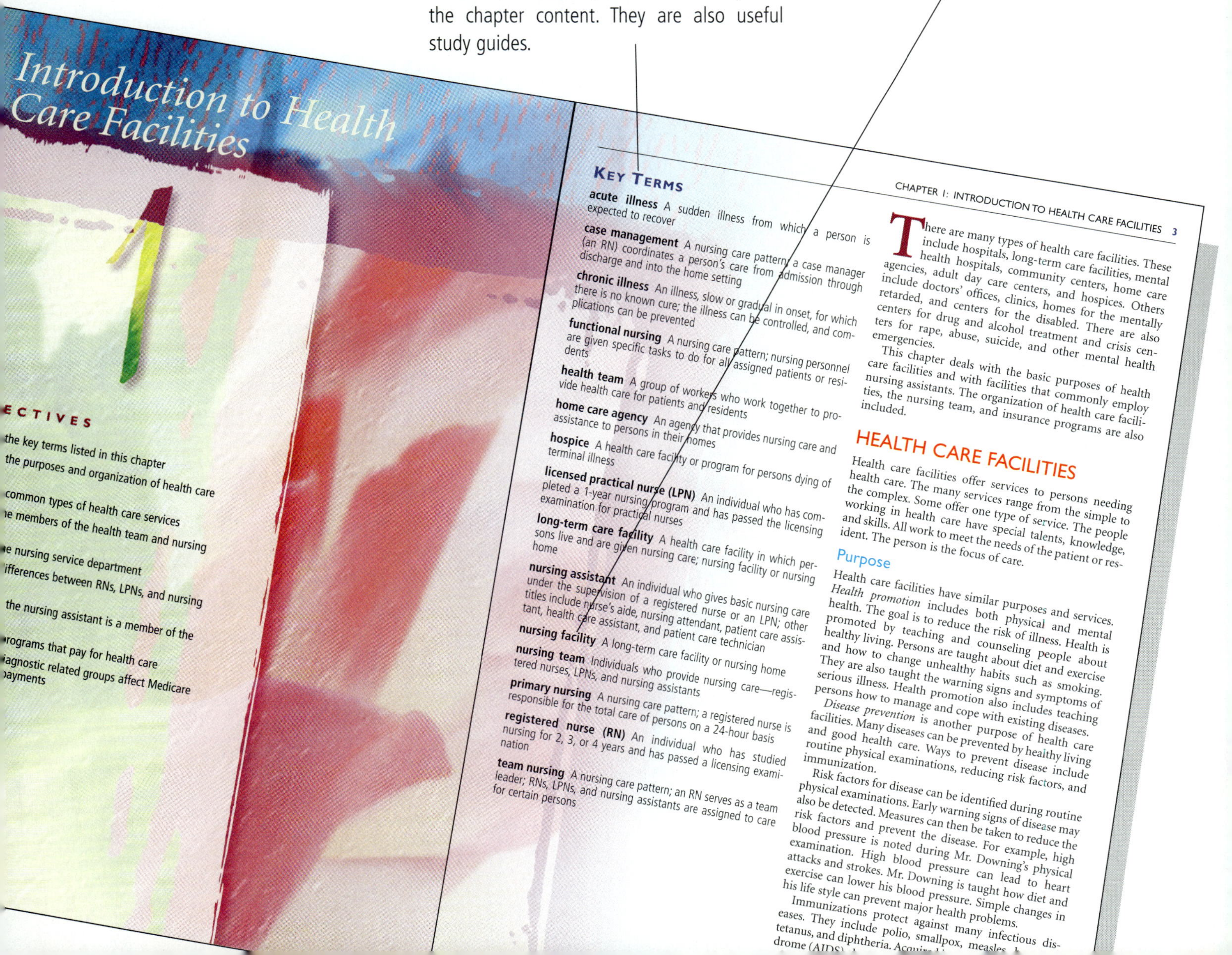
Introduction to Health Care Facilities

1

ECTIVES

the key terms listed in this chapter
the purposes and organization of health care
common types of health care services
he members of the health team and nursing
e nursing service department
ifferences between RNs, LPNs, and nursing
the nursing assistant is a member of the
rograms that pay for health care
iagnostic related groups affect Medicare
ayments

KEY TERMS

acute illness A sudden illness from which a person is expected to recover

case management A nursing care pattern; a case manager (an RN) coordinates a person's care from admission through discharge and into the home setting

chronic illness An illness, slow or gradual in onset, for which there is no known cure; the illness can be controlled, and complications can be prevented

functional nursing A nursing care pattern; nursing personnel are given specific tasks to do for all assigned patients or residents

health team A group of workers who work together to provide health care for patients and residents

home care agency An agency that provides nursing care and assistance to persons in their homes

hospice A health care facility or program for persons dying of terminal illness

licensed practical nurse (LPN) An individual who has completed a 1-year nursing program and has passed the licensing examination for practical nurses

long-term care facility A health care facility in which persons live and are given nursing care; nursing facility or nursing home

nursing assistant An individual who gives basic nursing care under the supervision of a registered nurse or an LPN; other titles include nurse's aide, nursing attendant, patient care assistant, health care assistant, and patient care technician

nursing facility A long-term care facility or nursing home

nursing team Individuals who provide nursing care—registered nurses, LPNs, and nursing assistants

primary nursing A nursing care pattern; a registered nurse is responsible for the total care of persons on a 24-hour basis

registered nurse (RN) An individual who has studied nursing for 2, 3, or 4 years and has passed a licensing examination

team nursing A nursing care pattern; an RN serves as a team leader; RNs, LPNs, and nursing assistants are assigned to care for certain persons

CHAPTER 1: INTRODUCTION TO HEALTH CARE FACILITIES 3

There are many types of health care facilities. These include hospitals, long-term care facilities, mental health hospitals, community centers, home care agencies, adult day care centers, and hospices. Others include doctors' offices, clinics, homes for the mentally retarded, and centers for the disabled. There are also centers for drug and alcohol treatment and crisis centers for rape, abuse, suicide, and other mental health emergencies.

This chapter deals with the basic purposes of health care facilities and with facilities that commonly employ nursing assistants. The organization of health care facilities, the nursing team, and insurance programs are also included.

HEALTH CARE FACILITIES

Health care facilities offer services to persons needing health care. The many services range from the simple to the complex. Some offer one type of service. The people working in health care have special talents, knowledge, and skills. All work to meet the needs of the patient or resident. The person is the focus of care.

Purpose

Health care facilities have similar purposes and services. *Health promotion* includes both physical and mental health. The goal is to reduce the risk of illness. Health is promoted by teaching and counseling people about healthy living. Persons are taught about diet and exercise and how to change unhealthy habits such as smoking. They are also taught the warning signs and symptoms of serious illness. Health promotion also includes teaching persons how to manage and cope with existing diseases.

Disease prevention is another purpose of health care facilities. Many diseases can be prevented by healthy living and good health care. Ways to prevent disease include routine physical examinations, reducing risk factors, and immunization.

Risk factors for disease can be identified during routine physical examinations. Early warning signs of disease may also be detected. Measures can then be taken to reduce the risk factors and prevent the disease. For example, high blood pressure is noted during Mr. Downing's physical examination. High blood pressure can lead to heart attacks and strokes. Mr. Downing is taught how diet and exercise can lower his blood pressure. Simple changes in his life style can prevent major health problems.

Immunizations protect against many infectious diseases. They include polio, smallpox, measles, tetanus, and diphtheria. Acqui... drome (AIDS)...

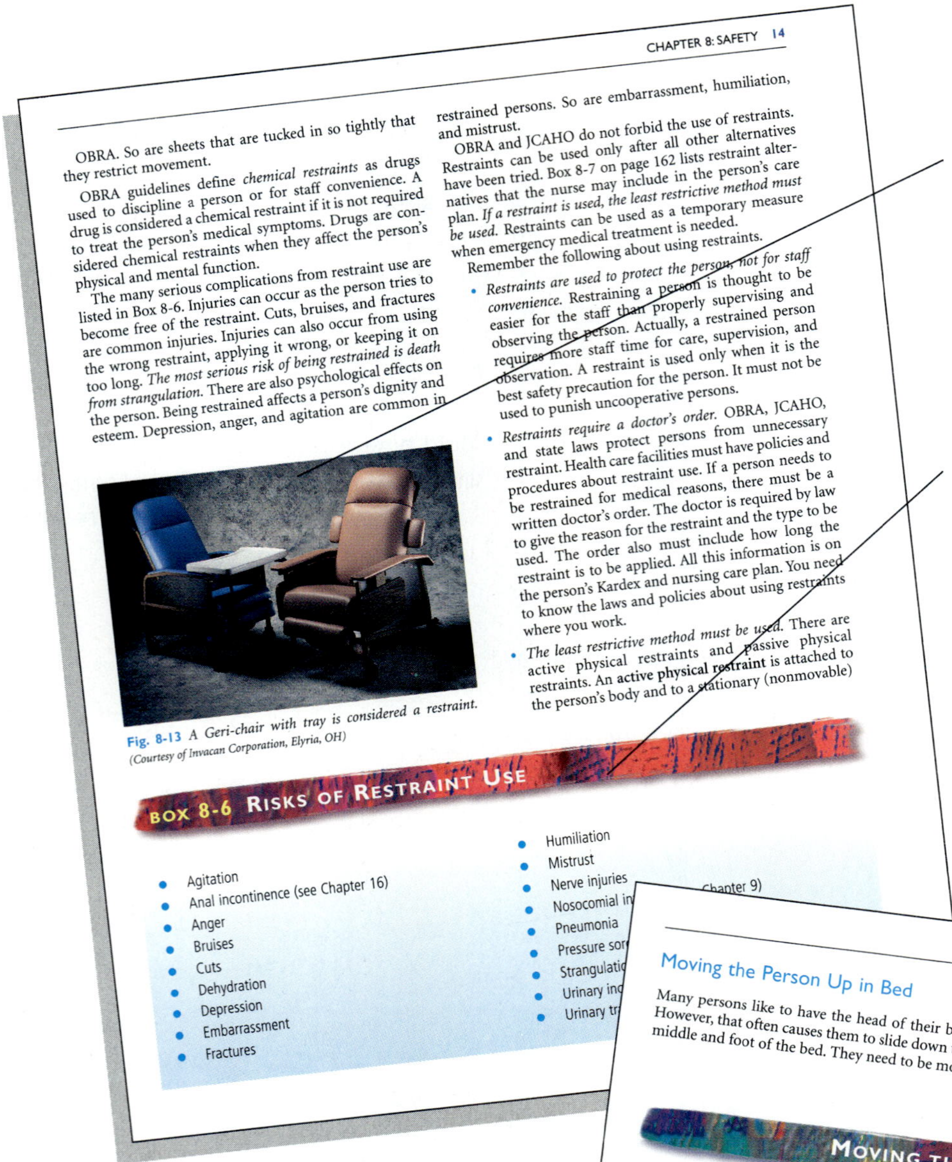
CHAPTER 8: SAFETY 14

OBRA. So are sheets that are tucked in so tightly that they restrict movement.

OBRA guidelines define *chemical restraints* as drugs used to discipline a person or for staff convenience. A drug is considered a chemical restraint if it is not required to treat the person's medical symptoms. Drugs are considered chemical restraints when they affect the person's physical and mental function.

The many serious complications from restraint use are listed in Box 8-6. Injuries can occur as the person tries to become free of the restraint. Cuts, bruises, and fractures are common injuries. Injuries can also occur from using the wrong restraint, applying it wrong, or keeping it on too long. *The most serious risk of being restrained is death from strangulation.* There are also psychological effects on the person. Being restrained affects a person's dignity and esteem. Depression, anger, and agitation are common in restrained persons. So are embarrassment, humiliation, and mistrust.

OBRA and JCAHO do not forbid the use of restraints. Restraints can be used only after all other alternatives have been tried. Box 8-7 on page 162 lists restraint alternatives that the nurse may include in the person's care plan. *If a restraint is used, the least restrictive method must be used.* Restraints can be used as a temporary measure when emergency medical treatment is needed.

Remember the following about using restraints.

- *Restraints are used to protect the person, not for staff convenience.* Restraining a person is thought to be easier for the staff than properly supervising and observing the person. Actually, a restrained person requires more staff time for care, supervision, and observation. A restraint is used only when it is the best safety precaution for the person. It must not be used to punish uncooperative persons.
- *Restraints require a doctor's order.* OBRA, JCAHO, and state laws protect persons from unnecessary restraint. Health care facilities must have policies and procedures about restraint use. If a person needs to be restrained for medical reasons, there must be a written doctor's order. The doctor is required by law to give the reason for the restraint and the type to be used. The order also must include how long the restraint is to be applied. All this information is on the person's Kardex and nursing care plan. You need to know the laws and policies about using restraints where you work.
- *The least restrictive method must be used.* There are active physical restraints and passive physical restraints. An **active physical restraint** is attached to the person's body and to a stationary (nonmovable)

Fig. 8-13 A Geri-chair with tray is considered a restraint. (*Courtesy of Invacan Corporation, Elyria, OH*)

BOX 8-6 RISKS OF RESTRAINT USE

- Agitation
- Anal incontinence (see Chapter 16)
- Anger
- Bruises
- Cuts
- Dehydration
- Depression
- Embarrassment
- Fractures
- Humiliation
- Mistrust
- Nerve injuries
- Nosocomial in… Chapter 9)
- Pneumonia
- Pressure sor…
- Strangulatio…
- Urinary inc…
- Urinary tr…

Color illustrations and photographs visually present a key idea, concept, or procedure step. They help you apply and remember the written material.

Boxes and tables contain important rules, principles, guidelines, signs and symptoms, and other information in a list format. They identify important information and are useful study guides for reviewing.

Procedures are written in a step-by-step format. They are divided into preprocedure, procedure, and postprocedure sections for easy studying.

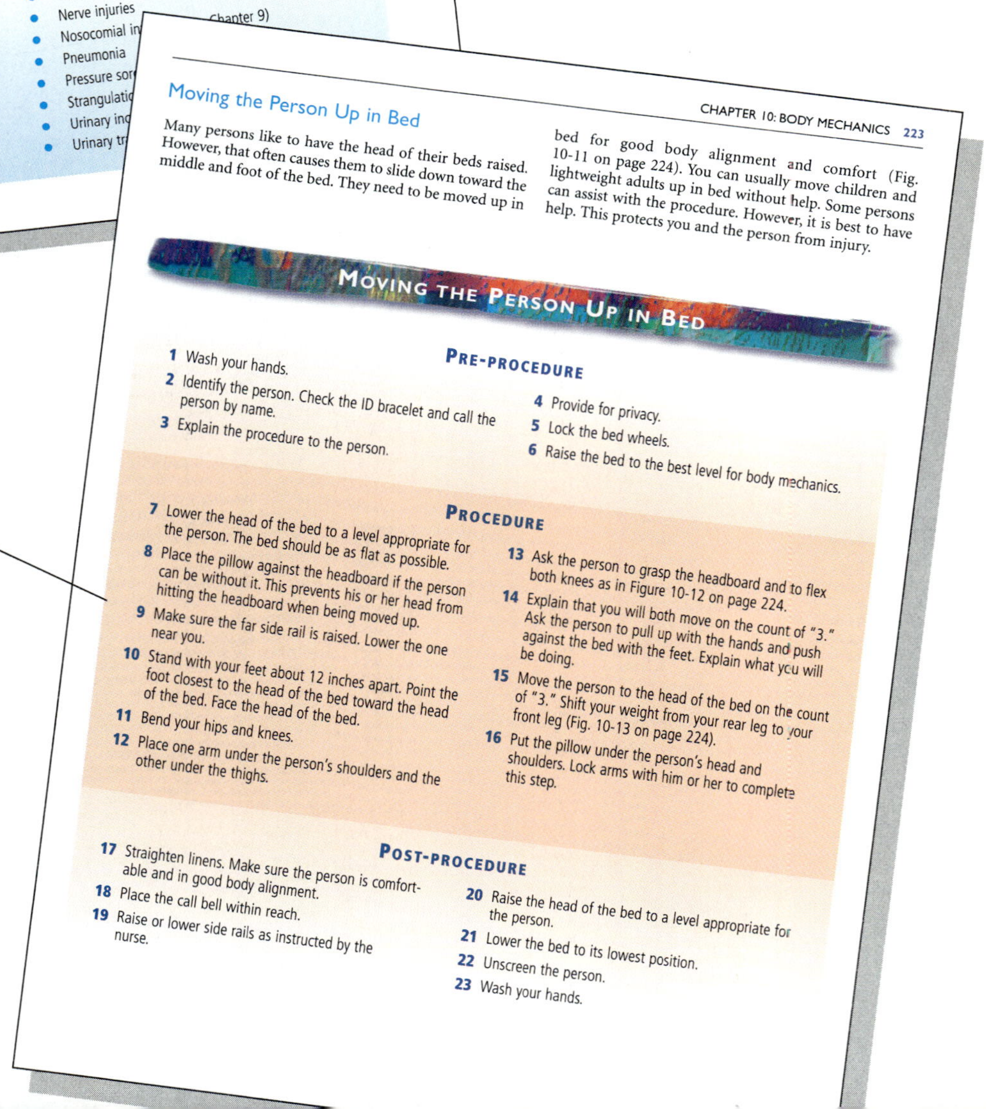
CHAPTER 10: BODY MECHANICS 223

Moving the Person Up in Bed

Many persons like to have the head of their beds raised. However, that often causes them to slide down toward the middle and foot of the bed. They need to be moved up in bed for good body alignment and comfort (Fig. 10-11 on page 224). You can usually move children and lightweight adults up in bed without help. Some persons can assist with the procedure. However, it is best to have help. This protects you and the person from injury.

MOVING THE PERSON UP IN BED

PRE-PROCEDURE

1 Wash your hands.
2 Identify the person. Check the ID bracelet and call the person by name.
3 Explain the procedure to the person.
4 Provide for privacy.
5 Lock the bed wheels.
6 Raise the bed to the best level for body mechanics.

PROCEDURE

7 Lower the head of the bed to a level appropriate for the person. The bed should be as flat as possible.
8 Place the pillow against the headboard if the person can be without it. This prevents his or her head from hitting the headboard when being moved up.
9 Make sure the far side rail is raised. Lower the one near you.
10 Stand with your feet about 12 inches apart. Point the foot closest to the head of the bed toward the head of the bed. Face the head of the bed.
11 Bend your hips and knees.
12 Place one arm under the person's shoulders and the other under the thighs.
13 Ask the person to grasp the headboard and to flex both knees as in Figure 10-12 on page 224.
14 Explain that you will both move on the count of "3." Ask the person to pull up with the hands and push against the bed with the feet. Explain what you will be doing.
15 Move the person to the head of the bed on the count of "3." Shift your weight from your rear leg to your front leg (Fig. 10-13 on page 224).
16 Put the pillow under the person's head and shoulders. Lock arms with him or her to complete this step.

POST-PROCEDURE

17 Straighten linens. Make sure the person is comfortable and in good body alignment.
18 Place the call bell within reach.
19 Raise or lower side rails as instructed by the nurse.
20 Raise the head of the bed to a level appropriate for the person.
21 Lower the bed to its lowest position.
22 Unscreen the person.
23 Wash your hands.

Spotlight on... are the success stories of nursing assistants. They were written by instructors and supervisors. They show that you and your role as a nursing assistant are important.

428 MOSBY'S TEXTBOOK FOR NURSING ASSISTANTS

are divided into columns. Patient or resident names are written down the left side of the page. The other columns are for times of day (such as 0800, 1200, 1600, 2000). Vital signs are recorded on the line in the column appropriate for the person and time. In some facilities, changed or abnormal vital signs are circled in red. Besides recording them, verbally report changed or abnormal vital signs to the nurse right away. The nurse or doctor compares the current measurements with previous ones.

BODY TEMPERATURE

Body temperature is the amount of heat in the body. It is a balance between the amount of heat produced and the amount lost by the body. Heat is produced as food is used for energy. It is lost through the skin, breathing, urine, and feces. Body temperature remains fairly stable. It is lower in the morning and higher in the afternoon and evening. Factors affecting body temperature include age, weather, exercise, pregnancy, the menstrual cycle, emotions, stress, and illness.

Normal Body Temperature

The Fahrenheit (F) and Centigrade or Celsius (C) scales are used to measure temperature. Common sites for measuring body temperature are the mouth, rectum, axilla (underarm), and ear (tympanic). Normal body temperature depends on the site.

- Oral—98.6° F (37° C)
- Rectal—99.6° F (37.5° C)
- Axillary—axillary temperature is 97.6° F (36.5° C)
- Tympanic—98.6° F (37° C)

A person may have a temperature higher or lower than these measurements. That temperature may be normal for that person.

Body temperature usually stays within a normal range. Normal ranges of body temperature for healthy adults are:

- Oral—97.6° to 99.6° F (36.5° to 37.5° C)
- Rectal—98.6° to 100.6° F (37.0° to 38.1° C)
- Axillary (underarm)—96.6° to 98.6° F (36.0° to 37.0° C)
- Tympanic (ear)—98.6° F (37° C)

The... are used to measure temperature. Glass ...rmometers are common in homes. So ...mometers. Electronic and tympanic ...common in hospitals and nursing

Spotlight On...

Heather R of Atlanta, Georgia, completed the nursing course at the Atlanta Job Corps Center. She then entered a work experience program in a doctor's office. During her work experience she was cross-trained to perform electrocardiograms, blood glucose tests, and venous punctures. After completing her work experience, Heather's interest is working as a home health aide.

Glass Thermometers

The glass thermometer (clinical thermometer) is a hollow glass tube with a mercury-filled bulb. When heated by the body, the mercury expands and rises in the tube. The mercury contracts and moves down the tube when cooled.

There are three types of glass thermometers. Each has a different bulb or tip (Fig. 18-1). Long- or slender-tip thermometers are used for oral and axillary temperatures. So are thermometers with stubby and pear-shaped tips. Rectal thermometers have stubby tips that are color coded in red. Glass thermometers have a Fahrenheit or Centigrade scale. Some have both scales.

Glass thermometers can be reused after disinfection. However, they have the following disadvantages:

- They take a long time to register—3 to 10 minutes depending on the site used. Oral temperatures take 2 to 3 minutes, rectal temperatures take at least 2 minutes, and axillary temperatures take 5 to 10 minutes.
- They break easily.
- When used orally, there is the danger of the person biting down on the thermometer and causing it to break. The broken glass can cut the mucous membranes of the mouth. Any swallowed mercury can cause mercury poisoning.
- Broken rectal thermometers can injure the rectum and colon.

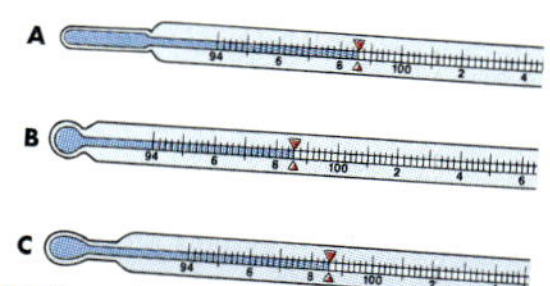

Fig. 18-1 *Types of glass thermometers.* ***A,*** *The long or slender tip.* ***B,*** *The stubby tip (rectal thermometer).* ***C,*** *The pear-shaped tip.*

Summaries at the end of the chapter identify important content and review what you have learned.

CHAPTER 2: THE NURSING ASSISTANT 41

SUMMARY

This chapter has presented many important considerations about your role as a nursing assistant. The important qualities and characteristics of nursing assistants and the importance of health, hygiene, and personal appearance have been presented. You also learned about the nursing assistant training and competency evaluation program, registry, and other OBRA requirements. You were also given information about how to find a job and how to work well with others.

An important part of this chapter is the legal and ethical aspects of your role. You have learned about what you can and cannot do both legally and ethically. What you do and how you do it affects you, your patients and residents, and your co-workers. All are affected both personally and legally. You have an important role, and you are a special person for wanting to be a nursing assistant. Use common sense, and act in a reasonable and careful manner. Respect your patients and residents, and enjoy your work!

REVIEW QUESTIONS

Circle the best answer.

1 Which is *false?*
- **a** Nurses supervise your work.
- **b** You assist nurses in giving care.
- **c** You must perform all tasks and procedures as directed by the nurse.
- **d** A job description serves as a guide for your roles and responsibilities.

2 All health care facilities have nursing assistants perform the same procedures and tasks.
- **a** True
- **b** False

3 Linda Ames is a nursing assistant. An RN asks her to perform the following functions. Which can she do?
- **a** Give Mr. Adams his medications
- **b** Supervise a co-worker
- **c** Take a telephone order from Dr. Gilson
- **d** Measure Ms. Parker's blood pressure

4 The doctor orders several laboratory tests for a resident. The resident wants to know why. Who is responsible for telling the resident?
- **a** The doctor
- **b** You are
- **c** The nurse
- **d** Any health team member

5 You are getting ready for work. Which should you *not* do?
- **a** Press and mend your uniform
- **b** Wear your name badge or photo ID
- **c** Wear jewelry
- **d** Style your hair so it is up and off the collar

6 Linda Ames applied for a job at West Bay Nursing Home. She got a copy of the nursing assistant job description. When should she ask questions about the job description?
- **a** After she completes the application
- **b** Before she completes the application
- **c** When her interview is scheduled
- **d** During the interview

7 Nursing assistant training and competency evaluation are required in all 50 states. What law requires this?
- **a** Civil law
- **b** Criminal law
- **c** Tort law
- **d** The Omnibus Reconciliation Act

8 Nursing assistant training programs must be at least
- **a** 75 hours
- **b** 16 hours
- **c** 3 weeks
- **d** 8 weeks

Continued.

Review questions are a useful study guide. They help you to review what you have learned. They can also be used when studying for a test or the competency evaluation. Answers are given at the back of the book beginning on page 748.

Contents

MOSBY'S TEXTBOOK FOR

Nursing Assistants

Introduction to Health Care Facilities

1

OBJECTIVES

- Define the key terms listed in this chapter
- Explain the purposes and organization of health care facilities
- Describe common types of health care services
- Identify the members of the health team and nursing team
- Describe the nursing service department
- Know the differences between RNs, LPNs, and nursing assistants
- Explain how the nursing assistant is a member of the nursing team
- Describe the programs that pay for health care
- Explain how diagnostic related groups affect Medicare and Medicaid payments

Key Terms

acute illness A sudden illness from which a person is expected to recover

case management A nursing care pattern; a case manager (an RN) coordinates a person's care from admission through discharge and into the home setting

chronic illness An illness, slow or gradual in onset, for which there is no known cure; the illness can be controlled, and complications can be prevented

functional nursing A nursing care pattern; nursing personnel are given specific tasks to do for all assigned patients or residents

health team A group of workers who work together to provide health care for patients and residents

home care agency An agency that provides nursing care and assistance to persons in their homes

hospice A health care facility or program for persons dying of terminal illness

licensed practical nurse (LPN) An individual who has completed a 1-year nursing program and has passed the licensing examination for practical nurses

long-term care facility A health care facility in which persons live and are given nursing care; nursing facility or nursing home

nursing assistant An individual who gives basic nursing care under the supervision of a registered nurse or an LPN; other titles include nurse's aide, nursing attendant, patient care assistant, health care assistant, and patient care technician

nursing facility A long-term care facility or nursing home

nursing team Individuals who provide nursing care—registered nurses, LPNs, and nursing assistants

primary nursing A nursing care pattern; a registered nurse is responsible for the total care of persons on a 24-hour basis

registered nurse (RN) An individual who has studied nursing for 2, 3, or 4 years and has passed a licensing examination

team nursing A nursing care pattern; an RN serves as a team leader; RNs, LPNs, and nursing assistants are assigned to care for certain persons

There are many types of health care facilities. These include hospitals, long-term care facilities, mental health hospitals, community centers, home care agencies, adult day care centers, and hospices. Others include doctors' offices, clinics, homes for the mentally retarded, and centers for the disabled. There are also centers for drug and alcohol treatment and crisis centers for rape, abuse, suicide, and other mental health emergencies.

This chapter deals with the basic purposes of health care facilities and with facilities that commonly employ nursing assistants. The organization of health care facilities, the nursing team, and insurance programs are also included.

HEALTH CARE FACILITIES

Health care facilities offer services to persons needing health care. The many services range from the simple to the complex. Some offer one type of service. The people working in health care have special talents, knowledge, and skills. All work to meet the needs of the patient or resident. The person is the focus of care.

Purpose

Health care facilities have similar purposes and services. *Health promotion* includes both physical and mental health. The goal is to reduce the risk of illness. Health is promoted by teaching and counseling people about healthy living. Persons are taught about diet and exercise and how to change unhealthy habits such as smoking. They are also taught the warning signs and symptoms of serious illness. Health promotion also includes teaching persons how to manage and cope with existing diseases.

Disease prevention is another purpose of health care facilities. Many diseases can be prevented by healthy living and good health care. Ways to prevent disease include routine physical examinations, reducing risk factors, and immunization.

Risk factors for disease can be identified during routine physical examinations. Early warning signs of disease may also be detected. Measures can then be taken to reduce the risk factors and prevent the disease. For example, high blood pressure is noted during Mr. Downing's physical examination. High blood pressure can lead to heart attacks and strokes. Mr. Downing is taught how diet and exercise can lower his blood pressure. Simple changes in his life style can prevent major health problems.

Immunizations protect against many infectious diseases. They include polio, smallpox, measles, hepatitis, tetanus, and diphtheria. Acquired immunodeficiency syndrome (AIDS) also is a major health problem. A great deal of research is still being done to find an AIDS vaccine.

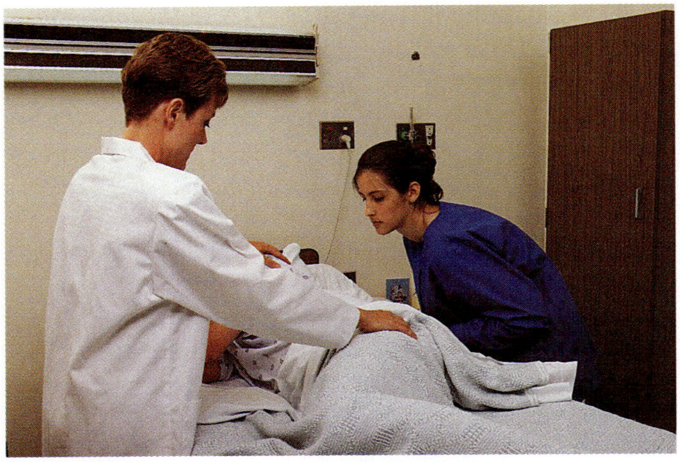

Fig. 1-1 *A nursing assistant helping an RN give patient care.*

Heart disease and cancer are among the leading causes of death today. AIDS also is a major health problem. Scientists are looking for the causes and cures of all these diseases as well as for ways to prevent them.

The *detection and treatment of disease* are primary purposes of most health care facilities. Diagnostic testing, physical examinations, surgery, emergency care, and medications are some methods used to detect and treat disease. Nurses are involved in disease detection by observing for signs and symptoms. Their role in disease treatment is to give nursing care and to carry out treatment measures ordered by the doctor. You assist nurses. Therefore, you also observe and care for persons (Fig. 1-1).

Rehabilitation, or restorative care, helps persons return to their highest possible level of physical and psychological functioning. In the past, rehabilitation focused on people with physical disabilities resulting from birth injuries, birth defects, or physical injuries. It is now understood that a person can have problems functioning psychologically, as well as physically, in everyday activities and at work. Rehabilitation helps persons learn or relearn the skills needed to live, work, and enjoy life.

Rehabilitation begins when a person first receives health care. Many health care workers are involved in helping the person become as independent as possible. The person is taught and encouraged to function without help.

Many health care facilities provide work-based learning experiences for students. The students may be studying to become nurses, doctors, x-ray and laboratory technicians, dieticians, or nursing assistants. These students also assist in health promotion, disease prevention, disease detection and treatment, and rehabilitation.

These purposes are all related and are hard to separate. For example, Mr. Downing enters a hospital emergency room with severe chest pain and difficulty breathing. After an examination and laboratory tests, the doctor makes the diagnosis of heart attack. Mr. Downing is admitted to the hospital for treatment. During treatment, he is given health teaching and counseling about the causes of a heart attack and about health habits that need changing. He is taught the importance of not smoking, eating a low fat diet, and getting regular exercise. The teaching and counseling are done to promote health and to prevent another heart attack. Mr. Downing is probably afraid of dying and worried about being unable to lead an active life. A rehabilitation program is planned in which activity begins slowly. Activity may progress to jogging or swimming. More teaching and counseling are provided about diet, medications, life-style, and activity. Mr. Downing and his family are encouraged to talk about their fears and concerns and are given help in learning to cope. Thus a successful rehabilitation program helps promote the person's health and may prevent another heart attack.

Types of Health Care Services

Nursing assistants work in many types of settings. Some work in doctors' offices. They perform basic functions and help with clerical duties. Nursing assistants may care for homebound persons in private homes. Most nursing assistants work in facilities providing the following services.

Hospital care Hospitals vary in size. Small community hospitals may have 25 to 50 beds while large medical centers have more than 500 beds (Fig. 1-2). Most large hospitals are in major cities or are part of colleges and universities. Hospital services include emergency care, surgery, nursing care, x-ray procedures and treatments, laboratory testing, respiratory therapy, physical therapy, occupational therapy, and speech therapy.

People of all ages may need hospital care. They go to have babies, for mental health problems, to have surgery, to heal broken bones, to diagnose and treat medical problems, or to die. Persons can have acute, terminal, or chronic illnesses. An **acute illness** begins suddenly and the person is expected to recover. A **terminal illness** eventually results in death (see Chapter 34). A **chronic illness** often begins slowly and has no cure. The illness can be controlled, and complications can be prevented with proper treatment.

The hospital stay may be very short, less than 24 hours. Others may last days, weeks, or months depending on the person's condition and illness. Outpatient services are very common. The person needs hospital services but does not have to stay overnight. Some surgeries, diagnostic procedures, and therapies do not require overnight stays.

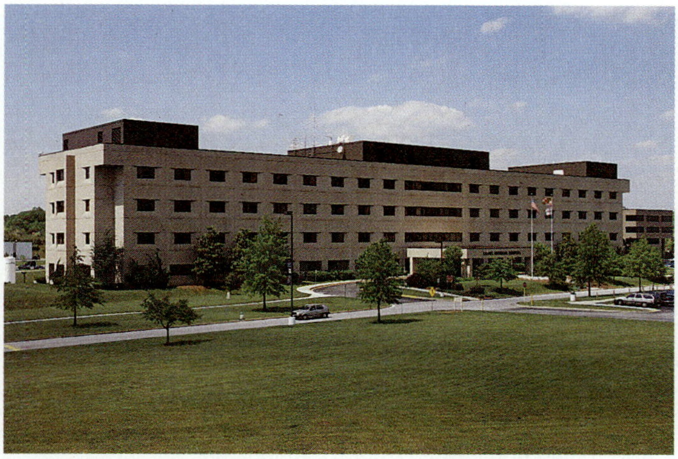

Fig. 1-2 *Community hospital. (Courtesy of Laurel Regional Hospital, Laurel, Maryland)*

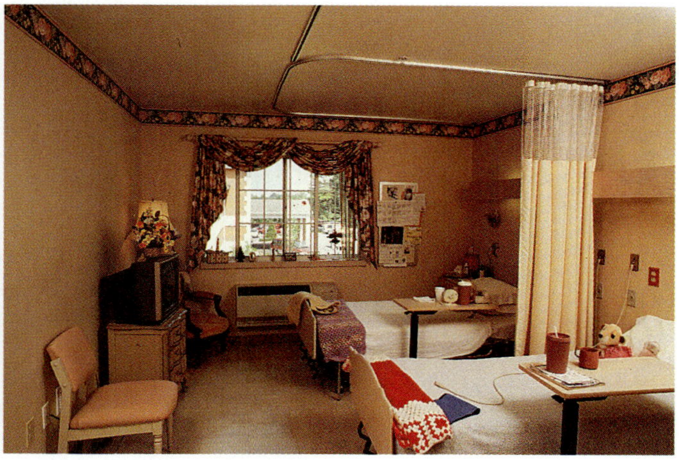

Fig. 1-3 *Room of a modern long-term care facility.*

Subacute care Hospital stays have shortened because of changes in insurance coverage. A person may no longer need hospital care, but may still need medical care or rehabilitation. Subacute care units are found in hospitals and long-term care facilities. There also are a growing number of separate facilities for subacute care. Persons needing subacute care may fully recover. Others may need long-term care.

Long-term care **Long-term care facilities** (nursing homes or nursing facilities) provide services to persons who cannot care for themselves at home but who do not need hospital care. Medical, nursing, dietary, recreational, rehabilitative, and social services are provided.

Persons in long-term care facilities are called residents, not patients. They are residents because the facility is their temporary or permanent home. Most residents are elderly, with chronic diseases, poor nutrition, or poor health. Long-term care facilities are designed to meet the special needs of the elderly (Fig. 1-3).

However, not all residents are elderly. Some residents are permanently disabled from accidents or diseases. They may need to live in a long-term care facility well before the age of 65. Other residents may be discharged early from hospitals because of insurance coverage (see Paying for Health Care, page 12). People are often discharged from hospitals when they are still sick or still recovering from surgery. Home care may be an option for some. Others may need the services of a long-term care facility.

Some residents become well enough to return home; others need nursing care until death. Long-term care facilities and the needs of residents are discussed in Chapter 7. Throughout this book, the term **nursing facility** is used when referring to long-term care facilities.

Mental health Mental health centers or hospitals specialize in the care and treatment of persons with mental illnesses. Persons may have difficulty dealing with events in life. Some are dangerous to themselves or others because of how they think and behave. Persons may be treated as outpatients. Others may need hospital care for a short time or for life. Mental health hospitals were once called *psychiatric hospitals.*

Home care **Home care agencies** provide care for persons in their homes. The agency may be part of a public health department or a private business. Many hospitals provide home care services. Services range from health teaching and supervision to bedside nursing care. Home care is an alternative to a nursing facility for some elderly persons and for those who are dying. Besides nursing care, agencies may provide social activities, physical therapy, rehabilitation, and food services. Home care and the role of the nursing assistant (home health care assistant) are discussed in Chapter 35.

Hospice care A **hospice** is a health care facility or program for those who are dying. The physical, emotional, social, and spiritual needs of the person and family are provided for in a setting that allows much freedom. Children and pets usually can visit at any time. Family and friends can take part in giving care. A hospice may be a separate facility or part of a hospital. Hospice care can also be provided in the person's home.

Health care systems Health care systems are forming all over the United States. A *health care system* involves health care agencies joining together as one provider of care. The system may include one or more hospitals, nursing facilities, home care agencies, hospice settings, and doctors. Some systems also have their own ambulance service. Medical supply stores are also common for persons needing to buy medical supplies for home care. The system may serve a community or a large geographic area.

BOX 1-1 Using a Health Care System

Dr. Moore is one of the doctors in a health care system that owns Mercy Hospital. The hospital has a subacute unit and operates LifeCare Ambulance Service, a home care agency, and a medical supply store. The system also operates Faircrest Nursing Home.

June Adams, aged 78, makes an appointment to see Dr. Moore. She complains of tightness in her chest, dizziness, and a "pounding heart beat." Dr. Moore admits her to Mercy Hospital. He asks Dr. Gills, another Mercy doctor and a heart specialist (cardiologist), to take over her care. While in the hospital she has a heart attack. A few days later she has a stroke and cannot move the left side of her body. She is given needed medical care. When her condition is stable, she is transferred to the subacute unit.

After several days in the subacute unit, Mrs. Adams has the choice of having home care or going to a nursing facility. She wants to go home. Her sister and her son and his wife want to help care for her. A nurse tells them about the need for a hospital bed, bedside commode, bedpan, wheelchair, and other equipment and supplies. They rent some items and buy the others at the medical supply store owned by Mercy Hospital.

The nurse arranges for Mrs. Adams to be transported home by LifeCare Ambulance Service. The nurse also works with Mercy Hospital's home care agency to provide home care services.

Mrs. Adams is at home. Every day a nursing assistant comes to bathe her and assist with other hygiene and grooming needs. A nurse visits three times a week. The nurse and nursing assistant work for Mercy Hospital's home care agency.

After being home a month, Mrs. Adams has another stroke. She is taken to Mercy Hospital by LifeCare Ambulance Service. After being in the hospital for 8 days, she is transferred to the subacute unit for rehabilitation. The second stroke has caused more disabilities. Dr. Gills advises Mrs. Adams and her family that home care may be difficult. He suggests she be admitted to a nursing home. Mrs. Adams and her family discuss the matter and agree with the need for a nursing home. The nurse then arranges for Mrs. Adams to be admitted to Faircrest Nursing Home. She is transferred there by LifeCare Ambulance Service.

A health care system intends to serve all health care needs. A person entering the system is referred to others in the system as needed. See Box 1-1 for an example of how the health care system can be used.

HOW A HEALTH CARE FACILITY IS ORGANIZED

Health care facilities have a governing or controlling body called the board of trustees or board of directors. The board makes sure that the facility gives good, safe care at the lowest possible cost. The board makes policies for the facility. An administrator manages the facility and reports directly to the board.

A group of directors assists the administrator in operating and managing the facility. The directors or department heads are responsible for specific areas (Fig. 1-4).

The director of nursing (DON) is responsible for the entire nursing staff. This includes the activities involved in providing safe nursing care. The nursing service department is discussed later in this chapter. Figure 1-4 shows a typical organizational chart of a health care facility.

The Health Team

The **health team** involves a group of workers whose skills and knowledge are directed to the total care of the person (Table 1-1 on pages 8 and 9). Their overall goal is to provide quality care. Members of the health team work together to meet the person's needs. Figure 1-5 (page 10) shows the person as the focus of all the health care workers.

Many health care workers are involved in the care of one person. Therefore, coordination of care is essential. A registered nurse (RN) is usually responsible for the coordination of care.

Nursing Service

Nursing service is a major department in a health care facility. The director of nursing is an RN, who may have a bachelor's or master's degree in nursing. Vice president of nursing, vice president of patient services, or other similar titles are used in some facilities. Nursing supervisors assist the director in managing and carrying out the responsibilities of the nursing department. Nursing supervisors are also RNs and may have college degrees.

Nursing supervisors are responsible for a work shift

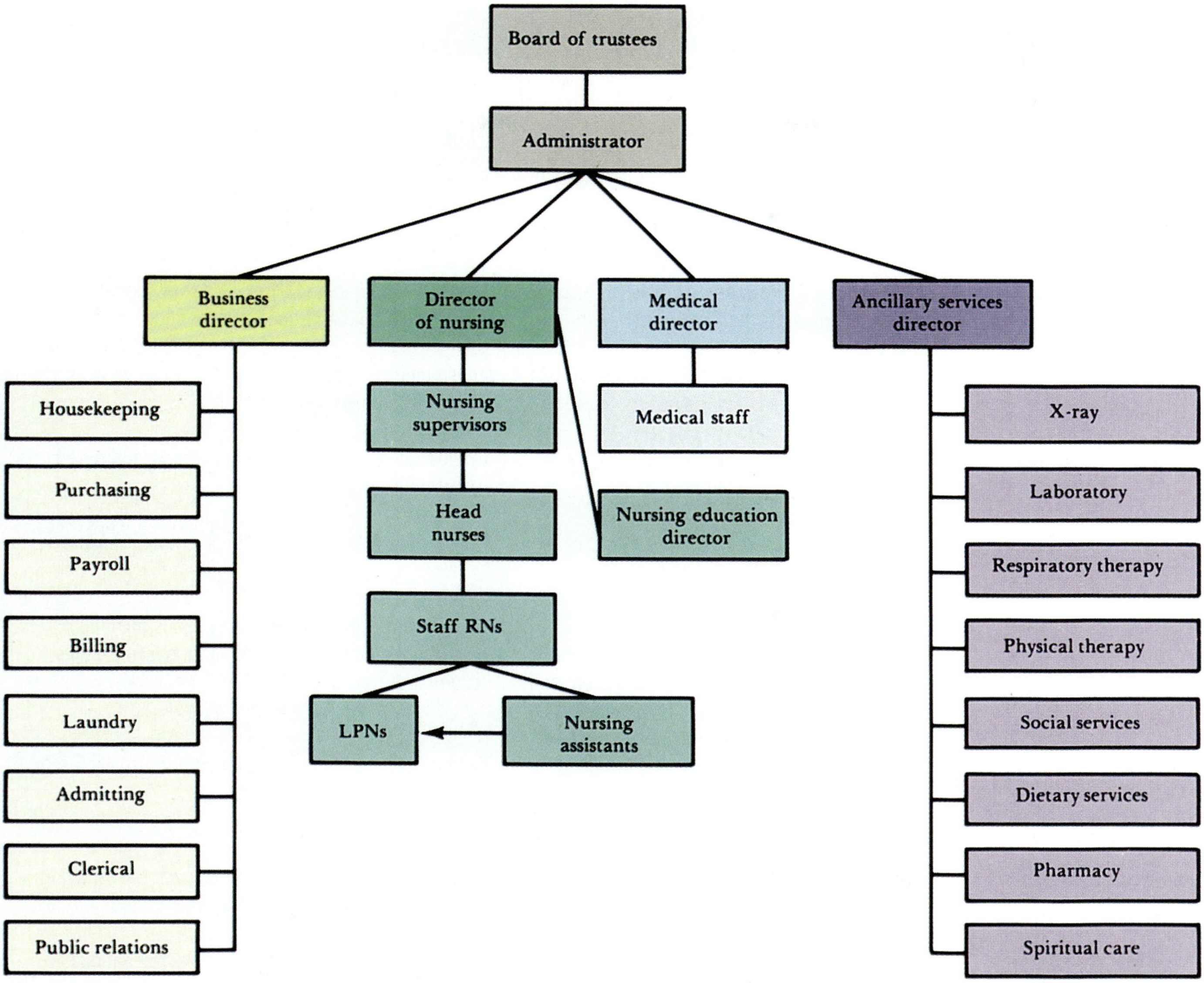

Fig. 1-4 *The organizational chart of a health care facility.*

or nursing area. The nursing areas may be surgical nursing units, medical nursing units, intensive care units, maternity departments, pediatric units, operating and recovery rooms, an emergency department, or a mental health nursing unit. These areas have head nurses or nurse managers. They are responsible for all patient or resident care and the actions of nursing personnel in their areas. Head nurses and nurse managers report to the nursing supervisors.

Each nursing area has RNs. They provide nursing care and assign and supervise the work of LPNs and nursing assistants. Staff RNs report to the head nurse or nurse manager. The LPN reports to the staff RN or to the head nurse or nurse manager. The nursing assistant reports to the RN or LPN supervising his or her work.

A nursing education department is also part of nursing service. A director of nursing education reports to the director of nursing. The director of nursing education is an RN, who may have a bachelor's or master's degree in nursing. RNs may be hired as nursing education instructors. They plan and present educational programs to nursing personnel so that current and safe care continues to be given.

Nursing Care Patterns

There are several ways to provide safe and effective nursing care. The nursing care pattern depends on the number of persons to be cared for, the available staff, and the cost. The most common patterns are presented.

Functional nursing focuses on tasks and jobs. Each nursing team member is assigned specific functions or tasks to do for all patients or residents. For example, one RN gives all medications. Another RN changes all dressings and gives all treatments. LPNs give baths, take vital

TABLE 1-1

MEMBERS OF THE HEALTH TEAM

Title	Description	Credentials
Activities Director	Works in nursing facilities; assesses, plans, and implements recreational needs of residents	Required training varies with state and/or facility policies; ranges from no required training to bachelor's degree
Audiologist	Tests hearing; prescribes hearing aids; and works with hearing impaired persons	Master's degree in audiology, 1 year of supervised employment, and a national examination
Chaplain	Works in all types of health care settings to assist patients and residents with their spiritual needs	Priest, minister, rabbi, sister, deacon, or other cleric with pastoral training
Dental Hygienist	Focuses on prevention of dental disorders; works under direction of a licensed dentist	Graduation from accredited dental hygiene program and state licensure
Dentist	Prevents and treats disorders and diseases of the teeth, gums, and oral structures	Doctor of Dental Science (DDS) and state licensure
Dietician	Assesses and plans for nutritional needs of patients and residents; teaches individuals and families about good nutrition, food selection, and preparation	Bachelor's degree; Registered Dieticians (RD) must pass national registration examination; some states require licensure
Licensed Practical/ Vocational Nurse (LPN/LVN)	Provides direct patient/resident care, including the administration of medications, under the direction of an RN	Graduate of a state-approved program (usually 1 year in length) and state licensure
Medical Laboratory Technician	Collects samples and performs laboratory tests on blood, urine, and other body fluids	Graduate of a 2-year program and national certifying examination; state licensure may be required
Medical Records Technician	Maintains medical records for legal and insurance purposes; transcribes medical reports, files records, and completes required reports	Graduates of two-year programs take the national Accredited Record Technician (ART) examination
Nursing Assistant	Assists RNs and LPNs/LVNs; gives direct bedside patient/resident care; must be supervised by a licensed nurse	Completion of state-approved training program (federal law requires at least 75 hours of training); successful completion of competency evaluation (written and skills test)
Occupational Therapist	Assists individuals to learn or regain the skills needed to perform activities of daily living; designs adaptive equipment for activities of daily living	Bachelor of Science degree in occupational therapy and national certification; state licensure may be required
Occupational Therapy Assistant	Performs tasks and services under supervision of occupational therapist	Graduation from accredited program (usually 2 years in length) and national certification; state licensure may be required
Pharmacist	Fills medication and prescription orders written by physician; monitors and evaluates drug interactions; consults with physicians and nurses regarding drug actions and interactions	Bachelor of Science in Pharmacy and state licensure

TABLE 1-1

MEMBERS OF THE HEALTH TEAM—CONT'D

Title	Description	Credentials
Physical Therapist	Assists persons with musculoskeletal problems; focuses on restoring function and preventing disability from illness or injury	Bachelor of Science in physical therapy and state licensure
Physical Therapy Assistant	Performs selected physical therapy tasks and functions under direction of physical therapist	Associate degree from accredited program; national certification required in many states
Physician (Doctor)	Diagnoses and treats diseases and injuries	Medical school graduation, residency, and National Board Examination; state licensure
Physician's Assistant	Assists physician in diagnosis and treatment of ill and injured persons; able to perform many medical tasks under direction of physician	Completion of required training program and national certification; state licensure may be required
Podiatrist	Prevents, diagnoses, and treats foot disorders	Doctor of Podiatric Medicine (DPM) and state and/or national board examination
Radiographer/Radiologic Technologist	Takes x-rays ordered by physician and processes film for viewing	Graduation from accredited program and National Registry Examination
Registered Nurse (RN)	Assesses, makes nursing diagnoses, plans, implements, and evaluates nursing care; supervises LPNs and nursing assistants	Graduate of state-approved nursing program with associate degree, diploma, or bachelor's degree; state licensure
Respiratory Therapist	Assists in treatment of lung and heart disorders; gives respiratory treatments and therapies ordered by physician	Graduation from a 1- or 2-year program and certification by National Board of Respiratory Therapy
Social Worker	Helps patients and families deal with social, emotional, and environmental issues affecting illness and recovery; coordinates community agencies to assist patient and family	Bachelor of Social Work (BSW) or Master of Social Work (MSW)
Speech-Language Therapist	Evaluates speech and language and treats persons with speech, voice, hearing, and communication disorders	Master's degree in speech/language pathology, 1 year supervised work experience, and national examination

signs, and weigh everyone. Nursing assistants make the beds, pass drinking water, and feed persons needing assistance. Functional nursing is uncoordinated and fragmented. Disadvantages to the person are many. They include interrupted rest, having to learn several names and titles of nursing staff, waiting to have total care completed, and frequent interruptions.

Team nursing involves a team of nursing personnel led by an RN. The RN determines the amount and kind of care needed by each person. The team leader assigns other RNs, LPNs, and nursing assistants to care for specific persons. Assignments are made according to the person's needs and the capabilities of the team members. The team members report back to the team leader about any observations made and the care given.

Primary nursing involves total care. The primary nurse is an RN who is responsible for the person's care on a 24-hour basis. Other RNs and LPNs give care when the primary nurse is off duty. The RN assesses, makes nursing diagnoses, plans, implements, and evaluates the person's care. The RN gives bedside nursing care and teaches and counsels the person and family. The RN also plans the

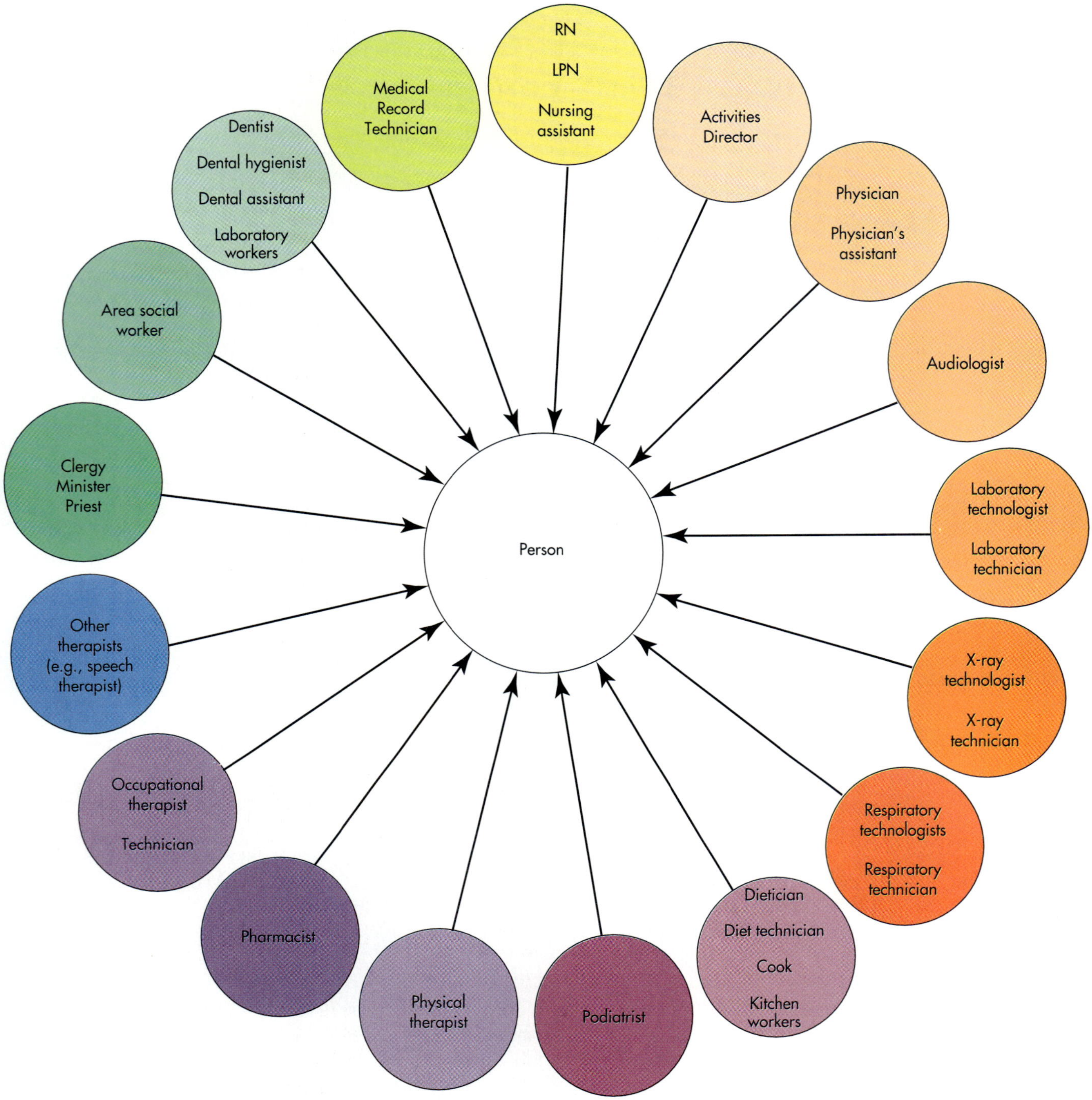

Fig. 1-5 *Members of the health team with the person as the focus of care.*

person's discharge. If necessary, home care or long-term care is arranged.

Case management is a newer nursing care pattern. It is similar to primary nursing. An RN serves as a case manager. The case manager coordinates the person's care from admission through discharge and into the home setting. The case manager communicates with the person's doctor and with the community agencies that may be needed for care. Case managers may work with the patients and residents of certain physicians. Others work only with persons who have certain health problems. For example, one case manager may work only with heart patients while another works only with cancer patients.

Spotlight On…

Alisa T-S of Atlanta, Georgia, is a nursing assistant who recently wrote the following award-winning essay.

Why I Am A Nursing Assistant

Nursing Assistants are the back bone of the nursing staff. My position as a nursing assistant is a very important role. A patient may need something as small as a cup of water and I am there to give it. A patient may need to cry and my shoulder is there to lean on. A patient may need to talk and my ears are there to listen. A patient may need help to and from the bathroom and I am there to assist them. As a nursing assistant, I am the one who carries out the duties that seem so small, but yet are so important.

I also play a big role in "Quality Care." This is what quality care means to me

Q = is for quality, because I give the best care that I am able to provide.
U = is for trying to understand what a patient might be going through.
A = is for the assurance a nursing assistant gives by listening to a patient's concerns.
L = is for the love I show by making every patient know I care.
I = is to show each patient that they are important.
T = is for the teamwork that I give to support the other nursing staff.
Y = is for yield, because I need to be careful with every decision I make.
C = is for the communication I try to establish with my patients.
A = is for applying myself 100% to each patient's needs.
R = is for the respect that each patient deserves.
E = is for the enthusiasm I feel seeing a patient recover back to good health.

My position has many rewards. It is not the salary that I earn. It is not the "Performance Award" that is given once a year. It is the self-satisfaction deep within myself. The feeling at the end of the day, knowing I have done my best and all that I can do. It is smiling at a patient and the patient smiles back. It is asking a patient how he is feeling and taking time to listen to his response. The greatest reward of all is to hear a patient telling another patient not to worry because I will take care of him. My reward may not be a big plaque that I can hang on the wall for people to admire and my reward may not be a trophy that sits on a mantelpiece for all my friends to see. My rewards are my "feelings" of being appreciated and needed by someone who is unable to do the small things for themselves.

A nursing assistant has many roles, even though they have great limitations. I may not be the one who passes out medication to make a patient feel better and I may not be the one who performs the surgery to take away the pain. So who am I. . . .I am the one who listens to a patient's problems no matter how big or small. I am the one who changes their sheets and the one who tucks their pillows underneath their head. I am also the one who gives them an extra blanket to keep them warm throughout the night. I AM PROUD OF WHO I AM AND PROUD OF WHAT I DO! So what was that question again? Why I am a nursing assistant? Because I care.

THE NURSING TEAM

The **nursing team** involves RNs, LPNs, and nursing assistants. Each has different roles and responsibilities as a result of the amount and kind of education received. All are concerned with the physical, social, emotional, and spiritual needs of patients and residents.

Registered Nurses

A **registered nurse** (RN) studies for 2 years at a community college, 2 or 3 years in a hospital-based diploma program, or 4 years at a college or university. Nursing and the biological, social, and physical sciences are studied. The graduate nurse takes a licensing examination offered by a state board of nursing. The examination must be passed for the nurse to become *registered* and receive a license to practice. RNs in the United States must be licensed by the state in which they practice. An RN practicing in Ohio must be licensed by the state of Ohio. If the RN wants to work in New York, a New York license must be obtained through an application process.

RNs assess, make nursing diagnoses, plan, implement, and evaluate nursing care (see Nursing Process, page 47). The RN identifies a person's nursing problems and develops a plan of care. The RN carries out the plan and evaluates its effectiveness on the person's condition. The person is helped to become more independent and is taught ways to stay or become healthy. Family teaching is also provided.

The RN is responsible for carrying out the doctor's orders. The RN may carry out the order or assign it to an LPN or a nursing assistant. RNs do not diagnose diseases or illnesses or prescribe treatments or medications. However, an RN can study to become a clinical nurse specialist or a nurse practitioner. Clinical nurse specialists and nurse practitioners are involved in diagnosing and prescribing.

RNs work as staff nurses, head nurses, nurse managers, supervisors, directors of nursing, and instructors. Their job opportunities depend on their amount and type of education, professional abilities, and experience.

Licensed Practical Nurses

A **licensed practical nurse** (LPN) completes 1 year of study in a hospital-based nursing program, community college, vocational school, or technical school. Some programs are 18 months long. Some public high schools offer 2-year practical nursing programs. In classroom and clinical settings, the study of nursing is emphasized. Students also study body structure and function, basic psychology, arithmetic, and communication skills. Graduates take a licensing examination for practical nursing. When the test is passed, the individual receives a license to practice and

BOX 1-2 NURSING ASSISTANT TITLES

- Certified Nursing Assistant
- Home Care Aide
- Home Health Aides
- Home Health Care Assistant
- Nurse Technicians
- Nurse's Aide
- Nursing Support Technician
- Patient Care Technician
- Patient Care Monitor
- Patient Care Attendant
- Patient Care Assistant
- Resident Care Specialist
- Resident Aides
- Support Partner

the title of *licensed practical nurse.* The title *licensed vocational nurse (LVN)* is used in some states. Like RNs, practical nurses must be licensed to practice nursing.

LPNs work under the supervision of RNs, licensed physicians, and licensed dentists. An LPN's responsibilities and functions are more limited than those of an RN. The LPN has less education in the biological, physical, and social sciences. LPNs can function with little supervision when the person's care is simple and the person's condition is stable. LPNs assist RNs in providing care to acutely ill persons and when complex procedures are required.

Nursing Assistants

Nursing assistants are employed in health care facilities to assist nurses in providing patient and resident care. There are many different titles for nursing assistants. The title depends on the setting and the nursing assistant's role. Some common titles are listed in Box 1-2. Under the direct supervision of RNs and LPNs, nursing assistants give basic nursing care. The nursing assistant as a member of the nursing team is discussed in greater detail in Chapter 2.

In 1987 the U.S. Congress passed the Omnibus Budget Reconciliation Act. The law is commonly called *OBRA.* This federal law applies to all 50 states. The law requires training for nursing assistants working in nursing facilities. It also requires a *competency evaluation.* This means that nursing assistants must prove that they have the knowledge and skills necessary to give safe care. Competency evaluation involves a written test and a skills test. Nursing assistant training and competency evaluation are discussed in Chapter 2.

Nursing assistant courses are conducted by community colleges, technical schools, and high school vocational programs. Others are offered by nursing education departments in health care facilities.

You may wish to continue your education to become an RN or LPN. Or you may want to work as another member of the health care team (see Table 1-1). Community colleges and 4-year colleges and universities can help you select the best program to meet your needs, abilities, and finances.

PAYING FOR HEALTH CARE

Hospital care and long-term care are very costly and can financially ruin the person and family. Even after the person goes home, bills may continue for doctor visits, medicines, medical supplies, and home care.

Most people cannot afford large medical bills. Some avoid medical care because they cannot pay. Others pay doctor bills even if they must go without food or needed medicine. Worry, fear, and emotional upset often occur when faced with the problem of paying for health care. If the person has insurance, part or all of the health care costs are usually covered.

Health care reform is a major focus today. The goals are to provide health care access to everyone and reduce the high cost of care. Government leaders have proposed many ways to reform health care. Efforts have already been made to reduce the cost of health care. Such efforts include managed care and prospective payment systems. More changes are likely in the future. Before managed care and prospective payment are presented, a general discussion of insurance programs is necessary.

- *Private insurance plans* are purchased by individuals and families. Depending on the plan, the insurance company pays for some or all health care costs.
- *Group insurance plans* cover individuals belonging to a group. Often employers have health insurance for employees under group coverage. The insurance premium is paid by the employee, the employer, or the employee and employer. Premiums are lower with group plans than with private insurance plans.
- *Medicaid* is a health insurance program sponsored by federal and state governments. Benefits, regulations, and eligibility requirements vary from state to state. Elderly people, the blind, the disabled, and low-income persons are usually eligible. Medicaid usually pays for hospital services, doctor fees, x-ray and laboratory tests, home care, family planning, dental and eye care, immunization and well-child clinics, and rehabilitation. There is no insurance premium to pay.

- *Medicare* is a health insurance plan administered by the Social Security Administration of the federal government. Benefits are for persons age 65 and older. Younger, disabled persons may also be eligible. Monthly premiums are paid by those who are insured. Medicare has two parts. Part A pays for some hospital costs up to certain amounts during a specified time period (see diagnostic related groups below). Long-term care and home care are included if certain regulations are met. Part B pays for some medical expenses such as doctors' office visits, diagnostic tests, and treatments. Part B may also cover physical therapy and rental of hospital equipment for home care. Medicare benefits and regulations are complex and change often. Local Social Security offices can provide information and answer questions.

Managed Care

Managed care deals with the delivery and payment of health care. To reduce health care costs, many insurance companies have contracts with doctors, hospitals, and health care delivery systems. The contracts generally call for reduced rates or discounts. The insured person uses those doctors and facilities providing the lower rates. If others are used, the care may be covered in part or not at all. Costs not covered by insurance must be paid by the person receiving the care.

Types of managed care Managed care limits the person's choice of where to go for health care. It also places limits on which doctors provide the care. Health maintenance organizations and preferred provider organizations (Box 1-3) are the two common types of managed care arrangements. As health care reform unfolds, new models are likely. While managed care generally involves private and group insurance plans, many states require managed care for Medicaid and Medicare participants.

Managed care as pre-approval for services Many insurance companies must approve the need for health care services. If the need is approved, the insurance company pays for the services. If pre-approval or precertification is not obtained, the person must pay for the health care. This pre-approval process and the monitoring of care is also called managed care. The purpose of managed care in this sense is to reduce unneeded medical and surgical services and procedures. The insurance company decides what to pay. Sometimes the insurance company decides where the person needs to go for the services, especially if there are contracts with an HMO or PPO.

Insurance companies have RNs who handle the pre-approval process. The process varies depending on the insurance plan. Pre-approval is usually needed for the types of services listed in Box 1-4.

BOX 1-3 Types of Managed Care

Health Maintenance Organization (HMO)—provides health care services for a prepaid fee. For the fee, persons receive all needed services offered by the organization. Some need only an annual physical examination, but others require hospital care. Whatever services are used, the cost is covered by the prepaid fee. HMOs emphasize preventing disease and maintaining health. Keeping someone healthy costs far less than treating illness.

Preferred Provider Organization (PPO)—is a group of doctors and hospitals that provides health care at reduced rates. Usually the arrangement is made between the PPO and an employer or an insurance company. Employees or those insured are given reduced rates for the services used. The person can choose any doctor or hospital in the PPO.

Prospective Payment Systems

Prospective payment systems limit the amount paid to hospitals by insurance companies, Medicare, and Medicaid. Prospective relates to *before* care. The amount to be paid for services is determined before the person enters the hospital.

Diagnostic related groups (DRGs) were legislated by U.S. Congress in 1983 to reduce Medicare and Medicaid costs. Before DRGs, Medicare and Medicaid paid for a certain amount of hospital costs. The amount was determined *after* the hospital stay. Under the DRG system, Medicare and Medicaid payments are determined *before* the person receives hospital care.

A diagnostic related group consists of specific diagnoses. The government has determined the length of stay and the cost of treating illnesses in the specific category. The hospital is paid the predetermined amount for Medicare and Medicaid persons. If the costs for treating the person are less than the DRG amount, the hospital keeps the extra money. If the costs are greater than the DRG amount, the hospital takes the loss.

Prospective payment has had a great effect on health care. Hospitals want to avoid financial loss from lengthy stays. As a result, persons are being discharged earlier than in the past. These persons are often still quite ill. Additional care in nursing facilities or home care is often required.

BOX 1-4 Health Care Needing Pre-Approval for Insurance Coverage

- Inpatient hospital care
- Skilled nursing care in a nursing facility
- Rehabilitation in a nursing facility
- Treatment in a psychiatric facility
- Treatment in a substance abuse facility
- Skilled home health care
- Private duty nursing
- Outpatient psychiatric care
- Outpatient substance abuse care
- Outpatient diagnostic testing for the
  *Back
  *Bladder
  *Colon
  *Heart
  *Intestines
  *Kidney
  *Stomach
- Outpatient surgery for disorders of the
  *Ear, nose, and throat
  *Female pelvis
  *Feet
  *Gallbladder
  *Hand or wrist
  *Heart
  *Knee
  *Rectum

Summary

This chapter has introduced various types of health care services, the general purposes and organization of health care facilities, and the health care workers involved in the person's care. Payment programs for health care were also presented. Whatever the size of the facility, the focus of care is still the patient or resident. All health team members work to meet the person's needs. You have an important place on the health team as RNs and LPNs supervise your work.

REVIEW QUESTIONS

Circle the best *answer.*

1 Helping a person return to the best possible physical and psychological functioning is known as
- **a** Detection and treatment of disease
- **b** Promotion of health
- **c** Rehabilitation
- **d** Disease prevention

2 The governing body of a health care facility is called the
- **a** Director of nursing
- **b** Health team
- **c** Board of trustees
- **d** Nursing team

3 A health care facility for dying persons is called
- **a** A hospice
- **b** A long-term care facility
- **c** An extended care facility
- **d** A hospital

4 The nursing team includes the following *except*
- **a** Registered nurses
- **b** Doctors
- **c** Nursing assistants
- **d** Licensed practical nurses

5 Members of the nursing team perform certain functions and tasks for all persons or residents. This is
- **a** Functional nursing
- **b** Primary nursing
- **c** Team nursing
- **d** Case management

6 These statements are about insurance programs. Which is *false?*
- **a** Preferred provider organizations (PPOs) provide health care at reduced rates.
- **b** Health maintenance organizations (HMOs) provide health care for a prepaid fee.
- **c** Medicare and Medicaid are government programs for anyone in need.
- **d** Diagnostic related groups (DRGs) affect Medicare and Medicaid payments.

Circle T *if the answer is true and* F *if the answer is false.*

7 **T F** Rehabilitation starts when the person is ready to be discharged from the health care facility.

8 **T F** The director of nursing is responsible for the entire nursing staff and the activities involved in providing safe nursing care.

9 **T F** Nursing supervisors are RNs or LPNs.

10 **T F** The nursing assistant is a member of both the health team and the nursing team.

11 **T F** Primary nursing and case management are similar nursing care patterns.

12 **T F** An LPN functions under the supervision of an RN, licensed physician, or licensed dentist.

13 **T F** An RN can diagnose health problems and prescribe the appropriate treatment.

14 **T F** A nursing assistant assists RNs and LPNs in providing nursing care.

Answers to these questions are on page 748.

The Nursing Assistant

2

OBJECTIVES

- Describe your role as a nursing assistant
- List the functions you can and cannot perform
- Explain why a job description is important
- Identify good health and personal hygiene practices
- Describe the practices for professional appearance
- Describe nursing assistant training and competency evaluation programs as required by OBRA
- Identify the information contained in the nursing assistant registry and other OBRA requirements
- Describe the ethical behavior of a nursing assistant
- Explain how you can prevent negligent acts
- Give examples of false imprisonment, defamation, assault, battery, and fraud
- Describe how to protect the right to privacy
- Explain the purpose of informed consent
- Identify your role in preparing and signing wills
- Describe the qualities and characteristics of a successful nursing assistant
- Explain what you should do to become employed
- Describe how you can work well with others to plan and organize work
- Explain cross-training as it relates to patient focused care

Key Terms

assault Intentionally attempting or threatening to touch a person's body without the person's consent

battery Unauthorized touching of a person's body without the person's consent

civil law Laws concerned with relationships between people; private law

crime An act that is a violation of a criminal law

criminal law Laws concerned with offenses against the public and society in general; public law

defamation Injuring a person's name and reputation by making false statements to a third person

empathy The ability to see things from another person's point of view

ethics Knowledge of what is right and wrong conduct

false imprisonment Unlawful restraint or restriction of a person's movement

fraud Saying or doing something to trick, fool, or deceive another person

invasion of privacy A violation of a person's right not to have his or her name, photograph, or private affairs exposed or made public without giving consent

law A rule of conduct made by a government body

legal That which pertains to a law

libel Defamation through written statements

malpractice Negligence by a professional person

negligence An unintentional wrong in which a person fails to act in a reasonable and careful manner and causes harm to a person or to the person's property

patient focused care (PFC) A delivery strategy that uses cross-trained staff and moves services from departments to the bedside

slander Defamation through oral statements

tort A wrong committed against a person or the person's property

will A legal statement of how a person's property is to be distributed after the person's death

Studying to become a nursing assistant is interesting and exciting. You will learn about things you may have wondered about. How is a bed made with a person in it? How is a person given a bath in bed? What is heard through a stethoscope? How do body organs function, and how are they related to each other?

First you need to understand what nursing assistants do. You may be told to do something that is not within the nursing assistant role. Therefore you need to know which functions you can and cannot perform. You must also know what is right and wrong behavior and your legal limitations in order to safely perform your job. Equally important is an understanding of the qualities and characteristics of a good nursing assistant and how to work well with others.

Soon you will look for a job. If you are already working, someday you may want a new job. You will learn how to complete a job application. You will also learn how to prepare for an interview.

ROLES, FUNCTIONS, AND RESPONSIBILITIES

As a nursing assistant, you perform basic nursing functions under the supervision of a nurse. Your work is supervised by RNs and LPNs. To help nurses provide safe and effective care, you must understand that nursing is a scientific and personal service given to patients and residents. You assist nurses in giving care. Often you function without a nurse physically present. At other times you help a nurse give bedside nursing care. The rules listed in Box 2-1 (page 18) should help you understand your role.

Nursing assistant functions and responsibilities vary among health facilities. *Responsibility* is the duty or obligation to perform some act or function and being able to answer for one's actions. The procedures in this textbook are performed by nursing assistants. Some are more complex and advanced than others.

You perform functions and procedures relating to personal hygiene, safety, nutrition, exercise, and elimination needs. Related functions include lifting and moving patients and residents, observing them, helping promote physical comfort, and collecting specimens (Fig. 2-1 on page 18). You may also assist with the admission and discharge of patients and residents, and measure temperatures, pulses, respirations, and blood pressures.

Your training prepares you to perform certain procedures. However, your employer may not allow nursing assistants to perform some of those procedures. Other facilities may want you to do things that you did not learn. You can perform additional procedures and tasks if:

BOX 2-1 RULES FOR THE NURSING ASSISTANT'S ROLE

- You are an assistant to the nurse.
- A nurse determines and supervises your work.
- You do not decide what should or should not be done for a patient or resident.
- If you do not understand directions or instructions, ask the nurse for clarification before going to the patient or resident.
- Perform no function or task that you have not been prepared to do or that you do not feel comfortable performing without a nurse's supervision.

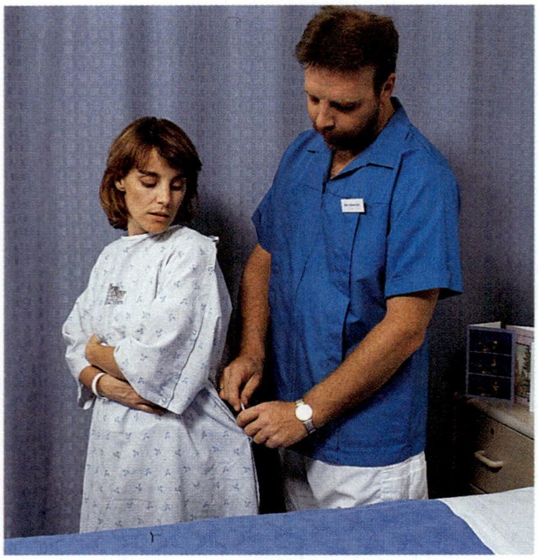

Fig. 2-1 *A nursing assistant helping a patient put on a robe.*

- You are given the necessary education and training
- You are given the necessary supervision
- The procedure or task is within the scope of nursing assistant practice in your state

Box 2-2 describes the limitations of the nursing assistant role. These are the functions, procedures, and tasks that nursing assistants never perform. You must understand what you *cannot* do as a nursing assistant.

Job Description

The job description lists your responsibilities and the functions your employer expects you to perform (Box 2-3 on pages 20-22). Always request a written job description when you apply for a job. Questions about the job description are asked during your job interview (see page 38). Before accepting a job you should tell the employer about any functions you do not know how to do. Also advise the employer of functions you are opposed to doing for moral or religious reasons. Have a clear understanding of what is expected of you before taking a job. Do not take a job that requires you to:

- Function beyond your educational limitations
- Perform acts that are against your moral or religious principles
- Act beyond the legal scope of your role

No one can force you to perform a function, task, or procedure that is beyond the legal scope of a nursing assistant. A nursing assistant's job may be threatened for refusing to follow a nurse's orders. Often the nursing assistant obeys out of fear. That is why you must understand the roles and responsibilities of nursing assistants. You also need to know which functions you can safely perform, the things you should never do, and your job description. Understanding the ethical and legal aspects of your role as a nursing assistant is equally important (see pages 25-29).

PERSONAL HEALTH, HYGIENE, AND APPEARANCE

The health team is an example to others. Patients, residents, families, and visitors expect the team to set a healthy example. A person has reason to question a nurse or doctor who smokes, especially when the person is told to stop smoking. As a health team member, you also set an example for others. Your personal health, appearance, and hygiene deserve careful attention.

Your Health

Feeling and looking healthy are important to you as a person, to the persons you care for, and to your employer. Patients, residents, and employers trust you. They believe you will give conscientious and effective care. To fulfill this trust you must be physically and mentally healthy. Otherwise you cannot function at your best.

BOX 2-2 Limitations of the Nursing Assistant Role

Never give medications. This includes medications given orally, rectally, by injection, or directly into the bloodstream through an intravenous line. There have been instances when a nurse has brought a medication to a person's room while the person was in the bathroom or busy with some activity. The nurse then told the nursing assistant to give the medication to the person later. In this situation (and other similar situations) the nursing assistant should respectfully but firmly refuse to follow the nurse's direction. Otherwise the nursing assistant would be performing a function and responsibility that is beyond the scope of nursing assistants.

Never insert tubes or objects into body openings or remove them from the body. You must not insert tubes into a person's bladder, esophagus, trachea, nose, ears, bloodstream, or body openings that have been surgically created. Exceptions to this rule are procedures in this textbook that you will study and practice with your instructor's supervision. For example, you may learn how to give enemas and insert rectal tubes.

Never take oral or telephone orders from physicians. You might answer the telephone or be near a doctor who wants to give you an order. You should politely give your name and title, ask the doctor to wait, and promptly find a nurse to speak with the doctor.

Never perform procedures that require sterile technique. With sterile technique, all objects that will be in contact with the person's body are free of all microorganisms. Sterile technique and procedures require skills, knowledge, and judgment beyond the training you will receive. You may assist the nurse during a sterile procedure. However, you will not perform the procedure yourself.

Never tell the patient, resident, or family the patient's or resident's diagnosis or medical or surgical treatment plans. The doctor is responsible for informing the patient, resident, or family about the diagnosis and treatment. Nurses may further clarify what the doctor has told the person and family.

Never diagnose or prescribe treatments or medications for anyone. Only doctors can diagnose and prescribe.

Never supervise other nursing assistants. Nurses are legally responsible for supervising the work of nursing assistants. You will not be trained or paid to supervise the work of others. Supervising other nursing assistants can have serious legal consequences.

Never ignore an order or request to do something that you cannot do or that is beyond the scope of nursing assistants. Promptly explain to the nurse why you cannot carry out the order or request. The nurse assumes you are doing what you were told to do unless you explain otherwise. Patient and resident care cannot be neglected.

Diet Good nutrition involves eating a balanced diet from the Food Guide Pyramid (see Chapter 17). Your daily diet should include the recommended number of servings from the following food groups:

- Bread, cereal, rice, and pasta group
- Vegetable group
- Fruit group
- Milk, yogurt, and cheese group
- Meat, poultry, fish, dry beans, eggs, and nuts group

Begin your day with a good breakfast. To maintain your weight, the number of calories taken in must balance your energy needs. To lose weight, caloric intake must be less than energy needs. Avoid foods from the fats, oils, and sweets group, salty foods, and crash diets.

Sleep and rest Adequate sleep and rest are needed to stay healthy and to do your job well. Most adults need about 7 hours of sleep daily. The amount varies with each person. Fatigue, lack of energy, and irritability mean you need more rest and sleep.

Body mechanics You will bend, carry heavy objects, and lift, move, and turn patients and residents. These activities place stress and strain on your body. You need to have good posture and learn to use your muscles effectively (see Chapter 10).

Exercise Exercise is important for muscle tone, circulation, and weight control. There are also psychological benefits. Walking, running, swimming, and biking are excellent forms of exercise. You will feel better physically

Text continued on page 23.

BOX 2-3 Nursing Assistant Job Description

JOB TITLE: Nursing Assistant
DEPARTMENT: Surgical/Ortho
GENERAL SUMMARY: The nursing assistant performs any combination of the following duties in the care of hospital patients, under direction of nursing staff:

- Answers call lights
- Bathes, dresses, and undresses patients
- Serves and collects food trays
- Feeds patients needing help
- Transports patients using wheelchairs or wheeled carts
- Assists patients to walk
- Drapes patients for examinations and treatments
- Remains with patients during examinations
- Holds instruments and adjusts lights during examinations
- Turns and repositions patients alone or with assistance to prevent pressure sores
- Changes bed linens
- Runs errands, directs visitors, and answers telephones
- Measures and records temperature, blood pressure, pulse, and respiration rates
- Measures and records fluid intake and output as directed
- Cleans and stores supplies
- Tidies patient rooms
- Gives enemas
- Transfers patients to and from bed
- Transports patients to other hospital areas using the bed, wheelchair, or stretcher
- Accompanies discharged patients to hospital exit
- Does not perform any procedure that requires licensing by the State of Illinois

CORPORATE PHILOSOPHY: It is the obligation of each employee of St. Joseph Medical Center to abide by and promote the Philosophy, Values, Mission and Vision of the Sisters of the Third Order of Saint Francis.

SKILLS OR SPECIALIZATION REQUIRED:

A. Education High school graduate or equivalent. Documented experience as a nursing assistant or completion of a nursing assistant training course. Registry status required.

B. Work experience Prior experience within the hospital environment is desired but not required. CPR skills are required.

C. Job knowledge Possess ability to perform duties as described in general summary. The applicant has an understanding of and practices patient confidentiality; displays problem identification and conflict resolution skills.

D. Skills and abilities

1. Communication skills
2. Organization and interpersonal skills
3. Able to operate selected hospital equipment
4. Good telephone skills
5. Understanding of aseptic technique and principles

PRINCIPAL DUTIES AND RESPONSIBILITIES: The following statements are intended to describe the essential elements, functions, and requirements of the position as defined by the ADA, *except* for those that begin with the word "may." The list should not be taken as an exhaustive list of all responsibilities, duties, and skills required of individuals assigned to this job. In accordance with the philosophy, objectives, and values of St. Joseph Medical Center and The Sisters of the Third Order of St. Francis, the nursing assistant assumes the following duties and responsibilities: she/he demonstrates through her/his care that returning the patient to his/her expected state of health and to maintain his/her safety, security, and dignity is a priority.

A. Patient care

1. Responds to emergency situations in accordance with established policies and procedures
2. Utilizes positive communication and interpersonal skills in performing duties
3. Provides psychological support
4. Provides nursing care under the direction of the nursing staff according to the Standards of Practice and Care, Nursing Service Policies and Procedures

B. Personal responsibilities

1. Demonstrates concern and respect for physical, spiritual, emotional, and economic needs of peers, co-workers, and other members of the health care team through collaborative work efforts, sharing ideas and resources, and a commitment to help each other to succeed
2. Promotes an atmosphere conducive to learning and orientation for nursing assistants by being a positive role model through personal actions
3. May assist in orientation of personnel as instructed by the Director of Surgical/Ortho

BOX 2-3 Nursing Assistant Job Description—cont'd

C. Material management

1. Assures accurate charging for all patient charge items
2. Cooperates in identifying and applying cost containment measures
3. Assists in maintaining equipment and department in optimal functioning order
4. Assists in ensuring that adequate supplies are available for the oncoming shift
5. Ensures that charges are recorded for all equipment
6. Maintains environment in a neat, safe manner, including patient environment

D. Communication

1. Reports any unusual occurrence or incident that occurs during her/his shift, according to policy
2. Keeps charge RN, supervisor, and/or unit director informed of patient condition changes or immediate problems on unit

E. Professional development

1. Makes improvements in the quality of nursing practice by participating in and utilizing Quality Improvement monitors
2. Participates in continuing education programs to maintain competence and gain additional skills that will enable him/her to broaden his/her scope of practice
3. Identifies areas for growth by establishing goals and actively works to achieve them
4. Supports, when possible, community organizations that seek to promote health needs of others (for example, cardiac screening)
5. Maintains documentation of attendance at inservices and continuing education programs
6. Conducts self in a professional manner at all times
7. Appears neat, clean, and dresses according to departmental dress code
8. Attends mandatory inservices
   a. Fire Safety
   b. Lifts and Carries
   c. Code Blue
   d. CPR
   e. Infection Control
9. Attends and contributes as indicated at department meetings
10. Demonstrates a willingness to learn new procedures
11. Works effectively with others, possessing tact, judgment, and diplomacy
12. Performs effectively in stressful situations
13. Is willing to work extra and/or other shifts
14. Is dependable as reflected in work attendance

PSYCHOLOGICAL CONSIDERATIONS: Some stress is experienced due to changing patient acuity, census fluctuations, and spontaneous reaction to situations as they arise. The dynamics of working closely with nurses, other health team members, and the public facilitates the stressful environment. Must display social sensitivity, acting suitably in all situations and adjusting behavior to fit the occasion and interpret how others are feeling. Behaviors must be flexible in response to changing situations to remain motivated with accuracy to reach a goal.

COGNITIVE SKILLS REQUIRED:

1. Ability to read and follow written English language as necessary (for example, policy and procedures for hospital and nursing)
2. Ability to follow verbal communications
3. Ability to understand written and spoken English, to remember and to understand the written and spoken word
4. Ability to organize and express thoughts in English words to others so they will understand
5. Ability to problem solve with a variety of variables, interpret instructions
6. Problem sensitivity: ability to prioritize nursing care based on changing conditions on the unit
7. Ability to communicate with all educational levels and display good human relations
8. Ability to learn technical material and equipment
9. Ability to prepare and label all specimens for laboratory analysis
10. Memorization: ability to remember words, numbers, procedures, and pieces of information
11. Ability to organize and maintain flexible scheduling to coordinate all job responsibilities

Continued.

BOX 2-3 Nursing Assistant Job Description—cont'd

12. Ability to perform duties in an atmosphere of frequent interruptions
13. Ability to practice effective time management

PHYSICAL REQUIREMENTS:

1. Must have normal or corrected vision in order to complete daily tasks
2. Must perform major visual functions, including acuity, depth perception, field of vision, accommodation, and color vision
3. Must be capable of hearing and speaking English in order to communicate with people on the phone and in person
4. Must be able to work in order to transport objects, equipment, and patients to various parts of the department and the hospital, including heavy but mobile equipment, some of which may weigh 100 pounds or more, which may be pushed or pulled on wheels
5. Must be able to stand for periods of time
6. Must be capable of maintaining body equilibrium to prevent falling when walking or standing
7. Must be capable of stooping, bending, kneeling, reaching, and squatting required during positioning patients and observations skills
8. Must be capable of carrying up to 50 pounds for transporting equipment and supplies; must be capable of moving and/or lifting patients from bed/wheelchair to the stretchers; moving devices are available; these patients may weigh up to or over 300 pounds
9. Must be capable of a wide range of hand, wrist, and finger motions, including pinching, grasping, and fingering required for tasks such as writing, answering phones, adjusting dials, using and carrying equipment and supplies, and positioning patients
10. Must be able to assist in properly positioning patients
11. Must be able to physically respond to emergency situations in accordance with established policies and procedures such as performing CPR
12. Must be able to coordinate eyes and hands, feet, or fingers rapidly and accurately in making precise movements with speed; must be able to make a movement response accurately and quickly

MEASUREMENTS FOR EQUIPMENT AND/OR SUPPLIES:

Height: may range from floor level to 7 feet
Weight: may range from several ounces to over 300 pounds
IV poles: 72 inches high, 2 pound force to move
Reach: to floor and up to 3 feet above or from body

PHYSIOLOGICAL CONSIDERATIONS: There is the potential for exposure to blood and body fluids, contagious and infectious diseases, including hepatitis and HIV virus. There is also the potential for exposure to chemicals such as cleaning solutions and medications. There may be noxious odors present. Personal protective equipment and supplies are readily available within the work environment, and the employee is expected to follow established hospital policy regarding use of protective equipment and supplies.

ENVIRONMENTAL CONSIDERATIONS: The normal work day is inside and protected from the elements. However, it may be necessary to exit the building to discharge patients. Temperature changes may be experienced in the work environment.

REPORTING RELATIONSHIPS: This position reports to the Director of the Surgical/Ortho Services or the Charge Nurse.

APPROVALS:

____
Department Manager/Director Date

____
Assistant Administrator Date

____
Human Resources Director Date

The above is intended to describe the general content of and requirements for the performance of this job. It is not to be construed as an exhaustive statement of duties, responsibilities or requirements.

____
Employee's Signature Date

*Modified from "St. Joseph Medical Center Job Description." Courtesy St. Joseph Medical Center, Bloomington, Illinois.

and more alert mentally when you exercise regularly. Do not begin a vigorous exercise program until you have consulted your doctor.

Your eyes Think for a moment what it would be like if you could not see. Loss of vision would mean major changes in how you live, work, and travel. Your eyes deserve special care and respect. Have your eyes examined and wear glasses or contact lenses as prescribed. Make sure you have enough light when reading or doing fine work.

Good vision is necessary in your work. Along with reading instructions, you will measure blood pressures and temperatures. These procedures involve fine measurements. Inaccurate readings can place patients and residents in danger.

Smoking Smoking has been linked to lung cancer, chronic lung diseases, and many heart and circulatory disorders. If you smoke, remember that cigarette smoke can be offensive to others. Smoke only in areas where smoking is allowed, and never smoke in or near patient and resident rooms. Many facilities have smoke-free environments. Smoke odors stay on a person's breath, hands, clothing, and hair. Therefore handwashing and good personal hygiene are essential. Wash your hands before and immediately after smoking and before giving care.

Drugs Drug abuse is a major problem in society. People can become physically and psychologically dependent on drugs. Drugs affect thinking, feeling, behavior, and functioning. Accidents, suicides, divorce, crime, and other tragic and violent events have been linked to drug abuse. Persons who are dependent on drugs may go to any length to obtain them.

Drugs that have an undesirable effect on your mind and body affect your ability to work effectively. A person who works under the influence of drugs places patients and residents in danger. You should take only drugs prescribed by a doctor and only in the way prescribed.

Alcohol At first alcohol produces feelings of well-being and stimulation. However, alcohol is a drug that has a depressant effect on the brain. Thinking, balance, coordination, and mental alertness are affected. Some people are physically or psychologically dependent on alcohol. They have an illness called alcoholism which can be treated and controlled with the person's desire and cooperation.

Moderate alcohol use is accepted by many people and religious groups. However, alcohol affects your mind and body. Therefore you must never report to work under the influence of alcohol or drink alcohol while working. The safety of your patients, residents, co-workers, and yourself must be considered.

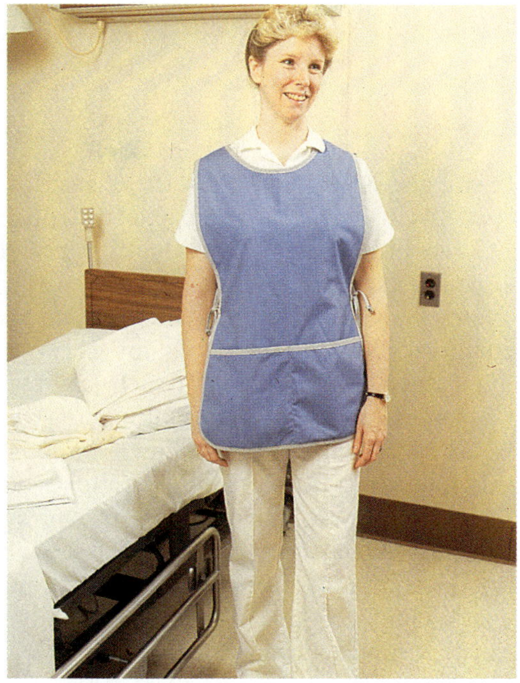

Fig. 2-2 *A well-groomed nursing assistant. Note the hairstyle and length and fit of the uniform.*

Hygiene You must pay careful attention to your personal cleanliness. Preventing offensive body and breath odors is important. You should bathe daily, use a deodorant or antiperspirant, brush your teeth after meals, and use a mouthwash regularly. Your hair should be clean and styled in an attractive and simple way. Fingernails should be clean, short, and neatly shaped.

Special hygiene measures are necessary during menstrual periods. Be sure to change tampons or sanitary napkins frequently, especially if flow is heavy. The genital area should be washed with soap and water at least twice a day. Handwashing is necessary after going to the bathroom, changing tampons or sanitary napkins, and washing the genital area.

Foot care prevents odors and infection. Feet should be bathed daily and dried thoroughly between the toes. Cut toenails straight across after bathing or soaking them in water.

Appearance Good health and personal hygiene practices help you look and feel well. Box 2-4 on page 24 describes practices and suggestions to help you look neat, clean, and professional (Fig. 2-2).

NURSING ASSISTANT TRAINING AND COMPETENCY EVALUATION

The care you give is very important to the health and welfare of patients and residents. Safe, effective, quality care is essential to protect them from harm. Until recently, only some states required nursing assistant training. Those states had laws requiring that individuals learn basic nursing knowledge and skills for employment as nursing assistants. The purpose of such training was to protect persons from unsafe and poor nursing care.

In 1987 the U.S. Congress passed the Omnibus Budget Reconciliation Act (OBRA). This law applies to all 50 states. One purpose of this law is to improve the quality of care given to residents of nursing facilities. The law requires education and competency evaluation for all nursing assistants employed in nursing facilities. This requirement ensures that nursing assistants have the necessary knowledge and skills to give safe care.

The Training Program

Every state has a nursing assistant training and competency evaluation program. State requirements vary. However, OBRA requires at least 75 hours of instruction. Sixteen of those hours must be supervised practical training. Such training occurs in a laboratory or clinical setting. The student actually performs nursing care and procedures on another person. This practical training (also called a clinical practicum or clinical experience) is supervised by a nurse. Usually the nurse is the course instructor.

The training program includes the knowledge and skills needed by nursing assistants to perform their roles and responsibilities. Areas to be studied include:

- Communication
- Infection control
- Safety and emergency procedures
- Residents' rights
- Basic nursing skills
- Personal care skills
- Feeding techniques
- Elimination procedures
- Skin care
- Transferring, positioning, and turning techniques
- Dressing
- Ambulating (walking) residents
- Range-of-motion exercises

BOX 2-4 Practices for a Professional Appearance

- Uniforms should fit well and be modest in length and style.
- Make sure your uniforms are clean, pressed, and mended. Wear a clean uniform daily.
- Wear your name badge or photo ID at all times when on duty.
- Underclothes should be clean, fit properly, and be changed daily. Because of perspiration, you may want to change underclothing more often during hot, humid weather and after vigorous exercise.
- Jewelry should not be worn while on duty. Most facilities let employees wear wedding rings; engagement rings may be allowed. Large rings and bracelets can scratch patients and residents. Necklaces, bracelets, and earrings can easily be pulled off by confused or combative persons, causing you physical injury. Young children also like to pull on jewelry.
- Stockings and socks should be clean, well-fitting, and changed daily. Do not roll stockings down or wear round garters. These practices interfere with circulation in the legs.
- Shoes should be comfortable, give needed support, and fit properly. Clean and polish shoes often to keep them white and neat. Wash laces and replace them as necessary.
- Nail polish should not be worn. Chipped nail polish provides a place for microorganisms to grow and multiply. Some facilities let employees wear clear nail polish.
- Hairstyles should be simple and attractive. Make sure your hair is off your collar and does not fall in your face. Use simple pins, combs, barrettes, and bands to keep long hair up and in place.
- Makeup should be modest in amount and moderate in color. Avoid a painted and severe appearance.
- Perfume, cologne, and after-shave lotions should not be worn. They may be offensive and nauseating to patients and residents. Some facilities let employees wear lightly scented colognes.

- Signs and symptoms of common diseases and conditions
- How to care for cognitively impaired residents (those who have problems with thinking and memory)

Competency Evaluation

The competency evaluation program includes a written test and a skills test. The *written* test involves multiple-choice questions with 4 possible answers. Some states also use true and false questions and matching questions. Each question has only 1 correct answer. The number of test questions varies from state to state. Some states have only 50 questions while others have more than 100. Your instructor can tell you how many questions are on your state's test. The test will probably be like the paper and pencil tests you take in your training program. Some states have computerized testing. The *skills* evaluation involves demonstrating nursing skills. You will perform certain skills learned in your training program.

The written and skills competency evaluations are taken after completing your training program. Your instructor tells you where the tests are given and helps you complete the application form. There is a fee for the competency evaluation. This fee is sent with your application. You are notified about the location and time of the tests after your application has been processed.

Preparation for the competency evaluation began the first day of your training program. If you listen, pay attention, study hard, and practice safe and effective care, you should do well on both the written and skills tests. If the first attempt was unsuccessful, you can retest. OBRA allows 3 opportunities to successfully complete the evaluation.

Nursing Assistant Registry

OBRA requires that each state have a nursing assistant registry. The registry is an official record or listing of persons who have successfully completed a state-approved nursing assistant training and competency evaluation program. The registry contains the following information about each nursing assistant:

- Full name, including maiden name and any married names
- Last known home address
- Social security number
- Last known employer, date hired, and date employment was terminated
- Date the competency evaluation was passed
- Information about findings of abuse, neglect, or dishonest use of property. Such information includes the nature of the offense and evidence supporting the finding. If a hearing was held, the date and its outcome are included. The individual has the right to include a statement disputing the finding. All of this information must remain in the registry for at least 5 years.

Registry information is requested by any facility or agency needing the information. The nursing assistant also receives a copy of all information relating to him or her in the registry. The copy is provided when first included in the registry and when information is changed or added. The nursing assistant can correct wrong information.

Other OBRA Requirements

OBRA also requires retraining and a new competency evaluation program for nursing assistants who have not worked for 2 consecutive years (24 months). For example, Linda Ames completed a training and competency evaluation. After working as a nursing assistant, she quit her job to go back to school. Three years later she decides to work as a nursing assistant again. According to OBRA, she has to take another training and competency evaluation program. This is to ensure that she has current knowledge and skills to give safe care. It does not matter how long she worked as a nursing assistant. What matters is how long she did *not* work.

Regular in-service education and performance reviews are other OBRA requirements. Nursing facilities must regularly provide educational programs to nursing assistants. The work of each nursing assistant must also be regularly evaluated. These requirements help ensure that nursing assistants have the knowledge and skills to give safe, effective care.

ETHICAL AND LEGAL CONSIDERATIONS

Situations occur in which you must decide what you should and should not do or what you can and cannot do. The problem may involve ethical or legal questions. What would you do if:

- A patient asks you to witness the signing of a will.
- A nurse tells you to "tie down" Mr. Green because he keeps trying to get out of bed.
- A friend's boss is one of your patients. The friend wants to know what is wrong with the patient.
- A family member is admitted to your nursing unit.

- A nurse told you to give Mrs. Andrews an enema. Mrs. Andrews refuses the procedure.
- You are helping an RN with a resident. She wants the room door open so that she can see when Dr. James arrives.
- You think another team member has abused a resident.

The following discussion will help you to decide what to do if these events or others happen.

Ethics

Ethics is the discipline concerned with what is right and wrong conduct. It involves morals and making choices or judgments about what should or should not be done. An ethical person behaves and acts in the right way.

Each professional group has a code of ethics. The code involves rules, or standards of conduct, that members of the group are to follow. The American Nurses Association (ANA) has a code of ethics for RNs. The National Federation of Licensed Practical Nurses (NFLPN) has one for LPNs. You should develop your own personal code of ethics. Consider the rules of conduct for nursing assistants in Box 2-5.

Legal Considerations

Legal considerations relate to laws. A **law** is a rule of conduct made by a government body such as the U.S. Congress or a state legislature. Laws protect the public welfare and are enforced by the government.

Criminal laws are concerned with offenses against the public and against society in general. A violation of a criminal law is called a **crime.** A person found guilty of a crime is fined or sent to prison. Murder, robbery, rape, and kidnapping are examples of crimes.

Civil laws deal with the relationships between people. Examples of civil laws are those that involve contracts and nursing practice. A person found guilty of breaking a civil law usually has to pay a sum of money to the injured person.

Torts

Tort comes from a French word meaning *wrong.* Torts are part of civil law. A tort is committed by an individual against another person or the person's property. Torts may be intentional or unintentional. Torts common to health care are presented below.

Unintentional Torts

Negligence is an unintentional wrong. The person did not mean or intend to cause harm. The negligent person failed to act in a reasonable and careful manner and thereby caused harm to the person or property of another. The person at fault failed to do what a reasonable and careful person would have done. Or he or she did what a reasonable and careful person would not have done. The negligent person may have to pay damages (that is, a sum of money) to the injured person.

Malpractice is negligence by professionals. A person has professional status because of training, education, and the type of service provided. Nurses, doctors, dentists, lawyers, and pharmacists are examples of professional people.

Box 2-6 gives some common examples of negligent acts committed by nursing assistants. As a nursing assistant, you are legally responsible *(liable)* for your own actions. What you do or do not do can lead to a lawsuit if harm results to the person or property of another. A nurse may direct you to do something that is beyond the legal scope of your role. Or you may be asked to do something for which you have not been prepared. Giving medications is

BOX 2-5 Rules of Conduct for Nursing Assistants

- Respect each patient or resident as an individual.
- Perform no act that is not within the legal scope of the nursing assistant.
- Perform no act for which you have not been adequately prepared.
- Take no drug without the prescription and supervision of a physician.
- Carry out the directions and instructions of the nurse to your best possible ability.
- Be loyal to your employer and co-workers.
- Act as a responsible citizen at all times.
- Recognize the limits of your role and knowledge.
- Keep patient and resident information confidential.
- Consider the patient's or resident's needs to be more important than your own.

an example. You may be told not to worry, that the nurse will take full responsibility if anything happens. The nurse will be held liable as your supervisor. However, in no way are you relieved of personal liability. *You are responsible for your own actions.*

You function under the direction and supervision of a nurse. However, there are times that you have a right and a duty to refuse to follow the nurse's directions. You should refuse to follow the nurse's order if:

- You are asked to do something that is beyond the legal scope of your role.
- You have not been prepared to perform the function safely.
- You know that the act or procedure may cause harm to the person.
- The nurse's directions or orders are unethical, illegal, or against the policies of the facility.
- Directions are unclear or incomplete.

You can protect the persons you care for and yourself from negligent acts by using common sense. Ask yourself if what you are doing is safe for the person.

Intentional Torts Intentional torts are acts that are meant to be harmful. Defamation (libel and slander), assault and battery, false imprisonment, invasion of privacy, and fraud are intentional torts.

Defamation is injuring the name and reputation of a person by making false statements to a third person. **Libel** is making false statements in print, writing, or through pictures or drawings. **Slander** is making false statements orally. You can protect yourself from defamation by never making false statements about a patient or resident, a co-worker, or any other person. Examples of defamation include:

- Implying or suggesting that a person has a sexually transmitted disease
- Saying that a patient is insane or mentally ill
- Implying or suggesting that a person is corrupt or dishonest

Assault and battery are intentional torts. They may result in both civil and criminal charges. **Assault** is intentionally attempting or threatening to touch a person's body without the person's consent. The person fears bodily harm. Threatening to "tie down" or restrain an uncooperative patient is an example of assault.

Battery is the actual touching of a person's body without the person's consent. Consent is the important factor in assault and battery. The person must consent to any procedure, treatment, or other act that involves touching the body. The person has the right to withdraw consent at any time.

Consent is more than a person's verbal okay or signature on a form. For consent to be valid, it must be *informed* consent. Informed consent is discussed on page 29.

You can protect yourself from being accused of battery. Explain to the person what is to be done and get the person's consent. The consent may be verbal, such as "yes" or "okay." Consent may be a gesture, such as a nod, turning over for a back rub, or holding out an arm so that the pulse can be taken.

False imprisonment is the unlawful restraint or restriction of a person's freedom of movement. Threat of restraint or actual physical restraint constitutes false imprisonment. Common examples of false imprisonment include:

- Preventing a person from leaving the facility
- Using unneeded restraints on a patient

BOX 2-6 Common Negligent Acts of Nursing Assistants

- The side rails have been ordered for a confused resident. The nursing assistant leaves the side rails down. The resident falls out of bed and breaks a hip.
- A patient is burned because a nursing assistant applied a warm water bottle that was too hot.
- A patient's dentures break after being dropped by the nursing assistant.
- A resident complains to the nursing assistant of chest pain and difficulty breathing. The complaints are not reported to the nurse. The patient has a heart attack and dies.
- A resident puts on the signal light. The nursing assistant goes past the room several times but does not answer the light. The resident goes into shock because of sudden, severe bleeding.

BOX 2-7 How to Protect the Person's Right to Privacy

- Keep all patient or resident information confidential. This includes information in the person's medical record (see Chapter 3).
- Make sure the person is covered when being moved in corridors.
- Screen the person as in Figure 2-3 and close the door when giving care. Also close drapes and window shades as appropriate.
- Expose only the body part involved in a treatment or procedure.
- Do not discuss the person or the person's treatment with anyone except the nurse supervising your work. "Shop talk" is a common cause of invasion of privacy.
- Ask visitors to leave the room when care must be given. Only personnel involved in the person's care should be present when care is given.
- Do not open the person's mail. Everyone has the right to send and receive mail unopened.
- Allow the person to visit with others and to use the telephone in private.

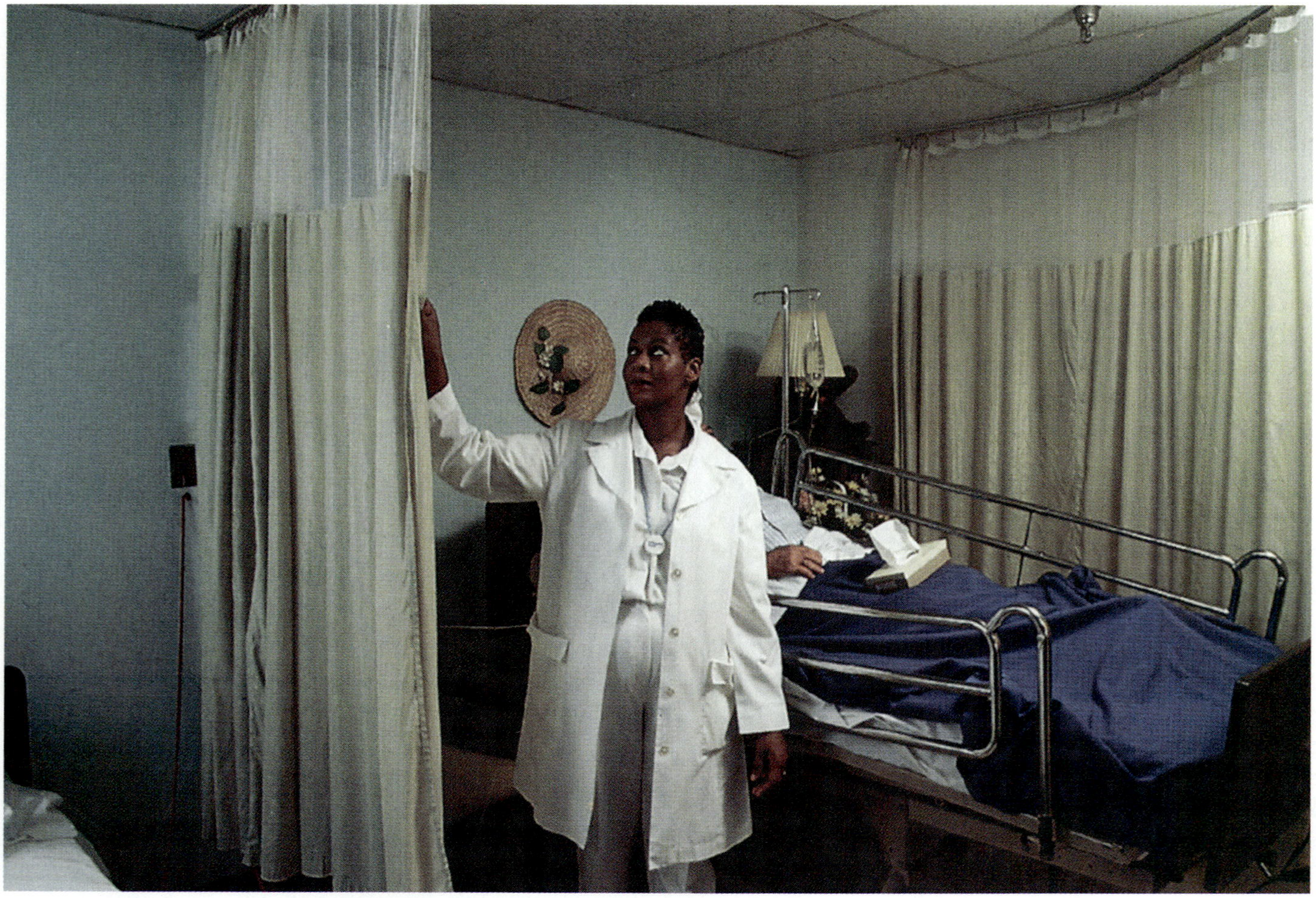

Fig. 2-3 *The nursing assistant protects the person's privacy by pulling the curtain around the bed.*

Invasion of privacy is another tort. Every person has the right not to have his or her name, photograph, or private affairs exposed or made public without having given consent. Violating this right is an invasion of privacy. You must treat patients and residents with respect and ensure their privacy. Only health workers involved in the person's care should see, handle, or examine the person's body. You can ensure the right to privacy by exercising the precautions listed in Box 2-7.

Fraud is saying or doing something to trick, fool, or deceive another person. The act is fraud if it does or could cause harm to a person or the person's property. Telling a patient, resident, or family that you are a nurse is fraud. Giving incomplete or inaccurate information on a job application is also fraud.

Informed Consent

Informed consent recognizes a person's right to decide what will be done to his or her body and who can touch his or her body. Consent is considered informed when the person clearly understands the reason for a treatment, what will be done, how it will be done, who will do it, and the expected outcomes. The person also must understand other treatment options and the effects of not having the treatment. The doctor is responsible for informing the person about all aspects of treatment.

Often consent must be given for persons under legal age (usually 18 years of age). Consent is given by a parent or legal guardian. Mentally incompetent persons also cannot give legal consent. Persons who are unconscious, sedated, or confused are not mentally competent to give legal consent. Persons with certain mental health disorders are also incompetent to give consent. Consent is given by a responsible party. The responsible party may be a husband, wife, son, daughter, or a legal representative. As with consent given by the patient or resident, consent by a parent, legal guardian, or other responsible party must be informed consent.

Consent is given when the person enters the health care facility. A form is signed giving general consent to treatment. Special consent forms are required for surgery and other complex and invasive procedures. The doctor is responsible for informing the person about all aspects of the surgery or procedure. The nurse may be given this responsibility. Nursing assistants are never responsible for obtaining written consent for general treatment or for surgery or special procedures.

Wills

A **will** is a legal statement of how a person wants property distributed after his or her death. A patient or resident may ask you to help prepare a will. You must politely refuse such a request. Explain that you do not have the knowledge or legal ability to prepare a will. Ask a nurse to speak to the person about contacting a lawyer.

Legally you can witness the signing of a will. However, many facilities have policies about staff members witnessing wills. Make sure you know the policy of your facility. Do not witness a person's will if you have been named in the will. To do so would prevent you from receiving what had been left to you. If you are a witness, you must be prepared to testify that the person was of sound mind when the will was signed. Also be prepared to testify that the person stated that the document being signed was the person's last will. Be sure to tell your supervisor that you were a witness to a person's will.

BECOMING EMPLOYED

The U.S. Department of Labor has predicted an increase of over 100,000 jobs for nursing assistants and home health aides between 1992 and 2005. These jobs are mainly in nursing facilities, home care agencies, and hospitals. Hospices, rehabilitation centers, and clinics also hire nursing assistants. Most jobs are in nursing facilities.

You can look for a job during your training program. Or you can wait until you have passed the competency test. If you already have a job, someday you may want to change to a different facility. Whenever you look for employment, you want to find the right job for you.

Finding a Job

You may already know where you want to work. If not, there are some simple ways to find out about job openings. One place is the *classified ad* sections of newspapers. The local *state employment service* is also a source. You may also hear about jobs from *people you know.* You can also directly *contact the facilities* where you would like to work. Phone book yellow pages have listings of health care facilities.

The facility for your student clinical experience is another place to look. The staff always looks at students as potential employees. They watch how students treat patients, residents, and co-workers. They look for the qualities and characteristics described on page 30. So you are really being considered for a job while still a student. This is one more reason to always function at your best. If that facility is not hiring, the staff may know of places looking for nursing assistants.

What Employers Look For

Before applying for a job or interviewing, think about what employers want in those they hire. If you had your own business, who would you want to hire? Answering that question helps you better understand the employer's point of view.

Employers want employees who:

- Are well groomed
- Are dependable
- Have the skills and training needed to do the job

Caring about others is a common trait of health team members. Caring enough to want to make the life of a person happier, easier, or less painful is an essential characteristic of a nursing assistant. There are certain traits, attitudes, and manners that allow one to perform the job

BOX 2-8 QUALITIES AND CHARACTERISTICS NEEDED BY THE NURSING ASSISTANT

Dependability The patient or resident and the nursing team rely on you to report to work on time and when scheduled. They also depend on you to perform duties and tasks as assigned and to keep obligations and promises.

Consideration You need to be considerate of the person's physical and emotional feelings. Patients, residents, and families must be treated gently and with kindness.

Cheerfulness You need to pleasantly greet and talk with patients, residents, and others. You cannot be moody, bad tempered, scornful or cutting, or unhappy when caring for patients or residents.

Empathy Empathy is being able to see things from the other person's point of view—to put yourself in the person's position. How would you feel if you had the person's problem?

Trustworthiness Patients, residents, and co-workers have confidence in you. They believe you will keep patient or resident information confidential. They trust that you will not gossip about patients, residents, co-workers, doctors, or the health team.

Respectfulness Patients and residents have rights, values, beliefs, and feelings. Although these may differ from yours, you must not criticize or condemn the person. The person is treated with respect and dignity at all times. Also show respect for supervisors and co-workers.

Courtesy You must be polite and courteous to patients, residents, families, visitors, and co-workers. People are addressed by title and name ("Mr. Johnson," "Ms. Poole," "Dr. Gilson"). Other courteous acts include explaining to the person what is going to be done before performing a procedure, saying "please" and "thank you," and not interrupting others unnecessarily.

Conscientiousness You must be careful, alert, and exact in following orders and instructions. You must give thorough care with knowledge and skill, and give your best possible effort.

Honesty You must be truthful, sincere, and genuine and show a true interest in the person. The amount and kind of care given, your observations, and any errors are to be reported truthfully and accurately.

Cooperation You must be willing to help and work with others. Cooperation is shown by working well with others and taking that "extra step" during busy and stressful times.

Enthusiasm Enthusiasm is being eager, interested, and excited about your work. What you are doing is important. If you are enthusiastic, you will want to gain more self-confidence, skill, and knowledge.

Self-awareness Being self-aware means knowing your own feelings, strengths, and weaknesses. You need to understand yourself before you can understand your patients or residents.

well. These are called *qualities and characteristics.* Along with caring, Box 2-8 describes the qualities and characteristics necessary for you to function effectively as a nursing assistant (Fig. 2-4).

Applicants who look good communicate many things to the employer. You have only one chance to make a good first impression. A well-groomed person is likely to get the job over someone who is sloppy and is wearing wrinkled or dirty clothes. Proper dress for an interview is discussed later in this section.

The importance of being dependable was discussed on page 30. Health care employers provide services to patients and residents. They need staff to be at work on time and when scheduled. Undependable people cause everyone problems. Other staff take on extra work. Fewer people give care to patients and residents. Quality of care can easily suffer. Supervisors spend time trying to find out if the person is coming to work. They also have to find someone else to cover for the absent employee. If you had your own business, you would want people to be at work when expected. Otherwise your business would be less efficient and productive.

Employers need to know that nursing assistant applicants are able to perform the skills required for the job. Also, OBRA requires that nursing facilities hire nursing assistants who have completed a state-approved training program. Home care agencies also require such training as do many hospitals. The employer must have proof that you have had the required training. If you have successfully completed the training, the employer knows you have the skills for the job. A certificate of course completion or a high school, college, or technical school transcript will document your training. Some employers accept a copy of an official grade report (report card). The

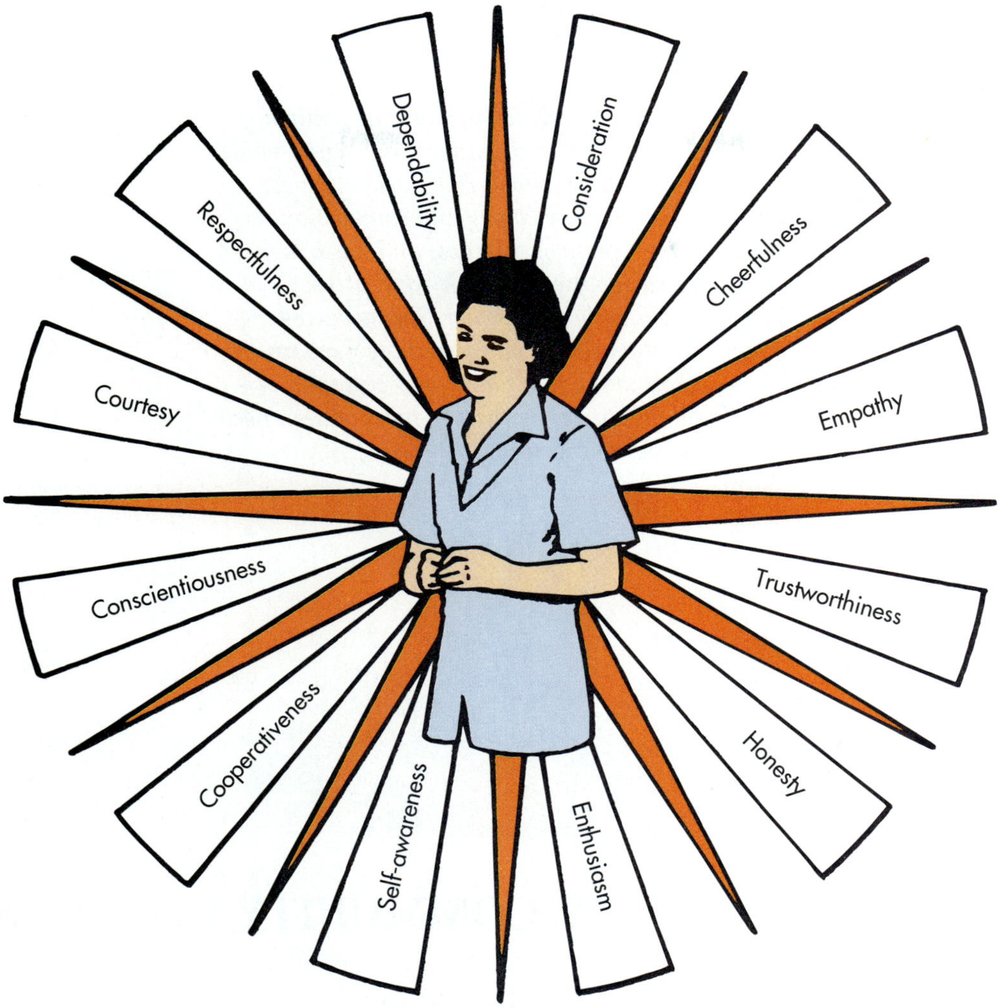

Fig. 2-4 *The qualities and characteristics of a successful nursing assistant.*

employer also checks your record in the state nursing assistant registry.

Many high school, college, and technical school programs give a certificate of course completion (Fig. 2-5 on page 32). The original is your personal property. Make several copies of the original certificate and then keep it in a safe place. Some employers accept a copy as proof of your training. Others make a copy of the original certificate. *Never give the original to the employer to keep.*

Job Applications

The facility will want you to complete a job application (Fig. 2-6 on pages 33-35). The application is obtained from the *personnel office* or *human resources office.* You may be asked to complete the application in the personnel office. Some facilities have you take the application with you and return it by mail or in person. Make sure you are well groomed when seeking or returning a job application. It may be your first chance to make a good impression.

The application asks for general information: your name, where you live, telephone number, the job you are applying for, how much you expect to earn, and when you can work. You will also be asked about your education, work experience, and any felony (criminal) convictions. Also be prepared to give the names, addresses, and telephone numbers of at least three references. Be sure to ask these references if it is okay if they are contacted by an employer.

Refer to the guidelines in Box 2-9 on page 36 when completing a job application. How you fill it out may mean the difference between getting or not getting the job. The application may also be your first chance to impress the employer. A neat, legible, complete application creates a better image than one that is sloppy or incomplete. Remember, employers use applications to screen out unqualified applicants.

The Job Interview

A job interview is the employer's chance to get to know and evaluate you. It is also a time for you to find out more about the facility. Remember, employers want people who are well groomed, dependable, and have the skills and

Text continued on page 36.

Spotlight On…

Terri D of Davenport, Iowa, *works as a nursing assistant in a hospital outpatient care center while she attends nursing school. Her nurse manager describes her as "very caring and compassionate. She displays a sense of calmness and has a high regard for each patient's dignity and privacy. Patients frequently request her. She has excellent communication skills and immediately reports observations to the RN. She is very customer oriented and prioritizes her care to meet patient needs. She is an asset to our unit."*

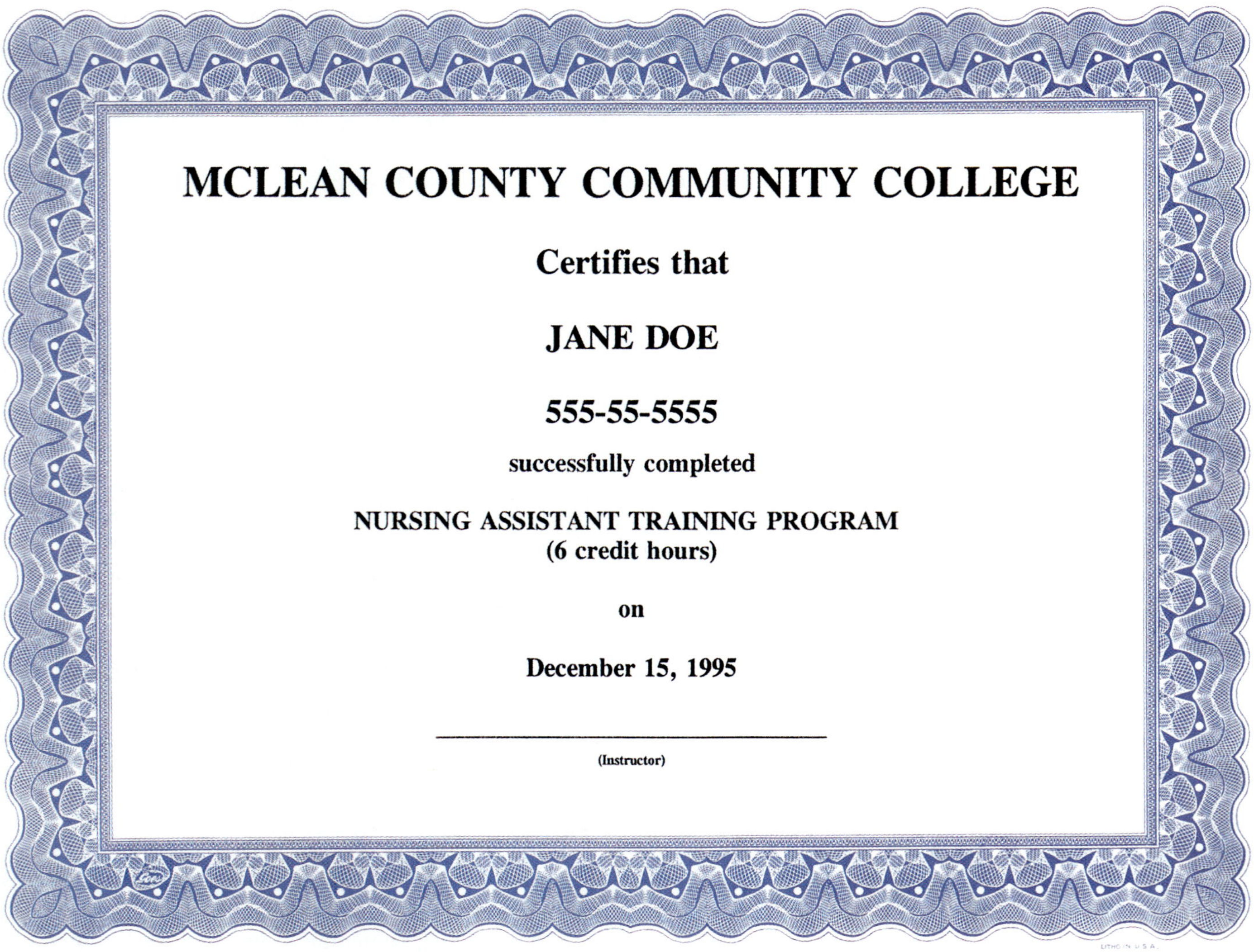

MCLEAN COUNTY COMMUNITY COLLEGE

Certifies that

JANE DOE

555-55-5555

successfully completed

NURSING ASSISTANT TRAINING PROGRAM
(6 credit hours)

on

December 15, 1995

____

(Instructor)

Fig. 2-5 *Certificate of completion for a nursing assistant training program.*

DATE

POSITION DESIRED

NAME LAST FIRST MIDDLE INITIAL

OSF℠
SAINT JOSEPH MEDICAL CENTER

2200 E. Washington Street, Bloomington, Illinois 61701
Phone (309) 662-3311

APPLICATION FOR EMPLOYMENT

St. Joseph Medical Center is an equal opportunity employer and does not discriminate because of age, sex, race, creed, color, religion, national origin, marital status, or disability.

PERSONAL

PLEASE PRINT

LAST NAME	FIRST NAME	MIDDLE INITIAL	SOCIAL SECURITY NO.
STREET ADDRESS, CITY, STATE, ZIP		TELEPHONE	AREA CODE
HAVE YOU EVER APPLIED HERE BEFORE? ☐ YES ☐ NO	WHEN?	FOR WHAT POSITION?	ALTERNATE TELEPHONE / AREA CODE
IF UNDER AGE 18, GIVE BIRTHDATE.	ARE YOU A U.S. CITIZEN OR AN ALIEN LEGALLY AUTHORIZED TO WORK IN THE U.S.A.? ☐ YES ☐ NO		
WERE YOU EVER IN OUR EMPLOYMENT? ☐ YES ☐ NO	IF YES, WHEN?	IN WHAT CAPACITY?	UNDER WHAT NAME DID YOU WORK?
DO YOU HAVE ANY RELATIVES WORKING AT ST. JOESPH MEDICAL CENTER? ☐ YES ☐ NO	IF YES, PLEASE LIST NAMES AND RELATIONSHIP		
HAVE YOU BEEN CONVICTED OF A FELONY? (A FELONY CONVICTION DOES NOT AUTOMATICALLY DISQUALIFY YOU FROM EMPLOYMENT). ☐ YES ☐ NO	IF YES, EXPLAIN:		

EMPLOYMENT DATA

ARE YOU WILLING TO WORK WEEKENDS AND/OR HOLIDAYS? ☐ YES ☐ NO	ARE YOU WILLING TO WORK OVERTIME IF REQUIRED? ☐ YES ☐ NO	CIRCLE DAYS YOU CAN WORK: MON. TUES. WED. THURS. FRI. SAT. SUN.	WHAT SHIFT ARE YOU WILLING TO WORK? 1ST 2ND 3RD ROTATION
ARE YOU APPLYING FOR: ☐ FULL-TIME ☐ PART-TIME ☐ EITHER ☐ TEMPORARY ☐ PRN ☐ SUMMER ONLY	IF APPLYING FOR PART-TIME, HOW MANY HOURS PER WEEK ARE YOU ABLE TO WORK?		

WHAT PROMPTED YOUR APPLICAITON?

☐ EMPLOYEE REFERRAL________________ ☐ OWN ACCORD________________

☐ NEWSPAPER________________ ☐ OTHER________________

STJOMC (Rev. 2/95) Med-Forms, Inc.™

Fig. 2-6 *A sample job application.* (Courtesy St. Joseph Medical Center, Bloomington, Illinois.)

Continued.

EDUCATION					
	NAME & ADDRESS OF SCHOOL	COURSE OF STUDY	CIRCLE LAST YEAR COMPLETED	DID YOU GRADUATE	LIST DEGREE OR DIPLOMA
HIGH SCHOOL			1 2 3 4	☐ YES ☐ NO	
COLLEGE			1 2 3 4	☐ YES ☐ NO	
OTHER					
IF NOW ATTENDING SCHOOL, PLEASE GIVE ANTICIPATED GRADUATION DATE.					

EMPLOYMENT HISTORY			
PRESENT OR MOST RECENT EMPLOYER	NAME OF EMPLOYER	STREET ADDRESS, CITY, STATE, ZIP	PHONE NUMBER
	WHAT NAME DID YOU WORK UNDER?	JOB TITLE	DATE OF EMPLOYMENT FROM: TO:
	REASON FOR LEAVING?	SUPERVISOR'S NAME	ENDING SALARY
	MAY WE CONTACT? ☐ YES ☐ NO IF NO, WHY?	DUTIES, SKILLS, EQUIPMENT USED:	
PREVIOUS EMPLOYERS LIST MOST RECENT FIRST	NAME OF EMPLOYER	STREET ADDRESS, CITY, STATE, ZIP	PHONE NUMBER
	WHAT NAME DID YOU WORK UNDER?	JOB TITLE	DATE OF EMPLOYMENT FROM: TO:
	REASON FOR LEAVING?	SUPERVISOR'S NAME	ENDING SALARY
	MAY WE CONTACT? ☐ YES ☐ NO IF NO, WHY?	DUTIES, SKILLS, EQUIPMENT USED:	
	NAME OF EMPLOYER	STREET ADDRESS, CITY, STATE, ZIP	PHONE NUMBER
	WHAT NAME DID YOU WORK UNDER?	JOB TITLE	DATE OF EMPLOYMENT FROM: TO:
	REASON FOR LEAVING?	SUPERVISOR'S NAME	ENDING SALARY
	MAY WE CONTACT? ☐ YES ☐ NO IF NO, WHY?	DUTIES, SKILLS, EQUIPMENT USED:	
	NAME OF EMPLOYER	STREET ADDRESS, CITY, STATE, ZIP	PHONE NUMBER
	WHAT NAME DID YOU WORK UNDER?	JOB TITLE	DATE OF EMPLOYMENT FROM: TO:
	REASON FOR LEAVING?	SUPERVISOR'S NAME	ENDING SALARY
	MAY WE CONTACT? ☐ YES ☐ NO IF NO, WHY?	DUTIES, SKILLS, EQUIPMENT USED:	

I HEREBY GIVE PERMISSION TO ST. JOSEPH MEDICAL CENTER TO CONTACT THE EMPLOYERS LISTED ABOVE TO OBTAIN ANY INFORMATION ST. JOSEPH MEDICAL CENTER DEEMS RELEVANT. I COMPLETELY RELEASE ST. JOSEPH MEDICAL CENTER AND THE PROVIDERS OF THE INFORMATION FROM ANY AND ALL LIABILITY ARISING OUT OF INQUIRIES MADE OR INFORMATION PROVIDED RELATIVE TO MY APPLICATION FOR EMPLOYMENT.

_______________________ DATE

_______________________ APPLICANT SIGNATURE

Fig. 2-6—cont'd *A sample job application.*

PLEASE NOTE ANY ADDITIONAL SKILLS, EXPERIENCE, OR TRAINING THAT YOU FEEL IS IMPORTANT. PLEASE INCLUDE EQUIPMENT OR COMPUTER SOFTWARE USED.

TYPING (APPROXIMATE SPEED: WPM)	SHORTHAND (APPROXIMATE SPEED: WPM)
WORD PROCESSING — CIRCLE ONE: BEGINNING INTERMEDIATE ADVANCED	TRANSCRIBING — CIRCLE ONE: BEGINNING INTERMEDIATE ADVANCED
COMPUTER EXPERIENCE — CIRCLE ONE: BEGINNING INTERMEDIATE ADVANCED	MEDICAL TERMINOLOGY — CIRCLE ONE: BEGINNING INTERMEDIATE ADVANCED

PROFESSIONAL LICENSES AND/OR CERTIFICATIONS

ARE YOU CURRENTLY: ☐ REGISTERED ☐ LICENSED ☐ CERTIFIED

ARE YOU ELIGIBLE FOR: ☐ REGISTRATION ☐ LICENSURE ☐ CERTIFICATION

IF LICENSED, REGISTERED OR CERTIFIED				
	TYPE	STATE ISSUED	DATE	NO.
	TYPE	STATE ISSUED	DATE	NO.
	TYPE	STATE ISSUED	DATE	NO.

IF THE JOB YOU ARE APPLYING FOR REQUIRES THE DRIVING OF A MOTOR VEHICLE WHILE ON DUTY, PLEASE PROVIDE THE FOLLOWING INFORMATION:

DRIVER'S LICENSE NO. ____________________ STATE ____________

EMPLOYMENT CONDITIONS

I understand that if I make any false statements, misrepresentations, or omissions on this application or during the hiring process, I may be refused employment or, if employed, I may be terminated regardless of when discovered. In consideration of my employment, I agree to conform to the rules, regulations and Philosophy and values of St. Joseph Medical Center. I understand this application is not intended to be a contract of employment. I understand that my employment can be terminated at any time and for any reason, at the option of either St. Joseph Medical Center or myself. I understand that no one other than the Administrator has any authority to enter into any agreement for employment for any specified period of time or to make any agreement contrary to the foregoing and that any such agreement must be in writing, signed by the Administrator, and notarized. I also understand that I will be required to complete a medical examination which may include a drug screen before beginning employment.

____________________ Date

____________________ Applicant Signature

Fig. 2-6—cont'd *A sample job application.*

BOX 2-9 Guidelines for Completing a Job Application

- Read the directions first and then follow them. The directions may ask you to use black ink and to print. Following directions is important on the job. Employers look at job applications to see how well applicants follow directions.
- Make sure your writing is neat and legible. A messy application creates a poor image. Writing must be legible so the employer has the correct information. You could miss out on getting a job if the employer cannot read your telephone number or address to contact you.
- Complete the entire application. If something does not apply to you, write "N/A" for nonapplicable or draw a line through the space. This tells the employer that you read the application and that you did not skip the item on purpose.
- Report any felony convictions as directed. Write "no" or "none" if you were arrested but not convicted. Some states require criminal background checks.
- Provide information about employment gaps. If there was a time when you did not work, the employer will wonder why. Provide this information so the employer has a good impression about your honesty. Some reasons include going to school, staying home to raise children, caring for an ill family member, or having been ill yourself.
- Give information about why you left a job, if asked. Be brief, but honest. Usually people leave a job for one that pays better or provides opportunities for advancement. Other reasons include those given above for employment gaps. If you were fired from a job, find a response that is honest but positive.
- Provide references as requested. Be prepared to give the names, titles, addresses, and telephone numbers of at least three references. You should have this information written down before completing an application. You may get the job faster or over a competing applicant if the employer can quickly check references. If they are missing or incomplete, the employer needs to wait for all of the information. This wastes your time and the employer's time. Also, the employer may wonder if you have something to hide if reference information is incomplete.
- Be honest in all your responses. Lying on an application is grounds for being fired. It may also constitute fraud.

training to do the job. You are evaluated in these three areas during the interview.

The interview may be at the time you complete the job application. Or the application may be reviewed first to see if you are qualified. Box 2-10 lists some of the questions that you may be asked. You should prepare answers to these questions ahead of time.

Your appearance is important. You must make a good impression. You need to be neat, clean, and well groomed (Fig. 2-7). Your dress is also important. Box 2-11 gives guidelines on how to dress for an interview.

You need to be on time. It shows the employer that you are dependable. If you have never been to the facility or do not know where it is, a *dry run* may be useful. Go to the facility some day before your interview. Note how much time it takes to get there and where to park. You might also ask where to find the personnel office. A dry run gives you an idea of how much time you need to get from your home to the personnel office.

When you arrive for the interview, give the receptionist your name and your purpose for being there. Also give the name of the interviewer. You may be asked to take a seat in the waiting area. Be sure to sit quietly in a professional manner. Do not smoke or chew gum. Use the time to go over the common interview questions and your answers. Remember, waiting may be part of the interview. The employer is likely to ask the receptionist about you—how you presented yourself when you arrived and what you did while waiting. You need to be polite and friendly at all times.

Be sure to greet the interviewer in a polite, courteous manner. A firm handshake is appropriate for both men

A

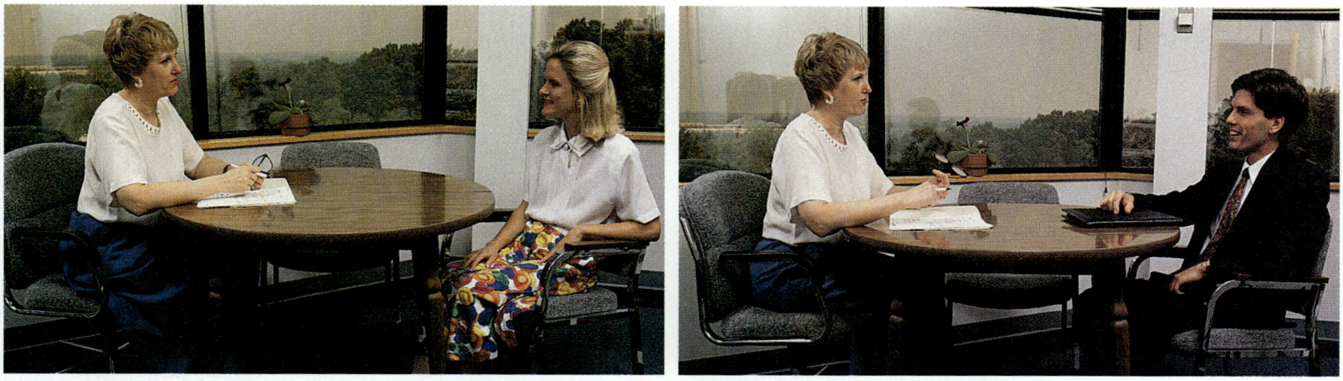

B

Fig. 2-7 *A, The nursing assistant is wearing a simple skirt and blouse for her interview. B, This man is wearing dark slacks, a shirt and tie, and a jacket for his interview.*

BOX 2-10 Common Interview Questions

- Please tell me about your career goals.
- What are you doing currently to achieve these goals?
- Describe what you consider to be *professional* nursing assistant behavior.
- Tell me about your last job.
- What would your supervisor and co-workers tell me about your dependability? Your skills? Your ability to adapt?
- Of all your responsibilities, which presented the most difficulty for you?
- How did you handle this difficulty?
- How do you set priorities?
- In what ways have your past experiences prepared you for this position?
- If there is one thing that you could change about your last job, what would it be?
- How do you handle problems with patients and co-workers?

BOX 2-11 Grooming and Dressing for an Interview

- Take a bath, brush your teeth, and wash your hair.
- Use a deodorant or antiperspirant.
- Make sure your hands and fingernails are clean.
- Apply makeup in a simple, attractive manner.
- Style your hair so that it is neat and attractive. You may want to wear it as you would for work.
- Do not wear jeans, shorts, tank tops, halter tops, or other casual clothing.
- Wear a simple dress, suit, or skirt and blouse (women). Men should wear a suit or dark slacks, shirt and tie, and a jacket.
- Make sure clothing is pressed and in good repair. Sew on loose buttons and mend garments as needed.
- Wear socks (men and women) or hose (women). Hose should be free of runs and snags.
- Make sure shoes are polished and in good repair.
- Avoid heavy perfumes, colognes, and aftershaves. A lightly scented fragrance is acceptable.
- Wear only simple jewelry that complements your clothes.
- Stop in the restroom when you arrive at the interview location. Check to make sure that your hair, makeup, and clothes are in place.

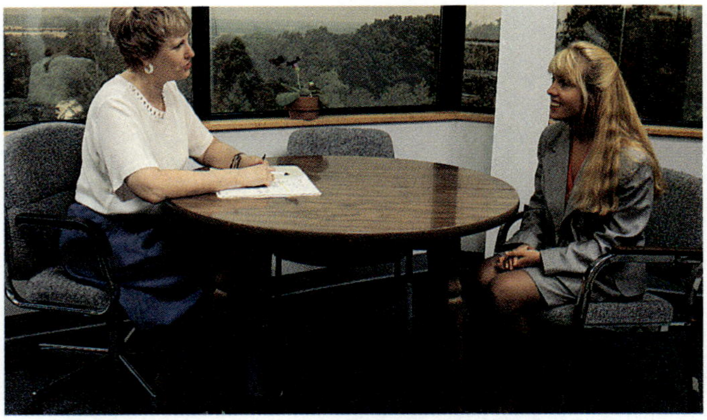

Fig. 2-8 *During the interview this nursing assistant is sitting with her back straight and her legs together. Her hands are clasped in front of her.*

and women. The interviewer should be addressed as Mr., Mrs., Ms., Miss, or doctor. You should remain standing until asked to take a seat. When sitting, use good posture and sit in a professional manner (Fig. 2-8). If the interviewer offers you a beverage, it is appropriate to accept. Be sure to thank the person.

Good eye contact with the interviewer is important. Look directly at the interviewer when answering or asking questions. Poor eye contact can communicate negative information. These include being shy, insecure, dishonest, or lack of interest. Also watch your body language (see Chapter 4). Body language relates to facial expressions, gestures, postures, and body movements. What you say is important during the interview. However, how you use and move your body also communicates a great deal. Avoid distracting habits such as biting your nails, playing with jewelry or clothing, and swinging your legs back and forth.

The interview may last 15 to 45 minutes. Answer honestly and to the best of your ability. Your answers should not be too short or too long. "Yes" and "no" answers give little information. You generally want to give a brief explanation of your response. At the end of the interview, you will have the chance to ask questions. You should ask questions about:

- Starting salary
- Work hours
- Job description
- New employee orientation program
- Benefits such as health and disability insurance, vacation, and continuing education
- Uniform requirements

You should also review the job description with the interviewer. If you have any questions, ask them at this time. Also advise the interviewer of any functions you cannot perform because of training, legal, ethical, or religious reasons. An honest discussion with the interviewer will prevent problems later.

The interviewer signals when the interview is over. You will be thanked for coming for the interview. You may be offered a job at this time. Or the interviewer may tell you when to expect a call. Follow-up is acceptable. Ask the interviewer when you can check on the status of your application. Before you leave, be sure to thank the interviewer and tell the person that you look forward to hearing from him or her.

A written thank you note is also advised (Fig. 2-9). This should be written the day of or the day after the interview. Your writing should be neat and legible. Use a computer or typewriter if your writing is hard to read. The thank you note should include:

- The date
- The interviewer's formal name using Mr., Mrs., Ms., Miss, or Dr.
- A short note that thanks the person for the interview, comments about the interview and the facility, and shows your eagerness to hear about the job
- Your signature using your first and last names

Be sure to accept the job that is best for you. You can apply several places and have an equal number of interviews. Take time to think about any offers before accepting one. If you have questions about the facility, be sure to ask them before accepting the job. Discussing the offer with a relative, friend, co-worker, or your instructor may help you with your decision.

Working With Others

You are a member of both the nursing and health teams. You will work closely with RNs, LPNs, and other nursing assistants. Your ability to work well with others affects how you function as a nursing assistant and the quality of care you give. Besides the ethical and legal considerations discussed in this chapter, the guidelines listed in Box 2-12 will help you to work well with others.

Planning and Organizing Your Work

Working well with others includes working in an organized and efficient way. You will give nursing care to patients or residents. You also will perform routine tasks on the nursing unit. Some assignments must be completed by a certain time. Other tasks or functions are to be done by the end of the shift. You must plan and organize

Text continued on page 40.

December 12, 1995

Dear Ms. Miller,

Thank you for the interview yesterday. I enjoyed meeting you and learning more about the hospital. I was impressed by the friendliness of the staff and would enjoy working in that environment.

Again, thank you. I look forward to hearing from you soon.

Sincerely,

Deborah R. Fendor

Fig. 2-9 *A sample thank you note written after an interview.*

BOX 2-12 Guidelines for Working With Other Members of the Nursing and Health Teams

- Understand the roles, functions, and responsibilities in your job description.
- Make sure you are familiar with the personnel and procedure manuals.
- Develop the desired qualities and characteristics of a nursing assistant.
- Report to work on time.
- Call the facility if you cannot report to work. Call as soon as possible, and give the reason for your absence.
- Practice good personal health and hygiene measures.
- Take pride in your appearance and follow the dress code of the facility.
- Act in an ethical and legal manner at all times.
- Follow the directions and instructions of the nurse supervising your work.
- Question unclear instructions and things you do not understand.
- Report patient or resident complaints and your observations to the nurse promptly.
- Help others willingly when asked.
- Do not waste supplies and equipment.
- Do not use the telephone, supplies, or equipment for your personal use.
- Follow the rules and regulations of the facility.
- Be accurate in measuring, reporting, and recording.
- Tell the nurse when you are leaving and when you return to the nursing unit.
- Do not discuss your personal problems with patients, residents, or families.
- Ask for any training that you might need.

BOX 2-13 PLANNING AND ORGANIZING YOUR WORK

- Discuss priorities with the RN or LPN when you receive your assignment.
- Know the routine of your shift and nursing unit.
- List care or procedures that are on a schedule. Some persons need to be turned or offered the bedpan every 2 hours.
- Estimate how much time is needed for each patient or resident, procedure, and task.
- Identify which tasks and procedures can be done while patients or residents are eating, visiting, or involved in activities or therapies.
- Plan care around meal times, visiting hours, and therapies. If working in a nursing facility, you must also consider daily recreation and social activities.
- Identify situations in which you will need help from a co-worker. Ask a co-worker to help you, and give the approximate time when you will need help.
- Schedule any equipment or rooms if necessary. Some facilities have only one shower or bathtub to a nursing unit. You will need to schedule the room for patient or resident use.
- Review the procedures to be performed and gather needed supplies beforehand.

your work to give safe, thorough care and to make good use of your time. The guidelines in Box 2-13 will help you to plan and organize your work.

CROSS-TRAINING

Patient focused care (PFC) is a health care trend in response to rising costs and concerns about quality. It is a delivery strategy that uses cross-trained staff and moves services from departments to the bedside. Staff members are used in efficient and productive ways. PFC reduces the number of people caring for each patient. Under other systems, a hospital patient may have contact with many employees from several departments such as physical therapy, respiratory therapy, cardiology, or radiology. The patient may also have contact with several staff members from one department.

For example, Dr. Gilson orders a blood test for Ms. Tyler. The nurse tells the unit secretary, who then calls the laboratory. The laboratory secretary tells a medical laboratory technician. The technician sends another staff member to Ms. Tyler's room to draw the blood sample. Five people have been involved so far.

With patient focused care, staff members on the nursing unit are cross-trained to perform basic skills also performed by other health team members. Nurses and nursing assistants may be cross-trained to draw blood (phlebotomy), take electrocardiograms (ECGs or EKGs), and perform basic physical therapy skills. With cross-training, the nurse or nursing assistant draws Ms. Tyler's blood when the order is given. The patient does not have to wait for laboratory staff to arrive, and fewer people are involved in one test. With cross-training the patient is served faster and with less staff.

Cross-training is not just for the nursing team. Housekeepers, unit secretaries, technicians, physical therapy assistants, and others can be cross-trained. They can be cross-trained for basic diagnostic and treatment services normally performed by certain departments. For example, Ms. Tyler asks the housekeeper to refill her water pitcher. Normally the housekeeper would have to find a nursing assistant or a nurse to fill the pitcher. Because the housekeeper has been cross-trained as a nursing assistant, she fills the water pitcher. The service was immediate and involved only one person. The housekeeper saved time by not having to find a member of the nursing team. The patient did not have to wait until a nursing team member could come to her bedside.

Your hospital may have patient focused care. You may be asked to take part in a cross-training program. Some may require that you be cross-trained before being hired. Generally, nursing assistants can be cross-trained to perform the following functions:

- Selected physical therapy measures (see Chapter 19)
- Phlebotomy techniques (see Chapter 24)
- EKG measurement (see Chapter 18)
- Basic dysrhythmia interpretation (see Chapter 18)
- General rehabilitation measures (see Chapter 26)
- General dietary services (see Chapter 17)

SUMMARY

This chapter has presented many important considerations about your role as a nursing assistant. The important qualities and characteristics of nursing assistants and the importance of health, hygiene, and personal appearance have been presented. You also learned about the nursing assistant training and competency evaluation program, registry, and other OBRA requirements. You were also given information about how to find a job and how to work well with others.

An important part of this chapter is the legal and ethical aspects of your role. You have learned about what you can and cannot do both legally and ethically. What you do and how you do it affects you, your patients and residents, and your co-workers. All are affected both personally and legally. You have an important role, and you are a special person for wanting to be a nursing assistant. Use common sense, and act in a reasonable and careful manner. Respect your patients and residents, and enjoy your work!

REVIEW QUESTIONS

Circle the best *answer.*

1 Which is *false?*

- **a** Nurses supervise your work.
- **b** You assist nurses in giving care.
- **c** You must perform all tasks and procedures as directed by the nurse.
- **d** A job description serves as a guide for your roles and responsibilities.

2 All health care facilities have nursing assistants perform the same procedures and tasks.

- **a** True
- **b** False

3 Linda Ames is a nursing assistant. An RN asks her to perform the following functions. Which can she do?

- **a** Give Mr. Adams his medications
- **b** Supervise a co-worker
- **c** Take a telephone order from Dr. Gilson
- **d** Measure Ms. Parker's blood pressure

4 The doctor orders several laboratory tests for a resident. The resident wants to know why. Who is responsible for telling the resident?

- **a** The doctor
- **b** You are
- **c** The nurse
- **d** Any health team member

5 You are getting ready for work. Which should you *not* do?

- **a** Press and mend your uniform
- **b** Wear your name badge or photo ID
- **c** Wear jewelry
- **d** Style your hair so it is up and off the collar

6 Linda Ames applied for a job at West Bay Nursing Home. She got a copy of the nursing assistant job description. When should she ask questions about the job description?

- **a** After she completes the application
- **b** Before she completes the application
- **c** When her interview is scheduled
- **d** During the interview

7 Nursing assistant training and competency evaluation are required in all 50 states. What law requires this?

- **a** Civil law
- **b** Criminal law
- **c** Tort law
- **d** The Omnibus Reconciliation Act

8 Nursing assistant training programs must be at least

- **a** 75 hours
- **b** 16 hours
- **c** 3 weeks
- **d** 8 weeks

Continued.

REVIEW QUESTIONS—CONT'D

9 The required competency evaluation is only a written test.

a True

b False

10 A nursing assistant in West Bay Nursing Home was found guilty of abusing a resident. She applies for a job at Meadow Springs Nursing Home. Where must information about the abuse be recorded?

a It will not be recorded; the information is confidential

b The state nursing assistant registry

c The job application

d The resident's record

11 Which is *true?*

a You should take drugs only under the advice and supervision of a doctor.

b Alcohol must never be consumed while on duty.

c Uncorrected eye problems can affect the person's safety.

d All of the above.

12 Laws are ethical standards of what is right and wrong conduct.

a True

b False

13 Which is *not* a crime?

a Negligence

b Murder

c Robbery

d Rape

14 A health care worker is guilty of negligence. The person can be sent to prison.

a True

b False

15 These statements are about negligence. Which is *true?*

a It is an unintentional tort.

b The negligent person did not act in a reasonable manner.

c Harm was caused to a person or a person's property.

d All of the above.

16 Nursing assistants are always responsible for their own actions.

a True

b False

17 The intentional attempt or threat to touch a person's body without the person's consent is

a Assault

b Battery

c Defamation

d False imprisonment

18 The illegal restraint of another person's movement is

a Assault

b Battery

c Defamation

d False imprisonment

19 Mr. Blue's photograph is made public without his consent. This is

a Battery

b Fraud

c Invasion of privacy

d Malpractice

20 Which will *not* protect the person's right to privacy?

a Getting the person's consent for treatment

b Screening the person when giving care

c Exposing only the body part involved in the treatment or procedure

d Asking visitors to leave the room when care is given

REVIEW QUESTIONS—CONT'D

21 You are responsible for obtaining the person's informed consent in writing.

a True

b False

22 You can be a witness to the signing of a will.

a True

b False

23 Lying on an employment application may be considered

a Negligence

b Fraud

c Libel

d Slander

24 When completing a job application you should do the following *except*

a Write neatly and clearly

b Provide references

c Give information about employment gaps

d Leave spaces blank that do not apply to you

25 Which of these qualities and characteristics do employers look for the most?

a Cooperation

b Courtesy

c Dependability

d Empathy

26 Empathy is

a Feeling sorry for patients or residents

b Seeing things from the other person's point of view

c Being polite to others

d All of the above

27 What should you wear to a job interview?

a A uniform

b Party clothes

c A simple dress or suit

d What is most comfortable

28 An employer wants proof that you completed a training program for nursing assistants. Which provides such proof?

a A transcript

b Certificate of course completion

c Nursing assistant registry

d All of the above

29 Nursing assistants can use the telephone and supplies of a facility for personal use.

a True

b False

30 You cannot report to work. You should call and give the employer the reason for your absence.

a True

b False

31 An RN or LPN plans and organizes your work.

a True

b False

32 You should be familiar with facility policy and procedure manuals.

a True

b False

33 Linda Ames has been a nursing assistant for 2 years. She is now attending a community college to become an RN. This is an example of cross-training.

a True

b False

34 Mercy Hospital uses cross-trained staff and places services at the bedside rather than in departments. This is

a Patient focused care

b Primary nursing

c Case management

d Managed care

Answers to these questions are on page 748.

Communicating in the Health Care Facility

3

OBJECTIVES

- Define the key terms listed in this chapter
- Explain why health team members need to communicate
- Describe the rules for effective communication
- Explain the purpose, parts, and information found in the medical record
- Describe your legal and ethical responsibilities if you have access to medical records
- Explain your role in the nursing process
- Identify information that can be collected about a person using sight, hearing, touch, and smell
- List the information that must be included when reporting to the nurse
- List the basic rules for recording
- Know how to use the 24-hour clock
- Describe the purpose of the Kardex
- Explain how computers are used in health care and how to protect the person's right to privacy when using computers
- Describe the rules for answering the telephone

Resident Name ______________________ I.D. Number ______________________

3.	PAST ROLES	a. Strong identification with past roles and life status	a.
		b. Expresses sadness/anger/empty feeling over lost roles/status ●[7]	b.
		c. *NONE OF ABOVE*	c.

SECTION H. MOOD AND BEHAVIOR PATTERNS

1.	SAD OR ANXIOUS MOOD	*(Check all that apply during last 30 days)*	
		a. **VERBAL EXPRESSIONS of DISTRESS** by resident (sadness, sense that nothing matters, hopelessness, worthlessness, unrealistic fears, vocal expressions of anxiety or grief) ●[8]	a.
		DEMONSTRATED (OBSERVABLE) SIGNS of mental DISTRESS	
		b. Tearfulness, emotional groaning, sighing, breathlessness ●[8]	b.
		c. Motor agitation such as pacing, handwringing or picking ●[8]	c.
		d. Failure to eat or take medications, withdrawal from self-care or leisure activities ●[8] ▲[14]	d.
		e. Pervasive concern with health ●[8]	e.
		f. Recurrent thoughts of death—e.g., believes he/she is about to die, have a heart attack ●[8]	f.
		g. Suicidal thoughts/actions ●[8]	g.
		h. *NONE OF ABOVE*	h.
2.	MOOD PERSISTENCE	Sad or anxious mood intrudes on daily life over last 7 days—not easily altered, doesn't "cheer up" 0. No 1. Yes ●[8]	
3.	PROBLEM BEHAVIOR	*(Code for behavior in last 7 days)* 0. Behavior not exhibited in last 7 days 1. Behavior of this type occurred less than daily 2. Behavior of this type occurred daily or more frequently	
		a. **WANDERING** (moved with no rational purpose; seemingly oblivious to needs or safety) 1 or 2 = ●[9]	a.
		b. **VERBALLY ABUSIVE** (others were threatened, screamed at, cursed at) 1 or 2 = ●[9]	b.
		c. **PHYSICALLY ABUSIVE** (others were hit, shoved, scratched, sexually abused) 1 or 2 = ●[9]	c.
		d. **SOCIALLY INAPPROPRIATE/DISRUPTIVE BEHAVIOR** (made disrupting sounds, noisy, screams, self-abusive acts, sexual behavior or disrobing in public, smeared/threw food/feces, hoarding, rummaged through others' belongings) 1 or 2 = ●[9]	d.
4.	RESIDENT RESISTS CARE	*(Check all types of resistance that occurred in the last 7 days)*	
		a. Resisted taking medications/injection	a.
		b. Resisted ADL assistance	b.
		c. *NONE OF ABOVE*	c.
5.	BEHAVIOR MANAGEMENT PROGRAM	Behavior problem has been addressed by clinically developed behavior management program. (Note: Do not include programs that involve only physical restraints or psychotropic medications in this category.) 0. No behavior problem 1. Yes, addressed 2. No, not addressed	
6.	CHANGE IN MOOD	Change in mood in last 90 days 0. No change 1. Improved 2. Deteriorated ▲[1]	
7.	CHANGE IN PROBLEM BEHAVIOR	Change in problem behavioral signs in last 90 days 0. No change 1. Improved 2. Deteriorated ●[1]	

SECTION I. ACTIVITY PURSUIT PATTERNS

1.	TIME AWAKE	*(Check appropriate time periods—last 7 days)* Resident awake all or most of time (i.e., naps no more than one hour per time period) in the:	
		a. Morning 7a.m.—Noon (or when resident wakes up) [a.]	c. Evening 5p.m.—10p.m. (or bedtime) [c.]
		b. Afternoon Noon—5p.m. [b.]	d. *NONE OF ABOVE* [d.]
2.	AVERAGE TIME INVOLVED IN ACTIVITIES	0. Most—(more than 2/3 of time) ▲[10] 1. Some—(1/3 to 2/3 time)	2. Little—(less than 1/3 of time) ▲[10] 3. None ▲[10]
3.	PREFERRED ACTIVITY SETTINGS	*(Check all settings in which activities are preferred)*	
		a. Own room [a.]	d. Outside facility [d.]
		b. Day/activity room [b.]	e. *NONE OF ABOVE* [e.]
		c. Inside NH/off unit [c.]	
4.	GENERAL ACTIVITIES PREFERENCES (adapted to resident's current abilities)	*(Check all specific preferences whether or not activity is currently available to resident)*	
		a. Cards/other games [a.]	f. Spiritual/religious activ. [f.]
		b. Crafts/arts [b.]	g. Trips/shopping [g.]
		c. Exercise/sports [c.]	h. Walking/wheeling outdoors [h.]
		d. Music [d.]	i. Watch TV [i.]
		e. Read/write [e.]	j. *NONE OF ABOVE* [j.]
5.	PREFERS MORE OR DIFFERENT ACTIVITIES	Resident expresses/indicates preference for other activities/choices. 0. No 1. Yes ●[10]	

SECTION J. DISEASE DIAGNOSES

Check only those diseases present that have a relationship to current ADL status, cognitive status, behavior status, medical treatments, or risk of death.** (Do not list old/inactive diagnoses.) **(If none apply, check the NONE OF ABOVE box)

1.	DISEASES	**HEART/CIRCULATION**	r. Manic depressive (bipolar disease) [r.]
		a. Arteriosclerotic heart disease (ASHD) [a.]	**SENSORY**
		b. Cardiac dysrhythmias [b.]	s. Cataracts [s.]
		c. Congestive heart failure [c.]	t. Glaucoma [t.]
		d. Hypertension [d.]	**OTHER**
		e. Hypotension [e.]	u. Allergies [u.]
		f. Peripheral vascular disease [f.]	v. Anemia [v.]
		g. Other cardiovascular disease [g.]	w. Arthritis [w.]
		NEUROLOGICAL	x. Cancer [x.]
		h. Alzheimer's [h.]	y. Diabetes mellitus [y.]
		i. Dementia other than Alzheimer's [i.]	z. Explicit terminal prognosis [z.]
		j. Aphasia [j.]	aa. Hypothyroidism [aa.]
		k. Cerebrovascular accident (stroke) [k.]	bb. Osteoporosis [bb.]
		l. Multiple sclerosis [l.]	cc. Seizure disorder [cc.]
		m. Parkinson's disease [m.]	dd. Septicemia [dd.]
		PULMONARY	ee. Urinary tract infection—in last 30 days ▲[14] [ee.]
		n. Emphysema/asthma/COPD [n.]	ff. *NONE OF ABOVE* [ff.]
		o. Pneumonia [o.]	
		PSYCHIATRIC/MOOD	
		p. Anxiety disorder [p.]	
		q. Depression [q.]	
2.	OTHER CURRENT DIAGNOSES AND ICD-9 CODES	260–263.9=●[12] 276.5=▲[14] 291.0–293.1=●[1]	
		a.	
		b.	
		c.	
		d.	
		e.	
		f.	

SECTION K. HEALTH CONDITIONS

1.	PROBLEM CONDITIONS	*(Check all problems that are present in last 7 days unless other time frame indicated)*	
		a. Constipation [a.]	j. Pain—resident complains or shows evidence of pain daily or almost daily [j.]
		b. Diarrhea ▲[14] [b.]	k. Recurrent lung aspirations in last 90 days [k.]
		c. Dizziness/vertigo ▲[14] [c.]	l. Shortness of breath [l.]
		d. Edema [d.]	m. Syncope (fainting) [m.]
		e. Fecal impaction [e.]	n. Vomiting ▲[14] [n.]
		f. Fever ▲[14] [f.]	o. *NONE OF ABOVE* [o.]
		g. Hallucinations/delusions [g.]	
		h. Internal bleeding ▲[14] [h.]	
		i. Joint pain [i.]	
2.	ACCIDENTS	a. Fell—past 30 days ●[11] [a.]	c. Hip fracture in last 180 days [c.]
		b. Fell—past 31-180 days ●[11] [b.]	d. *NONE OF ABOVE* [d.]

3 of 4 Rev. 3/91

Fig. 3-8—cont'd *Minimum data set (MDS).*

Continued.

Resident Name ______________________

3.	STABILITY OF CONDITIONS	a. Conditions/diseases make resident's cognitive, ADL, or behavior status unstable—fluctuating, precarious, or deteriorating.	a.
		b. Resident experiencing an acute episode or a flare-up of a recurrent/chronic problem.	b.
		c. *NONE OF THE ABOVE*	c.

SECTION L. ORAL/NUTRITIONAL STATUS

1.	ORAL PROBLEMS	a. Chewing problem [a.] b. Swallowing problem [b.] c. Mouth pain ●[15] d. *NONE OF ABOVE*	c. d.
2.	HEIGHT AND WEIGHT	***Record height (a) in inches and weight (b) in pounds.*** *Weight based on most recent status in* **last 30 days**; measure weight consistently ***in accord with standard facility*** practice—*e.g., in a.m. after voiding,* before meal, with shoes off, and in nightclothes. HT (in.) [a.] WT (lb.) [b.]	
		c. Weight loss (i.e., 5% + in last 30 days; or 10% in last 180 days) 0. No 1. Yes ●[12] ▲[14]	c.
3.	NUTRITIONAL PROBLEMS	a. Complains about the taste of many foods ●[12] [a.] b. Insufficient fluid; dehydrated ●[14] [b.] c. Did **NOT** consume all/almost all liquids provided **during last 3 days** ▲[14] [c.] d. Regular complaint of hunger ●[12] e. Leaves 25%+ food uneaten at most meals ●[12] ▲[14] f. *NONE OF ABOVE*	d. e. f.
4.	NUTRITIONAL APPROACHES	a. Parenteral/IV ▲[14] ●[12] [a.] b. Feeding tube ▲[14] ●[13] [b.] c. Mechanically altered diet ●[12] [c.] d. Syringe (oral feeding) ●[12] [d.] e. Therapeutic diet ●[12] f. Dietary supplement between meals g. Plate guard, stabilized built-up utensil, etc. h. *NONE OF ABOVE*	e. f. g. h.

SECTION M. ORAL/DENTAL STATUS

1.	ORAL STATUS AND DISEASE PREVENTION	a. Debris (soft, easily movable substances) present in mouth prior to going to bed at night ●[15]	a.
		b. Has dentures and/or removable bridge	b.
		c. Some/all natural teeth lost—does not have or does not use dentures (or partial plates) ●[15]	c.
		d. Broken, loose, or carious teeth ●[15]	d.
		e. Inflamed gums (gingiva), oral abscesses, swollen or bleeding gums, ulcers, or rashes ●[15]	e.
		f. Daily cleaning of teeth/dentures If not checked = ●[15]	f.
		g. *NONE OF ABOVE*	g.

SECTION N. SKIN CONDITION

1.	STASIS ULCER	(i.e., open lesion caused by poor venous circulation to lower extremities) 0. No 1. Yes	
2.	PRESSURE ULCERS	*(Code for highest stage of pressure ulcer)* 0. No pressure ulcers 1. Stage 1 A persistent area of skin redness (without a break in the skin) that does not disappear when pressure is relieved ●[12] ●[16] 2. Stage 2 A partial thickness loss of skin layers that presents clinically as an abrasion, blister, or shallow crater ●[12] ●[16] 3. Stage 3 A full thickness of skin is lost, exposing the subcutaneous tissues—presents as a deep crater with or without undermining adjacent tissue ●[12] ●[16] 4. Stage 4 A full thickness of skin and subcutaneous tissue is lost, exposing muscle and/or bone ●[12] ●[16]	
3.	HISTORY OF RESOLVED/CURED PRESSURE ULCERS	Resident has had a pressure ulcer that was resolved/cured in **last 90 days** 0. No 1. Yes	

I.D. Number ______________________

4.	SKIN PROBLEMS/CARE	a. Open lesions other than stasis or pressure ulcers (e.g., cuts)	a.
		b. Skin desensitized to pain/pressure/discomfort	b.
	If None Checked From C Thru G = ▲[16]	c. Protective/preventive skin care	c.
		d. Turning/repositioning program	d.
		e. Pressure-relieving beds, bed/chair pads (e.g., egg crate pads)	e.
		f. Wound care/treatment (e.g., pressure ulcer care, surgical wound)	f.
		g. Other skin care/treatment	g.
		h. *NONE OF ABOVE*	h.

SECTION O. MEDICATION USE

1.	NUMBER OF MEDICATIONS	(Record the number of *different medications used in the last 7 days; enter "0" if none used.)*	
2.	NEW MEDICATIONS	Resident has received new medications during the last 90 days 0. No 1. Yes	
3.	INJECTIONS	*(Record the number of days injections of any type received during the last 7 days.)*	
4.	DAYS RECEIVED THE FOLLOWING MEDICATION	(Record the number of days during last 7 days; *Enter "0" if not used; enter "1" if long-acting meds used less than weekly)*	
		a. Antipsychotics 1-7 = ▲[9] ▲[11] ▲[17]	a.
		b. Antianxiety/hypnotics 1-7 = ▲[9] ▲[11] ▲[17]	b.
		c. Antidepressants 1-7 = ▲[9] ▲[11] ▲[17]	c.
5.	PREVIOUS MEDICATION RESULTS	*(**SKIP this question** if resident currently receiving antipsychotics, antidepressants, or antianxiety/hypnotics—otherwise* ***code correct response for last 90 days)*** Resident has previously received psychoactive medications for a mood or behavior problem, and these medications were effective (without undue adverse consequences). 0. No, drugs not used 1. Drugs were effective 2. Drugs were not effective 3. Drug effectiveness unknown	

SECTION P. SPECIAL TREATMENTS AND PROCEDURES

1.	SPECIAL TREATMENTS AND PROCEDURES	SPECIAL CARE—*Check treatments received during the last 14 days.* a. Chemotherapy [a.] b. Radiation [b.] c. Dialysis [c.] d. Suctioning [d.] e. Trach. care [e.] f. IV meds g. Transfusions h. O_2 i. Other ________ j. *NONE OF ABOVE*	f. g. h. i. j.
		THERAPIES—Record the number of days *each of the following therapies was administered (for at least 10 minutes during a day) in the last 7 days:*	
		k. Speech—language pathology and audiology services	k.
		l. Occupational therapy	l.
		m. Physical therapy	m.
		n. Psychological therapy (any licensed professional)	n.
		o. Respiratory Therapy	o.
2.	ABNORMAL LAB VALUES	Has the resident had any **abnormal lab values during the last 90-day period?** 0. No 1. Yes 2. No tests performed	
3.	DEVICES AND RESTRAINTS	*Use the following code for last 7 days:* 0 Not used 1 Used less than daily 2 Used daily	
		a. Bed rails	a.
		b. Trunk restraint 1 or 2 = ▲[9] ●[18]	b.
		c. Limb restraint 1 or 2 = ▲[9] ●[18]	c.
		d. Chair prevents rising 1 or 2 = ▲[9] ●[18]	d.

● = Automatic Trigger ▲ = Potential Trigger

1 - Delirium
2 - Cognitive Loss/Dementia
3 - Visual Function
4 - Communication
5 - ADL Functional/Rehabilitation Potential
6 - Urinary Incontinence and Indwelling Catheter
7 - Psychosocial Well-Being
8 - Mood State
- Behavior Problems
10 - Activities
11 - Falls
12 - Nutritional Status
13 - Feeding Tubes
14 - Dehydration/Fluid Maintenance
15 - Dental Care
16 - Pressure Ulcers
17 - Psychotropic Drug Use
18 - Physical Restraints

4 of 4 Rev. 3/91

Fig. 3-8—cont'd *Minimum data set (MDS).*

FACE SHEET FOR NURSING FACILITY RESIDENT ASSESSMENT AND CARE SCREENING (MDS)

BACKGROUND INFORMATION/INTAKE AT ADMISSION

[ ] = Code the appropriate response [b.] = Check (✓) if response is applicable

I. IDENTIFICATION INFORMATION

1.	RESIDENT NAME ______ (First) (Middle Initial) (Last) ID# ______	
2.	DATE OF CURRENT ADMISSION	Month – Day – Year
3.	MEDICARE No. (SOC. SEC. or Comparable No. if no Medicare No.)	
4.	FACILITY PROVIDER NO.	Federal No.
5.	GENDER	1. Male 2. Female
6.	RACE/ETHNICITY	1. American Indian/Alaskan Native 2. Asian/Pacific Islander 3. Black, not of Hispanic origin 4. Hispanic 5. White, not of Hispanic origin
7.	BIRTHDATE	Month – Day – Year
8.	LIFETIME OCCUPATION	______
9.	PRIMARY LANGUAGE	Resident's primary language is a language other than English. 0. No 1. Yes ______ (Specify)
10.	RESIDENTIAL HISTORY PAST 5 YEARS	*(Check all settings resident lived in during 5 years prior to admission)* a. Prior stay at this nursing home [a.] b. Other nursing home/residential facility [b.] c. MH/psychiatric setting [c.] d. MR/DD setting [d.] e. *NONE OF ABOVE* [e.]
11.	MENTAL HEALTH HISTORY	Does resident's RECORD indicate any history of mental retardation, mental illness, or any other mental health problem? 0. No 1. Yes
12.	CONDITIONS RELATED TO MR/DD STATUS	***Check all conditions** that are related to MR/DD Status, that were manifested before age 22, and are likely to continue indefinitely.* a. Not Applicable—no MR/DD (Skip to Item 13) [a.] MR/DD with Organic Condition b. Cerebral palsy [b.] c. Down's syndrome [c.] d. Autism [d.] e. Epilepsy [e.] f. Other organic condition related to MR/DD [f.] g. MR/DD with no organic condition [g.] h. Unknown [h.]
13.	MARITAL STATUS	1. Never Married 2. Married 3. Widowed 4. Separated 5. Divorced
14.	ADMITTED FROM	1. Private home or apt. 2. Nursing facility 3. Acute care hospital 4. Other
15.	LIVED ALONE	0. No 1. Yes 2. In other facility
16.	ADMISSION INFORMATION AMENDED	***(Check all that apply)*** a. Accurate information unavailable earlier [a.] b. Observation revealed additional information [b.] c. Resident unstable at admission [c.]

II. BACKGROUND INFORMATION AT RETURN/READMISSION

1.	DATE OF CURRENT READMISSION	Month – Day – Year
2.	MARITAL STATUS	1. Never Married 2. Married 3. Widowed 4. Separated 5. Divorced
3.	ADMITTED FROM	1. Private home or apt. 2. Nursing facility 3. Acute care hospital 4. Other
4.	LIVED ALONE	0. No 1. Yes 2. In other facility
5.	ADMISSION INFORMATION AMENDED	***(Check all that apply)*** a. Accurate information unavailable earlier [a.] b. Observation revealed additional information [b.] c. Resident unstable at admission [c.]

III. CUSTOMARY ROUTINE (ONLY AT FIRST ADMISSION)

1. CUSTOMARY ROUTINE (Year prior to first admission to a nursing home) — ***(Check all that apply.** If all information UNKNOWN, check last box only.)*

CYCLE OF DAILY EVENTS	
a. Stays up late at night (e.g., after 9 pm)	a.
b. Naps regularly during day (at least 1 hour)	b.
c. Goes out 1+ days a week	c.
d. Stays busy with hobbies, reading, or fixed daily routine	d.
e. Spends most time alone or watching TV	e.
f. Moves independently indoors (with appliances, if used)	f.
g. *NONE OF ABOVE*	g.
EATING PATTERNS	
h. Distinct food preferences	h.
i. Eats between meals all or most days	i.
j. Use of alcoholic beverage(s) at least weekly	j.
k. *NONE OF ABOVE*	k.
ADL PATTERNS	
l. In bedclothes much of day	l.
m. Wakens to toilet all or most nights	m.
n. Has irregular bowel movement pattern	n.
o. Prefers showers for bathing	o.
p. *NONE OF ABOVE*	p.
INVOLVEMENT PATTERNS	
q. Daily contact with relatives/close friends	q.
r. Usually attends church, temple, synagogue (etc.)	r.
s. Finds strength in faith	s.
t. Daily animal companion/presence	t.
u. Involved in group activities	u.
v. *NONE OF ABOVE*	v.
w. UNKNOWN—Resident/family unable to provide information	w.

END

Signature and Date of RN Assessment Coordinator: ______

Signatures and Dates of Others Who Completed Part of the Assessment:

______ ______ ______

______ ______ ______

Form 1827HH BRIGGS, Des Moines, IA 50306 (800) 247-2343 PRINTED IN U.S.A. (9-90)

Fig. 3-8—cont'd *Minimum data set (MDS).*

BOX 3-1 Basic Observations of Patients and Residents

Ability to respond

- Is the person easy or difficult to arouse?
- Is the person able to give his or her name, the time, and the location when asked?
- Can the person identify others accurately?
- Can the person answer questions correctly?
- Can the person speak clearly?
- Are instructions followed appropriately?
- Is the person calm, restless, or excited?
- Is the person conversing, quiet, or talking a lot?

Movement

- Can the person squeeze your fingers with each hand?
- Can the person move arms and legs?
- Are the person's movements shaky or jerky?

Pain or discomfort

- Where is the pain located? (Ask the person to point to the pain.)
- Does the pain go anywhere else?
- What is the duration of the pain?
- How does the person describe the pain?
    - Sharp
    - Severe
    - Knifelike
    - Dull
    - Burning
    - Aching
    - Comes and goes
    - Depends on position
- Has medication been given?
- Did medication help relieve the pain? Is pain still present?
- Is the person able to sleep and rest?
- What is the position of comfort?

Skin

- Is the skin pale or flushed?
- Is the skin cool, warm, or hot?
- Is the skin moist or dry?
- What color are the lips and nails?
- Are there any sores or reddened areas?

Eyes, ears, nose, and mouth

- Is there drainage from the eyes?
- Are the eyelids closed?
- Are the eyes reddened?
- Does the person complain of spots, flashes, or blurring?
- Is the person sensitive to bright lights?
- Is there drainage from the ears?
- Can the person hear? Is repeating necessary? Are questions answered appropriately?
- Is there drainage from the nose?
- Can the person breathe through the nose?
- Is there breath odor?
- Does the person complain of a bad taste in the mouth?

Respirations

- Do both sides of the person's chest rise and fall with respirations?
- Is there noisy breathing?
- Is there difficulty breathing?
- What is the amount and color of sputum?
- What is the frequency of the person's cough? Is it dry or productive?

Bowels and bladder

- Is the abdomen firm or soft?
- Does the person complain of gas?
- What is the amount, color, and consistency of bowel movements?
- Does the person have pain or difficulty urinating?
- What is the amount of urine?
- Is the person able to control the passage of urine?
- What is the frequency of urination?
- What is the frequency of bowel movements?

the nurse plan. Other health workers may be involved. OBRA requires that the interdisciplinary health team plan care in nursing facilities (see Care Conferences, page 69).

Priorities relate to what is most important for the person. Maslow's theory of basic needs is useful for setting priorities (see Chapter 4). Maslow describes the needs that all humans have. The needs are arranged in order of importance. Some needs are required for life and survival, such as oxygen, water, and food. The needs necessary for life and survival must be met before all other needs. They have priority and must be done first.

Goals are then set. A **goal** is that which is desired in or by a person as a result of nursing care. Goals are aimed at the person's highest level of well-being and functioning:

BOX 3-1 Basic Observations of Patients and Residents—cont'd

Appetite

- Does the person like the diet?
- How much of the food on the tray is eaten?
- What are the person's food preferences?
- How much liquid was taken?
- What are the person's liquid preferences?
- How often does the person drink liquids?
- Is the person experiencing nausea?
- What is the amount and color of material vomited?
- Does the person have hiccups?
- Is the person belching?

Activities of daily living

- Can the person perform personal care without help?
  - Bathing?
  - Brushing teeth?
  - Combing and brushing hair?
  - Shaving?
- Does the person use the toilet, commode, bedpan, or urinal?
- Is the person able to feed self?
- Is the person able to walk?
- What amount and kind of assistance is needed?

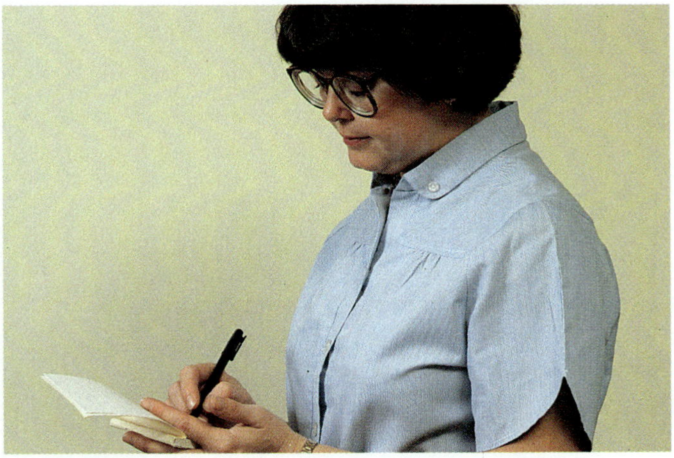

Fig. 3-9 *Nursing assistant writing down observations.*

physical, emotional, social, spiritual. Goals reflect health promotion, prevention of health problems, and rehabilitation.

Planning also includes choosing nursing interventions. An intervention is an action or measure. A **nursing intervention** is an action or measure taken by a nursing team member to help the person reach a goal. In this book, nursing intervention, nursing action, and nursing measure mean the same thing. A nursing intervention may be done without a doctor's order. Such actions involve only the nursing team. Some nursing measures involve other health team members. Nursing measures may come from a doctor's order. For example, a doctor orders that Mrs. Reece walk 50 yards two times a day. The nurse includes this order in her care plan.

The **nursing care plan** is a written guide about the care a person should receive. The plan has the person's nursing diagnoses and goals. It also has the measures or actions for each goal. There is a plan for each patient or resident. The nursing care plan is a communication tool. Nursing staff use the care plan to see what care to give. The plan helps ensure that the nursing team gives the same care.

In nursing facilities, OBRA requires the use of resident assessment protocols (RAPs) for developing care plans. The problems identified on the MDS (minimum data set) give **triggers** (clues) for the resident assessment protocols. RAPs are triggers and guidelines that help the team develop the resident's care plan (Fig. 3-11 on page 65). For example, the MDS shows that Mrs. Reece cannot do her activities of daily living (ADLs). This *triggers* the *RAPs,* which provide guidelines for actions to solve the problems. The *goal* is for Mrs. Reece to be independent in all ADLs. The actions to help Mrs. Reece reach the goal are as follows:

- Occupational therapy to work with the resident on ADLs
- Physical therapy to work with the resident on strengthening exercises daily
- A nursing staff member to walk the resident 50 feet twice daily

Some care plans are part of the person's chart or are part of the Kardex. Others are on computer. After it is written, the plan must be carried out. The plan may change if the person's nursing diagnoses change. Remember, nursing diagnoses may change as new information is gained during assessment. Carrying out nursing

Text continued on page 63.

BOX 3-2 Nursing Diagnoses Approved by the North American Nursing Diagnosis Association (NANDA)

- Activity Intolerance
- Activity Intolerance, Risk for
- Adaptive Capacity: Intracranial, Decreased
- Adjustment, Impaired
- Airway Clearance, Ineffective
- Anxiety
- Aspiration, Risk for
- Body Image Disturbance
- Body Temperature, Risk for Altered
- Breastfeeding, Effective
- Breastfeeding, Ineffective
- Breastfeeding, Interrupted
- Breathing Pattern, Ineffective
- Cardiac Output, Decreased
- Caregiver Role Strain
- Caregiver Role Strain, Risk for
- Communication, Impaired Verbal
- Confusion, Acute
- Confusion, Chronic
- Constipation
- Constipation, Colonic
- Constipation, Perceived
- Coping, Defensive
- Coping, Ineffective Community
- Coping, Ineffective Individual
- Decisional Conflict, (Specify)
- Denial, Ineffective
- Diarrhea
- Disuse Syndrome, Risk for
- Diversional Activity Deficit
- Dysreflexia
- Energy Field Disturbance
- Enhanced Community Coping, Potential for
- Environmental Interpretation Syndrome, Impaired
- Family Coping, Compromised: Ineffective
- Family Coping, Disabling: Ineffective
- Family Coping: Potential for Growth
- Family Processes, Altered
- Family Processed, Altered: Alcoholism
- Fatigue
- Fear
- Fluid Volume Deficit
- Fluid Volume Deficit, Risk for
- Fluid Volume Excess
- Gas Exchange, Impaired
- Grieving, Anticipatory
- Grieving, Dysfunctional
- Growth and Development, Altered
- Health Maintenance, Altered
- Health Seeking Behaviors (Specify)
- Home Maintenance Management, Impaired
- Hopelessness
- Hypothermia
- Hyperthermia
- Incontinence, Bowel
- Incontinence, Functional
- Incontinence, Reflex
- Incontinence, Stress
- Incontinence, Total
- Incontinence, Urge
- Infant Behavior, Disorganized
- Infant Behavior, Risk for Disorganized
- Infant Behavior, Potential for Enhanced Organized
- Infant Feeding Pattern, Ineffective
- Infection, Risk for
- Injury, Risk for
- Injury, Risk for Perioperative Positioning
- Knowledge Deficit (Specify)
- Loneliness, Risk for
- Memory, Impaired
- Neglect, Unilateral
- Noncompliance (Specify)
- Nutrition, Altered: Less than Body Requirements
- Nutrition, Altered: More than Body Requirements
- Nutrition, Altered: Potential for More than Body Requirements
- Oral Mucous Membrane, Altered
- Pain
- Pain, Chronic
- Parent/Infant/Child Attachment, Risk for Altered
- Parental Role Conflict
- Parenting, Altered
- Parenting, Risk for Altered
- Peripheral Neurovascular Dysfunction, Risk for
- Personal Identity Disturbance
- Physical Mobility, Impaired
- Poisoning, Risk for
- Post-Trauma Response
- Powerlessness
- Protection, Altered
- Rape-Trauma Syndrome
- Rape-Trauma Syndrome, Compound Reaction
- Rape-Trauma Syndrome, Silent Reaction

BOX 3-2 Nursing Diagnoses Approved by the North American Nursing Diagnosis Association (NANDA)—cont'd

- Relocation Stress Syndrome
- Role Performance, Altered
- Self-Care Deficit
  - Bathing/Hygiene
  - Feeding
  - Dressing/Grooming
  - Toileting
- Self-Esteem, Chronic Low
- Self-Esteem, Situational Low
- Self-Esteem Disturbance
- Self-Mutilation, Risk for
- Sensory/Perceptual Alterations (Specify) (Visual, Auditory, Kinesthetic, Gustatory, Tactile, Olfactory)
- Sexual Dysfunction
- Sexuality Patterns, Altered
- Skin Integrity, Impaired
- Skin Integrity, Risk for Impaired
- Sleep Pattern Disturbance
- Social Interaction, Impaired
- Social Isolation
- Spiritual Distress
- Spiritual Well-being, Potential for Enhanced
- Suffocation, Risk for
- Swallowing, Impaired
- Therapeutic Regimen, Ineffective Management Of: Community
- Therapeutic Regimen, Ineffective Management Of: Families
- Therapeutic Regimen, Effective Management Of: Individual
- Therapeutic Regimen, Effective Management Of (Individuals)
- Thermoregulation, Ineffective
- Thought Processes, Altered
- Tissue Integrity, Impaired
- Tissue Perfusion, Altered (Specify Type) (Renal, Cerebral, Cardiopulmonary, Gastrointestinal, Peripheral)
- Trauma, Risk for
- Urinary Elimination, Altered
- Urinary Retention
- Ventilation, Inability to Sustain Spontaneous
- Ventilatory Weaning Response, Dysfunctional
- Violence, Risk for: Self-directed or Directed at Others

(From North American Nursing Diagnosis Association: NANDA nursing diagnoses: definitions and classification 1995-1996, Philadelphia, 1994.)

measures and actions in the care plan is the implementation step of the nursing process.

Implementation

Implementation means to perform or carry out. The **implementation** step is performing or carrying out nursing measures in the nursing care plan (Fig. 3-12 on page 66). Care is given in this step.

Nursing measures may be simple or complex. The nurse assigns you measures that are simple and basic. You will learn to perform those measures during your training program. The measures and procedures in this book can be done by nursing assistants. The nurse may ask you to assist with more complex measures.

You need to chart the care given or report it to the nurse. This is done after giving care, not before. Also remember to report or record your observations. Observing is part of assessment. New observations may change the nursing diagnoses, causing changes in the nursing care plan. You need to know about any changes in the nursing care plan so you can give the correct care.

Observations are also used in the evaluation step of the nursing process.

Evaluation

Evaluation means to measure. The **evaluation** step involves measuring if the goals in the planning step have been met. The nurse evaluates to see what progress has been made. Goals may be met totally, in part, or not at all. Information from assessment is used for evaluation. Changes in nursing diagnoses, goals, and the care plan may result from evaluation.

The nursing process never ends. Nurses constantly collect information about the person. As the person's needs change, the nursing process changes. Nursing diagnoses, goals, and the care plan may change. You play an important part in the nursing process. You make and report observations. The nurse uses the information for nursing diagnoses, goals, and the care plan. You may help develop the care plan. In the implementation step, you perform nursing actions and measures written in the care plan. Your observations are used for the evaluation step.

The nursing process is used to organize nursing care and to solve the person's problems. It communicates the person's needs and care to the nursing team. Good communication between the nursing team and the person is needed.

Nursing Diagnosis	Goal	Intervention
Constipation related to lack of privacy	Patient will have regular bowel movements by 6/30	Ask patient to use call light when urge to have bowel movement is felt
		Answer call light promptly
		Assist patient to bathroom
		Close bathroom door for privacy
		Leave the room if the patient can be alone; tell the patient you are leaving and that you will return when he turns on the call light
Sleep pattern disturbance related to noisy environment	Patient will report a restful sleep by 6/29	Perform any necessary care measures before bedtime
		Close the door to the patient's room
		Turn off television or radio or keep volume low if patinet prefers
		Ask staff to avoid unnecessary talking outside the patient's room
		Ask staff to speak in low voices
		Turn off unneeded equipment

Fig. 3-10 *There is a goal for each nursing diagnosis and nursing measures for each goal.*

REPORTING AND RECORDING OBSERVATIONS

Reporting and recording are ways in which communication takes place among health team members. Both are accounts of what has been done for and observed about the person. **Reporting** is the verbal account of care and observations. **Recording** or **charting** is the written account of observations and care.

Reporting

You report patient or resident care and observations to the nurse. Reports must be prompt, thorough, and accurate. Always tell the nurse the person's name, room and bed number, and the time your observations were made or the care was given. Report only those things that you observed or did yourself. Reports are given as often as the person's condition requires or as often as requested by the nurse. Be sure to immediately report any changes from

Resident's Name:	Medical Record No.:

RESIDENT ASSESSMENT PROTOCOL SUMMARY

1. For each RAP area triggered, show whether you are proceeding with a care plan intervention.
2. Document problems, complications, and risk factors; the need for referral to appropriate health professionals; and the reasons for deciding to proceed or not to proceed to care planning. Documentation may appear anywhere the facility routinely keeps such information, such as problem sheets or nurses' progress notes.
3. Show location of this information.

	RAP PROBLEM AREA	CARE PLANNING DECISION (✓)		LOCATION OF INFORMATION
		PROCEED	NOT PROCEED	
1	DELIRIUM			
2	COGNITIVE LOSS/DEMENTIA			
3	VISUAL FUNCTION			
4	COMMUNICATION			
5	ADL FUNCTIONAL/ REHABILITATION POTENTIAL			
6	URINARY INCONTINENCE & INDWELLING CATHETER			
7	PSYCHOSOCIAL WELL-BEING			
8	MOOD STATE			
9	BEHAVIOR PROBLEMS			
10	ACTIVITIES			
11	FALLS			
12	NUTRITIONAL STATUS			
13	FEEDING TUBES			
14	DEHYDRATION/FLUID MAINTENANCE			
15	DENTAL CARE			
16	PRESSURE ULCERS			
17	PSYCHOTROPIC DRUG USE			
18	PHYSICAL RESTRAINTS			

Signature of RN Assessment Coordinator:		Date:	

Form 1833HH BRIGGS, Des Moines, IA 50306 (800) 247-2343 PRINTED IN U.S.A. **RESIDENT ASSESSMENT PROTOCOL SUMMARY**

Fig. 3-11 *Resident assessment protocols (RAPs). (Reprinted with permission of Briggs Corporation, Des Moines, IA.)*

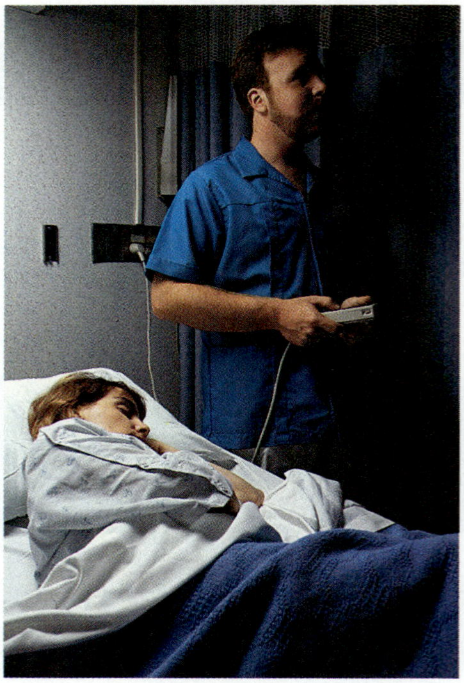

Fig. 3-12 *The nursing assistant carries out the measures in the care plan to help the person sleep. He turns off the television so the person can sleep.*

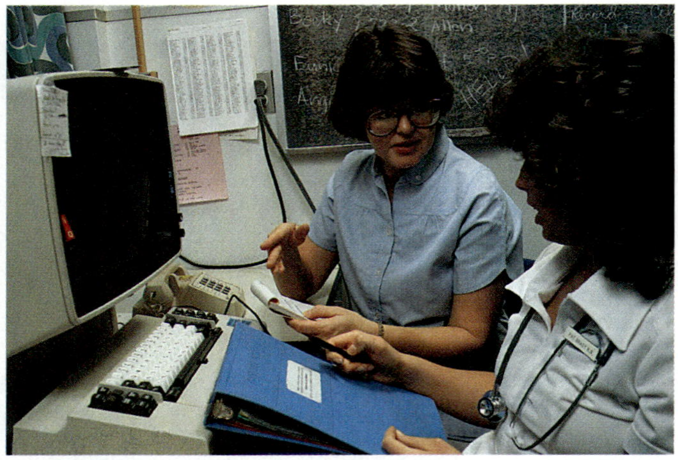

Fig. 3-13 *Nursing assistant uses notes when reporting.*

normal or changes in the person's condition. Use your written notes to give a specific, concise, and descriptive report (Fig. 3-13).

The nurse gives a report at the end of the shift to the nursing team of the oncoming shift (called the end-of-shift report). Information is shared about the care that has been given and the care that must be given to patients or residents. Information about the person's condition is also included. Some facilities have all nursing team members hear the end-of-shift report as they come on duty. Others have nursing assistants perform routine tasks while RNs and LPNs hear the report.

Recording

If allowed to record on the person's chart, you have an even greater responsibility to communicate clearly and thoroughly. Anyone who reads your charting should be able to tell:

- What you observed
- What you did
- The person's response

Be sure to follow the rules in Box 3-3 when recording.

Recording Time The 24-hour clock (military time or international time) is commonly used in health care (Fig. 3-14). This involves using a four-digit number for time. The first two digits are for the hour: 0100 = 1:00 AM; 1300 = 1:00 PM. The last two digits are for minutes: 0110 AM = 1:10 AM. With the 24-hour clock, 12-hour blocks of time and AM and PM abbreviations are not used.

As Table 3-1 on page 68 shows, using the 24-hour clock for morning times is easy. The hour is the same, but AM is not used. The PM times are harder if you have not used the system. For PM times, simply add 12 plus the clock time. If it is 2:00 PM, add 12 plus 2 for 1400. For 8:35 PM, add 12 and 835 for 2035.

Communication is better when using military time. The AM and PM abbreviations must be used with conventional clock time. Someone may forget to use AM or PM, or writing may be unclear. If this happens, the correct time is not communicated. Harm to the patient or resident could result if time is not accurately recorded. This is especially true if a treatment or medication is involved.

MEDICAL TERMINOLOGY AND ABBREVIATIONS

Use of medical terminology and abbreviations is common when communicating in health care. The terms seem strange and confusing at first. They also seem hard to learn and remember. You will learn medical words and abbreviations during your training. Soon you will understand and use them and will learn more as you work and gain experience.

Medical terms and abbreviations are presented throughout this book. Chapter 36 deals only with medical terminology and abbreviations. If a word or phrase is used that you do not understand, ask a nurse to explain its meaning. Otherwise, communication will not be effective. You may also want to buy a medical dictionary so you can learn new words.

BOX 3-3 Rules for Recording

- Always use ink.
- Include the date and the time whenever a recording is made. Record time using conventional time (AM or PM) or 24-hour clock time according to facility policy (see page 68).
- Make sure writing is legible and neat.
- Use only the abbreviations approved by the facility in which you are employed (see Chapter 36).
- Use correct spelling, grammar, and punctuation.
- Never erase or use correction fluid if you make an error. Cross out the incorrect part, write "error" over it, and rewrite the part. Some facilities use "mistaken entry" rather than "error." Follow facility policy for correcting errors.
- Sign all entries with your name and title as required by facility policy (for example, John Hayne, CNA).
- Do not skip lines. Draw a line through the blank space of a partially completed line or to the end of a page. This prevents others from recording in a space with your signature.
- Make sure each form on which you are writing is stamped with the person's name and other identifying information.
- Record only what you have observed and done yourself.
- Never chart a procedure or treatment until it has been completed.
- Be accurate, concise, and factual. Do not record judgments or interpretations.
- Record in a logical and sequential manner.
- Be descriptive. Avoid terms that have more than one meaning.
- Use the person's exact words whenever possible. Use quotation marks to show that the statement is a direct quote.
- Chart any changes from normal or changes in the person's condition. Also chart that you informed the nurse and the time you made the report (see Reporting, page 63).
- Do not omit information.
- Record safety measures such as raising side rails, assisting a person when up, or reminding someone not to get out of bed. This will help protect you if the person falls.

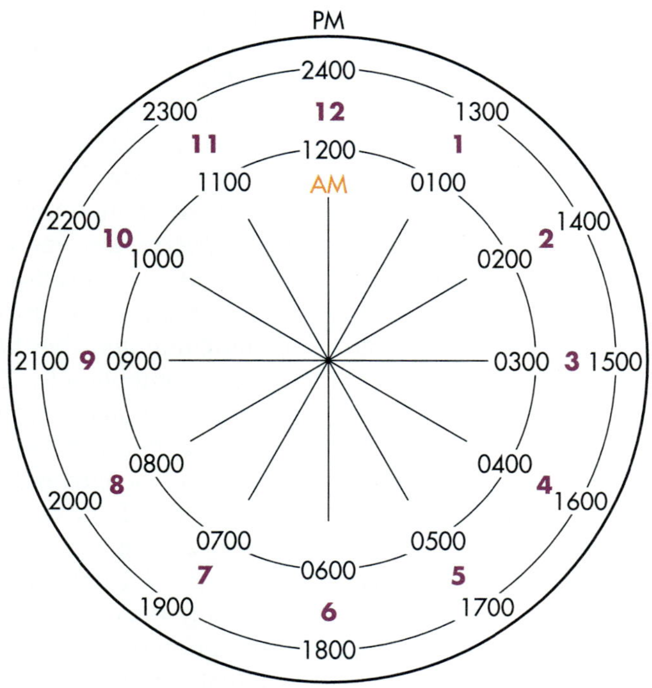

Fig. 3-14 *The 24-hour clock.*

TABLE 3-1

24-Hour Clock

Conventional time	24-Hour clock
1:00 AM	0100
2:00 AM	0200
3:00 AM	0300
4:00 AM	0400
5:00 AM	0500
6:00 AM	0600
7:00 AM	0700
8:00 AM	0800
9:00 AM	0900
10:00 AM	1000
11:00 AM	1100
12:00 noon	1200
1:00 PM	1300
2:00 PM	1400
3:00 PM	1500
4:00 PM	1600
5:00 PM	1700
6:00 PM	1800
7:00 PM	1900
8:00 PM	2000
9:00 PM	2100
10:00 PM	2200
11:00 PM	2300
12:00 midnight	2400 or 0000

COMPUTERS IN HEALTH CARE

As in other businesses and professions, computers are used in health care. Information systems collect, send, record, and store information. The information can be retrieved when needed. Medical records and care plans are on computer in many facilities. Instead of recording on the person's chart, health team members enter information into the computer (Fig. 3-15). Using a computer is easier, faster, and more efficient than writing on the chart. Recordings are more accurate, legible, and reliable.

Departments such as x-ray, the laboratory, dietary, and pharmacy communicate with the nursing unit by computer. Instead of sending a typed report by messenger for the medical record, the information is entered into the computer. The information can be accessed at the computer in the nurses' station or at the bedside. These computer systems provide communication links between departments. They reduce clerical work and telephone calls. Information is communicated with greater speed and accuracy.

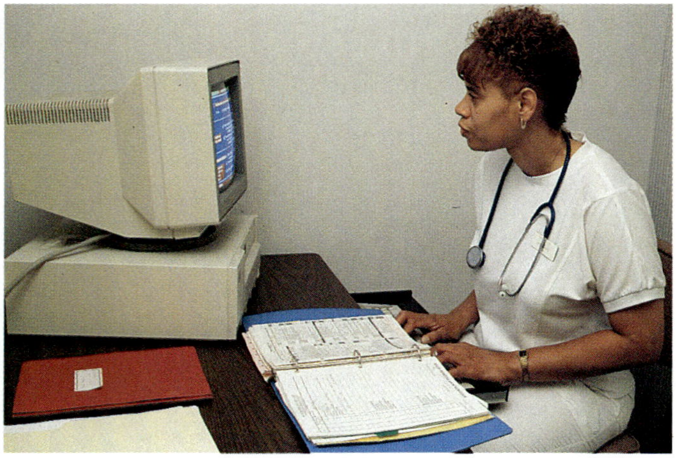

Fig. 3-15 *Nurse enters information into the computer.*

The computer is used for many other functions in health care. For example, computers are used to monitor certain measurements such as blood pressures, temperatures, heart rates, and heart function. The computer recognizes normal and abnormal measurements. When the abnormal is sensed, an alarm alerts the nursing staff. Monitoring by computer is accurate and increases early detection of life-threatening events.

Doctors can use computers when diagnosing. Signs and symptoms are entered into the computer. The computer asks questions and the doctor responds. Eventually the computer offers possible diagnoses. The doctor can also use the computer to prescribe medicines. The person's diagnosis is entered along with any requested information. The computer analyzes the information and suggests medicines and dosages. There are many other uses available.

Computers save time. Quality and safety of patient and resident care are increased. There are fewer things omitted from the medical record and fewer recording errors. Records are more complete and personnel more efficient.

Computers store vast amounts of information and are easy to access. Therefore the person's right to privacy must be protected. Only certain individuals are allowed to use the computer. They have their own codes (passwords) to access computer files. Usually nursing assistants do not use the computer. If you are allowed access, you must follow the ethical and legal considerations relating to privacy, confidentiality, and defamation (see Chapter 2). You also need to follow the rules in Box 3-4.

Using a computer is easy and fun. If you do not know how to use a computer, you should take time to learn. Eventually all health care facilities will have computerized information systems. Knowing how to use computers is a skill that makes you a good person to employ.

BOX 3-4 Rules to Protect Privacy When Using the Computer

- Do not tell anyone your password. If someone has your password, that person can access the computer under your name. If a record is altered, it would be hard to prove it was done by someone else since there is no handwriting to compare.
- Change your password on a regular basis.
- Follow the rules for recording listed in Box 3-3.
- Prevent others from seeing what is on the screen. Do not leave the computer unattended and log off after making an entry.
- Position equipment so that the screen cannot be seen in the hallway.
- Do not leave printouts where others can read them or pick them up.
- Destroy or shred any computer-printed worksheets.

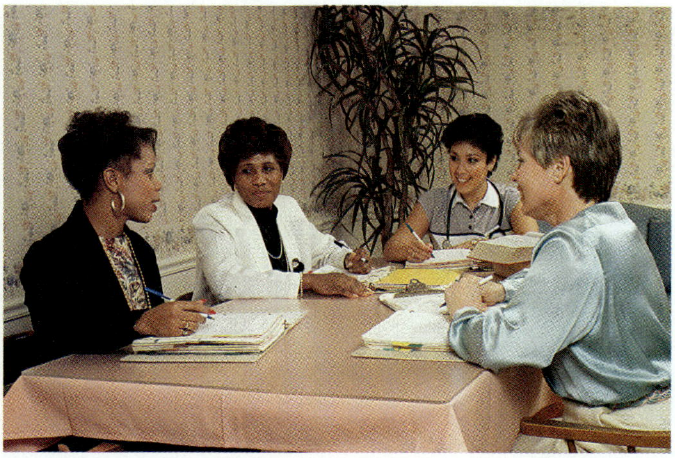

Fig. 3-16 *Members of the health team having a care conference.*

CARE CONFERENCES

A patient or resident care conference involves health team members sharing information and ideas about the person's care (Fig. 3-16). The purpose is to develop or revise a person's nursing care plan for effective care. Nursing assistants are usually included in the conference. They are encouraged to share suggestions and observations.

OBRA requires regular resident care conferences. These conferences are called the interdisciplinary care planning (IDCP) conference in nursing facilities. Members of the health team (called the interdisciplinary team by OBRA) involved in the person's care need to attend the conferences. They include an RN, other nursing staff members caring for the resident, the doctor, and other health team members as required to meet the person's needs.

TELEPHONE COMMUNICATIONS

Clerical personnel are hired to answer telephones on nursing units and in facilities. However, other staff may need to answer a phone. Often it is necessary to answer the phone in a person's room. Good telephone communication skills are essential. The caller cannot see you. But much information is given by your tone of voice, how clearly you speak, and your attitude. When answering the phone you must be as professional as if you were speaking to someone face-to-face.

Most facilities have policies about how telephones should be answered. You need to follow the policies where you work. The guidelines in Box 3-5 on page 70 can help you be professional and courteous when answering phones at work or at home.

CROSS-TRAINING OPPORTUNITIES

Receptionists and unit secretaries (ward clerks) use much of what you learned in this chapter. A receptionist answers the telephone and greets visitors. Information is also given about where to find patient or resident rooms and the various departments. A unit secretary or ward clerk works on a nursing unit. The person maintains the medical record, writes information on the Kardex, orders supplies, and communicates with members of the health team. Answering the phone, taking messages, and working with the computer are other responsibilities.

You may be asked to cross-train for one or both of these roles. Should you choose to do so, your job opportunities will be greater. You will also learn more about what these workers do. That will help you better understand and appreciate their roles and functions.

BOX 3-5 Guidelines for Answering Telephones

- Answer the call on the second ring if possible. This avoids excessive ringing of phones, which can disturb patients and residents. It also tells the caller that the staff is efficient.
- Do not answer the phone in a rushed or hasty manner. Take a deep breath before answering to avoid sounding breathless to the caller.
- Give a courteous greeting, identify the area, and give your name. For example: "Good morning. Three center. John Hayne." Or: "Good afternoon. Mrs. Reece's room. John Hayne speaking."
- Have a pencil and paper ready when you answer the phone. This lets you take a message for other staff or for the person or resident.
- Write down the caller's name. This way, you will not have to ask the caller to repeat his or her name during the call.
- Get the correct spelling of the caller's name. This lets you address the caller correctly and give correct messages.
- Write the following information when taking a message: the caller's name, date and time of the call, telephone number, and the message.
- Repeat the message and telephone number back to the caller. This helps you make sure you have the right information.
- Ask the caller to "Please hold" if necessary. You may have to place a caller on hold if you are taking another call, if another line is ringing, or if you cannot complete the conversation. However, find out who is calling first, then ask if the caller can hold. You do not want to put a caller with an emergency on hold.
- Do not lay the phone down or cover the receiver with your hand when you are not speaking to the caller. The caller may overhear confidential conversations.
- Return to a caller on hold within 30 seconds. It is impolite to keep a caller on hold. Ask if the caller can wait longer or if the call can be returned.
- Do not give confidential information to any caller. Remember that person and employee information are confidential. Refer such calls to a nurse.
- Transfer the call if appropriate. Tell the caller that you are going to transfer the call. Give the name of the department if appropriate. Give the caller the phone number in case the call gets disconnected or the line is busy.
- End the conversation politely. Thank the person for calling and say good-bye.
- Give the message to the appropriate person.

Spotlight On…

***Gwen H of Davenport, Iowa,** works as a nursing assistant on a neurology floor. Her nurse manager describes her as "kind, consistent, and self-directed. Her frequent checking on patients allows her to quickly identify the changes in their condition. She is very thorough with her care and always reports back to the RN. Efficiency and accuracy are important traits that Gwen possesses. Her good sense of humor also is appreciated by both her patients and co-workers."*

SUMMARY

Communication among health team members is essential for effective and coordinated patient and resident care. Verbal and written communication should be factual, concise, understandable, and presented in a logical order. Reports, the nursing process, the Kardex, medical record, and care conferences are ways in which health team members communicate with one another. Good telephone answering skills are also important when communicating in health care.

The traditional medical record presented in this chapter is being replaced in many facilities with computers. Regardless of the type of medical record used, remember that it is a legal document that contains highly personal and confidential information.

REVIEW QUESTIONS

Circle T *if the answer is true and* F *if the answer is false.*

1 T F Health team members communicate to provide effective and coordinated care to patients and residents.

2 T F Mrs. Reece is to be discharged from St. Jude's Medical Center. Her chart will be destroyed after she leaves the facility to protect her right to privacy.

3 T F The medical record cannot be used in a lawsuit because of the right to privacy.

4 T F Nursing assistants generally have access to the charts of all medical records in the facility.

5 T F Information is collected about a person using the senses.

6 T F Subjective data are signs noted when observing a person.

7 T F The nursing care plan lists the medications and treatments ordered by the doctor.

8 T F OBRA requires that hospitals use minimum data sets and resident assessment protocols.

9 T F Care conferences are held to develop or revise the person's nursing care plan.

Circle the best *answer.*

10 When communicating, you should do the following *except*

- **a** Use terms that have more than one meaning
- **b** Be brief and concise
- **c** Present information logically and in sequence
- **d** Give facts and be specific

11 These statements are about medical records. Which is *false?*

- **a** The record is used to communicate information about the person.
- **b** The record is a written account of the person's illness and response to treatment.
- **c** The record is a written account of care given by the health team.
- **d** Anyone working in the facility can read the medical record.

12 A person's blood pressure is measured 4 times a day. Where should the blood pressure be recorded?

- **a** Admission sheet
- **b** Graphic sheet
- **c** Flow sheet
- **d** Nurses' notes

REVIEW QUESTIONS—CONT'D

13 Where does the nurse describe the nursing care given?

- **a** Nursing care plan
- **b** Nurses' notes
- **c** Graphic sheet
- **d** Kardex

14 The nurse asks you to report your observations after giving care. What step of the nursing process is this?

- **a** Assessment
- **b** Nursing diagnosis
- **c** Planning
- **d** Implementation

15 You are asked to carry out the measures in the nursing care plan. What step of the nursing process is this?

- **a** Nursing diagnosis
- **b** Planning
- **c** Implementation
- **d** Evaluation

16 Which statement is *true?*

- **a** The nursing process is done without the person's involvement.
- **b** The nursing assistant is responsible for the nursing process.
- **c** The nursing process is used to communicate with the nursing team about the person's care.
- **d** The nursing process is only used in hospitals.

17 The nursing care plan

- **a** Is written by the physician
- **b** Consists of actions nursing personnel should take to help a person
- **c** Is the same for all persons
- **d** Is also called the Kardex

18 When recording information you should do the following, *except*

- **a** Use ink
- **b** Include the date and time
- **c** Erase if you make an error
- **d** Sign all entries with your name and title

19 These statements are about recording. Which is *false?*

- **a** Use the person's exact words when possible.
- **b** Record only what you have observed and done yourself.
- **c** Do not skip lines.
- **d** To save time, chart a procedure before it is completed.

20 In the evening you note that the clock says 9:26. In 24-hour clock time this is recorded as

- **a** 9:26 PM
- **b** 926
- **c** 0926
- **d** 2126

21 These statements are about computers in health care. Which is *false?*

- **a** Computers are used to collect, send, record, and store information.
- **b** The person's privacy must be protected.
- **c** All employees have the same password.
- **d** Computers link one department to another.

22 You answer a person's phone. How should you answer?

- **a** "Good morning. Mrs. Reece's room."
- **b** "Good morning. Third floor."
- **c** "Hello."
- **d** "Good morning. Mrs. Reece's room. John Hayne speaking."

Answers to these questions are on page 748.

Understanding The Persons You Care For

4

OBJECTIVES

- Define the key terms listed in this chapter
- Identify the parts that make up the whole person
- Describe the basic needs identified by Abraham Maslow
- Explain how culture and religion influence health and illness
- Identify the psychological and social effects of illness
- Describe persons cared for in health care facilities
- Identify patient rights as outlined in the American Hospital Association's *A Bill of Rights*
- Identify the elements needed for effective communication
- Describe how verbal and nonverbal communication are used
- Explain the techniques and barriers to effective communication
- Explain why family and visitors are important to patients and residents
- Identify the courtesies nursing assistants should give to patients, residents, and visitors

KEY TERMS

body language Facial expressions, gestures, posture, and body movements that send messages to others

culture The values, beliefs, habits, likes, dislikes, customs, and characteristics of a group that are passed from one generation to the next

esteem The worth, value, or opinion one has of a person

geriatrics The branch of medicine concerned with the problems and diseases of old age and the elderly

need That which is necessary or desirable for maintaining life and mental well-being

nonverbal communication Communication that does not involve words

obstetrics The branch of medicine concerned with the care of women during pregnancy, labor, and childbirth, and for the 6 to 8 weeks after birth

paraphrasing Restating the person's message in your own words

pediatrics The branch of medicine concerned with the growth, development, and care of children ranging in age from the newborn to the adolescent

psychiatry The branch of medicine concerned with the diagnosis and treatment of people with mental health problems

religion Spiritual beliefs, needs, and practices

self-actualization Experiencing one's potential

verbal communication Communication that uses the written or spoken word

The patient or resident is the most important person in the health facility. Age, religion, nationality, culture, education, occupation, and life-style are some factors that make each patient or resident a unique person. The person must be treated as a human being, as one who is valuable, important, and special. You must also treat the person as someone who thinks, acts, and makes decisions.

You will care for many patients and residents. Each is a person. Each has fears, needs, and rights. This chapter will help you understand and communicate with the persons you serve, help, and care for.

CARING FOR THE PERSON

In a busy facility, it is often easy to forget that the person lying in the bed is someone who lives, works, loves, and has fun. Things are done to and for the person. The person is told what to eat and when to eat, sleep, bathe, have visitors, sit in a chair, walk, and use the bathroom. Easily forgotten is the fact that the person once did these things without help. No wonder patients and residents often complain that doctors, nurses, nursing assistants, and other staff treat them as things, not as people.

Too often the person is treated as a physical disease or problem: "the gallbladder in 310" rather than "Sally Jones in 310." Most patients and residents have physical problems. However, to provide effective care, you must be aware of the whole person.

The whole person has physical, social, psychological, and spiritual parts. The parts are woven together and cannot be separated (Fig. 4-1). Each part relates to and depends on the others. As a social being, a person speaks

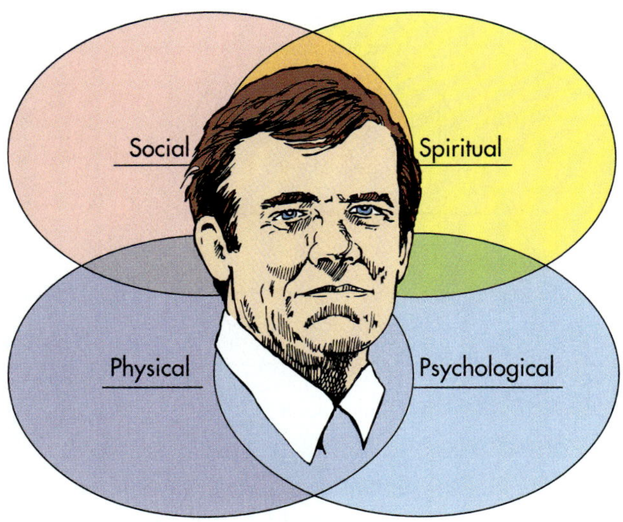

Fig. 4-1 *A person is a physical, psychological, social, and spiritual being. The parts overlap and cannot be separated.*

and communicates with others. Physically, the brain, mouth, tongue, lips, and throat structures must function for speech. Communication is also highly psychological because it involves the thinking and reasoning abilities of the mind. Considering only the physical part is ignoring the person's ability to think, make decisions, and interact with others. It also ignores the person's experiences, joys, sorrows, and needs.

NEEDS

A **need** is that which is necessary or desirable for maintaining life and mental well-being. According to Abraham Maslow, a famous psychologist, certain basic needs must be met for a person to survive and function. These needs are arranged in order of importance (Fig. 4-2). Lower-level needs must be met before the higher-level needs. These basic needs are, from the lowest level to the highest level:

- Physiological or physical needs
- The need for safety and security
- The need for love and belonging
- Esteem needs
- The need for self-actualization

People normally meet their own needs every day. When they cannot, it is usually because of disease, illness, or injury. When ill, they usually seek help from doctors, nurses, and other health team members.

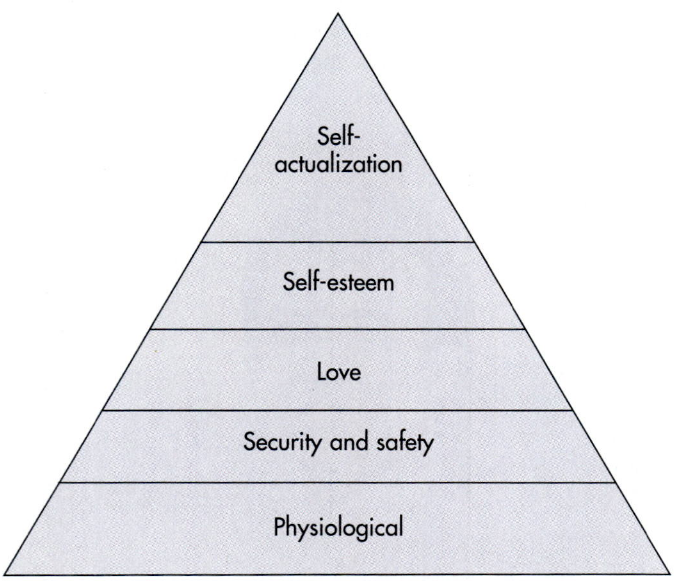

Fig. 4-2 *Basic needs for life as described by Maslow. These needs, from the lowest to the highest level, are physiological needs, the need for safety and security, the need for love and belonging, the need for esteem, and the need for self-actualization.*

Physiological Needs

Humans share many physiological needs with other life forms such as animals, fish, and plants. The physical needs required for life are oxygen, food, water, elimination, and rest. These needs are the most important for survival. They must be met before higher-level needs.

A person dies within minutes without oxygen. People can survive longer without food or water but begin to feel weak and ill within a few hours. If the kidneys or intestines do not function normally, poisonous wastes build up in the bloodstream. If the problem is not corrected, the person dies. Without enough rest and sleep, a person becomes exhausted.

You assist nurses to help patients and residents meet their physical needs. You must truly appreciate these physical needs. Most people take them for granted until a problem occurs. How do you feel when you have difficulty breathing or when you are choking? How do you react when thirsty, hungry, or tired?

The Need for Safety and Security

Safety and security needs relate to the need for protection from harm, danger, and fear. Many people find certain medical and nursing procedures to be harmful or dangerous. This is not surprising. Many procedures involve frightening equipment, require entering the body, and cause pain or discomfort. Patients and residents feel safer and more secure if they understand the procedure. They should know:

- Why a procedure is to be done
- Who will do it
- How it will be performed
- What sensations or feelings to expect

The Need for Love and Belonging

The need for love and belonging relates to love, closeness, affection, belonging, and meaningful relationships with others. There have been many cases in which patients or residents have been slow to recover or have died because of lack of love and belonging. This is particularly true of children and the elderly. The person's need for love and belonging can be met by family, friends, and health workers.

The Need for Esteem

Esteem is the worth, value, or opinion one has of a person. Esteem needs relate to thinking well of yourself and of being thought well of by others. People often lack esteem when ill or injured. Think about the following:

- How does a father feel when he cannot work and support his family because of an illness?
- Does a woman who has had a breast removed feel pretty and whole?
- Does a person with a leg amputation feel complete and attractive?

The Need for Self-Actualization

Self-actualization means experiencing one's potential. It involves learning, understanding, and creating to the limit of a person's capacity. This is the highest need. Rarely, if ever, is it totally met. Most people constantly try to learn and understand more. The need for self-actualization can be postponed and life will continue.

CULTURE AND RELIGION

Culture is defined as the characteristics of a group of people—the language, values, beliefs, habits, likes, dislikes, and customs—that are passed from one generation to the next. The person's culture influences health beliefs and practices. Culture also influences behavior during illness.

You will care for people from different cultural backgrounds. Besides caring for Americans of various nationalities, you may care for people from other cultures and countries. These people have family practices, food preferences, hygiene habits, and clothing styles that are different from yours. The person may also speak and understand a foreign language. Some cultural groups have beliefs about the causes and cures of illnesses. They may perform certain rituals aimed at ridding the body of disease. Many have beliefs and rituals about dying and death.

Box 4-1 lists the top 10 countries of origin of persons who have immigrated to the United States. This list is based on data gathered through 1992 by the U.S. Department of Immigration and Naturalization Services. Box 4-2 on page 78 gives general information about the health care beliefs of the people of these countries. Throughout this chapter and this book, information about the cultural beliefs and practices of these peoples will be given as appropriate.

Religion relates to spiritual beliefs, needs, and practices. Like culture, a person's religion influences health and illness practices. Religions may have beliefs and practices relating to daily living habits, behaviors, relationships with others, diet, healing, days of worship, birth and birth control, medical treatments, and death.

Many people rely on religion for support, comfort, and strength during illness. They may want to pray and observe certain religious practices. A visit from their spiritual leader or adviser may be appreciated. If a person asks that a member of the clergy visit, promptly report the request to the nurse. Make sure the person's room is neat and orderly, and place a chair by the bed. Ensure privacy during the visit.

BOX 4-1 TOP TEN COUNTRIES OF ORIGIN OF IMMIGRANTS TO THE UNITED STATES*

Mexico	22%
Vietnam	8%
Philippines	6.3%
Former Soviet Union	4.5%
Dominican Republic	4.3%
Mainland China	4%
India	3.8%
El Salvador	2.7%
Poland	2.6%
United Kingdom	2.1%

*Information based on data gathered through the 1992 U.S. Department of Immigration and Naturalization Services.

The nursing process reflects the person's culture and religion. The nurse and the person plan measures that include the person's cultural and religious practices. You must show respect and accept the person's culture and religion. When you meet people from other cultures or religions, take advantage of the opportunity to learn about their beliefs and practices. This will help you to understand the person and give better care.

Individuals may not follow every belief and practice of their culture or religion. Remember, each person is unique. Do not judge patients and residents by your own standards.

BEING SICK

If people could choose between health or illness, surely health would be chosen. Unfortunately, people do become ill and injured. Besides physical problems from illness, there are some psychological and social effects.

The person may be unable to perform normal activities such as working, going to school, preparing meals, doing house or yard work, and taking part in sports or hobbies. Daily activities bring personal satisfaction, worth, and contact with others. Most people are frustrated and angry when unable to perform them. These feelings may become even greater if others must perform routine functions for the person.

Text continued on page 79.

BOX 4-2 Top Ten Countries of Origin of Immigrants to the United States:* Health Care Beliefs

Country	Health Care Beliefs
Mexico	Acute sick care only. Health is believed to be a matter of choice or God's will. Disease influenced by hot and cold imbalances. Males are viewed as being healthier than females or children. Pain or the appearance of blood used in determining severity of illness.
Vietnam	Acute sick care only. Practices such as pinching or scratching the area let the *bad winds* or the unhealthy air currents out of the body and restore health-producing marks or red lines. Medicine to restore the yin-yang balance and the hot-cold equilibrium is important.
Philippines	Health promotion is important. Mental illness is highly disgraceful. The evil eye can be cast upon someone through the eyes or the mouth.
Former Soviet Union	Health promotion is important. Maternal and child care encouraged. Health care addresses acute problems. Rehabilitation is not emphasized.
Dominican Republic	Hot/cold balance theory is a factor in the cause of disease.
Mainland China	Health promotion is important. Attribute an upset in body energy to the cause of disease. Health is a state of spiritual and physical harmony with nature; health and illness are not separate but part of a lifelong continuum. Some resist surgery because of a religious belief that they do not own their physical bodies, that the soul or spirit will escape from the body and be lost forever if surgery is performed. Drawing blood may be resisted because of the belief that blood does not regenerate; blood is perceived as the source of life. Stigma attached to mental illness.
India	Acute sick care only. Diseases are believed to be caused by an upset in body balance.
El Salvador	Fresh air, sleep, and good nutrition are important health practices.
Poland	Acute sick care.
United Kingdom	Acute sick care; health promotion is important.

*Information based on data gathered through 1992 by the U.S. Department of Immigration and Naturalization Services.
From Geissler EM: *Pocket guide to cultural assessment,* St Louis, 1994, Mosby–Year Book.

Sick people have many fears and anxieties. There is fear of death, disability, chronic illness, and loss of function. Some explain why they are afraid. Others keep their feelings to themselves. They fear being laughed at for being afraid. A person with a broken leg may fear having a limp or not walking again. A person having surgery might be afraid of cancer. These fears and anxieties are normal and expected. You need to appreciate how people are affected by illness. Think about how you would feel and react if you had the person's illness and problems. That will help you to have empathy for the person.

We expect sick people to behave in a certain way. We expect them to see a doctor, stay in bed, and need others for care and comfort. These dependent behaviors are accepted so that the person can get well. When recovery is delayed or does not occur, the normal psychological and social effects of illness become greater.

Culture and religion are also factors in how people think and behave when ill. Box 4-3 on page 80 lists the common sick care practices for persons from the top ten countries of origin of people who have immigrated to the United States. Remember, the information given in Box 4-3 is only general information.

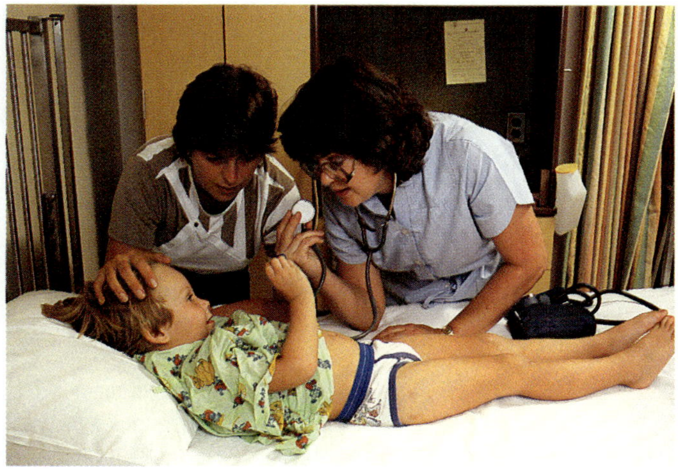

Fig. 4-3 *The nursing assistant giving care to a sick child.*

PERSONS YOU WILL CARE FOR

Patients and residents are grouped in health facilities according to problems, needs, and age. There are areas for children, persons with medical problems, those having surgery, people with mental health problems, and those needing long-term care. Nursing staff in each area are familiar with the persons' problems. They have the knowledge and skill to give the best care possible. There is also equipment and supplies to meet the persons' needs.

The following sections focus on hospital patients. Long-term care residents are discussed in Chapter 7.

Obstetrical Patients

Obstetrics is the branch of medicine concerned with the care of women during pregnancy, labor, and childbirth, and during the 6 to 8 weeks after birth. Obstetrical patients are seen in clinics or doctors' offices during pregnancy. When labor begins, these women usually are admitted to the obstetrical (maternity) department.

Pregnancy, labor, and childbirth are normal and natural events. There usually are no problems or complications. However, complications can occur at any time from the beginning of pregnancy through the 6 to 8 weeks after childbirth.

Newborns

Newborns are generally cared for in the nursery near the maternity department. Nursing staff care for the babies and take them to their mothers for feedings. Most hospitals have *rooming-in* programs that let the mother care for the infant in her room. Similar programs have the mother care for the baby during the day; at night the newborn is in the nursery.

Pediatric Patients

Pediatrics is the branch of medicine concerned with the growth, development, and care of children ranging in age from the newborn to the adolescent. Pediatric patients may be healthy or sick. Children may be seen in clinics, doctors' offices, or at home. When hospital care is needed, children are admitted to a pediatric unit. The unit is designed and equipped to meet the needs of children and parents. The child's physical, safety, and emotional needs are major concerns of nursing staff (Fig. 4-3).

Medical Patients

Medical patients are usually adults with illnesses, diseases, or injuries that do not need surgery. They may have acute, chronic, or terminal illnesses. Examples are infections, strokes, or heart attacks. Various therapies, medications, and treatments help these patients meet their basic needs.

Surgical Patients

Surgical patients are those being prepared for or who have had surgery. Surgeries range from simple to very complex procedures. An appendectomy (removal of the appendix) is a simple surgery. Open-heart and brain surgery are complex. Some surgeries are done on an out-patient basis.

The needs of preoperative patients usually involve physical preparation and teaching about what to expect after surgery. Patients are also helped to deal with their fears and anxieties about the need for and the outcome of the operation. Patient needs after surgery relate to relieving pain and discomfort, preventing complications,

BOX 4-3 Top Ten Countries of Origin of Immigrants to the United States:* Sick Care Practices

Country	Sick Care Practices
Mexico	Biomedical; magical and religious; and traditional. Common beliefs include: *mal ojo*—evil eye, *empacho*—bolus of food stuck to stomach wall, *susto*—result of a traumatic emotional experience, *mal puesto*—hex or illness imposed by another.
Vietnam	Magical and religious; eastern medicine. Herbal medicine important; most are classified as *cool,* while most western medicines are considered *hot.* Traditionally, illness is dealt with through self-care and self-medication. Folk remedies include variations of acupuncture, massage, herbal remedies, and dermabrasive practices (cupping, pinching, rubbing, and burning).
Philippines	Biomedical; and magical and religious. Combination of home remedies, professional providers, and traditional healers. Fatalism accompanies beliefs that ghosts and spirits control life and death. Taking the powers of the gods is believed to have a cause and effect relationship to subsequent bad happenings.
Former Soviet Union	Biomedical; holistic, folk, and western medical practices.
Dominican Republic	Magical and religious; traditional.
Mainland China	Holistic and traditional. Traditional health care includes cupping, acupuncture, and herbal medicine.
India	Biomedical and traditional. Spiritual values influence most aspects of life and death.
El Salvador	Biomedical.
Poland	Biomedical; magical and religious; folk. Older generations believe in the evil eye *(Szatan)* and in prayer and wearing religious medals and scapulars to help protect them against illness. Folk healers and miracle workers are also sought.
United Kingdom	Biomedical.

*Information based on data gathered through 1992 by the U.S. Department of Immigration and Naturalization Services.
From Geissler EM: *Pocket guide to cultural assessment,* St Louis, 1994, Mosby–Year Book.

and adjusting to body changes caused by surgery. Chapter 25 deals with patients having surgery.

Psychiatric Patients

Psychiatry is the branch of medicine concerned with the diagnosis and treatment of people with mental health problems. These persons may be treated in doctors' offices, clinics, general hospitals, or psychiatric hospitals. Their problems vary from mild to severe mental and emotional disorders. Some function normally but need help making some decisions or coping with life stresses. Others are severely disturbed. They cannot perform simple functions such as eating, bathing, or dressing. Special precautions and treatments may be necessary if patients are dangerous to themselves or others.

Geriatric Patients

Geriatrics is the branch of medicine concerned with the problems and diseases of old age and the elderly. Aging is a normal process, not an illness or disease. Many elderly people enjoy good health. Others suffer from acute or

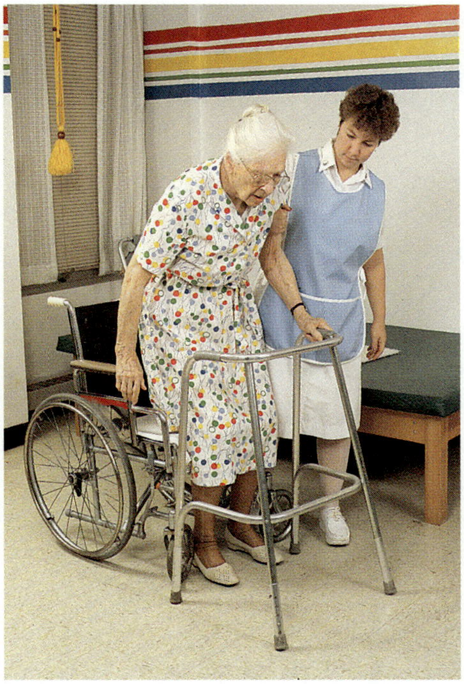

Fig. 4-4 *This elderly person lives in a nursing facility.*

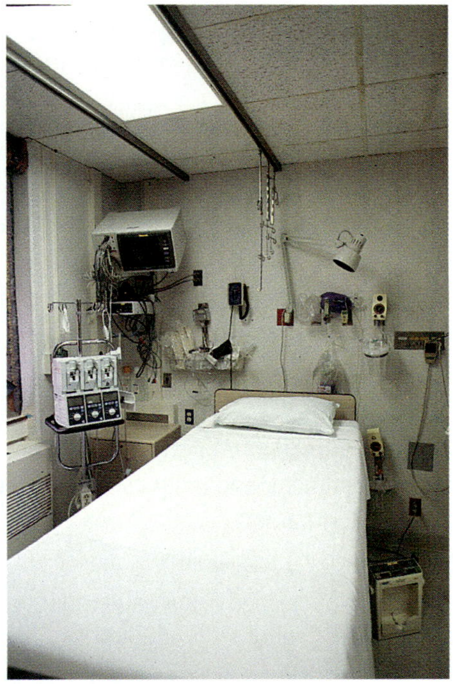

Fig. 4-5 *A general view of the design and equipment in a coronary care unit.*

chronic illnesses or from degenerative diseases common in the elderly.

Some body changes normally occur because of the aging process. There are also social and psychological changes. The physical, psychological, and social changes of aging are presented in Chapter 7. Sometimes the changes are so severe that the person may have to reside in a nursing facility (Fig. 4-4).

Patients in Special Care Areas

Some patients have special problems, are seriously ill, or are in life-and-death situations. They need special care and equipment. Special care units are designed and equipped to treat and prevent life-threatening problems and complications. These special care areas include intensive care units, coronary care units (Fig. 4-5), surgical intensive care units, neonatal intensive care units, kidney dialysis units, burn units, and emergency rooms. The nurses in these areas have had special education and training. They are prepared to meet the patient's complex needs and to operate technical equipment.

PATIENT AND RESIDENT RIGHTS

In 1973 the American Hospital Association (AHA) issued *A Patient's Bill of Rights.* The idea of patient rights came about when people demanded more information about their health problems and treatment. They also demanded better care at lower costs and greater involvement in decisions about their care and treatment. Patients were not willing to be viewed as helpless and unknowing people who accepted the doctor's advice without question.

A Patient's Bill of Rights has an ethical and legal basis. The right to privacy and informed consent are involved. Although the relationship between the doctor and the patient is stressed, there are important messages for the health team. The basic points of *A Patient's Bill of Rights* are presented in Box 4-4 on page 82.

The Omnibus Budget Reconciliation Act of 1987 (OBRA) outlines the rights of residents in nursing facilities. They are presented in Chapter 7.

COMMUNICATING WITH PATIENTS AND RESIDENTS

Several elements are necessary for effective communication between you and the patient or resident.

- You must understand and respect the patient or resident as a person.
- The person must be viewed as more than a disease or an illness. The person is a physical, psychological, social, and spiritual human being.
- You must appreciate the problems and frustrations the person is experiencing as a result of being sick.
- You need to recognize and respect the person's rights.
- You must respect the person's religion and culture.

BOX 4-4 PATIENT RIGHTS

Consideration and respect

- To be treated as a person and be given kind and thoughtful care.
- Personal values, beliefs, cultural practices, and personality are considered when planning and providing care.

Information

- To receive information from the doctor about the diagnosis, treatment, and prognosis in terms the patient can understand.
- Unfamiliar medical terminology is avoided.
- An interpreter is needed if the patient does not understand or speak English.
- The nearest relative or legal guardian is informed of the patient's diagnosis, treatment, and prognosis if it is considered unwise to tell the patient.

Informed consent

- To receive information and explanations about any treatments or procedures.
- The doctor must provide information about treatment purpose, risks, alternatives, and probable length of incapacitation.
- The patient should be told the name of the person who will perform the treatment or procedure.
- (Informed consent is discussed in Chapter 2.)

Refusing treatment

- To refuse treatment.
- The patient does not have to consent to each treatment or procedure recommended by the doctor.
- The doctor must inform the patient of the risks to life and health involved in refusing the treatment.

Privacy

- To have the patient's body, record, care, and personal affairs kept private.
- The right to privacy is still protected after death.
- (The right to privacy is discussed in Chapter 2.)

Confidentiality

- To expect that information will be shared with other health workers in a wise and careful manner.
- All health workers must recognize the confidential nature of patient information. (Some patients are very sensitive about their health problems and personal relationships.)

Hospital services

- To expect that the hospital can provide needed services.
- After immediate needs are met, the patient may be transferred to another facility that is better equipped to handle the patient's problems and needs.
- The patient is to be informed of the reason for the transfer and of other alternatives.

Information on the hospital's relationship to educational and health care institutions

- To be informed of any relationships with schools and other health care facilities.
- Patients have the right to know about these relationships and to know the names of students or other persons providing or involved in their care.

Information on research and human experimentation

- To receive information and explanations about research for making an informed decision about participating.
- The patient's consent must be obtained before involvement in human experimentation or research.
- The patient may refuse to participate.

Continuing care

- To be informed of the care needed after discharge.
- The patient must be given written information about the times and locations of appointments with doctors.

The patient's bill

- To examine bills and receive an explanation of the items in the bill.
- This right exists even if the bill is to be paid by an insurance company or the government.

Hospital rules and regulations

- To be informed of any rules and regulations applying to conduct as a patient.
- The patient and family may be given a pamphlet that explains the rules and regulations.

The rules for communication discussed in Chapter 3 apply when you are communicating with patients and residents.

- Use words that have the same meaning to both you and the person.
- Avoid using medical terminology and other words that are unfamiliar to the person.
- Communicate in a logical and orderly manner. Do not allow your thoughts to wander.
- Be specific and factual when presenting information.
- Be brief and concise.

Verbal and nonverbal methods of communication are used when relating to patients and residents. You need to understand how to use both methods for effective communication with them.

Verbal Communication

Words are used in **verbal communication**. The words may be spoken or written. Verbal communication is used to converse with patients or residents, to find out how they are feeling physically and emotionally, and to share information with them.

Most verbal communication involves the spoken word. Shouting, whispering, and mumbling cause ineffective communication. You need to:

- Control the loudness and tone of your voice
- Speak clearly, slowly, and distinctly
- Avoid using slang or vulgar words
- Repeat information as needed
- Ask one question at a time and wait for the answer; do not ask several questions at once

The written word is used when persons cannot speak or hear. If a person cannot speak, provide a way for the person to send messages. A Magic slate, paper and pencil, an electronic talking aid, picture board, or a communication board can be used (Fig. 4-6). Write messages

A B C D

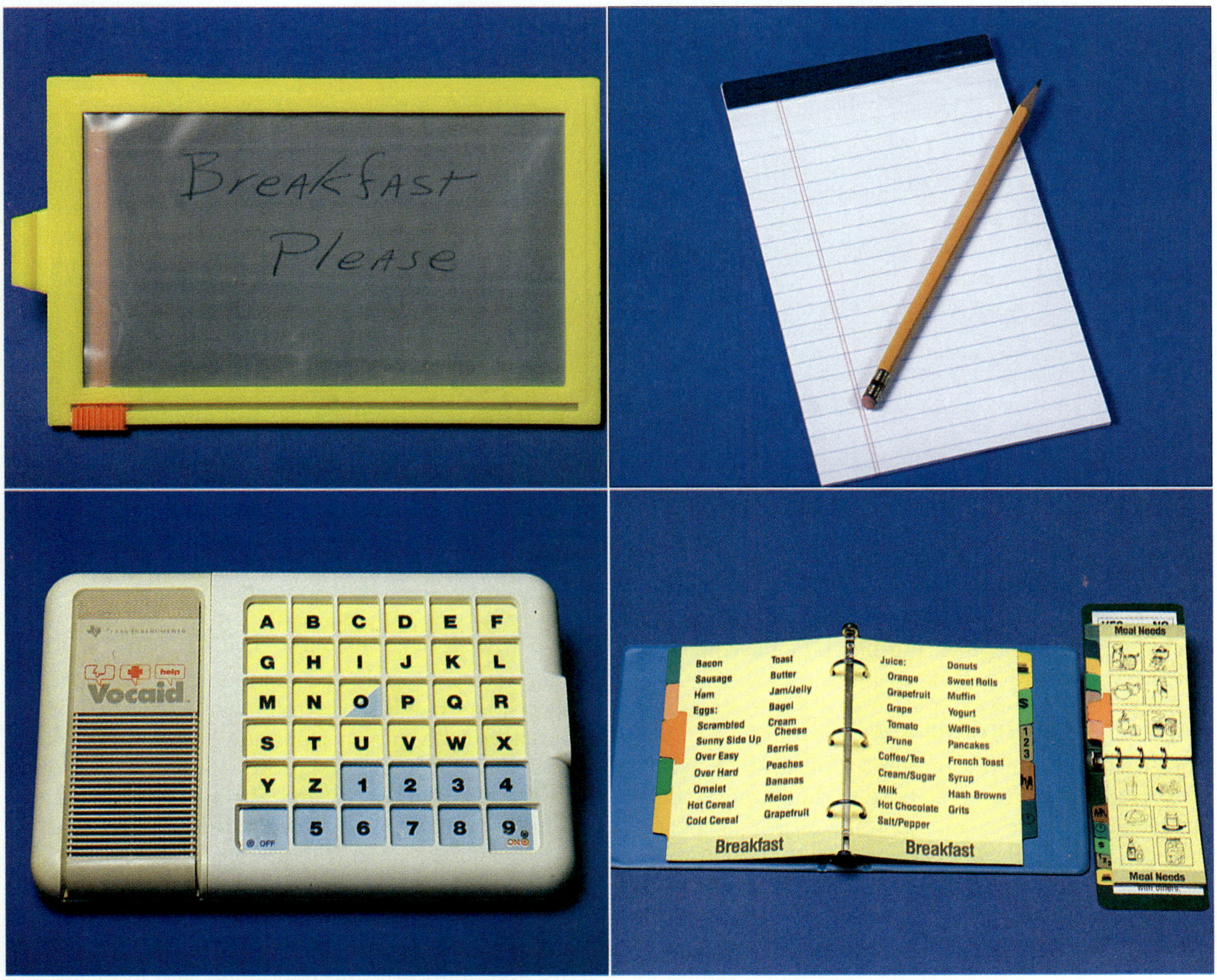

Fig. 4-6 *A, A Magic slate. B, Paper and pencil, C, Electronic talking aid. D, Communication board.*

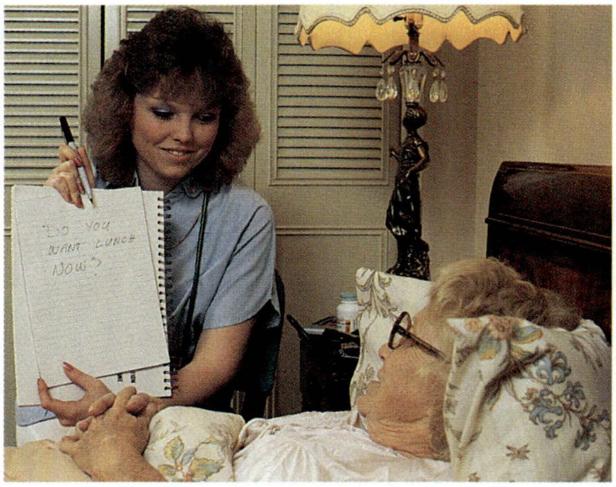

Fig. 4-7 *The nursing assistant writing a note to a person who has a hearing difficulty.*

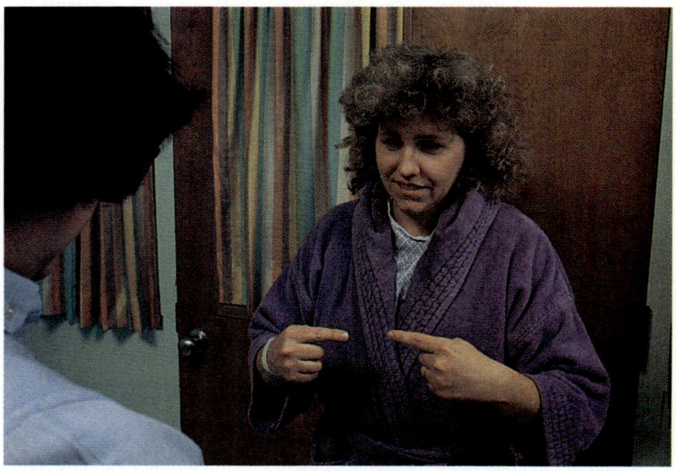

Fig. 4-8 *A person using sign language to communicate.*

to communicate with deaf persons or those with severe hearing problems (Fig. 4-7). Deaf persons may use sign language to communicate (Fig. 4-8) (see Chapter 27).

Communication between you and the person should be kept on a professional level. You should not become personally involved with patients or residents.

Nonverbal Communication

Nonverbal communication does not involve words. Gestures, facial expressions, posture, body movements, touch, and smell are examples of how messages are sent and received without words. Nonverbal messages are considered to be a more accurate reflection of a person's feelings. They are usually involuntary and hard to control. A person may say one thing but act in a different way. Therefore you need to watch the person's eyes, the way hands are held or moved, gestures, posture, and other actions.

Touch Touch is a very important form of nonverbal communication. Comfort, caring, love, affection, and reassurance can be conveyed by touch. Touch means different things to different people. The meaning depends on the person's age, culture (Box 4-5), gender (male or female), and life experiences. Although some people do not like to be touched, do not be afraid to use touch to convey caring and warmth. Patients and residents are often comforted by having their hands held.

Body Language People send messages to you through their **body language.** Body language includes:

- Posture
- Gait
- Facial expressions
- Eye contact
- Hand movements
- Gestures
- Body movements
- Appearance (dress, hygiene, and adornments such as jewelry, perfume, and cosmetics)

A person with slumped posture is probably not feeling well or happy. A person may deny having pain but protects the affected body part by standing, lying, or sitting in a certain way.

You also send messages to others by the way you act and move. Your facial expressions, the way you stand or sit, how you walk, and how you look at the person are some of the ways you communicate with another. Your body language should show interest and enthusiasm about your work and caring and respect for the person. Be sure to control body language in relation to odors from excretions or the person's body. Many odors are beyond the person's control. The person's embarrassment and humiliation increase if you react to the odor.

Techniques for Effective Communication

Certain techniques help you communicate with patients, residents, and families. The techniques result in a better relationship with these persons and help you gain more information for the nursing process. Such information is used for the assessment and evaluation steps of the nursing process. As you communicate with the person, you also find out about the person's likes and dislikes. These are useful when the nurse plans care.

Listening Listening means being attentive to the person's verbal and nonverbal communication. You must use the

BOX 4-5 Top Ten Countries of Origin of Immigrants to the United States:* Touch Practices

Country	Touch Practices
Mexico	Touch is used often. Touching people while complimenting them neutralizes the power of the evil eye in some believers.
Vietnam	The head is considered the seat of the soul and should not be touched. Only the elderly are allowed to touch the heads of young children. Touching persons of the same sex is acceptable. The female breast is accepted as the means of infant feeding. The lower torso is extremely private. The area between the waist and knees is kept covered, even in private. Handshaking has wide acceptance with men but not with women. A man will not extend his hand in handshake to a woman or a superior. Sisters and brothers do not touch or kiss each other.
Philippines	Some parts of the country believe that the evil eye can be neutralized on a child by putting a bit of saliva on the finger and making the sign of the cross on a child's forehead when giving a compliment. Touch is stressed.
Former Soviet Union	Three kisses on the cheek for greeting and for farewells are common. Touch is an important part of nonverbal communication.
Dominican Republic	No information.
Mainland China	Chinese do not like to be touched by strangers. Nod or slight bow given when introduced.
India	Men may shake hands with other men but not with women. Instead, the man places his palms together and bows slightly. Bare upper arms or shoulders are considered indecent.
El Salvador	No information.
Poland	Hugging and kissing on the cheek are acceptable between sexes.
United Kingdom	The English have generally low touch practices.

*Information based on data gathered through 1992 by the U.S. Department of Immigration and Naturalization Services.
From Geissler EM: *Pocket guide to cultural assessment,* St Louis, 1994, Mosby–Year Book.

senses of sight, hearing, touch, and smell. You must concentrate on what the person is saying. You also must observe nonverbal clues. The person's nonverbal communication can support what is being said. Or it can show opposite feelings. For example, Mr. Hart says he is happy to be going to a nursing home so his daughter does not have to stay home to care for him. However, you note tears in his eyes and he looks away from you. His verbal says happy, but his nonverbal shows sadness.

Listening requires that you care and have interest. The following guidelines are important:

- Face the person.
- Have good eye contact with the person. See Box 4-6 on page 86 for the eye contact practices of other cultures.
- Lean toward the person (Fig. 4-9 on page 86). Do not sit back with your arms crossed.
- Respond to the person. Nod your head. Say "uh huh," "mmm," and "I see." Repeat what the person says and ask questions.
- Avoid the barriers to effective communication (see page 87).

BOX 4-6 Top Ten Countries of Origin of Immigrants to the United States:* Eye Contact Practices

Country	Eye Contact Practices
Mexico	Sustained direct eye contact is rude, immodest, or dangerous for some. *Mal ojo* (evil eye) is the result of admiration. Women and children are thought to be more susceptible to *mal ojo;* therefore children may avoid direct eye contact.
Vietnam	Blinking means only that a message has been received. Looking directly into another's eyes when talking is considered disrespectful.
Philippines	Some may fear eye contact. However, if it is established, it is important to return and to maintain eye contact.
Former Soviet Union	Direct, sustained eye contact is the norm.
Dominican Republic	No information.
Mainland China	Gazing around and looking to one side when listening to another are polite. With the elderly, direct eye contact is used.
India	No information.
El Salvador	No information.
Poland	Direct eye contact is made.
United Kingdom	Staring is believed to be a part of good listening. Understanding is indicated by blinking the eyes.

*Information based on data gathered through 1992 by the U.S. Department of Immigration and Naturalization Services.
From Geissler EM: *Pocket guide to cultural assessment,* St Louis, 1994, Mosby–Year Book.

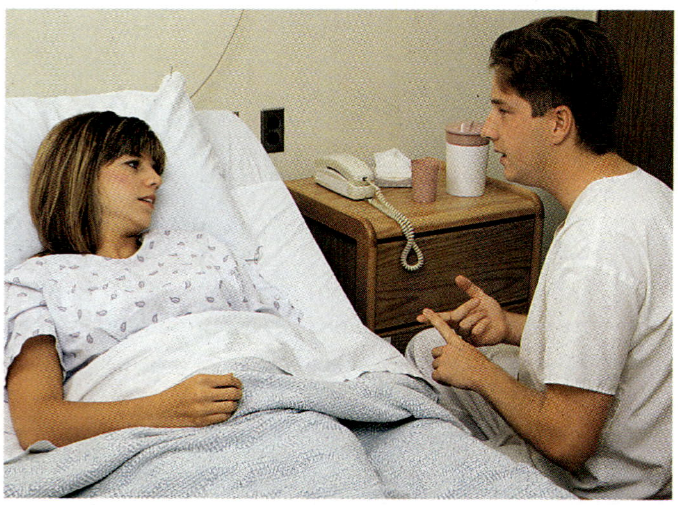

Fig. 4-9 *The nursing assistant shows he is listening by facing the person, having good eye contact, and leaning toward the person.*

Paraphrasing **Paraphrasing** is restating the person's message in your own words. You use fewer words than the person did to send the message. For example:

Mr. Hart: My wife left here crying after she spoke with the doctor. I don't know what he said to her.

Nursing assistant: You don't know why your wife was crying.

Mr. Hart: He must have told her that I have a tumor.

Paraphrasing serves three purposes:

- It shows you are listening.
- It gives the person the opportunity to see if you understand the message sent.
- It promotes further communication because the person generally responds to your statement.

Direct questions Direct questions focus on specific information. There is something you need to know and you ask the person. Some direct questions have "yes" or "no" answers. Others require the person to give more information. For example:

Nursing assistant: Mr. Hart, do you want to shave this morning?

Mr. Hart: Yes.

Nursing assistant: Mr. Hart, when would you like to shave and have your bath?

Mr. Hart: Could we start in about 15 minutes? I'd like to call my son first.

Nursing assistant: Yes, we can start in 15 minutes. Did you have a bowel movement today, Mr. Hart?

Mr. Hart: No.

Nursing assistant: You said you didn't eat well this morning. Can you tell me what you ate?

Mr. Hart: I only had toast and coffee. I just don't feel like eating this morning.

Open-ended questions Open-ended questions lead or invite the person to share thoughts, feelings, or ideas. The person is able to choose what to talk about. Answers require more than a "yes" or "no." However, the person controls what is talked about and how much information is given. Consider these examples:

- "What do you like about living with your daughter?"
- "Tell me about your grandson."
- "What was your wife like?"
- "What do you like about being retired?"

In these examples, the nursing assistant chose a topic. However, the person can choose how to answer the question. Responses to open-ended questions generally are longer and give more information than direct questions.

Clarifying Clarifying gives you the chance to make sure you understand the message. You can ask the person to repeat the message, say you do not understand, or restate the message. For example:

- "Could you say that again?"
- "I'm sorry, Mr. Hart. I don't understand what you mean."
- "Are you saying that you want to go home?"

Focusing Focusing is dealing with a specific topic. It may be useful when a person rambles or wanders in thought. For example, Mr. Daley talks at length about his favorite foods and places to eat. You need to know why he did not feel like eating breakfast. Therefore, you focus the conversation on breakfast by saying: "Let's talk about today's breakfast. You said you didn't feel like eating."

Silence Silence is a very powerful way to communicate. Sometimes, especially during times of sadness, you do not need to say anything. Just being there is enough to show you care. At other times, silence allows you or the person time to think, organize thoughts, or choose words. Silence may be useful when difficult decisions must be made. It is also useful when the person is upset and needs time to regain control. Silence on your part shows caring and respect for the person's situation and feelings.

Though silence is very useful, sometimes pauses or long periods of silence are uncomfortable. Do not think that you need to talk when the person is silent. Silence may be what is needed. Dealing with silence becomes easier as you gain experience as a nursing assistant.

Barriers to Effective Communication

Communication may fail for many reasons. You and the person must use and understand the same language. If not, messages are not accurately interpreted.

Changing the subject is another barrier to communication. Either you or the person may change the subject when the topic causes one or both to be uncomfortable. Avoid changing the subject whenever possible.

Giving your opinion usually tells the person that you are judging his or her values, behavior, or feelings. Let others express their feelings and concerns without adding your opinion, making a judgment, or jumping to conclusions.

Another barrier is talking a lot when others are silent or speak infrequently. Excessive talking is usually due to nervousness and being uncomfortable with silence. Silences have meaning. Acceptance, rejection, fear, or the need for quiet and time to think are conveyed by silence.

Listening is very important for effective communication. Communication is blocked if you fail to listen with interest and sincerity. Do not pretend to listen. This causes inappropriate responses and conveys a lack of interest and caring. You may also miss important complaints of pain, discomfort, or other abnormal sensations that must be reported to the nurse.

Pat answers such as "Don't worry," "Everything will be okay," and "Your doctor knows best" block communication. These make patients and residents feel that their concerns, feelings, and fears are being ridiculed and are not important to you or the nursing team.

Illness can affect communication. Speech and body movements are affected by some central nervous system disorders. The person may be unable to speak. Some disorders affect movement, which interferes with nonverbal communication.

BOX 4-7 Top Ten Countries of Origin of Immigrants to the United States:* Family Roles in Hospital Care

Country	Family Roles in Hospital Care
Mexico	The male should be consulted before health care decisions are made and should be included in any counseling sessions. Culturally, a mother is not allowed the authority to give consent for her child's treatment. Family decisions overrule decisions made by health care providers. Women may not give care at home if that care involves touching adult male genitalia.
Vietnam	The patient is considered a person who needs to be taken care of by all family members.
Philippines	A child may feel an obligation to the parent who is ill and spend hours giving care. The family may decide to give physical care.
Former Soviet Union	Family members usually bathe, feed, and comfort the patient, as well as change bed linen.
Dominican Republic	No information.
Mainland China	A family member may be given leave from work to care for an aged relative. The family traditionally remains with the patient during hospitalization. They supply food and assist with feeding, bathing, and keeping the patient comfortable.
India	No information.
El Salvador	No information.
Poland	Parents may wish to be involved in caring for their hospitalized child.
United Kingdom	No information.

*Information based on data gathered through 1992 by the U.S. Department of Immigration and Naturalization Services.
From Geissler EM: *Pocket guide to cultural assessment,* St Louis, 1994, Mosby–Year Book.

THE FAMILY AND VISITORS

Family, relatives, and friends can help meet the person's needs for safety and security, love and belonging, and esteem. They can offer support and comfort and can lessen loneliness. Some also help with the person's care. They may help with meals, bathing, brushing and combing hair, and other care. Often a recovery is influenced by the presence or absence of significant family members or friends. Box 4-7 describes family roles in hospital care for some cultural groups.

The person should be able to visit with family and friends in private and without unnecessary interruptions (Fig. 4-10). Sometimes care must be given when visitors are present. You should politely ask them to leave the

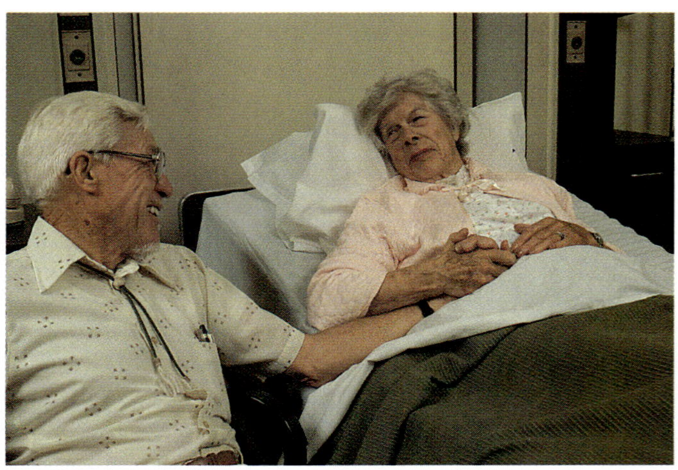

Fig. 4-10 *A patient visiting with family.*

Spotlight On…

Wendy B of Pontiac, Illinois, *works as a nursing assistant in a hospital-based hospice program. Her caring, dedication, and high standards of care make her patients' remaining months as comfortable and enjoyable as possible. The wife of one of Wendy's patients expressed her feelings this way: "Wendy was the sunshine in many dreary, gloomy days of our life. She not only gave excellent care to my husband, but answered my questions and helped me to cope with my husband's illness and death. She gave me a shoulder to lean on."*

room and show them where they can wait comfortably. Do not expose the person's body in front of visitors. Promptly tell visitors when they may return to the room.

Family and visitors must be treated with courtesy and respect. They may be very concerned and frightened about the person's condition. They also need support and understanding of the nursing team. However, do not discuss the person's condition with them. Refer their questions to the nurse.

Visitors often have questions about visiting rules. The number of visitors allowed and the visiting hours vary among facilities. Often they depend on the person's age or condition. Parents of a hospitalized child can usually visit as often and as long as they want. The family members of a person in a critical care unit are usually allowed only short visits. Dying persons can usually have family members present at the bedside constantly. You need to know your facility's visiting policies and the special considerations allowed for individual patients or residents. Visitors may also have questions about the location of the chapel, gift shop, business office, lounge, or cafeteria. You must know the location, special rules, and hours of these facilities.

Sometimes a family member or friend negatively affects the person. If the person is upset or tired because of a visitor, report your observations to the nurse. The nurse can then speak with the visitor about the person's needs.

SUMMARY

People are physical, psychological, spiritual, and social beings. They have certain basic needs necessary for life: physiological needs, the need for safety and security, love and belonging, esteem, and self-actualization. When people cannot meet their own needs, they usually seek health care services.

Culture and religion are important factors in health and illness. Beliefs, values, habits, diet, and health and illness practices may relate to a person's culture or religion. Try to become aware of the beliefs and practices of the major cultures and religions in your community.

Being sick affects the whole person. How a person handles illness is influenced by religion, culture, family, the person's basic personality, the seriousness of the illness, and the speed of recovery. The person may have many fears and anxieties about illness, basic needs, and being able to function normally again. You need to have empathy for your patients and residents if you are to provide effective care.

Patients and residents may have different problems, but all have the same basic needs and the same rights. Verbal and nonverbal communication is used by everyone—patients, residents, health workers, families, and other visitors. Remember that the strongest and truest messages are usually sent nonverbally. Observe facial expressions, gestures, and body language for clues about the person's feelings. Try to control your own nonverbal communication so you do not send the person negative messages. Use touch to communicate understanding, comfort, and caring to the person. Avoid blocking communication by being aware of the common barriers to effective communication. Instead, use the techniques of listening, paraphrasing, direct and open-ended questioning, clarifying, focusing, and silence.

Family members and visitors are important to the person. They can help meet the person's basic needs and influence recovery. Treat them with respect and courtesy.

REVIEW QUESTIONS

Circle the best *answer.*

1 Sally Jones had surgery to remove her gallbladder. You must be concerned

a Only with what is on her nursing care plan

b With her physical, safety and security, and esteem needs

c With her as a physical, psychological, social, and spiritual person

d Only with her cultural and religious needs

2 Of the following basic needs, which is the most essential?

a Self-actualization

b Esteem needs

c Love and belonging

d Safety and security

3 You are assigned to four residents. Based on Maslow's theory of basic needs, which person's needs must be met first?

a Mr. Hart who wants another blanket

b Miss Parks who asks you to read her mail to her

c Ms. Street who asks for more water

d Mr. Hill who is crying

4 Sally Jones said she was afraid of surgery. She said "I don't know what they are going to do to me." What basic need is not being met?

a Physical needs

b The need for safety and security

c The need for love and belonging

d Esteem needs

5 Mr. Hart is a resident of a nursing facility. He wants a little vegetable garden out behind the facility garage. What need does this relate to?

a Self-actualization

b Esteem needs

c Love and belonging

d Safety and security

6 Which is *false?*

a A person's cultural background probably influences health and illness practices.

b Dietary practices may be influenced by both culture and religion.

c A person's religious and cultural practices are not allowed in the health care facility.

d A person may not follow all of the beliefs and practices of his or her religion or culture.

7 Fears and anxieties about being sick are normal reactions.

a True

b False

8 Which is true?

a An obstetrical patient is one who is pregnant, in labor, giving birth, or who has given birth during the previous 6 to 8 weeks.

b Pediatrics is concerned only with sick children.

c Geriatric persons suffer from a disease commonly known as aging.

d All of the above.

9 As a patient, Sally Jones has the right to

a Considerate and respectful care

b Information about her diagnoses, treatment, and prognoses

c Refuse treatment

d All of the above.

10 The right to privacy is protected after death.

a True

b False

11 Which is false?

a Verbal communication involves the written or spoken word.

b Verbal communication is the truest reflection of a person's feelings.

c Messages can be sent by facial expressions, gestures, posture, body movements, appearance, and eye contact.

d Touch means different things to different people.

REVIEW QUESTIONS—CONT'D

12 To communicate with Sally Jones you should

a Use medical words and phrases

b Change the subject often to show you care about her interests and concerns

c Give your opinion when she is sharing fears and concerns

d Be quiet when she is silent

13 You and Sally Jones are talking. You do the following. Which might mean that you are not listening?

a You sit facing her.

b You have good eye contact with her.

c You sit with your arms crossed.

d You ask her questions.

14 You and Sally Jones are talking about her surgery. Which is a direct question?

a"Do you feel better now?"

b "Tell me what your plans are for home."

c "What will you do when you get home?"

d "You said that you will be off work for awhile."

15 Sally Jones wants to take a shower. You say "You would like a shower." This is

a Focusing

b Clarifying

c Paraphrasing

d An open-ended question

16 Focusing is a useful communication tool when

a A person is rambling

b You want to make sure you understand the message

c You want the person to share thoughts and feelings

d You need certain information

17 Which will not block communication?

a "Don't worry."

b "Everything will be just fine."

c "This is a good hospital."

d "Why are you crying?"

18 Sally Jones has many visitors. Which is true?

a Family and friends can help meet her basic needs.

b Privacy should be allowed.

c Visitors should be politely asked to leave the room when care must be given.

d All of the above

Answers to these questions are on page 748.

Body Structure and Function

5

OBJECTIVES

- Define the key terms listed in this chapter
- Identify the basic structures of the cell, and explain how cells divide
- Describe four types of tissue
- Identify the structures of each body system
- Describe the functions of each body system

KEY TERMS

artery A blood vessel that carries blood away from the heart

capillary A tiny blood vessel; food, oxygen, and other substances pass from the capillaries to the cells

cell The basic unit of body structure

digestion The process of physically and chemically breaking down food so that it can be absorbed for use by the cells

hemoglobin The substance in red blood cells that carries oxygen and gives blood its color

hormone A chemical substance secreted by the glands into the bloodstream

menstruation The process in which the lining of the uterus breaks up and is discharged from the body through the vagina

metabolism The burning of food for heat and energy by the cells

organ Groups of tissues with the same function

peristalsis Involuntary muscle contractions in the digestive system that move food through the alimentary canal

respiration The process of supplying the cells with oxygen and removing carbon dioxide from them

system Organs that work together to perform special functions

tissue A group of cells with the same function

vein A blood vessel that carries blood back to the heart

NOTE: Students are responsible for only those terms mentioned in the text. Additional terms used in labeling figures throughout this chapter are for illustrative purposes only.

As a nursing assistant, you will help patients and residents meet their basic needs. Their bodies do not work at peak efficiency because of illness, disease, or injury. You will provide care and perform procedures to promote comfort, healing, and recovery. A basic knowledge of the body's normal structure and function will help you understand certain signs and symptoms, reasons for care, and purposes of procedures. This knowledge should result in safer and more efficient patient and resident care.

CELLS, TISSUES, AND ORGANS

The basic unit of body structure is the **cell.** Each cell has the same basic structure. However, the function, size, and shape of cells may be different (Fig. 5-1 on page 94). Cells are so small that a microscope is needed to see them. Cells need food, water, and oxygen to live and perform their functions.

The cell and its basic structures are shown in Figure 5-2 on page 94. The *cell membrane* is the outer covering that encloses the cell and helps it hold its shape. The *nucleus* is the control center of the cell; it directs the cell's activities. The nucleus is in the center of the cell. The *cytoplasm* is the portion of the cell that surrounds the nucleus. Cytoplasm contains many smaller structures that perform cell functions. The *protoplasm,* which means "living substance," refers to all of the structures, substances, and water within the cell. Protoplasm is a semiliquid substance much like an egg white.

Chromosomes are threadlike structures within the nucleus. Each cell has 46 chromosomes. Chromosomes contain *genes.* Genes control the physical and chemical traits inherited by children from their parents. Inherited traits include height, eye color, and skin color.

Besides controlling cell activities, the nucleus is responsible for cell reproduction. Cells reproduce by dividing in half. The process of cell division is called *mitosis.* Cell division is needed for growth and repair of body tissues. During mitosis, the 46 chromosomes arrange themselves in 23 pairs. As the cell divides, the 23 pairs of chromosomes are pulled in half. The two new cells are identical, and each contains 46 chromosomes (Fig. 5-3 on page 94).

The cells are the body's building blocks. Groups of cells with similar functions combine to form **tissues.** The body has four basic types of tissue:

- *Epithelial tissue* covers internal and external body surfaces. Tissue that lines the nose, mouth, respiratory tract, stomach, and intestines is epithelial tissue. So are the skin, hair, nails, and glands.
- *Connective tissue* anchors, connects, and supports other body tissues. Connective tissue is found in every part of the body. Bones, tendons, ligaments, and cartilage are connective tissue. Blood is a form of connective tissue.
- *Muscle tissue* allows the body to move by stretching and contracting. There are three types of muscle tissue (see page 96).
- *Nerve tissue* receives and carries impulses to the brain and back to body parts.

Groups of tissues form **organs.** An organ performs one or more functions. Examples of organs include the heart, brain, liver, lungs, and kidneys. **Systems** are formed by

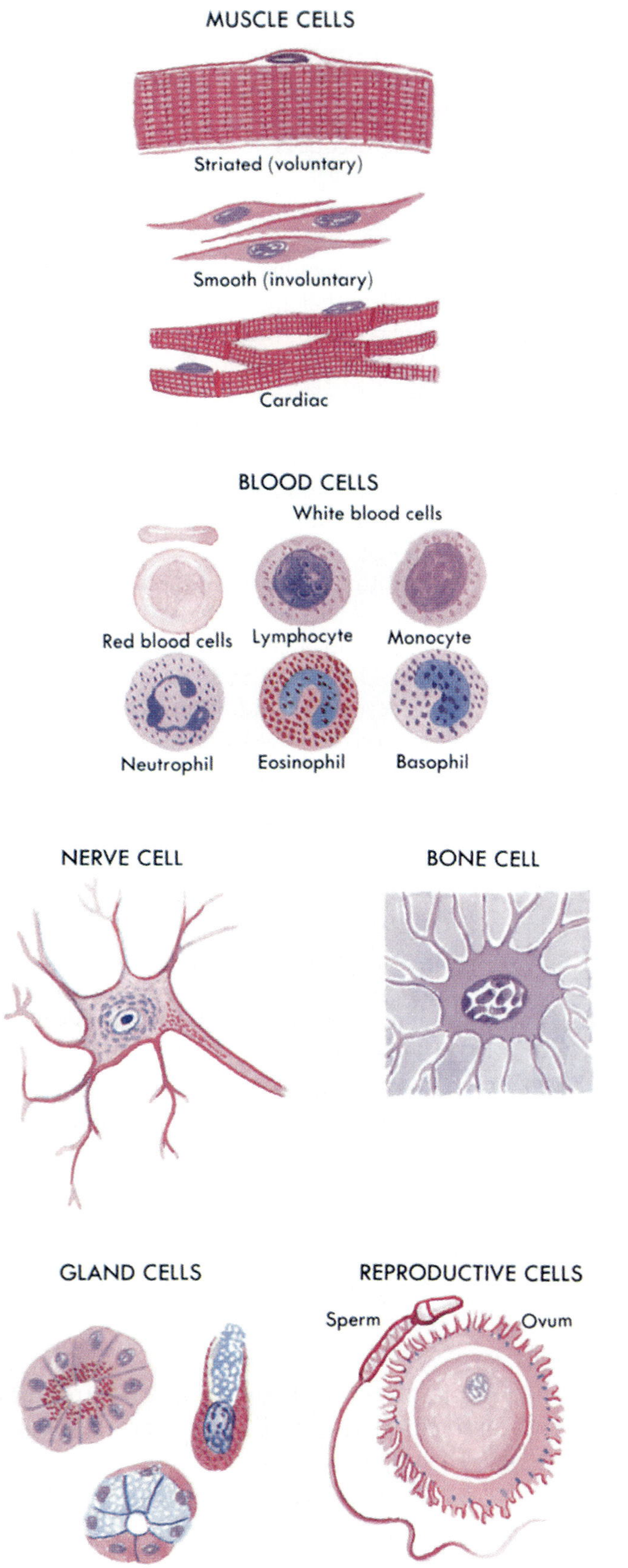

Fig. 5-1 *The different types of cells. (From Thibodeau GA: Anatomy and physiology, St Louis, 1987, Mosby–Year Book.)*

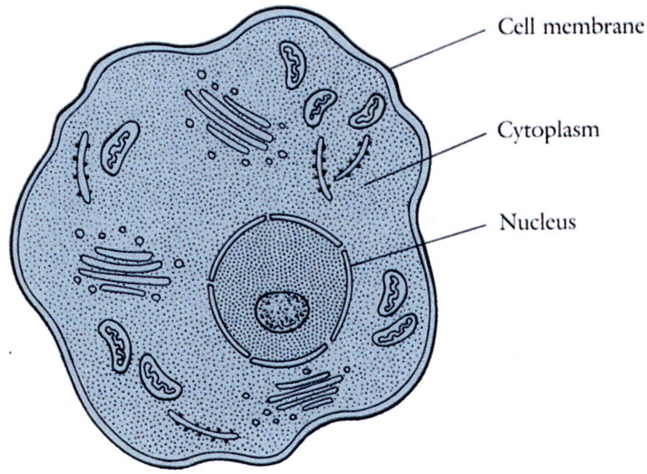

Fig. 5-2 *Parts of a cell.*

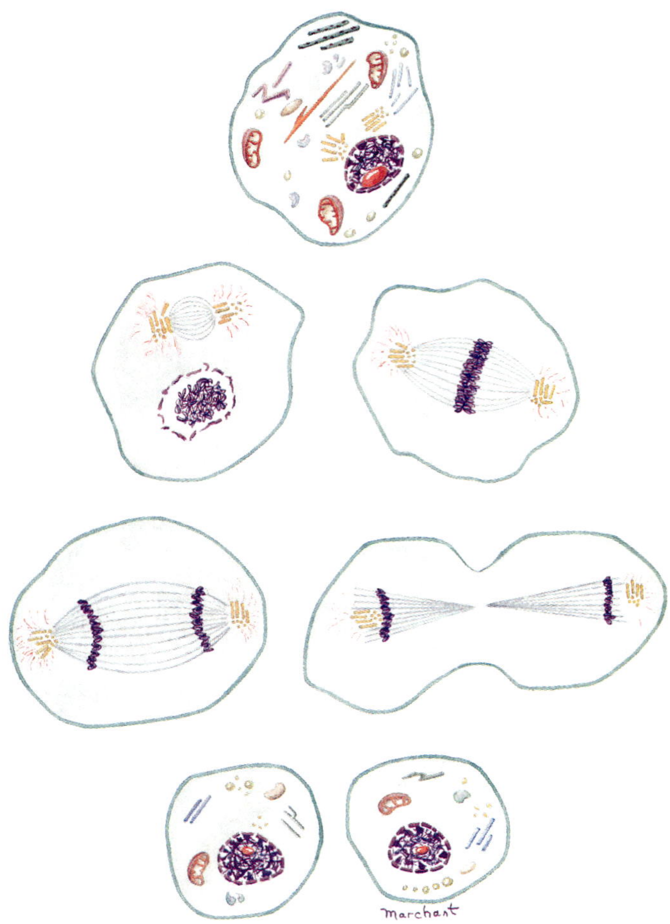

Fig. 5-3 *Cell division.*

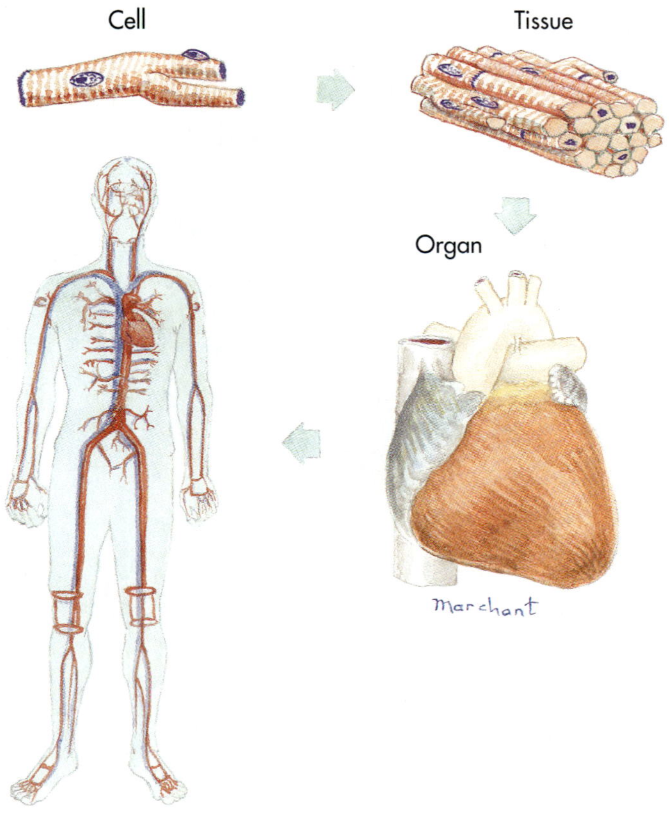

Fig. 5-4 *Organization of the body.*

organs that work together to perform special functions (Fig. 5-4).

THE INTEGUMENTARY SYSTEM

The *integumentary system,* or skin, is the largest system of the body. *Integument* means covering. The skin is the body's natural covering. Skin is made up of epithelial, connective, and nerve tissue, as well as oil and sweat glands. There are two skin layers: the epidermis and the dermis (Fig. 5-5 on page 96). The *epidermis* is the outer layer; it contains living and dead cells. The dead cells were once deeper in the epidermis and were pushed upward as other cells divided. Dead cells constantly flake off and are replaced by living cells. Living cells also die and flake off. Living cells of the epidermis contain *pigment.* Pigment gives skin its color. The epidermis has no blood vessels and few nerve endings. The *dermis* is the inner layer of the skin and is made up of connective tissue. Blood vessels, nerves, sweat and oil glands, and hair roots are found in the dermis.

Oil and *sweat glands, hair,* and *nails* are considered appendages of the skin. The entire body, except the palms of the hands and soles of the feet, is covered with hair. The hair of the nose, eyes, and ears protects these organs from dust, insects, and other foreign objects. Nails protect the tips of fingers and toes. Nails help fingers pick up and handle small objects. Sweat glands help the body regulate temperature. Sweat consists of water, salt, and a small amount of wastes. Sweat is secreted through pores in the skin. The body is cooled as sweat evaporates. Oil glands lie near hair shafts. They secrete an oily substance into the space near the hair shaft. Oil travels to the skin surface, helping to keep the hair and skin soft and shiny.

The skin has many important functions. It is the protective covering of the body. Bacteria and other substances are prevented from entering the body. The skin prevents excessive amounts of water from leaving the body and protects organs from injury. Nerve endings in the skin sense both pleasant and unpleasant stimulation. There are nerve endings over the entire body. The body is protected because cold, pain, touch, and pressure can be sensed. The skin helps regulate body temperature. Blood vessels dilate (widen) when temperature outside the body is high. More blood is brought to the body surface for cooling during evaporation. When blood vessels constrict (narrow), the body retains heat because less blood reaches the skin.

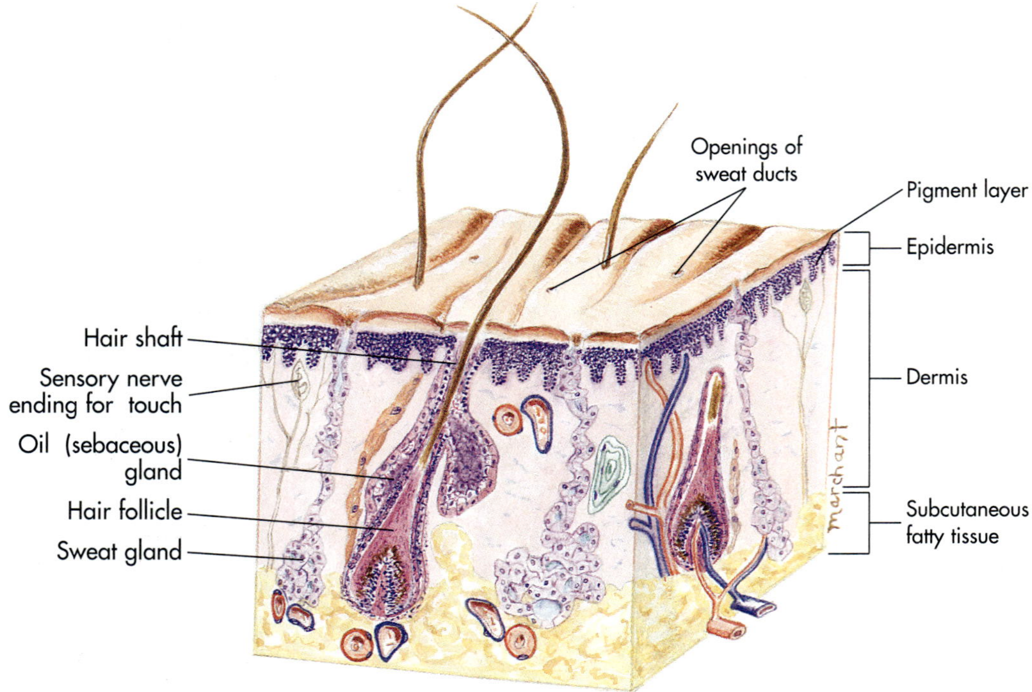

Fig. 5-5 *Layers of the skin.*

THE MUSCULOSKELETAL SYSTEM

The musculoskeletal system provides the framework for the body and allows the body to move. This system also protects and gives the body shape. Besides bones and muscles, the system has ligaments, tendons, and cartilage.

Bones

The human body has 206 bones (Fig. 5-6). There are four types of bones:

- *Long bones* bear the weight of the body. Leg bones are long bones.
- *Short bones* allow skill and ease in movement. Bones in the wrists, fingers, ankles, and toes are short bones.
- *Flat bones* protect the organs. Such bones include the ribs, skull, pelvic bones, and shoulder blades.
- *Irregular bones* are the vertebrae in the spinal column. They allow various degrees of movement and flexibility.

Bones are hard, rigid structures that are made up of living cells. They are covered by a membrane called *periosteum.* Periosteum contains blood vessels that supply bone cells with oxygen and food. Inside the hollow centers of the bones is a substance called *bone marrow.* Blood cells are manufactured in the bone marrow.

Joints

A *joint* is the point at which two or more bones meet. Joints allow movement (joint movement is discussed in Chapter 19). *Cartilage* is the connective tissue at the end of long bones. Cartilage cushions the joint so that bone ends do not rub together. The *synovial membrane* lines the joints. The membrane secretes *synovial fluid.* Synovial fluid acts as a lubricant so the joint can move smoothly. Bones are held together at the joint by strong bands of connective tissue called *ligaments.*

There are three types of joints (Fig. 5-7 on page 98):

- *Ball-and-socket* joint allows movement in all directions. It is made up of the rounded end of one bone and the hollow end of another bone. The rounded end of one fits into the hollow end of the other. The joints of the hips and shoulders are ball-and-socket joints.
- *Hinge joint* allows movement in one direction. The elbow is a hinge joint.
- *Pivot joint* allows turning from side to side. The skull is connected to the spine by a pivot joint.

Muscles

There are more than 500 muscles in the human body (Figs. 5-8 and 5-9 on pages 99 and 100). Some are voluntary, and others are involuntary. *Voluntary* muscles can be consciously controlled. Muscles that are attached to bones *(skeletal muscles)* are voluntary. Arm muscles do not work

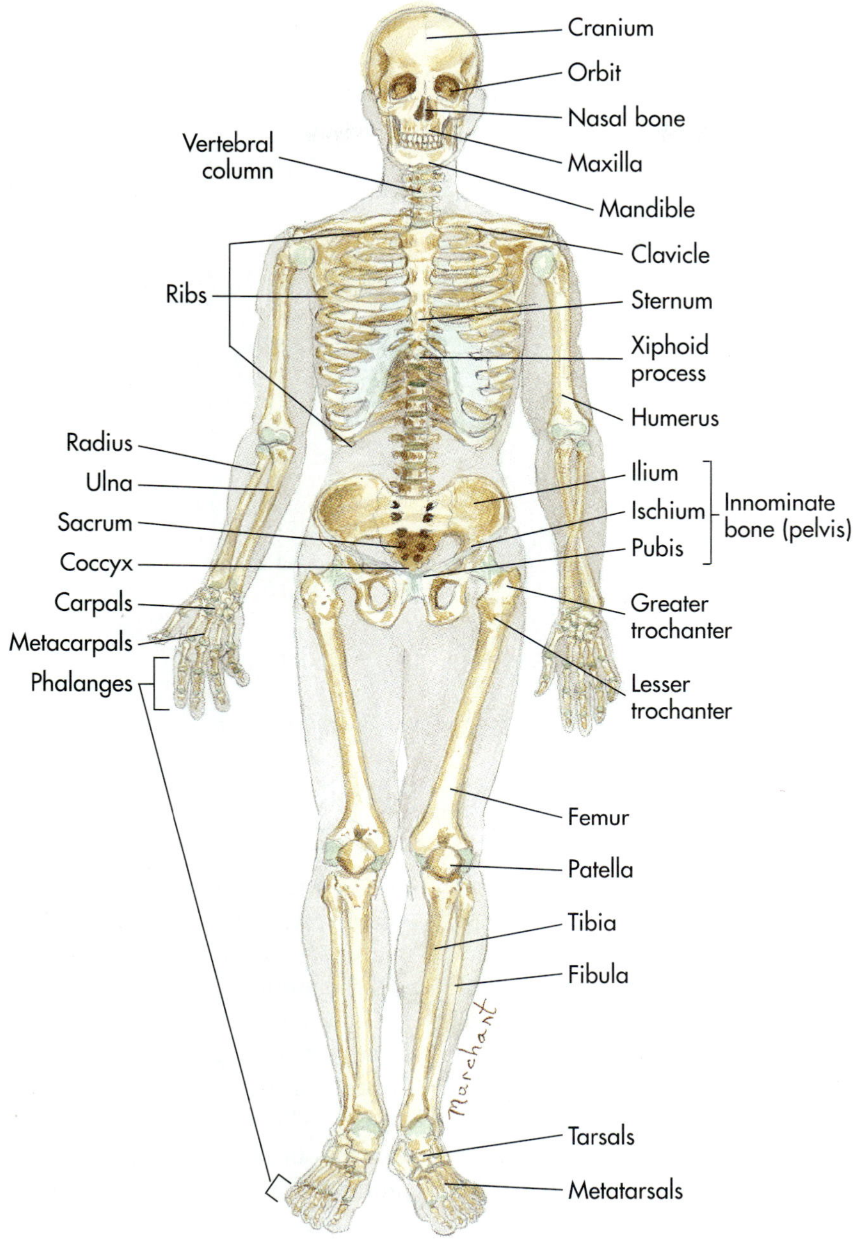

Fig. 5-6 *Bones of the body.*

unless you move your arm; likewise for leg muscles. Skeletal muscles are *striated,* that is, they look striped or streaked. *Involuntary muscles* work automatically and cannot be consciously controlled. Involuntary muscles control the action of the stomach, intestines, blood vessels, and other body organs. Involuntary muscles are also called *smooth muscles.* They look smooth, not streaked or striped. *Cardiac muscle* is in the heart. Although it is an involuntary muscle, it has the striated appearance of skeletal muscle.

Muscles perform three important body functions:

- Movement of body parts
- Maintenance of posture
- Production of body heat

Strong, tough connective tissues called *tendons* connect muscles to bones. When muscles contract (shorten), tendons at each end of the muscle cause the bone to move. The body has many tendons; the Achilles tendon is shown in Figure 5-9. Some muscles constantly contract to maintain the body's posture. When muscles contract, they burn food for energy, resulting in the production of heat. The greater the muscular activity, the greater the amount of heat produced in the body. Shivering is a way the body produces heat when exposed to cold. The shivering sensation is from rapid, general muscle contractions.

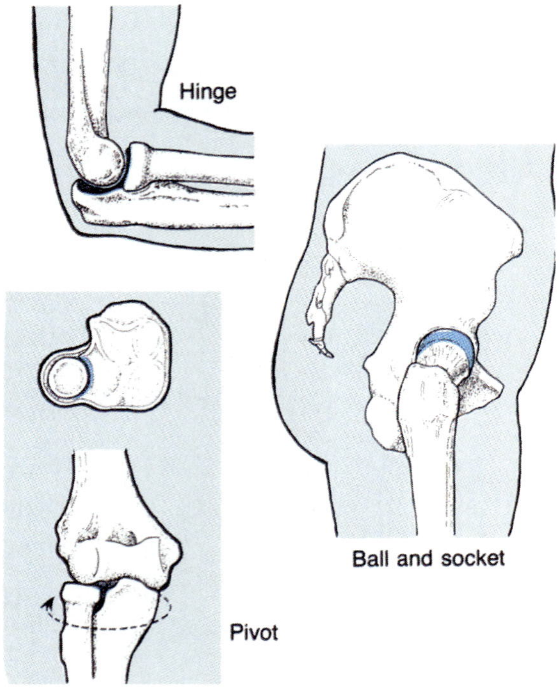

Fig. 5-7 *Types of joints.* *(Modified from Austrin M: Young's learning medical terminology step by step, ed 8, St Louis, 1995, Mosby–Year Book.)*

THE NERVOUS SYSTEM

The nervous system controls, directs, and coordinates body functions. The two main divisions of the nervous system are the *central nervous system* (CNS) and the *peripheral nervous system.* The central nervous system consists of the *brain* and *spinal cord* (Fig. 5-10 on page 101). The peripheral nervous system involves the *nerves* throughout the body (Fig. 5-11 on page 101). Nerves carry messages or impulses to and from the brain. Nerves are connected to the spinal cord. The nerve cell *(neuron)* is the basic unit of the nervous system (Fig. 5-12 on page 102). Threadlike projections from the cytoplasm of the neuron are called *nerve fibers.* Nerve fibers that bring impulses to the cell are called *dendrites.* Fibers that carry impulses away from neurons are called *axons.* A neuron usually has only one axon. Dendrites may be short or as long as 3 feet.

Receptors or *end-organs* are inside and outside of the body. Each receptor is attached to a neuron by a dendrite. A stimulus is received by the receptor and travels to the brain. Stimuli include heat, cold, touch, smell, hearing, vision, balance, hunger, and thirst. If the body or body part must respond to the stimulus, the brain sends an impulse through the neurons to the proper muscles and glands.

Nerves are easily damaged and take a long time to heal. Some nerve fibers have a protective covering called a *myelin sheath.* The myelin sheath also insulates the nerve fiber. Nerve fibers covered with myelin can conduct impulses faster than those fibers without the protective covering.

The Central Nervous System

The central nervous system consists of the brain and spinal cord. The brain is covered by the skull. The three main parts of the brain are the *cerebrum,* the *cerebellum,* and the *brainstem* (Fig. 5-13 on page 102).

The cerebrum is the largest part of the brain. It is the center of thought and intelligence. The cerebrum is divided into two halves called the right and left *hemispheres.* The right hemisphere controls movement and activities of the left side of the body. The left hemisphere controls the right side. The outside of the cerebrum is called the *cerebral cortex.* The cerebral cortex controls the highest functions of the brain. These include reasoning, memory, consciousness, speech, voluntary muscle movement, vision, hearing, sensation, and other activities.

The cerebellum regulates and coordinates body movements. The smooth movements of voluntary muscles and balance are possible because of control by the cerebellum. Injury to the cerebellum results in jerky movements, loss of coordination, and muscle weakness.

The brainstem connects the cerebrum to the spinal cord. There are three important structures within the brainstem: the *midbrain, pons,* and *medulla.* The midbrain and pons relay messages between the medulla and the cerebrum. The medulla is directly below the pons. Heart rate, breathing, the size of blood vessels, swallowing, coughing, and vomiting are some functions controlled by the medulla. The brain is connected to the spinal cord at the lower end of the medulla.

Text continued on page 102.

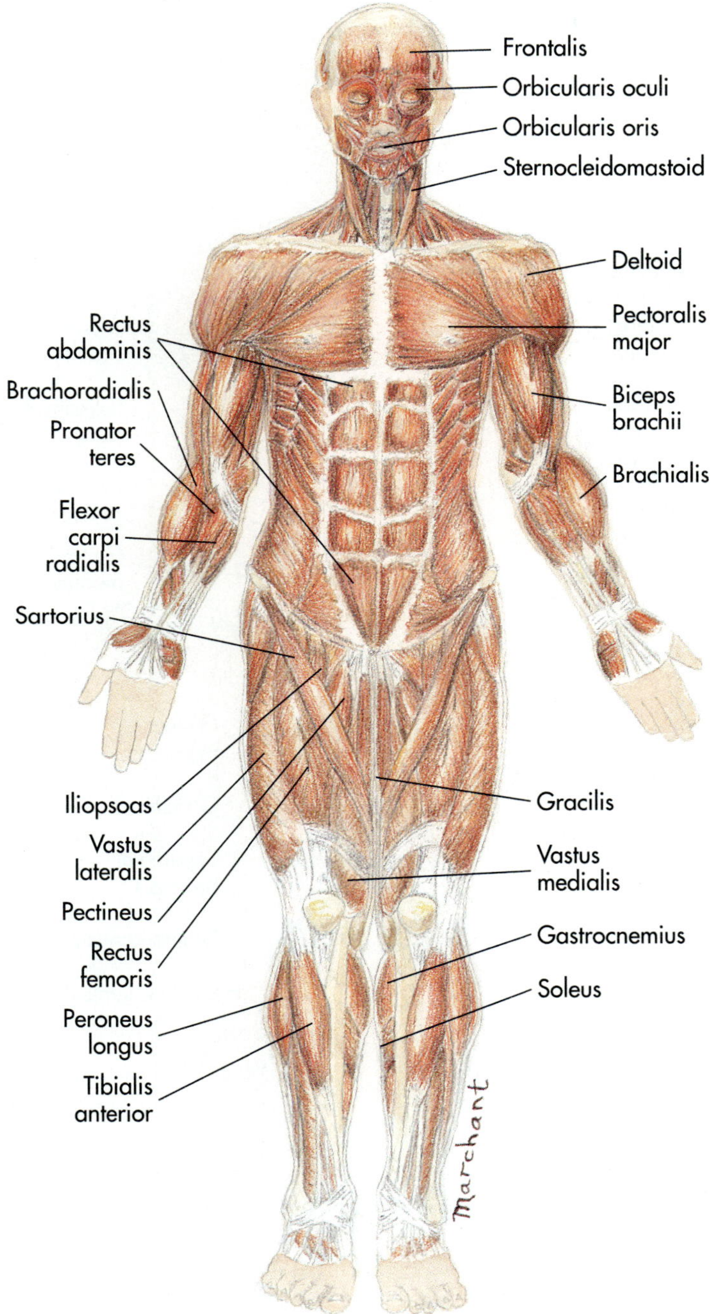

Fig. 5-8 *Anterior view of the muscles of the body.*

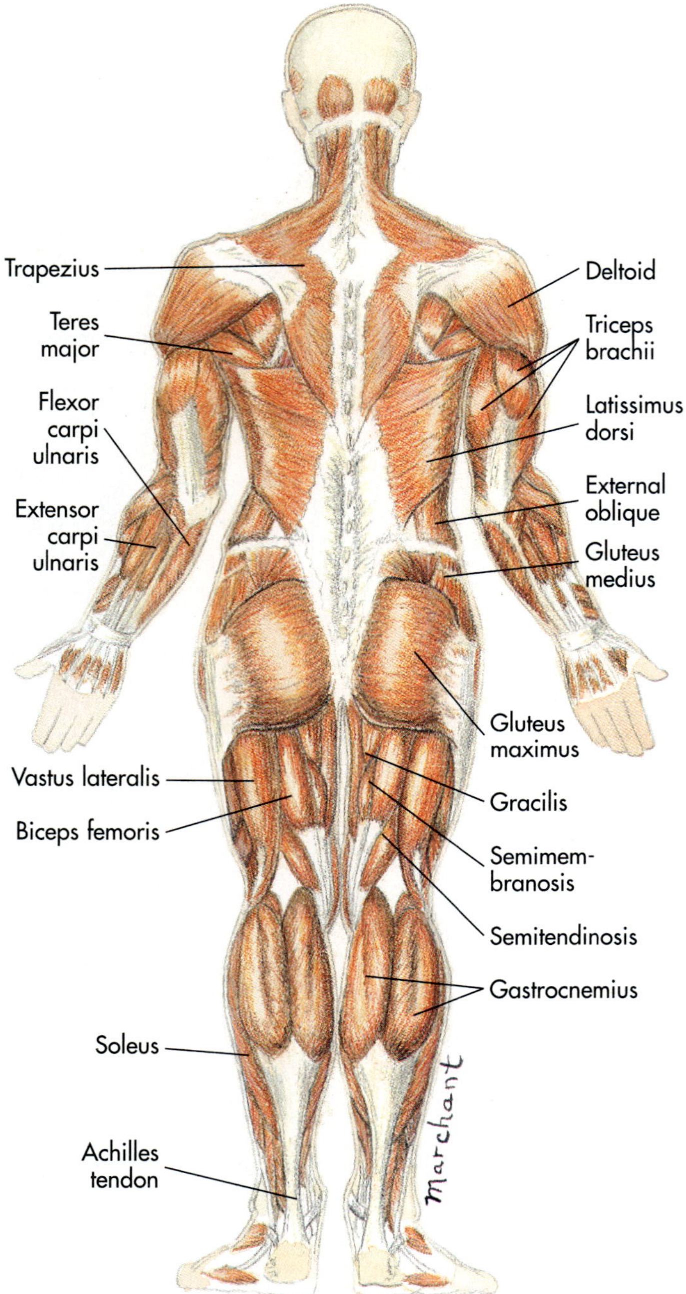

Fig. 5-9 *Posterior view of the muscles of the body.*

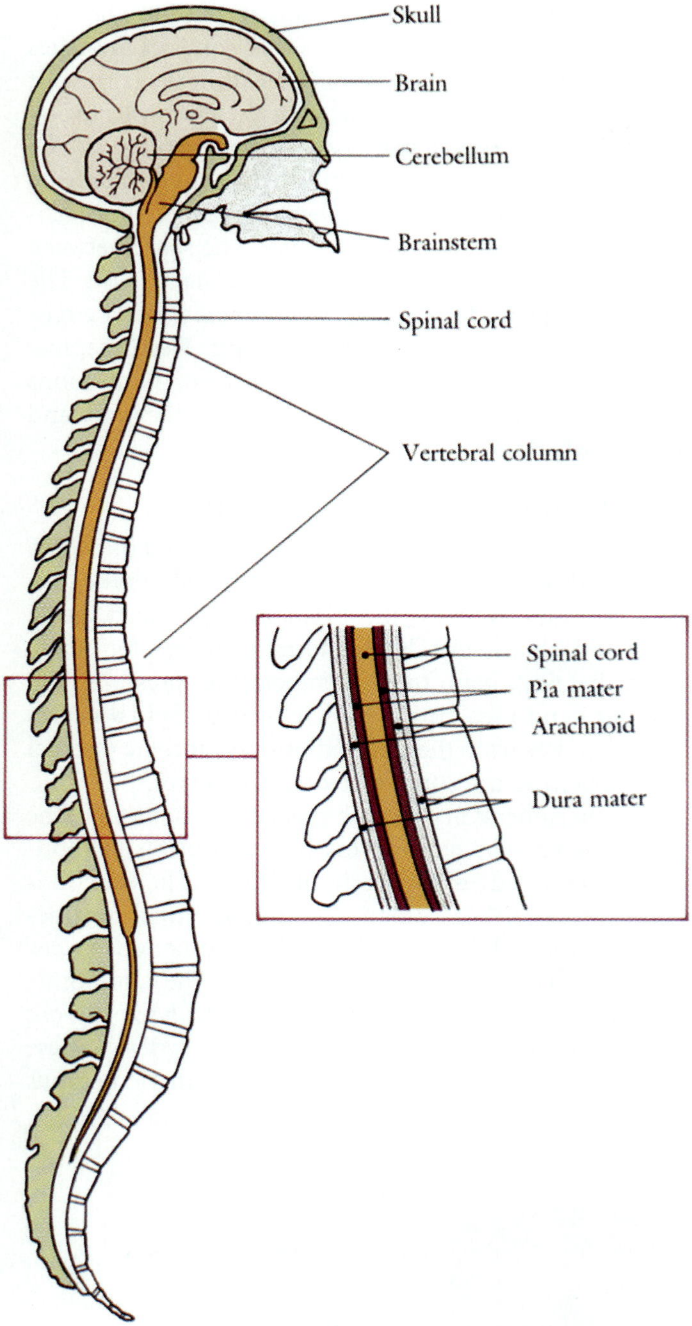

Fig. 5-10 *Central nervous system.*

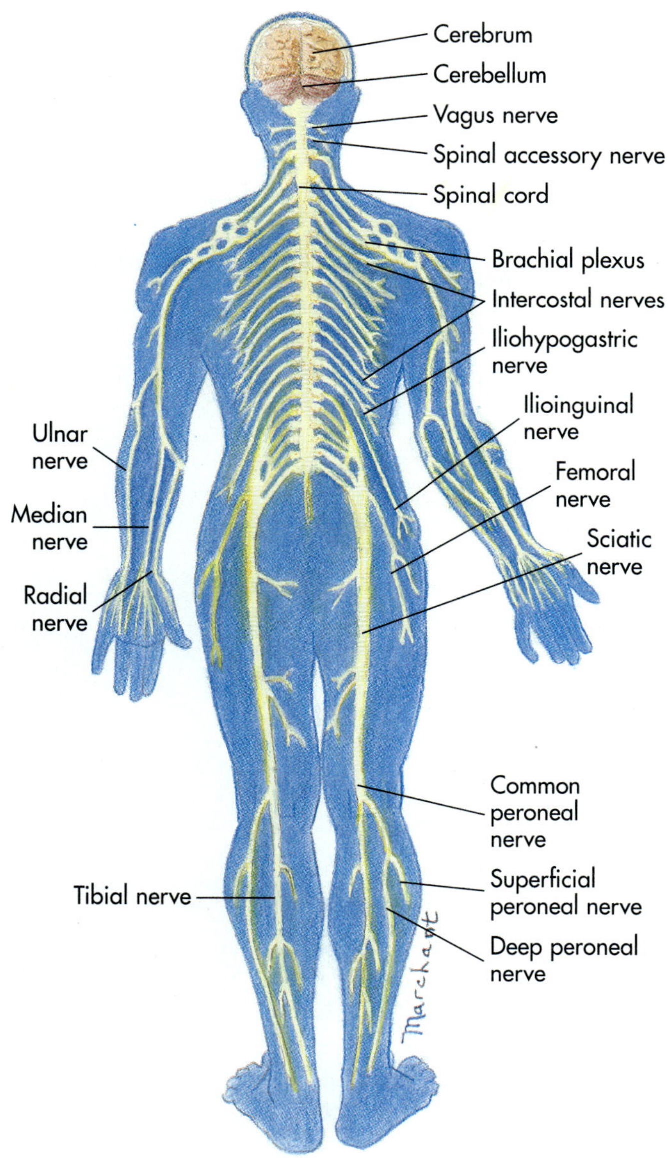

Fig. 5-11 *Peripheral nervous system.*

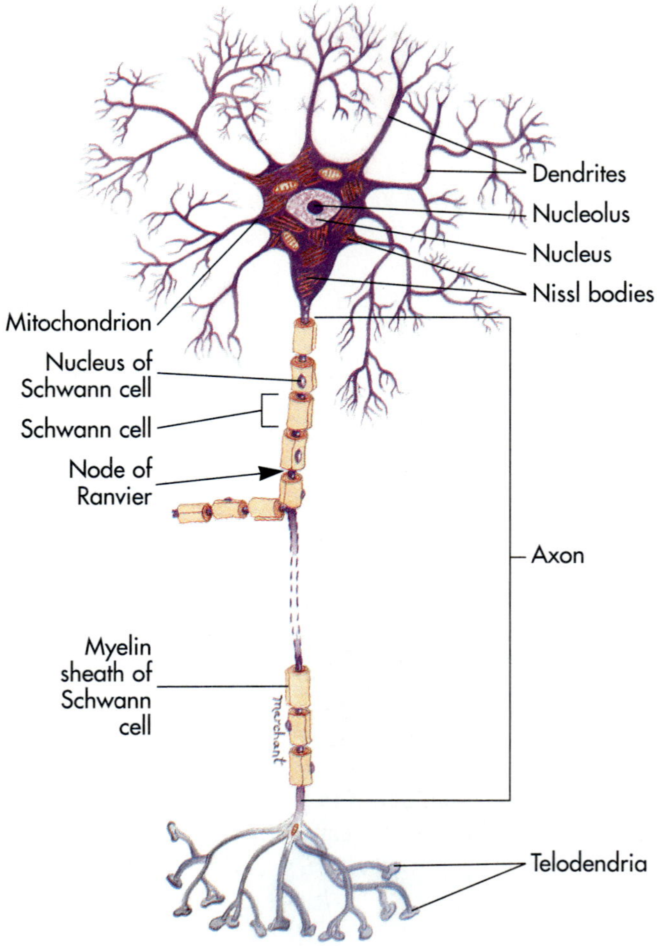

Fig. 5-12 *A neuron.*

The spinal cord lies within the spinal column. The cord is about 18 inches long. Pathways that conduct messages to and from the brain are contained within the cord.

The brain and spinal cord are covered and protected by three layers of connective tissue called *meninges.* The outer layer lies next to the skull. It is a tough covering called the *dura mater.* The middle layer is called the *arachnoid.* The inner layer is the *pia mater.* The space between the middle and inner layers is the *arachnoid space.* The space is filled with fluid called *cerebrospinal fluid.* It circulates around the brain and spinal cord. Cerebrospinal fluid protects the central nervous system. It cushions shocks that could easily injure structures of the brain and spinal cord.

The Peripheral Nervous System

The peripheral nervous system has twelve pairs of *cranial nerves* and 31 pairs of *spinal nerves.* Cranial nerves conduct impulses between the brain and the head, neck, chest, and abdomen. They conduct impulses for smell, vision, hearing, pain, touch, temperature, pressure, and voluntary and involuntary muscle control. Spinal nerves carry impulses from the skin, extremities, and the internal body structures not supplied by cranial nerves.

Some peripheral nerves with special functions form the *autonomic nervous system.* This system controls involuntary muscles and certain body functions. The functions include the heartbeat, blood pressure, intestinal contractions, and glandular secretions. These functions occur automatically without conscious effort. The autonomic nervous system is divided into the *sympathetic nervous system* and the *parasympathetic nervous system.* These divisions balance one another. The sympathetic nervous

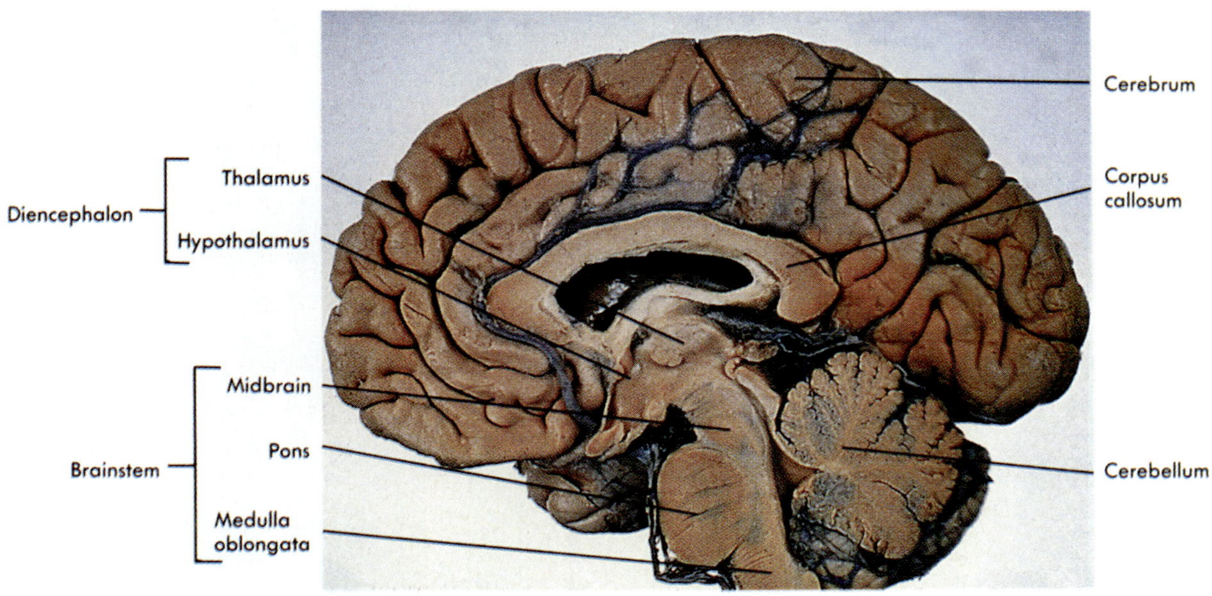

Fig. 5-13 The brain. *(From Vidic B, Suarez FR: Photographic atlas of the human body, St Louis, 1984, Mosby–Year Book.)*

system tends to speed up functions. The parasympathetic nervous system slows them down. When you are angry, frightened, excited, or exercising, the sympathetic nervous system is stimulated. The parasympathetic system is activated when you relax or when the sympathetic system has been under stimulation for too long.

The Sense Organs

The five major senses are sight, hearing, taste, smell, and touch. Receptors for taste are in the tongue and are called *taste buds.* Receptors for smell are in the nose. Touch receptors are found in the dermis, especially in the toes and fingertips.

The eye Receptors for vision are in the eyes. The eye is a delicate organ that can be easily injured. Bones of the skull, eyelids and eyelashes, and tears protect the eyes from injury. Eye structures are shown in Figure 5-14. The eye has three layers:

- The *sclera,* the white of the eye, is the outer layer. It is made of tough connective tissue.
- The *choroid* is the second layer. Blood vessels, the *ciliary muscle,* and the *iris* make up the choroid. The iris gives the eye its color. The opening in the middle of the iris is the *pupil.* Pupil size varies with the amount of light entering the eye. The pupil constricts (narrows) in bright light and dilates (widens) in dim or dark places.
- The *retina* is the inner layer of the eye. Receptors for vision and the nerve fibers of the optic nerve are contained in the retina.

Light enters the eye through the *cornea.* The cornea is the transparent part of the outer layer that lies over the eye. Light rays pass to the *lens,* which lies behind the pupil. The light is then reflected to the retina and carried to the brain by the optic nerve.

The *aqueous chamber* separates the cornea from the lens. The chamber is filled with a fluid called *aqueous humor.* The fluid helps the cornea keep its shape and position. The *vitreous body* is behind the lens. The vitreous body is a gelatin-like substance that supports the retina and maintains the shape of the eye.

The ear The ear is a sense organ that functions in hear-ing and balance. It is divided into the *external ear, middle ear,* and *inner ear.* Ear structures are shown in Figure 5-15 on page 104.

The external ear (outer part) is called the *pinna* or *auricle.* Sound waves are guided through the external ear into the *auditory canal.* Glands in the auditory canal secrete a waxy substance called *cerumen.* The auditory canal extends about 1 inch to the *eardrum.* The eardrum *(tympanic membrane)* separates the external and middle ear.

The middle ear is a small space that contains the *eustachian tube* and three small bones called *ossicles.* The eustachian tube connects the middle ear and the throat. Air enters the eustachian tube so that there is equal pressure on both sides of the eardrum. The ossicles amplify sound received from the eardrum and transmit the sound to the inner ear. The three ossicles are:

- The *malleus,* which looks like a hammer
- The *incus,* which resembles an anvil
- The *stapes,* which is shaped like a stirrup

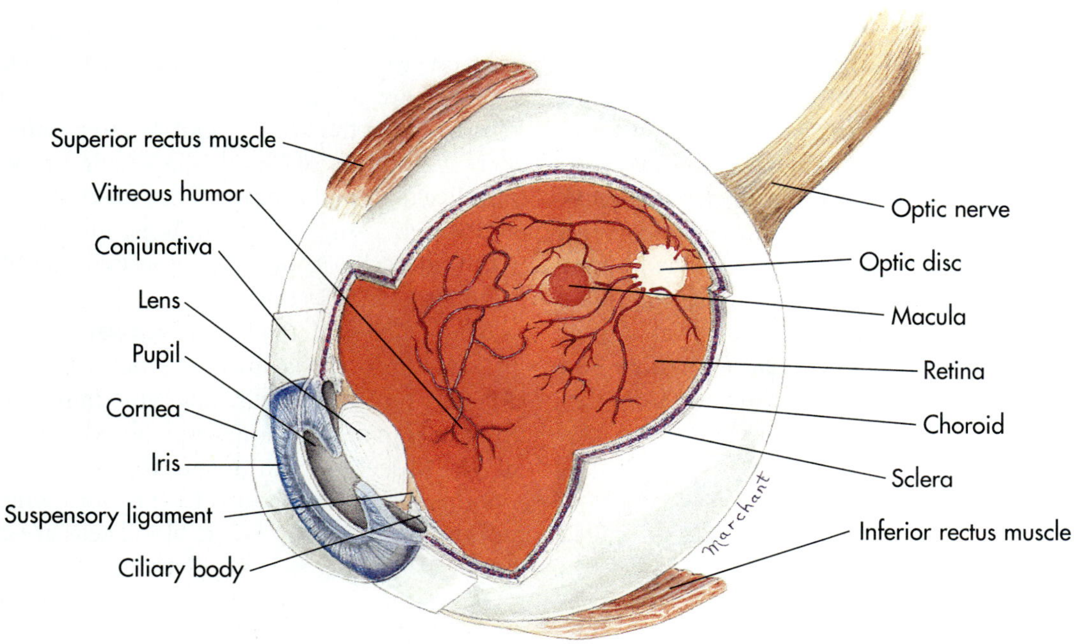

Fig. 5-14 *The eye.*

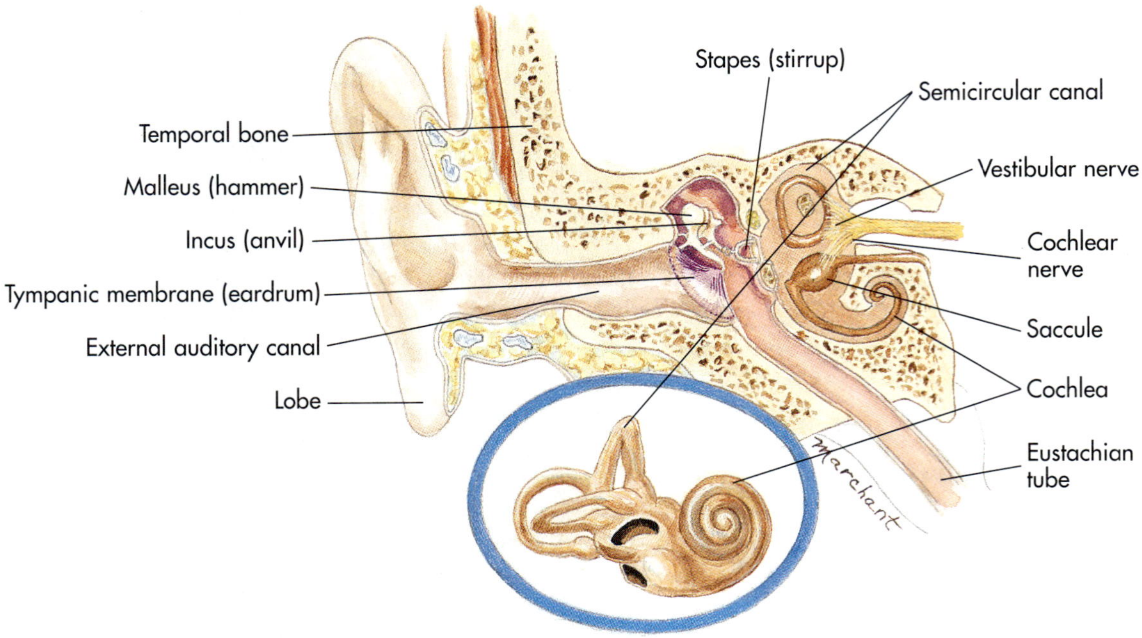

Fig. 5-15 *The ear.*

The inner ear consists of the *semicircular canals* and the *cochlea.* The cochlea, which looks like a snail shell, contains fluid. The fluid carries sound waves received from the middle ear to the *auditory nerve.* The auditory nerve then carries the message to the brain.

The three semicircular canals are involved with balance. They sense the head's position and changes in position, and send messages to the brain.

THE CIRCULATORY SYSTEM

The circulatory system is made up of the blood, heart, and blood vessels. The heart pumps blood through the blood vessels. The circulatory system has many important functions. Blood carries food, oxygen, and other substances to the cells. Blood also removes waste products from cells. Regulation of body temperature is aided by the blood and blood vessels. Heat from muscle activity is carried by the blood to other body parts. Blood vessels in the skin dilate if the body needs to be cooled. They constrict if heat should be kept in the body. The circulatory system also produces and carries cells that defend the body from disease-causing microorganisms.

The Blood

The blood consists of blood cells and a liquid called *plasma.* Plasma is mostly water. It carries blood cells to other body cells. Plasma also carries other substances needed by cells for proper functioning. Food (proteins, fats, and carbohydrates), hormones (see The Endocrine System, page 113), and chemicals are among the many substances carried in the plasma. Waste products are also carried in the plasma.

Red blood cells are called *erythrocytes.* They give the blood its red color because of a substance in the cell called **hemoglobin.** As red blood cells circulate through the lungs, hemoglobin picks up oxygen. The hemoglobin carries oxygen to the cells. When the blood is bright red, hemoglobin in the red blood cells is saturated (filled) with oxygen. As blood circulates through the body, oxygen is given to the cells. The cells release carbon dioxide (a waste product), which is picked up by the hemoglobin. Red blood cells saturated with carbon dioxide make the blood look dark red.

There are about 25 trillion (25,000,000,000,000) red blood cells in the body. About $4^1/_2$ to 5 million cells are in a cubic milliliter of blood (the size of a tiny drop). These cells live for 3 or 4 months. They are destroyed by the liver and spleen as they wear out. Bone marrow produces new red blood cells. About 1 million new red blood cells are produced every second.

White blood cells, called *leukocytes,* are colorless. They protect the body against infection. There are 5,000 to 10,000 white blood cells in a cubic milliliter of blood. At the first sign of infection, white blood cells rush to the site of the infection and begin to multiply rapidly. The number of white blood cells increases when there is an infection in the body. White blood cells are also produced by the bone marrow. They live about 9 days.

Platelets (thrombocytes) are necessary for the clotting of blood. They are also produced by the bone marrow. There are about 200,000 to 400,000 platelets in a cubic milliliter of blood. A platelet lives about 4 days.

The Heart

The heart is a muscle. It pumps blood through the blood vessels to the tissues and cells. The heart lies in the middle to lower part of the chest cavity toward the left side (Fig. 5-16). The heart is hollow and has three layers (Fig. 5-17):

- The *pericardium* is the outer layer. It is a thin sac covering the heart.
- The *myocardium* is the second layer. This layer is the thick muscular portion of the heart.
- The *endocardium* is the inner layer. The endocardium is the membrane lining the inner surface of the heart.

The heart has four chambers (see Fig. 5-17). Upper chambers receive blood and are called the *atria*. The right atrium receives blood from body tissues. The *left atrium* receives blood from the lungs. Lower chambers are called ventricles. Ventricles pump blood. The *right ventricle* pumps blood to the lungs for oxygen. The *left ventricle*

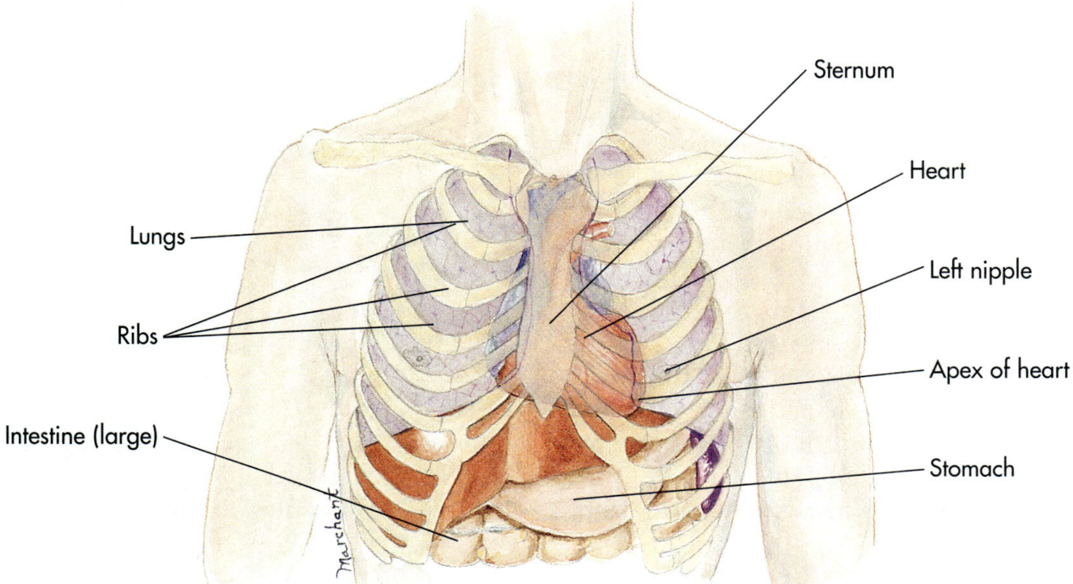

Fig. 5-16 *Location of the heart in the chest cavity.*

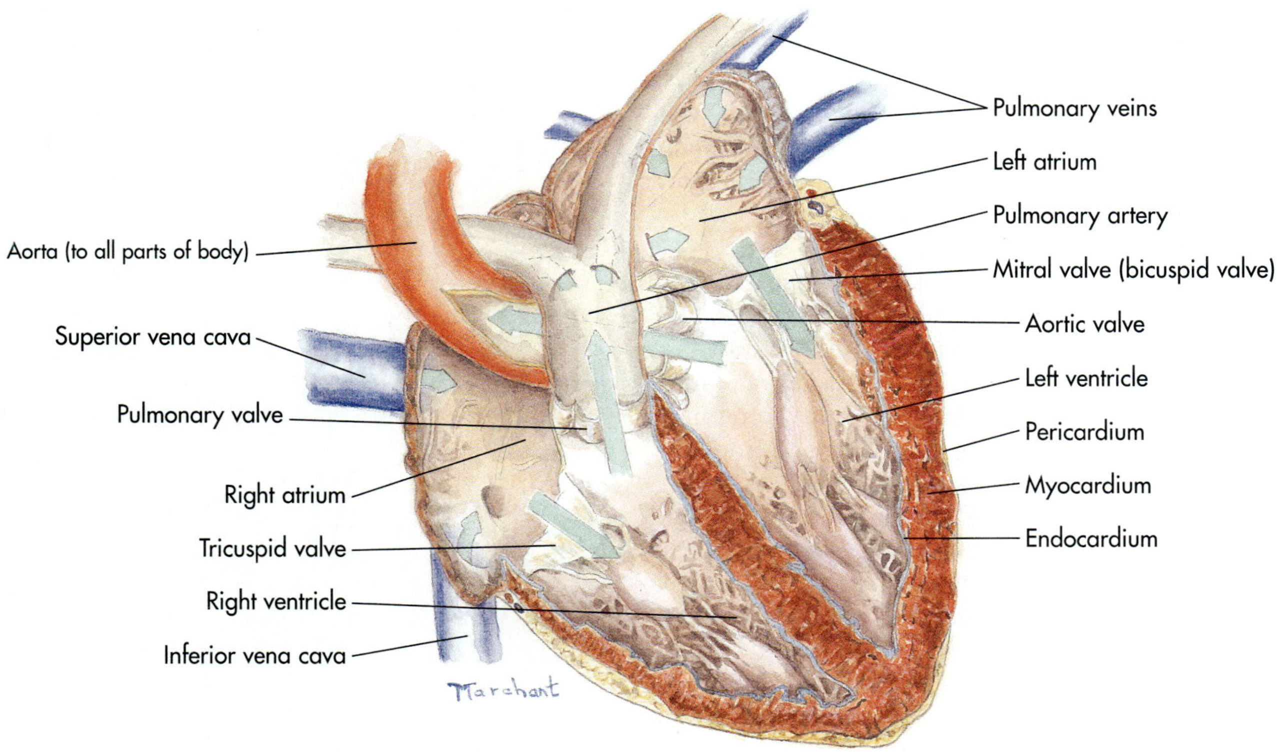

Fig. 5-17 *Structures of the heart.*

pumps blood to all parts of the body. *Valves* are located between the atria and ventricles. The valves allow blood to flow in one direction. They prevent blood from flowing back into the atria from the ventricles. The *tricuspid valve* is between the right atrium and right ventricle. The *mitral valve (bicuspid valve)* is between the left atrium and left ventricle.

There are two phases of heart action. During *diastole,* the resting phase, heart chambers fill with blood. During *systole,* the working phase, the heart contracts. Blood is pumped through the blood vessels when the heart contracts.

The Blood Vessels

Blood flows to body tissues and cells through the blood vessels. There are three groups of blood vessels: arteries, capillaries, and veins. **Arteries** carry blood away from the heart. Arterial blood is rich in oxygen. The *aorta* is the largest artery. The aorta receives blood directly from the left ventricle. The aorta branches into other arteries that carry blood to all parts of the body (Fig. 5-18). These arteries branch into smaller parts within the tissues. The smallest branch of an artery is an *arteriole.* Arterioles connect with blood vessels called **capillaries.** Capillaries are very tiny vessels. Food, oxygen, and other substances pass from capillaries into the cells. Waste products, including carbon dioxide, are picked up from cells by the capillaries. Waste products are carried back to the heart by the veins.

Veins return blood to the heart. They are connected to the capillaries by *venules.* Venules are small veins. Venules begin branching together to form veins. The many branches of veins also branch together as they near the heart to form two main veins (Fig. 5-18). The two main veins are the *inferior vena cava* and the *superior vena cava.* Both empty into the right atrium. The inferior vena cava carries blood from the legs and trunk. The superior vena cava carries blood from the head and arms. Venous blood is dark red in color because it contains little oxygen and a lot of carbon dioxide.

Blood flow through the circulatory system is diagrammed in Figure 5-17 and can be summarized as follows. Venous blood, poor in oxygen, empties into the right atrium. Blood flows through the tricuspid valve into the right ventricle. The right ventricle pumps blood into the lungs to pick up oxygen. Oxygen-rich blood from the lungs enters the left atrium. Blood from the left atrium passes through the mitral valve into the left ventricle. The left ventricle pumps the blood to the aorta, which branches off to form other arteries. The arterial blood is carried to the tissues by arterioles and to the cells by capillaries. The cells and capillaries exchange oxygen and nutrients for carbon dioxide and waste products. Capillaries connect with venules. Venules carry blood that contains carbon dioxide and waste products. The venules form veins. Veins return blood to the heart.

THE RESPIRATORY SYSTEM

Oxygen is needed for survival. Every cell needs oxygen. Air contains about 20% oxygen, enough to meet body needs under normal conditions. The respiratory system brings oxygen into the lungs and eliminates carbon dioxide. The process of supplying the cells with oxygen and removing carbon dioxide from them is called **respiration.** Respiration involves *inhalation* (breathing in) and

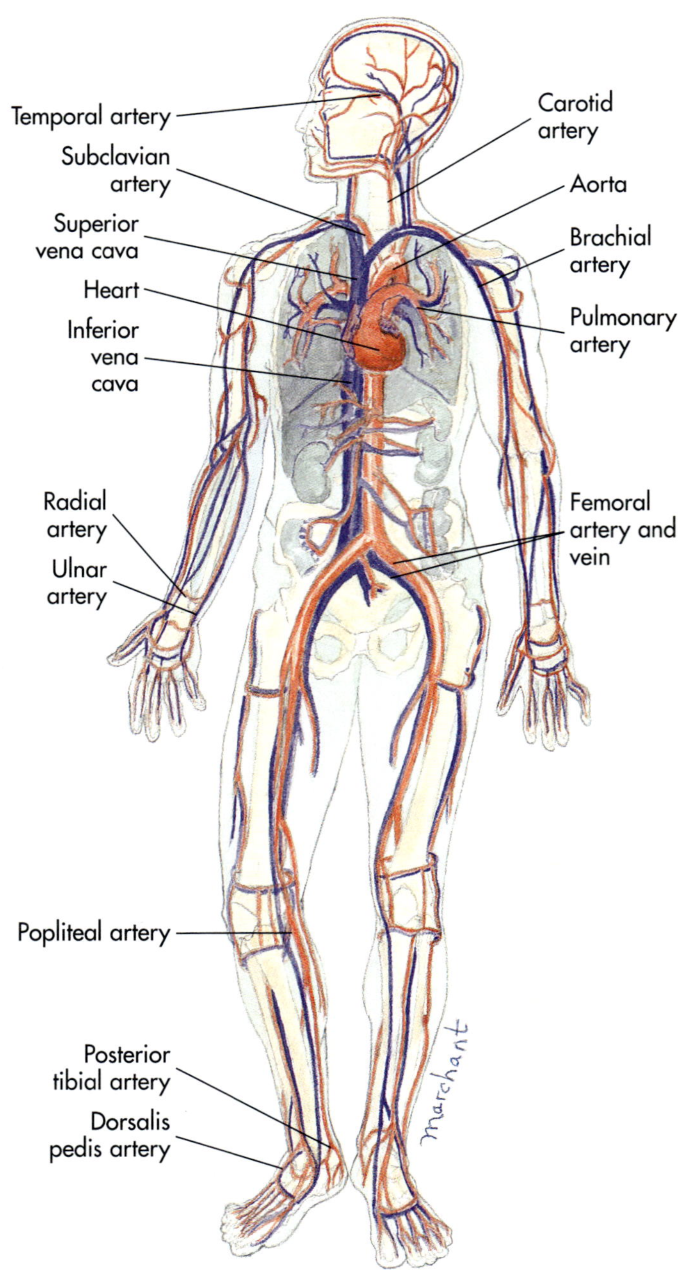

Fig. 5-18 *Arterial and venous systems.*

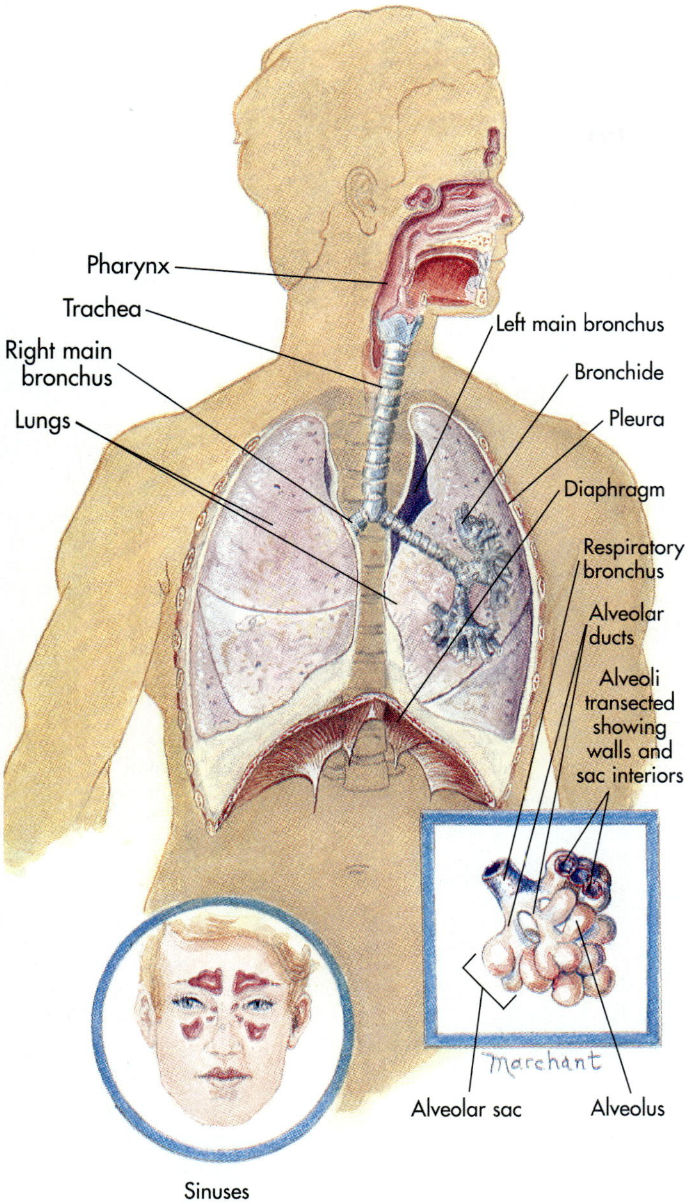

Fig. 5-19 *Respiratory system.*

exhalation (breathing out). The terms *inspiration* (breathing in) and *expiration* (breathing out) are also used. The respiratory system is shown in Figure 5-19.

Air enters the body through the *nose.* The air then passes into the *pharynx* (throat), a tube-shaped passageway for both air and food. Air passes from the pharynx into the *larynx* (the voice box). A piece of cartilage called the *epiglottis* acts like a lid over the larynx. The epiglottis prevents food from entering the airway during swallowing. During inhalation the epiglottis lifts up to let air pass over the larynx. Air passes from the larynx into the *trachea* (the windpipe). The trachea divides at its lower end into the *right bronchus* and *left bronchus.* Each bronchus enters a lung. Upon entering the lungs, the bronchi further divide several times into smaller branches called *bronchioles.* Eventually the bronchioles subdivide and end in tiny one-celled air sacs called *alveoli.* Alveoli look like small clusters of grapes. They are supplied by capillaries. Oxygen and carbon dioxide are exchanged between the alveoli and capillaries. Blood in the capillaries picks up oxygen from the alveoli. Then the blood is returned to the left side of the heart and pumped to the rest of the body. Alveoli pick up carbon dioxide from the capillaries for exhalation.

The lungs are spongy tissues filled with alveoli, blood vessels, and nerves. Each lung is divided into lobes. The right lung has three lobes, the left lung has two. The lungs are separated from the abdominal cavity by a muscle called the *diaphragm.* Each lung is covered by a two-layered sac called the *pleura.* One layer is attached to the lung and the other to the chest wall. The pleura secretes a very thin fluid that fills the space between the layers. The fluid prevents the layers from rubbing together during inhalation and exhalation. A bony framework consisting of the ribs, sternum, and vertebrae protects the lungs.

THE DIGESTIVE SYSTEM

The digestive system breaks down food physically and chemically so it can be absorbed for use by the cells. This process is called **digestion.** The digestive system is also called the *gastrointestinal system (GI system).* The system also eliminates solid wastes from the body. The digestive system consists of the *alimentary canal (GI tract)* and the accessory organs of digestion (Fig. 5-20 on page 108). The alimentary canal is a long tube extending from the mouth to the anus. Its major parts are the mouth, pharynx, esophagus, stomach, small intestine, and large intestine. The accessory organs of digestion are the teeth, tongue, salivary glands, liver, gallbladder, and pancreas.

Digestion begins in the *mouth.* The mouth is also called the *oral cavity.* The oral cavity receives food and prepares it for digestion. Using chewing motions, the *teeth* cut, chop, and grind food into smaller particles for digestion and swallowing. The *tongue* aids in chewing and swallowing. *Taste buds* on the tongue's surface contain nerve endings. Taste buds allow sweet, sour, bitter, and salty tastes to be sensed. *Salivary glands* in the mouth secrete *saliva.* Saliva moistens food particles for easier swallowing and begins the digestion of food. During swallowing, the tongue pushes food into the pharynx.

The *pharynx* (throat) is a muscular tube. The act of swallowing is continued as the pharynx contracts. Contraction of the pharynx pushes food into the *esophagus.* The esophagus is a muscular tube about 10 inches long. It extends from the pharynx to the stomach. Involuntary muscle contractions called **peristalsis** move food down the esophagus into the stomach.

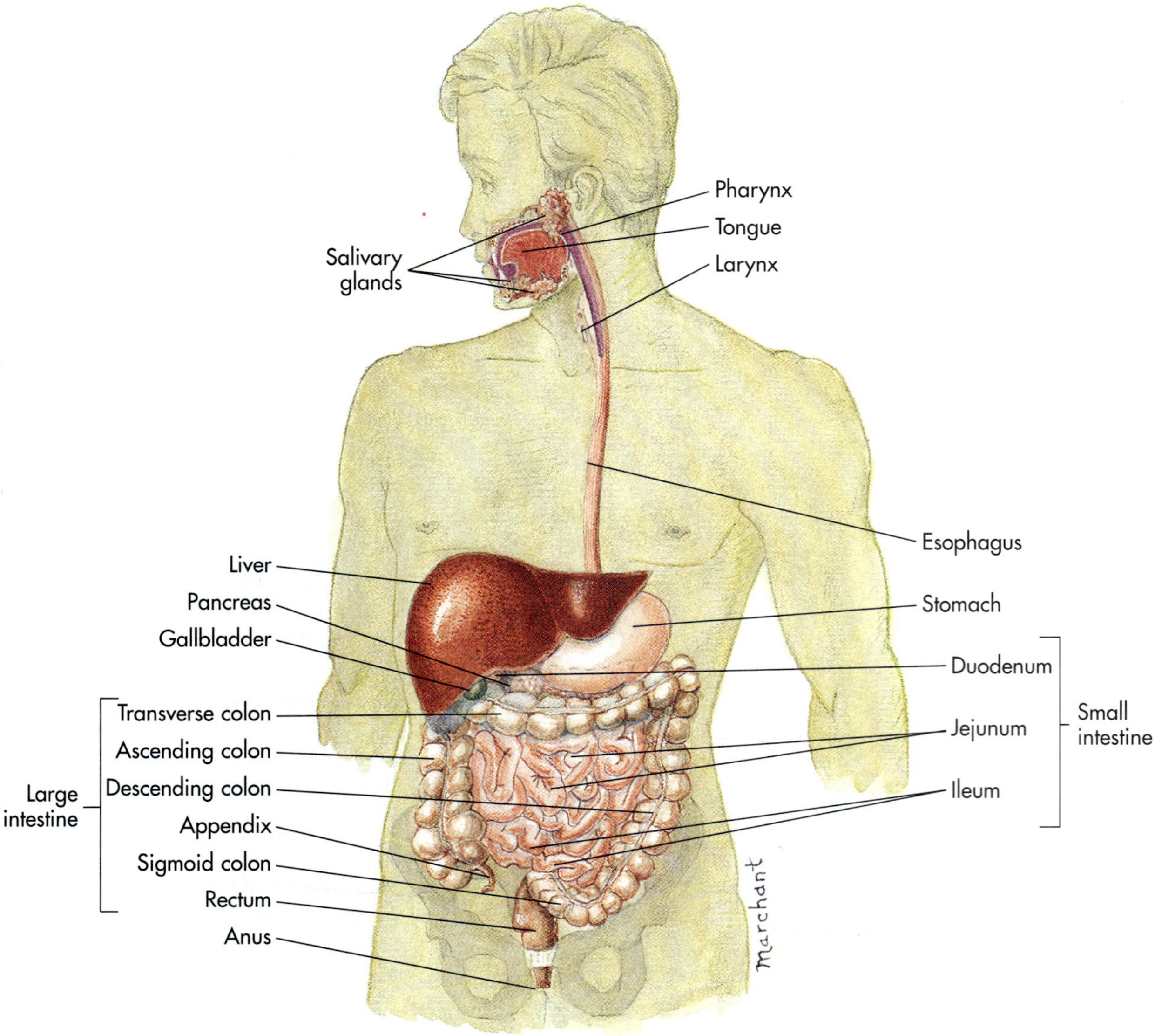

Fig. 5-20 *Digestive system.*

The *stomach* is a muscular, pouchlike sac in the upper left portion of the abdominal cavity. Strong stomach muscles stir and churn food to break it up into even smaller particles. The stomach is lined with a mucous membrane containing glands that secrete *gastric juices.* Food is mixed and churned with the gastric juices to form a semiliquid substance called *chyme.* Through peristalsis, the chyme is pushed from the stomach into the small intestine.

The *small intestine* is about 20 feet long and has three parts. The first part is the *duodenum.* In the duodenum, more digestive juices are added to the chyme. One is called *bile.* Bile is a greenish liquid produced by the *liver* and stored in the *gallbladder.* Juices from the *pancreas* and small intestine are also added to the chyme. The digestive juices chemically break down food so that it can be absorbed.

Peristalsis moves the chyme through the two remaining portions of the small intestine: the *jejunum* and the *ileum.* Tiny projections called *villi* line the small intestine. Villi absorb the digested food into the capillaries. Most of the absorption of food takes place in the jejunum and ileum.

Some chyme remains undigested. The undigested chyme passes from the small intestine into the *large intestine (large bowel* or *colon).* The colon absorbs most of the water from the chyme. The remaining semisolid material is called *feces.* Feces consist of a small amount of water, solid wastes, and some mucus and germs. These are the waste products of digestion. Feces pass through the colon into the *rectum* by peristalsis. Feces pass out of the body through the *anus.*

THE URINARY SYSTEM

Wastes are removed from the body through the respiratory system, the digestive system, and the skin. The digestive system rids the body of solid wastes. The lungs rid the body of carbon dioxide. Water and other substances are contained in sweat. There are other waste products in the blood as a result of body cells burning food for energy. The functions of the urinary system are to remove waste products from the blood and to maintain water balance within the body. The structures of the urinary system are shown in Figure 5-21.

The *kidneys* are two bean-shaped organs in the upper abdomen. They lie against the muscles of the back on each side of the spine. They are protected by the lower edge of the rib cage.

Each kidney has over a million tiny *nephrons* (Fig. 5-22). The nephron is the basic working unit of the kidney. Each nephron has a *convoluted tubule,* which is a tiny coiled tubule. Each convoluted tubule has a *Bowman's capsule* at one end. The capsule partially surrounds a cluster of capillaries called a *glomerulus.* Blood passes through the glomerulus and is filtered by the capillaries. The fluid portion of the blood is squeezed into the Bowman's capsule. The fluid then passes into the tubule. Most of the water and other necessary substances are reabsorbed by the blood and recirculated in the body. The rest of the fluid and the waste products form *urine* in the tubule. Urine flows through the tubule to a *collecting tubule.* All of the collecting tubules within the millions of nephrons drain into the *renal pelvis* within the kidney.

A tube, called the *ureter,* is attached to the renal pelvis of the kidney. Each ureter is about 10 to 12 inches long. The ureters carry urine from the kidneys to the *bladder.* The bladder is a hollow muscular sac situated toward the front in the lower part of the abdominal cavity. Urine is stored in the bladder until the desire to urinate is felt. The need to urinate usually occurs when there is about half a pint (250 ml) of urine in the bladder. Urine passes from the bladder through the *urethra.* The opening at the end of the urethra is the *meatus.* Urine passes from the body through the meatus. Urine is a clear yellowish fluid.

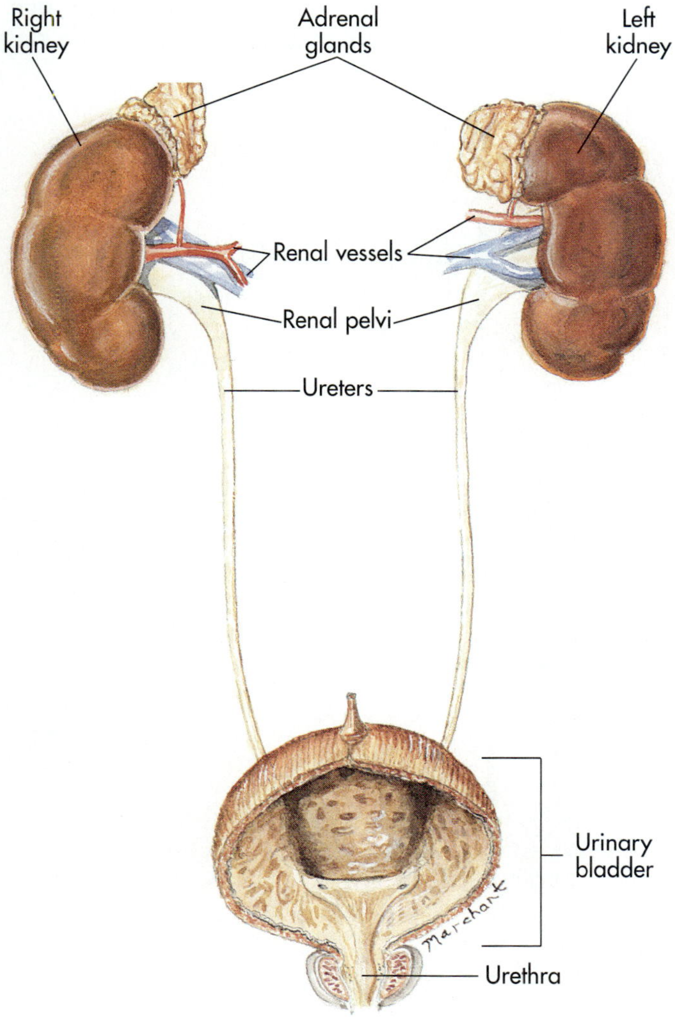

Fig. 5-21 *Urinary system.*

THE REPRODUCTIVE SYSTEM

Human reproduction results from the union of a female sex cell and a male sex cell. Structures of the male and female reproductive systems are different. The differences allow for the process of reproduction.

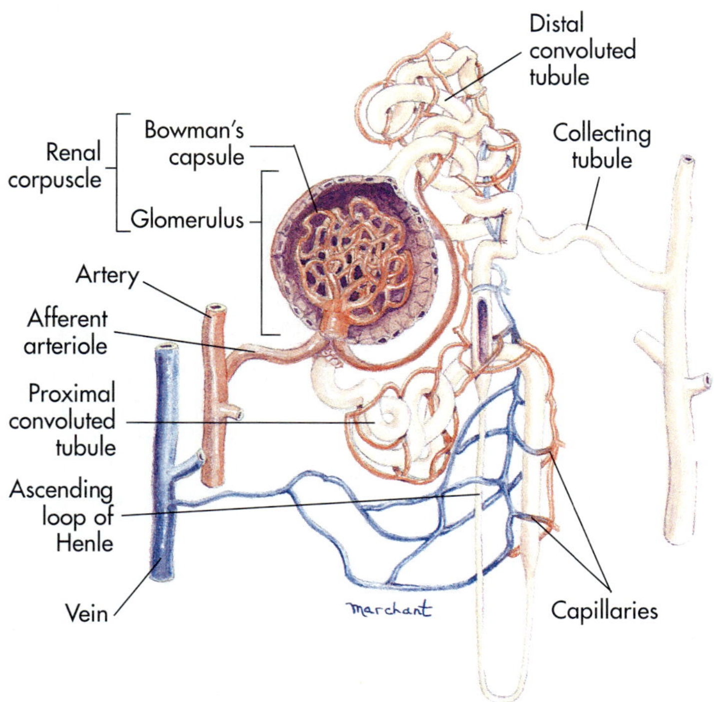

Fig. 5-22 *A nephron.*

The Male Reproductive System

The structures of the male reproductive system are shown in Figure 5-23. The *testes (testicles)* are the male sex glands. Sex glands are also called *gonads*. The two testes are oval or almond-shaped glands. Male sex cells are produced in the testes. Male sex cells are called *sperm* cells. *Testosterone*, the male hormone, is also produced in the testes. This hormone is needed for the functioning of the reproductive organs and for the development of the male's secondary sex characteristics (see Chapter 6). The testes are suspended between the thighs in a sac called the *scrotum*. The scrotum is made of skin and muscle.

Sperm travel from the testis to the *epididymis*. The epididymis is a coiled tube on top and to the side of the testis. From the epididymis, sperm travel through a tube called the *vas deferens*. Eventually each vas deferens joins a *seminal vesicle*. The two seminal vesicles store sperm and produce *semen*. Semen is a fluid that carries sperm from the male reproductive tract. The ducts of the seminal vesicles unite to form the *ejaculatory duct*. The ejaculatory duct passes through the prostate gland.

The *prostate gland*, shaped like a doughnut, lies just below the bladder. The gland secretes fluid into the semen. As the ejaculatory ducts leave the prostate they join the *urethra*, which also runs through the prostate. The urethra is the outlet for both urine and semen. The urethra is contained within the penis.

The *penis* is outside of the body and has *erectile* tissue. When a man becomes sexually excited, blood fills the erectile tissue. This causes the penis to become enlarged, hard, and erect. The erect penis can enter the vagina of the female reproductive tract. The semen, which contains sperm, is then released into the female vagina.

The Female Reproductive System

The structures of the female reproductive system are shown in Figure 5-24. The female gonads are two almond-shaped glands called *ovaries*. There is an ovary on each side of the uterus in the abdominal cavity. The ovaries contain *ova* or eggs. Ova are the female sex cells. One ovum (egg) is released monthly during the woman's reproductive years. Release of an ovum from an ovary is called *ovulation*. The ovaries also secrete the female hormones *estrogen* and *progesterone*. These hormones are needed for the functioning of the reproductive system and the development of secondary sex characteristics in the female (see Chapter 6).

When an ovum is released from an ovary, it travels through a *fallopian tube*. There are two fallopian tubes, one on each side. The tubes are attached at one end to the

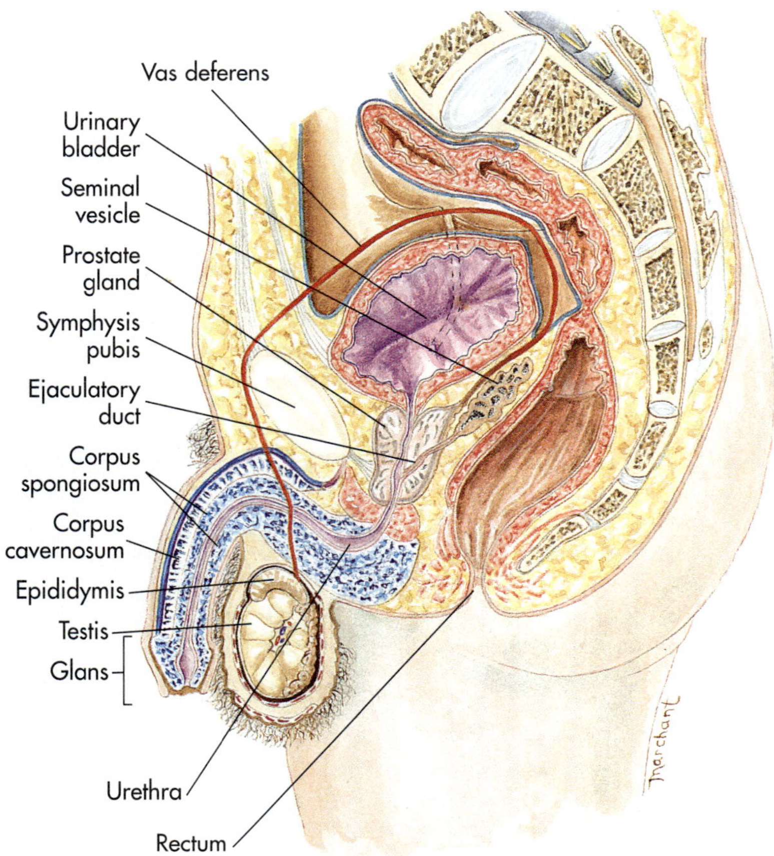

Fig. 5-23 *Male reproductive system.*

uterus. The ovum travels through the fallopian tube to the *uterus.* The uterus is a hollow, muscular organ shaped like a pear. The uterus is in the center of the pelvic cavity behind the bladder and in front of the rectum. The main part of the uterus is the *fundus.* The neck or narrow section of the uterus is the *cervix.* Tissue lining the uterus is called the *endometrium.* There are many blood vessels in the endometrium. If sex cells from the male and female unite into one cell, that cell implants into the endometrium, where it grows into a baby. The uterus serves as a place for the unborn baby to grow and receive nourishment.

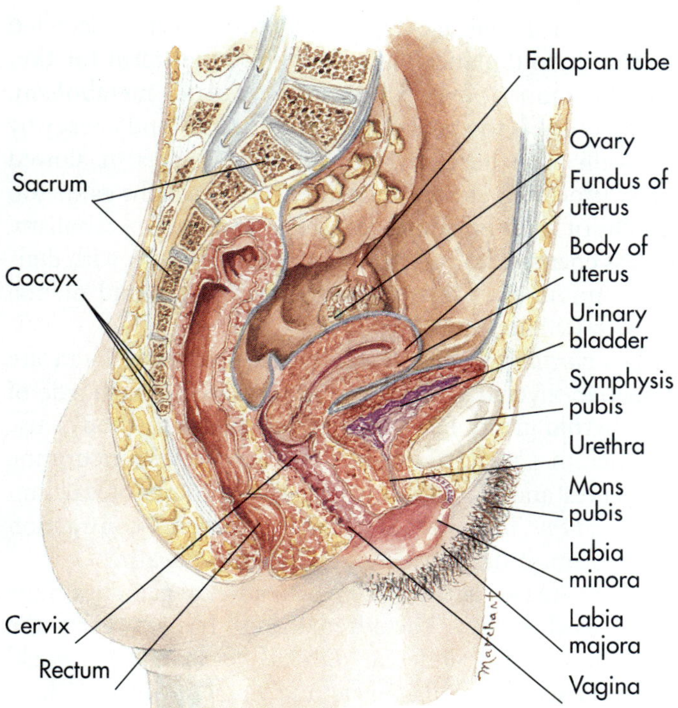

Fig. 5-24 *Female reproductive system.*

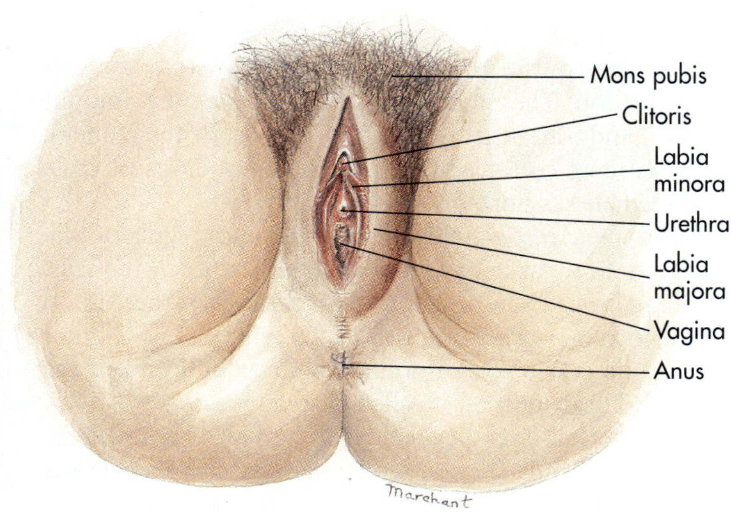

Fig. 5-25 *External female genitalia.*

The cervix of the uterus projects into a muscular canal called the *vagina.* The vagina opens to the outside of the body and is located just behind the urethra. The vagina receives the penis during sexual intercourse and serves as part of the birth canal. Glands in the vaginal wall keep it moistened with secretions. In young girls, the external vaginal opening is partially closed by a membrane called the hymen. The hymen ruptures when the female has intercourse for the first time.

The external genitalia of the female are referred to as the *vulva* (Fig. 5-25). The *mons pubis* is a rounded fatty pad over a bone called the *symphysis pubis.* The mons pubis is covered with hair in the adult female. The *labia majora* and *labia minora* are two folds of tissue on each side of the vaginal opening. The *clitoris* is a small organ composed of erectile tissue. The clitoris becomes hard when sexually stimulated.

The *mammary glands (breasts)* are considered organs of reproduction because they secrete milk after childbirth. The glands are located on the outside of the chest. They are made up of glandular tissue and fat (Fig. 5-26). The milk drains into ducts that open onto the nipple.

Menstruation The endometrium is rich in blood to nourish the cell that grows into an unborn baby *(fetus).* If pregnancy does not occur, the endometrium breaks up and is discharged through the vagina to the outside of the

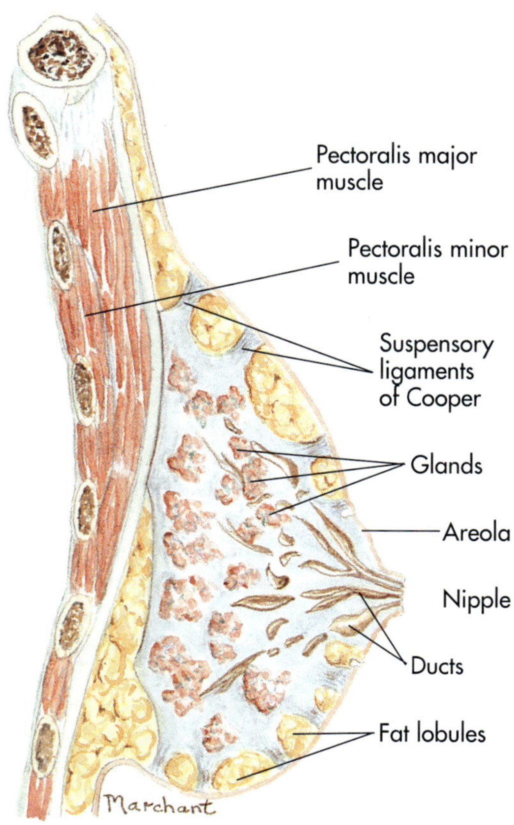

Fig. 5-26 *The female breast.*

body. This process is called **menstruation.** Menstruation occurs about every 28 days. Therefore, it is also called the *menstrual cycle.*

The first day of the cycle begins with menstruation. Blood flows from the uterus through the vaginal opening. Menstrual flow usually lasts 3 to 7 days. Ovulation occurs during the next phase of the cycle. An ovum matures in an ovary and is released. Ovulation usually occurs on or about the fourteenth day of the cycle. Meanwhile, estrogen and progesterone (the female hormones) are secreted by the ovaries. These hormones cause the endometrium to thicken for possible pregnancy. If pregnancy does not occur, the hormones decrease in amount. Blood supply to the endometrium decreases because of the decrease in hormones. The endometrium breaks up and is discharged through the vagina. Another menstrual cycle begins.

Fertilization

For reproduction to occur, a male sex cell (sperm) must unite with a female sex cell (ovum). The uniting of the sperm and ovum into one cell is called *fertilization.* A sperm has 23 chromosomes, and an ovum has 23 chromosomes. When the two cells unite, the fertilized cell has 46 chromosomes.

During intercourse, millions of sperm are deposited in the vagina. Sperm travel up the cervix, through the uterus, and into the fallopian tubes. If a sperm and an ovum unite in a fallopian tube, fertilization occurs and results in pregnancy. The fertilized cell travels down the fallopian tube to the uterus. After a short time, the fertilized cell implants in the thick endometrium and grows during pregnancy.

THE ENDOCRINE SYSTEM

The endocrine system is made up of glands called the *endocrine glands* (Fig. 5-27). The endocrine glands secrete chemical substances called **hormones** into the bloodstream. Hormones regulate the activities of other organs and glands in the body.

The *pituitary gland* is called the *master gland.* About the size of a cherry, it is at the base of the brain behind the eyes. The pituitary gland is divided into the anterior pituitary lobe and the posterior pituitary lobe. The *anterior pituitary lobe* secretes important hormones. *Growth hormone* is needed for the growth of muscles, bones, and other organs. Adequate amounts of growth hormone are needed throughout life to maintain normal-sized bones and muscles. Growth will be stunted if a baby is born with deficient amounts of the growth hormone. Too much of the hormone causes excessive growth.

Thyroid-stimulating hormone (TSH) is also secreted by the anterior pituitary lobe. The thyroid gland requires thyroid-stimulating hormone for proper functioning. *Adrenocorticotropic hormone* (ACTH) is another hormone secreted by the anterior lobe. This hormone stimulates the adrenal gland. The anterior lobe also secretes hormones that regulate the growth, development, and function of the male and female reproductive systems.

The *posterior pituitary lobe* secretes *antidiuretic hormone* (ADH) and *oxytocin.* Antidiuretic hormone prevents the kidneys from excreting excessive amounts of water. Oxytocin causes the uterine muscles to contract during childbirth.

The *thyroid gland,* shaped like a butterfly, is in the neck in front of the larynx. *Thyroid hormone* (TH) is secreted by the thyroid gland. Thyroxine is another term for thyroid hormone. Thyroid hormone regulates **metabolism.** Metabolism is the burning of food for heat and energy by the cells. Too little thyroid hormone results in slowed body processes, slowed movements, and weight gain. Too much of the hormone causes increased metabolism, excess energy, and weight loss. If a baby is born with deficient amounts of thyroid hormone, physical and mental growth will be stunted.

The *parathyroid glands* secrete *parathormone.* There are four parathyroid glands. Two are located on each side of the thyroid gland. Parathormone regulates the body's use of calcium. Calcium is needed for the proper functioning of nerves and muscles. Insufficient amounts of calcium cause *tetany.* Tetany is a state of severe muscle contraction and spasm. If untreated, tetany can cause death.

There are two *adrenal glands.* An adrenal gland is on the top of each kidney. The adrenal gland has two parts: the *adrenal medulla* and the *adrenal cortex.* The adrenal medulla secretes *epinephrine* and *norepinephrine.* These hormones stimulate the body to quickly produce energy during emergencies. Heart rate, blood pressure, muscle power, and energy all increase. The adrenal cortex secretes three groups of hormones that are essential for life. The *glucocorticoids* regulate metabolism of carbohydrates. They also control the body's response to stress and inflammation. The *mineralocorticoids* regulate the amount of salt and water that is absorbed and lost by the kidneys. The adrenal cortex also secretes small amounts of male and female sex hormones.

The *pancreas* secretes *insulin.* Insulin regulates the amount of sugar in the blood available for use by the cells. Insulin is needed for sugar to enter the cells. If there is too little insulin, sugar cannot enter the cells. If sugar cannot enter the cells, excess amounts of sugar build up in the blood. This condition is called *diabetes mellitus.*

The *gonads* are the glands of human reproduction. Male sex glands (testes) secrete *testosterone.* Female sex glands (ovaries) secrete *estrogen* and *progesterone.*

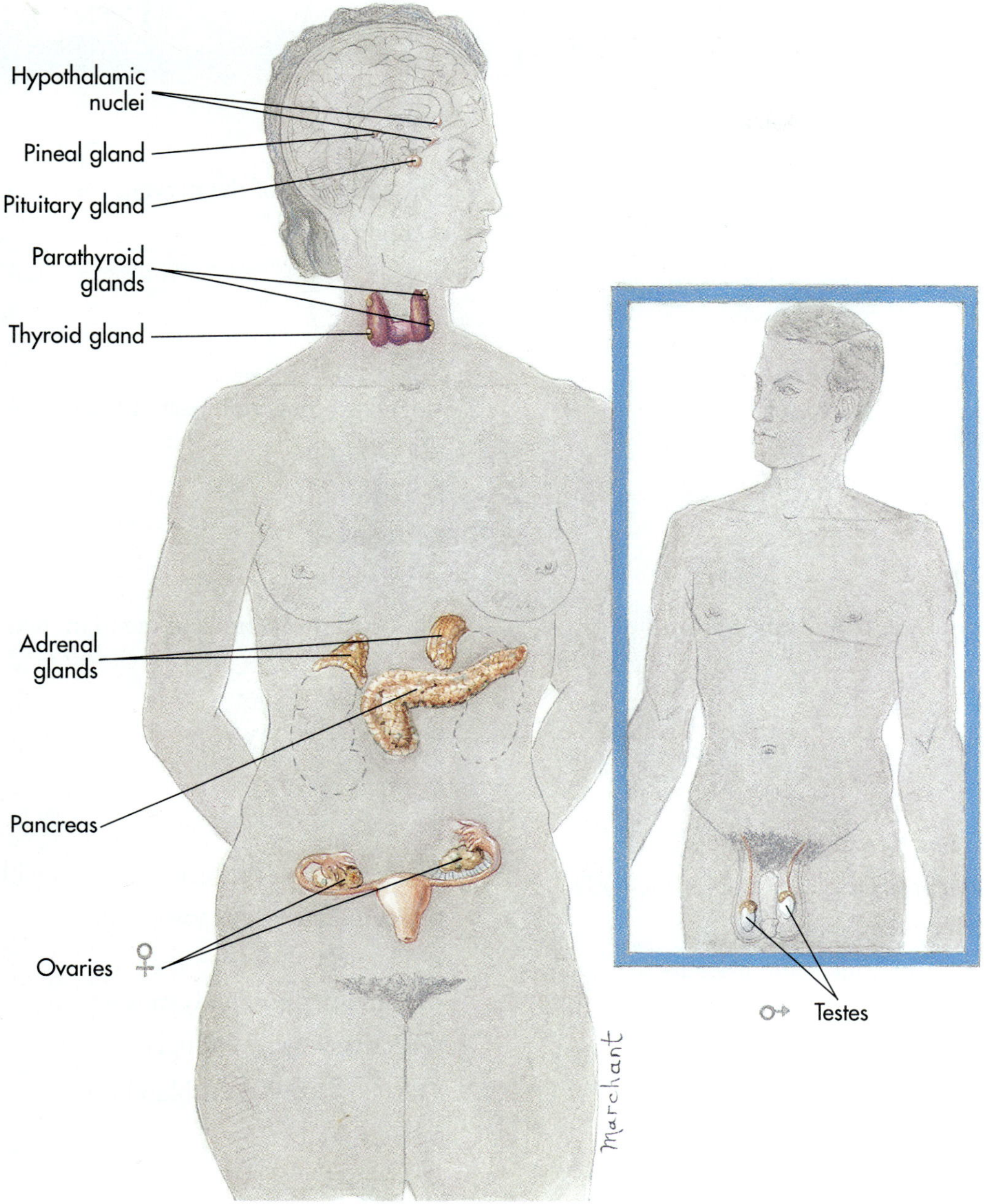

Fig. 5-27 *Endocrine system.*

Summary

The human body has several systems. Each system has its own structures and functions. The body systems are related to and dependent on each other for proper functioning and survival. Injury to or disease of one part of the system affects the entire system and the whole body. You may need to refer to this chapter as you study other chapters in this book and as you learn basic nursing procedures. Each procedure involves a person's body and your body. You need to have a basic understanding of the body's structure and function to give safe and effective care.

Review Questions

Circle the best *answer.*

1 The basic unit of body structure is the
a Cell
b Neuron
c Nephron
d Ovum

2 Organs are formed by groups of
a Cells
b Tissues
c Systems
d Chromosomes

3 The outer layer of the skin is called the
a Dermis
b Epidermis
c Integument
d Myelin

4 Which is *not* a function of the skin?
a Providing the protective covering for the body
b Regulating body temperature
c Sensing cold, pain, touch, and pressure
d Providing the shape and framework for the body

5 Which part allows movement?
a Bone marrow and periosteum
b Synovial membrane
c Joints
d Ligaments

6 Skeletal muscles
a Are under involuntary control
b Appear smooth
c Are under voluntary control
d Appear striped and smooth

7 Muscles are connected to bones by
a Cartilage
b Ligaments
c Nerve fibers
d Tendons

8 The basic unit of the nervous system is the
a Brain
b Spinal cord
c Neuron
d Nephron

9 Which is not a main part of the brain?
a Cerebrum
b Pons
c Brainstem
d Cerebellum

10 The highest functions of the brain take place in the
a Cerebral cortex
b Medulla
c Brainstem
d Spinal nerves

11 Besides hearing, the ear is involved with
a Regulating body movements
b Balance
c Smoothness of body movements
d Controlling involuntary muscles

12 The liquid part of the blood is the
a Hemoglobin
b Red blood cell
c Plasma
d Alveolus

13 Which part of the heart pumps blood to the body?
a Right atrium
b Right ventricle
c Left atrium
d Left ventricle

14 Which carry blood away from the heart?
a Capillaries
b Veins
c Venules
d Arteries

Review Questions—cont'd

15 Oxygen and carbon dioxide are exchanged
- **a** In the bronchi
- **b** Between the alveoli and capillaries
- **c** Between the lungs and the pleura
- **d** In the trachea

16 The process of digestion begins in the
- **a** Mouth
- **b** Stomach
- **c** Small intestine
- **d** Colon

17 Food is made easier to swallow by
- **a** Bile
- **b** Gastric juices
- **c** Chyme
- **d** Saliva

18 Most food absorption takes place in the
- **a** Stomach
- **b** Small intestine
- **c** Colon
- **d** Large intestine

19 Urine is formed by the
- **a** Jejunum
- **b** Kidneys
- **c** Bladder
- **d** Liver

20 Urine passes from the body through
- **a** The ureters
- **b** The urethra
- **c** The anus
- **d** Nephrons

21 The male sex gland is called the
- **a** Penis
- **b** Semen
- **c** Testis
- **d** Scrotum

22 The male sex cell is the
- **a** Semen
- **b** Ovum
- **c** Gonad
- **d** Sperm

23 The female sex gland is the
- **a** Ovary
- **b** Fallopian tube
- **c** Uterus
- **d** Vagina

24 The discharge of the lining of the uterus is called
- **a** The endometrium
- **b** Ovulation
- **c** Fertilization
- **d** Menstruation

25 The endocrine glands secrete substances called
- **a** Hormones
- **b** Mucus
- **c** Semen
- **d** Insulin

26 The master gland of the body is the
- **a** Endocrine gland
- **b** Pituitary gland
- **c** Thyroid gland
- **d** Adrenal gland

Answers to these questions are on page 748.

Growth and Development

6

OBJECTIVES

- Define the key terms listed in this chapter
- Understand the principles of growth and development
- Identify the stages of growth and development and the normal age ranges for each stage
- Identify the developmental tasks of the infant, toddler, and preschooler
- Describe the normal growth and development of infants, toddlers, and preschoolers
- Identify the developmental tasks of middle childhood, late childhood, and adolescence
- Describe the normal growth and development of middle childhood, late childhood, and adolescence
- Identify the developmental tasks of young, middle, and late adulthood
- Describe the normal growth and development of young and middle adulthood

KEY TERMS

development Changes in a person's psychological and social functioning

developmental task That which the person must complete during a stage of development

growth The physical changes that can be measured and that occur in a steady, orderly manner

menarche The time when menstruation first begins

menopause The time when menstruation stops

primary caregiver The person in the child's environment who is mainly responsible for providing or assisting with the child's basic needs

puberty The period when the reproductive organs begin to function and secondary sex characteristics appear

reflex An involuntary movement

You will care for people in different stages of development. A basic understanding of growth and development helps you give better care. Patient and resident needs are also easier to understand. This chapter presents the basic changes that occur in normal, healthy persons from birth through old age.

Human growth and development is presented in nine stages. Age ranges and normal characteristics are given for each stage. Only basic descriptions are given. The stages overlap. Therefore, it is hard to see clear-cut endings and beginnings of the stages. You need to be aware that the rate of growth and development varies among individuals.

Growth and development theories generally involve the two-parent family. In our society, many households have only one parent. Single parents are common because of divorce and unmarried mothers keeping their babies. Often children are raised by a relative while the mother works or attends school. Also, many divorced fathers gain or share child custody.

Primary caregiver is used in this chapter where *mother* or *father* would have been used. The **primary caregiver** is that person in the child's environment who is mainly responsible for providing or assisting with the child's basic needs. The primary caregiver may be a mother, father, grandparent, aunt, uncle, or court-appointed guardian. The words *parent* and *parents* are used in this chapter. However, another primary caregiver may have the parent role.

PRINCIPLES

Growth is the physical changes that are measured and that occur in a steady and orderly manner. Growth is measured in height and weight. Growth is also measured in the changes in physical appearance and body functions that occur as a person grows older.

Development relates to changes in psychological and social functioning. A person behaves and thinks in certain ways in different stages of development. A 2-year-old thinks in simple terms and needs a primary caregiver for many basic needs. A 40-year-old thinks in complex ways and meets most basic needs without help from others.

Growth and development affect the entire person. Although each is defined, growth and development:

- Overlap
- Are dependent on each other
- Occur at the same time

For example, an infant cannot say simple syllables (development) until the physical structures needed for speech are strong enough (growth). The basic principles of growth and development are:

- Growth and development occur from the moment of fertilization until death.
- The process proceeds from the simple to the complex. A baby learns to sit before standing, to stand before walking, and to walk before running.
- Growth and development occur in specific directions:
  1. From the head to the foot—babies learn to hold up their heads before they learn to sit. After learning to sit, they learn to stand.
  2. From the center of the body outward—babies control shoulder movements before they control hand movements.
- There is a sequence, order, and pattern to growth and development. Certain **developmental tasks** must be completed during each stage. A stage cannot be skipped. Each stage lays the foundation for the next stage.
- The rate of growth and development is uneven rather than at a set pace. Growth is more rapid during infancy. Also, children have growth spurts. Some children develop rapidly; others develop slowly.
- Each stage of growth and development has its own characteristics and developmental tasks.

INFANCY (BIRTH TO 1 YEAR)

Infancy is the first year of life. Rapid physical, psychological, and social growth and development occur during this time. The developmental tasks of infancy are:

- Learning to walk
- Learning to eat solid foods
- Beginning to talk and communicate with others
- Beginning to have emotional relationships with primary caregivers, brothers, and sisters
- Developing stable sleep and feeding patterns

The *neonatal period* of infancy is the first 4 weeks after birth. A baby is called a *neonate* or a *newborn* during this time.

The average newborn is 19 to 21 inches long and weighs 7 to 8 pounds at birth. Boys are usually longer and weigh more than girls. Birth weight usually doubles by the age of 5 to 6 months and triples by the first birthday. Babies are usually 20 to 30 inches long at the end of the first year.

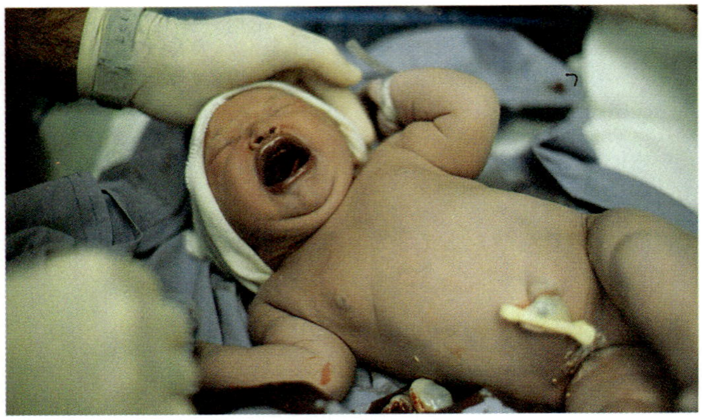

Fig. 6-1 *A newborn.*

The newborn's head is large compared to the rest of the body. The skin is wrinkled, and the baby appears red. Arms and legs seem short compared with the trunk, and the abdomen is large and round. Eyes are a deep blue. The newborn has fat, pudgy cheeks, a flat nose, and a receding chin (Fig. 6-1).

The central nervous system is not well developed. Movements are uncoordinated and without purpose. Babies can see at birth, although vision is not clear. They seem attracted to patterns. As babies develop, they prefer colors. Babies hear well. They are startled by loud noises and soothed by soft sounds. Babies respond better to female than to male voices. Infants react to touch, and the senses of smell and taste are developed.

Newborns have certain **reflexes** (involuntary movements). These reflexes decline and then disappear as the central nervous system develops.

- The *Moro reflex (startle reflex)* occurs when a baby is frightened by a loud noise or sudden movement. The arms are thrown apart, the legs extend, and the head is thrown back.
- The *rooting reflex* is stimulated when the infant's cheek is touched at or near the mouth. The baby's head turns toward the touch. The rooting reflex is necessary for feeding; it helps guide the baby's mouth to the nipple.
- The *sucking reflex* is produced by touching the cheeks or side of the lips.
- The *grasping reflex* occurs when the palm of an infant's hand is stimulated, causing the fingers to close around the object (Fig. 6-2). This reflex begins to decline around the second month and disappears by the third month.

Infants sleep most of the time during the first few weeks of life. They awaken when hungry and fall asleep right after eating. The time between feedings lengthens as infants grow and develop. Infants also stay awake more and sleep less as growth and development occur.

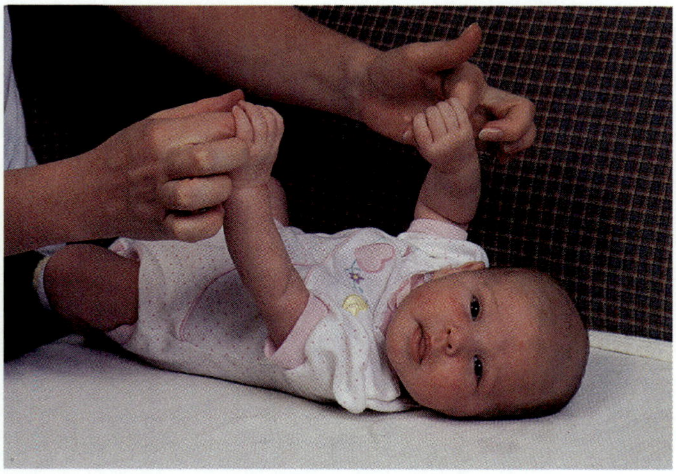

Fig. 6-2 *The grasping reflex.*

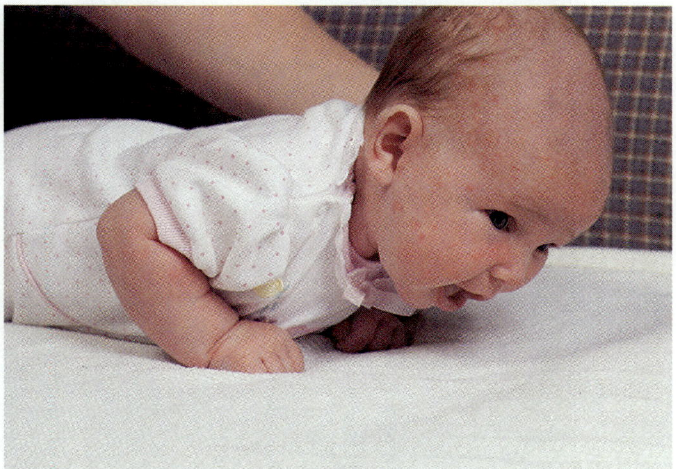

Fig. 6-3 *The 1-month-old infant can lift its head when lying on the stomach.*

Body movements of newborns are uncoordinated and without purpose. They are generally involuntary. As the central nervous system and muscular system develop, infants develop specific, voluntary, and coordinated movements. Newborns cannot hold their heads up. At 1 month, infants can hold their heads up when held and can lift and turn their heads when lying on their stomachs (Fig. 6-3). At two months they can smile and follow objects with their eyes (Fig. 6-4). The grasping reflex is declining in the 2-month-old infant.

Three-month-old infants can raise their heads and shoulders when lying on their stomachs (Fig. 6-5 on page 120). They can sit for a short while when supported and can hold a rattle. The grasping reflex has disappeared. Infants 4 months of age should be able to roll over. They can sit up if supported and may sleep all night. The Moro and rooting reflexes have disappeared. Tears are shed when crying. A rattle is held with both hands, objects are put in the mouth, and the infant babbles when spoken to. At 5 months, infants can grasp objects and play with their toes. Teeth start to come through (Fig. 6-6 on page 120).

Six-month-old infants usually have two lower front teeth and start to chew and bite finger foods. They can hold a bottle for feeding and can sit alone for a short time (Fig. 6-7 on page 120). At 7 months the upper teeth start to erupt. Babies respond to their names, can say "dada," and show a fear of strangers. At age 8 months, infants may be able to stand when holding onto something. They react to the word "no." Infants at this age do not like to be dressed or have diapers changed. Nine-month-old infants crawl (Fig. 6-8 on page 120) and more upper teeth appear.

At 10 months, most infants can walk around while holding on to furniture (Fig. 6-9 on page 120). They understand the words "bye-bye," "mama," and "dada." They smile when looking into a mirror. Infants at 11 months of age may begin to take steps and can hold a

A

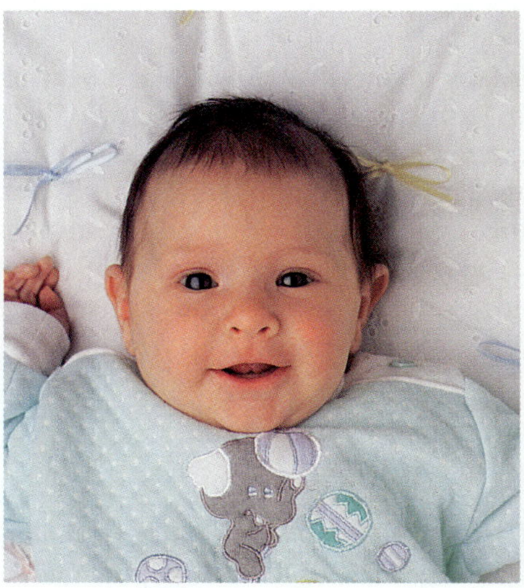

B

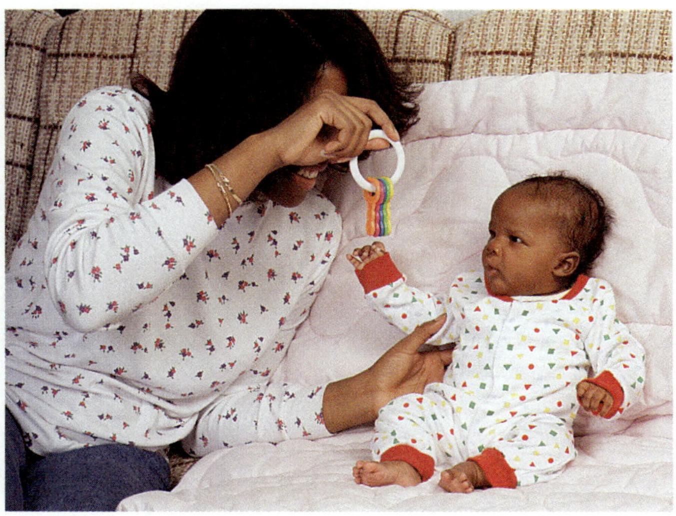

Fig. 6-4 *A 2-month-old child. **A,** Child smiles. **B,** Child follows objects with the eyes.*

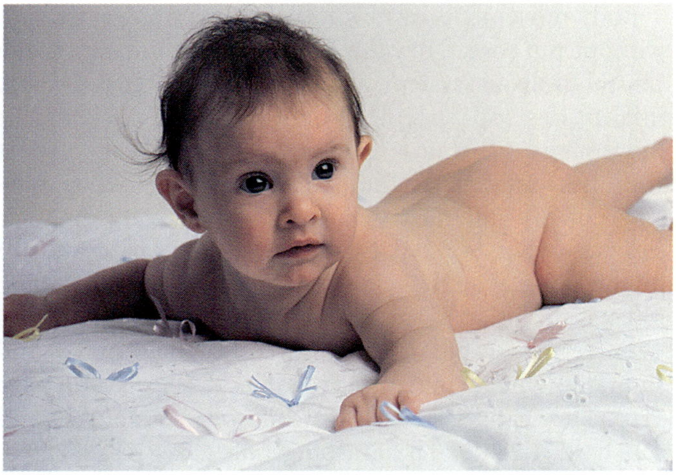

Fig. 6-5 The 3-month-old child can raise its head and shoulders.

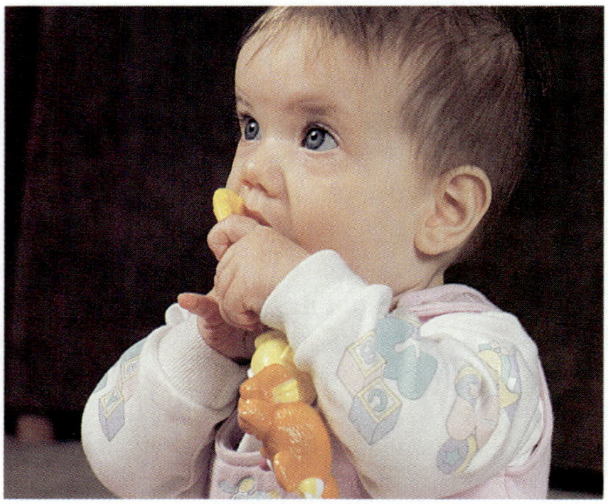

Fig. 6-6 The 5-month-old child puts objects into its mouth as teeth begin to erupt.

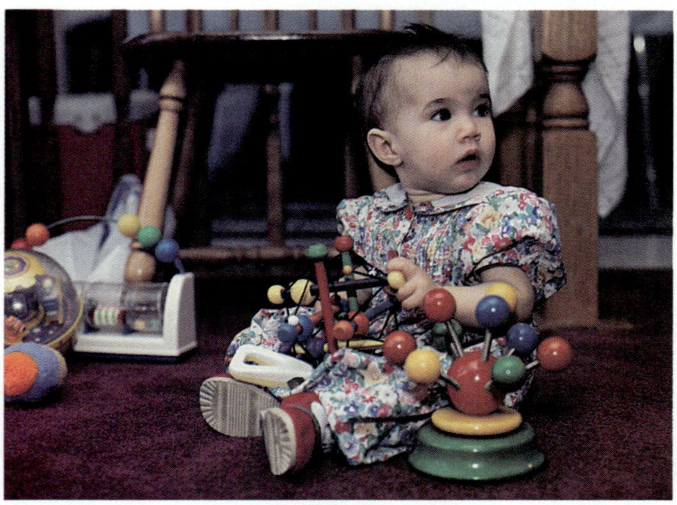

Fig. 6-7 A 6-month-old child can sit alone for a short time.

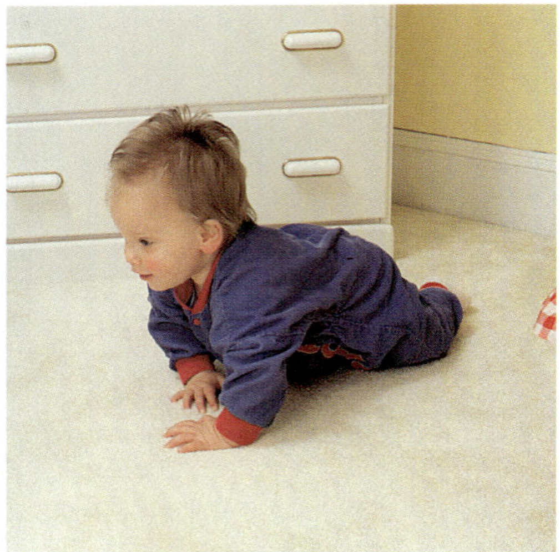

Fig. 6-8 A 9-month-old child is able to crawl.

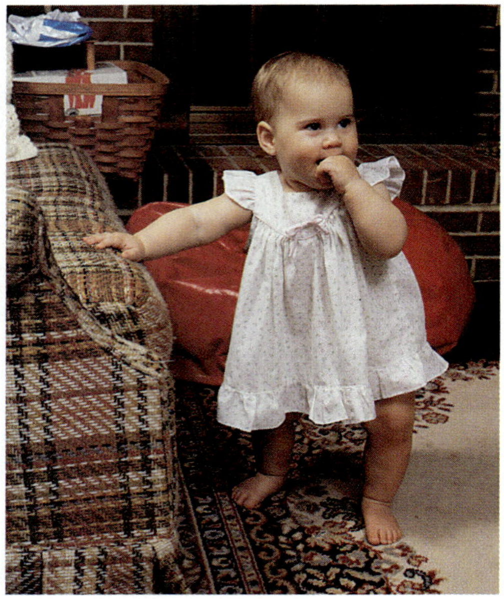

Fig. 6-9 A 10-month-old child can walk while holding onto furniture.

crayon. Many infants start to walk at 1 year of age. They can hold a cup for drinking. One-year-olds know more words, can say "no," and shake their heads for "no."

During the first 6 months, the infant's diet is mainly breast milk or formula. Solid foods are usually added at five to six months. These solid foods are usually strained fruits and vegetables. Junior foods are added during the eighth and ninth months. A 1-year-old can eat table foods.

TODDLERHOOD (1 TO 3 YEARS)

Physical growth during the second year of life is not as rapid as during infancy. The developmental tasks during this period are:

- Tolerating separation from the primary caregiver
- Gaining control of bowel and bladder function
- Using words to communicate with others
- Becoming less dependent on the primary caregiver

Because of the need to assert independence, the toddler years have been called the "terrible two's." The ability to move about and walk increases. So does the child's curiosity. Toddlers get into anything and everything. Whatever can be reached is touched, smelled, and tasted. As toddlers become more coordinated, they start to climb. They soon learn that things look different and can be seen better from above than from below. The toddler's new and increasing skills allow exploration of the environment. The child ventures farther away from the primary caregiver. The toddler also discovers that some things can be done without the primary caregiver's help. By the age of 3 years the toddler can run, jump, climb, ride a tricycle, and walk up and down stairs.

Hand coordination also increases, giving toddlers new skills. The need to feel, smell, and taste things is reflected in their increasing ability to feed themselves. They progress from eating with their fingers to using a spoon (Fig. 6-10). Toddlers can drink from cups. Hand coordination lets toddlers scribble, build towers with blocks, string beads, and turn book pages. Right- or left-handedness is seen during the second year.

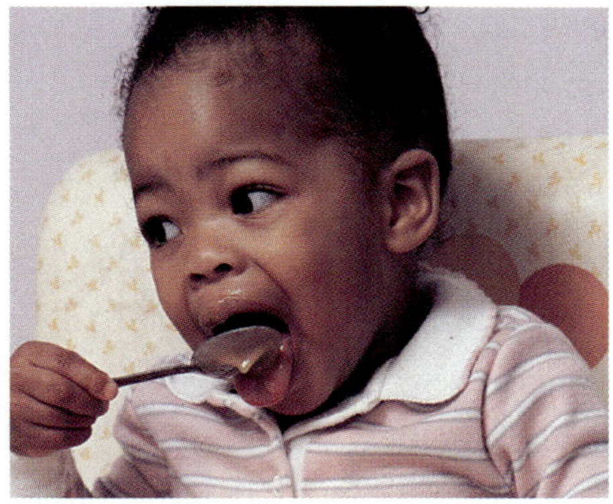

Fig. 6-10 *A toddler is able to use a spoon.*

Toilet training is a major developmental task for toddlers. Bowel and bladder control is related to central nervous system development. Children must be psychologically and physically ready for toilet training. They are usually ready around 18 to 20 months. The process starts with bowel control. Bowel control is easier because the frequency of bowel movements per day is less than urination. By age 2, toddlers are usually capable of bladder control during the day. By 3 years of age, toddlers achieve bladder control during the night.

Speech and language skills increase. Speech becomes clearer, and vocabulary increases. Words are learned by imitating others. Toddlers understand more words than they use. They are capable of 2- or 3-word sentences. By 3 years of age, children can speak in short sentences.

The ability to play increases. The child plays alongside other children but does not play with them. There is no sharing of toys with others. This is because the toddler is very possessive and does not understand sharing. The word "mine" is often used.

Temper tantrums and saying "no" are common during this stage. When disciplined the toddler often kicks and screams. The temper tantrum is the child's way of objecting to having independence challenged. The use of "no" can frustrate primary caregivers. Almost every request may be answered "no," even if the toddler is following the request.

Another developmental task is tolerating separation from the primary caregiver. As toddlers start to explore their environments, they tend to venture away from primary caregivers. However, when discomfort, frustration, or injury occur, they quickly return to primary caregivers or cry for their attention. If the primary caregiver is consistently present whenever needed, a child learns that the primary caregiver will be there and feels secure. Thus toddlers learn to tolerate brief periods of separation.

PRESCHOOL (3 TO 6 YEARS)

The preschool years (early childhood) are from the ages of 3 to 6. Children grow taller but gain little weight during this stage. Preschoolers are thinner, more coordinated, and more graceful than toddlers. The developmental tasks of the preschool years include:

- Increasing the ability to communicate and understand others
- Performing self-care activities
- Learning the differences between the sexes and developing sexual modesty
- Learning right from wrong and good from bad
- Learning to play with others
- Developing family relationships

The 3-Year-Old

Three-year-olds become more coordinated. They can:

- Walk on tiptoe
- Balance on one foot for a few seconds
- Run, jump, and climb with ease

- Draw circles and crosses
- Put on shoes
- Dress themselves
- Manage buttons
- Wash their hands
- Brush their teeth (Fig. 6-11)
- Feed themselves
- Pour from a bottle
- Help set the table without breaking dishes

Most three-year-olds know about 1,000 words, imitate new words, and ask questions constantly. They also talk constantly, even if no one is listening. Sentences are brief, usually only 3 or 4 words. Three-year-olds can name body parts, family members, friends, and animals. They like talking dolls and musical toys.

Play is important. Three-year-olds play in small groups with 2 or 3 other children and share toys. They play simple games and learn to follow simple rules. Three-year-olds may have imaginary playmates and may imitate adults during play. Coloring books and crayons, scissors and paper, and playing "house" and "dress-up" are enjoyed by 3-year-olds (Fig. 6-12).

At 3 years old, children know that there are two sexes. They know that male and female bodies are different. They also know their own sex. Little girls may wonder how the penis works and why they do not have one. Little boys may wonder how girls can urinate without a penis.

Children 3 years of age begin to understand time. They may speak of the past, present, and future. "Yesterday" and "tomorrow" are still somewhat confusing. Children may be afraid of the dark and need a night-light in the bedroom.

Three-year-olds are less fearful of strangers. They can tolerate separation from primary caregivers for short periods. They are less jealous than toddlers are of a new baby. Things are done to please primary caregivers at this age.

The 4-Year-Old

Four-year-olds can hop, skip, and throw and catch a ball. Hand coordination also increases. They can lace shoes, draw faces, copy a square, and they try to print letters. They can bathe with some help and can usually tend to toileting needs with help.

Vocabulary increases to about 1,500 words. The child continues to ask many questions and tends to exaggerate when telling stories. The 4-year-old can sing simple songs, repeat four numbers, count to three, and name a few colors.

Children 4 years of age may tend to physically attack others. They also tease, tattle, tell fibs, and may call other children names. They are more impatient and may blame an imaginary playmate when in trouble. Bragging, telling tales about family members, and showing off are seen in 4-year-olds. They can run simple errands and can play cooperatively with other children. Four-year-olds are proud of their accomplishments but have mood swings.

Children in this age group enjoy playing "dress-up," wearing costumes, and telling and hearing stories. They like to draw and make things. Imagination, drama, and imitation of adults are seen during play (Fig. 6-13). They play in groups of two or three and tend to be bossy. Playing "doctor and nurse" is common as curiosity about the opposite sex continues.

Four-year-olds have a strong preference for the primary caregiver of the other sex. Rivalries with brothers and sisters are seen, especially when younger children take the 4-year-old's possessions. Rivalries also occur when older children have more and different privileges. Family mem-

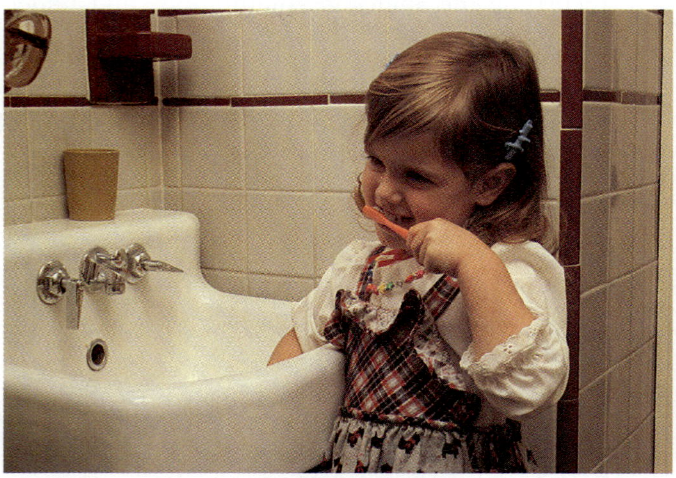

Fig. 6-11 *A 3-year-old has increased coordination.*

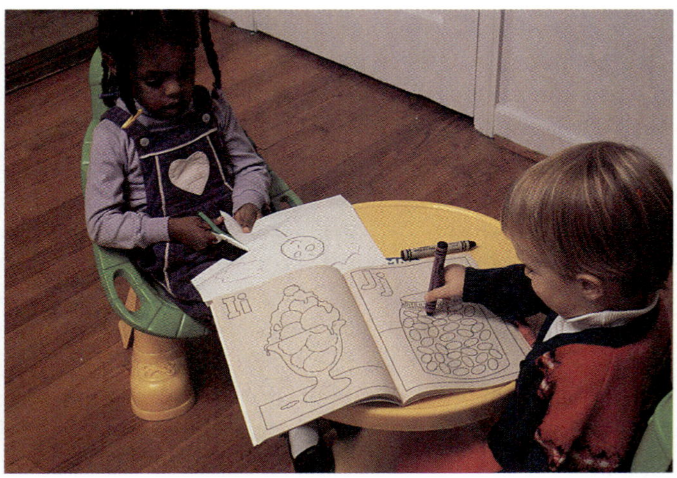

Fig. 6-12 *Three-year-olds enjoy cutting paper and using coloring books and crayons.*

bers are often the focus of the child's frustrations and aggressive behavior. Some 4-year-olds try to run away from home.

The 5-Year-Old

Coordination continues to develop. Five-year-olds can jump rope, skate, tie shoelaces, dress, and bathe. They can use a pencil well and copy diamond and triangle shapes. They can print a few letters and numbers and their first names. Drawings of people include the body, head, arms, legs, and feet.

The ability to communicate also increases. Vocabulary consists of about 14,000 words. Sentences have 6 to 8 words. They ask fewer questions than before, but questions have more meaning. They may want definitions for unfamiliar terms and take part in conversations. Four or more colors, coins, days of the week, and months can be named. They specify what they draw and give detailed descriptions of their drawings.

Five-year-olds are more responsible and truthful, and they quarrel less than before. There is greater awareness of rules and an eagerness to do things the right way. They have manners, are independent, and can be trusted within limits. Five-year-olds have fewer fears but may have nightmares and dreams. They are also proud of their accomplishments.

Simple number and word games are enjoyed by 5-year-olds. Although they may cheat to win, they like rules and try to follow them. They imitate adults during play and have a greater interest in watching television. They also enjoy activities with the primary caregiver of the same sex (Fig. 6-14). Such activities include cooking, housecleaning, shopping, yard work, and sports.

The child of 5 years tolerates brothers and sisters well. Although younger children may be considered a nuisance, 5-year-olds usually protect them.

MIDDLE CHILDHOOD (6 TO 8 YEARS)

Preschoolers may have been to nursery school and kindergarten. However, middle childhood is the time for school. Children enter the world of peer groups, games, and learning. The developmental tasks of middle childhood are:

- Developing the social and physical skills needed for playing games
- Learning to get along with other children of the same age and background (peers)
- Learning behaviors and attitudes appropriate to one's own sex
- Learning basic reading, writing, and arithmetic skills
- Developing a conscience and morals
- Developing a good feeling and attitude about oneself

The 6-Year-Old

The 6-year-old grows about 2 inches taller and gains 3 to 6 pounds. Baby teeth are lost, and replacement with permanent teeth begins. Children are very active and are skilled at running, jumping, skipping, hopping, and riding a bicycle. They seem to have a need to be constantly on the go. Sitting is tolerated for only a short time.

Six-year-olds enter the first grade and the world of school, activities, and other children. Children this age are often described as bossy, opinionated, charming, argumentative, and "know-it-alls." They have set ways of doing things and like to have their own way. They may have temper tantrums. Six-year-olds play well with children of both sexes. However, they begin to prefer

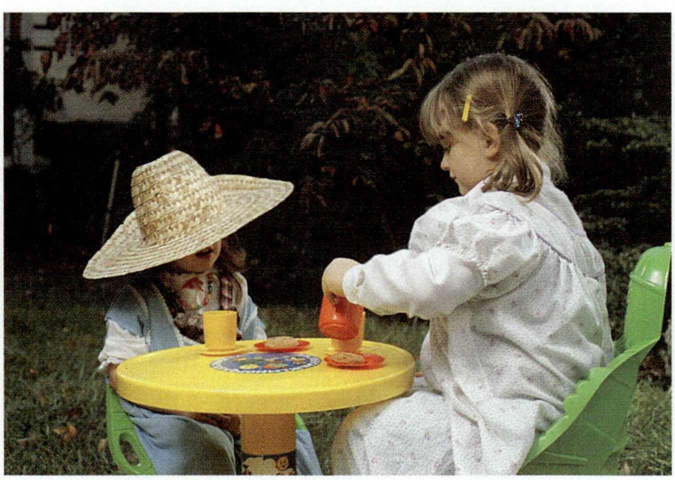

Fig. 6-13 *Four-year-olds play "dress-up" and imitate adults.*

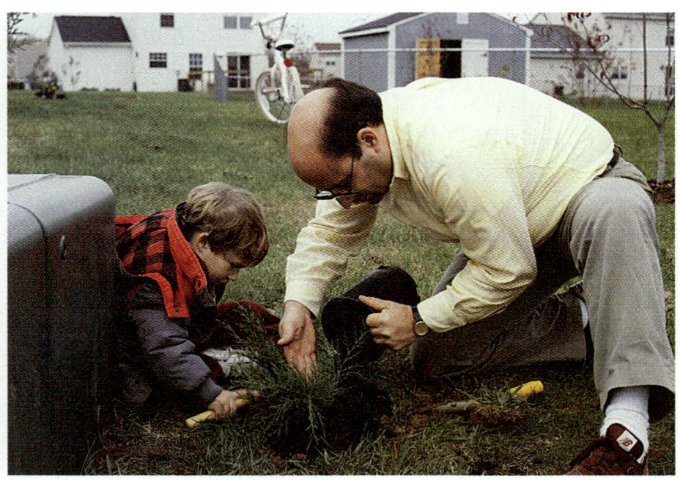

Fig. 6-14 *Five-year-olds enjoy doing things with the parent of the same sex.*

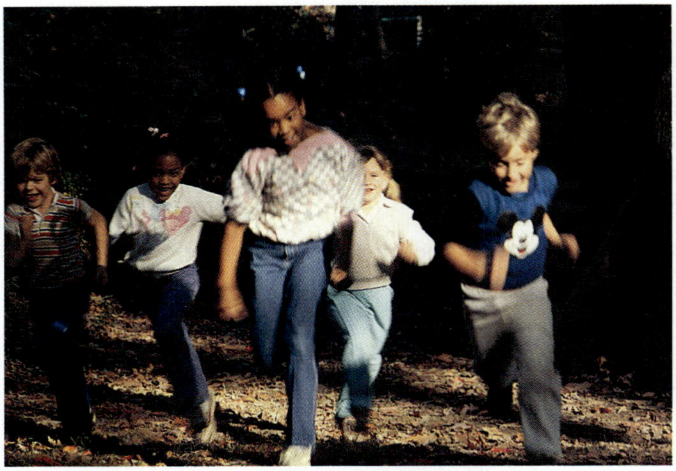

Fig. 6-15 *Six-year-olds play with children of both sexes but begin to prefer playing with children of the same sex.*

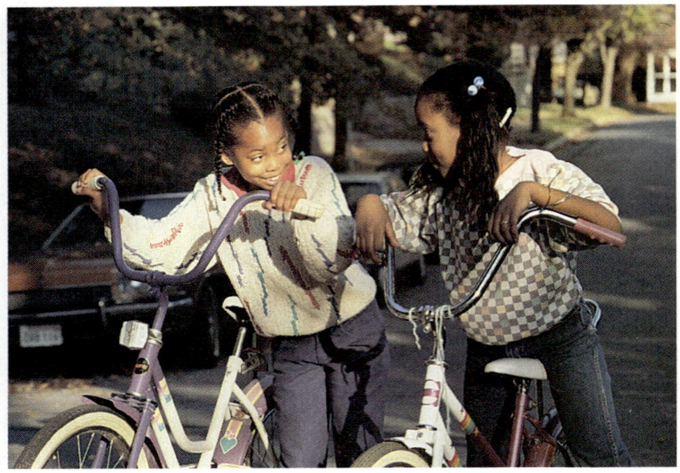

Fig. 6-16 *Seven-year-olds enjoy biking.*

playing with children of the same sex (Fig. 6-15). There is more sharing with others, and the child may have a "best friend." A child may cheat to win or leave a game before it is over to avoid losing. Tattling is common.

Six-year-olds have a vocabulary of about 16,500 words. They know the alphabet and begin to read and spell. They can communicate thoughts and feelings better than before.

Play interests range from rough play to quiet activities such as playing with cards, paints, clay, and checkers. Collections are started of odds and ends rather than specific things like stamps, rocks, or butterflies. More active play includes tag, hide-and-seek, playing with balls, skating, and playing in mud or sand.

The 7-Year-Old

Seven-year-olds grow about 2 inches in height. The average 7-year-old weighs about 49 to 56 pounds and is 47 to 49 inches tall. Hand coordination increases. Children learn to write rather than print. They are quieter than 6-year-olds and spend much time alone. They are more serious, less stubborn, and more concerned about being well-liked. Seven-year-olds are more aware of themselves, their bodies, and the reactions of others. They do not like to be teased or criticized and are sensitive about how others treat them. They like going to school, learning, and reading. They worry about the second grade being too hard. There are concerns about grades and what the teacher thinks about them. Reading skills increase, and the child can tell time.

Play includes swimming, biking, collecting and trading objects, playing ball and games with rules, and working puzzles and magic tricks (Fig. 6-16). Children this age play in groups. However, boys prefer to play with boys and girls prefer to play with girls. They may join scouting groups, such as the Cub Scouts or Brownies.

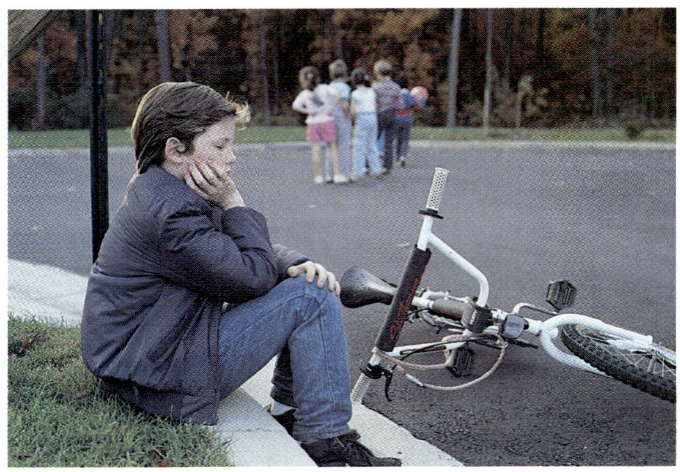

Fig. 6-17 *Belonging to a peer group is important to the 8-year-old.*

The 8-Year-Old

The 8-year-old enters the third grade. Growth in height and weight continues. More permanent teeth appear. The child continues to be physically active. Movements are faster and more graceful.

Peer group activities and opinions are important to the 8-year-old. Being accepted and included in peer groups are important for the needs of love and belonging and esteem (Fig. 6-17). Children this age get along with adults. However, they prefer the fads, opinions, and activities of peer groups. Boys and girls play separately. Their interests relate to group games, collections, television, and movies. An 8-year-old may belong to a "secret" club.

Eight-year-olds have been described as defensive, opinionated, practical, and outgoing. Advice is freely given to others. However, they do not accept criticism well. They often do household tasks such as vacuuming, cooking, and yard work, but expect to be paid. They expect to have more privileges than younger brothers and sisters.

Learning continues. They are curious about science, history, and other places and countries. They enjoy school, especially because it provides social opportunities with peers. Eight-year-olds become daring in the classroom. They may pass notes and throw spitballs or paper airplanes when they think the teacher is not looking. Despite these acts of mischief, they are mannerly, relate well to adults, and can take part in adult conversations. They are also friendly and affectionate.

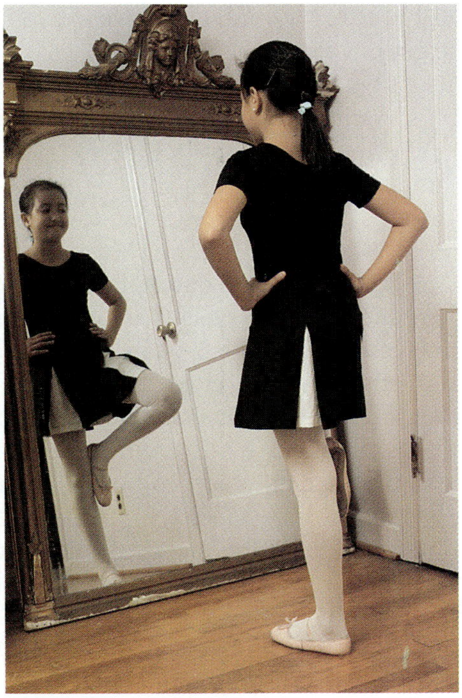

Fig. 6-18 *Movements are smooth and graceful in late childhood.*

LATE CHILDHOOD (9 TO 12 YEARS)

Late childhood is also called preadolescence. The person is between leaving childhood and dependency on others and entering adolescence. The developmental tasks of late childhood are similar to those of middle childhood. However, a preadolescent is expected to show more refinement and maturity in achieving the following tasks:

- Becoming independent of adults and learning to depend on oneself
- Developing and keeping friendships with peers
- Understanding the physical, psychological, and social roles of one's sex
- Developing moral and ethical behavior
- Developing greater muscular strength, coordination, and balance
- Learning how to study

Boys grow about 1 inch a year. Girls grow about 2 inches per year. Boys gain about $3^1/_2$ to 4 pounds each year. Girls gain between 4 and 5 pounds each year. Girls are usually taller than boys during late preadolescence. Many permanent teeth erupt.

Body movements are more graceful and coordinated (Fig. 6-18). There is greater muscular strength and increased physical skill. Skill in team sports is very important to boys in late childhood.

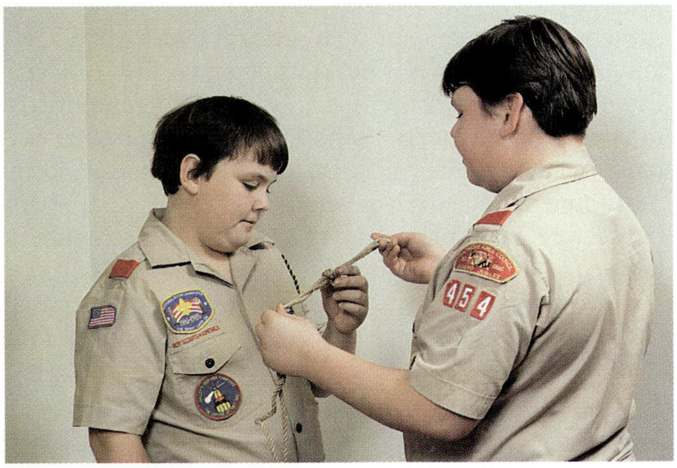

Fig. 6-19 *Organized activities are important in late childhood.*

Body changes occur as the onset of puberty nears. In girls the pelvis becomes broader, fat appears on the hips and chest, and the budding of breasts occurs. Boys show fewer signs of maturing sexually during this time. Genital organs begin to grow in size. However, secondary sex characteristics, such as deepening of the voice or growth of facial hair, are not seen until about 13 or 14 years of age.

These children must have factual sex education. Information about sex is shared among friends, although the information is often incomplete and inaccurate. Parents and children may be uncomfortable discussing sex with each other and may avoid the subject. When children do ask questions, honest and complete answers must be given in terms the children can understand.

Peer groups are the center of preadolescent activities. The group begins to affect the child's attitudes and behavior. Preference for companions of the same sex continues. Boys need to show their strength and toughness and may give each other nicknames. Membership in "secret" clubs continues to be important. Boys join organized team sports and scouting groups (Fig. 6-19).

Arguments between boys and girls are common, and boys often tease girls.

Associations between girls are stronger than those seen among boys. Writing and passing notes in class and talking on the telephone for long periods are frequent activities among girls.

Preadolescents are more aware of the mistakes and weaknesses of adults. They do not accept the standards and rules of adults without question. Rebellion against adults is common. Disagreements between parents and children increase, although the parents continue to be important for the child's development.

By the age of 12 the child uses about 7,000 words in conversation and understands about 50,000 words in reading. Use of the dictionary, encyclopedia, and other reference books increases. Girls are generally better than boys are in the use of words, writing, and memorizing. Boys are often better in arithmetic. Interest in science, history, and geography continues in both sexes. Girls often enjoy reading romantic books and stories. Boys usually prefer science fiction, mysteries, and adventure stories.

ADOLESCENCE (12 TO 18 YEARS)

Adolescence is a time of rapid growth and psychological and social maturity. The stage begins with puberty. **Puberty** is the period during which the reproductive organs begin to function and the secondary sex characteristics appear. The age at the onset of puberty and the beginning of adolescence varies. Girls experience puberty between the ages of 10 and 14. Most boys reach puberty between the ages of 12 and 16.

Because the age of puberty varies, adolescence ranges from the ages of 12 to 18 years. The developmental tasks of adolescence include:

- Accepting changes in the body and appearance
- Developing appropriate relationships with males and females of the same age
- Accepting the male or female role appropriate for one's age
- Becoming independent from parents and adults
- Developing morals, attitudes, and values needed for functioning in society

The onset of puberty in girls is marked by **menarche,** the beginning of menstruation. Secondary sex characteristics appear. These include:

- Increase in breast size
- Appearance of pubic and axillary (underarm) hair
- Slight deepening of the voice
- Widening and rounding of the hips

During late childhood, male sex organs begin to increase in size. This growth continues during adolescence. Puberty in boys is signaled by nocturnal emissions ("wet dreams"). During sleep (nocturnal) the penis becomes erect and semen is released (emission). Other secondary sex characteristics appear. These include:

- Appearance of facial hair and growth of a beard
- Pubic and axillary hair
- Hair on the arms, chest, and legs
- Deepening of the voice
- Increases in neck and shoulder size

Adolescence is also marked by a growth spurt. Boys grow an average of 4 to 12 inches and gain 15 to 60 pounds. They usually stop growing between the ages of 18 and 21. Some continue to grow until about age 25. Girls grow an average of 2 to 8 inches and gain between 15 and 50 pounds. They usually stop growing between the ages of 17 and 18. Some continue to grow until about age 21.

Adolescence is often described as the awkward stage. Awkwardness and clumsiness are due to the uneven growth of muscles and bones. The adolescent develops coordination and graceful body movements as the growth of muscles and bones evens out.

Teenagers often have difficulty accepting the changes in appearance. Some girls are embarrassed about breast development, especially if breast size is very large or small. Some are embarrassed about wearing a bra. Others wear tight sweaters so the breasts are noticed. Genital size may be a concern of boys. Height is also a problem to many teenagers. Boys do not like being short because it limits play in such sports as basketball and football. They do not like being a great deal shorter than their peers. Tall girls may feel embarrassed about being different and taller than other girls and boys.

Emotional reactions vary from high to low. Adolescents can be happy one moment and sad the next. Predicting a reaction to a comment or event is difficult. Teenagers can control their emotions better later in this stage. Older adolescents (15- to 18-year-olds) can still become sad and depressed. However, they can better control the time and place of their emotional reactions.

Adolescents need to become independent of adults, especially their parents. They must learn to function, make decisions, and act in a responsible manner without adult supervision. Many teenagers work toward this independence by:

- Having part-time jobs
- Babysitting
- Going to dances and parties
- Dating
- Joining school clubs and organizations
- Shopping without an adult
- Staying home alone

However, judgment and reasoning are not always sound. They still need guidance, discipline, and emotional and financial support from parents. Arguments and disagreements with parents are common, especially when restrictions and limitations are set on behavior and activities. Teenagers would rather be with peers than do things with parents and other family members. Adolescents tend to confide in and seek advice from adults other than their parents.

Teenage interests and activities reflect the need to become independent, to develop relationships with the opposite sex, and to act like males or females. Both sexes are interested in parties, dances, and other social activities. Clothing, makeup, and hairstyles are important. A teenager may babysit or get a part-time job to have extra money for clothes, makeup, and hair- and skin-care products. Parents and teenagers rarely agree about clothing styles. Teenagers may spend a lot of time experimenting with makeup and hairstyles. They may also spend a lot of time talking to friends on the phone, listening to music, and reading teen magazines (Fig. 6-20).

Dating begins during adolescence. Although the age when dating begins varies, there is usually a dating pattern. "Crowd" dates are common in the seventh and eighth grades. They are usually related to school activities, such as a dance or basketball game. The same group of girls just happens to be with the same group of boys during these social events. In the ninth grade, pairing off is common during crowd dating. The tenth grade is usually when boy-girl couples go to social events together and then join other couples. Double dating occurs in the eleventh grade. Dates involve one couple during the twelfth grade, although there is some double dating.

Many difficult decisions and conflicts result as the adolescent matures physically, psychologically, and emotionally. Parents and teenagers often disagree about dating. Parents worry that dating will lead to sexual activities and pregnancy. Teenagers usually do not understand or appreciate their parents' concern. "Going steady" helps meet the teenager's need for security, love and belonging, and esteem. Teenagers sometimes have difficulty controlling their sexual urges and considering the consequences of being sexually active.

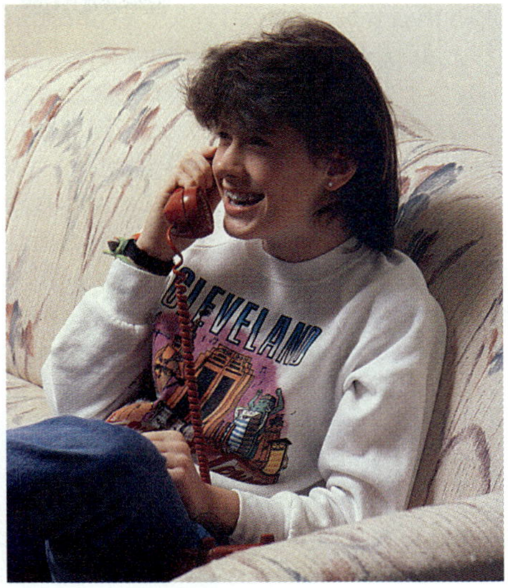

Fig. 6-20 *Adolescents enjoy talking on the phone.*

Adolescents begin to think about careers and what to do after high school graduation. Interests, skills, and talents are some factors that influence the choice of further education and getting a job. Adolescents also need to develop morals, values, and attitudes for living in society. They need to develop a sense about what is good and bad, right and wrong, and important and unimportant. Parents, peers, culture, religion, television, school, and movies are among the many factors influencing teenagers. Drug abuse, unwanted pregnancy, alcoholism, and criminal acts are common problems of troubled adolescents.

YOUNG ADULTHOOD (18 TO 40 YEARS)

Psychological and social development continue during young adulthood. There is little physical growth. Adult height has been reached. Body systems are fully developed. Developmental tasks of young adulthood include:

- Choosing education and an occupation
- Selecting a marriage partner
- Learning to live with the husband or wife
- Becoming a parent and raising children
- Developing a satisfactory sex life

Education and occupation are so closely related that they can rarely be separated. A young adult may choose to be a teacher, nurse, doctor, lawyer, computer programmer, nursing assistant, truck driver, mechanic, or one of many other occupations. Most jobs require specific knowledge and skills. The amount and kind of education needed depends on the career choice. Most adults find that job choices are greater with adequate educational preparation. Employment is necessary for economic independence and for supporting a family.

Some adults remain single. Most marry at least once. The many reasons for marriage include love, emotional security, wanting a family, sex, wanting to leave an unhappy home life, social status, companionship, and money. Some marry to feel wanted, needed, and desirable. Many factors also affect selecting a marriage partner. They include age, religion, interests, education, race, personality, and of course, love. Some marriages are happy and successful while others are not. There are no guarantees that a marriage will work. Therefore the two people will have to work together to build a marriage based on trust, respect, caring, and friendship.

The married couple must learn to live together. Habits, routines, meal preparation, and pastimes may need to be changed or adjusted to "fit" the other person's needs. They must learn how to solve problems and make decisions together. They need to work toward the same goals. Open and honest communication helps create a successful marriage (Fig. 6-21).

Couples also need to develop a satisfactory sex life. Sexual frequency, desires, practices, and preferences vary. Understanding and accepting the other person's needs are necessary for a satisfying and intimate relationship.

Most couples decide to have children. With modern birth control methods, the number of children and when to have them can be planned. However, many pregnancies are unplanned. Most couples have a child during the first few years of marriage; some wait several years before starting a family. Other couples decide not to have children. Some have difficulty or cannot have children because of physical problems in the husband or wife. Those couples having children need to agree on child-rearing practices and discipline methods. They will need to adjust to the child. They will also need to adjust to the child's need for time, energy, and parental attention.

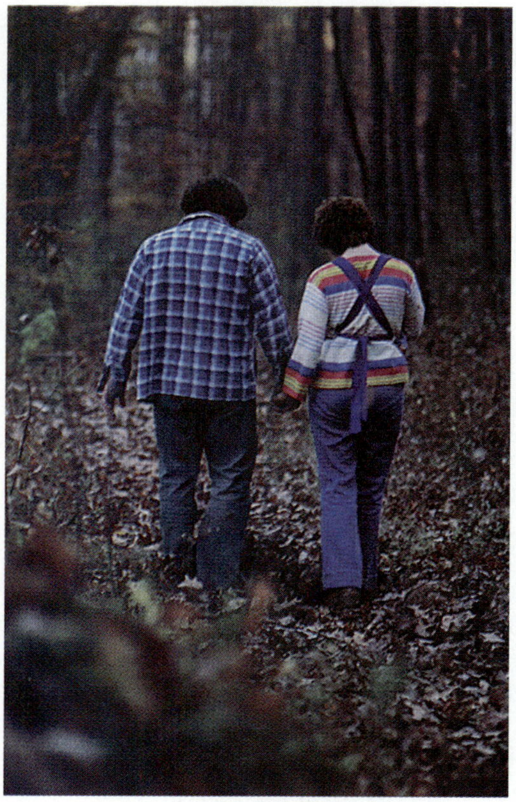

Fig. 6-21 *Communication is necessary for a successful marriage and a satisfactory sex life.*

MIDDLE ADULTHOOD (40 TO 65 YEARS)

This stage of development is more stable and comfortable. Children are usually grown and have moved away. Husbands and wives now have time to spend alone together. There are fewer worries about children and money. The developmental tasks of middle adulthood relate to:

- Adjusting to physical changes
- Having grown children
- Developing leisure-time activities
- Relating to aging parents

Several physical changes occur during middle adulthood. They may be very gradual and go unnoticed, or they may be seen early. People in their early forties may feel energetic and able to function as they did in their twenties. However, energy and endurance begin to slow down. Weight control becomes a problem as metabolism and physical activities slow down. Facial wrinkles and gray hair appear. The need for eyeglasses is common. Hearing loss may begin. Menstruation stops between the ages of 42 and 55; this is called **menopause.** Ovaries stop secreting hormones, and the woman can no longer have children. Many diseases and illnesses can develop. The disorders can become chronic or life threatening.

Children leave home for college, marry, move to homes of their own, and start their own families. Adults have to cope with letting children go, being in-laws, and becoming grandparents. Parents must let children lead their own lives. However, they need to be available for emotional support in times of need.

Middle-aged adults often discover spare time when the demands of parenthood decrease. Hobbies and pastimes such as gardening, fishing, painting, golfing, volunteer work, and membership in clubs and organizations are sources of pleasure (Fig. 6-22). Hobbies and pastimes become even more important after retirement and during late adulthood.

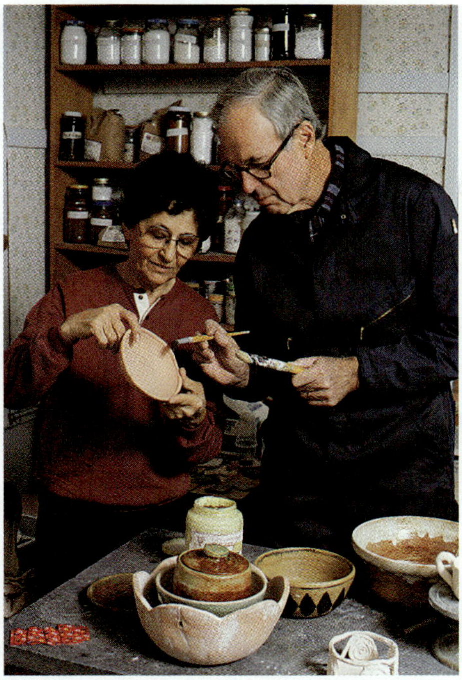

Fig. 6-22 *Middle-aged adults usually have more time for hobbies.*

Middle-aged adults may have parents who are aging and developing poor health. Responsibility for aging parents may begin during this stage. Middle-aged adults often have to deal with the death of parents.

LATE ADULTHOOD (65 YEARS AND OLDER)

Many physical, psychological, and social changes occur during later adulthood. People in this stage of development are often referred to as the elderly.

Chapter 7 describes the changes that occur in the elderly, as well as the care they may require. The developmental tasks of the elderly are:

- Adjusting to decreased physical strength and loss of health
- Adjusting to retirement and reduced income
- Coping with the death of a husband or wife
- Developing new friends and relationships
- Preparing for one's own death

SUMMARY

Growth and development continue throughout life and affect the whole person. There are nine stages:

- Infancy (birth to 1 year)
- Toddlerhood (1 to 3 years)
- Preschool (3 to 6 years)
- Middle childhood (6 to 8 years)
- Late childhood (9 to 12 years)
- Adolescence (12 to 18 years)
- Young adulthood (18 to 40 years)
- Middle adulthood (40 to 65 years)
- Late adulthood (65 years and older)

Each has its own age range, characteristics, and developmental tasks. The developmental tasks of one stage must be accomplished before the next stage is entered. There is an orderly pattern to the process. However, the rate of growth and development varies from person to person.

The knowledge and understanding gained from this chapter can be applied in work and personal situations. Everyday life puts you in contact with people of different ages and levels of development. A basic knowledge of growth and development helps you better understand individuals. A 2-year-old's temper tantrum can be dealt with better. The changes of puberty and an adolescent's unpredictable behavior are more understandable. Perhaps you can be more sensitive to the worries, concerns, and needs of adults of different ages.

Review Questions

Circle the best *answer.*

1 Changes in psychological and social functioning are called
- **a** Growth
- **b** Development
- **c** A reflex
- **d** A stage

2 Which is *false?*
- **a** Growth and development occur from the simple to the complex.
- **b** Growth and development occur in an orderly pattern.
- **c** Growth and development occur at specific rates.
- **d** Each stage has its own characteristics.

3 The stage of infancy is the first
- **a** 4 weeks of life
- **b** 3 months of life
- **c** 6 months of life
- **d** Year of life

4 Which reflexes are needed for feeding in the infant?
- **a** The Moro and startle reflexes
- **b** The rooting and sucking reflexes
- **c** The grasping and Moro reflexes
- **d** The rooting and grasping reflexes

5 Crawling begins at about
- **a** 5 months
- **b** 6 months
- **c** 7 months
- **d** 8 months

6 Solid foods are usually given to a baby during the
- **a** Fifth or sixth month
- **b** Seventh or eighth month
- **c** Ninth or tenth month
- **d** Eleventh or twelfth month

7 Toilet training begins
- **a** During infancy
- **b** During the toddler years
- **c** When the primary caregiver is ready
- **d** At the age of 3

8 The toddler can
- **a** Use a spoon and cup
- **b** Ride a bike
- **c** Help set the table
- **d** Name parts of the body

9 Playing with other children begins during
- **a** Infancy
- **b** The toddler years
- **c** The preschool years
- **d** Middle childhood

10 Tattling, fibbing, and teasing are commonly seen at age
- **a** 3
- **b** 4
- **c** 5
- **d** 6

11 Loss of baby teeth usually begins at the age of
- **a** 4
- **b** 5
- **c** 6
- **d** 7

12 Which is *not true* of the 7-year-old?
- **a** The child learns to write.
- **b** The child spends a lot of time alone.
- **c** The child does not like school.
- **d** The child is able to tell time.

REVIEW QUESTIONS—CONT'D

13 Peer group activities become more important at the age of

a 6

b 7

c 8

d 9

14 Most information about sex is exchanged between

a Children and teacher

b Teacher and parents

c Parents and children

d Members of a peer group

15 Reproductive organs begin to function and secondary sex characteristics appear during

a Late childhood

b Preadolescence

c Puberty

d Early adulthood

16 Which is *false?*

a Boys reach puberty earlier than girls.

b Most girls reach puberty between the ages of 12 and 13.

c Menarche marks the onset of puberty in girls.

d A growth spurt occurs during adolescence.

17 Dating usually begins

a During late childhood

b With "crowd" dating

c With "pairing off"

d During late adolescence

18 Adolescence is a time when parents and children

a Talk openly about sex

b Express love and affection

c Disagree

d Do things as a family

19 Which is *not* a developmental task of young adulthood?

a Adjusting to changes in the body and in physical appearance

b Selecting a marriage partner

c Choosing an occupation

d Becoming a parent

20 Middle adulthood is from about

a 25 to 35 years

b 30 to 40 years

c 40 to 50 years

d 40 to 65 years

21 Middle adulthood is a time when

a Families are started

b Physical energy and free time are gained

c Children are grown and leave home

d People need to prepare for death

Answers to these questions are on page 749.

Care of the Elderly

7

OBJECTIVES

- Define the key terms listed in this chapter
- Describe the effects of retirement
- Identify the changes in social relationships that elderly people may experience
- Describe how death of a spouse can affect the survivor
- Describe the changes that occur in the body's systems during aging and the care that is required
- Describe the causes, effects, and behaviors of confusion
- Describe housing alternatives for the elderly
- Explain the requirements of the Omnibus Budget Reconciliation Act of 1987
- Describe resident rights and how to promote a resident's quality of life
- Explain what is meant by elderly abuse and the signs of elderly abuse
- Explain what to do if you suspect elderly abuse

KEY TERMS

geriatrics The care of aging people

gerontology The study of the aging process

The number of people older than 65 years of age is increasing every day. People live longer and are healthier than ever before. Today most people can expect to live into their 70s. Earlier in this century, most people died in their 50s. There also have been steady increases in the number of 70-, 80-, 90-, and 100-year-olds. Many of these persons continue to live healthy and happy lives in their own homes. Others live with another relative.

Gerontology is the study of the aging process. **Geriatrics** is the care of the aged. Aging, or growing old, is a normal process. Normal changes occur in body structure and function. Because of these changes, the elderly have special needs. They are also at greater risk for illness, chronic diseases, and injuries.

PSYCHOLOGICAL AND SOCIAL EFFECTS OF AGING

Physical, psychological, and social changes occur as a person grows older. Graying hair, wrinkles, and slow movements are physical reminders of growing old. Retirement and death of a spouse, relatives, and friends are social reminders. American society values youth and beauty. This emphasis can make aging a painful process socially, psychologically, and physically.

Retirement

Most people look forward to retiring. People usually retire at the age of 65. Some retire earlier. Others work until the age of 70. Retirement is a reward for a lifetime of hard work. The person has earned the right not to work and can now relax and enjoy life (Fig. 7-1). Travel, leisure, and doing whatever one wants are retirement "benefits" (Fig. 7-2). Many people enjoy retirement. Others are not as fortunate. Retirement is often a person's first real experience with aging. Some must retire because of chronic disease or disability. Poor health and medical expenses can make enjoying retirement very difficult.

Working has social and psychological effects. Work helps meet the basic needs of love, belonging, and self-esteem. Personal satisfaction and usefulness result from working. There is pride in a day's work or a job well done. Friendships develop, and day-to-day events are shared with co-workers. Leisure activities, recreation, and com-

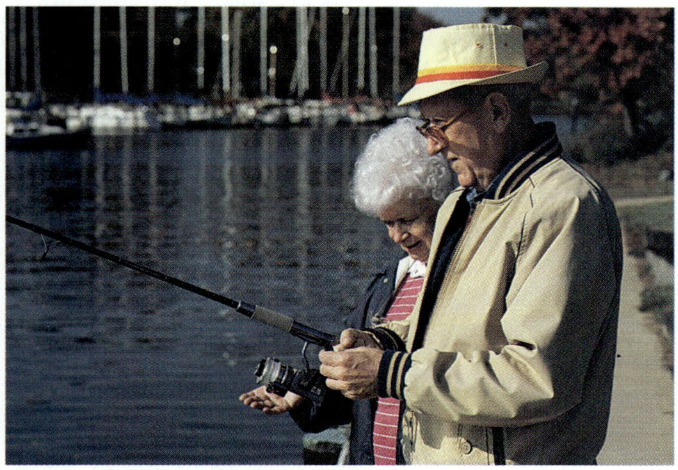

Fig. 7-1 *A retired couple enjoying fishing together.*

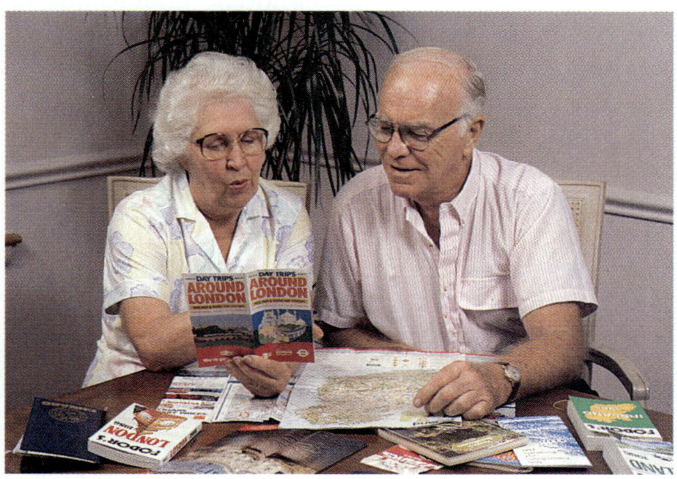

Fig. 7-2 *An elderly couple plan a vacation.*

panionship often involve co-workers. Some people need work for psychological and social fulfillment. Retirement can be hard for them. Some retired people have part-time jobs or do volunteer work. Such activities promote usefulness and well-being.

Reduced income Retirement usually means reduced financial income. Retirement income is often less than one half of the person's working income. The monthly social security check may be the only money. Even that has not kept pace with the high cost of living.

Unfortunately, retirement and aging do not mean fewer expenses. There may still be rent or mortgage payments. Food, clothing, gas and electricity, water bills, and taxes are other expenses. Car expenses, home repairs, medicine, and health care are additional costs. So are entertainment and gifts for children, grandchildren, and other family and friends.

Reduced income may force certain changes. Some retirees limit social and leisure activities because of less money for entertainment. Moving to cheaper housing may be necessary. Some elderly live with children or other relatives. Food choices may change. A person may buy cheaper brands of food, clothes, and household items. Some cannot afford health care or needed medicines. Some retirees are forced to rely on children or other relatives for money or needed items.

Retirement causes severe financial problems for many people. However, some have planned for retirement through savings, investments, retirement plans, and insurance. Their retirement years are financially comfortable.

Social Relationships

Social relationships change throughout life. Children grow up, leave home, and have their own families. Many live far away from parents. Elderly friends and relatives move away, die, or are disabled. Yet most elderly people have regular contact with children, grandchildren, brothers and sisters, nieces and nephews, and other relatives and friends. However, many elderly are lonely. Separation from children and lack of companionship with people their own age are common causes of loneliness in the elderly (Fig. 7-3).

Many elderly people adjust to these changes. Hobbies, church and community activities, and new friends help prevent loneliness. Being a grandparent can be a source of great love and enjoyment (Fig. 7-4). Being included in family activities helps prevent loneliness. It also allows the elderly person to feel useful and wanted (Fig. 7-5).

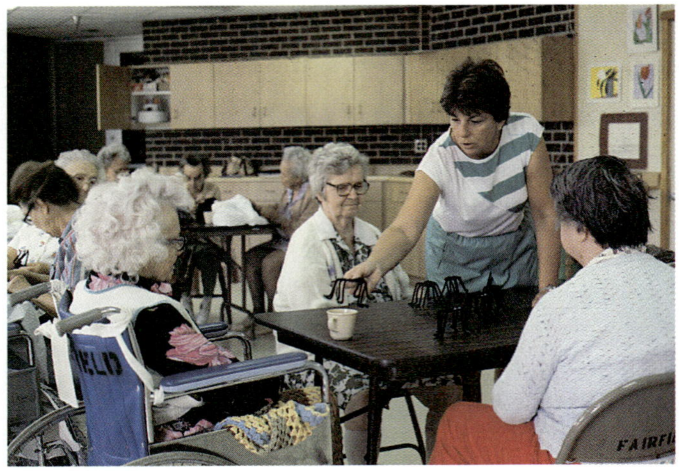

Fig. 7-3 *Elderly people enjoy companionship with people their own age.*

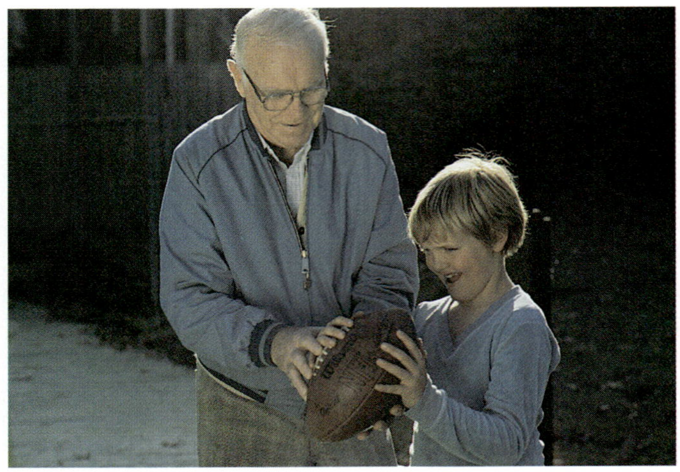

Fig. 7-4 *An elderly man plays with his grandchild.*

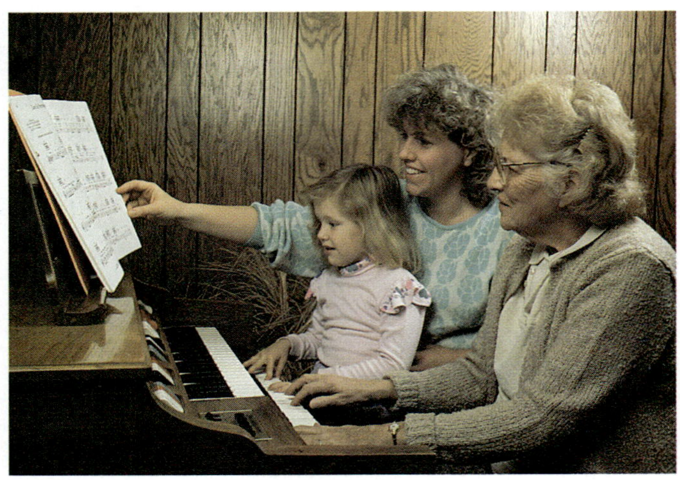

Fig. 7-5 *An elderly woman is included in family activities.*

Some elderly persons speak and understand a foreign language. Communication occurs with family and friends who speak the same language. These relatives and friends may move away or die. Greater loneliness and isolation for the foreign-speaking person may result. The person may not have anyone to talk to and may not be understood by others. In addition, the person's cultural values and practices may not be understood or recognized.

Some elderly people are cared for by their children. Parents and children change roles. Instead of the parent caring for the child, the child cares for the parent. This role change and dependency on a child can make the elderly person feel more secure. However, others feel unwanted, in the way, and useless. Some feel a loss of dignity and self-respect. Tensions may develop between the child, parent, and other family members in the household. Tension can be from the lack of privacy and disagreements. Criticisms about housekeeping, childrearing, cooking, and friends are other common causes of tension.

Death of a Spouse

As a couple grows older, the chances increase that one partner will die. Women live longer than men. Therefore becoming a widow is a reality for many women.

A person may try to psychologically prepare for the death of a partner. When death occurs, the loss of the spouse is devastating. No amount of preparation is ever enough for the emptiness and changes that result. The person loses more than a husband or wife. A friend, lover, companion, and confidant are also lost. The grief felt by the surviving spouse may be very great. Serious physical and mental health problems can result. The surviving spouse may lose the will to live or attempt suicide.

PHYSICAL EFFECTS OF AGING

Certain physical changes are a normal part of aging and occur in everyone (Table 7-1 on page 136). The rate and degree of change vary with each person. Influencing factors include diet, general health, exercise, stress, environment, and heredity. Many changes are gradual and may go unnoticed for a long time. The physical changes of aging result in a slowing down of body processes. Energy level and body efficiency decline. The normal changes of aging may be accompanied by changes caused by disease, illness, or injury.

The Integumentary System

The skin loses its elasticity and fatty tissue layer. As a result, the skin sags. Folds, lines, and wrinkles appear. Dry skin develops because of decreases in oil and sweat glands. Skin breakdown and pressure sores are dangers (see Chapter 13).

Loss of fatty tissues beneath the skin increases sensitivity to cold. Sweaters, lap blankets, socks, and extra blankets are often needed for warmth. Elderly people must be protected from drafts and extreme cold. Thermostat settings may need to be higher than normal.

Dry skin is easily damaged and causes itching. Daily showers or tub baths are avoided. Usually a complete bath is taken twice a week. Partial baths are taken on the other days. This bathing schedule will maintain hygiene. Only mild soaps are used. Often soap is not used on the arms, legs, back, chest, and abdomen. Lotions, oils, and creams prevent drying and itching.

Nails become thick and tough. Feet usually have poor circulation. A nick or cut can lead to a serious infection. Amputation of a part of the foot or leg may be necessary to fight the infection. Nail and foot care are described in Chapter 14.

An elderly person may complain of cold feet. Socks help. Hot water bottles and heating pads are not used because the risk of burns is great. Fragile skin, poor circulation, and decreased sensitivity to heat and cold increase the risk of burns.

White or gray hair is a common sign of aging. Men lose a lot of hair. Hair thins on both men and women. Thinning occurs on the head, in the pubic area, and under the arms. Growth of facial hair may occur in women. Hair tends to be drier because of decreased scalp oils. Brushing helps stimulate circulation and oil production. Shampooing frequency depends on personal preference. Usually shampooing is less frequent than when younger. Shampooing should be done as often as necessary for cleanliness and comfort.

The Musculoskeletal System

As aging progresses, there is gradual muscle atrophy (shrinking) and decreasing strength. Bones become brittle and can break easily. Joints become stiff and painful. These changes result in a gradual loss of height, loss of strength, and decreased mobility.

Activity and diet can help slow down the rate of these changes. Elderly persons need to be as active as possible. Bathing, dressing and undressing, grooming, and other daily activities are forms of physical activity. Range-of-motion exercises (Chapter 19) are also helpful. The diet should be high in protein, calcium, and vitamins. Because bones can break easily, the person must be protected from injury. Measures to prevent falls must be practiced (Chapter 8). The person is turned and moved gently and carefully. A person may need support and assistance when getting out of bed and in walking.

TABLE 7-1

PHYSICAL CHANGES DURING THE AGING PROCESS

System	Changes
Integumentary	Skin becomes less elastic Fatty tissue layer is lost Skin thins and sags Skin is fragile and easily injured Folds, lines, and wrinkles appear Decreased secretion of oil and sweat glands Dry skin develops Itching Increased sensitivity to cold Nails become thick and tough Whitening or graying hair Loss or thinning of hair Facial hair in some women
Musculoskeletal	Muscle atrophy Decreasing strength Bones become brittle; can break easily Joints become stiff and painful Gradual loss of height Decreased mobility
Nervous	Vision and hearing decrease Decreased senses of taste and smell Reduced sense of touch Reduced sensitivity to pain Reduced blood flow to the brain Progressive loss of brain cells Shorter memory Forgetfulness Slowed ability to respond Confusion Dizziness Changes in sleep patterns
Cardiovascular	Heart pumps with less force Arteries narrow and are less elastic Less blood flows through narrowed arteries Weakened heart has to work harder to pump blood through narrowed vessels
Respiratory	Respiratory muscles weaken Lung tissue becomes less elastic Difficulty breathing Decreased strength for coughing
Digestive	Decreased saliva production Difficulty in swallowing Decreased appetite Decreased secretion of digestive juices Fried and fatty foods difficult to digest Indigestion Loss of teeth Decreased peristalsis causing flatulence and constipation
Urinary	Reduced blood supply to kidneys Kidneys atrophy Kidney function decreases Poisonous substances can build up in the blood Urine becomes concentrated Urinary frequency and urgency may occur Urinary incontinence may occur The need to urinate at night may occur

The Nervous System

The loss of vision and hearing are discussed in Chapter 27. Loss of taste and smell are discussed on page 137. Often the sense of touch and sensitivity to pain are also reduced in the elderly. Injuries and diseases that normally cause severe pain may go unnoticed. They may cause only minor discomforts. Heat, cold, and pressure on bony areas may not be felt. Therefore the elderly must be protected from injury. Safety measures are practiced when applying heat or cold. The skin is carefully inspected for signs of breakdown. Good skin care and the measures to prevent pressure sores are practiced.

Blood flow to the brain is reduced. There is also a progressive loss of brain cells. These changes affect personality and mental function. Memory is often shorter, and forgetfulness increases. The ability to respond is slowed. Confusion, dizziness, and fatigue may also occur. Elderly people often remember events from long ago better than recent events. Many elderly people are mentally active and involved in current events. They show fewer personality and mental changes. Care of the confused person is described in Chapter 30.

Less sleep is needed. Loss of energy and decreased blood flow cause fatigue. Usually the elderly rest or nap during the day. They usually go to bed early and get up early. Their sleep periods are shorter.

The Cardiovascular System

The heart muscle becomes less efficient. Blood is pumped through the body with less force. These changes may not cause problems when the person is resting. Activity, exercise, excitement, and illness increase the body's need for oxygen and nutrients. The heart may be unable to meet these needs.

Arteries lose their elasticity and become narrow. Less blood flows through them, causing poor circulation in many parts of the body. As a result, a weakened heart has to work harder to pump blood through the narrowed vessels.

The elderly person needs rest periods during the day. Daily activities should be planned to avoid overexertion. The person should not walk long distances, climb many stairs, or carry heavy objects. Personal care items, the television, telephone, and other frequently used items should be in handy places.

A moderate amount of daily exercise helps to stimulate circulatory, respiratory, digestive, and musculoskeletal functions. Exercise also helps to prevent the formation of thrombi (blood clots) in the leg veins. Many elderly persons engage in exercise programs. Activities include golf, walking, biking, dancing, tennis, swimming, and other forms of exercise. Active or passive range-of-motion exercises are necessary if the person is confined to bed (Chapter 19). Some people have more severe cardiovascular changes. Doctors may order certain exercises and activity limitations.

The Respiratory System

Respiratory muscles weaken. Lung tissue becomes less elastic and more rigid. Often lung changes are not obvious at rest. However, difficulty in breathing *(dyspnea)* may occur with activity. The person may not have enough strength to cough and clear the upper airway of secretions. Respiratory infections and diseases may develop. These can be life-threatening to the elderly.

Normal breathing must be promoted. Heavy bed linens should not cover the chest. They can prevent normal chest expansion. Turning, repositioning, and deep breathing help prevent respiratory complications that may result from bed rest. Breathing is usually easier in semi-Fowler's position (Chapter 11). The person should be as active as possible.

The Digestive System

Many changes occur in the gastrointestinal system. Difficulty swallowing *(dysphagia)* often occurs from decreases in the amount of saliva. Taste and smell become dulled and decrease appetite. Secretion of digestive juices decreases. As a result, fried and fatty foods are hard to digest and may cause indigestion. Loss of teeth and ill-fitting dentures affect chewing. This results in digestion problems. Certain foods are avoided because they are hard to chew. Usually high-protein foods such as meat are avoided. Decreased peristalsis results in slower emptying of the stomach and colon. Flatulence and constipation are common because of decreased peristalsis (see Chapter 16).

Dry, fried, and fatty foods should be avoided. This helps swallowing and digestion problems. Good oral hygiene and denture care improve the ability to taste. People may not have natural teeth or dentures. Their food is pureed or ground. Avoiding high-fiber foods may be necessary even though they help prevent constipation. Foods high in fiber are hard to chew and can irritate the intestines. High-fiber foods include apricots, celery, and fruits and vegetables with skins and seeds. Foods that provide soft bulk are often ordered for those with chewing difficulties or constipation. These foods include whole-grain cereals and cooked fruits and vegetables.

Aging requires certain dietary changes. Elderly people need fewer calories than younger persons. Energy levels and daily activity levels are lower. Additional fluids are needed for kidney function. Foods that prevent constipation and musculoskeletal changes need to be included in the diet. The diet should also include enough protein for tissue growth and repair. However, protein may be lacking in the diets of the elderly. Foods that are high in protein are generally the most expensive.

The Urinary System

During aging, kidney function decreases. A reduced blood supply causes the kidneys to atrophy (shrink). Poisonous substances can build up in the blood and cause serious health problems. Urine becomes more concentrated because the elderly usually do not drink enough fluids.

Bladder muscles weaken. Bladder size decreases, causing the bladder to hold less urine. Urinary frequency or urgency may occur. Some have urinary incontinence (inability to control the passage of urine from the bladder). Many elderly people have to go to the bathroom several times during the night.

The doctor may order increased fluid intake to promote kidney function. Intake should include water, fruit juices, and milk. Other beverages preferred by the person should be provided. Most fluids should be ingested before 1800 (5:00 PM). This reduces the need to urinate during the night. Bladder training programs may be necessary for those with urinary incontinence. Indwelling catheters are sometimes needed. Urinary elimination is discussed in Chapter 15.

HOUSING ALTERNATIVES

Most elderly persons live in their own homes. Some choose to give up their homes; others are forced to do so. Reduced income, taxes, home repairs, and the inability to do yard work are influencing factors. Some elderly people retire to warmer climates. Others no longer want a large home when children are gone. Some cannot care for themselves. There are housing alternatives that meet the needs of the elderly.

Living with Family

Sometimes elderly brothers, sisters, and cousins live together. They provide companionship for each other. They can also share living expenses. They can care for each other during illness or disability. One may have the role of caregiver if the other is ill or disabled.

Some elderly people live with their adult children. The elderly parent (or parents) moves in with the child or the child moves into the parent's home. As discussed earlier in this chapter, living with a child can help the elderly person feel safe and secure. The elderly parent may be healthy, may need some supervision, or may be ill or disabled. The adult child may be a caregiver if the elderly parent is ill or disabled. Many children choose to care for a parent so a nursing home is not required. They want to try being a caregiver first. A nursing home is an option if they find that the level of care needed cannot be provided.

As explained on page 134, living with an adult child is a social change for the elderly. The parent, adult child, and the child's family all need to adjust. Sleeping arrangements may change if there is not an extra bedroom. If the parent is very ill, a hospital bed may be needed. It may need to be placed in a living room or dining room.

The adult child's family still needs time alone. Other brothers, sisters, and family members may help give care. *Respite care* may be needed. Respite means a break, rest, or lull. Respite care is when the person is admitted to a nursing facility or home care is obtained for a few days or weeks. Caregivers can have a vacation, rest, or simply take a break from the stress of giving care. Community and church groups may have volunteers who can help give care.

Adult day care centers Adult children may still need to work even though the elderly parent cannot be left alone. Adult day care centers provide meals, supervision, and activities for the elderly. Some provide transportation from home to the center.

Eligibility requirements vary. Some may require that the person be able to walk using a cane or walker if needed. Others allow wheelchairs. Most require that the person be capable of some self-care activities.

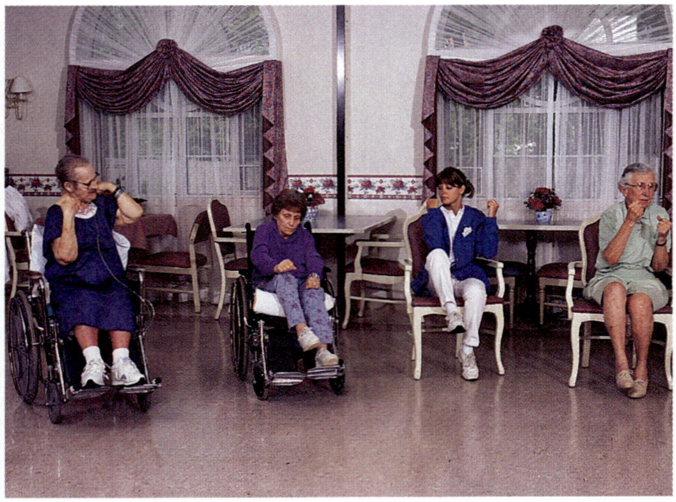

Fig. 7-6 *Members of this adult day care center are involved in an exercise program.*

Many activities are available. Cards, board games, movies, crafts, dancing, walks, and lectures are some examples (Fig. 7-6). Some provide bowling and swimming. The activities are all supervised and assistance given as needed.

Apartments

Apartments have some advantages for the elderly. Maintenance, yard work, snow removal, and major appliance repair are the landlord's responsibility. The elderly person is independent. Personal belongings are kept. However, rent can be costly. Utility bills are another expense. Many elderly persons enjoy gardening and yard work (Fig. 7-7). Apartment living usually does not provide those opportunities.

Residential Hotels

Some cities have residential hotels. Private rooms or efficiency apartments can be rented. Food services may include a dining room, cafeteria, or room service. Recreational activities and emergency medical services may be provided. Most hotels are close to shopping areas, churches, and other civic services. Residential hotels and apartments have similar disadvantages.

Senior Citizen Housing

State and federal funds have helped to build housing for senior citizens. An elderly person or couple can live independently in an apartment near people of the same age. The buildings have wheelchair access, handrails, elevators, and other safety measures. Apartments may be furnished. Appliances are arranged to meet the special

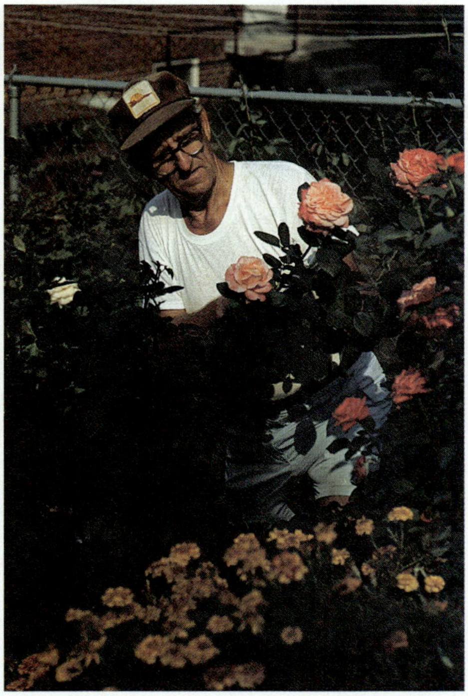

Fig. 7-7 *This man enjoys gardening. Apartment living usually does not provide opportunities for gardening or other yard work.*

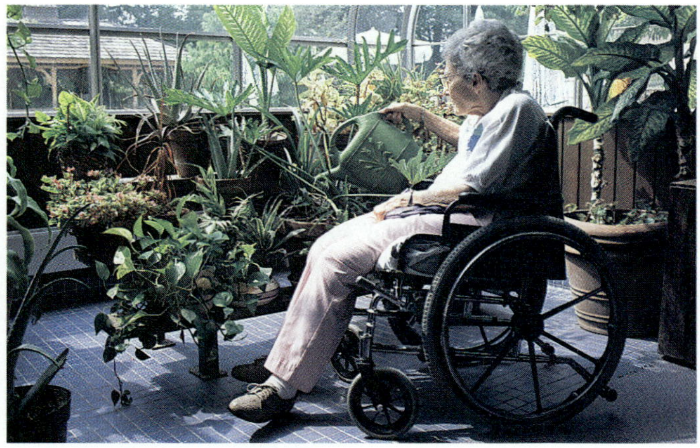

Fig. 7-8 *The atmosphere of a nursing facility is similar to that of a home.*

needs of the elderly. Many services are available. There is usually a dining room and a nurse or doctor on call. A daily telephone call is made to check on each tenant. Transportation is usually available to church, the doctor, or shopping areas. The elderly pay monthly rent. However, the rent is usually less than that for a regular apartment if government funds are involved.

Nursing Facilities

Nursing facilities are housing alternatives for the elderly who can no longer care for themselves. Nursing facilities offer different levels of care. Some merely provide room, food, and laundry services. Others provide nursing, rehabilitation, dietary, recreational, social, and religious services.

Some persons remain in nursing facilities for the rest of their lives. Others stay until able to return home. The nursing facility is the person's temporary or permanent home. The surroundings are as homelike as possible (Fig. 7-8). The person is a resident, not a patient.

Nursing facilities are designed to meet the special needs of the elderly. Physical changes of aging and safety needs (see Chapter 8) are considered in facility design and construction.

Nursing facilities may be privately owned or operated by the government. In either case, state and federal agencies monitor the care given. State and federal standards required by law must be followed. Periodic inspections may be expected or unannounced.

Most nursing facilities receive Medicare or Medicaid funds. Such facilities must meet the requirements of the Omnibus Budget Reconciliation Act of 1987 (OBRA). Unannounced surveys are conducted to determine if nursing facilities are meeting OBRA requirements. Funding will not occur if the many requirements are not met. OBRA requirements are described throughout this book. Box 7-1 on page 140 lists the OBRA requirements for a facility's physical environment.

Independent living units Independent living units are a new trend. A wing of the facility has small apartments. Elderly persons or couples live in the units. They perform self-care activities and take their own medications. Food services are available, and help is nearby if needed. However, each person takes care of himself or herself. Little supervision or assistance is needed.

Hospital long-term care units Many hospitals have long-term care units. These units are for persons who still need skilled care but not to the extent required previously. At one time these persons were transferred to nursing facilities. Now they can receive skilled care on the long-term care unit. Some eventually go home. Others may go to nursing facilities.

BOX 7-1 OBRA Facility Environment Requirements

Sufficient space and equipment

- Dining space with easy access and appropriate tables and chairs
- Program areas with easy access; appropriate exercise and other equipment
- Recreational areas with easy access and sufficient space for movement and storage of equipment and supplies
- Toilet facilities with easy access and located nearby
- Functional and comfortable furniture for residents, families, and visitors
- Tables of proper height and chairs that facilitate comfort and ease of sitting and standing for residents
- Halls with handrails and easy access for wheelchairs, walkers, and other space and safety needs

Quality of life and comfort in the environment

- Clean and orderly halls, dining, health services, program and recreational areas, bathroom facilities
- Odor-free environment
- Temperature between 71°–81° F
- Acceptable noise level
- Adequate ventilation and humidity
- No glare from environment and proper lighting
- Music, television as requested by the resident or family
- Paint color or wallpaper appealing to residents
- Pest-free, hazard-free environment
- Resident's needs and independence are accommodated
- Clean, soft, and adequate linens for resident
- Posted signs to identify nonsmoking areas

Resident rooms

- See Chapter 11

Safety

- See Chapter 8

From Jaffe MS: *The OBRA guidelines for quality improvement,* El Paso, 1993, Skidmore-Roth.

OBRA REQUIREMENTS

The Omnibus Budget Reconciliation Act of 1987 is concerned with the quality of life, health, and safety of residents. Nursing facilities must provide care in a manner and in an environment that maintains or improves each resident's quality of life, health, and safety. Nursing assistant training and competency evaluation are OBRA requirements (see Chapter 2). Many other requirements must be met as well.

Resident Rights

Nursing facility residents have certain rights under federal and state laws. Residents have rights as citizens of the United States. They also have rights relating to their everyday lives and care in a nursing facility. Nursing facilities must protect and promote resident rights. Residents must be free to exercise their rights without facility interference. Some residents are incompetent (not able) and cannot exercise their rights. Legal representatives exercise rights for them.

Nursing facilities must inform residents of their rights. They must be informed orally and in writing. Such information is given before or during admission to the facility. It must be given in the language used and understood by the resident.

Resident rights that relate to your roles and responsibilities are discussed here.

Information The right to information means access to all records relating to the resident. Such records include the resident's medical record, contracts, incident reports, and financial records. The request for any record can be oral or written. The record must be available within 24 hours of the request. The facility has 2 working days to provide requested photocopies.

The resident or legal representative also has the right to be fully informed of the person's total health condition. Such information must be given in language the person can understand. Interpreters may be needed for those speaking a language other than English. Sign language or other aids may be needed for those with hearing impairments.

The resident or legal representative must also have information about the resident's doctor. This includes the doctor's name, specialty, and how to contact the doctor.

You need to report any request for information to the nurse. Remember, you *do not* give the information described above to the resident or family (see Chapter 2).

Refusing treatment The resident has the right to refuse treatment. Like hospital patients, the resident also has the right to refuse to take part in research. OBRA defines treatment as care provided to relieve symptoms, improve functional level, or maintain or restore health. A person who does not give consent or refuses treatment cannot be given the treatment. However, the facility must find out what the resident is refusing and why. Through teaching and clarifying, the facility should try to educate the person about the treatment, problems from not having the treatment, and other treatment choices. Although the resident may refuse a specific treatment, the facility must provide all other services. Changes in the resident's care plan may be needed.

Advance directives are also part of the right to refuse treatment. They include living wills or other instructions about life support. Advance directives are discussed in Chapter 34.

Like requests for information, you need to report any treatment refusal to the nurse.

Privacy and confidentiality The rights to privacy and confidentiality were discussed in Chapter 2. They were also presented under the Patient's Bill of Rights in Chapter 4. OBRA also provides for privacy and confidentiality.

Residents have the right to personal privacy. The resident's body must not be exposed unnecessarily. Only those workers directly involved in care, treatments, or examinations should be present. The resident must give consent for others to be present. For example, a student wants to observe a procedure or treatment. The resident's consent is needed for the student to be an observer. A resident also has the right to use the bathroom in private. Privacy must be maintained for personal care activities as well.

Residents also have the right to visit with others in private. They have the right to visit in an area where they cannot be seen or heard by others. The facility must try to provide private space when it is requested. Offices, chapels, dining rooms, meeting rooms, activity rooms, and conference rooms can be used if available.

The right to visit in privacy also involves telephone conversations (Fig. 7-9). Residents also have the right to send and receive mail without interference by others. Letters sent and received by the resident must not be opened by others without the resident's permission. Mail must be delivered to the resident within 24 hours of its delivery to the facility.

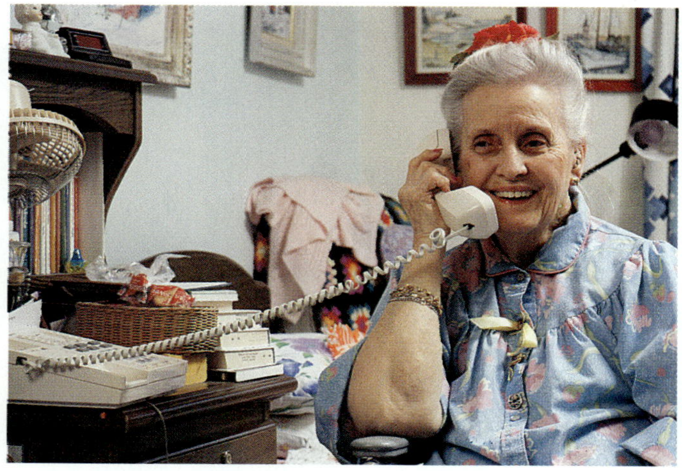

Fig. 7-9 *A resident talking privately on a telephone.*

Information about the resident's care, treatment, and condition must be kept confidential. Medical and financial records are also confidential. The resident must give consent for them to be released to other facilities or persons. However, consent is not needed for the release of medical records when the resident is being transferred to another facility. Records can also be released without the resident's consent when they are required by law or for insurance purposes.

Throughout this book you are reminded to provide privacy. You are also reminded to keep information about the person confidential. Providing for privacy and keeping medical and personal information confidential show respect for the person and protect the person's dignity.

Personal choice OBRA requires that residents be free to choose their own doctors. They also have the right to participate in planning their own care and treatment. This means that residents have the right to make decisions about their own care and treatment. It also means that residents have the right to choose activities, schedules, and care based on their personal preferences. For example, residents have the right to choose when to get up and go to bed, what to wear, how to spend their time, and what to eat (Fig. 7-10 on page 142). They are also free to choose companions and visitors inside and outside of the nursing facility.

Personal choice is important for quality of life, dignity, and self-respect. The individual's personal preference is emphasized throughout this book. You are reminded to allow the person's preferences whenever it is safely possible.

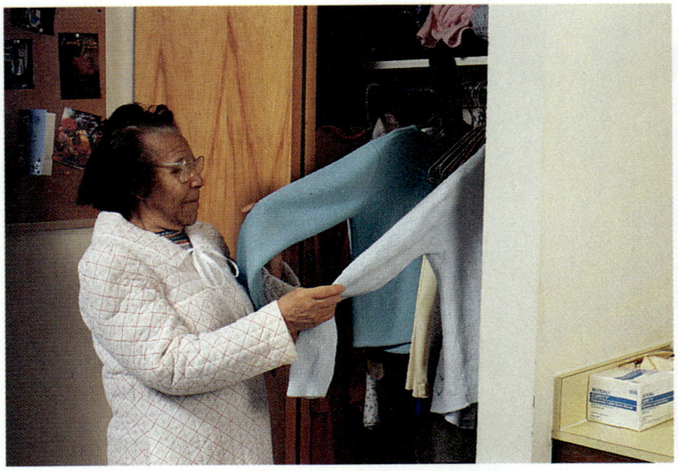

Fig. 7-10 *A resident choosing what clothing to wear.*

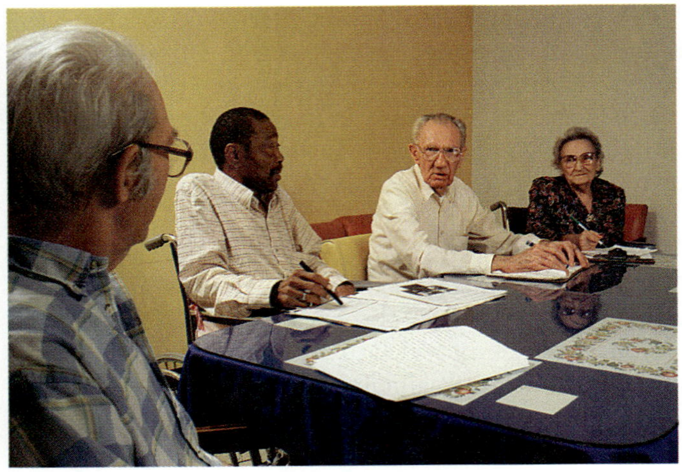

Fig. 7-11 *Residents at a group meeting.*

Disputes and grievances Residents have the right to voice concerns, questions, and complaints about treatment or care. The dispute or grievance may involve another resident. It may be about treatment or care that was not given. The facility must promptly try to correct the situation. The resident must not be punished in any way for voicing the dispute or grievance.

Work The resident has rights that relate to performing work for the facility. The resident does not work to receive care, items, or other things or privileges. There is no requirement that the resident must perform services for the facility.

However, the resident *can* work or perform services if the desire or need for work is part of the resident's care plan. The resident may be used to being quite active—gardening, repairing things, building things, sewing, mending, cooking. The resident may want to work. Another resident may need to work for rehabilitation or activity purposes. In either case, the desire for work or the need for work should become part of the resident's care plan.

The care plan should specify:

- The reason for the work—desire or need
- What work will be done
- If the services are paid or voluntary

Participation in resident and family groups Residents have the right to take part in resident and family groups. This means that residents have the right to form groups (Fig. 7-11). And a resident's family has the right to meet with the families of other residents. These groups can discuss concerns and offer ideas to improve quality of life in the facility. They can also plan activities for residents and families. Or the groups can provide support and reassurance for group members. Residents also have the right to take part in social, religious, and community activities. They have the right to assistance in getting to and from activities of their choice.

Care and security of personal possessions Residents have the right to keep and use personal items. This includes clothing and some furnishings. Available space and the health and safety of other residents can affect the type and amount of personal property allowed. A person's property must be treated with care and respect. Though the items may not have value to you, they are important to the resident. They also relate to personal choice, dignity, and quality of life.

The facility must take reasonable measures to protect the person's property. Items must be labeled with the resident's name. And the facility must investigate reports of lost, stolen, or damaged items. Police help is sometimes needed. The resident and family will probably be advised not to keep jewelry and other expensive items in the facility.

You must protect yourself and the facility from being accused of stealing a resident's property. Do not go through a resident's closet, drawers, purse, or other space without the person's knowledge and consent. Have another worker with you and the resident or legal representative present if you must inspect closets and drawers. The worker serves as a witness to your activities.

Freedom from abuse, mistreatment, and neglect OBRA states that residents have the right to be free from verbal, sexual, physical, or mental abuse. Elderly abuse is discussed on page 143.

Residents also have the right to be free from involuntary seclusion. Involuntary seclusion is separating the resident from others against his or her will. It can also mean keeping the person confined to a certain area or away from his or her room without consent. If the person is incompetent, involuntary seclusion occurs against the legal representative's consent.

No one can abuse, neglect, or mistreat the resident. This includes facility staff, volunteers, staff from other agencies or groups, other residents, family, visitors, and legal guardians. Nursing facilities must have policies and procedures for investigating suspected or reported cases of resident abuse. Also, nursing facilities cannot employ persons who have been convicted of abusing, neglecting, or mistreating other individuals.

Freedom from restraints Residents have the right not to have body movements restricted. Body movements can be restricted by the application of restraints or the administration of certain drugs. Some drugs can restrain the person because they affect mood, behavior, and mental function. Sometimes residents need to be restrained to protect them from harming themselves or others. A doctor's order is necessary for restraints to be used. Restraints cannot be used for the convenience of the staff or to discipline a resident. Restraints are discussed in Chapter 8.

Quality of Life

OBRA requires that nursing facilities care for residents in a manner that promotes dignity, self-worth, and physical, psychological, and emotional well-being. Protecting resident rights is one way to promote quality of life. Personal choice, privacy, participation in group activities, having personal property, and freedom from restraint show respect for the person.

The resident is also spoken to in a polite and courteous manner (see Chapter 4). Giving good, honest, and thoughtful care enhances the resident's quality of life.

Box 7-2 on page 144 lists actions which show concern for the person's dignity and privacy. These actions are required by OBRA. Surveyors check to make sure that these actions are demonstrated in the care of residents.

Activities Activities are important for a resident's quality of life. OBRA requires that nursing facilities provide activity programs that meet the interests and physical, mental, and psychosocial needs of each resident. Such activities must allow personal choice and promote physical, intellectual, social, and emotional well-being. Many facilities also provide religious services for spiritual health. You will assist residents to and from activity programs. You may also be assigned to help residents with activities.

Environment The environment of the facility must also promote quality of life. The environment must be clean and safe and be as home-like as possible. Allowing the resident to have personal possessions enhances quality of life. It allows personal choice and promotes a homelike environment. The safe environment is discussed in Chapter 8. The furniture and equipment in a resident's room are discussed in Chapter 11. Information relating to temperature and sound levels is also discussed.

ABUSE OF THE ELDERLY

Elderly abuse has become more evident in today's society. Abuse is defined as having one or more of the following elements:

- Willful causing of injury
- Unreasonable confinement
- Intimidation
- Punishment
- Deprivation of goods or services needed for physical, mental, or psychosocial well-being

With abuse, one or more of these elements result in physical harm, pain, or mental anguish. Protection against abuse extends to persons in a coma. The abuser is usually a family member or a person caring for the elderly individual. There are different forms of abuse.

- *Physical abuse* involves hitting, slapping, kicking, pinching, and beating. It also includes corporal punishment—punishment inflicted directly on the body, such as beatings, lashings, or whippings. Neglect is also physical abuse. It may involve depriving the person of needed medical services or treatment. Neglect is also failure to provide food, clothing, hygiene, and other basic needs. In nursing facilities, neglect includes but is not limited to leaving a person lying or sitting in urine or feces, isolating residents in their rooms or other locations, and failing to answer call bells.
- *Verbal abuse* is the use of oral or written words or statements that speak badly of, sneer at, criticize, or condemn the resident. OBRA guidelines also include unkind gestures under verbal abuse.
- *Involuntary seclusion* is confining the person to a specific area. Elderly people have been locked in closets, basements, attics, and other spaces.
- *Financial abuse* is when the elderly person's money is used by another person.
- *Mental abuse* includes humiliation, harassment, and threats of being punished or deprived of needs such as food, clothing, care, a home, or a place to sleep.
- *Sexual abuse* is when the person is harassed about sex or is attacked sexually. The person may be forced to perform sexual acts out of fear of punishment or physical harm.

BOX 7-2 OBRA Required Actions to Promote the Resident's Dignity and Privacy

Courteous and dignified interactions with residents

- Use appropriate tone of voice
- Use good eye contact when interacting with the resident
- Stand or sit close enough to the resident as appropriate
- Use proper name and title of resident
- Obtain resident's attention before interacting with the resident
- Use touch if approved by the resident
- Respect the resident's social status and listen with interest to what the resident is saying
- Do not yell, scold, or embarrass the resident

Courteous and dignified care to residents

- Groom hair, beards, and nails as the resident wishes
- Assist with dressing in clothing appropriate to time of day and resident's personal choice
- Promote resident independence and dignity in dining
- Respect resident's private space and property
- Assist with ambulation and transfer without interfering with independence
- Assist with bathing and personal hygiene preferences without interfering with independence
  *Neat, clean appearance of resident
  *Clean shaven or groomed beard
  *Nails trimmed and clean
  *Dentures, hearing aid, glasses, and other prostheses used as appropriate
  *Clothing clean and properly fitted and fastened
  *Shoes and hose properly applied and fastened
  *Extra clothing for warmth as needed such as sweater or lap blanket

Privacy and self-determination of residents

- Drape properly during personal care and procedures to avoid exposure and embarrassment
- Drape properly in chair
- Use curtains or screens during personal care and procedures
- Close door to room during care and procedures or as resident desires
- Knock on door before entering and wait to be asked in
- Provide privacy during doctor examination with draping and curtains or screen
- Close bathroom door when used by resident

Maintain personal choice and independence

- Resident smokes in designated areas
- Resident participates in activities according to interests
- Resident is involved in scheduling activities and care
- Resident gives input into plan of care regarding preferences and independence
- Resident involved in room or roommate change

From Jaffe MS: *The OBRA guidelines for quality improvement,* El Paso, 1993, Skidmore-Roth.

BOX 7-3 Signs of Elderly Abuse

- Living conditions are unsafe, unclean, or inadequate.
- Personal hygiene is lacking. The person is unclean, and clothes are dirty.
- Weight loss; there are signs of poor nutrition and inadequate fluid intake.
- Frequent injuries; circumstances behind the injuries are strange or seem impossible.
- Old and new bruises are seen.
- The person seems very quiet or withdrawn.
- The person seems fearful, anxious, or agitated.
- The person does not seem to want to talk or answer questions.
- The person is restrained or locked in a certain area for long periods of time. Toilet facilities, food and water, and other necessary items cannot be reached.
- Private conversations are not allowed. The caregiver is present during all conversations.
- The person seems anxious to please the caregiver.
- Medications are not taken properly. Medications are not purchased, or too much or too little medication is taken.
- Visits to the emergency room may be frequent.
- The person may go from one doctor to another. Some people do not have a doctor.

Abused elderly people may be seen in their homes, hospitals, or nursing facilities. Often the abuse is unrecognized. There are many signs of elderly abuse. The abused person may show only some of the signs listed in Box 7-3.

OBRA and state laws require the reporting of elderly abuse. If abuse is suspected, it must be reported. Where and how to report suspected abuse varies in each state. If you need to report suspected abuse, you must give as much information as possible. The reporting agency takes action based on the information given. They act immediately if there is a life-threatening situation. Sometimes the help of police or the courts is necessary.

Helping the abused elderly is not always easy or possible. The abuse may never be reported or recognized, or the investigating agency may be unable to gain access to the person. Sometimes the elderly are abused by their children. A victim may want to protect the child. Some victims are embarrassed or believe the abuse is deserved. A victim may be afraid of what will happen. He or she may think that the present situation is better than no care at all. Some people fear not being believed if they report the abuse themselves.

Elderly abuse is an unfortunate situation. You may suspect that a person is being abused. If so, discuss the situation and your observations with the nurse. Give as much information as possible. The nurse then contacts the appropriate members of the health team. The agency that investigates elderly abuse in your community is also contacted.

Spotlight On…

Ron C of Albuquerque, New Mexico, *made a difference with a 90-year-old woman and her daughter. The woman needed an operation to repair her fractured hip. Prior to surgery it was important to get advance directives. The daughter said she could not speak to her mother about such things because she was afraid it would frighten her mother as well as take away her hope that the surgery would be successful. Along with the nurse manager, Ron presented the information to the woman. His tender, sensitive, and understanding manner toward her created an atmosphere of caring. The woman, with her daughter at her bedside, was then able to make her decisions.*

Protecting Residents from Abuse

OBRA requires that nursing facilities not employ persons who have been convicted of abuse, neglect, or mistreatment of persons in a nursing facility, hospital, home agency, or other health care facility. Before hiring a person, the facility must thoroughly check the applicant's past work history. All references must be checked and efforts made to find out about any past criminal prosecutions. For nursing assistant job applicants, the employer must also check the nursing assistant registry for any findings about abuse, neglect, mistreatment of residents or misappropriation (misuse, stealing) of their property. For nurses or other staff, the appropriate licensing authority must be contacted.

The facility must take certain actions if there is suspected abuse within the facility.

- The incident must be immediately reported to the facility administrator and to other officials as required by federal and state laws.
- All claims of abuse must be thoroughly investigated.
- The facility must prevent further potential for abuse while the investigation is in progress.
- Investigation results must be reported to the facility administrator and to other officials as required by federal and state laws within 5 days of the incident.
- Corrective action must be taken if the claim is found to be true.

SUMMARY

Aging is a normal process. Body functions slow down and become less efficient. Many persons function independently. They enjoy life with a loving spouse, family, and friends. For others aging can be difficult, painful, and lonely. Loved ones die or move away. The physical changes of aging, disease, and illness make even the most simple, everyday tasks difficult or impossible. Income may not cover monthly living expenses. There may be little or no money for medical bills and medicines. Leaving a lifelong home for a nursing home is often the only choice.

Many people dread living in a nursing home. However, OBRA serves to protect nursing facility residents. Some of the many OBRA requirements relate to resident rights and the quality of life.

Some elderly are abused. Their needs and problems present additional concerns. You must be alert to the possibility that a person is being abused. You can help the victim by discussing the situation with a nurse as soon as possible.

You need to understand the physical, psychological, and social changes that accompany aging. Imagine yourself being old. Put yourself in the place of the elderly person. The aged person depends on you for assistance in meeting basic needs. You can more effectively meet these needs if you can appreciate the person's situation. Patience, tolerance, and kindness are needed when working with the elderly. Their behaviors, habits, and body changes may seem unusual. However, they still need love and the companionship of others. You can help bring happiness and cheer to the elderly.

Review Questions

Circle the best *answer.*

1 Retirement usually results in

a Lowered income

b Physical changes from aging

c Companionship and usefulness

d Financial security

2 Elderly people may experience loneliness because

a Children may have moved away

b Friends and relatives may have died or moved

c Of difficulties in communicating with others

d All of the above

3 When elderly people live with their children they often feel

a Independent

b Wanted and a part of things

c Useless

d Dignified

4 Death of a spouse results in the loss of a

a Friend

b Lover

c Companion

d All of the above

5 Changes occur in the skin. Care should include all of the following *except*

a Providing extra blankets for warmth

b Applying lotion

c Using soap daily

d Providing good skin care

6 An elderly person has cold feet. You should

a Provide socks

b Apply a hot water bottle

c Soak the feet in hot water

d Apply a heating pad

7 Changes occur in the musculoskeletal system during the aging process. Which is *false?*

a Bones become brittle and can break easily.

b Bed rest is needed because of loss of strength.

c Joints become stiff and painful.

d Range-of-motion exercises help to slow down the rate of the musculoskeletal changes.

8 Reduced blood supply to the brain can result in

a Confusion

b Dizziness

c Fatigue

d All of the above

9 Changes occur in the nervous system. Which is *true?*

a More sleep is needed than when younger.

b Recent events are remembered better than past events.

c Sensitivity to pain is reduced.

d Confusion occurs in every elderly person.

10 Arteries lose their elasticity and become narrow. These changes result in

a A slower heart rate

b Lower blood pressure

c Poor circulation to many parts of the body

d A decrease in the amount of blood in the body

11 An elderly person has cardiovascular changes. Care includes the following *except*

a Placing personal items in a convenient location

b A moderate amount of daily exercise

c Planning activities to avoid exertion

d Walking long distances

REVIEW QUESTIONS—CONT'D

12 Respiratory changes occur with aging. Which is *false?*

- **a** Heavy bed linens prevent normal chest expansion.
- **b** The person is turned and repositioned frequently if on bed rest.
- **c** The side-lying position is best for breathing when there are respiratory changes.
- **d** The person should be as active as possible.

13 The elderly should avoid dry foods because of

- **a** Decreases in saliva
- **b** Loss of teeth or ill-fitting dentures
- **c** Decreased amounts of digestive juices
- **d** Decreased peristalsis

14 Changes occur in the gastrointestinal system. The elderly person should avoid

- **a** Cooked fruits and vegetables
- **b** Foods high in protein
- **c** Apricots and celery
- **d** All of the above

15 The doctor has ordered an increased fluid intake for an elderly person. You should

- **a** Give most of the fluid before 1800 (5:00 PM)
- **b** Provide mostly water
- **c** Start a bladder training program
- **d** Insert an indwelling urinary catheter

16 You are working in a nursing facility. You must

- **a** Open a resident's mail
- **b** Choose what the resident will wear
- **c** Provide for the resident's privacy
- **d** Search the resident's closet and drawers

17 Who decides how a resident's hair should be styled?

- **a** The resident
- **b** The nurse
- **c** The nursing assistant
- **d** The family

18 Which statement is *false?*

- **a** Residents can offer suggestions to improve the facility.
- **b** Residents can be restrained to prevent them from leaving the facility.
- **c** Residents must be free from abuse, neglect, and mistreatment.
- **d** Allowing personal choice is important for the resident's quality of life.

19 Which is *not* a sign of elderly abuse?

- **a** Stiff joints and joint pain
- **b** Old and new bruises
- **c** Poor personal hygiene
- **d** Frequent injuries

20 You suspect a patient has been abused. What should you do?

- **a** Tell the family.
- **b** Call a state agency.
- **c** Tell a nurse of your suspicion.
- **d** Ask the patient if he or she has been abused.

Answers to these questions are on page 749.

Safety

8

OBJECTIVES

- Define the key terms listed in this chapter
- Explain why some people cannot protect themselves
- Identify safety precautions for infants and children
- Identify safety measures that prevent home accidents
- Identify common safety hazards in health care facilities
- Explain why a person must be identified before receiving care
- Describe how to accurately identify a person
- Describe the safety measures that prevent falls
- Explain the purpose of restraints and the safety rules for use
- Explain when restraints can be used
- Identify the information to report to the nurse when restraints are used
- Describe common equipment-related accidents and how they can be prevented
- Identify the accidents and errors that need to be reported
- Describe the safety measures related to fire prevention and the use of oxygen
- Know what to do if there is a fire
- Give examples of natural and man-made disasters
- Perform the procedures described in this chapter

Key Terms

active physical restraint A restraint attached to the person's body and to a stationary (nonmovable) object; movement and access to one's body are restricted

coma A state of being unaware of one's surroundings and being unable to react or respond to people, places, or things

disaster A sudden catastrophic event in which many people are injured and killed, and property is destroyed

ground That which carries leaking electricity to the earth and away from the electrical appliance

hemiplegia Paralysis on one side of the body

paraplegia Paralysis from the waist down

passive physical restraint A restraint near but not directly attached to the person's body; it does not totally restrict freedom of movement and allows access to certain body parts

quadriplegia Paralysis from the neck down

restraint Any item, object, device, garment, material, or chemical that restricts a person's freedom of movement or access to one's body

suffocation Termination of breathing that results from lack of oxygen

Safety is a basic need. Everyone wants to be safe when driving a car, taking a walk, or when receiving health care. People need to be safe from accidents and dangers. Homes and health care facilities are thought to be free of dangers and hazards. This is not true. Many accidental injuries occur in the home. Some cause death. Accidents also occur in health care facilities.

You must practice safety at home and in everyday activities. When caring for patients or residents, you need to practice ordinary safety precautions and the other safety measures presented in this chapter.

THE SAFE ENVIRONMENT

In a safe environment, a person has a low risk of illness or injury. The person feels safe and secure both physically and psychologically. There is little risk of infection, falling, burns, poisoning, or other injuries. The person is comfortable in relation to temperature, noise, and smells. There is enough light and room to move about safely. The person and the person's property are safe from fire and intruders. The person is not afraid and has few worries and concerns.

FACTORS AFFECTING PERSONAL SAFETY

You need to know about any factors that increase a person's risk of an accident. This is so you can provide for the person's safety. Age, poor vision, and loss of hearing are some factors described in this section. Some people cannot protect themselves. They rely on others for safety.

Age

Children and the elderly need to be protected from injury. Infants are helpless. They depend on others for protection. Young children have not learned what is safe and what are dangers. They normally explore their surroundings, put objects in their mouths, and touch and feel new things. As a result they may fall, eat or drink poisonous substances, choke, be burned, and have other accidents. The safety precautions listed in Box 8-1 on page 152 are practiced when caring for infants and children. The safety measures that apply to falls (page 154), burns (page 156), poisoning (page 156), and suffocation (page 156) are also practiced.

BOX 8-1 SAFETY PRACTICES FOR INFANTS AND CHILDREN

- Do not leave infants or young children unattended. They must be supervised when in strollers, walkers, high chairs, infant seats, bathtubs, wading pools, or when playing outside.
- Use the safety strap to fasten a child in a high chair.
- Do not let children play on curbs or behind parked cars. They should not play in piles of leaves or snow where there is heavy traffic.
- Check children in cribs often.
- Make sure crib side rails are up and locked in place.
- Keep one hand on a child lying in a crib, on a scale, or on a table if you must look away for a moment (Fig. 8-1).
- Place safety plugs in electrical outlets (Fig. 8-2). The plugs prevent children from sticking their fingers or small objects into the openings.
- Keep cords and electrical equipment out of the reach of children.
- Keep childproof caps on medicine containers and household cleaners.
- Store household cleaners and medicines in locked storage areas that are beyond the reach of children (Fig. 8-3).
- Supervise any child who is in or near water. Keep bathroom doors closed to prevent drowning in toilets or bathtubs. Keep buckets empty and upside down except when in use.
- Do not prop baby bottles on a rolled towel or blanket. Hold the baby and bottle during feedings.
- Keep plastic bags and wraps away from children because of the danger of suffocation.
- Use guardrails at the top and bottom of stairs to prevent small children from climbing up and down stairs.
- Use federally approved car restraints (Fig. 8-4).
- Protect the child from falls (page 154).
- Protect the child from poisoning (page 156).
- Protect the child from burns (page 156).
- Protect the child from choking and suffocating (page 156).

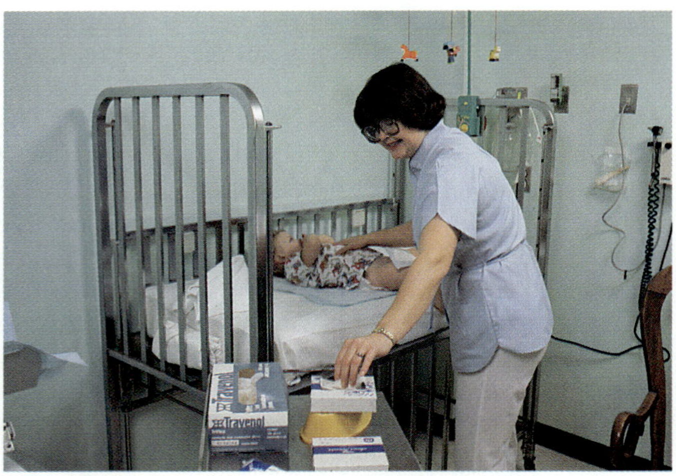

Fig. 8-1 *One hand is kept on the child while the nursing assistant momentarily looks away.*

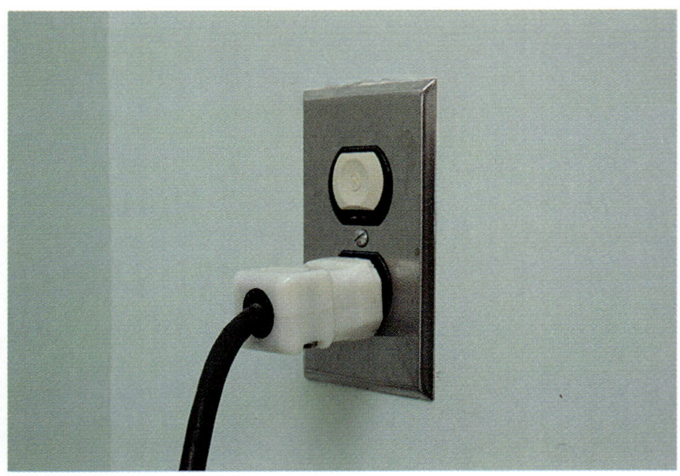

Fig. 8-2 *Safety plug in an electrical outlet.*

Many elderly people are at risk for accidents because of physical changes due to aging. Movements are slower and less steady. Balance may be affected, causing the person to fall easily. The person may be unable to move quickly and suddenly to avoid dangerous situations. Other factors make the elderly prone to accidents and injuries. They include decreased sensitivity to heat and cold, poor vision, hearing problems, and a decreased sense of smell. Confusion, poor judgment, memory problems, and disorientation are other factors.

A 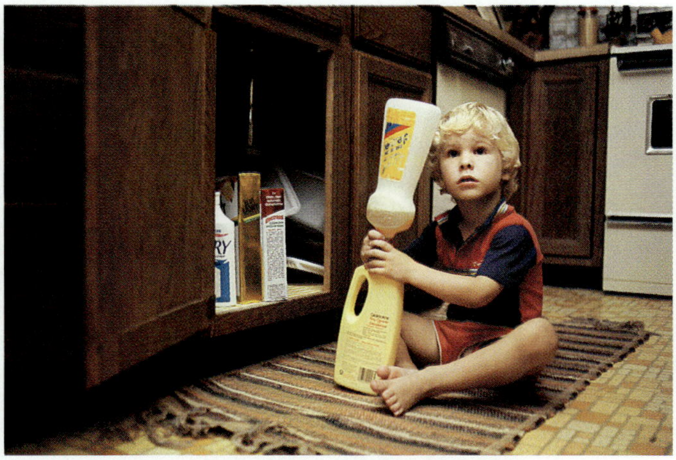 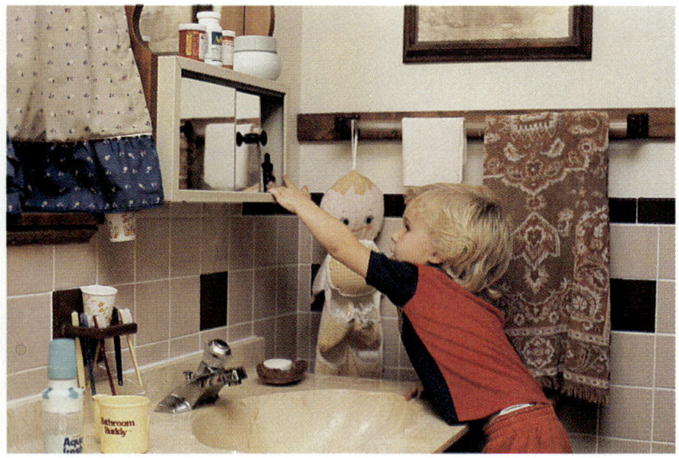 B

Fig. 8-3 *A, Household cleaners are within a child's reach when placed in cabinets under the sink. They should be kept in high, locked cabinets that are not used to store food.* ***B,*** *The bathroom medicine chest holds many medicine containers. Like household products, they should be in high, locked places out of the reach of children.*

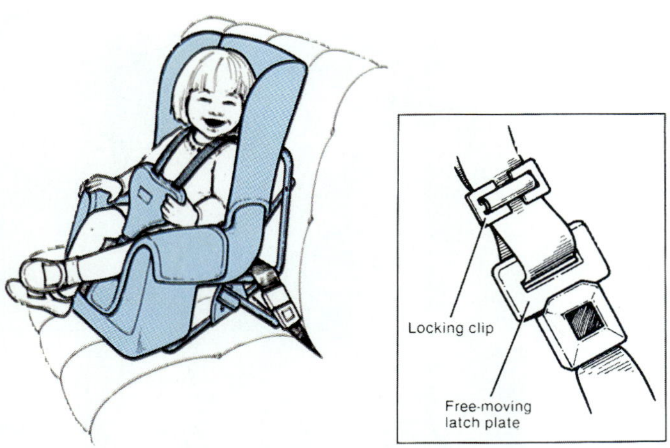

Fig. 8-4 *Child in a car restraint.* *(Courtesy of Whaley LF, Wong DL: Essentials of pediatric nursing, 1993, St Louis, Mosby–Year Book.)*

Awareness of Surroundings

People must be aware of their surroundings to protect themselves from injury. Some persons are not aware. They are unconscious or in a **coma.** A person in a coma cannot react or respond to people, places, or things. The person relies on others for protection.

Confusion and disorientation occur in some elderly people and in persons with certain diseases and injuries. These people have a reduced awareness of their surroundings. They may not understand what is happening to and around them. Confused and disoriented people can be dangerous to themselves and others.

Vision

People with poor vision have difficulty seeing. They are at risk for falling or tripping because of toys, rugs, furniture, or electrical cords in their paths. They may also have problems reading labels on medicines, cleaners, and other containers. Taking the wrong medicine, the wrong dose, or poisoning can result from not being able to read labels.

Hearing

Hearing-impaired persons have problems hearing warning signals. Fire alarms, emergency vehicle sirens, weather warnings, and tornado sirens may not be heard. These people may not know of the need to move to a safe place or away from an emergency vehicle. They may have problems hearing oncoming cars and car horns.

Smell and Touch

The senses of smell and touch can be affected by age and illness. If smell is reduced, there may be problems smelling smoke or gas. Persons with a reduced sense of touch are easily burned. They have difficulty sensing between heat and cold.

Paralysis

Paraplegic persons are paralyzed from the waist down. **Quadriplegic** persons are paralyzed from the neck down. Those with **hemiplegia** are paralyzed on one side of the body. These people may be unable to sense pain, heat, or cold. They may be aware of their surroundings and danger, but unable to move to safety.

Medications

Medications have different side effects on different people. Loss of balance, reduced awareness, confusion, disorientation, drowsiness, and loss of coordination are some of the many side effects. These sensations may be new and frightening to the person. The person may be fearful, uncooperative, or act in unusual ways as a result.

SAFETY IN THE HOME

Most home accidents can be prevented. Common sense and simple safety measures can prevent accidental injuries. If you provide home care, check to see that measures have been taken to prevent accidents in the home. The nurse is consulted if there are safety hazards.

Falls

Falls are the most common home accidents, especially among the elderly. Most falls occur in bedrooms and bathrooms. They are usually due to slippery floors, throw rugs, poor lighting, cluttered floors, furniture that is out of place, pets underfoot, and slippery bathtubs and showers. The measures in Box 8-2 can prevent falls in the home. They also prevent falls in hospitals and nursing facilities.

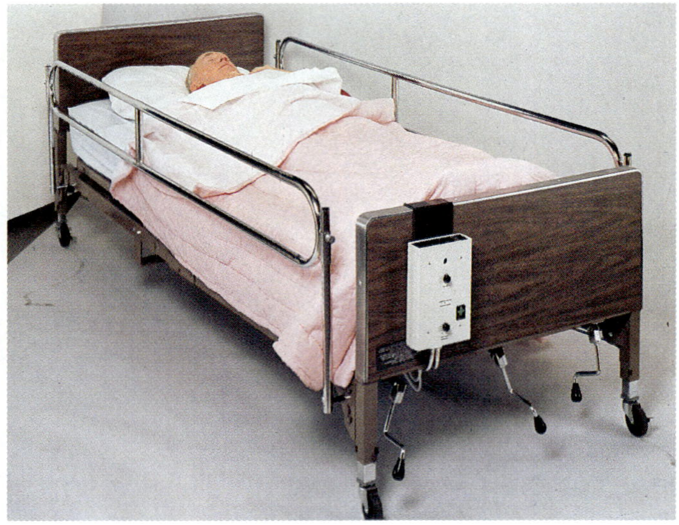

Fig. 8-5 *Weight-sensitive alarm.* (Courtesy of Posey Co., Arcadia, CA)

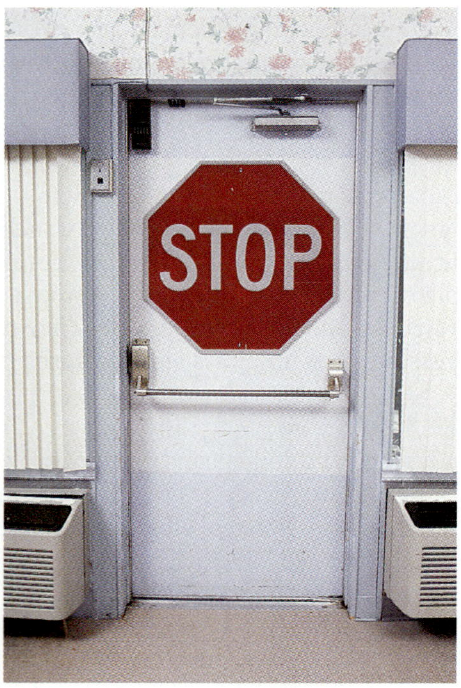

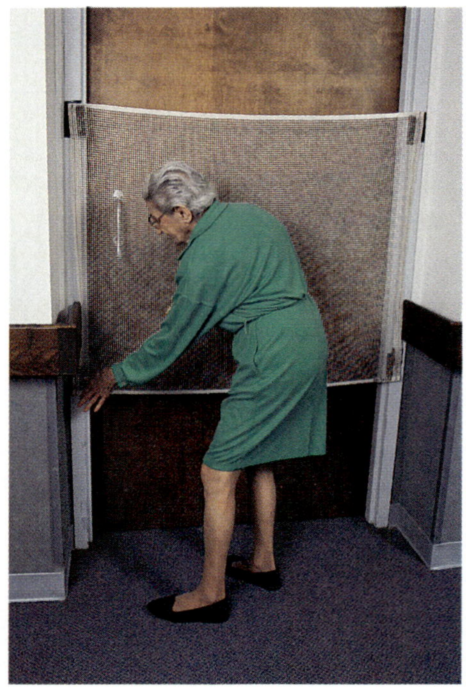

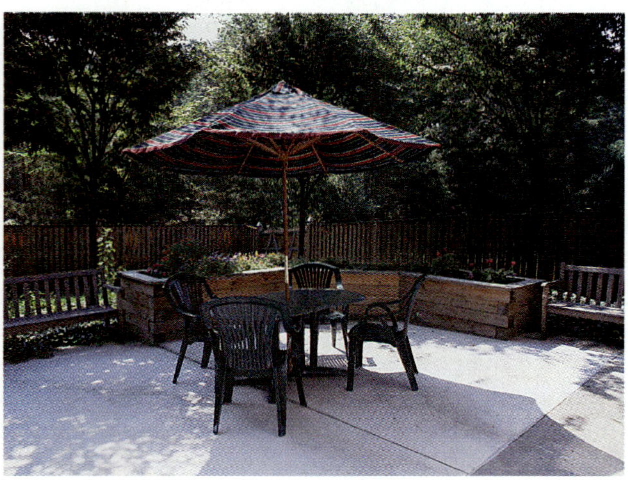

Fig. 8-6 *Barriers prevent wandering.*

BOX 8-2 Safety Measures to Prevent Falls

- Good lighting in rooms, hallways, and bathrooms
- Light switches within reach and easy to find; this includes light switches in bathrooms
- Night-lights in bedrooms, hallways, and bathrooms
- Hand rails on both sides of stairs and in bathrooms
- Safety rails and grab bars in showers, tubs, and next to the toilet
- Wall-to-wall carpeting or carpeting that is tacked down; avoid scatter, area, and throw rugs
- One-colored floor coverings; bold designs can cause dizziness in the elderly
- Nonglare, nonslip floor surfaces
- Nonskid wax on hardwood, tiled, or linoleum floors
- Uncluttered floors and stairs that are free of toys, electrical cords, and other items that can cause tripping; bathroom floors should also be uncluttered
- Floors free of spills and excess furniture
- Electric and extension cords kept out of the way
- Furniture arrangements that allow for easy movement
- Rearranging furniture is avoided
- Chairs with armrests that give support when sitting and standing
- Telephone and lamp at the bedside
- Nonslip surfaces or nonslip bathmats in tubs and showers
- Nonskid shoes and slippers
- Clothing that fits properly and is not loose or dragging on the floor

Additional measures for persons at risk of falling

- Call bells are answered promptly; the person may need immediate assistance or may not wait for help
- The call bell is always within the person's reach; the person is taught how to use the bell and is encouraged to call for help whenever help is needed (see Chapter 11)
- The person is asked to call for assistance when help is needed in getting out of bed or a chair or when walking
- Frequent checks are made on persons with poor judgment or memory
- The person is in a room close to the nurses' station
- Family and friends are asked to visit during busy times and during the evening and night shifts
- Companionship is provided; arrangements are made for sitters, companions, or volunteers to be with the person
- Electronic warning devices are used, such as weight-sensitive alarms for beds and chairs (Fig. 8-5)
- Explanations are given often about medical devices and treatments
- Sensory overload and sleep deprivation are prevented (see Chapter 20)
- Pillows or wedge pads or seats keep the person correctly positioned (see Chapter 10)
- The bed is close to the floor; it may be necessary to place the mattress on the floor
- Nonslip strips are on the floor next to the bed and in the bathroom
- The bedpan, urinal, or commode is offered or the person is assisted to the bathroom at regular times
- Distraction techniques are used: television, radio, soft music
- Companionship is provided
- A warm drink, soft lights, or a back massage is used to calm the agitated person
- Barriers prevent wandering (Fig. 8-6)
- The bed is in the lowest horizontal position, except when giving bedside nursing care; the distance from the bed to the floor is reduced if the person falls or gets out of bed
- Side rails are kept up, if ordered, when the bed is raised
- The person wears nonskid shoes or slippers rather than soft bedroom slippers
- Crutches, canes, and walkers have nonskid tips, which prevent slipping or skidding on floors
- Wheelchair brakes are in working order
- Wheels of beds, wheelchairs, and stretchers are locked when transferring persons
- Caution is used when turning corners, entering corridor intersections, and going through doors; a person coming from the opposite direction could be injured
- A safety check is made of the room after visitors leave; they may have lowered a side rail, removed the call bell, moved a walker out of reach, or brought an item that could present dangers to the person

BOX 8-3 Safety Measures to Prevent Burns

- Keep matches out of the reach of children
- Supervise the play of children
- Never leave children at home alone
- Teach children fire safety, fire prevention measures, and the dangers of fire
- Turn handles of pots on stoves so they do not point outward where people stand and walk (Fig. 8-7)
- Supervise the smoking of adults who cannot protect themselves
- Do not allow smoking in bed
- Keep space heaters and materials that can catch fire away from children
- Measure the temperature of bath water (see Chapter 13)
- Do not leave children unattended in bathtubs; they may turn on the hot water
- Supervise children who are eating to prevent spills of hot foods; also supervise persons who are eating in bed and the elderly who are at risk for spilling
- Apply warm applications correctly (see Chapter 23)
- Use electrical appliances correctly

Burns

Burns are a leading cause of death, especially among children and the elderly. Common causes of home fires are smoking in bed, spilling hot liquids, children playing with matches, charcoal grills, fireplaces, and stoves (Fig. 8-7). Box 8-3 lists safety measures to prevent burns.

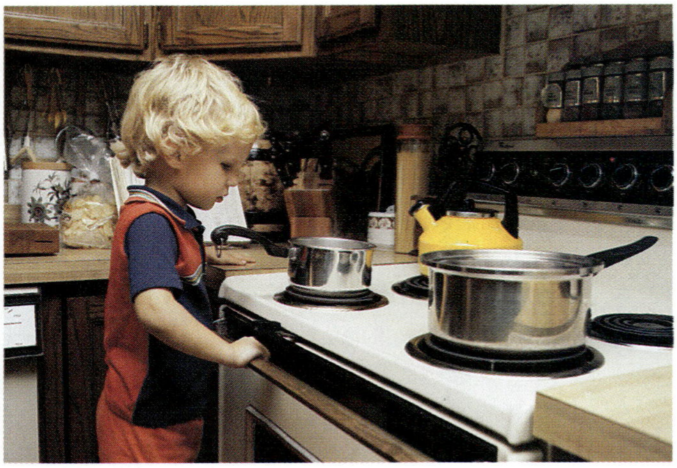

Fig. 8-7 *This child is in danger of being burned from hot water. Other burns could result if the stove is hot. Pot handles should be turned inward.*

Poisoning

Accidental poisoning is another major cause of death. Children are often victims. Aspirin and household products are the most common poisons. Poisoning in adults may be accidental from carelessness or poor vision when reading labels. Poisoning can also occur from taking too much medication. Confused or disoriented persons can forget that medication was already taken. Or they take more medication than the amount ordered. Sometimes poisoning is a suicide attempt. Box 8-4 lists the measures that prevent poisoning.

Suffocation

Suffocation is the termination of breathing that results from lack of oxygen. Death occurs if the person does not start breathing. Common causes of suffocation include choking on an object, drowning, inhaling gas or smoke, strangulation, and electrical shock. Carbon monoxide poisoning also results in the lack of oxygen. The person breathes in air filled with carbon monoxide rather than oxygen. Faulty exhaust systems on cars and damaged furnaces and chimneys are common causes of carbon monoxide poisoning. Safety measures to help prevent suffocation are:

- Take small bites of food and chew food slowly and thoroughly
- Make sure dentures fit properly
- Have exhaust systems on cars checked regularly
- Have gas odors promptly investigated by competent repairmen
- Have furnaces and chimneys inspected when persons in the same dwelling have signs and symptoms of carbon monoxide poisoning: headache, confusion,

BOX 8-4 Measures to Prevent Poisoning

- Keep childproof caps on all medicine containers and household products
- Label all medicine containers and household products clearly
- Store medicines and poisonous materials in a place that is high, locked, and out of the reach of children
- Store medicines and poisonous materials in their original containers and not in food containers
- Keep medicines out of purses where children may find them
- Make sure there is good lighting for reading labels
- Keep poisonous houseplants out of the reach of children
- Teach children not to eat plants, unknown foods, or leaves, stems, seeds, berries, nuts, or bark
- Place poison warning stickers ("Mr. Yuk") on household cleaners and toxic substances (Fig. 8-8)
- Never call medicine candy
- Read labels and follow directions on household products and other toxic substances
- Keep emergency phone numbers by the telephone: poison control center, police, ambulance, hospital, and doctor

Fig. 8-8 *The "Mr. Yuk" warning sticker is placed on poisonous products. (Courtesy of Children's Hospital, Pittsburgh Poison Center, Pittsburgh, PA)*

difficulty breathing, dizziness, sleepiness, or cherry-pink skin
- Open doors and windows if gas odors or signs and symptoms of carbon monoxide poisoning are noticed
- Rest for at least 1 hour after eating and before strenuous activity or swimming
- Make sure all electrical cords and appliances are in good repair
- Dispose of plastic bags (including those from dry cleaners) properly

SAFETY IN THE HEALTH CARE FACILITY

Safety hazards also exist in health care facilities. The measures that promote safety in the home also apply in health care facilities. Additional safety measures also are needed because similar and different kinds of dangers are present.

Identifying the Patient or Resident

You will care for many patients or residents while on duty. Each has different treatments, therapies, and activity limits. Patients and residents must be protected from infections, falls, and equipment accidents. Safety also means giving the right care to the right person. A person's life and health can be threatened if the wrong care is given.

Hospital patients and some nursing facility residents receive identification (ID) bracelets when admitted to the facility (Fig. 8-9 on page 158). Information on the bracelet includes the person's:

- Name
- Room and bed number
- Age
- Sex (male, female)
- Religion
- Doctor
- Facility name
- Allergies

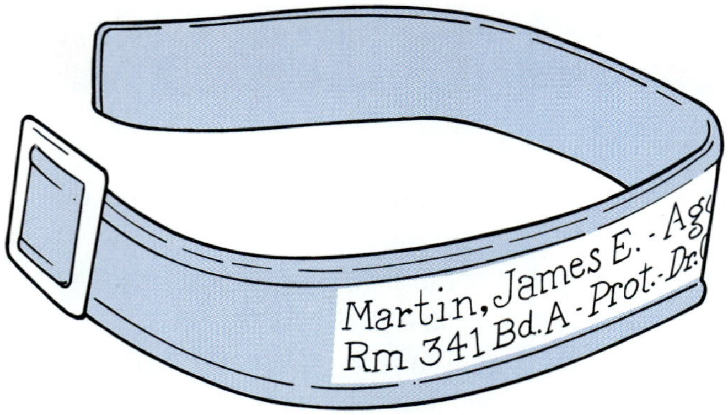

Fig. 8-9 *Patient identification bracelet.*

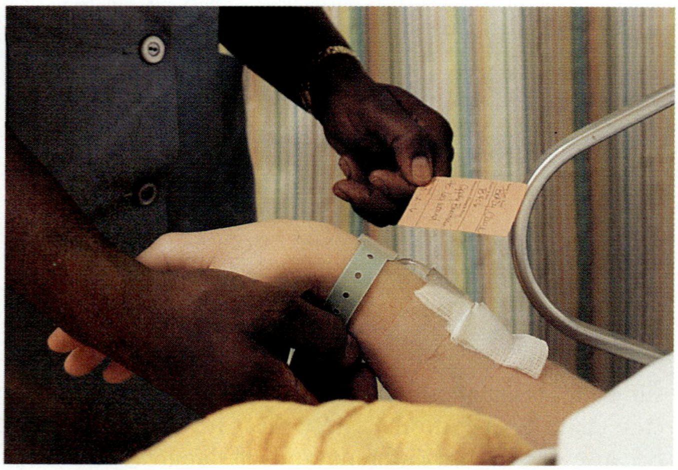

Fig. 8-10 *The nursing assistant comparing the patient's ID bracelet with a treatment card to accurately identify the patient.*

The ID bracelet is used to identify the person before giving care. Some facilities have treatment cards for each treatment or therapy ordered by the doctor. To identify the person, the identifying information on the treatment card is compared with that on the ID bracelet (Fig. 8-10). Comparing the treatment card and the ID bracelet helps ensure that care is given to the right person. Assignment sheets can be used for the same purpose if treatment cards are not used.

Also call the person by name when checking the ID bracelet. Calling the person by name is a courtesy that is given as the person is being touched and before care is given. However, calling the person by name is not a reliable way to identify the person. Confused, disoriented, drowsy, hearing-impaired, or distracted persons may answer to any name.

Nursing facility residents may not wear ID bracelets because the facility is their home. People do not wear ID bracelets in their homes. Some nursing facilities use an identification system that involves photographs. The resident's photograph is taken at the time of admission and placed in the person's medical record for identification purposes. You may work in a facility that uses photographs for identification. If so, you must learn to use the system safely.

Preventing the Spread of Microorganisms

Infection is a major hazard in health care facilities. Infections are caused by microorganisms that are easily spread from one person to another. Illness increases a person's risk of infection. The infection adds to that person's health problems. Chapter 9 describes how to prevent infection.

Preventing Falls

Falls are common safety problems in health care facilities. Besides the factors that affect the ability of persons to protect themselves, patients and residents have other problems that can cause falls. Weakness from illness, a strange environment, and sleeping in a strange bed and room increase the risk of falling. Many medications have side effects that can lead to falls. Such side effects include:

- Low blood pressure when standing or sitting
- Drowsiness
- Fainting
- Dizziness
- Poor muscle coordination
- Unsteadiness
- Frequent urination
- Confusion and disorientation
- Visual impairment

The risk of falling increases with age. Most falls are in persons between the ages of 65 and 85. Persons who have fallen before are at greater risk of falling in the health care facility. Research has shown that most falls occur in the evening, between 1800 (6:00 PM) and 2100 (9:00 PM). Falls are also more likely to occur during the change of shift: between 0600 (6:00 AM) and 0800 (8:00 AM) and between 1400 (2:00 PM) and 1600 (4:00 PM).

The need to urinate is a major cause of falls. For example, Mrs. Ford has an urgent need to urinate. She puts on her call bell but thinks she cannot wait. She tries to get up herself and falls.

The general safety measures to prevent falls must be practiced (see Box 8-2). Additional safety measures may be needed for hospital patients, nursing facility residents, or persons receiving home care (see Box 8-2). Side rails and hand rails are safety devices used to prevent falls. At one time using restraints was a common practice.

BOX 8-5 Factors Increasing the Risk of Falls

- A history of falls
- Poor vision
- Confusion
- Disorientation
- Decreased mobility
- Joint pain and stiffness
- Muscle weakness
- Low blood pressure
- Problems with balance
- Medications
- Depression
- Weakness
- Strange surroundings
- Poor judgment
- Memory problems

However, restraints can cause falls. Now restraints are used only when other measures fail.

Hospitals and nursing facilities have fall prevention programs. These programs involve measures to prevent falls in all patients or residents. Some persons have an even greater risk of falling. Box 8-5 lists the factors that increase a person's risk of falling. The nursing assessment reveals the factors that affect the person's risk of falling. The nursing care plan has measures for the person's specific risk factors. The nurse may include several of the measures listed in Box 8-2 in the person's nursing care plan.

Side rails Hospital beds have side rails which can be raised or lowered. They are locked in place by levers, latches, or buttons. They protect the person from falling out of bed. The person can use the side rails to move and turn in bed. Side rails can be half, three quarters, or the full length of the bed (Fig. 8-11). If the half length is used (see Fig. 12-3, p. 266), there are usually two rails on each side. One is for the upper part of the bed and the other for the lower part.

Side rails are necessary for persons who are unconscious, sedated with medication, confused, or disoriented. Side rails are kept up at all times for these persons, except when giving bedside nursing care. The nurse tells you which patients or residents require side rails.

Many people are embarrassed by the use of side rails. They feel like children. Nurses decide if side rails are needed for adults who are physically and mentally stable. Some facilities do not require side rails if the person signs a statement releasing the facility from responsibility for falls. If a person objects to side rails, report the concern to the nurse. Patients and residents must be protected physically. However, their esteem, dignity, and quality of life must also be protected.

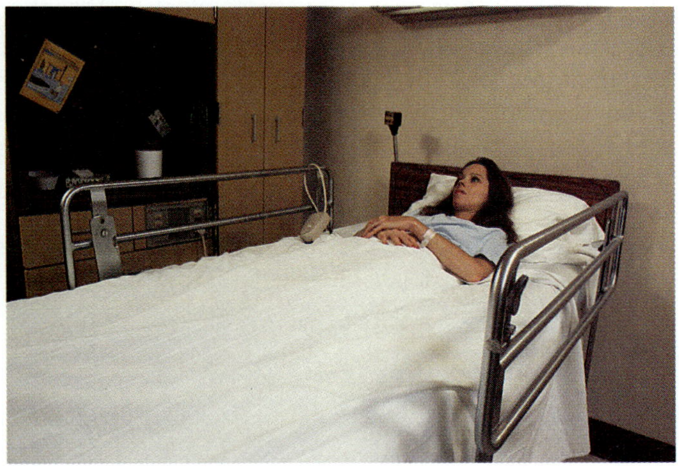

Fig. 8-11 *Hospital bed with side rails locked in the raised position.*

Side rails keep people from getting out of bed. Therefore, they are considered restraints under OBRA. They are not used without consent from the person or the person's legal representative. Restraints and OBRA requirements are discussed on page 160.

The procedures in this book include using side rails. This is done to help you to remember their importance and how to use them correctly. If a person uses his or her right not to have side rails, they are not used. You can then omit the steps asking you to lower the side rail at the beginning of the procedure and to raise the side rails at the end of the procedure. *However, whenever the bed is raised to give care or perform a procedure, the side rails must be raised to prevent the person from falling. The right not to use side rails applies only when the bed is in its lowest position. Be sure to explain to the person why the side rails are being used.*

Hand rails and grab bars Hand rails are in hallways (Fig. 8-12), stairways, and bathrooms (see Fig. 11-17, page 260) in nursing facilities and hospitals. If home care is required, hand rails may be installed in bathrooms and other parts of the home.

Hand rails provide support for persons who are weak or unsteady when walking. They also provide support for sitting down on or getting up from a toilet. Grab bars are along bathtubs for use in getting in and out of the tub.

Restraints (Protective Devices)

A **restraint** is any item, object, device, garment, material, or chemical that restricts a person's freedom of movement or access to one's body. Restraints are used only as a last resort to protect persons from harming themselves or others. Restraints are classified as physical or chemical.

Restraints can cause serious injury and even death. Therefore OBRA and the Joint Commission on Accreditation of Health Care Organizations (JCAHO) have guidelines about use of restraints. The Food and Drug Administration (FDA) also has issued warnings about restraints. OBRA states that residents have the right to be free from restraint (see Chapter 7). No physical or chemical restraint can be used to discipline a person or for staff convenience. According to OBRA guidelines, to discipline a person means to take any action that punishes or penalizes the person. Convenience is any action that

- Controls the person's behavior
- Requires less effort by the facility
- Is not in the person's best interests

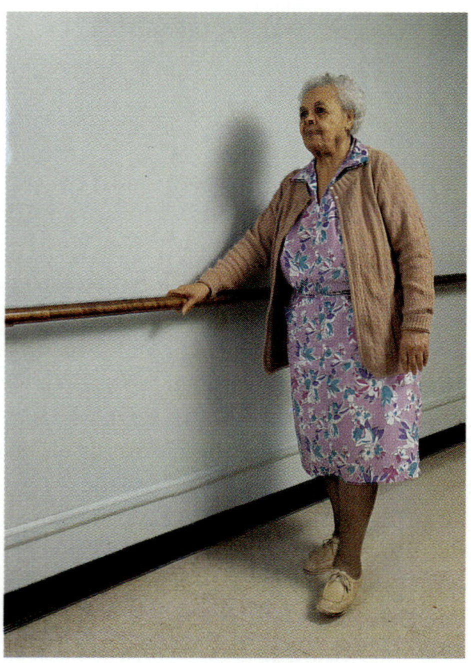

Fig. 8-12 *An elderly woman using the hand rails for support when walking.*

OBRA allows restraints only "to ensure the physical safety of the resident or of other residents." Many nursing facilities are restraint free and more are becoming so.

What does it mean to ensure the physical safety of the person or others? It means that persons are protected from *harming* themselves or others. Certain behaviors can be harmful to the person or to others in the area. They include:

- Getting out of bed, a chair or wheelchair, or a stretcher when assistance is required
- Crawling over side rails or the foot of the bed
- Interfering with treatment (pulling out tubes, removing dressings, or disconnecting equipment)
- Wandering in or away from the facility
- Agitated or combative behavior toward staff, family, or other patients or residents

Restraints were often used to prevent falls. However, research has shown that restraints actually cause falls. Falls occur when persons try to get free of the restraints. Thus restrained persons are at risk for falls. Research has shown that more serious injuries occur from falls in restrained persons than in nonrestrained persons.

Certain persons were more commonly restrained than others. Restraints were common in persons with physical problems who also were confused, showed poor judgment, or had behavior problems. Elderly persons were more likely to be restrained than younger persons. *Now, all other alternatives must be tried before restraints can be used.*

Physical restraints have been defined by law. The definition includes the following key points:

- May be any manual method, physical or mechanical device, material or equipment
- Are attached to or next to the person's body
- Cannot be easily removed by the person
- Restrict freedom of movement or access to one's body

If used, the restraint confines the person to a bed or chair or prevents movement of a body part. Restraints can be applied to the chest, waist, elbows, wrists, hands, or legs. Commercial restraints are made of cloth or leather. Certain furniture or barriers also prevent free movement. Geriatric chairs (Geri-chairs) or chairs with attached trays are examples (Fig. 8-13). Such chairs are often used for persons who need support to sit up. Positioning any chair so close to a wall that the person cannot move is another form of restraint. Side rails are also restraints under

OBRA. So are sheets that are tucked in so tightly that they restrict movement.

OBRA guidelines define *chemical restraints* as drugs used to discipline a person or for staff convenience. A drug is considered a chemical restraint if it is not required to treat the person's medical symptoms. Drugs are considered chemical restraints when they affect the person's physical and mental function.

The many serious complications from restraint use are listed in Box 8-6. Injuries can occur as the person tries to become free of the restraint. Cuts, bruises, and fractures are common injuries. Injuries can also occur from using the wrong restraint, applying it wrong, or keeping it on too long. *The most serious risk of being restrained is death from strangulation.* There are also psychological effects on the person. Being restrained affects a person's dignity and esteem. Depression, anger, and agitation are common in restrained persons. So are embarrassment, humiliation, and mistrust.

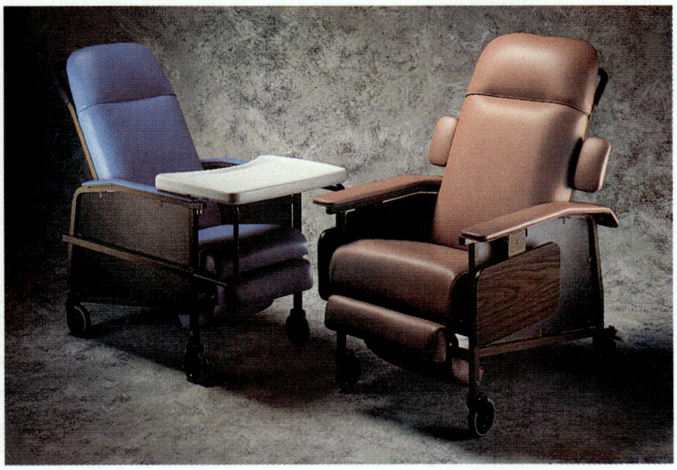

Fig. 8-13 *A Geri-chair with tray is considered a restraint.* *(Courtesy of Invacare Corporation, Elyria, OH)*

OBRA and JCAHO do not forbid the use of restraints. Restraints can be used only after all other alternatives have been tried. Box 8-7 on page 162 lists restraint alternatives that the nurse may include in the person's care plan. *If a restraint is used, the least restrictive method must be used.* Restraints can be used as a temporary measure when emergency medical treatment is needed.

Remember the following about using restraints.

- *Restraints are used to protect the person, not for staff convenience.* Restraining a person is thought to be easier for the staff than properly supervising and observing the person. Actually, a restrained person requires more staff time for care, supervision, and observation. A restraint is used only when it is the best safety precaution for the person. It must not be used to punish uncooperative persons.
- *Restraints require a doctor's order.* OBRA, JCAHO, and state laws protect persons from unnecessary restraint. Health care facilities must have policies and procedures about restraint use. If a person needs to be restrained for medical reasons, there must be a written doctor's order. The doctor is required by law to give the reason for the restraint and the type to be used. The order also must include how long the restraint is to be applied. All this information is on the person's Kardex and nursing care plan. You need to know the laws and policies about using restraints where you work.
- *The least restrictive method must be used.* There are active physical restraints and passive physical restraints. An **active physical restraint** is attached to the person's body and to a stationary (nonmovable)

BOX 8-6 Risks of Restraint Use

- Agitation
- Anal incontinence (see Chapter 16)
- Anger
- Bruises
- Cuts
- Dehydration
- Depression
- Embarrassment
- Fractures
- Humiliation
- Mistrust
- Nerve injuries
- Nosocomial infection (see Chapter 9)
- Pneumonia
- Pressure sores (see Chapter 13)
- Strangulation
- Urinary incontinence (see Chapter 15)
- Urinary tract infection

BOX 8-7 ALTERNATIVES TO RESTRAINTS

- Diversion activities: television, videos, music, games, books, relaxation tapes, etc.
- Pillows and positioning aids
- Meeting food, fluid, and elimination needs
- Visits by family, friends, and volunteers
- Arranging for companions and sitters
- Spending time with the person
- Reminisce with the person
- Allowing wandering in a safe area
- Exercise program
- Outdoor time
- Jobs or tasks the person consents to
- Electronic warning devices on beds and doors
- Measures to prevent falls (see Box 8-2)
- Reclining chairs
- Frequent observation
- Moving the person closer to the nurses' station
- Frequent explanations about required medical equipment or devices
- Orienting confused individuals to person, time, and place
- Good lighting
- Consistent staff assignments
- Promoting uninterrupted sleep

object. It restricts the person's movement or access to one's body. Vest, leg, arm, wrist, hand, and some belt restraints are physical restraints. A **passive physical restraint** is near but not directly attached to the person's body. It does not totally restrict freedom of movement and allows access to certain body parts. The quick-release belt is a passive physical restraint. Passive physical restraints are the least restrictive. Belts are less restrictive than vests. For example, Mrs. Ford feels that both legs are intact even though the left one was amputated. She often tries to get up without asking for help. The quick-release lap belt reminds her to ask for help. In addition, she can release the belt herself.

- *Restraints are used only after trying other methods to control or protect the person.* The nurse uses the nursing process to identify the person's needs and problems and to plan care measures. Goals and the nursing care plan center on the person's needs and problems. The nursing measures also must protect the person's dignity and promote quality of life. Some people are at risk for harming themselves or others. Therefore the nursing care plan must include measures to protect the person and to prevent the person from harming others. Remember, restraints diminish the person's dignity and quality of life. They can be used only after other measures fail to provide needed protection. Many of the measures to prevent falls are alternatives to the use of restraints (see Box 8-2).
- *Unnecessary restraint is false imprisonment (see Chapter 2).* If you are told to apply a restraint, you must clearly see and understand the need. If not, politely ask for an explanation. If you apply a restraint unnecessarily, you may be charged with false imprisonment.
- *Restraints require the person's informed consent.* The person must be informed of the reason for the restraint. The person is told how the restraint will help the planned medical treatment. The person must also be informed of problems that could occur from being restrained. If the person cannot give informed consent, the person's legal representative must be given the necessary information. Either the person or legal representative must give consent. If it is not given, the restraint cannot be used. The doctor or nurse is responsible for providing the necessary information and obtaining the informed consent.
- *Restraints must be used according to the manufacturer's instructions.* The manufacturer gives specific instructions on how to apply and secure the restraint. Failure to follow such instructions could affect the person's safety. You could be found negligent for improperly applying or securing a restraint.

- *The restrained person's basic needs must be met by the nursing team.* The restraint should be snug and firm, but not tight. A tight restraint may interfere with circulation and breathing. The person must be comfortable. Movement of the restrained part must be possible to a limited and safe extent. The person is checked at least every 15 minutes. Food, fluid, and elimination needs must also be met.
- *Restraints may have to be applied rapidly.* They must be applied with enough help to protect the person and staff from injury. Persons in immediate danger of harming themselves or others need to be restrained quickly. Combative and agitated people can hurt themselves and the staff when restraints are being applied. Enough staff members are needed to complete the task safely and efficiently.
- *A person may become more confused or agitated after being restrained.* Whether confused or alert, people are aware of restricted body movements. The person may try to get out of the restraint or struggle or pull at it. Many restrained persons beg anyone who passes by to set them free or to help release them. These behaviors are often viewed as signs of confusion. Confused persons may become more confused because they do not understand what is happening to them. Persons who are restrained need repeated explanations and reassurance. Spending time with the person often has a calming effect.
- *The person's quality of life must be protected.* Restraints should be used for as short a time as possible. The person's care plan shows how restraint use will slowly be reduced. The goal is to meet the person's needs using as little restraint as possible. Besides meeting physical needs, you must also meet the person's psychosocial needs. You can meet these needs by visiting with the person, explaining the purpose of the restraints, and taking residents to activities.

Safety rules Though used to protect the person, restraints can be dangerous. The person must be observed often. Complications from being restrained must be prevented, such as interferences with breathing and circulation. You should practice the safety measures in Box 8-8 on page 164 when caring for a restrained person.

BOX 8-8 SAFETY MEASURES FOR USING RESTRAINTS

- Use the type of restraint specified by the nurse and the care plan. The nurse selects the least restrictive device.
- Never apply any restraint unless you have been instructed in its proper use. Demonstrate proper application to the nurse before using it on any person.
- Use the correct size. The nurse will tell you what size to use.
- Use only commercial restraints that have manufacturer instructions for use. Read the manufacturer's warning labels.
- Follow manufacturer's instructions for application. There are many different types of restraints. Some are safe for bed, chair, and wheelchair use. Others can be used only with certain equipment.
- Do not use sheets, towels, tape, rope, straps, bandages, or other items to restrain a person.
- Use intact restraints. There should be no tears, frayed edges, missing loops or straps, or other damage.
- Do not use restraints to position a person on a toilet.
- Follow facility policies and procedures when applying restraints.
- Position the person in good body alignment before applying the restraint (see Chapter 10).
- Pad bony areas and skin that may be injured by a restraint. The padding protects the body parts from pressure and injury.
- Apply the restraint securely enough to protect the person. It should be snug but allows some movement of the restrained part. Make sure that the person can breathe easily if a restraint is applied to the chest. You should be able to slide an open, flat hand between the restraint and the person's body (Fig. 8-14).
- Criss-cross vest restraints in front (Fig. 8-15). Do not criss-cross restraints in the back unless part of the manufacturer's instructions. Criss-crossing vests in the back can cause death from strangulation.
- Tie restraints according to facility policy. The policy should follow the manufacturer's instructions. The knot must be easily released in an emergency. Quick-release knots often are used (Fig. 8-16). Some restraints have quick-release buckles.
- Secure straps out of the person's reach.
- Secure the restraint to the moveable part of the bed frame or to the bed springs (see Fig. 8-16). Never secure the restraint to the side rails. Restraints are not secured to side rails because the person can reach them to release knots or buckles. Also, the person can be injured when side rails are raised and lowered. For chairs, straps are secured to the wheelchair or the chair frame (Fig. 8-17).
- Make sure full side rails are up when using a vest or belt restraint. The side rails should be padded (Fig. 8-18). The person could accidentally fall off the bed and strangle on the restraint if the side rails are not up. If half or three-quarter length side rails are used, the person could get caught between them (Fig. 8-19 on page 166).
- Position the person in a chair so the hips are well to the back of the chair. If a belt restraint is used, apply it at a 45-degree angle over the hips (Fig. 8-20 on page 166).
- Do not use back cushions when a person is restrained in a chair. If the cushion moves out of place, there will be slack in the straps. Strangulation could result if the person slides down forward or down from the extra slack (Fig. 8-21 on page 167).
- Check the person's circulation every 15 minutes if wrist or leg restraints have been applied. You should feel a pulse at a pulse site below the restraint. Fingers or toes should be warm and pink.
- Notify the nurse immediately if:
  *You cannot feel a pulse
  *Fingers or toes are cold, pale, or blue in color
  *The person complains of pain, numbness, or tingling in the restrained part
  *The skin is red or damaged
- Check the person every 15 minutes to make sure he or she is safe and comfortable. Also check the position of the restraint, especially the front and back.
- Keep scissors in your pocket. In an emergency, cutting the tie is faster than untying the knot. Never leave scissors at the bedside or where they can be reached by a patient or resident.
- Remove the restraint and reposition the person every 2 hours. Skin care is given and range-of-motion exercises are done at this time.
- Make sure the person's basic needs are met. The person must receive food and fluids. Offer a drink of water often to prevent dehydration. Help the person to the toilet or offer the bedpan or urinal every 2 hours.
- Make sure the call bell is always within the person's reach.
- Chart each time the restraint is released, the observations made, and the care given.

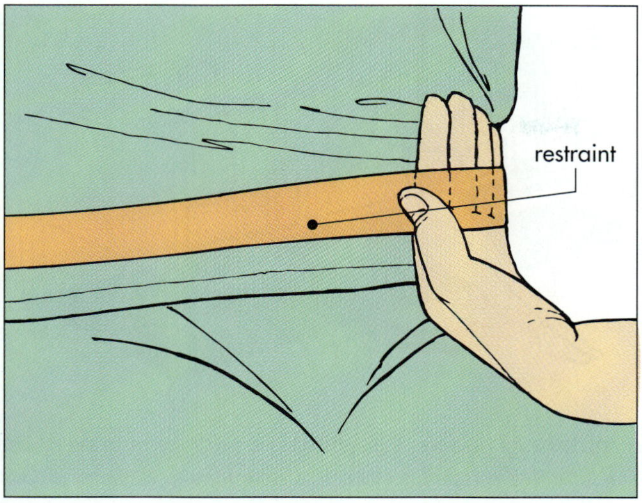

Fig. 8-14 *A flat hand should be able to slide between the restraint and the person.*

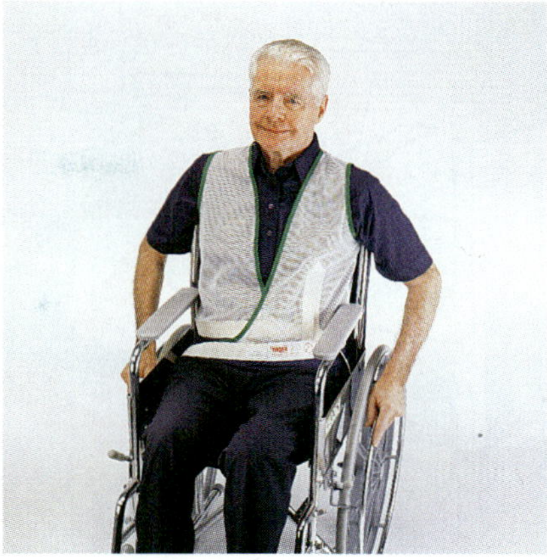

Fig. 8-15 *Vest restraint criss-crosses in front.* (*Courtesy of Posey Co., Arcadia, CA*)

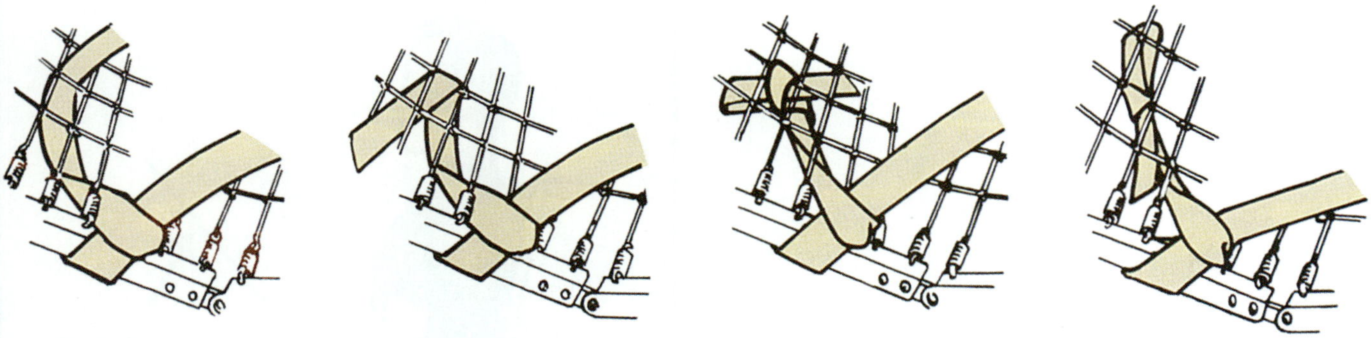

Fig. 8-16 *The Posey quick-release tie.* (*Courtesy of Posey Co., Arcadia, CA*)

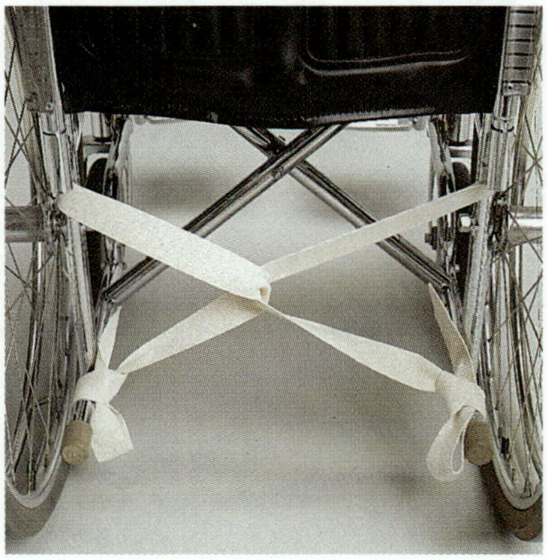

Fig. 8-17 *The restraint straps are secured to the chair frame of the wheelchair using a quick-release tie.* (*Courtesy of Posey Co., Arcadia, CA*)

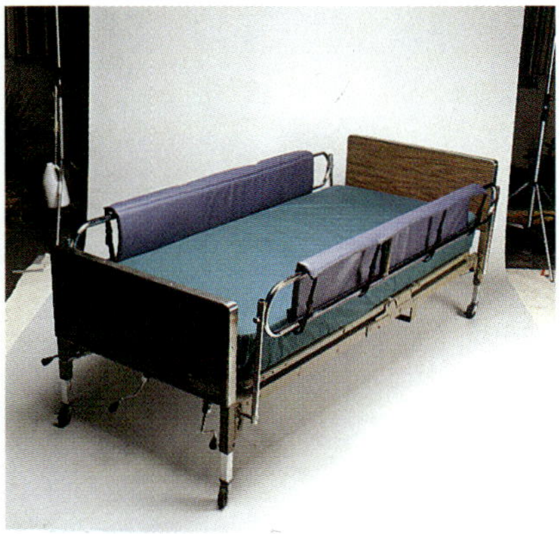

Fig. 8-18 *Padded side rails.* (*Courtesy of Posey Co., Arcadia, CA*)

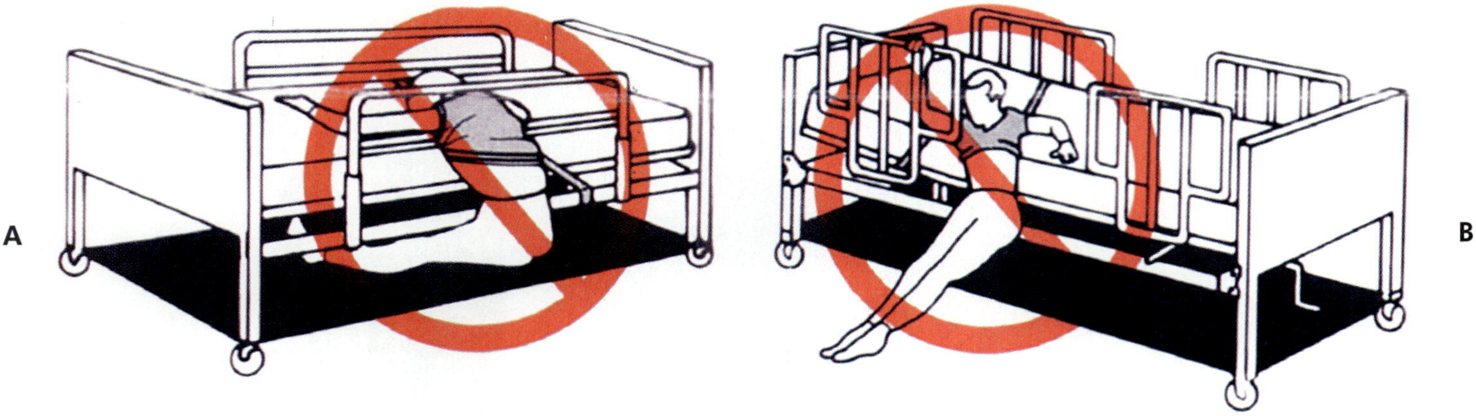

Fig. 8-19 *A, Full-length side rails should be used with a vest or belt restraint. The side rails should be padded to prevent the resident from getting caught between the rails. B, Half-length side rails are dangerous for the restrained person.* (Courtesy of Posey Co, Arcadia, CA)

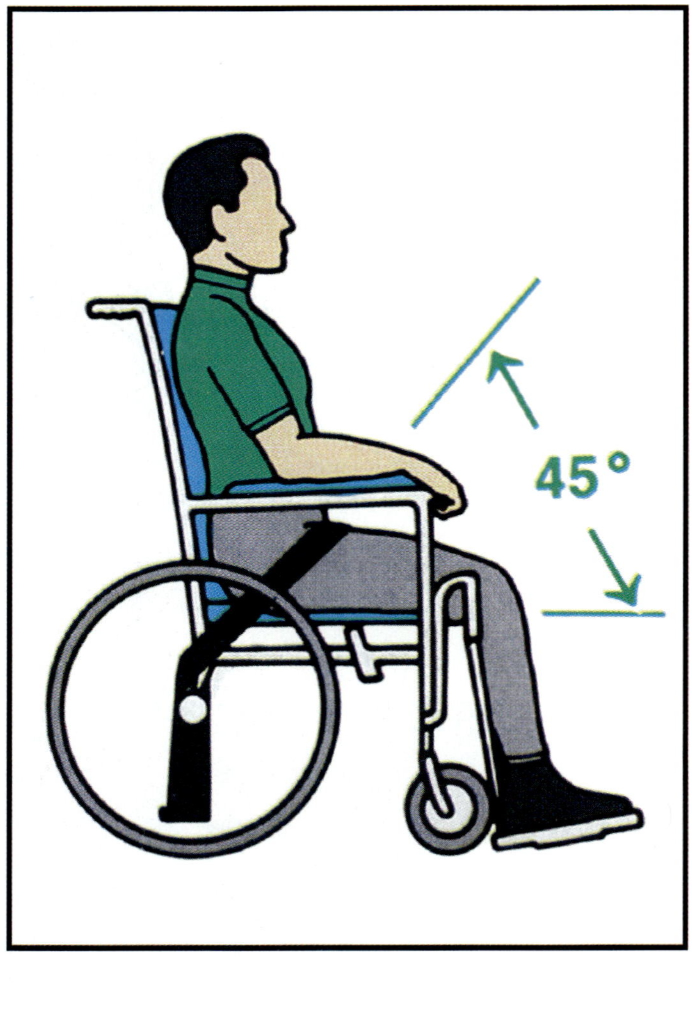

Fig. 8-20 *The safety belt is at a 45-degree angle over the person's hips.* (Courtesy of Posey Co, Arcadia, CA)

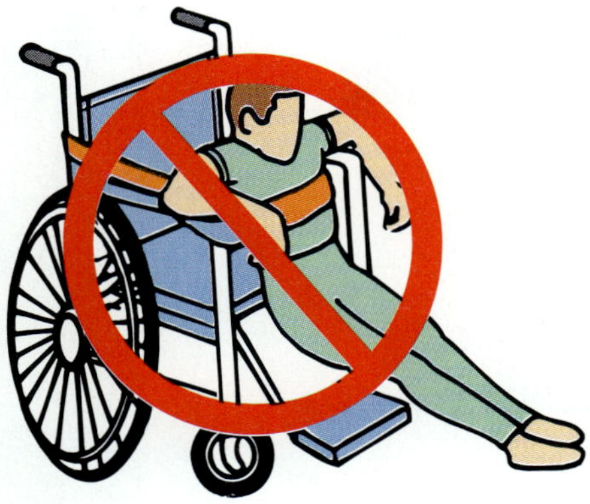

Straps to prevent sliding should always be over the thighs—NOT around the waist or chest. Straps should be at a 45° angle and secured to the chair under the seat, not behind the back. They should be snug but comfortable and not restrict breathing. If a belt or vest is too loose or applied around the waist, the patient may slide partially off the seat—resulting in the possible suffocation and death.

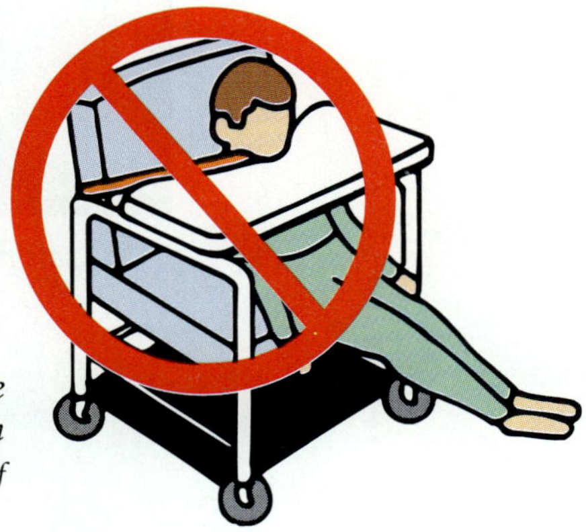

Tray tables (with or without a belt or vest) pose potential danger if the patient should slide partly under the table and become caught. This could result in suffocation and death. Make sure the patient's hips are positioned at the back of the chair—this may necessitate the use of an anti-slide material (Posey Grip), a pommel cushion, or a restrictive device if the patient shows any tendency to slide forward.

Fig. 8-21 *Strangulation could result if the person slides down forward or down from the extra slack in the restraint.* (Courtesy of Posey Co, Arcadia, CA)

Reporting and recording Certain information about restraints must be in the person's medical record. You may be instructed to apply restraints or be assigned to care for a restrained person. The following must be reported to the nurse:

- The type of restraint applied
- The time of application
- The time of removal
- The type of care given when the restraint was removed
- The color and condition of the person's skin
- Whether a pulse is felt in the restrained extremity
- Complaints of pain, numbness, or tingling in the restrained part

Wrist restraints Wrist restraints are also called hand restraints. They are used to limit the movement of an arm.

Applying Wrist Restraints

Pre-procedure

1. Get the wrist restraints.
2. Wash your hands.
3. Identify the person. Check the ID bracelet and call the person by name.
4. Explain the procedure to the person.
5. Provide for privacy.

Procedure

6. Make sure the person is comfortable and in good body alignment (see Chapter 10).
7. Apply the restraint following the manufacturer's instructions. Make sure the soft part is toward the skin (Fig. 8-22).
8. Make sure the restraint is snug but not tight. You should be able to slide two fingers under the restraint (Fig. 8-23).
9. Tie the ends to the moveable part of the bed frame or to the bed springs. Use a knot approved by the facility.
10. Repeat steps 7, 8, and 9 for the other wrist.

Post-procedure

11. Place the call bell within the person's reach.
12. Unscreen the person.
13. Wash your hands.
14. Check the person and the restraints at least every 15 minutes. Check the pulse, color, and temperature of the restrained wrist or ankle. Report your observations to the nurse.
15. Do the following at least every 2 hours:
    - Remove the restraints.
    - Reposition the person.
    - Meet the person's needs for food, fluids, and elimination.
    - Give skin care.
    - Perform range-of-motion exercises.
    - Reapply the restraints.
16. Report your observations to the nurse. Include the care given when the restraints were removed.

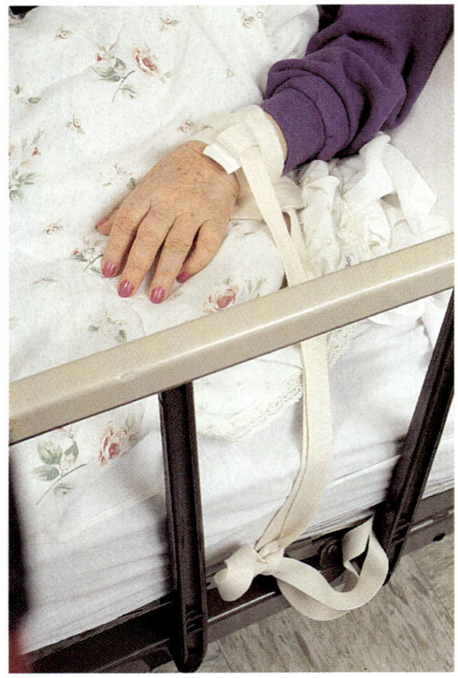

Fig. 8-22 *The soft part of the restraint is toward the skin.*

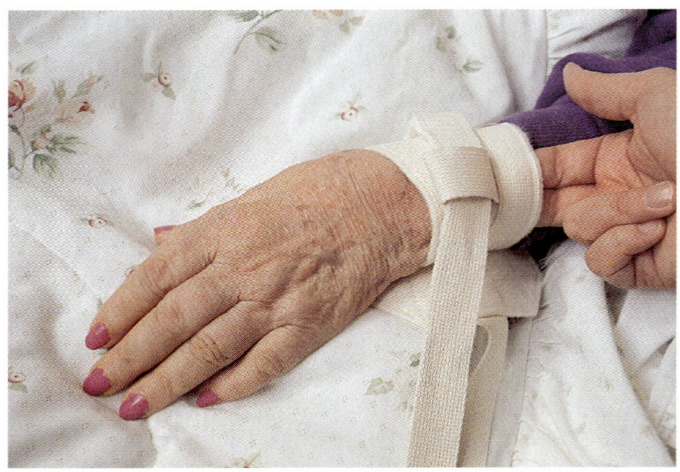

Fig. 8-23 *Two fingers should be able to fit between the restraint and the wrist.*

Mitt restraints A person's hands are placed in mitt restraints. They prevent use of the fingers but do not prevent hand, wrist, or arm movements. Mitt restraints are thumbless and prevent the person from scratching, pulling out tubes, or removing dressings. The person may be given a hand roll to grasp so the fingers are kept in a normal position. Hand rolls are not needed with padded mitts (Fig. 8-24).

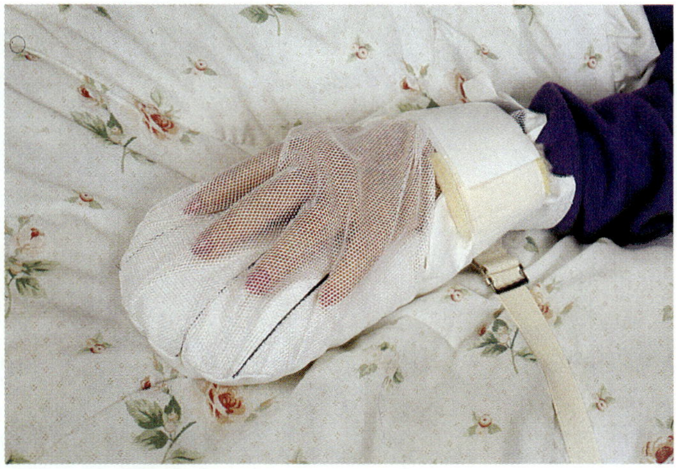

Fig. 8-24 *Padded mitt restraint.* *(Courtesy of Posey Co, Arcadia, CA)*

Applying Mitt Restraints

Pre-procedure

1. Collect the following equipment:
   - Two mitt restraints
   - Two washcloths or two commercial hand rolls if the mitts are not padded
   - Tape if wash cloths are used
2. Make the hand rolls as in Figure 8-25 or use commercial ones.
3. Wash your hands.
4. Identify the person. Check the ID bracelet and call the person by name.
5. Explain the procedure to the person.
6. Provide for privacy.

Procedure

7. Make sure the person's hands are clean and dry.
8. Give the person a hand roll to grasp if a padded mitt is not used.
9. Apply the mitt restraint (Fig. 8-26) following the manufacturer's instructions.
10. Tie the ends to the movable part of the bed frame or to the bed springs. Use a knot approved by the facility.
11. Repeat steps 8, 9, and 10 for the other hand.

Post-procedure

12. Place the call bell within the person's reach.
13. Unscreen the person.
14. Wash your hands.
15. Check the person and the restraints at least every 15 minutes.
16. Do the following at least every 2 hours:
    - Remove the restraints.
    - Reposition the person.
    - Meet the person's needs for food, fluids, and elimination.
    - Give skin care.
    - Perform range-of-motion exercises.
    - Reapply the restraints.
17. Report your observations to the nurse. Include the care given when the restraints were removed.

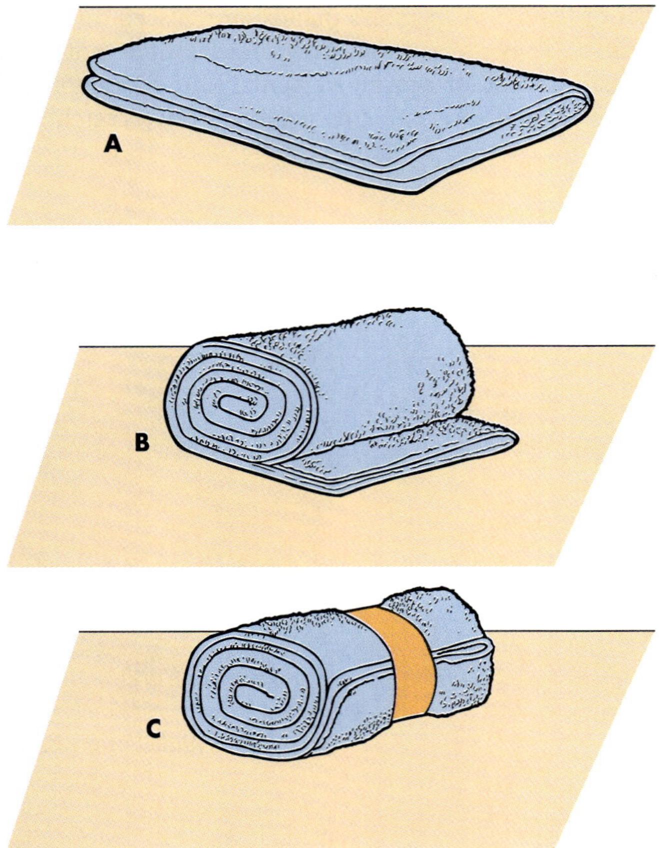

Fig. 8-25 *Make a hand roll from a washcloth.* **A,** *Fold the washcloth in half.* **B,** *Roll up the washcloth.* **C,** *Tape the rolled washcloth.*

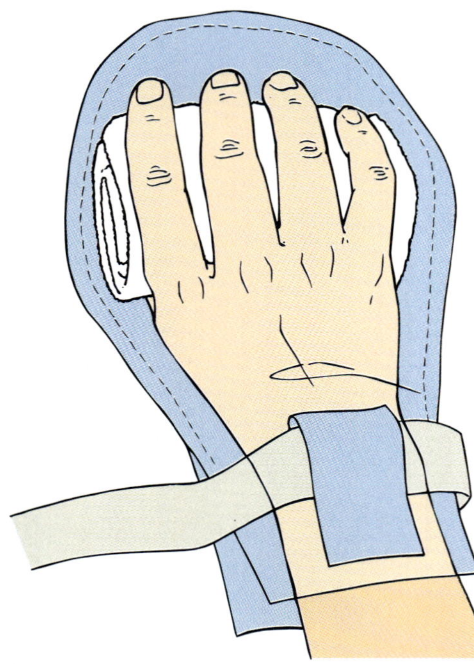

Fig. 8-26 *Mitt restraint. Person is holding a hand roll.*

Applying a Vest Restraint

Pre-procedure

1. Collect the following:
   - Vest restraint (the nurse tells you the size)
   - Pads for the side rails
2. Get assistance if needed.
3. Wash your hands.
4. Identify the person. Check the ID bracelet and call the person by name.
5. Explain the procedure to the person.
6. Provide for privacy.

Procedure

7. Put the pads on the side rails if the person is in bed.
8. Assist the person to a sitting position (if he or she is lying down) by locking arms with the person (see page 164).
9. Apply the restraint with your free hand. Remember to follow the manufacturer's instructions. The vest crosses in front.
10. Make sure there are no wrinkles in the front or back of the restraint.
11. Help the person lie down if he or she is in bed.
12. Bring the ties through the slots.
13. Make sure the person is comfortable and in good body alignment (see Chapter 10).
14. Secure the straps to the movable part of the bed frame, the bed springs, or to the chair or wheelchair. Use a facility approved knot.
15. Make sure you can slide a flat hand under the restraint (see Fig. 8-14). Adjust the straps as needed. The restraint should be snug but not tight.

Post-procedure

16. Place the call bell within the person's reach.
17. Raise the side rails.
18. Unscreen the person.
19. Wash your hands.
20. Check the person and the restraint at least every 15 minutes.
21. Do the following at least every 2 hours:
    - Remove the restraint.
    - Reposition the person.
    - Meet the person's needs for food, fluids, and elimination.
    - Give skin care.
    - Perform range-of-motion exercises.
    - Reapply the restraint.
22. Report your observations to the nurse. Include the care given when the restraint was removed.

Vest restraints Vest restraints are applied to the chest. They are active physical restraints. The person with a vest restraint cannot get out of bed or out of a chair. The person's arms are put through the sleeves so the vest crosses in front (see Fig. 8-15). The vest must *never* cross in the back. If it crosses in the back, there is only a small neck opening at the front. If the person slides down in the bed or chair, strangulation can occur from the small neck opening. *Vest restraints always cross in the front.* The restraint is always applied over a gown, pajamas, or clothes.

The vest restraint procedure is included in this book. However, vest restraints carry great risks to the person's life. Death can occur from strangulation. If the person becomes caught in the restraint, it can become so tight that the person's chest cannot expand to inhale air. The person quickly suffocates and dies. Correct application of a restraint is always important. In the case of vest restraints it is critical. Therefore, you are advised to only assist the nurse in its application. It is best that the nurse assume full responsibility for the application of a vest restraint.

Applying a Belt Restraint

Pre-procedure

1. Obtain a belt restraint. The nurse tells you the size.
2. Get assistance if needed.
3. Wash your hands.
4. Identify the person. Check the ID bracelet and call the person by name.
5. Explain the procedure to the person.
6. Provide for privacy.

Procedure

7. Assist the patient to a sitting position (if he or she is lying down) by locking arms with the person (see page 164).
8. Apply the restraint with your free hand. Follow the manufacturer's instructions.
9. Make sure there are no wrinkles in the front or back of the restraint.
10. Bring the ties through the slots in the belt.
11. Help the person lie down if he or she is in bed.
12. Make sure the person is comfortable and in good body alignment (see Chapter 10).
13. Secure the straps to the movable part of the bed frame, the bed springs, or to the chair or wheelchair. Use a facility approved knot.

Post-procedure

14. Place the call bell within the person's reach.
15. Unscreen the person.
16. Wash your hands.
17. Check the person and the restraint at least every 15 minutes.
18. Do the following at least every 2 hours:
    - Remove the restraint.
    - Reposition the person.
    - Meet the person's needs for food, fluids, and elimination.
    - Give skin care.
    - Perform range-of-motion exercises.
    - Reapply the restraint.
19. Report your observations to the nurse. Include the care given when the restraint was removed.

Belt restraints The belt restraint (Fig. 8-27) is used for the same reasons as the vest restraint. The belt is applied around the waist and secured to the bed or chair. The belt is applied over clothes, a gown, or pajamas. There are many different types of belt restraints. The quick-release type can be released by the person. Therefore, it is less restrictive than the types that can only be released by a staff member.

Elbow restraints Elbow restraints prevent infants and small children from bending their elbows. They prevent children from scratching and touching incisions or pulling out tubes. A long-sleeved shirt is worn so the restraint can be secured in place with safety pins. Both arms are restrained to achieve the desired effect.

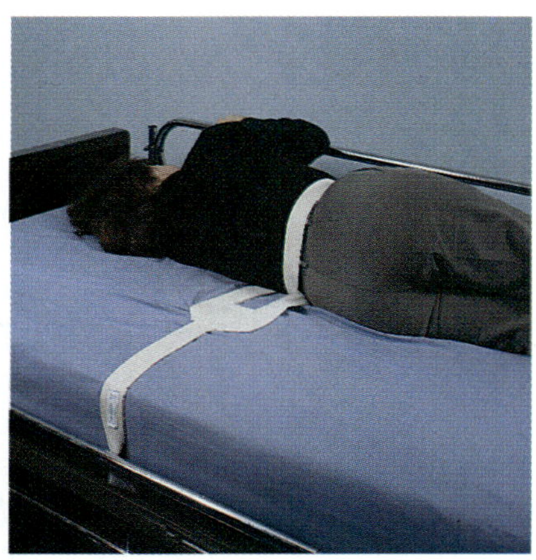

Fig. 8-27 *Roll belt.* *(Courtesy of Posey Co, Arcadia, CA)*

Applying Elbow Restraints

Pre-procedure

1. Collect the following:
   - Two elbow restraints
   - Tongue depressors
   - Safety pins
2. Insert the tongue depressors into the slots (Fig. 8-28).
3. Wash your hands.
4. Identify the child. Check the ID bracelet and call the child by name.
5. Explain the procedure to the child and parents.
6. Provide for privacy.

Procedure

7. Wrap the restraint around the child's elbow.
8. Tie the strings around the arm.
9. Pin the restraint to the child's shirt to prevent the restraint from sliding down the arm. The pins should point down and away from the child as in Figure 8-29.
10. Repeat steps 7, 8, and 9 to apply the other restraint.

Post-procedure

11. Place the call bell within the child's or parents' reach.
12. Unscreen the child.
13. Wash your hands.
14. Check the child and the restraints often.
15. Do the following at least every 2 hours:
    - Remove the restraint.
    - Reposition the child.
    - Meet the child's needs for food, fluids, and elimination.
    - Give skin care.
    - Perform range-of-motion exercises.
    - Reapply the restraint.
16. Report your observations to the nurse. Include the care given when the restraint was removed.

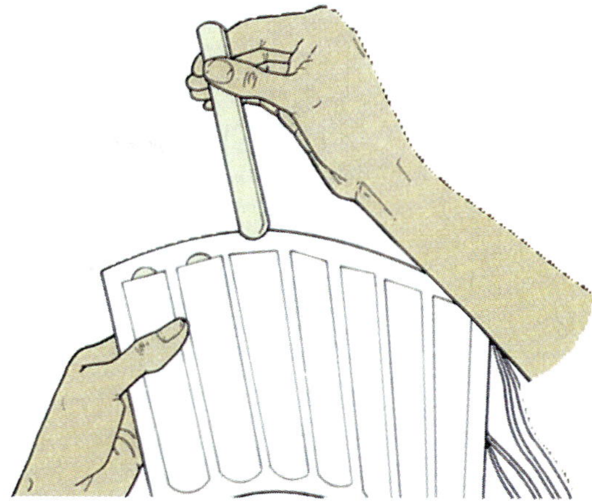

Fig. 8-28 *Tongue depressors keep the elbow restraint rigid.*

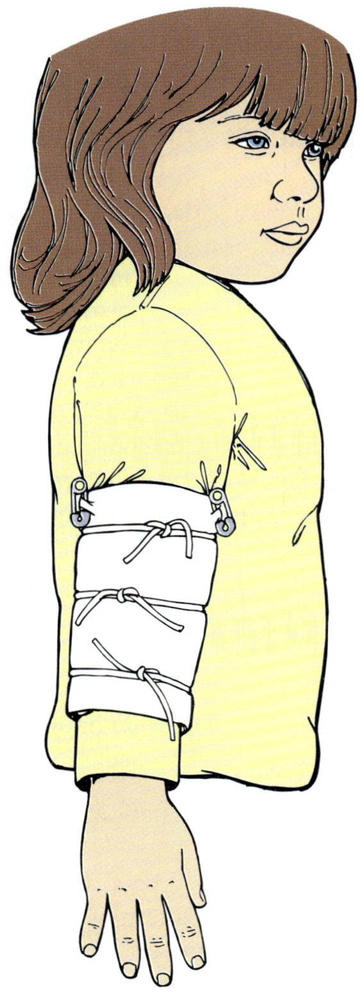

Fig. 8-29 *An elbow restraint is secured to the shirt with safety pins. The pins should point down and away from the child.*

Equipment Accidents

Glass and plastic items are inspected before use. They are checked for cracks, chips, and sharp or rough edges. All these can cause cuts, stabs, or scratches. Damaged equipment is not used or given to patients or residents. Instead, take the item to the nurse, point out the defect, and discard the item as instructed. The bloodborne pathogen standard is followed when discarding such items (see Chapter 9).

Electric equipment must function properly and be in good repair. Frayed cords (Fig. 8-30) and overloaded electrical outlets (Fig. 8-31) can cause electrical shocks that may result in death. Fires may also result. Frayed cords and equipment that does not function properly must be repaired by a trained person.

Three-pronged plugs (Fig. 8-32) are used on all equipment. Two prongs carry electrical current and the third prong is the ground. A **ground** carries leaking electricity to the earth and away from the item. If a ground is not used, leaking electricity can be conducted to a person and cause electrical shocks and possible death. Any shock received while using a piece of equipment must be immediately reported. The item is sent for repair immediately. Obtain a new item to give the required care.

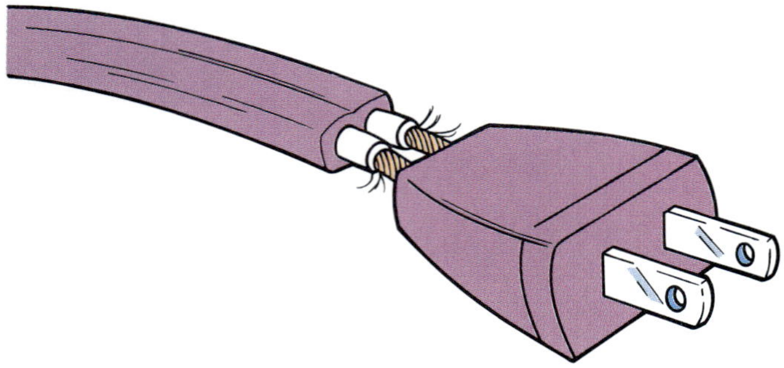

Fig. 8-30 *A frayed electric wire.*

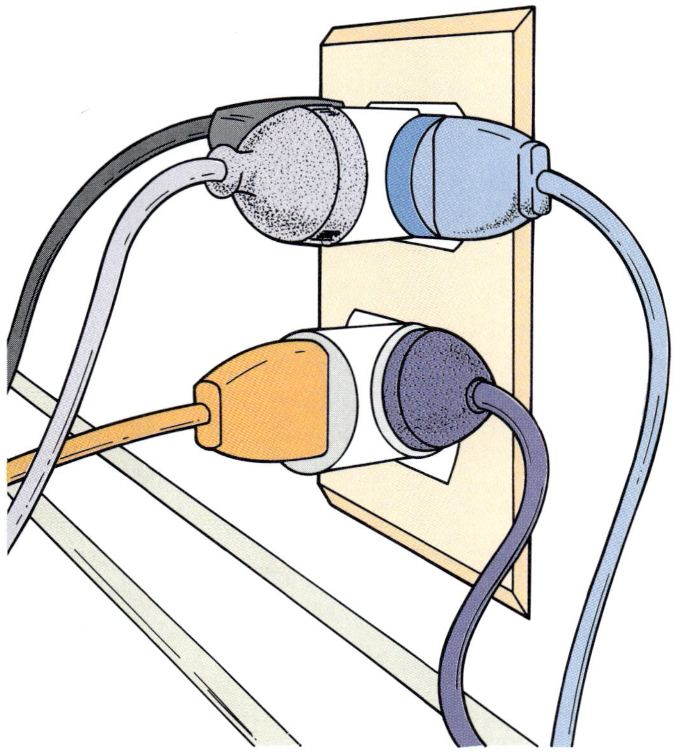

Fig. 8-31 *An overloaded electrical outlet.*

Reporting Accidents and Errors

Accidents and errors are reported immediately to your supervisor. This includes accidents involving patients, residents, visitors, or staff. You must report errors in care. Such errors include giving a person a wrong treatment, giving a treatment to the wrong person, or forgetting to give a treatment. Broken items owned by the person, such as dentures or eyeglasses, are reported. Loss of a person's money or clothing is also reported.

The facility requires a written report about the accident or error. This is called an *incident report.* The report is completed as soon as possible after the accident or error. The following information is required:

- Names of those involved
- Date and time of the accident or error
- Location of the accident or error
- A complete description of what happened
- Names of witnesses
- Any other requested information

Incident reports are reviewed by a committee of health care workers. They look for a pattern of accidents or errors. For example, are falls occurring on the same shift and on the same unit? Are patients or residents reporting lost or missing items on the same shift or same unit? The committee may recommend new policies or procedures to prevent the same situation from occurring in the future.

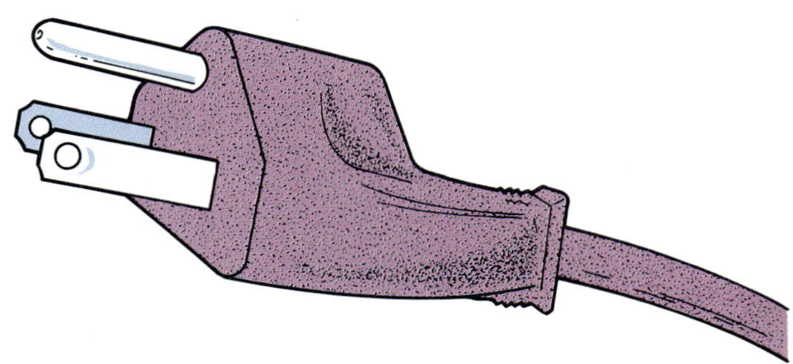

Fig. 8-32 *A three-pronged plug.*

FIRE SAFETY

Faulty electrical equipment and wiring, overloaded electrical circuits, and smoking are major causes of fire. Fire is a constant danger. The entire health team is responsible for preventing fires and for acting quickly and responsibly in the event of a fire.

Fire and the Use of Oxygen

Three things are needed to start and maintain a fire:

- A spark or flame
- A material that will burn
- Oxygen

Air has a certain amount of oxygen. However, some people need more oxygen than is available in the air. Doctors order supplemental oxygen for these persons. Supplemental oxygen is supplied in portable oxygen tanks, through wall outlets, or through air concentrators (see Chapter 24). Because oxygen is needed for fires, special safety precautions are practiced where oxygen is being given and stored. Such measures are needed in all health care settings, including private homes.

- "No Smoking" signs are placed on the person's door and near the bed.
- Patients, residents, and visitors are politely reminded not to smoke in the person's room.
- Smoking materials (cigarettes, cigars, and pipes), matches, and lighters are removed from the room.
- Electrical equipment is turned off *before* being unplugged. Sparks occur when electrical appliances are unplugged while turned on.
- Wool blankets and synthetic fabrics that cause static electricity are removed from the person's room. The person wears a cotton gown or pajamas. Health care workers should wear cotton uniforms.
- Electrical equipment is removed from the person's room. This includes electric razors, heating pads, and radios.
- Materials that ignite easily are removed from the person's room. These include oil, grease, alcohol, and nail polish remover.

Many facilities have no-smoking policies and are smoke-free environments. No smoking is allowed inside the buildings. Signs are posted on all entry doors. However, some people ignore such policies. If a person is receiving supplemental oxygen, it is important to remind the person and any visitors about the need for no smoking. Such reminders also are important when home care is given.

Fire Prevention

Fire prevention measures have been described in relation to children, burns in the home, equipment-related accidents, and the use of oxygen. These and other fire safety measures are summarized in Box 8-9.

What To Do if a Fire Occurs

Every facility has policies and procedures for what to do if there is a fire. You must know the policies and procedures for your facility. Also know the location of fire alarms, fire extinguishers, and emergency exits. Fire drills are held

BOX 8-9 FIRE PREVENTION MEASURES

- Follow the fire safety precautions involved in the use of oxygen.
- Smoke only in areas where smoking is allowed.
- Be sure all ashes, cigars, and cigarettes are extinguished before emptying ashtrays.
- Provide ashtrays to persons who are allowed to smoke.
- Empty ashtrays into a metal container partially filled with sand or water. Do not empty ashtrays into plastic containers or wastebaskets lined with paper or plastic bags.
- Supervise the smoking of persons who cannot protect themselves. This includes persons who are confused, disoriented, or sedated.
- Follow safety practices when using electrical equipment.
- Supervise the play of children, and keep matches out of their reach.

periodically in all facilities to practice emergency fire procedures.

The following practices are usually carried out by the health team when there is a fire:

- Sound the nearest fire alarm.
- Notify the switchboard operator of the exact location of the fire. Call 911 or the local fire department for a home fire.
- Move patients or residents who are in the immediate area of the fire to a safe place.
- Turn off any oxygen or electrical equipment being used in the general area of the fire.
- Close all doors and windows.
- Use a fire extinguisher on a small fire that has not spread to a larger area.
- Clear equipment from all regular and emergency exits.
- Do not use elevators if there is a fire.

You should be able to use a fire extinguisher. Fire departments give demonstrations on the use of fire extinguishers to health care employees. These demonstrations are given once or twice a year. Some facilities require all employees to demonstrate use of a fire extinguisher.

There are different extinguishers for different kinds of fires: oil and grease fires; electrical fires; and paper and wood fires. A general procedure for using a fire extinguisher follows.

Using a Fire Extinguisher

Procedure

1. Pull the fire alarm.
2. Get the nearest fire extinguisher.
3. Carry the extinguisher upright.
4. Take the extinguisher to the fire.
5. Remove the safety pin (Fig. 8-33, A).
6. Push the top handle down (Fig. 8-33, B).
7. Direct the hose at the base of the fire (Fig. 8-33, C).

A

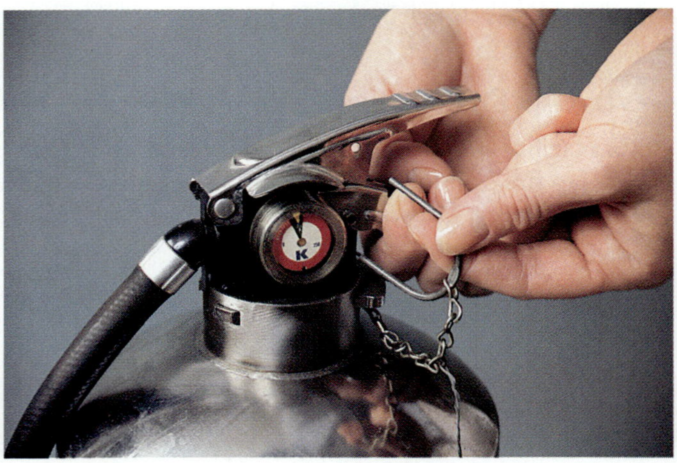

B

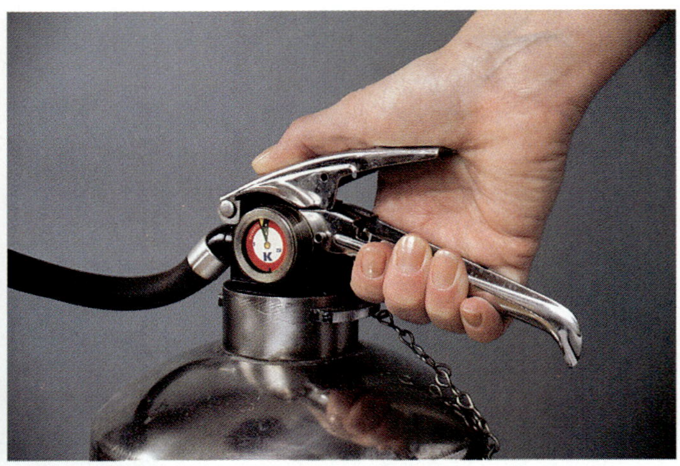

C

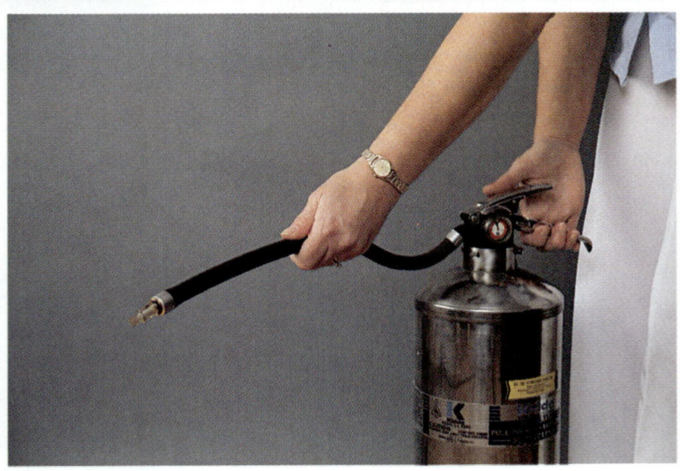

Fig. 8-33 *A, The safety pin of the fire extinguisher is removed. B, The top handle is pushed down. C, The hose is directed at the base of the fire.*

DISASTERS

A **disaster** is a sudden catastrophic event. Many people are injured and killed, and property is destroyed. Disasters may be natural: tornadoes, hurricanes, blizzards, earthquakes, volcanic eruptions, and floods. Man-made disasters include auto, bus, train, and airplane accidents; fires; nuclear power plant accidents; riots; explosions; and wars.

Local communities, fire and police departments, hospitals, and nursing facilities have disaster plans. You should know the disaster plan where you work and the disaster plan of the community where you live and work.

Disaster plans include policies and procedures to deal with great numbers of people who will be brought to the facility for treatment. The plan generally provides for the discharge of patients and residents who can go home. Certain personnel are assigned to the emergency department. Others are assigned to take extra equipment to the emergency area and to transport persons from the initial treatment area. Off-duty personnel may be called in to work.

A disaster may damage the facility. Therefore the disaster plan includes policies and procedures for evacuating the facility.

SUMMARY

Most accidents can be prevented. Knowing common safety hazards and accidents, knowing who needs protection, and using common sense promote safety. Remember, infants, young children, and the elderly have a greater risk of accidents than healthy people in other age groups.

Similar accidents happen in homes and health care facilities. However, even older children, teenagers, and young and middle-aged adults are at greater accident risk when in health care facilities. Illness, medications, strange surroundings, and special equipment increase the risk of accidental injury. As a nursing assistant, you need to practice safety precautions, use side rails as instructed, and encourage patients and residents to use hand rails.

Identifying patients and residents before giving care is very important. The person's life and health can be seriously threatened if the wrong care is given or if care is omitted. Use the ID bracelet to accurately identify the person. Having two people on the same nursing unit with the same last name is not uncommon. They may even have the same first and last names.

If restraints are ordered, they must be used to protect the person or to prevent the person from harming others. All other alternatives must have been tried first. When a restraint is needed, the least restrictive method must be used. The person is checked often to make sure that breathing and circulation are normal. Remember, the restrained person depends on others for meeting basic needs. Also remember that you can be charged with false imprisonment if a person is restrained unnecessarily.

Fire is a safety hazard. Safety precautions for smoking and electrical equipment help prevent fires. Extra precautions are needed when oxygen is used. People who smoke present added fire safety concerns. Be sure you know where to find fire alarms, fire extinguishers, and emergency exits and what to do if there is a fire. The safety precautions and measures that are taken for fires in the health care facility also apply to fire safety in the home.

REVIEW QUESTIONS

Circle the best *answer.*

1 A safe environment is one in which a person feels safe both physically and psychologically.

- **a** True
- **b** False

2 Why is age a factor in safety?

- **a** Young children have not learned what is safe and what is dangerous.
- **b** Infants are helpless.
- **c** Physical changes from aging can affect balance and movements.
- **d** All of the above.

3 Mrs. Ford's nursing assessment shows the following. Which is not a risk for accidents?

- **a** The need for eyeglasses
- **b** Hearing impairment
- **c** Memory problems
- **d** Oriented to person, time, and place

4 Mrs. Ford's roommate is in a coma. This means that the roommate

- **a** Is alert and oriented
- **b** Cannot react or respond to people, places, and things
- **c** Is aware of her surroundings
- **d** Is paralyzed on one side of her body

5 You are assigned to the pediatric unit. Which measure is unsafe?

- **a** Check children in cribs often.
- **b** Keep one hand on a child in a crib if you need to look away.
- **c** Prop a baby bottle on a rolled towel or blanket.
- **d** Keep plastic bags away from children.

6 You are providing home care. There are three children in the home all under the age of 5 years. Which is unsafe?

- **a** Using a safety strap to fasten the 18-month-old in a high chair
- **b** Letting the 4-year-old take her own bath
- **c** Keeping the bathroom door closed when it is not in use
- **d** Supervising the children when they are playing

7 Which statement is *false?*

- **a** Childproof caps are needed only on medicine containers.
- **b** Household cleaners should be kept in locked storage areas out of the reach of children.
- **c** Safety plugs in electrical outlets protect children from electrical shocks.
- **d** All of the above.

8 A paraplegic is paralyzed

- **a** From the waist down
- **b** From the neck down
- **c** On the right side of the body
- **d** On the left side of the body

9 Safety measures are needed so Mrs. Ford does not fall. Which is unsafe?

- **a** Nonglare, waxed floors
- **b** One-color floor coverings
- **c** Safety rails and grab bars in the bathroom
- **d** Nonskid shoes

10 Mrs. Ford often tries to get up without help. What should you do?

- **a** Remind her to use her call bell when she needs help.
- **b** Check on her often.
- **c** Help her to the bathroom at regular intervals.
- **d** All of the above.

11 Burns can be caused by

- **a** Smoking, especially smoking in bed
- **b** Leaving children unattended or home alone
- **c** Bath water that is too hot and applying warm applications incorrectly
- **d** All of the above.

REVIEW QUESTIONS—CONT'D

12 These statements are about poisoning. Which is *false?*

a Poisonous products should be clearly labeled, have the "Mr. Yuk" sticker, and be stored in their original containers.

b Poisonings occur in adults because of poor lighting when reading labels.

c Medicines are kept in purses to keep them from children.

d Some houseplants are poisonous.

13 Suffocation can be prevented by keeping electrical cords and appliances in good repair.

a True

b False

14 The person is called by name to accurately identify the person before giving care.

a True

b False

15 These statements are about falls. Which is *false?*

a Persons between the ages of 65 and 85 are at risk of falling.

b Falls are more likely to occur during the evening hours.

c Restraints prevent falls.

d The need to urinate is a major cause of falls.

16 These statements are about side rails. Which is *true?*

a Side rails are restraints under OBRA.

b Side rails are always raised when the bed is raised.

c Consent is needed for the use of side rails.

d All of the above.

17 Mrs. Ford's roommate is in a coma. Side rails are required for her safety.

a True

b False

18 These statements are about restraints. Which is *false?*

a A restraint restricts freedom of movement or access to one's body.

b Restraints require a nurse's order.

c Restraints are used only to prevent persons from harming themselves or others.

d Some drugs are chemical restraints.

19 Mrs. Ford still tries to get up without help. Restraints are considered during a care conference. Which is *false?*

a She must consent to their use.

b The least restrictive method must be used.

c Other measures do not need to be tried if she consents to the use of restraints.

d All of the above.

20 The following can occur because of restraints. Which is the most serious?

a Fractures

b Strangulation

c Pressure sores

d Urinary tract infection

21 These statements are about restraints. Which is *false?*

a Unnecessary restraint is false imprisonment.

b Restraints are applied so that they are tight.

c You should be able to feel a pulse in the wrist if the arm and hand are restrained.

d Restraints are removed every 2 hours to reposition the person and give care.

22 A belt restraint is applied to a person in bed. Where should you tie the straps?

a To the side rails

b To the head board

c To the movable part of the bed frame

d None of the above.

23 You have been instructed to apply a restraint. Which action is *unsafe?*

a You decide the type and size of restraint to use.

b The manufacturer's instructions are followed.

c The person is first positioned in good alignment.

d The restraint is applied so there is some movement of the body part.

24 A vest restraint is ordered. Which statement is *false?*

a The vest should criss-cross in back.

b You should be able to slide a flat hand under the restraint.

c The restraint is tied according to facility policy.

d The side rails must be padded.

REVIEW QUESTIONS—CONT'D

25 Mrs. Ford has a belt restraint. How often should you check her and the position of the restraint?

- **a** Every 15 minutes
- **b** Every 30 minutes
- **c** Every hour
- **d** Every 2 hours

26 Restrained persons can meet their own needs for food, fluids, and elimination.

- **a** True
- **b** False

27 Elbow restraints prevent children from scratching and touching incisions.

- **a** True
- **b** False

28 To prevent equipment accidents, you should

- **a** Fix broken equipment
- **b** Use two-pronged plugs to ground electrical equipment
- **c** Check glass and plastic items for damage
- **d** All of the above.

29 You gave Mrs. Ford the wrong treatment. Which is *true?*

- **a** The error is reported to the nurse at the end of the shift.
- **b** Action is taken only if Mrs. Ford was injured.
- **c** You will be found guilty of negligence.
- **d** An incident report must be completed.

30 All the following are needed to start a fire *except*

- **a** A spark or flame
- **b** A material that will burn
- **c** Oxygen
- **d** Carbon monoxide

31 The fire alarm sounds. The following are done *except*

- **a** Turning off oxygen
- **b** Using elevators
- **c** Closing doors and windows
- **d** Moving patients or residents to a safe place

32 Many people are injured and killed and property is destroyed in a disaster.

- **a** True
- **b** False

Answers to these questions are on page 749.

Preventing Infection

9

OBJECTIVES

- Define the key terms listed in this chapter
- Explain the difference between nonpathogens and pathogens
- Identify what microorganisms need to live and grow
- List the signs and symptoms of infection
- Explain the chain of infection
- Describe nosocomial infection and the persons at risk
- Explain the differences between medical asepsis, surgical asepsis, disinfection, and sterilization
- Describe practices of medical asepsis
- Describe common methods of disinfection and sterilization
- Explain how to care for equipment and supplies
- Explain the purpose of Standard and Transmission-Based Precautions and their effects on the person
- Describe the types of Transmission-Based Precautions and the general rules for maintaining them
- Carry out Standard and Transmission-Based Precautions
- Explain the Bloodborne Pathogen Standard
- Perform the procedures in this chapter

KEY TERMS

asepsis Being free of disease-producing microorganisms

autoclave A pressurized steam sterilizer

biohazardous waste Items contaminated with blood, body fluids, or body substances and that may be harmful to others; *bio* means life and *hazardous* means dangerous or harmful

carrier A human being or animal that is a reservoir for microorganisms but does not have signs and symptoms of infection

clean technique Medical asepsis

communicable disease A disease caused by pathogens that are easily spread; a contagious disease

contagious disease Communicable disease

contamination The process by which an object or area becomes unclean

disinfection The process by which pathogens are destroyed

germicide A disinfectant applied to skin, tissues, or inanimate objects

host The environment in which microorganisms live and grow; reservoir

immunity Protection against a specific disease

infection A disease state that results from the invasion and growth of microorganisms in the body

medical asepsis The practices used to remove or destroy pathogens and to prevent their spread from one person or place to another person or place; clean technique

microbe A microorganism

microorganism A small (micro) living plant or animal (organism) that cannot be seen without the aid of a microscope; a microbe

nosocomial infection An infection acquired after admission to a health care facility

nonpathogen A microorganism that does not usually cause an infection

normal flora Microorganisms that usually live and grow in a certain location

pathogen A microorganism that is harmful and capable of causing an infection

personal protective equipment Specialized clothing or equipment (gloves, gown, mask, goggles, face shield) worn for protection against a hazard

reservoir The environment in which microorganisms live and grow; the host

spore A bacterium protected by a hard shell that forms around the microorganism

surgical asepsis The practices that keep equipment and supplies free of all microorganisms; sterile technique

sterile The absence of all microorganisms

sterile technique Surgical asepsis

sterilization The process by which all microorganisms are destroyed

vaccination The administration of a vaccine to produce immunity

vaccine A preparation containing weakened or dead microorganisms

Infection is a major safety and health hazard. Some infections are minor and cause short illnesses. Others are serious and can cause death, particularly in infants and the elderly. The health team must protect patients, residents, and themselves from infection. This is done by preventing the spread of the cause of the infection.

MICROORGANISMS

A **microorganism (microbe)** is a small (micro) living plant or animal (organism) that cannot be seen without a microscope. Microbes are everywhere. They are in the air, food, mouth, nose, respiratory tract, stomach, intestines, and on the skin. They are in the soil and water, and on animals, clothing, and furniture. Some microbes cause infections and are considered harmful. They are called **pathogens. Nonpathogens** are microorganisms that do not usually cause an infection.

Types of Microorganisms

There are five general types of microorganisms.

- *Bacteria* are microscopic plant life that multiply rapidly. They consist of one cell and are often called *germs.*
- *Fungi* are plants that live on other plants or animals. Mushrooms, yeasts, and molds are common fungi.
- *Protozoa* are microscopic one-celled animals.
- *Rickettsiae* are microscopic forms of life found in the tissues of fleas, lice, ticks, and other insects. They are transmitted to humans by insect bites.
- *Viruses* are extremely small microscopic organisms that grow in living cells.

Requirements of Microorganisms

Microorganisms need a reservoir to live and grow. The **reservoir** or **host** is the environment in which the microorganism lives and grows. The reservoir can be a person, a plant, an animal, the soil, food, water, or other material. The microbe must get *water* and *nourishment* from the reservoir. Most microbes need *oxygen* to live. Others cannot live where there is oxygen. A *warm* and *dark* environment is needed. Most microbes grow best at body temperature and are destroyed by heat and light.

Normal Flora

Normal flora refers to microorganisms that usually live and grow in a certain area. Certain microbes are found in the respiratory tract, in the intestines, on the skin, and in other sites outside the body. They are nonpathogens when in or on a natural reservoir. When a nonpathogen is transmitted from its natural site to another site or host, it becomes a pathogen. *Escherichia coli* is normally found in the large intestine. If the *E. coli* enters the urinary system, it can cause an infection.

INFECTION

An **infection** is a disease state resulting from the invasion and growth of microbes in the body. It may be local or systemic. A *local infection* is in a specific body part. A *systemic infection* involves the whole body. The person with an infection has certain signs and symptoms. Some or all of the signs and symptoms listed in Box 9-1 are present. Pathogens can be present without causing an infection. The development of an infection depends on many factors.

BOX 9-1 Signs and Symptoms of Infection

- Fever
- Pain or tenderness
- Fatigue
- Loss of appetite
- Nausea
- Vomiting
- Diarrhea
- Rash
- Sores on mucous membranes
- Redness and swelling of a body part
- Discharge or drainage from the infected area

The Chain of Infection

The chain of infection (Fig. 9-1) is a process involving a:

- Source
- Reservoir
- Portal of exit
- Method of transmission
- Portal of entry
- Susceptible host

For an infection to develop, there must be a **source.** The source is a pathogen that can cause disease. The pathogen must have a *reservoir* where it can grow and multiply. Humans and animals are among the reservoirs for microbes. If they do not have signs and symptoms of infection, they are **carriers.** Carriers can pass the pathogen on to others. The pathogen must be able to leave the reservoir. In other words, it must have a *portal of exit.* Exits in the human body are the respiratory, gastrointestinal, urinary, and reproductive tracts, breaks in the skin, and the blood.

When a pathogen leaves the reservoir, it must be *transmitted* to another host for an infection to develop. Methods of transmission include direct contact, air (airborne droplets from coughing or sneezing), food, water, animals, and insects. Microbes can also be transmitted by eating and drinking utensils, dressings, and equipment for personal care and hygiene (see Fig. 9-2 on page 186). The pathogen must then enter the body through a *portal of entry.* Portals of entry are the same as the exits. Whether the pathogen grows and multiplies depends on a *susceptible host* (a person at risk for infection). The human body has the natural ability to protect itself from infection. A person's ability to resist infection is related to age, nutritional status, stress, fatigue, general health, medications, and the presence of disease or injury.

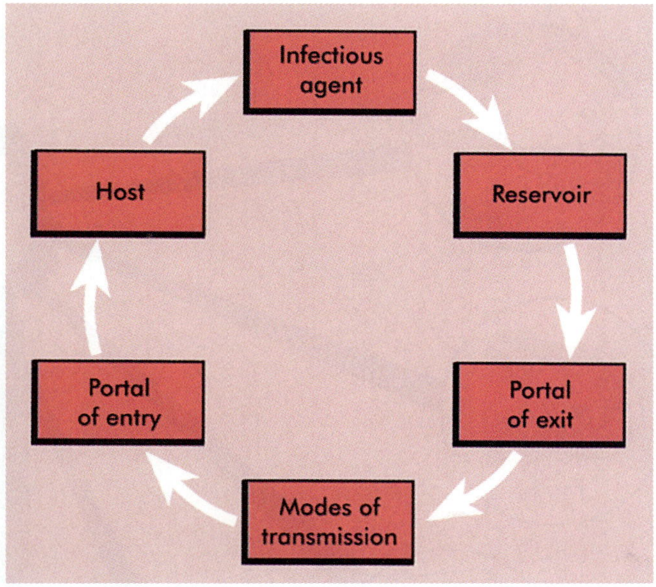

Fig. 9-1 *The chain of infection.* (From Potter PA, Perry AG: *Fundamentals of nursing: concepts, process, and practice,* ed 3, St Louis, 1993, Mosby–Year Book.)

Nosocomial Infection

Persons can develop infections after admission to a health care facility. A **nosocomial infection** is an infection acquired after admission to a health care facility. *Nosocomial* comes from the Greek word for hospital. Nosocomial infections also can occur in long-term care, rehabilitation, and other health care facilities.

Nosocomial infections are caused by normal flora or by microbes transmitted to the person from another source. As explained earlier, normal flora become pathogens when transmitted from their natural location to another site or host. The example was given of *E. coli* entering the urinary system. Incorrect or inadequate wiping after bowel movements can cause *E. coli* to enter the urinary system. *E. coli* can also be transmitted to other body areas by the hands. Feces (bowel movements) contain *E. coli.* If handwashing is not thorough, *E. coli* are transmitted to any body part touched by the hands.

Nosocomial infections occur from many sources. Treatments, therapies, and diagnostic procedures are sources of infection. Microbes can enter the body if the equipment used has not been properly handled, cleaned, disinfected, or sterilized (see page 189). Microbes can also be transferred from one person to another. Caregivers can transfer microbes from one patient or resident to another. They can also transfer microbes from themselves to patients or residents. The most common sites for nosocomial infections are the urinary system, wounds, respiratory system, and the bloodstream.

Patients and residents are at high risk for infection. They are already weak from disease or injury. They may have surgical wounds or other open skin areas. Infants and the elderly cannot fight infections as well as other persons. Therefore the health team must prevent the spread of infection. Medical and surgical asepsis, isolation precautions, and the Bloodborne Pathogen Standard all help prevent nosocomial infections.

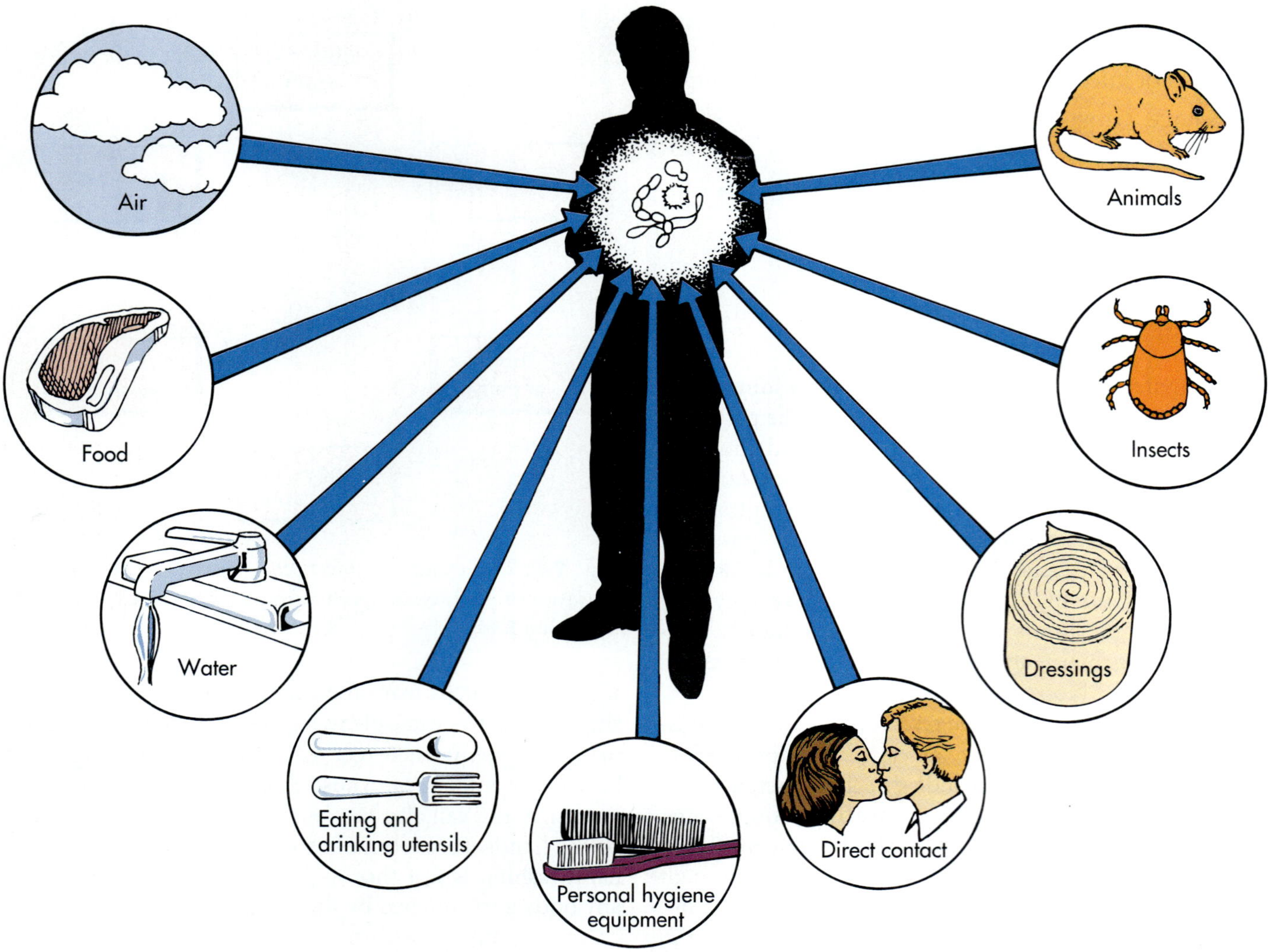

Fig. 9-2 *Methods by which microorganisms can be spread.*

ASEPSIS

Asepsis is being free of disease-producing microorganisms. Because microbes are everywhere, there must be practices to achieve asepsis. **Medical asepsis (clean technique)** is the practices used to remove or destroy pathogens and to prevent their spread from one person or place to another person or place. The number of pathogens is reduced. **Disinfection** is the process by which pathogens are destroyed.

No microoganisms can be present during surgery, whenever the body is entered, or when there are open wounds (cuts, burns, surgical incisions). During surgery the skin is cut or the surgeon inserts instruments into the respiratory, gastrointestinal, urinary, or reproductive systems. All these are portals of entry for microorganisms. To prevent infection, surgical asepsis is used. **Surgical asepsis (sterile technique)** is the practice that keeps equipment and supplies free of all microorganisms. **Sterile** means the absence of *all* microorganisms, both pathogenic and nonpathogenic. **Sterilization** is the process in which *all* microorganisms are destroyed. In other words, both pathogens and nonpathogens are destroyed.

Contamination is the process by which an object or area becomes unclean. In medical asepsis, an object or area is *clean* when it is free of pathogens. Therefore the object or area is contaminated if pathogens are present. Likewise, a sterile object or area is contaminated when pathogens or nonpathogens are present.

Common Aseptic Practices

Aseptic practices are followed in the home, community, and health care facilities. Their purpose is to break the chain of infection. Some common ways to prevent the spread of microorganisms are:

- Washing your hands after urinating, having a bowel movement, or changing tampons or sanitary napkins or pads
- Washing your hands after contact with any body fluid or substance, whether it is your own or another person's; body fluids and substances include blood, saliva, vomitus, urine, feces, vaginal discharge, mucus, semen, wound drainage, pus, respiratory secretions, and other secretions and excretions
- Washing your hands before handling, preparing, or eating food
- Washing fruits and raw vegetables before eating or serving them
- Providing individual toothbrushes, drinking glasses, towels, washcloths, and other personal care items for each family member
- Covering the nose and mouth when coughing, sneezing, or blowing the nose
- Bathing, washing hair, and brushing teeth regularly
- Washing cooking and eating utensils with soap and water after use
- Observing sanitation practices such as garbage disposal and sewage treatment

Handwashing

Handwashing with soap and water is the easiest and most important way to prevent the spread of infection. The hands are used in almost every activity and are easily contaminated. Microbes on the hands can be spread to other persons or objects if handwashing is not practiced. *Your hands must be washed before and after giving care.* The rules for handwashing are in Box 9-2.

BOX 9-2 RULES OF HANDWASHING

- Wash your hands under warm running water.
- Hand-operated faucets are contaminated. Use paper towels to turn water on and off (Fig. 9-3 on page 188). The paper towel prevents the clean hand from becoming contaminated again. A clean paper towel is used for each faucet.
- Although soap dispensers are found in health care facilities, bar soap is common in homes. When bar soap is used, it is held during the entire procedure. When the procedure is completed, the soap is rinsed under running water. Rinsing removes microcrobes. After rinsing, bar soap is dropped into the soap dish. Do not touch the soap dish during or after the handwashing procedure. (Because bar soap may be used in home care, the handwashing procedure on page 188 includes bar soap.)
- Your hands and forearms are held lower than your elbows throughout the procedure. If your hands and forearms are held up, dirty water runs from the hands to the elbows, contaminating those areas.
- Attention is given to areas often missed during handwashing: the thumbs, knuckles, sides of the hands, little fingers, and under the nails. A nail file or orange stick is used to clean under the fingernails (Fig. 9-4 on page 188).
- Check facility policy for how long you should wash your hands. At least a 10- to 15-second hand wash is required. Your judgment is important. You know what your hands have touched and where your hands have been. If the person has an infection, the possibility of contamination is greater. Follow these guidelines for handwashing.
  - *2 minutes before caring for any person at the beginning of your shift
  - *10 to 15 seconds before caring for another person
  - *1 minute or longer if your hands are contaminated with blood, body fluids, secretions, or excretions
  - *1 to 2 minutes if you have given care to a person with an infection
- Use a lotion after handwashing to prevent chapping and drying of the skin. Skin breaks can occur in chapped and dry skin. Remember, breaks in the skin are portals of entry for microorganisms.

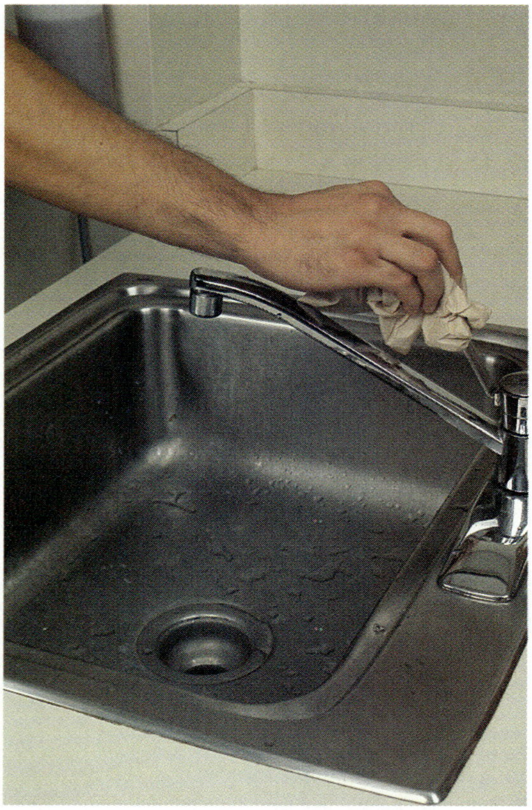

Fig. 9-3 *A paper towel is used to turn the faucet off.*

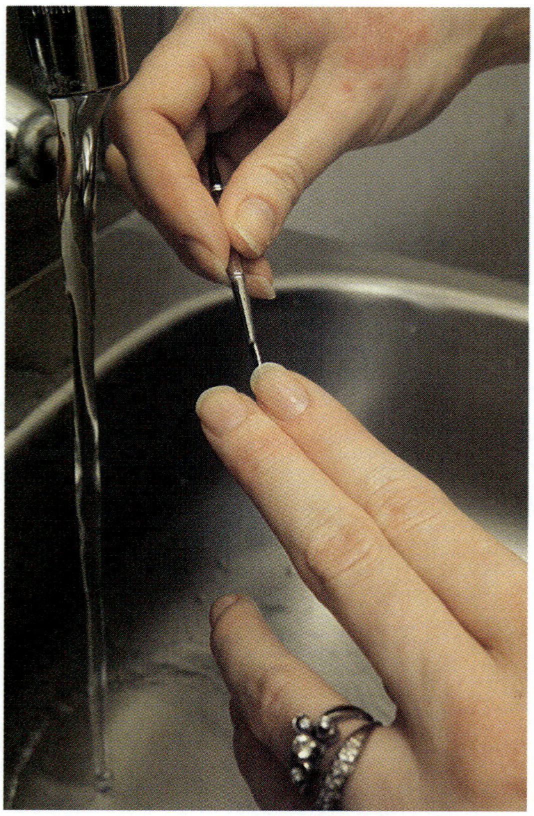

Fig. 9-4 *An orange stick is used to clean under the fingernails.*

Handwashing

Procedure

1. Make sure that soap, paper towels, orange stick or nail file, and a wastebasket are available. Collect missing items.
2. Push your watch up 4 to 5 inches. Also push up uniform sleeves.
3. Stand away from the sink so your clothes do not touch the sink. The soap and faucet must be easy to reach (Fig. 9-5).
4. Turn on the faucet using a paper towel.
5. Adjust the water until it feels warm and comfortable.
6. Toss the used paper towel into the wastebasket.
7. Wet your wrists and hands thoroughly under running water. Keep your hands lower than your elbows during the procedure (see Fig. 9-5).
8. Apply about 1 teaspoon of soap to your hands. Rinse bar soap before use.
9. Rub your palms together and interlace your fingers to work up a good lather (Fig. 9-6). This step should last at least 10 seconds.
10. Wash each hand and wrist thoroughly, and clean well between the fingers. Clean well under the fingernails by rubbing the tips of your fingers against your palms (Fig. 9-7).
11. Continue washing for 1 to 2 minutes, if needed.
12. Use a nail file or orange stick to clean under the fingernails (see Fig. 9-4). This step is necessary for the first handwashing of the day and if your hands are highly soiled.
13. Rinse your wrists and hands well. Water should flow from the arms to the hands.
14. Repeat steps 8 through 13, if needed.
15. Return bar soap to its dish (if bar soap is used).
16. Dry your wrists and hands with paper towels. Pat dry.
17. Discard the paper towels.
18. Turn off the faucet with a clean paper towel to avoid contaminating your hand. Use a clean paper towel for each faucet.
19. Toss paper towels into the wastebasket.

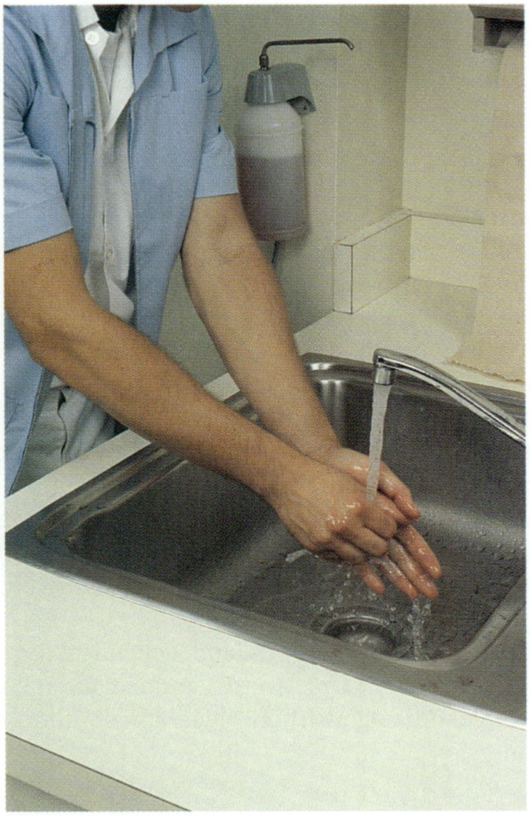

Fig. 9-5 *The nursing assistant stands so that his uniform does not touch the sink. He can reach the soap and water. Hands are lower than the elbows.*

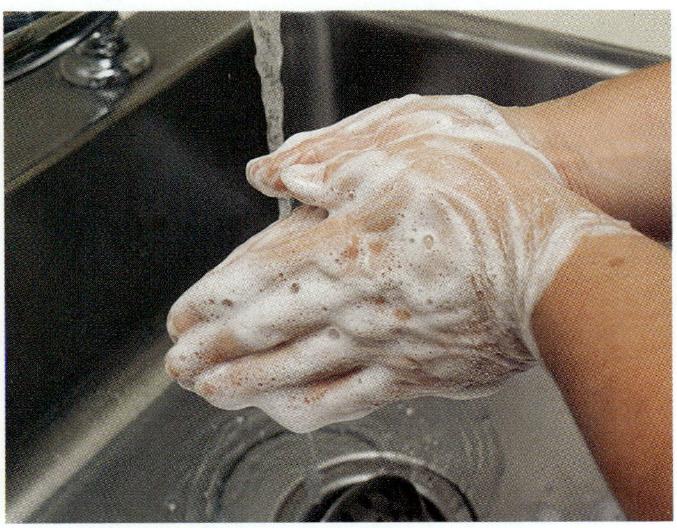

Fig. 9-6 *The palms are rubbed together to work up a good lather.*

Care of Supplies and Equipment

Facilities have supply departments that buy, disinfect, sterilize, and distribute equipment. Many items are disposable. Disposable items are used once for a person and then discarded. However, some disposable items are used many times by the same person. Examples include disposable bedpans, urinals, wash basins, thermometers, water pitchers, and drinking cups. Disposable equipment helps reduce the spread of infection.

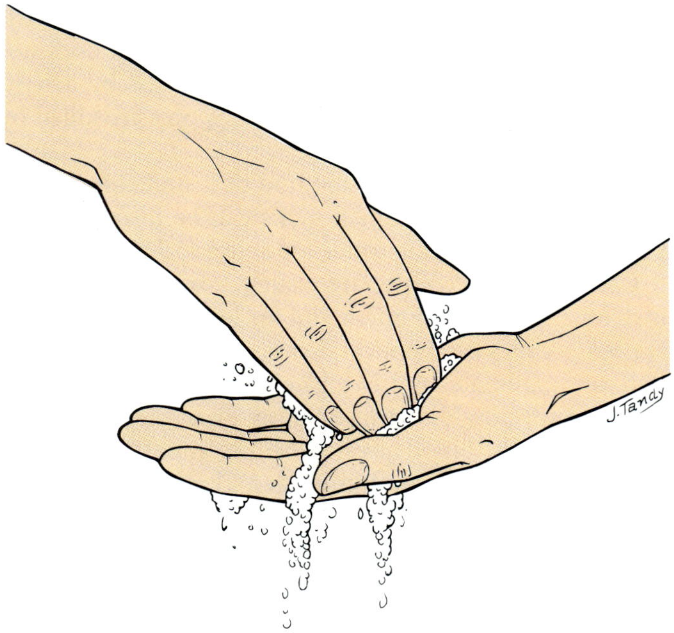

Fig. 9-7 *The tips of the fingers are rubbed against the palms to clean underneath the fingernails.*

Large and costly equipment is usually not disposable. It is disinfected or sterilized before use by any person. Before disinfection or sterilization, equipment is cleaned.

Cleaning Cleaning removes debris, reduces the number of microbes present, and removes organic material. Organic material includes any body fluid or body substance. The guidelines listed below are followed when cleaning equipment.

- Wear personal protective equipment (gloves, a mask, a gown, and protective eyewear) when cleaning equipment contaminated with a body fluid or substance.
- Rinse the item in cold water first to remove organic material. Heat causes organic material to become thick, sticky, and hard to remove.
- Use soap and hot water to wash the item.
- Scrub thoroughly.
- Use a brush if necessary.
- Rinse the item in warm water.
- Dry the item.
- Disinfect or sterilize the item.
- Disinfect equipment and the sink used in the cleaning procedure.
- Discard the personal protective equipment.

Disinfection Disinfection is the process in which pathogens are destroyed. However, disinfection does not destroy spores. **Spores** are bacteria protected by a hard shell that forms around the microbe. Spores are killed by extremely high temperatures.

Boiling water is a simple method of disinfection. It can be done in the home. Small items can be disinfected by placing them in boiling water for at least 15 minutes.

Chemical disinfectants are usually used for cleaning instruments and equipment and for housekeeping. There are many types of chemical disinfectants. Some are used only on inanimate (not living) objects. They are used to clean nondisposable items such as glass thermometers, metal bedpans, blood pressure cuffs, and stethoscopes. They are also used on commodes, chairs, countertops, wheelchairs, stretchers, and room furniture after the person has been discharged. Some disinfectants are applied to skin, tissues, and inanimate objects. These are called **germicides.** Alcohol is a common germicide.

Disinfectants can burn and irritate the skin. You should wear *waterproof* gloves when using a disinfectant to prevent skin irritation. General purpose utility gloves or rubber household gloves are worn. Do not wear disposable gloves when using disinfectants. Specific chemical disinfectants may have special precautions for use or storage. Ask the nurse about procedures for a specific disinfectant.

Sterilization Sterilization procedures destroy all nonpathogens, pathogens, and spores. Very high temperatures are used. Remember, microbes grow best at body temperature and are destroyed by heat.

You may learn to sterilize equipment when *steam under pressure* is the method used. An **autoclave** (Fig. 9-8) is a pressurized steam sterilizer. It is used to sterilize metal objects such as surgical instruments, basins, bedpans, and urinals. Glass and surgical linens are also sterilized in autoclaves. Plastic and rubber items are not placed in autoclaves because they are destroyed by high temperatures. Pressure cookers used to prepare food can sterilize objects in the home. Steam under pressure usually sterilizes objects in 30 to 45 minutes.

Radiation, liquid chemicals, and a chemical gas may be used for sterilizing. Unless cross-trained for the central supply area, nursing assistants generally do not use these methods.

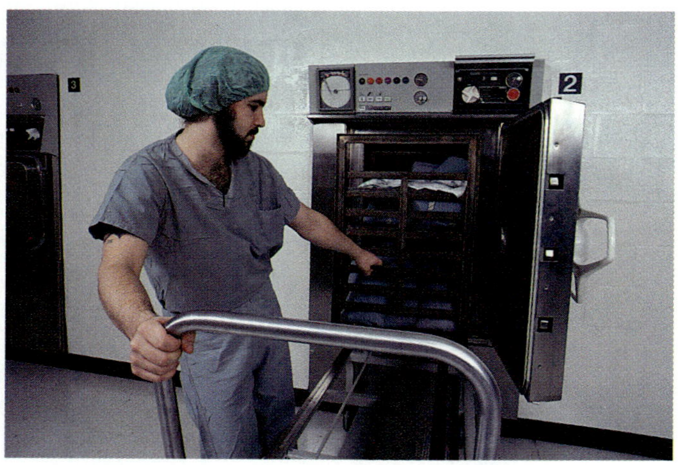

Fig. 9-8 *An autoclave.*

Other Aseptic Measures

Handwashing, cleaning, disinfection, and sterilization are important aseptic measures. However, other aseptic measures are practiced to prevent the spread of infection and microorganisms. These measures, listed in Box 9-3, break the chain of infection. They are required in health care facilities to protect patients, residents, visitors, and health workers. The measures can also be used in the home and in everyday activities.

BOX 9-3 Aseptic Measures

- Hold equipment and linens away from your uniform or clothes (Fig. 9-9).
- Prevent the movement of dust. Do not shake linens and other equipment. Use a damp cloth to dust furniture.
- Clean from the cleanest area to the dirtiest. This prevents soiling a clean area.
- Clean away from your body. If you dust, brush, or wipe toward yourself, microorganisms will be transmitted to your skin, hair, and clothing.
- Flush urine and feces down the toilet.
- Pour contaminated liquids directly into sinks or toilets. Avoid splashing onto other areas.
- Avoid sitting on a person's bed. You will pick up microorganisms and transfer them to the next surface that you sit on.
- Make sure all persons have their own personal hygiene equipment.
- Do not take equipment from one person's room to use for another person. Even if the item has not been used, do not take it from one room to another.
- Use leakage-resistant bags for soiled tissues, linen, and other materials.
- Keep tables, countertops, wheelchair trays, and other surfaces clean and dry.
- Label bottles with the person's name and the date the bottle was opened.
- Keep bottles and fluid containers tightly capped or covered.
- Provide for the person's hygiene needs (see Chapter 13). Body areas contaminated with feces, urine, blood, pus, and other body fluids, secretions, and excretions need to be washed with soap and water.
- Wear personal protective equipment as needed (see pages 193-201).

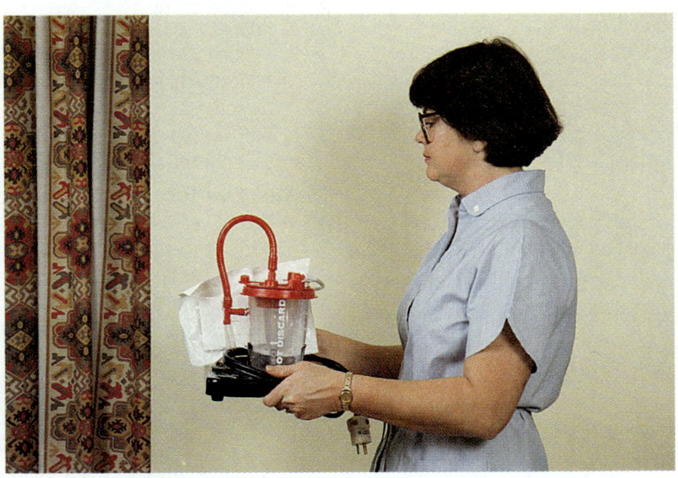

Fig. 9-9 *Equipment is held away from the uniform.*

ISOLATION PRECAUTIONS

Sometimes other measures are needed to prevent the spread of microorganisms. Barriers are set up to prevent the escape of pathogens. The pathogens are kept within a certain area, usually the person's room.

In January 1996, the Centers for Disease Control and Prevention (CDC) released new guidelines for isolation precautions. The new guidelines recognize the importance of all body fluids, secretions, and excretions in the transmission of pathogens. Two tiers of precautions are practiced: Standard Precautions and Transmission-Based Precautions. *The new guidelines replace previous CDC recommendations for isolation precautions.*

Purpose

Isolation precautions prevent the spread of a **communicable** or **contagious disease.** Communicable diseases are caused by pathogens that are spread easily. Common communicable diseases are measles, mumps, chicken pox, syphilis, gonorrhea, and acquired immunodeficiency syndrome (AIDS) (see Chapter 28). Persons may have respiratory, wound, skin, gastrointestinal, or blood infections that are highly contagious. Special precautions are needed for these persons. Pathogens causing these infections must be kept in one area. That protects staff, visitors, and other patients or residents from the infection.

Clean Versus Dirty

Isolation precautions are based on *clean* and *dirty*. Clean refers to areas or objects that are uncontaminated. Uncontaminated areas are free of pathogens. Dirty areas or objects are contaminated. If a clean area or object is in contact with something *dirty*, the clean item is now dirty. *Clean* and *dirty* also depend on how the pathogen is spread.

Standard Precautions

Standard Precautions are designed to reduce the risk of spreading pathogens from both known and unknown infections. They prevent the spread of infection from

- Blood
- All body fluids, secretions, and excretions (except sweat) even if blood is not visible
- Nonintact skin (skin that has open breaks)
- Mucous membranes

Standard Precautions are used in the care of all persons. These precautions are listed in Box 9-4.

Transmission-Based Precautions

Some persons have infections that require precautions in addition to the Standard Precautions. The additional precautions depend on how the pathogen is spread. Table 9-1 on page 194 describes the Transmission-Based Precautions. You must understand how certain infections are spread (see Fig. 9-2). This helps you understand the different types of Transmission-Based Precautions.

BOX 9-4 STANDARD PRECAUTIONS

Hand Washing

- Wash your hands after touching blood, body fluids, secretions, excretions, and contaminated items. Hands are washed even if gloves were worn.
- Wash your hands immediately after removing gloves and between patient or resident contacts. Also wash your hands whenever indicated to avoid transferring microbes to other persons or environments.
- Wash your hands between tasks and procedures on the same person. This prevents cross-contamination of different body sites.
- Use plain soap for routine hand washing. (Other agents may be needed in certain situations. The nurse will tell you what to use.)

Gloves

- Wear gloves when touching blood, body fluids, secretions, excretions, and contaminated items.
- Put on clean gloves just before touching mucous membranes and nonintact skin.
- Change gloves between tasks and procedures on the same person after contacting material that may be highly contaminated.
- Remove gloves promptly after use. Remove gloves before touching noncontaminated items and surfaces and before going to another person.
- Wash your hands immediately after removing gloves. This prevents the transfer of microorganisms to other persons or environments.

Masks, Eye Protection, and Face Shields

- Wear masks, eye protection, and face shields during procedures and care activities that are likely to cause splashes or sprays of blood, body fluids, secretions, and excretions. Masks, eye protection, and face shields protect the mucous membranes of the mouth, eyes, and nose from splashes or sprays (Fig. 9-10).

Gowns

- Wear a gown during procedures and care activities that are likely to cause splashes or sprays of blood, body fluids, secretions, or

BOX 9-4 Standard Precautions—continued

excretions. The gown protects the skin and prevents soiling of clothing.

- Remove a soiled gown as promptly as possible.
- Wash your hands after gown removal to prevent the transfer of microorganisms to other persons or environments.

Patient-Care Equipment

- Handle used patient-care equipment carefully. Equipment may be soiled with blood, body fluids, secretions, and excretions. Prevent skin and mucous membrane exposure and contamination of clothing. Also prevent the transfer of microorganisms to other persons and environments.
- Do not use reusable equipment for the care of another person until the item has been cleaned and disinfected or sterilized.
- Discard disposable (single-use) items properly.

Environmental Control

- Follow facility procedures for the routine care, cleaning, and disinfection of surfaces. This includes environmental surfaces, side rails, bedside equipment, and other frequently touched surfaces.

Linen

- Follow facility policy for handling, transporting, and processing used linen that is soiled with blood, body fluids, secretions, or excretions. Prevent skin and mucous membrane exposures and contamination of clothing. Transfer of microorganisms to other persons and environments must be prevented.

Occupational Health and Bloodborne Pathogens*

- Prevent injuries when using needles, scalpels, and other sharp instruments or devices.
- Prevent injuries when handling sharp instruments after procedures and when cleaning used instruments.
- Prevent injuries when disposing of used needles.
- Never recap used needles. Do not manipulate them using both hands or use any technique that involves directing the needle point toward any body part. Use a one-handed "scoop" technique or a mechanical device that holds the needle sheath.
- Do not remove used needles from disposable syringes by hand.
- Do not bend, break, or otherwise manipulate used needles by hand.
- Place used disposable syringes and needles, scalpel blades, and other sharp items in puncture-resistant containers.
- Place reusable syringes and needles in a puncture-resistant container for transport to the reprocessing area.
- Use resuscitation devices when mouth-to-mouth resuscitation is indicated (Chapter 33).

Patient Placement

- A private room is used if the person: contaminates the environment; does not or cannot assist in maintaining hygiene or environmental control.
- Follow the nurse's instructions if a private room is not available.

**Nursing assistants do not use needles, syringes, or scalpels in patient or resident care. Information about the proper handling of these items is included to provide the entire scope of Standard Precautions.*

A

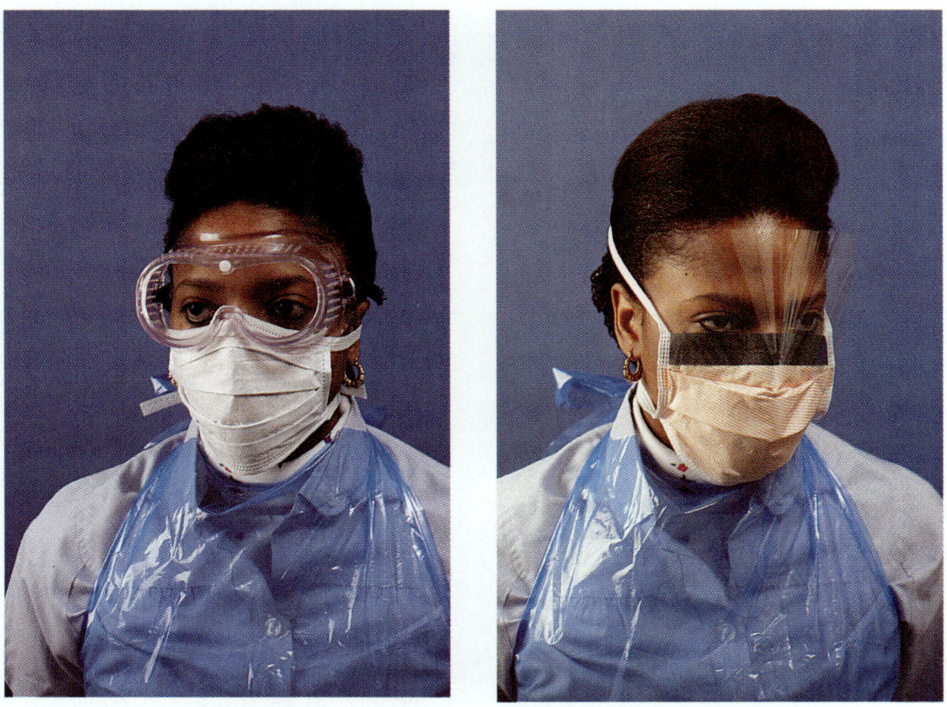

B

Fig. 9-10 ***A,*** *Mask and goggles protect the eyes from splashing body fluids.* ***B,*** *A face shield protects the eyes and mucous membranes of the mouth. Note that a plastic apron is worn to protect the uniform from soiling.*

TABLE 9-1

TRANSMISSION - BASED PRECAUTIONS

Airborne Precautions

For known or suspected infections involving microorganisms that are transmitted by airborne droplets—measles, chicken pox, tuberculosis

Practices:

- Standard Precautions are followed.
- A private room is preferred.
- Keep the room door closed and the person in the room.
- Wear respiratory protection (tuberculosis respirator) when entering the room of a person with known or suspected tuberculosis.
- Do not enter the room of a person with known or suspected measles or chicken pox if you are susceptible to these diseases.
- Wear respiratory protection (mask) if you must enter the room of a person with known or suspected measles or chicken pox if you are susceptible to these diseases. (Respiratory protection is not indicated for persons who are immune to measles or chicken pox.
- Limit moving and transporting the person from the room. The person wears a mask if moving or transporting from the room is necessary.

Droplet Precautions

For known or suspected infections involving microorganisms that are transmitted by droplets generated by coughing, sneezing, talking, or procedures—meningitis, pneumonia, epiglottitis, diphtheria, pertussis (whooping cough), influenza, mumps, rubella, streptococcal pharyngitis, or scarlet fever

Practices:

- Standard Precautions are followed.
- A private room is preferred.
- Wear a mask when working within 3 feet of the person. (Wear a mask on entering the room if required by facility policy.)
- Limit moving and transporting the person from the room. The person wears a mask if moving or transporting from the room is necessary.

Contact Precautions

For known or suspected infections involving microorganisms that can be transmitted by direct contact with the person (hand or skin-to-skin contact that occurs during care activities) or indirect contact (touching surfaces or patient-care items in the person's room)—gastrointestinal, respiratory, skin, or wound infections

Practices:

- Standard Precautions are followed.
- A private room is preferred.
- Wear gloves when entering the room.
- Change gloves after having contact with infective material that may contain high concentrations of microorganisms.
- Remove gloves before leaving the person's room.
- Wash your hands immediately with an agent specified by the nurse.
- Make sure your hands do not touch potentially contaminated surfaces or items after removing gloves and hand washing.
- Wear a gown on entering the room if you will have substantial contact with the person, environmental surfaces, or items in the room.
- Wear a gown on entering the room if the person is incontinent or has diarrhea, an ileostomy, a colostomy, or wound drainage not contained by a dressing.
- Remove the gown before leaving the person's room. Make sure your clothing does not contact potentially contaminated surfaces in the person's room.
- Limit moving or transferring the person from the room. Maintain precautions if the person is moved or transferred from the room.

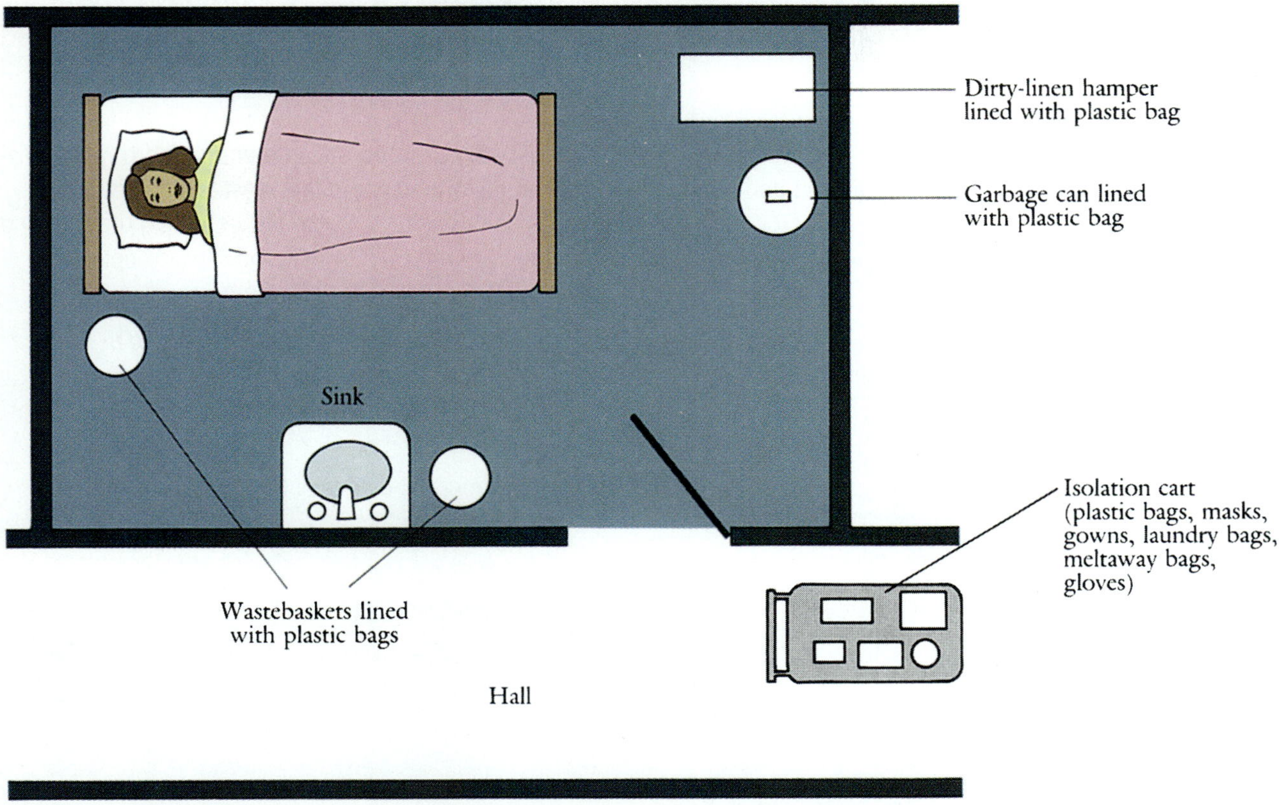

Fig. 9-11 *Setup for isolation precautions.*

The person's room When isolation precautions are ordered, the person is separated from others. A private room is preferred. If necessary, a semiprivate room is used. The room must have hand washing and toilet facilities. The unit includes items needed for meeting basic needs (Fig. 9-11). Equipment for measuring temperature, pulse, and blood pressure is kept in the room (see Chapter 18). Besides a waste basket, there are containers for laundry and trash.

There is a cabinet, bedside stand, or cart outside the room. This is used to store supplies needed for isolation precautions: gowns, gloves, masks, protective eyewear, plastic bags, laundry bags, and trash bags. A sign is placed on the outside of the room door. It states the precautions being practiced.

BOX 9-5 Rules for Isolation Precautions

- Collect all needed equipment before entering the room. This reduces the number of trips in and out of the room.
- Floors are contaminated. So is any object that is on the floor or that falls to the floor.
- Floor dust is contaminated. Mops wetted with a disinfectant solution are used for cleaning. A wet mop keeps dust down.
- Drafts are prevented. Pathogens are carried in the air by drafts.
- Paper towels are used to handle contaminated items. This keeps the hands or gloves clean.
- Items removed from the room are bagged in leakage-resistant bags.
- Double bagging is done if the outer part of the bag is or can be contaminated. See page 203 for double bagging.
- Disposable dishes, eating utensils, and trays are discarded in the appropriate waste container in the person's room. Reusable dishes, eating utensils, and trays are returned to the food service department.
- Do not touch your hair, nose, mouth, eyes, or other body parts when caring for a person in isolation.
- If your hands become contaminated, they must not touch any clean area or object.
- Wash your hands if they become contaminated.
- Place clean items or objects on paper towels.
- Do not shake linen.
- Use paper towels to turn faucets on and off.
- Tell the nurse if you have any cuts, open skin areas, a sore throat, vomiting, or diarrhea.

General rules Maintaining isolation precautions can be difficult. Facility policies may differ from those in this text. The rules in Box 9-5 are a guide for giving safe care when isolation precautions are used.

Special Procedures

Isolation precautions may require wearing gloves, a gown, a mask, or protective eyewear. Double bagging may be needed when removing linens, trash, and equipment from the area. Special measures are needed to collect specimens and to transport persons on isolation precautions.

Gloves Disposable gloves act as a barrier between the person and the worker. The skin is a natural barrier that prevents microbes from entering the body. However, small skin breaks on the hands and fingers are common. Some are very small and hard to see. Gloves give added protection. They protect the worker from pathogens in the person's blood, body fluids, secretions, and excretions. Patients and residents are also protected from microorganisms that may be on the worker's hands.

Gloves are worn whenever contact with blood is likely. They are also worn when contact with infected material is likely. Contact may be direct. Or contact may be with equipment or surfaces that may be contaminated with blood or infective material. Gloves are also worn whenever you put your hands into the person's mouth. Other body fluids and body substances may contain blood or be infected. Therefore you must wear gloves whenever there is likely to be contact with blood or with body fluids, body substances, or mucous membranes that may contain blood or be infected. This includes saliva, vomitus, urine, feces, vaginal discharge, mucus, semen, wound drainage, pus, respiratory secretions, and other secretions and excretions.

Disposable gloves are easy to put on. No special technique is required. However, you must not tear the gloves when putting them on. Carelessness, long fingernails, and rings can tear gloves. Torn gloves are discarded. Blood, fluids, secretions, and excretions can enter the glove through the tear. This contaminates the hand. Remember the following about wearing gloves.

- A new pair is needed for every patient or resident.
- Torn, cut, or punctured gloves are removed immediately and discarded. Wash your hands and put on a new pair.
- Gloves are worn once and discarded.
- New gloves are needed whenever gloves become contaminated with infected material. More than one pair of gloves may be needed for a procedure.
- Gloves are pulled up to cover the wrists. If a gown is worn, the gloves must cover the cuffs (Fig. 9-12).
- When gloves are removed, the inside part will be on the outside. The inside of the gloves is considered *clean.*

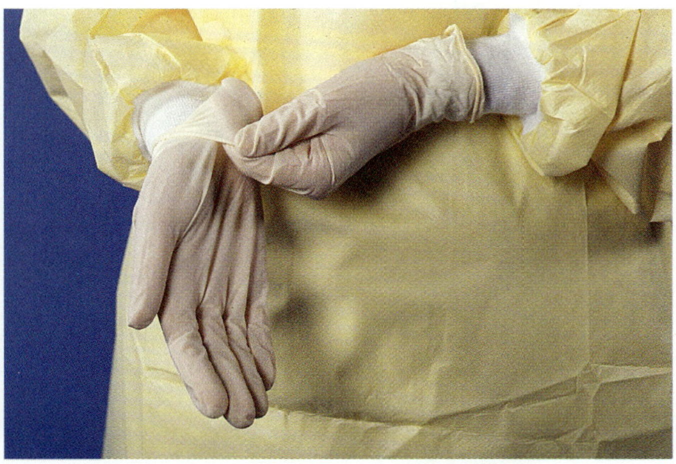

Fig. 9-12 *The gloves cover the cuffs of the gown.*

REMOVING GLOVES

PROCEDURE

1. When both hands are still gloved, be sure that only glove touches glove. Gloves should not touch skin on the wrists or arms.
2. Remove one glove by grasping it just below the cuff (Fig. 9-13, A on page 198).
3. Pull the glove down over your hand so it is inside out (Fig. 9-13, B).
4. Hold the removed glove with your other gloved hand.
5. Reach inside the other glove with the first two fingers of your ungloved hand (Fig. 9-13, C).
6. Pull the glove down (inside out) over your hand and the other glove (Fig. 9-13, D).
7. Discard the gloves in the appropriate container.
8. Wash your hands.

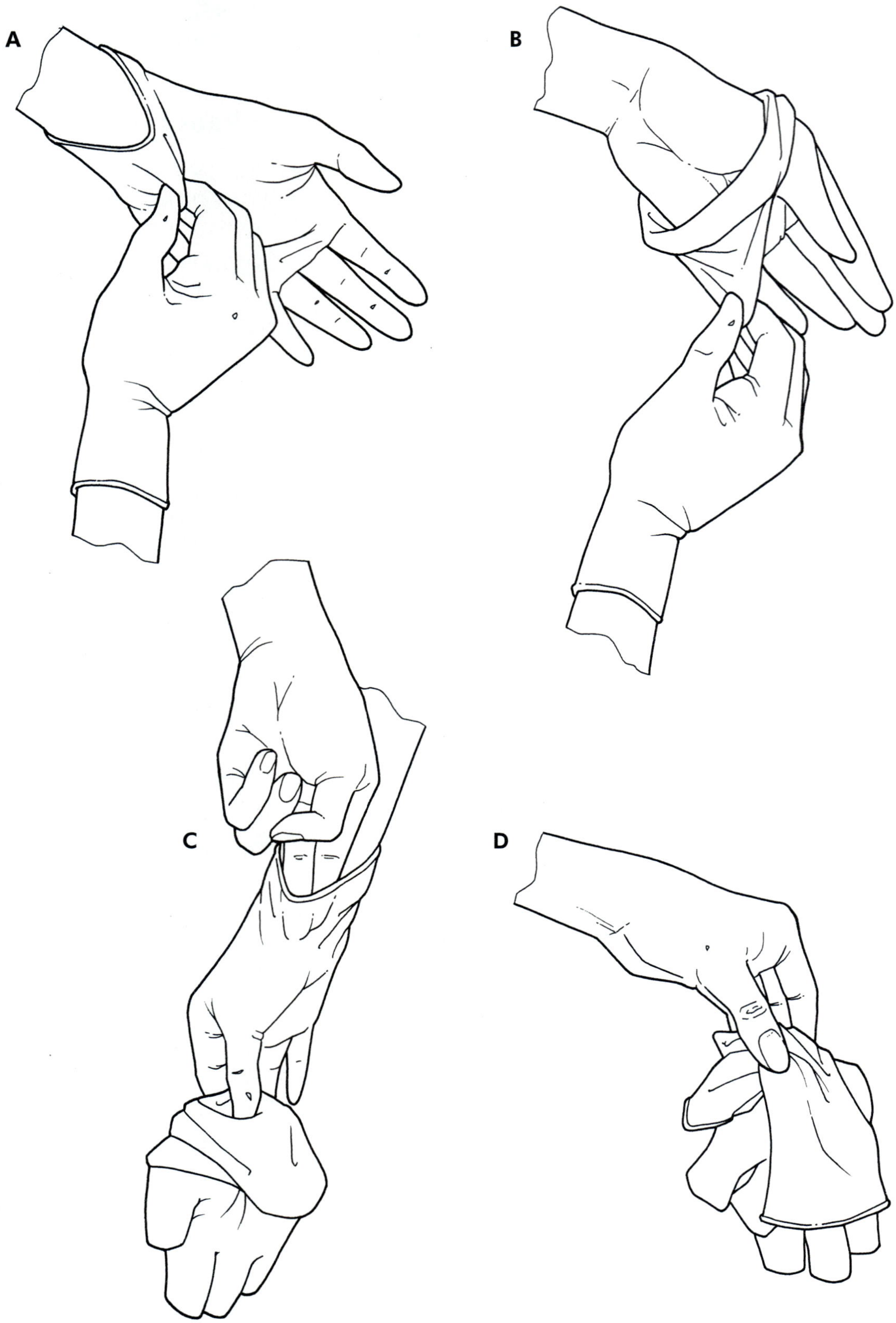

Fig. 9-13 *Removing gloves.* ***A,*** *The glove is grasped below the cuff.* ***B,*** *The glove is pulled down over the hand. The glove is inside out.* ***C,*** *The fingers of the ungloved hand are inserted inside the other glove.* ***D,*** *The glove is pulled down and over the hand and glove. The glove is inside out.*

Gowns Gowns keep clothing free from the person's pathogenic microorganisms. Gowns also protect the **person** from microbes that may be on the clothing of staff and visitors who enter the room. They also prevent soiling of clothing when giving care. Gowns are never worn outside the person's room.

Gowns must be long enough and large enough to completely cover clothing. The sleeves are long with tight cuffs. The gown opens at the back, where it is tied at the neck and waist. The inside and the neck of the gown are *clean.* The outside and waist strings are contaminated.

Some facilities use plastic aprons (see Fig. 9-11). Gowns are worn when the arms and wrists must be protected from soiling or contact with blood, body fluids, secretions, and excretions. They are also worn when splashing or splattering are possible. Gowns and aprons are used once. A wet gown is contaminated. If it becomes wet, the gown is removed and a dry one put on.

Disposable gowns are made of paper; reusable gowns are made of cloth. Disposable gowns are discarded after use. Reusable gowns are laundered before being used again.

Gowning Technique

Procedure

1. Remove your watch and all jewelry.
2. Roll up long sleeves of your uniform.
3. Wash your hands.
4. Put on a face mask if required.
5. Pick up a clean gown. Hold it out in front of you so it can unfold. Do not shake the gown.
6. Put your hands and arms through the sleeves of the gown (Fig. 9-14, A on page 200).
7. Make sure the gown completely covers the front of your uniform. The gown should be snug at the neck.
8. Tie the strings at the back of the neck (Fig. 9-14, B on page 200).
9. Overlap the back of the gown. Your uniform must be completely covered. The gown should be snug (Fig. 9-14, C on page 200) and should not hang loosely.
10. Tie the waist strings at the back.
11. Put on the gloves.
12. Provide necessary patient or resident care.
13. Remove and discard the gloves.
14. Remove the gown as follows:
    - **a.** Untie the waist strings.
    - **b.** Wash your hands.
    - **c.** Untie the neck strings. Do not touch the outside of the gown.
    - **d.** Pull the gown down from the shoulder.
    - **e.** Turn the gown inside out as it is removed. Hold the gown at the inside shoulder seams and bring your hands together (Fig. 9-14, D on page 200).
15. Roll up the gown away from you, keeping it inside out.
16. Discard the gown in the appropriate container.
17. Wash your hands.
18. Remove the face mask and discard it.
19. Wash your hands.
20. Open the door using a paper towel. Discard it in the wastebasket inside the room as you leave.

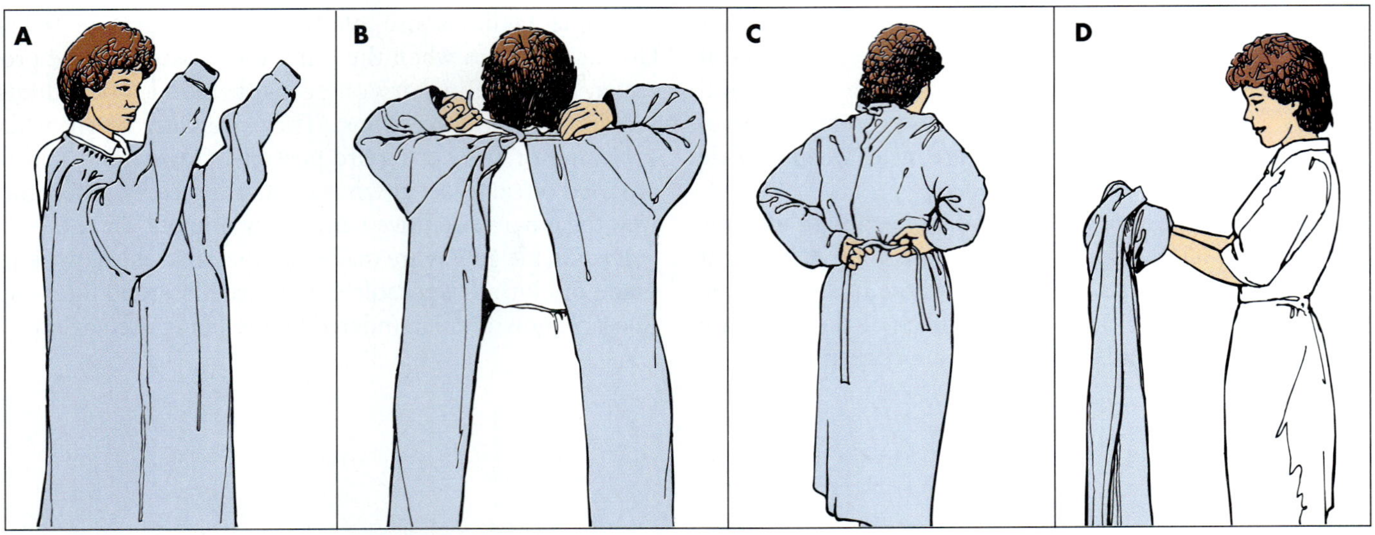

Fig. 9-14 *Gowning technique.* ***A,*** *The arms and hands are put through the sleeves.* ***B,*** *The strings are tied at the back of the neck.* ***C,*** *The gown is overlapped in the back so that the entire uniform is covered.* ***D,*** *The gown is turned inside out as it is removed.*

Wearing a face mask Face masks prevent the spread of microbes from the respiratory tract. Masks may be worn by patients or residents, visitors, or health care workers. Disposable masks are used. If a mask becomes wet or moist from breathing, it is contaminated. A new mask is applied when contamination occurs.

The mask should be snug over the nose and mouth. Hands are washed before putting on a mask. When removing the mask, first remove your gloves and wash your hands before undoing the ties. Only the ties are touched during removal. The front of the mask is considered contaminated.

WEARING A FACE MASK

PROCEDURE

1. Wash your hands.
2. Pick up the mask by its upper ties. Do not touch the part that will cover your face.
3. Position the mask over your nose. Your nose and mouth must be covered (Fig. 9-15, A).
4. Place the upper strings over your ears. Tie the strings in the back toward the top of your head (Fig. 9-15, B).
5. Tie the lower strings at the back of your neck (Fig. 9-15, C). Make sure the lower part of the mask is under your chin.
6. Pinch the metal band around your nose if you wear glasses. The top of the mask should be snug over your nose and under the bottom edge of the glasses.
7. Wash your hands.
8. Provide necessary care. Avoid coughing, sneezing, and unnecessary talking while wearing the mask.
9. Change the mask if it becomes moist or contaminated.
10. Remove the mask as follows:
    - **a.** Remove the gloves.
    - **b.** Untie the lower strings.
    - **c.** Untie the top strings.
    - **d.** Hold the top strings and remove the mask.
    - **e.** Bring the strings together. The inside of the mask will fold together (Fig. 9-15, D). Avoid touching the inside of the mask.
11. Discard the mask in the appropriate container.
12. Wash your hands.

A B C D

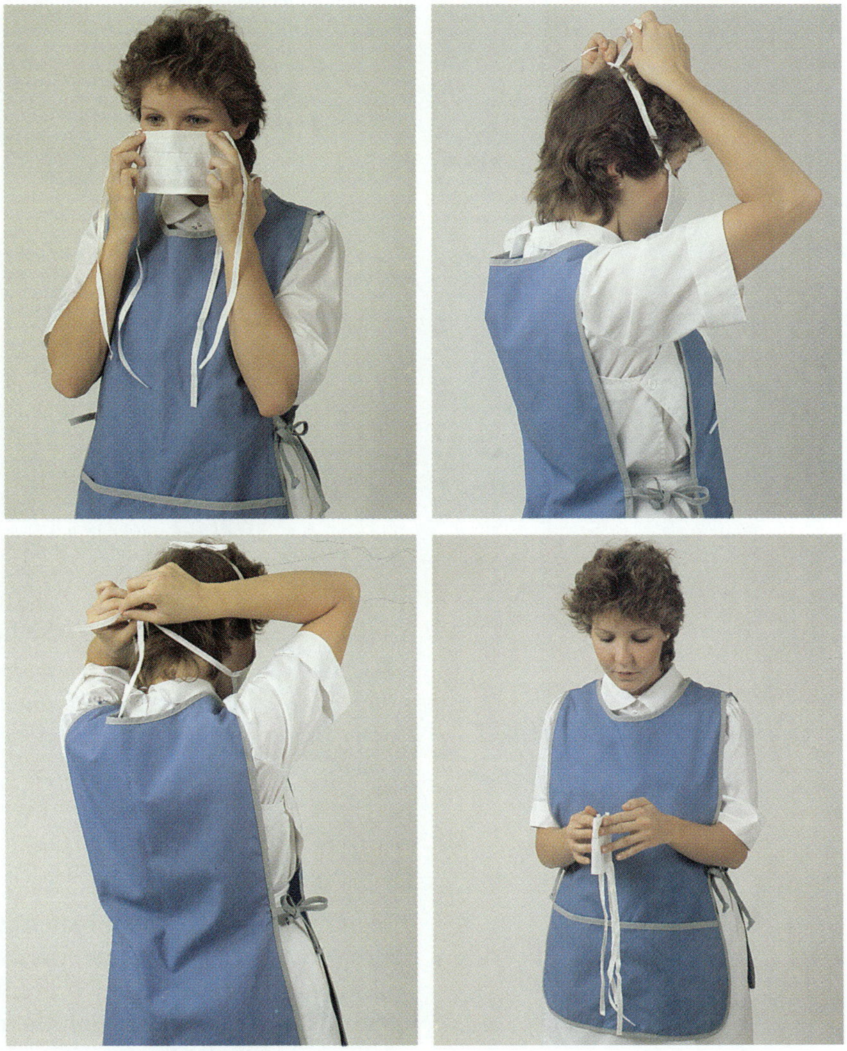

Fig. 9-15 ***A,*** *The mask is positioned so that mouth and nose are covered.* ***B,*** *The upper strings are tied on the back of the head.* ***C,*** *The lower strings are tied at the neck.* ***D,*** *The strings of the face mask are brought together so that the inside of the mask will be folded together after being removed.*

Protective eyewear Goggles or face shields (see Fig. 9-10) are worn when splashing or splattering is likely. They are worn with face masks. Together the mask and protective eyewear protects your eyes, nose, and mouth from splashing or splattering blood or oral fluids. Such protection may be needed when giving care, cleaning instruments, or disposing of contaminated fluids. Remember, if the mask becomes wet, it must be changed.

Disposable eyewear is discarded after use. Reusable eyewear is cleaned before being used for another patient or resident. It is washed with soap and water. Then a facility approved disinfectant is used.

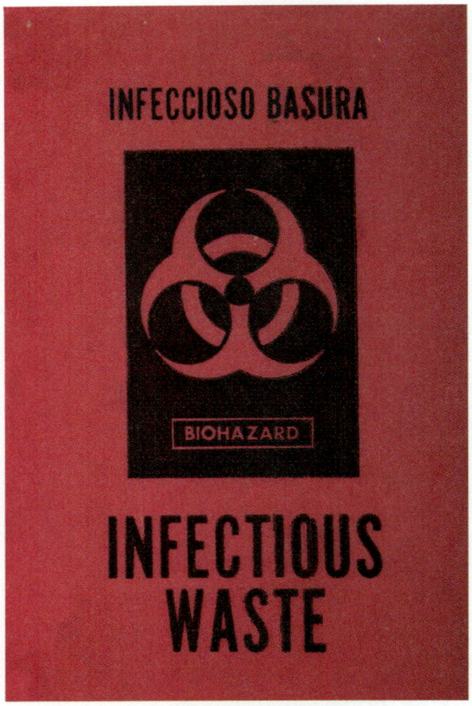

Fig. 9-16 *Trash container with the* BIOHAZARD *symbol.*

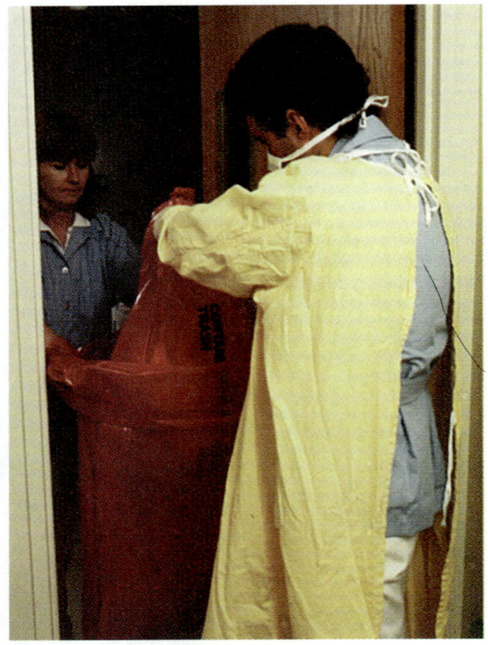

Fig. 9-18 *Two nursing assistants double bagging equipment. One nursing assistant is in the room inside the doorway. The other is outside the room. The "dirty" bag is placed inside the "clean" bag.*

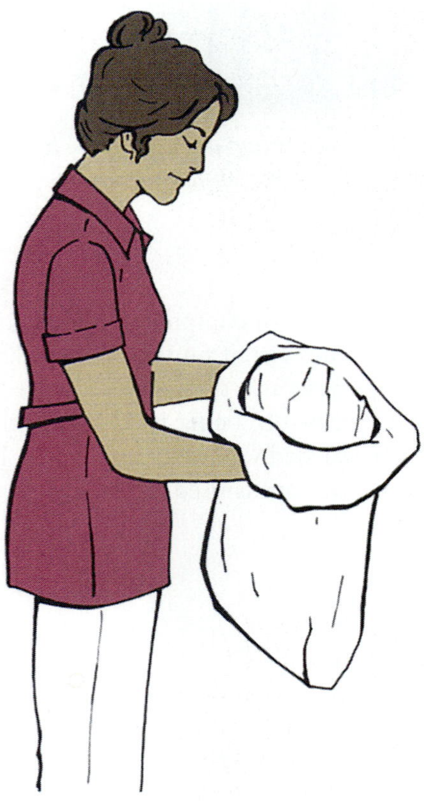

Fig. 9-17 *A cuff is made on the clean bag.*

Bagging articles Contaminated items are bagged before being removed from the person's room. Leak-proof plastic bags are used. They prevent leaking, and microorganisms cannot pass through them.

Trash is usually placed in a biohazardous waste container (Fig. 9-16). **Biohazardous waste** refers to items that are contaminated with the person's blood, body fluids, or body substances and that may be harmful to others. *Bio* means life and *hazardous* means dangerous or harmful.

Linen is bagged, labeled, and handled according to facility policy. You should know your facility's policy regarding the handling of contaminated waste, linen, and equipment.

A single bag is usually adequate. Double bagging involves placing contaminated items in two bags. However, the CDC no longer recommends double bagging unless the outside of the bag is soiled. Two workers are needed for double bagging. One worker is inside the room and the other is at the doorway outside the room. The worker in the room places contaminated items into a bag. The bag is then sealed securely. The worker outside the room holds open another bag that is considered clean. A wide cuff is made on the clean bag to protect the hands from contamination (Fig. 9-17). The worker inside the room stands at the doorway and places the contaminated bag into the clean bag (Fig. 9-18).

The following guidelines apply to bagging items:

- Separate bags are used for linens, glass, dry garbage, wet garbage, and equipment being returned to the central supply department.
- The contents of the bag (linens, dry garbage, wet garbage) are marked on the bag. Dry garbage consists of paper and disposable items. Dressings and leftover food are examples of wet garbage.
- Discard leftover food into the wet garbage container.
- Seal each bag with string or tape.
- Label the bag as required by facility policy.

Double Bagging

Procedure

1. Ask a co-worker to help you. The co-worker stands outside the room.
2. Place soiled linen, equipment, supplies, and wet garbage in the appropriate containers. The containers should be lined with leak-proof plastic bags.
3. Seal the bags securely with ties.
4. Ask your co-worker to make a wide cuff on the clean bag and then hold it wide open. The cuff protects the hands from contamination (see Fig. 9-17).
5. Place the contaminated bag into the clean bag held by your co-worker. Do not touch the outside of the clean bag.
6. Ask your co-worker to seal the clean bag. Also have the bag labeled according to facility policy.
7. Repeat steps 4, 5, and 6 as needed for other contaminated bags.
8. Ask your co-worker to take or send the bags to the appropriate department for disposal, disinfection, or sterilization.

Collecting specimens You may be asked to collect a urine, stool, or sputum specimen. These procedures are presented in later chapters. However, you need to know that special precautions are taken when collecting specimens from persons on isolation precautions.

The container is labeled according to facility policy. Then the container and lid are placed on a paper towel in the person's bathroom. Gloves are worn. The outside of the container must not be contaminated when the specimen is collected or transferred from collecting receptacle to the container. The lid must be put on securely. The double bagging procedure is followed if required by facility policy to remove the specimen from the room. No part of the lid or container can be touched by bare hands. Warning labels are applied according to facility policy.

Transporting persons Patients and residents on isolation precautions usually do not leave their rooms. Sometimes special treatments or diagnostic studies are needed. The person may have to be transported to another area of the facility. Procedures for transporting vary among facilities. Some require transporting the person by bed. This prevents contaminating wheelchairs and stretchers that are used by other persons. Other facilities allow the use of wheelchairs or stretchers.

The following guidelines will help you safely transport persons on isolation precautions. Besides the person's own physical safety, a safe transport means that other staff and visitors are protected from the infection.

- The person wears a clean gown or pajamas.
- Persons on Airborne and Droplet Precautions wear masks. They are given tissues and a leak-proof bag. Used tissues are placed in the bag.
- You wear a gown, mask, and gloves as required by the isolation precaution.
- An extra layer of sheets is placed on the stretcher or wheelchair. This provides protection against draining body fluids.
- Do not let anyone else on the elevator. This reduces exposure to the infection.
- Staff in the area where the person is taken are alerted to the isolation precautions. They need to wear gowns, masks, protective eyewear, and gloves as needed.
- The stretcher or wheelchair is disinfected after use.

Psychological Impact of Isolation Precautions

The person has needs for love, belonging, and self-esteem. Too often these needs go unmet when isolation precautions are used. Visitors and staff may need to wear gowns, masks, protective eyewear, and gloves. The extra effort needed before entering the room, being unsure of what can and cannot be touched, and the fear of getting the disease often cause people to avoid the person. Loneliness, feeling unloved and unwanted, and rejection can occur.

Self-esteem can easily suffer. Besides dealing with illness, the person knows the disease is contagious and can be spread to others. The person may feel dirty, unclean, and undesirable. Unfortunately, visitors and health care workers may unknowingly make the person feel ashamed and guilty for having a contagious disease.

The nurse can help the person, visitors, and the health team understand the need for isolation precautions and their psychological effects on the person. You can help meet the person's need for love, belonging, and self-esteem. The following actions will be helpful. However, objects that become contaminated with infected material must be disinfected or discarded.

- Remember, the pathogen is undesirable, not the person.
- Treat the person with respect, kindness, and dignity.
- Provide newspapers, magazines, and other reading materials.
- Provide hobby materials if possible.
- Make sure there is a clock in the room.
- Encourage the person to telephone family and friends.
- Provide a current television guide.
- Organize your work so you can stay in the room to visit with the person.
- Say hello from the doorway often.

BLOODBORNE PATHOGEN STANDARD

The number of people infected with the AIDS virus (HIV) and hepatitis B virus (HBV) is increasing (see Chapter 28). Health workers care for these people. Therefore health workers are at risk for exposure. The Bloodborne Pathogen Standard is intended to protect workers from exposure. The standard is a regulation of the Occupational Safety and Health Administration (OSHA). OSHA is part of the U.S. Department of Labor. Box 9-6 contains the definitions used by OSHA's Bloodborne Pathogen Standard.

The AIDS and hepatitis B viruses are found in the blood. They are disease-producing pathogens. Therefore they are bloodborne pathogens. The viruses exit the body through blood and are transmitted to others by blood. The virus can also be transmitted by other *potentially infectious materials* (see Box 9-6). Such materials are contaminated with blood or with a body fluid, secretion, or excretion that may contain blood. Potentially infectious materials may also include needles, suction equipment, soiled linens, dressings, and other equipment and items used in the person's care.

Exposure Control Plan

Employers must have a written exposure control plan. The plan identifies those workers who have a risk of occupational exposure. That is, they may be exposed to blood or to other potentially infectious materials. Those at risk usually include nurses, nursing assistants, surgical personnel, central supply staff, laundry staff, housekeepers, physical therapists, laboratory staff, and others. The plan also includes the actions to take when there is an exposure incident.

Staff at risk for exposure must receive free information and training. Training must occur upon employment. Then training is done every year. Training is also required for new or changed procedures and tasks that involve exposure to bloodborne pathogens. OSHA requires that training include:

- An explanation of the Bloodborne Pathogen Standard and where to get a copy
- The causes, signs, and symptoms of bloodborne diseases
- How bloodborne pathogens are transmitted
- An explanation of the exposure control plan and where to get a copy
- How to know which tasks might cause occupational exposure
- The use and limitations of safe work practices, engineering controls, and personal protective equipment
- Information on the hepatitis B vaccination
- Who to contact and what to do in an emergency
- Information on reporting an exposure incident, postexposure evaluation, and follow-up.
- Information on warning labels and color coding

Preventive Measures

Preventive measures help reduce the risk of occupational exposure. OSHA measures include hepatitis B vaccination and Standard Precautions.

Hepatitis B vaccination Hepatitis B is an inflammatory disease of the liver. It is caused by the hepatitis B virus (HBV). HBV is usually transmitted by blood and sexual contact. The hepatitis B vaccine is given to produce immunity against hepatitis B. Having **immunity** means that a person has protection against a specific disease and will not get or be affected by the disease. A **vaccination** involves giving a **vaccine** to produce immunity. A vaccine is a preparation containing dead or weakened microorganisms. There are vaccines for many diseases, including

BOX 9-6 Bloodborne Pathogen Standard Definitions

blood Human blood, human blood components, and products made from human blood

bloodborne pathogens Pathogenic microorganisms that are present in human blood and can cause disease in humans; these pathogens include, but are not limited to, hepatitis B virus (HBV) and human immunodeficiency virus (HIV)

contaminated The presence or reasonably anticipated presence of blood or other potentially infectious materials on an item or surface

contaminated laundry Laundry soiled with blood or other potentially infectious materials or that may contain sharps

contaminated sharps Any contaminated object that can penetrate the skin including, but not limited to, needles, scalpels, broken glass, broken capillary tubes, and exposed ends of dental wires

decontamination The use of physical or chemical means to remove, inactivate, or destroy bloodborne pathogens on a surface or item to the point where they can no longer transmit infectious particles and the surface or item is safe for handling, use, or disposal

engineering controls Controls that isolate or remove the bloodborne pathogen hazard from the workplace (sharps disposal containers, self-sheathing needles)

exposure incident A specific eye, mouth, other mucous membrane, nonintact skin, or parenteral contact with blood or other potentially infectious materials that results from the performance of an employee's duties

handwashing facilities The adequate supply of running water, soap, single-use towels, or hot-air drying machines

HBV Hepatitis B virus

HIV Human immunodeficiency virus

occupational exposure Reasonably anticipated skin, eye, mucous membrane, or parenteral contact with blood or other potentially infectious materials that may result from the performance of an employee's duties

other potentially infectious materials

- The following human body fluids: semen, vaginal secretions, cerebrospinal fluid, synovial fluid, pleural fluid, pericardial fluid, peritoneal fluid, amniotic fluid, saliva in dental procedures, any body fluid that is visibly contaminated with blood, and all body fluids in situations where it is difficult or impossible to differentiate between body fluids
- Any tissue or organ (other than intact skin) from a human (living or dead)
- HIV-containing cell or tissue cultures, organ cultures, and HIV- or HBV-containing culture medium or other solutions; and blood, organs, or other tissues from experimental animals infected with HIV or HBV

parenteral Piercing mucous membranes or the skin barrier through events such as needlesticks, human bites, cuts, and abrasions

personal protective equipment Specialized clothing or equipment worn by an employee for protection against a hazard

regulated waste

- Liquid or semiliquid blood or other potentially infectious materials
- Contaminated items that would release blood or other potentially infectious materials in a liquid or semiliquid state if compressed
- Items that are caked with dried blood or other potentially infectious materials that are capable of releasing these materials during handling
- Contaminated sharps; and pathological and microbiological wastes containing blood or other potentially infectious materials

source individual Any person (living or dead) whose blood or other potentially infectious materials may be a source of occupational exposure to employees; examples include, but are not limited to

- Hospital and clinical patients
- Clients in institutions for the developmentally disabled
- Trauma victims
- Clients of drug and alcohol treatment facilities
- Residents of hospices and nursing homes
- Human remains
- Persons who donate or sell blood or blood components

sterilize The use of a physical or chemical procedure to destroy all microbial life, including spores

work practice controls Controls that reduce the likelihood of exposure by altering the way the task is performed measles, mumps, polio, and smallpox. The microorganisms in the vaccine depend on the disease. The polio vaccine contains microorganisms that cause polio. The hepatitis B vaccine contains the virus causing hepatitis B. It provides immunity against hepatitis B.

The hepatitis B vaccination involves 3 injections (shots). The second injection is given 1 month after the first one. The third injection is given 6 months after the second one. The vaccination can be given before or after exposure to the HBV.

Employers must make the hepatitis B vaccination available to employees within 10 working days of being hired. The employee must also receive training about the vaccination. The vaccination is free to the employee. The cost is paid for by the employer.

An employee can refuse the vaccination. If so, the employee must sign a statement saying that the vaccine is being refused. An employee who refuses the vaccine may request and obtain the vaccination at a later date.

Standard Precautions Standard Precautions were presented on pages 192-193. *All* human blood and other potentially infectious materials are treated as if they are infectious for HIV and HBV.

Methods of Control

Methods of control required by OSHA include engineering and work practice controls, personal protective equipment, and housekeeping measures.

Engineering and work practice controls Engineering and work practice controls are used to control the transmission of HIV and HBV. *Engineering controls* reduce employee exposure in the workplace. The hazard is removed or isolated, or the worker is isolated from the exposure. Special containers for contaminated sharps (needles, broken glass) remove and isolate the hazard from workers. There are also special containers for blood specimens and other body fluid specimens such as urine. All special containers must be puncture-resistant and leakproof. The containers are color coded in red or labeled with the BIOHAZARD symbol (see Fig. 9-16).

Work practice controls reduce the risk of exposure. All procedures involving blood or other potentially infectious materials must be done in a way that minimizes splattering, splashing, and spraying. Producing droplets must also be avoided. OSHA has identified the following work practice controls. The controls address the handling of needles and sharp instruments. Nursing assistant responsibilities do not include the use of needles or sharp instruments. However, such work practice controls are included here so you are aware of how such items should be handled.

- Do not eat, drink, smoke, apply cosmetics or lip balm, or handle contact lenses in areas of occupational exposure.
- Do not store food or drink in refrigerators or other areas where blood or potentially infectious materials are kept.
- Wash hands when gloves are removed and as soon as possible after skin contact with blood or other potentially infectious materials.
- Never recap, bend, or remove needles by hand unless the employer can show that no method is possible or that such action is required by a specific medical procedure. When recapping, bending, or removing contaminated needles is required by medical procedure, this must be done by mechanical means (use of forceps) or a one-handed technique.
- Never shear or break contaminated needles.
- Discard contaminated needles and sharps instruments in containers that are closable, puncture-resistant, and leakproof. The containers must be color coded red or labeled with the BIOHAZARD symbol. Containers must be upright and not allowed to overfill.

Personal protective equipment **Personal protective equipment** is specialized clothing or equipment worn by an employee for protection against a hazard. Gloves, goggles, face shields, masks, laboratory coats, gowns, shoe covers, and surgical caps are personal protective equipment. They help prevent occupational exposure to infectious materials. Personal protective equipment meets OSHA's standards if it does not permit blood or other potentially infectious material to pass through. Blood or other potentially infectious materials must not reach the worker's clothes, undergarments, skin, eyes, mouth, or other mucous membranes.

Personal protective equipment must be free to the worker. The worker does not buy or pay for personal protective equipment. Correct sizes must be available. The employer is responsible for making sure the equipment is properly cleaned, laundered, repaired, replaced, or discarded.

Personal protective equipment is used whenever occupational exposure may occur. OSHA also requires the following precautions for safe handling and use of personal protective equipment.

- Remove protective equipment before leaving the work area and after a garment becomes contaminated.
- Place used protective equipment in designated areas or containers when being stored, washed, decontaminated, or discarded.

- Wear gloves when it can be expected that there will be contact with blood or other potentially infectious materials. Gloves are also worn when handling or touching contaminated items or surfaces. Gloves are replaced if worn, punctured, or contaminated.
- Never wash or decontaminate disposable gloves for reuse.
- Discard utility gloves when they show signs of cracking, peeling, tearing, puncturing, or deteriorating. Utility gloves may be decontaminated for reuse if they will not be ruined in the process.

Housekeeping The Bloodborne Pathogen Standard requires that the facility be kept clean and sanitary. The employer must have a cleaning schedule. The schedule must include the methods of decontamination to be used and the tasks and procedures to be done.

Equipment Contaminated equipment must be cleaned and decontaminated. So must contaminated work surfaces. Such work surfaces are decontaminated with an appropriate disinfectant:

- Upon completion of procedures
- Immediately when there is obvious contamination
- After any spill of blood or other potentially infectious material
- At the end of the work shift when surfaces have become contaminated since the last cleaning

Reusable bins, pails, and cans must be inspected and decontaminated. There must be a schedule for such inspection and decontamination procedures. A brush and dustpan are used to clean up broken glass. Tongs can also be used. You must never pick up broken glass with your hands, not even if wearing gloves. Broken glass is discarded into a puncture-resistant container.

Waste Federal, state, and local laws regulate the removal of waste from the facility. The Bloodborne Pathogen Standard requires special measures when discarding contaminated sharps and other *regulated waste.* Regulated waste includes:

- Liquid or semiliquid blood or other potentially infectious materials
- Items contaminated with blood or other potentially infectious materials
- Items caked with blood or other potentially infectious materials
- Contaminated sharps (such as needles, sharp instruments, broken glass)

Closable, puncture-resistant, and leakproof containers are required for regulated waste. Containers must be color coded in red or labeled with the BIOHAZARD symbol.

Laundry The employer is responsible for laundering contaminated items. Some facilities have their own laundry. Others use a commercial laundry. OSHA requires that the following procedures be followed for contaminated laundry.

- Handle contaminated laundry as little as possible.
- Wear gloves or other appropriate personal protective equipment when handling contaminated laundry.
- Bag contaminated laundry where it was used.
- Mark laundry bags or containers with the BIOHAZARD symbol if the laundry is sent offsite.
- Place wet contaminated laundry in leakproof containers before transporting. The containers should be color coded in red or labeled with the BIOHAZARD symbol.

Exposure Incidents

The exposure control plan must include the procedure for evaluating exposure incidents. An *exposure incident* occurs while performing duties of employment. It is a specific eye, mouth, other mucous membrane, nonintact skin, or parenteral contact with blood or other potentially infectious materials. OSHA defines *parenteral* as piercing mucous membranes or the skin barrier. Such piercing can occur through needlesticks, human bites, cuts, and abrasions.

Exposure incidents are reported at once. Medical evaluation and follow-up are free to the employee. This includes required laboratory tests. The employee's blood is collected for HBV and HIV testing. However, the employee may refuse such testing. If so, the blood sample is kept for at least 90 days. Testing can still be done if the employee changes his or her mind.

Confidentiality is very important. The employee must be informed of the results of the evaluation. The employee is also told of any medical conditions resulting from the exposure incident that may need further treatment. The person performing the evaluation provides a written opinion to the employer. The employer must give the employee a copy of the opinion within 15 days after the evaluation has been completed.

The source individual's blood is tested for HIV or HBV. The *source individual* is the person whose blood or body fluids are the source of an exposure incident. Test results are to be made available to the exposed employee. State laws vary about releasing such information. The employer must inform the employee about any laws affecting the source's identity and test results.

CROSS-TRAINING OPPORTUNITIES

Other health workers are involved in infection control. They work in the central supply department and the housekeeping department. Infection control measures and the Bloodborne Pathogen Standard are followed. Personal protective equipment is worn as needed. You may be asked to cross-train to work in one or both of these areas.

Central Supply

Staff in the central supply department disinfect and sterilize supplies and equipment. These procedures may be done for new items bought by the facility. Used equipment and supplies are also disinfected or sterilized before being used for another person. Central supply staff also make sure that each nursing unit is stocked with items needed for care. They also bring special equipment to nursing units as requested.

Housekeeping

The housekeeping staff cleans patient or resident rooms, the nursing units, hallways, bathrooms, and other departments and parts of the facility. They have special cleaning methods and procedures for cleaning and disinfecting floors, furniture, bathrooms, and equipment.

SUMMARY

Preventing the spread of infection is the responsibility of every health worker. You must be conscientious about your work. Your employer and your patients and residents assume that you will practice medical asepsis to prevent the spread of microorganisms and infection. One act of carelessness can spread microorganisms and endanger the person's safety. The reverse is also true. You can develop the same infection as the person if you do not practice medical asepsis or required isolation precautions. The simple procedure of handwashing before and after patient or resident contact significantly reduces the spread of microorganisms.

REVIEW QUESTIONS

Circle T *if the answer is true and* F *if the answer is false.*

1 T F A pathogen can cause an infection.

2 T F Microorganisms are not pathogenic in their natural environments.

3 T F An infection results from the invasion and growth of microorganisms in the body.

4 T F The source of an infection is a pathogen.

5 T F A microorganism must enter the body of a susceptible host for an infection to develop.

6 T F Sterilization is the same as clean technique.

7 T F An item is sterile if nonpathogens are present.

8 T F The hands and forearms are held up during the handwashing procedure.

9 T F You should clean under the fingernails when washing your hands.

10 T F Paper towels are used to turn faucets on and off during the handwashing procedure.

11 T F Disposable items help reduce the spread of infection.

12 T F Unused items in a person's room can be used for another person.

13 T F OSHA requires that employees receive free information and training about bloodborne pathogens.

14 T F A person has immunity against hepatitis B. The person will develop the disease.

REVIEW QUESTIONS—CONT'D

Circle the best *answer.*

15 The pathogens in Mr. Morgan's wound need the following to grow *except*

a Water

b Nourishment

c Oxygen

d Light

16 Microorganisms grow best in an environment that is

a Warm and dark

b Warm and light

c Cool and dark

d Cool and light

17 The person with an infection may have

a Fever, nausea, vomiting, rash, and/or sores

b Pain or tenderness, redness, and/or swelling

c Fatigue, loss of appetite, and/or a discharge

d All of the above.

18 Microbes enter and leave the body through the

a Respiratory tract and/or breaks in the skin

b Gastrointestinal system and/or the blood

c Reproductive system and/or urinary system

d All of the above

19 A nosocomial infection occurs

a Before admission to the facility

b After admission to the facility

c Only in infants and the elderly

d Only in hospitals

20 Mr. Morgan is at risk for a nosocomial infection. You can prevent nosocomial infections by the following *except*

a Handwashing before and after giving him care

b Practicing Standard Precautions

c Following the Bloodborne Pathogen Standard

d Sterilizing all items used for care

21 The process of sterilization

a Destroys spores

b Is used to clean furniture

c Can be used for plastic and rubber items

d All of the above.

22 To practice infection control, you should do the following *except*

a Use a damp cloth to dust furniture

b Sit on the person's bed

c Clean away from the body or uniform

d Clean from the cleanest area to the dirtiest

23 When cleaning equipment, you should

a Rinse the item in cold water before cleaning

b Wash the item with soap and hot water

c Use a brush if necessary

d All of the above

24 Which is used to sterilize equipment?

a Handwashing

b Boiling water

c An autoclave

d Chemical disinfectants

25 Isolation precautions

a Prevent infection

b Destroy pathogens

c Keep pathogens within a specific area

d Destroy pathogens and nonpathogens

26 A *clean* area

a Has been rinsed with water

b Is contaminated with pathogens

c Is free of pathogens

d Has no obvious dirt

27 Standard Precautions

a Are used for all patients and residents

b Prevent the spread of pathogens through the air

c Require gowns, masks, and gloves

d All of the above

REVIEW QUESTIONS—CONT'D

28 Gloves are worn when in contact with Mr. Morgan's
- **a** Blood
- **b** Body fluids
- **c** Secretions or excretions
- **d** All of the above

29 Droplet Precautions prevent the
- **a** Person from coming in contact with pathogens
- **b** Spread of pathogens found in wounds
- **c** Spread of pathogens through fecal material
- **d** Spread of pathogens from coughing and sneezing

30 Which statement about isolation precautions is *false?*
- **a** Floors are contaminated.
- **b** Paper towels are used to handle contaminated objects.
- **c** Specimens are double bagged.
- **d** Hands are washed only when leaving the room.

31 Which part of the gown is *clean?*
- **a** The neck strings
- **b** The waist strings
- **c** The sleeves
- **d** The back

32 The face mask
- **a** Can be reused
- **b** Is considered clean on the inside
- **c** Is contaminated when it becomes moist
- **d** Should fit loosely over the nose and mouth so the person can breathe

33 Mr. Morgan is on Contact Precautions. Which is *false?*
- **a** A mask is worn.
- **b** A gown is worn for contact with infected material.
- **c** Gloves are worn.
- **d** Protective eyewear is worn if splattering of blood or body fluids is likely.

34 Mr. Morgan is on Contact Precautions. Which will *not* help him psychologically?
- **a** Treating him with respect, kindness, and dignity
- **b** Providing reading materials
- **c** Encouraging him to telephone family and friends
- **d** Finishing your work in the room quickly

35 When putting on personal protective equipment, what order is followed?
- **a** Gloves, mask, gown
- **b** Mask, gloves, gown
- **c** Mask, gown, gloves
- **d** Gown, mask, gloves

36 Work practice controls reduce the risk of exposure to bloodborne pathogens. Which is *false?*
- **a** Hands are washed when gloves are removed
- **b** Sharp objects are discarded into containers with the BIOHAZARD symbol
- **c** Food and blood can be stored in the same places
- **d** You cannot eat or drink in areas of occupational exposure

37 Proper use of personal protective equipment involves the following *except*
- **a** Washing disposable gloves for reuse
- **b** Removing protective equipment before leaving the work area
- **c** Discarding cracked or torn utility gloves
- **d** Wearing gloves when touching contaminated items or surfaces

38 When are contaminated work surfaces cleaned?
- **a** After completing a procedure
- **b** Immediately when there is obvious contam-ination
- **c** After blood or other potentially infectious material is spilled
- **d** All of the above

Answers to these questions are on page 749.

Body Mechanics

10

OBJECTIVES

- Define the key terms in this chapter
- Explain the purpose and rules of using good body mechanics
- Identify comfort and safety measures for lifting, turning, and moving persons in bed
- Explain the purpose of a transfer belt
- Identify the comfort and safety measures for using a stretcher to transport a person
- Explain why good body alignment and position changes are important
- Identify the comfort and safety measures for positioning persons in bed
- Position persons in the basic bed positions and in a chair
- Perform the procedures described in this chapter

KEY TERMS

base of support The area on which an object rests

body alignment The way in which body parts are aligned with one another; posture

body mechanics Using the body in an efficient and careful way

dorsal recumbent position The back-lying or supine position

Fowler's position A semisitting position; the head of the bed is elevated 45 to 60 degrees

friction The rubbing of one surface against another

gait belt A transfer belt

lateral position The side-lying position

logrolling Turning the person as a unit in alignment with one motion

posture The way in which body parts are aligned with one another; body alignment

shearing When skin sticks to a surface and the muscles slide in the direction the body is moving

side-lying position The lateral position

Sims' position A side-lying position in which the upper leg is sharply flexed so that it is not on the lower leg and the lower arm is behind the person

supine position The back-lying or dorsal recumbent position

transfer belt A belt used to hold onto a person during a transfer or when walking with the person; a gait belt

You will move patients and residents often. A person may be moved or turned in bed or transferred from the bed to a chair, wheelchair, or stretcher. These and other activities require correct use of your body to protect yourself from injury. Using your body correctly also protects patients and residents from the dangers of not being held or supported properly.

Box 10-1 on page 214 contains a review of the musculoskeletal system's structure and function. For more detailed information, see Chapter 5.

BODY MECHANICS

Body mechanics means using the body in an efficient and careful way. It involves good posture, balance, and the strongest and largest muscles to perform work. Fatigue, muscle strain, and injury can result from improper use and positioning of the body during activity or rest. You must be concerned with the person's and your own body mechanics. Risk of injury is reduced by using good body mechanics.

The major movable body parts are the head, trunk, arms, and legs. **Posture (body alignment)** is the way body parts are aligned with one another. Good body alignment (posture) allows the body to move and function with strength and efficiency. Good alignment is necessary when standing, sitting, or lying down.

The **base of support** is the area on which an object rests. The feet provide the base of support when standing. A good base of support is needed for balance. For example, it is hard to balance on one foot for a long time. Standing with your feet apart gives a wider base of support. The wider base of support gives a balanced and stable feeling. Therefore a wide base of support gives more balance and stability (Fig. 10-3 on page 216).

The strongest and largest muscles are in the shoulders, upper arms, hips, and thighs. These muscles are used to lift and move heavy objects. If smaller and weaker muscles are used, strain and exertion is placed on them. That causes fatigue and injury. Use the strong thigh and hip muscles for lifting and moving. This is done by bending your knees or squatting to lift a heavy object (Fig. 10-4 on page 217). Do not bend from the waist when lifting. Bending from the waist places strain on the small muscles of the back. Holding items close to your body and base of support involves upper arm and shoulder muscles (Fig. 10-5 on page 217). If the object is held away from the body, strain is placed on smaller muscles in the lower arms.

Text continued on page 218.

BOX 10-1 MUSCULOSKELETAL SYSTEM: REVIEW OF BODY STRUCTURE AND FUNCTION

The musculoskeletal system provides the framework for the body and allows the body to move. It also protects and gives the body shape.

BONES

Bones are hard, rigid structures that are made up of living cells. *Long bones* (leg bones) bear the weight of the body. *Short bones* allow skill and ease in movement. Bones in the wrists, fingers, ankles, and toes are short bones. *Flat bones* protect the organs. Such bones include the ribs, skull, pelvic bones, and shoulder blades. *Irregular bones* are the vertebrae in the spinal column. They allow various degrees of movement and flexibility.

JOINTS

A *joint* is the point at which two or more bones meet. Joints allow movement (joint movement is discussed in Chapter 19). There are three types of joints (Fig. 10-1). A *ball-and-socket* joint allows movement in all directions. The joints of the hips and shoulders are ball-and-socket joints. A *hinge joint* allows movement in one direction. The elbow and knee are hinge joints. A *pivot joint* allows turning from side to side. The skull is connected to the spine by a pivot joint.

MUSCLES

There are more than 500 muscles in the human body (Fig. 10-2). *Voluntary* muscles can be consciously controlled. Muscles that are attached to bones *(skeletal muscles)* are voluntary. Arm muscles do not work unless you move your arm; likewise for leg muscles. *Involuntary muscles* work automatically and cannot be consciously controlled. Involuntary muscles control the action of the stomach, intestines, blood vessels, and other body organs. *Cardiac muscle* is in the heart. It is an involuntary muscle.

Muscles perform three important body functions:

- Movement of body parts
- Maintenance of posture
- Production of body heat

Some muscles constantly contract to maintain the body's posture. When muscles contract, they burn food for energy, resulting in the production of heat. The greater the muscular activity, the greater the amount of heat produced in the body. Shivering is a way the body produces heat when exposed to cold. The shivering sensation is from rapid, general muscle contractions.

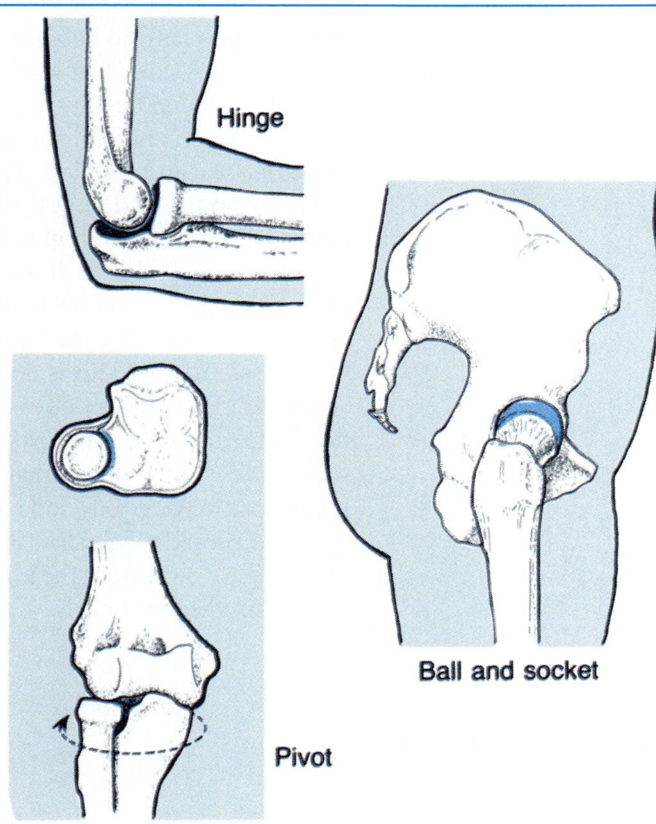

Fig. 10-1 *Types of joints.* *(Modified from Austrin M: Young's learning medical terminology step by step, ed 8, St Louis, 1994, Mosby–Year Book.)*

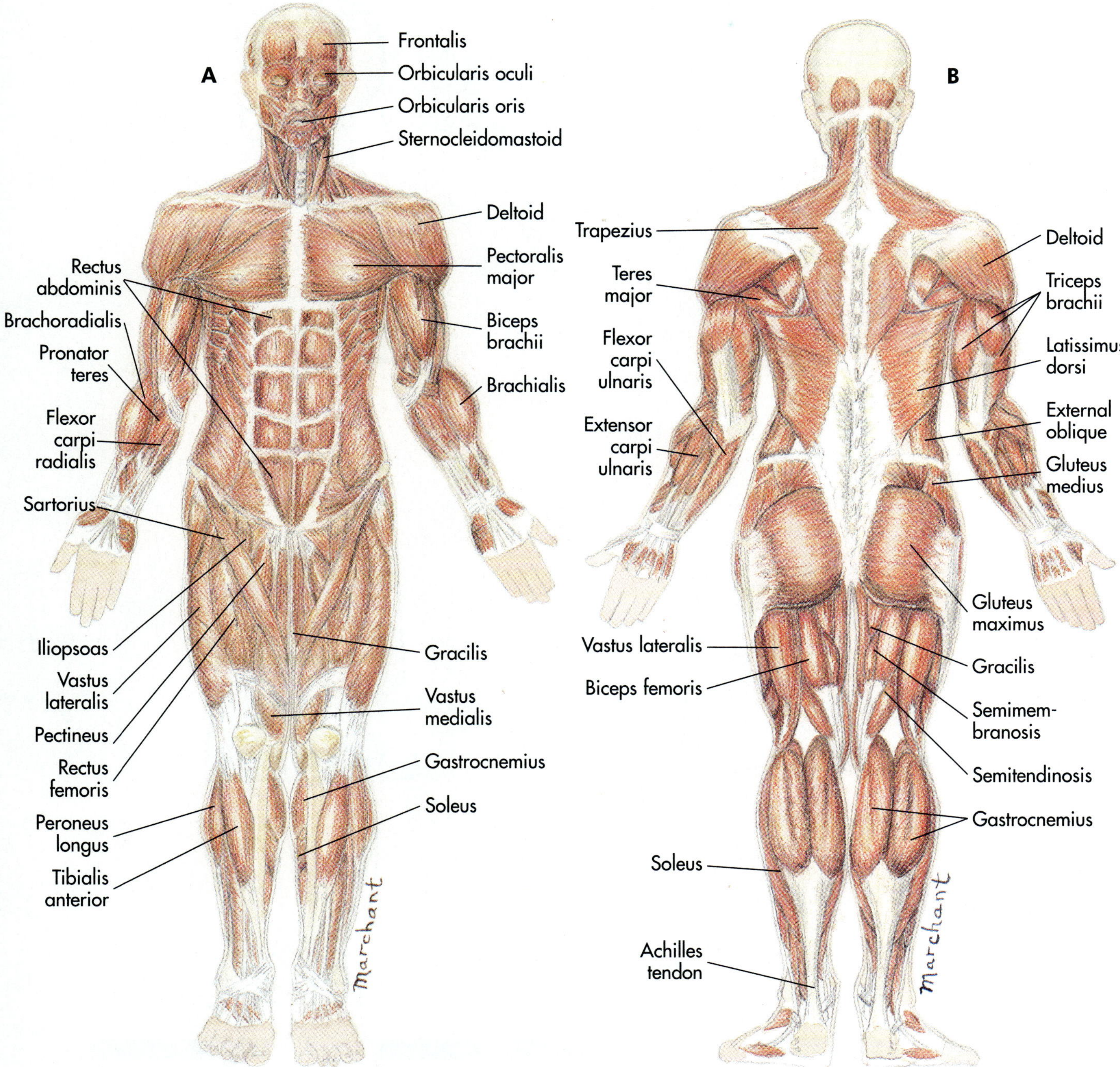

Fig. 10-2 ***A,*** *Anterior view of muscles.* ***B,*** *Posterior view of muscles.*

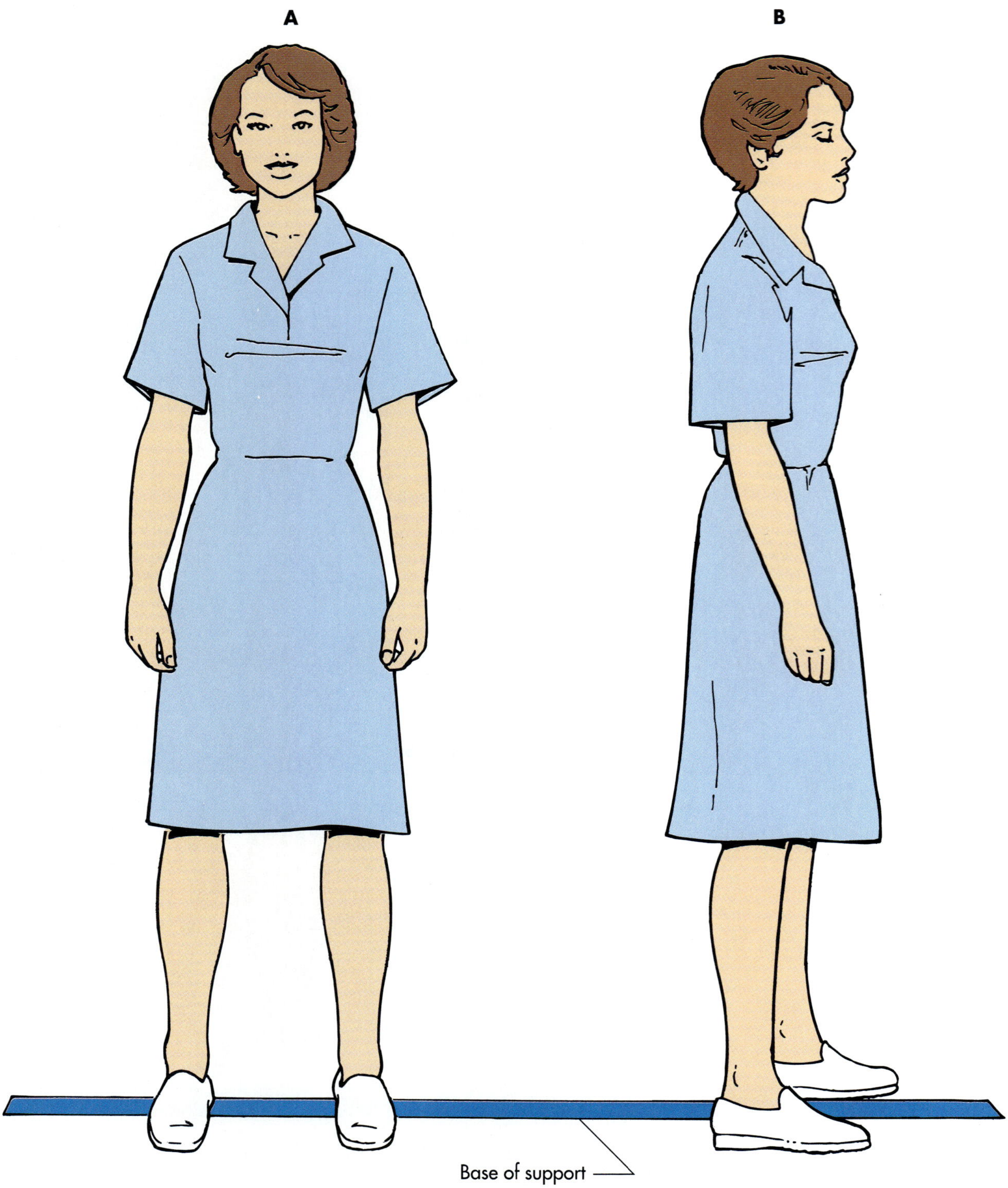

Fig. 10-3 ***A,*** *Anterior view of an adult in good body alignment with feet apart for a wide base of support.* ***B,*** *Lateral view of an adult with good posture and alignment.*

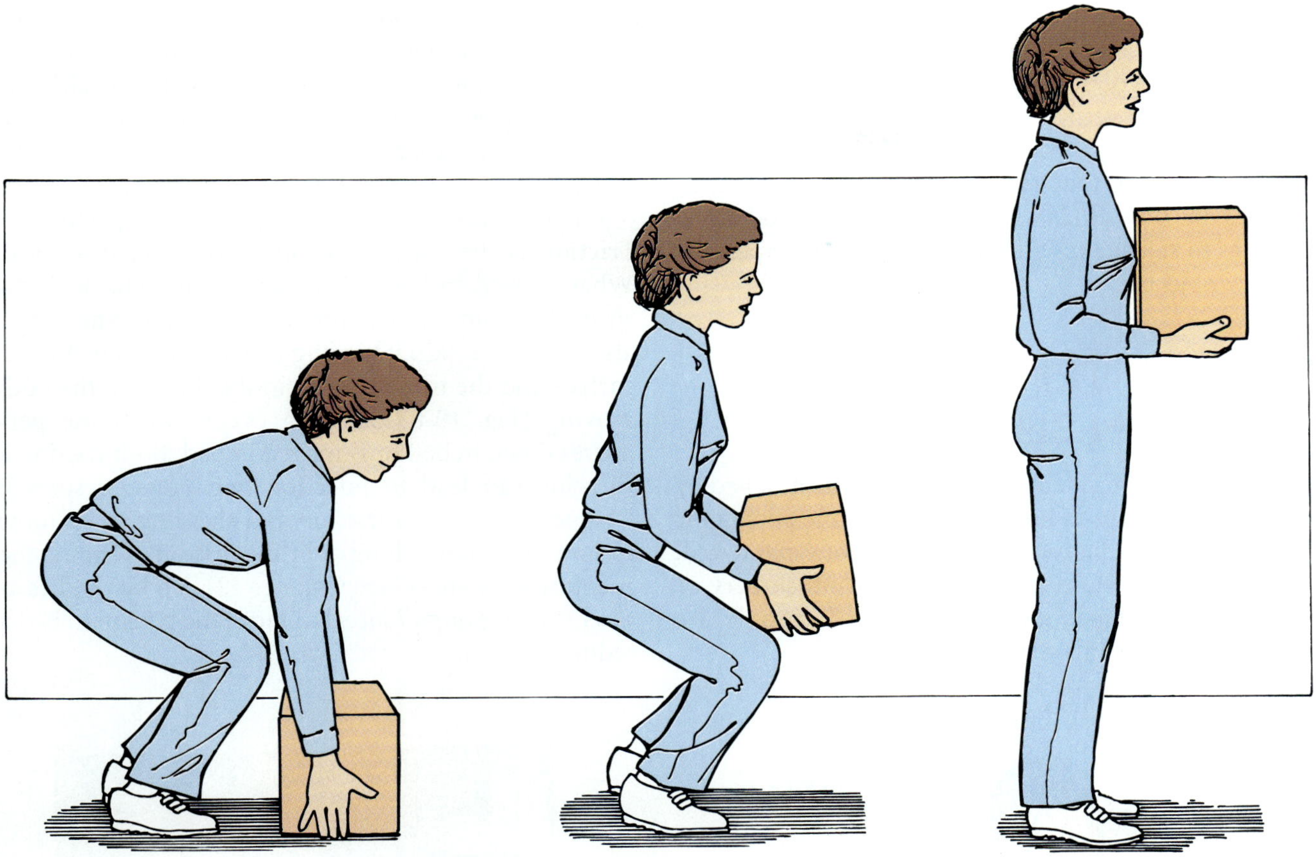

Fig. 10-4 *Picking up a box using good body mechanics.*

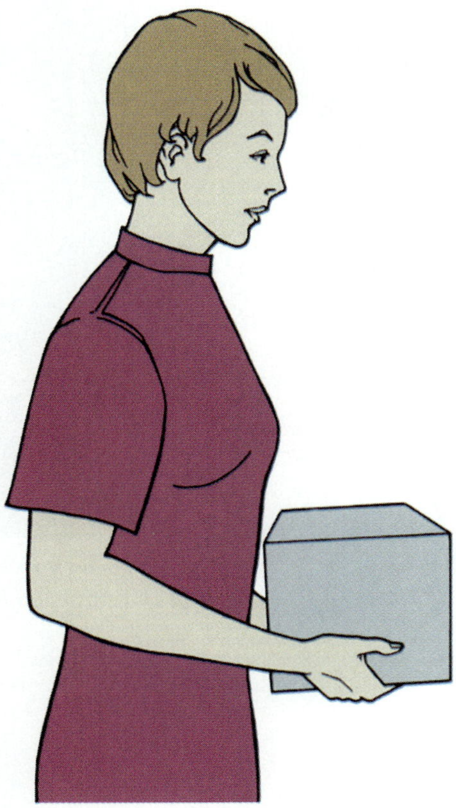

Fig. 10-5 *The box is carried close to the body and base of support.*

General Rules

You should use good body mechanics in all activities. Cleaning, laundry, getting in and out of a car, picking up a baby, mowing the yard, and shoveling snow are some of the many activities that require good body mechanics. The rules in Box 10-2 will help you use good body mechanics to safely and efficiently lift and move persons and heavy objects.

LIFTING AND MOVING PERSONS IN BED

Some patients and residents can move and turn in bed by themselves. Others need help from at least one person for position changes. Those who are unconscious, paralyzed, on complete bed rest, in a cast, or weak from surgery or disease need assistance. Sometimes 2 or 3 people are needed. Mechanical lifts may be used.

The rules of body mechanics are followed when moving and lifting persons in bed. The person is protected from injury by being kept in good body alignment. The person is positioned in good body alignment after being moved. Proper positioning is described on pages 246-250.

Friction must be reduced to protect the person's skin. **Friction** is the rubbing of one surface against another. When moved in bed, the person's skin rubs against the sheet. This can scratch and injure the skin. **Shearing** can also injure the skin. Shearing is when the skin sticks to a surface and the muscles slide in the direction the body is moving (Fig. 10-8) Shearing occurs when the person moves down in bed or is moved in bed. Both friction and shearing can lead to infection and pressure sores (see Chapter 13). Reduce friction and shearing when moving persons in bed by rolling or lifting instead of sliding them. A cotton drawsheet (see Chapter 12) can be used as a *lift sheet (turning or pull sheet)* to move the person in bed and reduce friction.

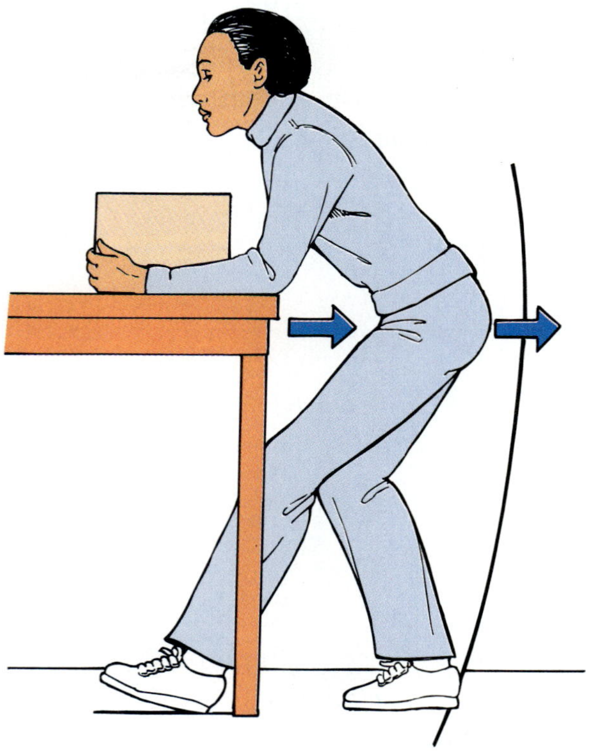

Fig. 10-6 *Move your rear leg back when pulling an item.*

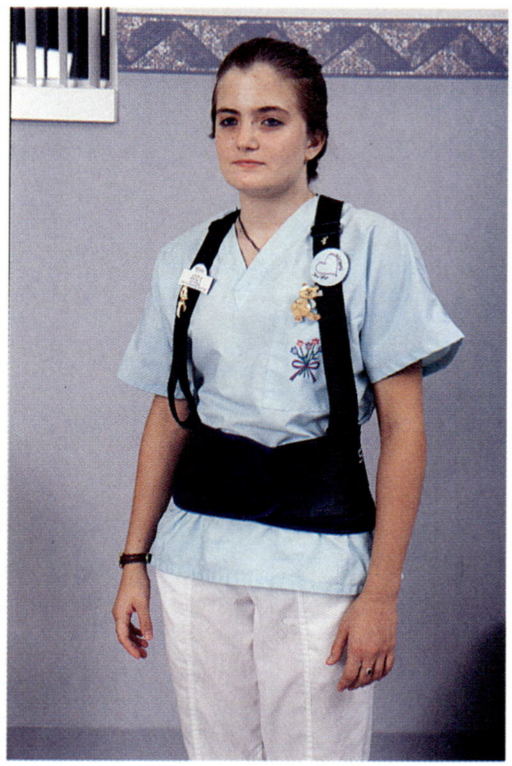

Fig. 10-7 *The nursing assistant is wearing a body support. It helps in using good body mechanics.*

BOX 10-2 Rules for Body Mechanics

- Make sure your body is in good alignment and that you have a wide base of support.
- Use the stronger and larger muscles of your body. They are in the shoulders, upper arms, thighs, and hips.
- Keep objects close to your body when you lift, move, or carry them.
- Avoid unnecessary bending and reaching. If possible, have the height of the bed and overbed table level with your waist when giving care. Adjust the bed and table to the proper height (see Chapter 11).
- Face the area in which you are working. This prevents unnecessary twisting.
- Push, slide, or pull heavy objects whenever you can rather than lifting them.
- Widen your base of support when pushing or pulling. Move your front leg forward when pushing an item. Move your rear leg back farther when pulling an item (Fig. 10-6 on opposite page).
- Use both hands and arms to lift, move, or carry heavy objects.
- Turn your whole body when you change the direction of your movement. You need to move your feet in the direction of the turn.
- Work with smooth and even movements. Avoid sudden or jerky motions.
- Get help form a co-worker if the person cannot assist with being turned or moved.
- Get help from a co-worker to move heavy objects or persons.
- Bend your hips and knees to lift heavy objects from the floor (see Fig. 10-2, B). Straighten your back as the object reaches thigh level. Your leg and thigh muscles will work to raise the item off the floor and to waist level.
- Do not lift objects higher than chest level. Do not lift above your shoulders. Use a step stool if you must reach an object that is higher than chest level.
- Wear a body support (Fig. 10-7 on opposite page) to help you use good body mechanics.

Other comfort and safety measures are considered before moving persons in bed.

- Consult the nurse for any limits or restrictions in positioning or moving the person. These may be a doctor's order or in the care plan.
- Decide how to move the person and how many helpers you need.
- Get enough co-workers to help *before* starting the procedure.
- Keep the person covered and screened to protect the right to privacy.
- Protect any tubes or drainage containers connected to the person.

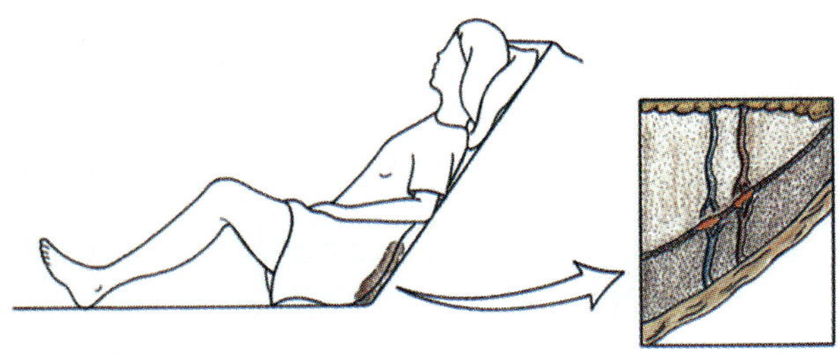

Fig. 10-8 *When the head of the bed is raised to a sitting position, skin on the buttocks stays in place. However, internal structures move forward as the person slides down in bed. Skin is pinched between the mattress and hip bones. (From Potter PA, Perry AG:* Fundamentals of nursing, *ed 3, St Louis, 1993, Mosby–Year Book.)*

Raising the Person's Head and Shoulders

You may have to raise the person's head and shoulders to tie the back of a gown, to turn or remove a pillow, or to give care. The head and shoulders are easily and safely raised by locking arms with the person. You may need help if a person is heavy or hard to move. Figure 10-9 shows the procedure being done by one person. Figure 10-10 on page 222 shows the procedure with 2 members of the nursing team.

RAISING THE PERSON'S HEAD AND SHOULDERS

PRE-PROCEDURE

1 Wash your hands.
2 Identify the person. Check the ID bracelet and call the person by name.
3 Explain the procedure to the person.
4 Provide for privacy.
5 Lock the bed wheels.
6 Raise the bed to the best level for body mechanics.

PROCEDURE

7 Make sure the far side rail is raised. Lower the one near you.
8 Ask the person to put the near arm under your near arm and behind your shoulder. His or her hand should rest on your shoulder. If you are standing on the right side, the person's right hand rests on your right shoulder (Fig. 10-9, A).
9 Put your arm near the person under his or her arm near you. Your hand will be on the person's shoulder.
10 Put your free arm under the person's neck and shoulders (Fig. 10-9, B).
11 Help the person pull up to a sitting or semisitting position on the count of "3" (Fig. 10-9, C).
12 Use the arm and hand that supported the neck and shoulders to straighten or remove the pillow, tie the gown, or provide other care (Fig. 10-9 D).
13 Help the person lie down. Provide support with your locked arm. Support his or her neck and shoulders with your other arm.

POST-PROCEDURE

14 Make sure the person is comfortable and in good body alignment.
15 Place the call bell within reach.
16 Raise or lower side rails as instructed by the nurse.
17 Lower the bed to its lowest position.
18 Unscreen the person.
19 Wash your hands.

Text continued on page 223.

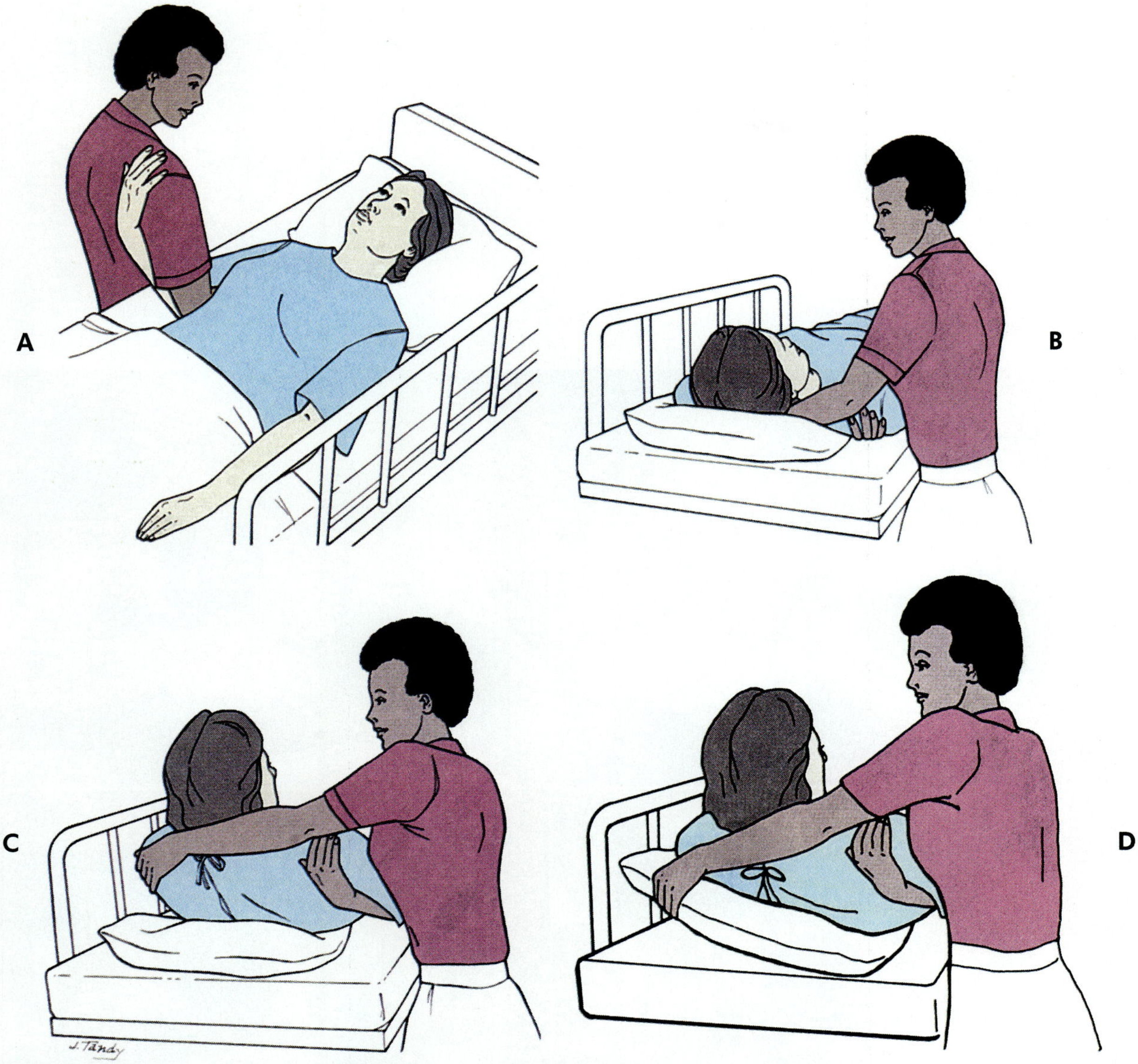

Fig. 10-9 *Raise the person's head and shoulders by locking arms with the person.* ***A,*** *The person's near arm is under the nursing assistant's near arm and behind the shoulder.* ***B,*** *The far arm of the nursing assistant is under the person's neck and shoulders. The near arm is under the person's near arm.* ***C,*** *The person is raised to a semisitting position by locking arms.* ***D,*** *The nursing assistant lifts the pillow while the person is raised in a semisitting position.*

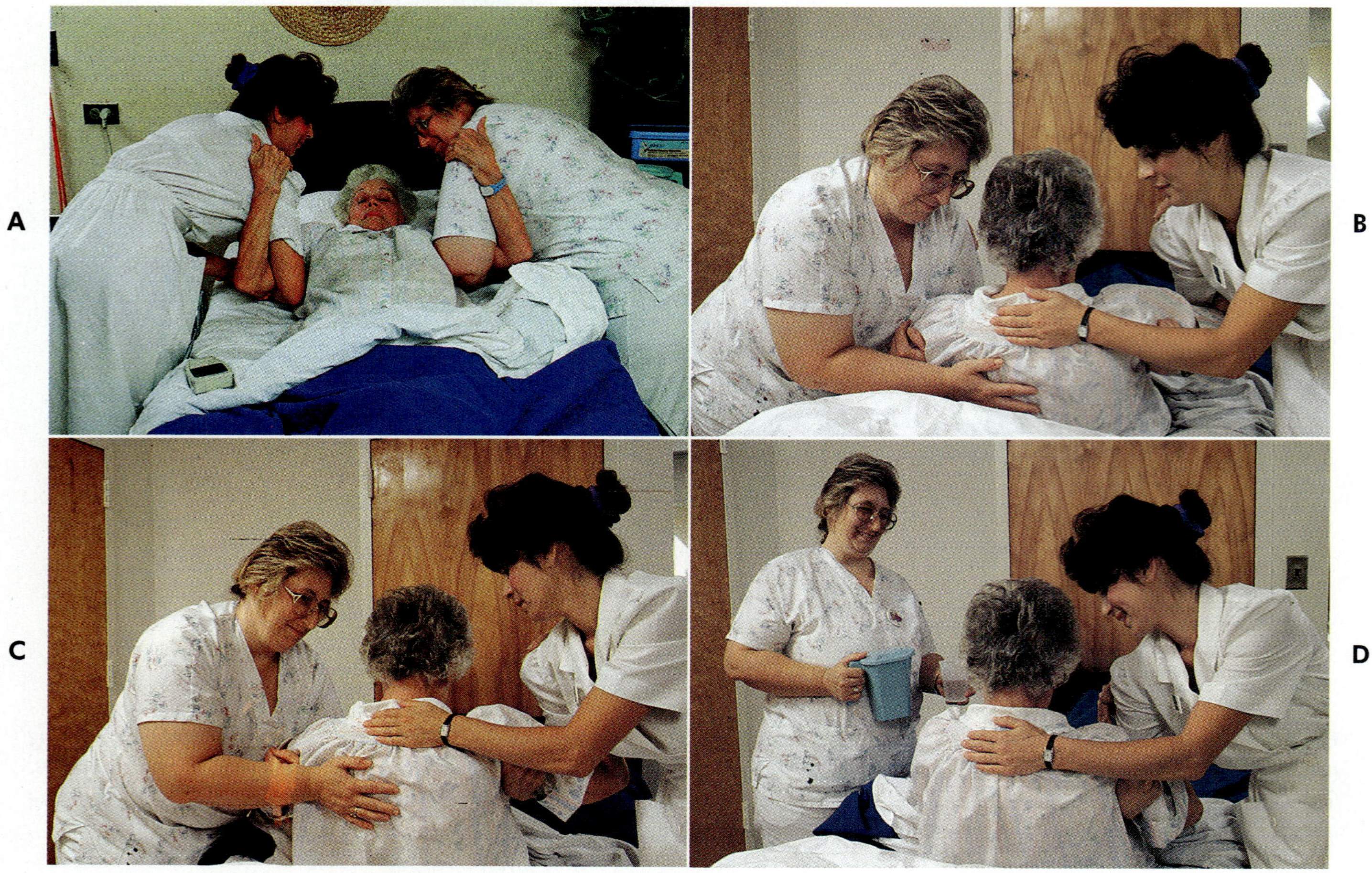

Fig. 10-10 ***A,*** *The two nursing assistants lock arms with the person.* ***B,*** *The nursing assistants have their arms under the person's head and neck.* ***C,*** *The nursing assistants raise the person to a semisitting position.* ***D,*** *One nursing assistant supports the person in the semisitting position while the other gives care.*

Moving the Person Up in Bed

Many persons like to have the head of their beds raised. However, that often causes them to slide down toward the middle and foot of the bed. They need to be moved up in bed for good body alignment and comfort (Fig. 10-11 on page 224). You can usually move children and lightweight adults up in bed without help. Some persons can assist with the procedure. However, it is best to have help. This protects you and the person from injury.

Moving the Person Up in Bed

Pre-procedure

1. Wash your hands.
2. Identify the person. Check the ID bracelet and call the person by name.
3. Explain the procedure to the person.
4. Provide for privacy.
5. Lock the bed wheels.
6. Raise the bed to the best level for body mechanics.

Procedure

7. Lower the head of the bed to a level appropriate for the person. The bed should be as flat as possible.
8. Place the pillow against the headboard if the person can be without it. This prevents his or her head from hitting the headboard when being moved up.
9. Make sure the far side rail is raised. Lower the one near you.
10. Stand with your feet about 12 inches apart. Point the foot closest to the head of the bed toward the head of the bed. Face the head of the bed.
11. Bend your hips and knees.
12. Place one arm under the person's shoulders and the other under the thighs.
13. Ask the person to grasp the headboard and to flex both knees as in Figure 10-12 on page 224.
14. Explain that you will both move on the count of "3." Ask the person to pull up with the hands and push against the bed with the feet. Explain what you will be doing.
15. Move the person to the head of the bed on the count of "3." Shift your weight from your rear leg to your front leg (Fig. 10-13 on page 224).
16. Put the pillow under the person's head and shoulders. Lock arms with him or her to complete this step.

Post-procedure

17. Straighten linens. Make sure the person is comfortable and in good body alignment.
18. Place the call bell within reach.
19. Raise or lower side rails as instructed by the nurse.
20. Raise the head of the bed to a level appropriate for the person.
21. Lower the bed to its lowest position.
22. Unscreen the person.
23. Wash your hands.

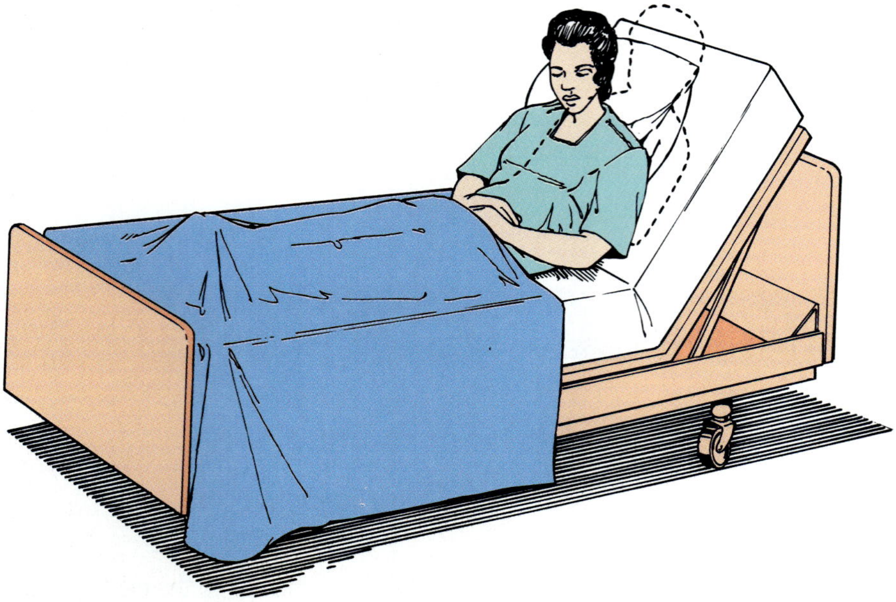

Fig. 10-11 *A person in poor body alignment after sliding down in bed.*

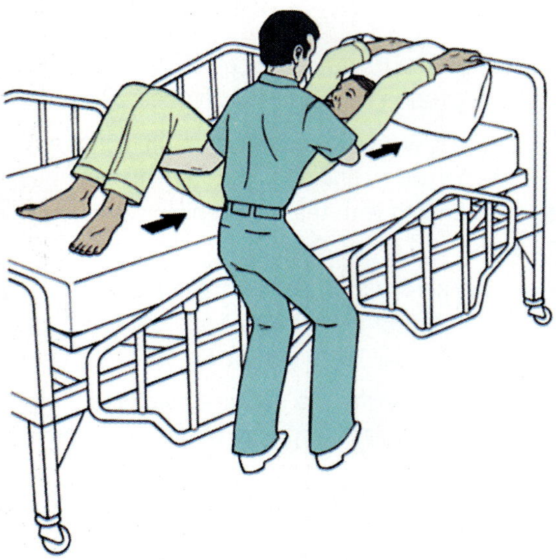

Fig. 10-12 *The person grasps the headboard and flexes the knees to assist in being moved up. The nursing assistant has one arm under the person's shoulder and the other under the thighs.*

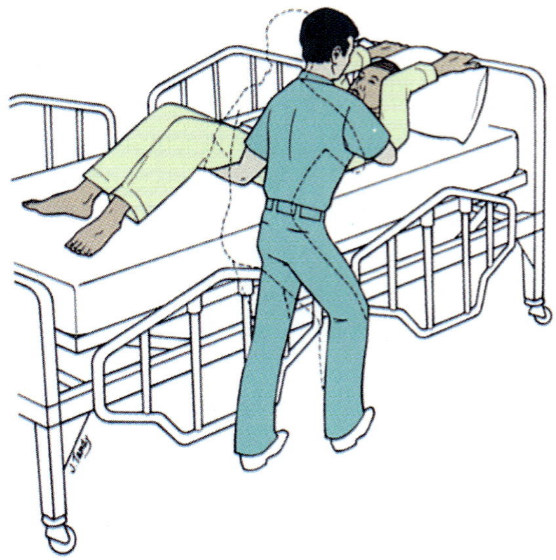

Fig. 10-13 *The person is moved up in bed as the nursing assistant's body weight is shifted from the rear leg to the front leg.*

Moving the Person Up in Bed With Assistance

Assistance is needed when a person cannot help with being moved up in bed. At least two people are needed to move heavy persons and those weak from surgery or disease. Be sure to ask for help before starting the procedure. Remember to cooperate if a co-worker asks you to help with care.

Moving the Person Up in Bed with Assistance

Pre-procedure

1 Ask a co-worker to help you.

2 Wash your hands.

3 Identify the person. Check the ID bracelet and call the person by name.

4 Explain the procedure to the person.

5 Provide for privacy.

6 Lock the bed wheels.

7 Raise the bed to the best level for body mechanics.

Procedure

8 Lower the head of the bed to a level appropriate for the person. The bed should be as flat as possible.

9 Place the pillow against the headboard if the person can be without it. This prevents his or her head from hitting the headboard when being moved up.

10 Stand on one side of the bed. Have your helper stand on the other.

11 Lower the side rails.

12 Stand with a wide base of support. Point the foot near the head of the bed toward the head of the bed. Face that direction.

13 Bend your hips and knees.

14 Place one arm under the person's shoulder and one arm under the buttocks. Your helper does the same. Grasp each other's forearms.

15 Have the person flex both knees (Fig. 10-14).

16 Explain that you and your helper will move on the count of "3." The person should push against the bed with the feet if able.

17 Move the person to the head of the bed on the count of "3." Shift your weight from your rear leg to your front leg (Fig. 10-15).

18 Repeat steps 12 through 17 if necessary.

Post-procedure

19 Put the pillow under the person's head and shoulders. Straighten linens. Make sure the person is comfortable and in good body alignment.

20 Place the call bell within reach.

21 Raise or lower side rails as instructed by the nurse.

22 Raise the head of the bed to a level appropriate for the person.

23 Lower the bed to its lowest position.

24 Unscreen the person.

25 Wash your hands.

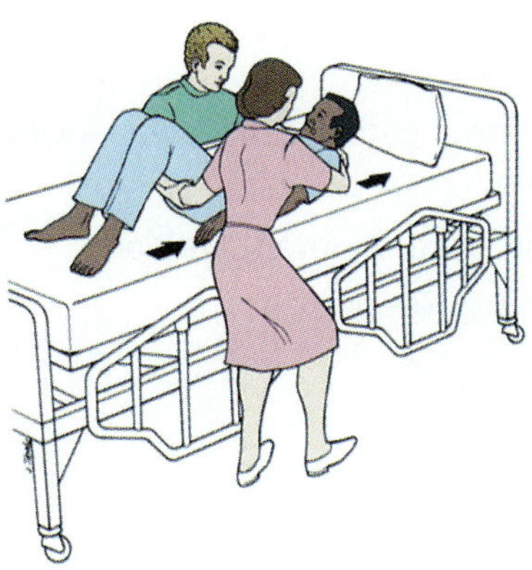

Fig. 10-14 *A person is moved up in bed by two nursing assistants. Each has one arm under the person's shoulder and the other under the buttocks. They have locked arms under the person. The person's knees are flexed.*

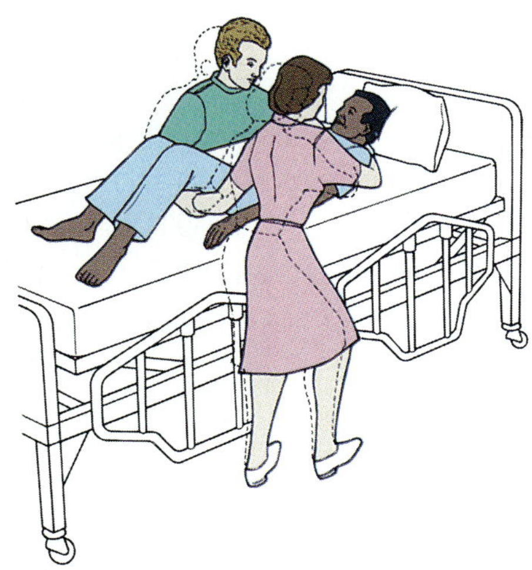

Fig. 10-15 *A person is moved up in bed as nursing assistants shift their weight from the rear leg to the front leg.*

Moving the Person Up in Bed Using a Lift Sheet

With the help of a co-worker, you can easily and safely move a person up in bed using a lift sheet (turning sheet). Friction and shearing are reduced, and the person is lifted more evenly. A flat sheet folded in half or a drawsheet is used for the lift sheet. The lift sheet is placed under the person. It extends from the shoulders to above the knees. Certain persons are moved up in bed with a lift sheet. They include those who are unconscious, paralyzed, recovering from spinal surgery, or who have spinal cord injuries. Long-term care residents should be moved with lift sheets.

MOVING THE PERSON UP IN BED USING A LIFT SHEET

PRE-PROCEDURE

1. Ask a co-worker to help you.
2. Wash your hands.
3. Identify the person. Check the ID bracelet and call the person by name.
4. Explain the procedure to the person.
5. Provide for privacy.
6. Lock the bed wheels.
7. Raise the bed to the best level for body mechanics.

PROCEDURE

8. Lower the head of the bed to a level appropriate for the person. It should be as flat as possible.
9. Place the pillow against the headboard if the person can be without it.
10. Stand on one side of the bed. Your helper stands on the other side.
11. Lower the side rails.
12. Stand with a broad base of support. Point the foot near the head of the bed toward the head of the bed. Face that direction.
13. Roll the sides of the lift sheet up close to the person (Fig. 10-16).
14. Grasp the rolled up lift sheet firmly near the person's shoulders and buttocks.
15. Bend your hips and knees.
16. Slide the person up in bed on the count of "3" (Fig. 10-17). Shift your weight from your rear leg to your front leg.
17. Unroll the lift sheet.

POST-PROCEDURE

18. Put the pillow under the person's head and shoulders. Straighten linens. Make sure the person is comfortable and in good body alignment.
19. Place the call bell within reach.
20. Raise or lower side rails as instructed by the nurse.
21. Raise the head of the bed to a level appropriate for the person.
22. Lower the bed to its lowest position.
23. Unscreen the person.
24. Wash your hands.

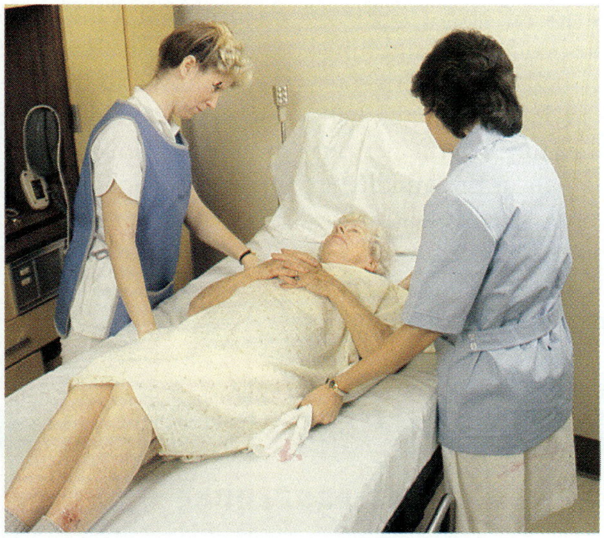

Fig. 10-16 *The turning sheet is rolled up close to the person.*

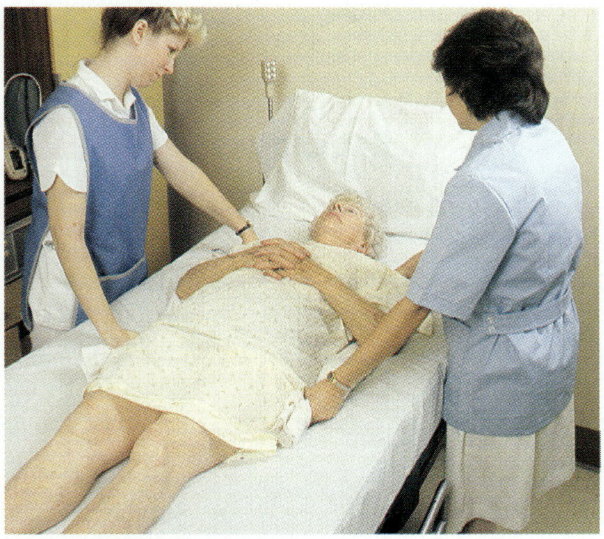

Fig. 10-17 *Two nursing assistants move a person up in bed with a turning sheet. The turning sheet is rolled close to the person and held near the shoulders and buttocks.*

Moving a Person to the Side of the Bed

Persons are moved to the side of the bed for repositioning and for certain procedures such as a bed bath. A person in the middle of the bed is moved to the side of the bed before being turned. Otherwise, after turning, the person lays on the side of the bed rather than in the middle. A person should lie in the middle of the bed to allow for good body alignment.

Sometimes you have to reach over the person to give care. Good body mechanics can be used if reaching is reduced and if the person is close to you.

The person should be in the back-lying position when being moved to the side of the bed. The person is moved in segments. This can be done by one person. A lift sheet is used for persons with spinal cord injuries, those recovering from spinal surgery, the very elderly, and arthritic persons. Two staff members are needed when a lift sheet is used to move a person to the side of the bed.

Moving the Person to the Side of the Bed

Pre-procedure

1 Ask a co-worker to help you if a lift sheet will be used.
2 Wash your hands.
3 Identify the person. Check the ID bracelet and call the person by name.
4 Explain the procedure to the person.
5 Provide for privacy.
6 Lock the bed wheels.
7 Raise the bed to the best level for body mechanics.

Procedure

8 Lower the head of the bed to a level appropriate for the person. The bed should be as flat as possible.
9 Stand on the side of the bed to which you will move the person.
10 Make sure the far side rail is raised. Lower the one near you.
11 Stand with your feet about 12 inches apart and with one foot in front of the other. Flex your knees.
12 Cross the person's arms over the person's chest.
13 *Method 1:* Moving the person in segments
- a Place your arm under the person's neck and shoulders. Grasp the far shoulder.
- b Place your other arm under the midback.
- c Move the upper part of the person's body toward you. Rock backward and shift your weight to your rear leg (Fig. 10-18, A).
- d Place one arm under the person's waist and one under the thighs.
- e Rock backward to move the lower part of the person's body toward you (Fig. 10-18, B).
- f Repeat the procedure for the legs and feet as in Figure 10-18, C. Your arms should be under his or her thighs and calves.

Method 2: Moving the person with a lift sheet
- a Roll the side of the lift sheet up close to the person.
- b Grasp the rolled up lift sheet near the person's shoulders and buttocks.
- c Rock backward on the count of "3," moving the person toward you. Your helper rocks backward slightly and then forward toward you while keeping the arms straight (Fig. 10-19).
- d Unroll the lift sheet.

Post-procedure

14 Make sure the person is comfortable, in good body alignment, and positioned as directed by the nurse. Reposition the pillow under his or her head and shoulders.
15 Place the call bell within the person's reach.
16 Raise or lower side rails as instructed by the nurse.
17 Lower the bed to its lowest position.
18 Unscreen the person.
19 Wash your hands.

Text continued on page 230.

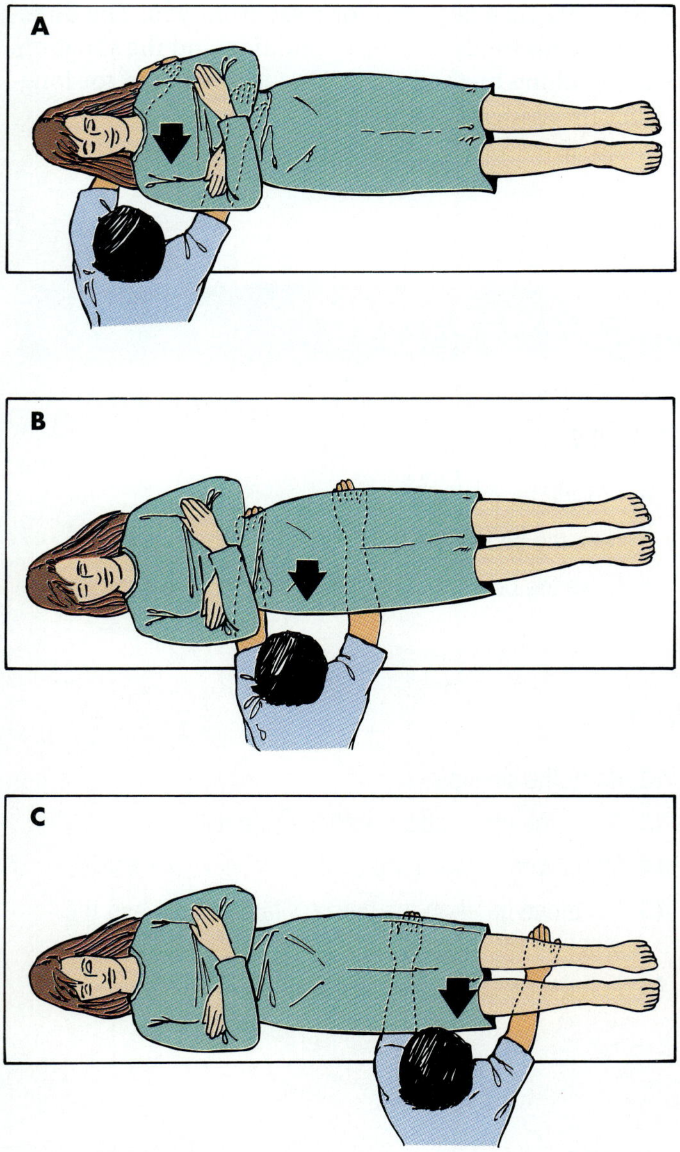

Fig. 10-18 *A, The person is moved to the side of the bed in segments. The upper part is moved first as the nursing assistant has one arm under the person's neck and shoulders and the other under the middle of the back.* ***B,*** *The nursing assistant has one arm under the waist and the other under the thighs to move the person's lower body to the side of the bed.* ***C,*** *The person's legs and feet are moved to the side of the bed. The nursing assistant has one arm under the person's thighs and the other under the calves.*

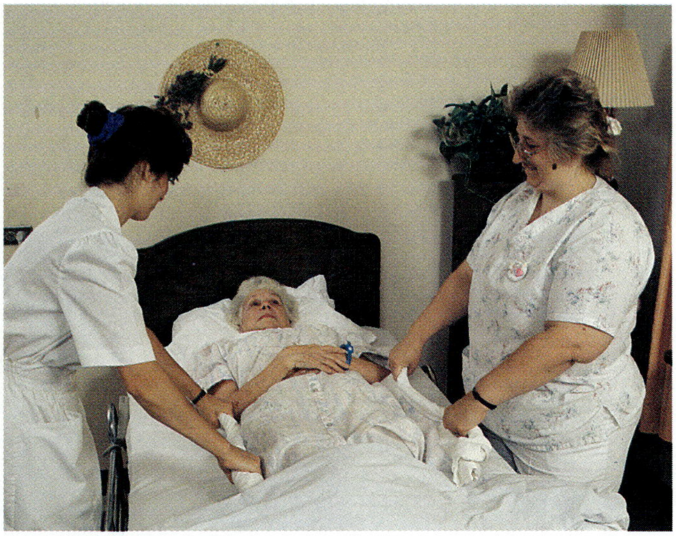

Fig. 10-19 *Two workers use a lift sheet to move a person to the side of the bed. The lift sheet lifts some of the person's weight off the bed. Friction is reduced as the person is moved.*

Turning Persons

Persons are turned onto their sides to prevent the complications from bed rest and to receive care. Certain medical and nursing procedures require the side-lying position. Persons are turned toward or away from you. The direction depends on the person's condition and the situation. The logrolling method (page 226) is often used for long-term care residents.

Turning the Person Toward You

Pre-procedure

1 Wash your hands.
2 Identify the person. Check the ID bracelet and call the person by name.
3 Explain the procedure to the person.
4 Provide for privacy.
5 Lock the bed wheels.
6 Raise the bed to the best level for body mechanics.

Procedure

7 Lower the head of the bed to a level appropriate for the person. The bed should be as flat as possible.
8 Stand on the side of the bed opposite to where you will turn the person. Make sure the far side rail is up.
9 Lower the side rail near you.
10 Move the person to the side near you.
11 Cross the person's arms over the person's chest. Cross the leg near you over the far leg.
12 Raise the side rail.
13 Go to the other side. Lower the side rail.
14 Stand with a wide base of support. Flex your knees.
15 Place one hand on the person's far shoulder and the other on the far hip.
16 Roll the person toward you gently (Fig. 10-20).

Post-procedure

17 Make sure the person is comfortable and in good body alignment (Fig. 10-21):
   - **a** Position a pillow against the back for support.
   - **b** Put a pillow under the head and shoulder.
   - **c** Place a pillow in front of the bottom leg. Place the top leg on top of the pillow in a flexed position.
   - **d** Support the arm and hand with a small pillow.

18 Place the call bell within reach.
19 Raise or lower side rails as instructed by the nurse.
20 Lower the bed to its lowest position.
21 Unscreen the person.
22 Wash your hands.

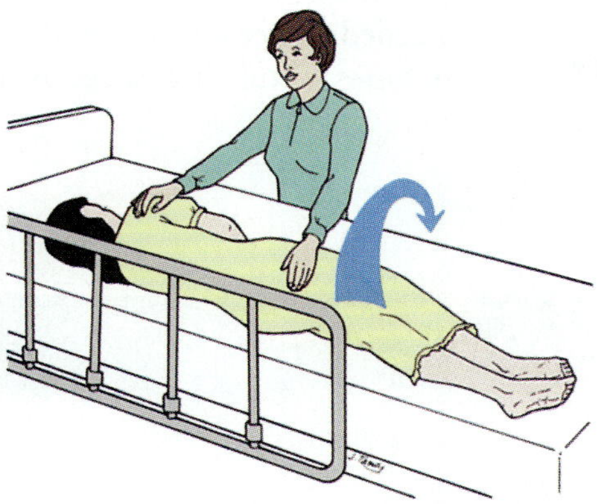

Fig. 10-20 *The person is turned toward the nursing assistant. The person's arms and legs are crossed, and the nursing assistant has one hand on the person's far shoulder and the other on the far hip.*

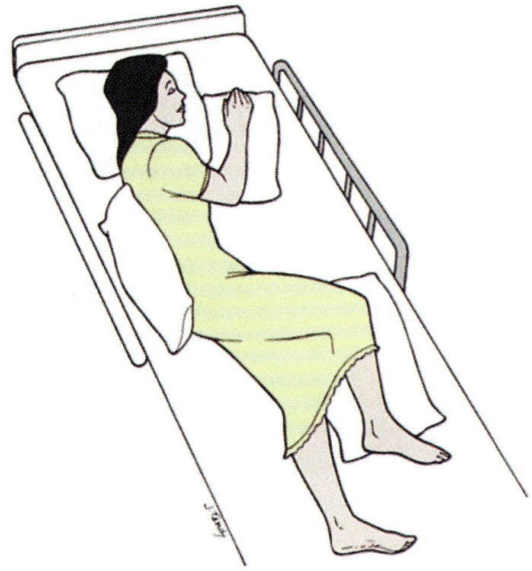

Fig. 10-21 *The person is positioned on the side in the middle of the bed. A pillow is in front of the bottom leg with the top leg on a pillow in the flexed position; a pillow is against the back; a small pillow supports the arm and hand; there is a pillow under the head and shoulder.*

Turning the Person Away From You

Pre-procedure

1 Follow steps 1 through 11 in *Turning the Person Toward You* (see page 230).

Procedure

2 Stand with a wide base of support. Flex your knees.

3 Place one hand on the person's shoulder and the other on the buttock near you.

4 Push the person gently toward the other side of the bed (Fig. 10-22). Shift your weight from your rear leg to your front leg.

Post-procedure

5 Make sure the person is comfortable and in good body alignment. Use pillows to support the person as in Figure 10-21. (See *Turning the Person Toward You,* step 17.)

6 Raise or lower side rails as instructed by the nurse.

7 Place the call bell within the person's reach.

8 Lower the bed to its lowest position.

9 Unscreen the person.

10 Wash your hands.

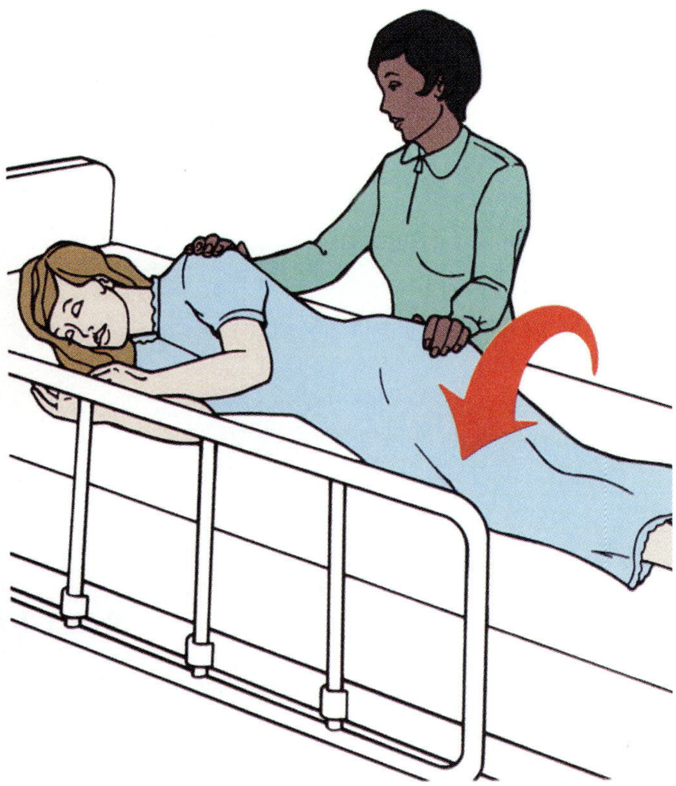

Fig. 10-22 *The person is turned away from the nursing assistant. The person's arms and legs are crossed, and the nursing assistant has one hand on the person's shoulder and the other on the person's buttock.*

Logrolling

Logrolling is turning the person as a unit, in alignment, with one motion. The spine is kept straight. Persons with spinal cord injuries or those recovering from spinal surgery must keep their spines straight at all times. Rolling over in one motion keeps the back in straight alignment when the person is turned. This method is often used for long-term care residents.

Two workers are needed. Three are needed if a person is tall or heavy. Sometimes a turning sheet is used for logrolling.

Logrolling a Person

Pre-procedure

1. Ask a co-worker to help you.
2. Wash your hands.
3. Identify the person. Check the ID bracelet and call the person by name.
4. Explain the procedure to the person.
5. Provide for privacy.
6. Lock the bed wheels.
7. Raise the bed to the best level for body mechanics.

Procedure

8. Make sure the bed is flat.
9. Make sure the side rail is up on the side to which the person will be turned.
10. Stand on the other side. Lower the side rail.
11. Move the person as a unit to the side of the bed near you. Use the turn sheet.
12. Place the person's arms across the chest. Place a pillow between the knees (Fig. 10-23, A).
13. Raise the side rail. Go to the other side and lower the side rail.
14. Position yourself near the shoulders and chest. Your helper should stand near the buttocks and thighs.
15. Stand with a broad base of support. One foot should be in front of the other.
16. Ask the person to hold his or her body rigid.
17. Roll the person toward you as in Fig. 10-23, A, or use a turn sheet as in Fig. 10-23, B. Make sure the person is turned as a unit.

Post-procedure

18. Make sure the person is comfortable and in good body alignment. Use pillows.
    - **a** One pillow against the back for support.
    - **b** One pillow under the head and neck if allowed.
    - **c** One pillow or folded bath blanket between the legs.
    - **d** A small pillow under the arm and hand.
19. Place the call bell within reach.
20. Raise or lower side rails as instructed by the nurse.
21. Lower the bed to its lowest position.
22. Unscreen the person.
23. Wash your hands.

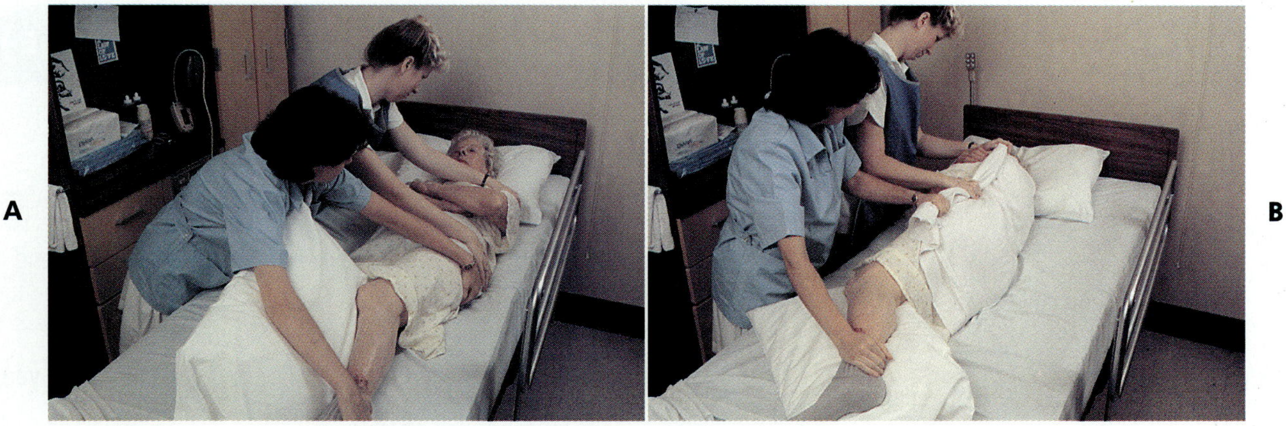

Fig. 10-23 *Logrolling. **A,** There is a pillow between the person's legs, and the arms are crossed on the chest. The person is on the far side of the bed. **B,** A turning sheet is used to logroll a person.*

SITTING ON THE SIDE OF THE BED

Persons are helped to sit on the side of the bed *(dangle)* for many reasons. Some increase activity in stages. They progress from bed rest to sitting on the side of the bed and then to sitting in a chair. Walking in the room and then in the hallway are the next steps. Surgical patients are allowed to sit on the side of the bed (dangle) some time after surgery. While dangling their legs, these patients cough, deep breathe, and move their legs back and forth and in circles to stimulate circulation. Other reasons for the procedure include preparing a person to walk or for transfer to a chair or wheelchair.

Two workers may be needed. If there is a problem with balance or coordination, the person must be supported. The person should lie down if a feeling of faintness occurs. Certain observations are made while the person is sitting on the side of the bed:

- Take pulse and respirations
- Observe for difficulty in breathing
- Observe for pallor or cyanosis
- Note complaints of dizziness or lightheadedness

Text continued on page 236.

Helping the Person Sit on the Side of the Bed (Dangle)

Pre-procedure

1 Explain the procedure to the person.
2 Collect:
- Robe and nonskid slippers or shoes
- Paper or sheet

3 Wash your hands.
4 Identify the person. Check the ID bracelet and call the person by name.
5 Decide what side of the bed to use.
6 Move furniture to provide moving space for you and the person.
7 Provide for privacy.
8 Position the person in a side-lying position facing you.
9 Lock the bed wheels.
10 Raise the bed to the best level for body mechanics.

Procedure

11 Prepare the person to get out of bed:
- a Fanfold top linens to the foot of the bed.
- b Place the paper or sheet under the person's feet to protect the bottom linen from slippers or shoes.
- c Put slippers or shoes on the person.

12 Raise the side rail if the bed is manually operated. Stand near the person's waist if the bed is electric. This protects the person from falling out of bed.
13 Raise the head of the bed so that the person is in a sitting position.
14 Lower the side rail.
15 Stand by the person's hips. Turn on a diagonal so you face the far corner of the foot of the bed.
16 Slide one arm under the person's neck and shoulders. Grasp the far shoulder. Place your other hand under the thighs near the knees (Fig. 10-24).
17 Pivot toward the foot of the bed while you pull the person's feet and legs over the edge of the bed. As the legs go over the edge of the mattress, the trunk will be upright (Fig. 10-25).
18 Ask the person to push both fists into the mattress (Fig. 10-26 on page 236). This supports the person in the sitting position.
19 Do not leave the person alone. Provide support if necessary.
20 Ask how the person feels. Check pulse and respirations. Help the person lie down if necessary.
21 Help the person put on a robe.
22 Lower the bed to its lowest position if the person is to get out of bed.
23 Reverse the procedure to return the person to bed.
24 Lower the head of the bed after the person has returned to bed. Help him or her move to the center of the bed.
25 Remove the shoes/slippers and the paper/sheet used to protect linen.

Post-procedure

26 Make sure the person is comfortable and in good body alignment. Cover the person.
27 Place the call bell within reach.
28 Lower the bed to its lowest position.
29 Return the robe and shoes/slippers to their proper place.
30 Return furniture to its proper location.
31 Unscreen the person.
32 Wash your hands.
33 Report the following to the nurse:
- How well the activity was tolerated
- The length of time dangled
- Pulse and respiratory rates
- The amount of assistance needed
- Other observations or complaints made

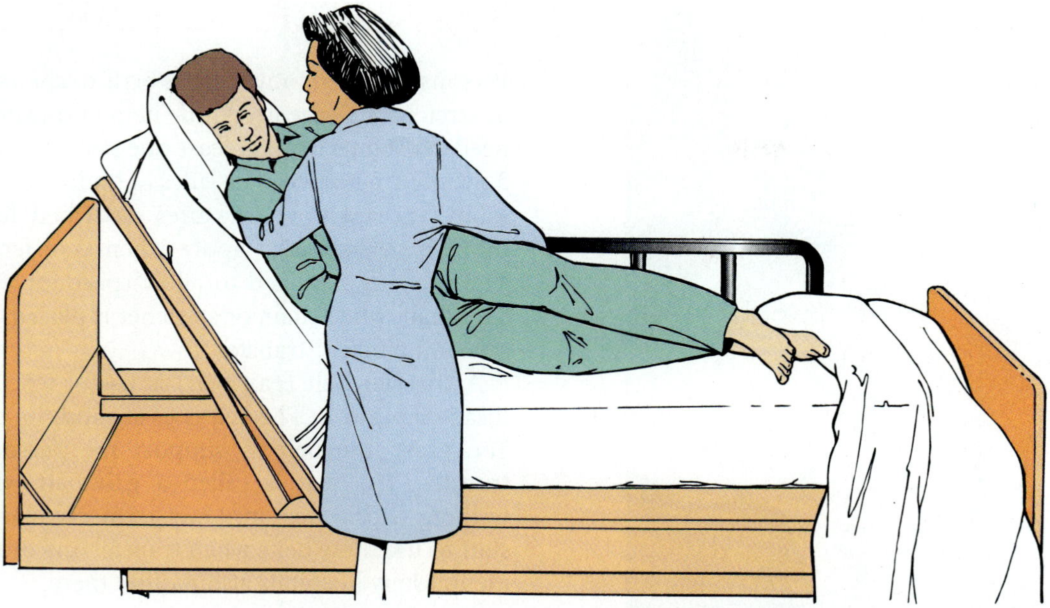

Fig. 10-24 *The nursing assistant has one arm under the person's neck and shoulders and is grasping the far shoulder. Her other hand is under the thighs near the knees.*

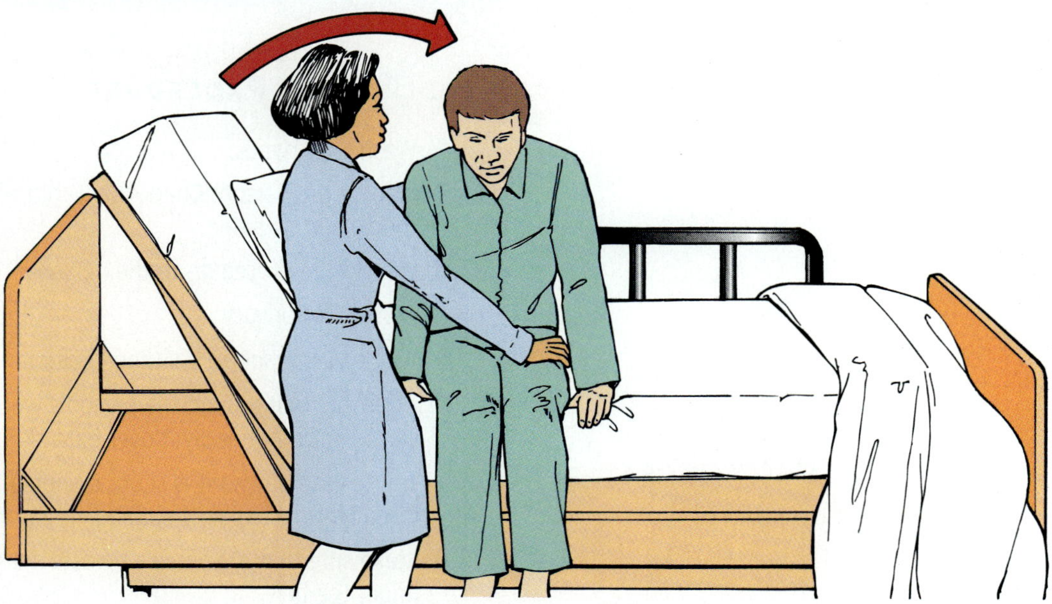

Fig. 10-25 *The nursing assistant pivots toward the foot of the bed while pulling the person's feet and legs over the edge of the bed. As the legs go over the edge of the mattress, the trunk will be upright.*

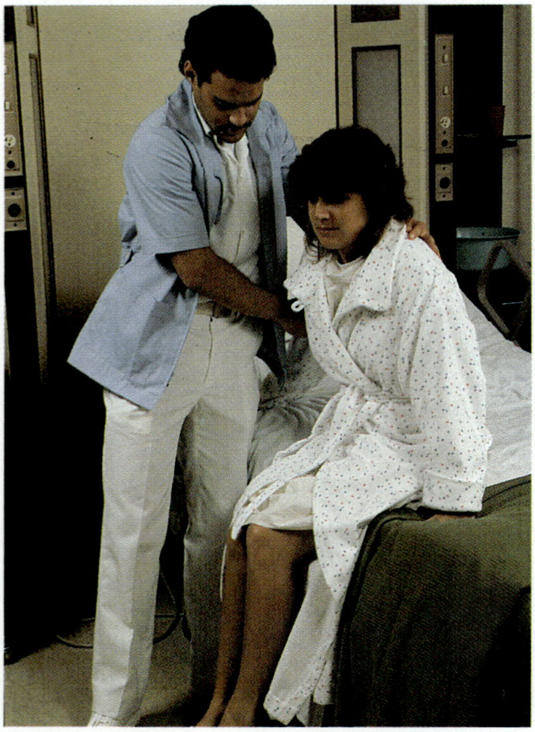

Fig. 10-26 *The person is supporting herself with the fists pushed into the mattress.*

TRANSFERRING PERSONS

Persons are often moved from beds to chairs, wheelchairs, or stretchers. Some need little help in transferring. Others need assistance from at least one person. Sometimes 2 or 3 people are needed. The rules of body mechanics and the safety and comfort measures described for lifting and moving persons also apply when transferring persons. The room is arranged to allow space for a safe transfer. The chair, wheelchair, or stretcher is placed correctly for a safe and efficient transfer.

A **transfer belt** (gait belt) is useful when transferring disabled persons. The belt goes around the person's waist. You grasp the belt to support the person during the transfer. The belt is called a **gait belt** when used for walking with a person. Long-term care facilities require staff to use these belts when transferring or walking a resident. Many hospitals also require them.

APPLYING A TRANSFER (GAIT) BELT

PROCEDURE

1. Wash your hands.
2. Identify the person. Check the ID bracelet and call the person by name.
3. Explain the procedure to the person.
4. Provide for privacy.
5. Assist the person to a sitting position.
6. Apply the belt around the person's waist over clothing. Do not apply it over bare skin.
7. Tighten the belt so it is snug. It should not cause discomfort or impair breathing.
8. Make sure that a woman's breasts are not caught under the belt.
9. Place the buckle either off center in the front or in the back for the person's comfort (Fig. 10-27).

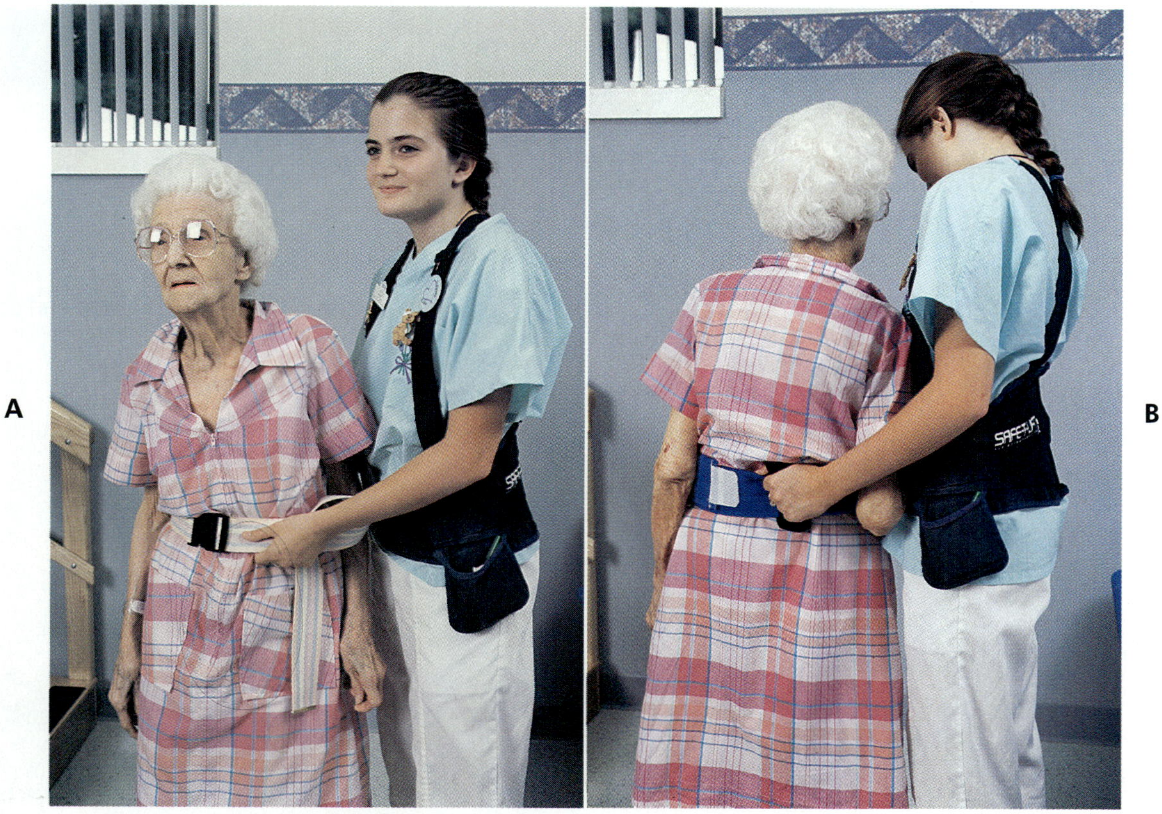

Fig. 10-27 *Transfer (safety) belt.* ***A,*** *The belt is positioned off center in the front.* ***B,*** *The belt buckle is positioned at the back.*

Transferring a Person to a Chair or Wheelchair

Safety is very important when transferring a person to a chair or wheelchair. Falls must be prevented. The person wears shoes with nonskid soles to prevent sliding or slipping on the floor. The chair or wheelchair must be sturdy enough to support the person's weight. The number of workers needed for a transfer depends on the person's physical capabilities, condition, and size. The person should assist in the transfer whenever possible to help increase muscle strength.

Most wheelchairs and bedside chairs have vinyl seats and backs. Vinyl holds body heat, causing the person to be warm and perspire. You can cover the back and seat with a folded bath blanket. This increases the person's comfort when in the chair.

The person is helped out of bed on his or her strong side. If the left side is weak and the right side strong, get the person out of bed on the right side. When transferring, the strong side moves first and pulls the weaker side along. Transfers from the weak side are awkward and unsafe.

The nurse may ask you to take the person's pulse before and after the transfer. The person may have been on bed rest or may tire with even a little exertion. The pulse rate gives some information about how the activity was tolerated. Also observe and report if the person tires easily, complains of weakness or being lightheaded, has pain or discomfort, or has difficulty breathing (dyspnea). Also report the amount of help needed and how the person helped in the transfer.

Text continued on p. 242.

Transferring a Person to a Chair or Wheelchair

Pre-procedure

1 Explain the procedure to the person.

2 Collect:
- Wheelchair or arm chair
- One or two bath blankets
- Robe and shoes
- Paper or sheet
- Transfer (gait) belt if needed
- Pillow

3 Wash your hands.

4 Identify the person. Check the ID bracelet and call the person by name.

5 Provide for privacy.

6 Decide which side of the bed to use. Move furniture to provide moving space.

Procedure

7 Place the chair at the head of the bed. The chair back must be even with the headboard (Fig. 10-28).

8 Place a folded bath blanket on the seat. Lock the wheelchair wheels and raise the footrests.

9 Make sure the bed is in the lowest position and the bed wheels are locked.

10 Fanfold top linens to the foot of the bed.

11 Place the paper or sheet under the person's feet. Put shoes on the person.

12 Help the person dangle. Make sure his or her feet touch the floor.

13 Help the person put on a robe.

14 Apply the transfer belt if it will be used.

15 Help the person stand. Use this method if using a transfer belt:

a Stand in front of the person.

b Have the person place his or her fists on the bed by the thighs.

c Make sure the person's feet are flat on the floor.

d Have the person lean forward.

e Grasp the transfer belt at each side.

f Brace your knees against the person's knees and block his or her feet with your feet (Fig. 10-29).

g Ask the person to push the fists down on the bed and to stand on the count of "3." Pull the person into a standing position as you straighten your knees (Fig. 10-30 on page 240).

16 Use this method if a transfer belt is not used.

a Stand in front of the person.

b Have the person place the fists on the bed by the thighs.

c Make sure the person's feet are flat on the floor.

d Place your hands under his or her arms. Your hands should be around the shoulder blades (Fig. 10-31 on page 240).

e Have the person lean forward.

f Brace your knees against the person's knees, and block his or her feet with your feet.

g Ask the person to push the fists into the bed and to stand on the count of "3." Pull the person up into a standing position as you straighten your knees.

17 Support the person in the standing position. Hold the transfer belt or keep your hands around the person's shoulder blades. Continue to block the person's feet and knees with your feet and knees. This helps prevent falling.

18 Turn the person so he or she can grasp the far arm of the chair. The legs will touch the edge of the chair as in Figure 10-32 on page 240.

19 Continue to turn the person until the other armrest is grasped.

20 Lower him or her into the chair as you bend your hips and knees (Fig. 10-33 on page 240). The person assists by leaning forward and bending the elbows and knees.

21 Make sure the buttocks are to the back of the seat. Position the person in good alignment.

TRANSFERRING A PERSON TO A CHAIR OR WHEELCHAIR—CONT'D

PROCEDURE—CONT'D

22 Position the feet on the wheelchair footrests.

23 Cover the person's lap and legs with a bath blanket. The blanket must be off the floor and the wheels.

24 Remove the transfer belt if used.

25 Position the chair as the person prefers.

POST-PROCEDURE

26 Make sure the call bell and other necessary items are within reach.

27 Unscreen the person.

28 Wash your hands.

29 Report the following to the nurse:

- The pulse rate if taken
- How well the activity was tolerated
- Complaints of lightheadedness, pain, discomfort, difficulty breathing, weakness, or fatigue
- The amount of assistance required to transfer the person

30 Reverse the procedure to return the person to bed.

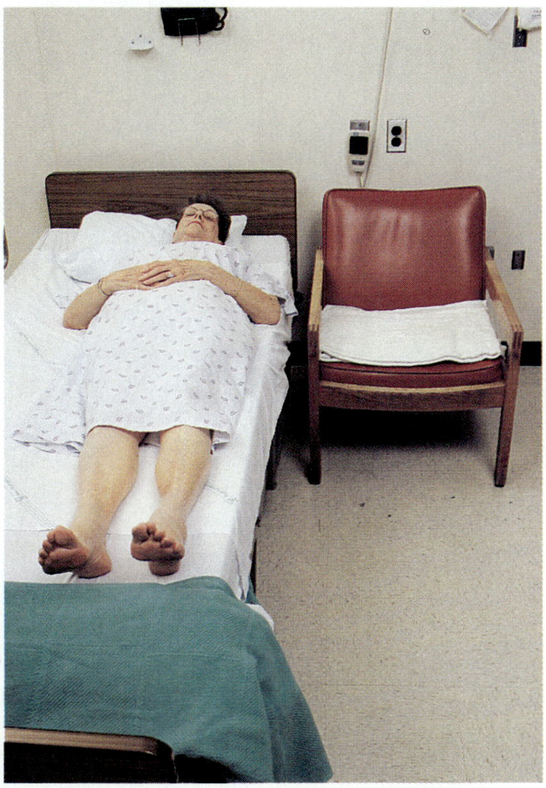

Fig. 10-28 *The chair is positioned next to and even with the headboard.*

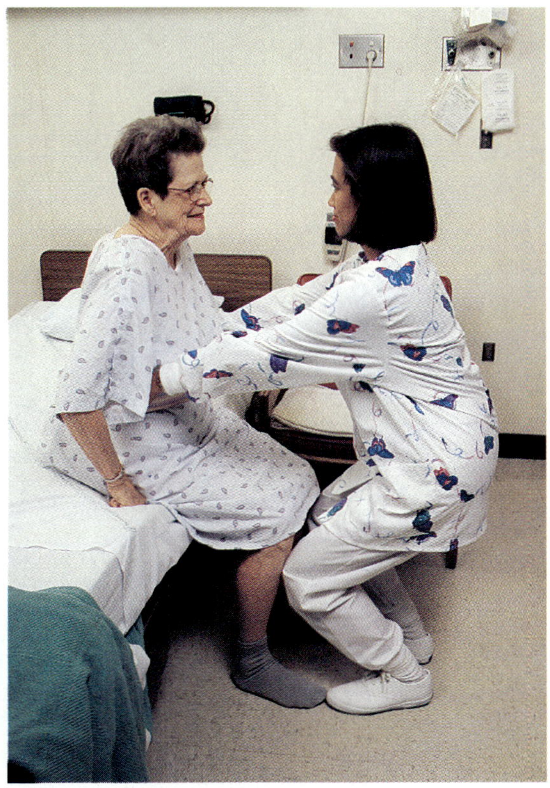

Fig. 10-29 *Prevent the person from sliding or falling by blocking the person's knees and feet with your own knees and feet.*

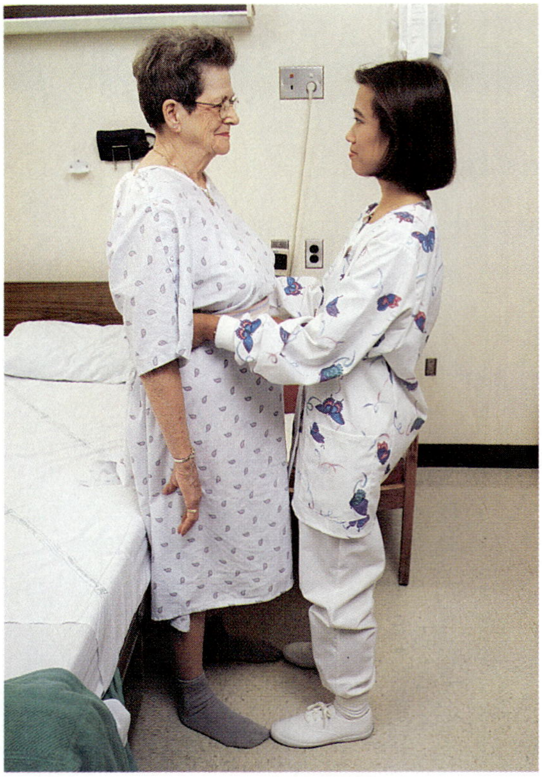

Fig. 10-30 *The person is pulled up to a standing position and supported by holding the transfer belt and blocking the person's knees and feet.*

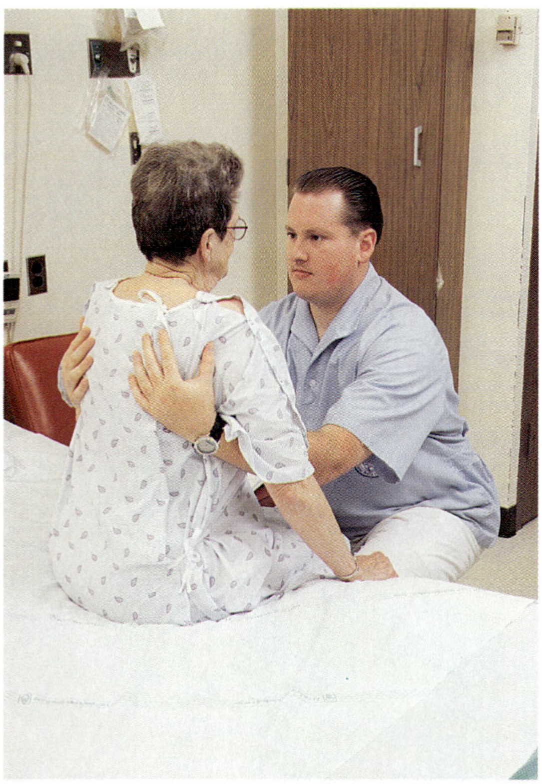

Fig. 10-31 *A person being prepared to stand. The hands are placed under the person's arms and around the shoulder blades.*

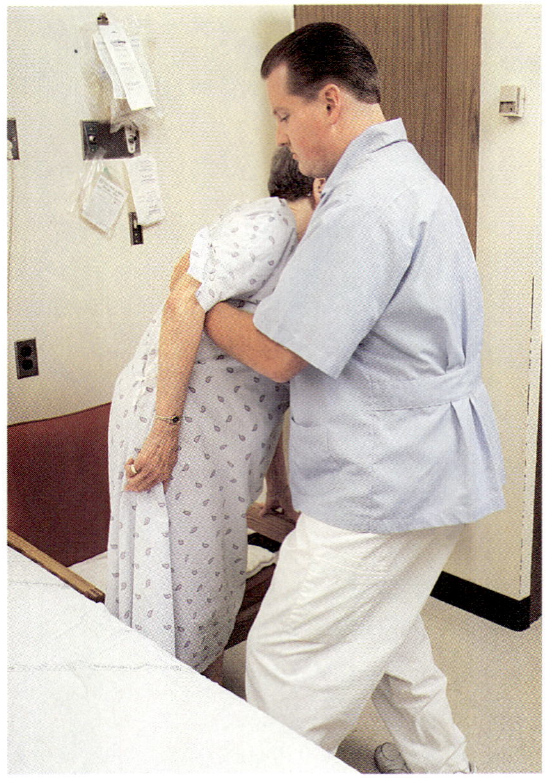

Fig. 10-32 *The person is supported as she grasps the far arm of the chair. The legs are against the chair.*

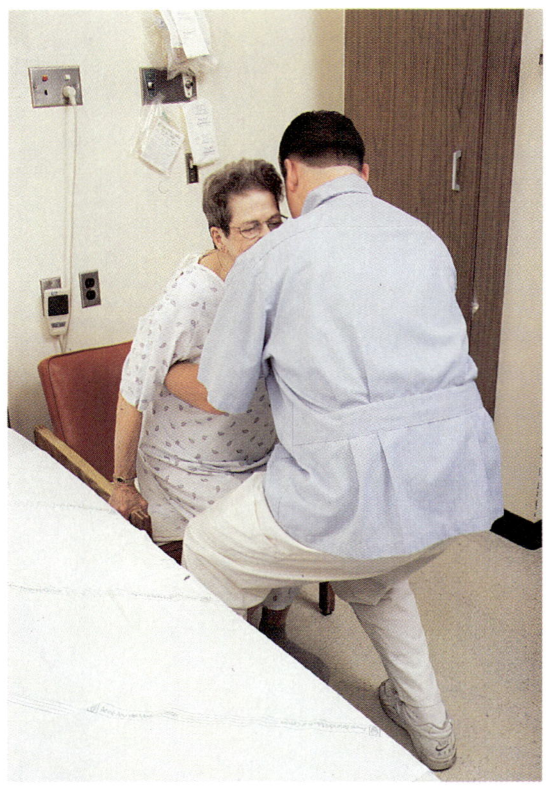

Fig. 10-33 *The person holds the arm rests, leans forward, and bends the elbows and knees while being lowered into the chair.*

Transferring a Person to a Wheelchair (Two Workers)

Pre-procedure

1. Ask a co-worker to help you.
2. Explain the procedure to the person.
3. Collect:
   - Wheelchair with removable armrests
   - Bath blankets
   - Shoes
   - Cushion if used
4. Wash your hands.
5. Identify the person. Check the ID bracelet and call the person by name.
6. Provide for privacy.
7. Determine which side of the bed to use. Move furniture to provide moving space.

Procedure

8. Fanfold top linens to the foot of the bed.
9. Assist the person to the side of the bed near you. Help him or her to a sitting position by raising the head of the bed.
10. Place the wheelchair at the side of the bed, even with the person's hips.
11. Remove the armrest near the bed. Put the cushion or a folded bath blanket on the seat.
12. Lock wheelchair and bed wheels.
13. Stand behind the wheelchair. Put your arms under the person's arms and grasp the forearms (Fig. 10-34, A on page 242).
14. Have your assistant grasp the person's thighs and calves (Fig. 10-34, B on page 242).
15. Bring the person toward the chair on the count of "3." Lower him or her into the chair as in Figure 10-35 on page 242.
16. Make sure the buttocks are to the back of the seat. Position the person in good alignment.
17. Put the armrest back on the wheelchair.
18. Put the shoes on the person. Position the feet on the footrests.
19. Cover the person's lap and legs with a bath blanket. The blanket must be off the floor and wheels.
20. Position the chair as the person prefers.

Post-procedure

21. Make sure the call bell and other necessary items are within reach.
22. Unscreen the person.
23. Wash your hands.
24. Report the following to the nurse:
    - The pulse rate if taken
    - Complaints of lightheadedness, pain, discomfort, difficulty breathing, weakness, or fatigue
    - How well the activity was tolerated
25. Reverse the procedure to return the person to bed.

A

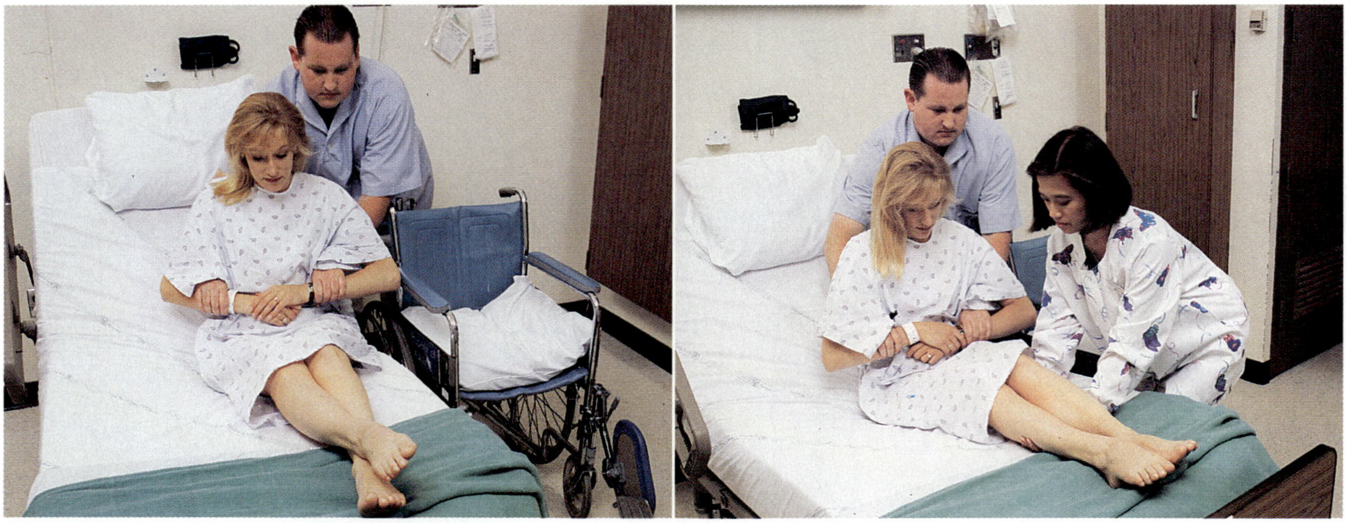

B

Fig. 10-34 *A, Grasp the person's forearms by putting your arms under the person's arms.* ***B,*** *The thighs and calves are held to support the lower extremities during a transfer.*

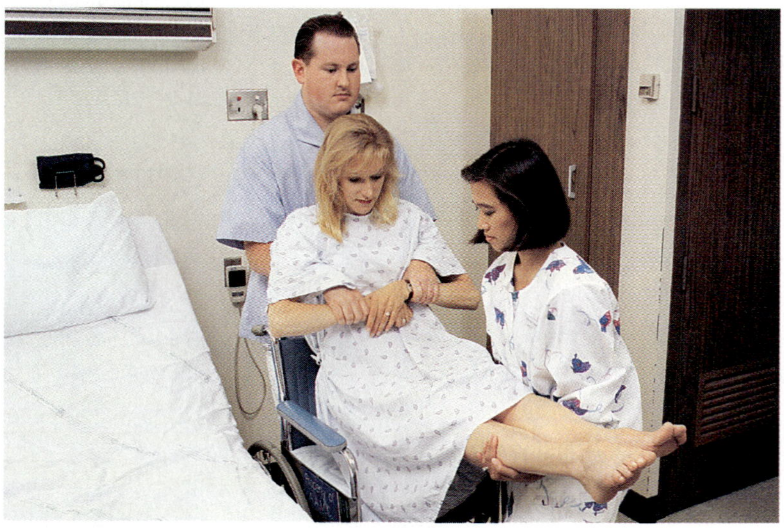

Fig. 10-35 *The person is supported while being lowered into the chair.*

Mechanical Lifts

Mechanical lifts are used to transfer disabled persons. A person may be transferred to a chair, stretcher, bathtub, shower chair, toilet, whirlpool, or car. Before using a lift, make sure it is working. You need to compare the person's weight and the lift's weight limit. Do not use the lift if a person's weight exceeds its capacity.

At least two people are needed to transfer a person with a mechanical lift. The manufacturer's instructions are followed for a safe transfer. The following procedure is used as a guide.

Text continued on page 245.

Using a Mechanical Lift

Pre-procedure

1 Ask a co-worker to help you.
2 Explain the procedure to the person.
3 Collect:
   - Mechanical lift
   - Arm chair or wheelchair
   - Slippers
   - Bath blanket
4 Wash your hands.
5 Identify the person. Check the ID bracelet and call the person by name.
6 Provide for privacy.

Procedure

7 Center the sling under the person (Fig. 10-36 on page 244). Turn him or her from side to side as if making an occupied bed to position the sling (see Chapter 12). Position the sling according to the manufacturer's instructions.
8 Place the chair at the head of the bed. It should be even with the headboard and about 1 foot away from the bed. Place a folded bath blanket in the chair.
9 Lock the bed wheels and lower the bed to its lowest position.
10 Raise the lift so it can be positioned over the person.
11 Position the lift over the person (Fig. 10-37, A on page 244).
12 Lock the lift wheels in position.
13 Attach the sling to the swivel bar (Fig. 10-37, B).
14 Raise the head of the bed to a sitting position.
15 Cross the person's arms over the chest. Let him or her hold onto the straps or chains, but not the swivel bar.
16 Pump the lift high enough until the person and sling are free of the bed (Fig. 10-37, C).
17 Ask your co-worker to support the legs as you move the lift and person away from the bed (Fig. 10-37, D).
18 Position the lift so that the person's back is toward the chair.
19 Lower the person into the chair. (Follow the manufacturer's instructions for lowering the lift.) Guide the person into the chair as in Figure 10-37, E.
20 Lower the swivel bar to unhook the sling. Leave the sling under the person unless otherwise indicated.
21 Put the slippers on the person. Position the feet on the footrests if a wheelchair is used.
22 Cover the person's lap and legs with a bath blanket. The blanket must be off the floor and wheels.
23 Position the chair as the person prefers.

Post-procedure

24 Make sure the call bell and other necessary items are within reach.
25 Wash your hands.
26 Report the following to the nurse:
   - The pulse rate if taken
   - Complaints of lightheadedness, pain, discomfort, difficulty breathing, weakness, or fatigue
   - How well the activity was tolerated
27 Reverse the procedure to return the person to bed.

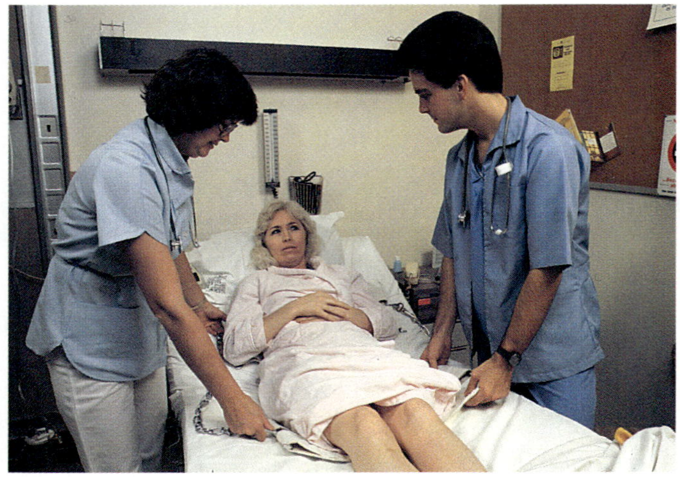

Fig. 10-36 *The sling of the mechanical lift is positioned under the person. The lower edge of the sling is behind the person's knees.*

A

B

C

D

E

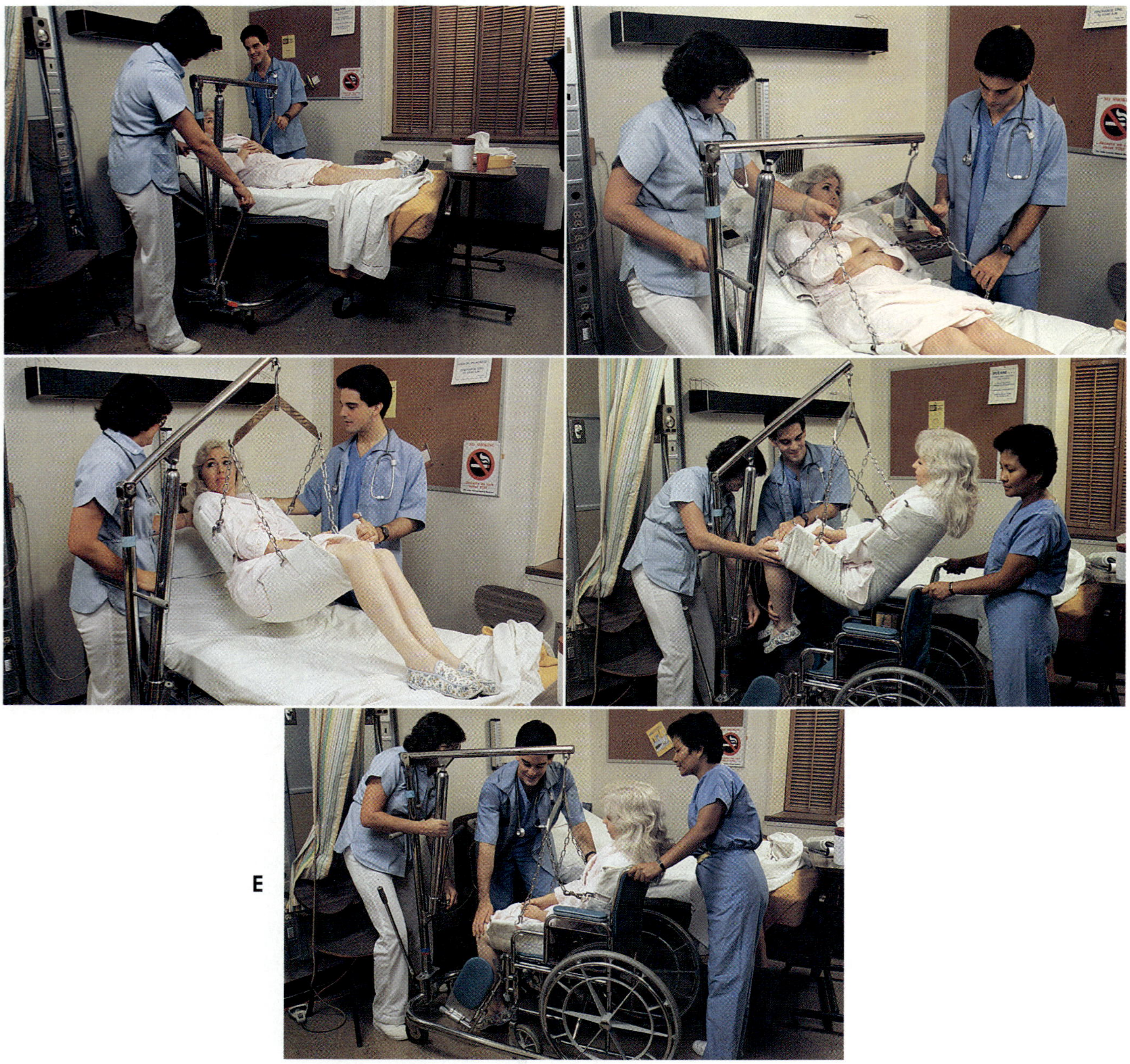

Fig. 10-37 *A, The lift is positioned over the person and the legs of the lift are spread to widen the base of support.* ***B,*** *The sling is attached to a swivel bar.* ***C,*** *The lift is raised until the sling and person are off of the bed.* ***D,*** *The person's legs are supported as the person and lift are moved away from the bed.* ***E,*** *The person is guided into a chair.*

Moving the Person to a Stretcher

Persons are transferred to stretchers for transport to other areas. Stretchers are used for persons who cannot sit up, those who must remain in a lying position, and for seriously ill persons. The stretcher is covered with a folded flat sheet or bath blanket. A pillow and extra blankets are available. With the nurse's permission, raise the head of the stretcher to a sitting or semisitting position. This increases the person's comfort.

Safety straps are used when the person is on the stretcher. The stretcher's side rails are kept up during the transport. Move the person feet first so the helper at the head of the stretcher can watch the person's breathing and color during the transport. A person on a stretcher is never left unattended.

A drawsheet can be used to transfer a person from the bed to a stretcher. At least 3 workers are needed for a safe transfer. Remember to keep the person in good body alignment and to use good body mechanics.

Transferring a Person to a Stretcher

Pre-procedure

1 Ask two co-workers to help you.
2 Explain the procedure to the person.
3 Collect:
- Stretcher covered with a sheet or bath blanket
- Bath blanket
- Pillow(s) if needed

4 Wash your hands.
5 Identify the person. Check the ID bracelet and call the person by name.
6 Provide for privacy.
7 Raise the bed to its highest level.

Procedure

8 Cover the person with a bath blanket. Fanfold top linens to the foot of the bed.
9 Loosen the cotton drawsheet on each side.
10 Lower the head of the bed so it is as flat as possible.
11 Lower the side rail on the side to which the person will be moved.
12 Ask your co-workers to help move the person to the side of the bed with the drawsheet.
13 Go to the other side of the bed. Lower the side rail. Protect the person from falling by holding the far arm and leg.
14 Have the co-workers position the stretcher next to the bed and stand behind the stretcher (Fig. 10-38 on page 246).
15 Lock the wheels of the bed and stretcher.
16 Roll up and grasp the drawsheet at the hip and mid-chest levels.
17 Ask your helpers to roll up and grasp the drawsheet. This supports the entire length of the person's body.
18 Transfer the person to the stretcher on the count of "3" by lifting and pulling him or her (Fig. 10-39 on page 246). Make sure the person is centered on the stretcher.
19 Place a pillow or pillows under the person's head and shoulders if allowed.
20 Make sure the person is covered and comfortable.
21 Fasten safety straps. Raise the side rails.
22 Unlock the stretcher's wheels. Transport the person.

Post-procedure

23 Wash your hands.
24 Report the following to the nurse:
- The time of the transport
- Where the person was transported to
- Who accompanied him or her
- How the transfer was tolerated

25 Reverse the procedure to return the person to bed.

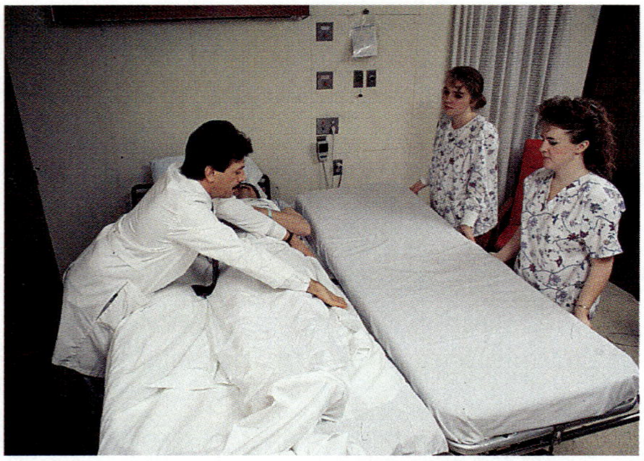

Fig. 10-38 *The stretcher is against the bed and is held in place by two nursing assistants.*

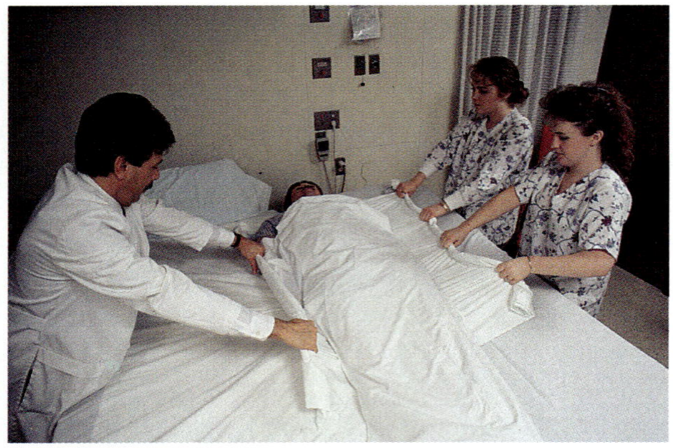

Fig. 10-39 *The person is transferred from the bed to a stretcher by workers using a drawsheet.*

POSITIONING

The person must be properly positioned when in bed or sitting in a chair. Physical comfort and well-being are promoted with regular position changes and good alignment. Breathing is easier and circulation is promoted. Proper positioning also helps prevent many complications. These include pressure sores (see Chapter 13) and contracture deformities (see Chapter 19). Some persons must be repositioned every hour or every 2 hours.

The doctor may order a certain position for a person. A doctor may also restrict a person from a certain position. The following guidelines help you to safely position patients and residents.

- Consult with the nurse about position changes for a person.
- Know how often to turn a person and to what positions.
- Use good body mechanics.
- Ask a co-worker to help you if indicated.
- Explain the procedure to the person.
- Be gentle when moving the person.
- Provide for privacy.
- Place the call bell within the person's reach after positioning.

Basic Positions for the Person in Bed

Good body alignment and position changes are essential for persons confined to bed. Many persons can change positions alone. Others need some help. Some depend entirely on nursing personnel for position changes.

Fowler's position Fowler's position involves raising the head of the bed to a semisitting position. The head of the bed is raised 45 to 60 degrees. Good alignment for Fowler's position involves keeping the spine straight, supporting the head with a small pillow, and supporting the arms with pillows (Fig. 10-40). A small pillow may be placed under the lower back. Small pillows may also be placed under the thighs and ankles. A footboard may be used (see Chapter 19). The nurse tells you where to place pillows for the person.

Persons with heart and respiratory disorders usually breathe more easily in Fowler's position. Persons receiving tube feedings need the head of their beds raised. Eating, watching television, visiting, and reading are easier in Fowler's position.

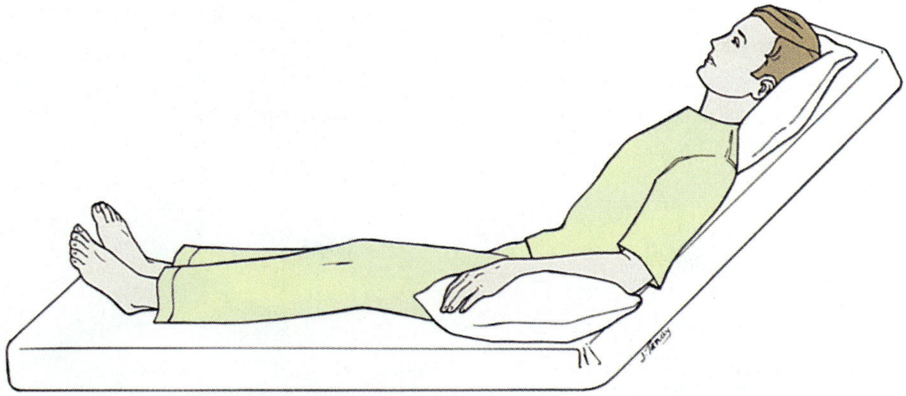

Fig. 10-40 *Fowler's position. Pillows are used to maintain alignment.*

Supine position The **supine (dorsal recumbent)** position is the back-lying position. Good alignment involves having the bed flat, supporting the head and shoulders on a pillow, and placing the arms and hands at the person's sides. The arms may be supported with regular-size pillows. The hands may be supported on small pillows with the palms down as in Figure 10-41. A small pillow may be placed under the ankles.

The nurse may ask you to place a folded or rolled towel under the lower part of the back. A small pillow may be placed under the person's thighs if requested by the nurse.

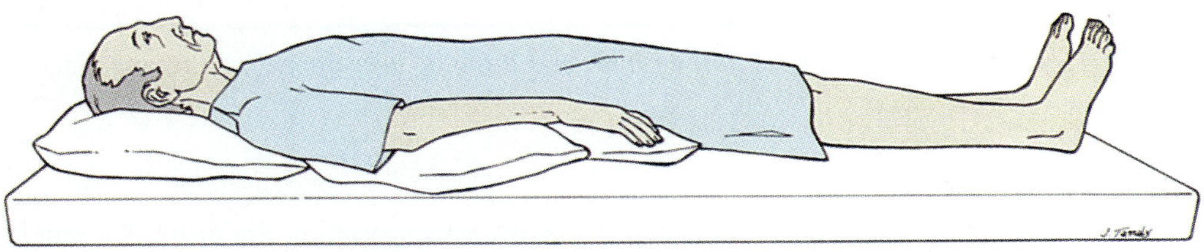

Fig. 10-41 *Person in supine position.*

Prone position Persons in the **prone position** lie on their abdomens with their heads turned to one side. Position the person in good alignment by placing a small pillow under the head, one under the abdomen, and one under the lower legs (Fig. 10-42). The arms are flexed at the elbows with the hands near the head. Persons can also be positioned so their feet hang over the end of the mattress (Fig. 10-43). If feet hang over the mattress, a pillow is not used under the lower legs.

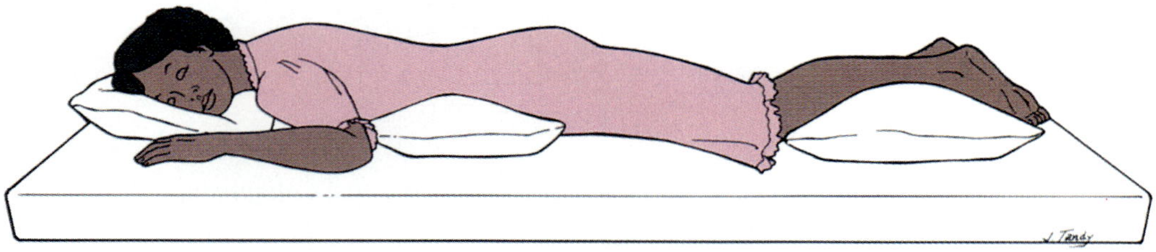

Fig. 10-42 *Person in prone position.*

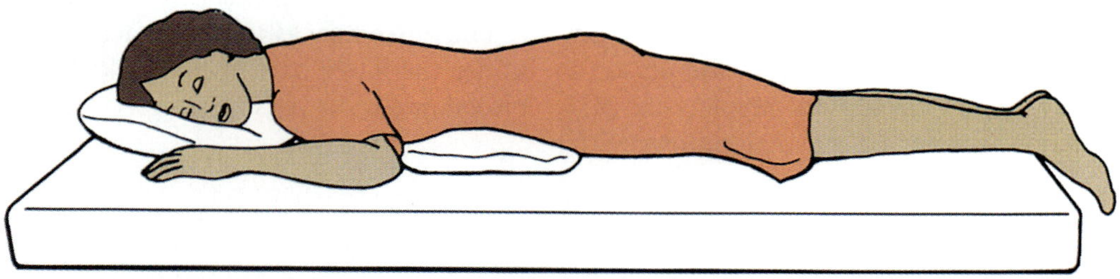

Fig. 10-43 *Person in prone position with the feet hanging over the edge of the mattress.*

Lateral position A person in the **lateral (side-lying) position** lies on one side or the other (Fig. 10-44). Good alignment includes placing a pillow under the head and neck and supporting the upper leg and thigh with pillows. A small pillow is placed under the upper hand and arm, and a pillow is positioned against the person's back.

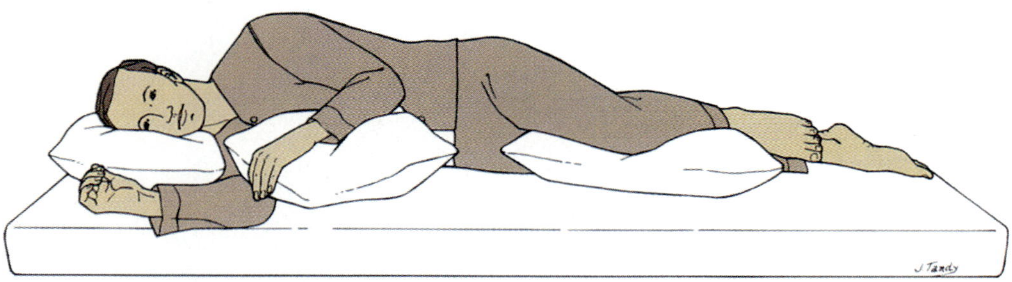

Fig. 10-44 *Person in lateral position with pillows used for support.*

Sims' position The **Sims' position** is a side-lying position. The upper leg is sharply flexed so it is not on the lower leg, and the lower arm is behind the person (Fig. 10-45). Good alignment involves placing a pillow under the person's head and neck, supporting the upper leg with a pillow, and placing a pillow under the upper arm and hand.

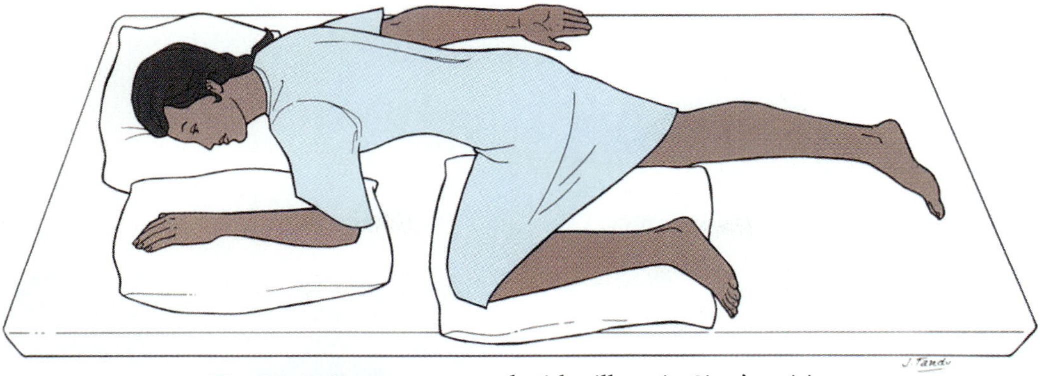

Fig. 10-45 *Person supported with pillows in Sims' position.*

Positioning in a Chair

Persons who sit in chairs must be able to hold their upper bodies and heads erect. Poor alignment results if the person cannot stay upright. The person's back and buttocks are against the back of the chair. Feet are flat on the floor or on the wheelchair footrests. Backs of the knees and calves are slightly away from the edge of the seat (Fig. 10-46). With the nurse's permission, you may put a small pillow between the person's lower back and the chair. (*Remember,* a pillow is not used behind the back if restraints are used.) This supports the lower back. Paralyzed arms are positioned on pillows. Wrists are positioned at a slight upward angle (Fig. 10-47).

Persons may need postural supports and positioners. Postural supports help keep persons in good body alignment (Fig. 10-48 on page 250). Sometimes restraints are used for postural support (Fig. 10-49 on page 250). The rules and safety measures for restraints apply when they are used as postural supports (see Chapter 8).

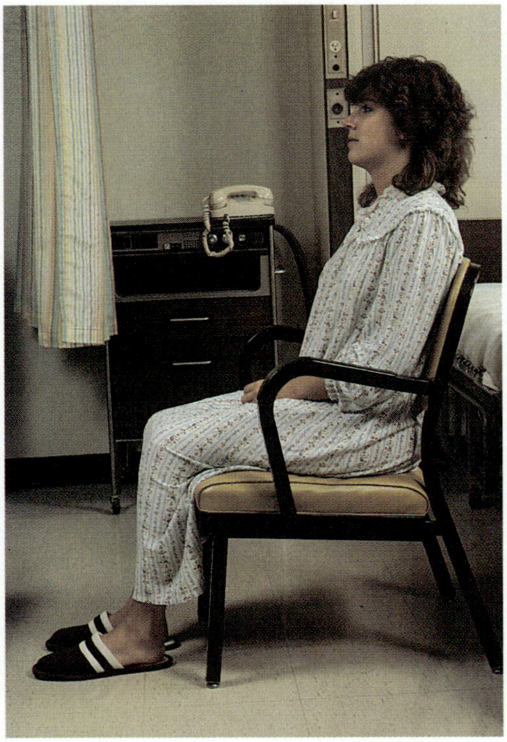

Fig. 10-46 *Person positioned in a chair. The person's feet are flat on the floor, the calves do not touch the chair, and the back is straight and against the back of the chair.*

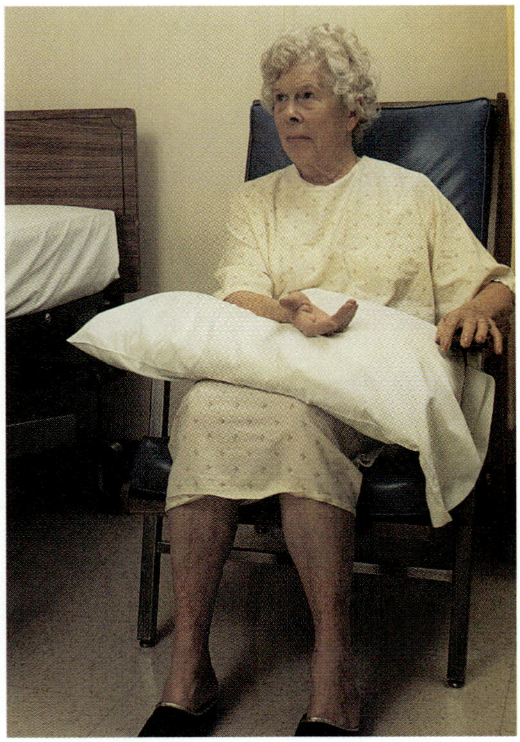

Fig. 10-47 *A pillow is used to support the paralyzed arm. Note that the wrist is at a slight upward angle.*

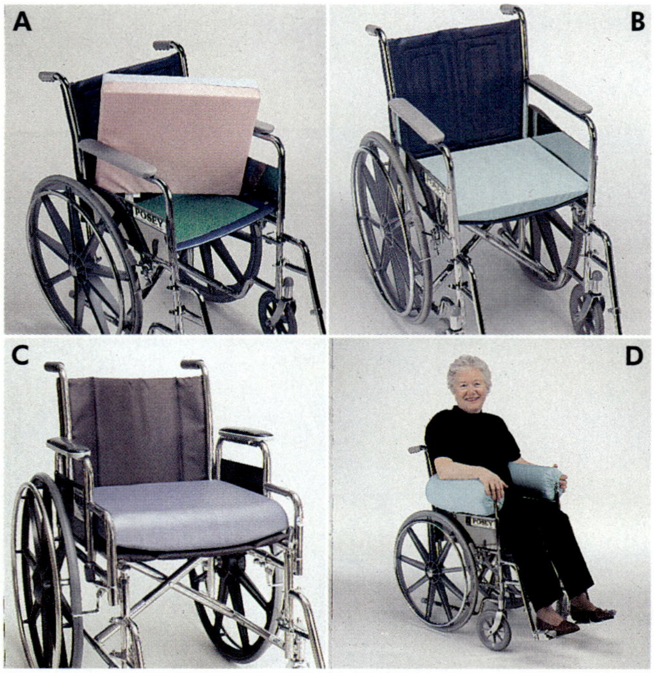

Fig. 10-48 *Postural supports.* ***A,*** *Wedge cushion.* ***B,*** *Wheelchair foundation.* ***C,*** *Molding foam cushion.* ***D,*** *Lateral stabilizers.* (Courtesy of Posey, Arcadia, CA.)

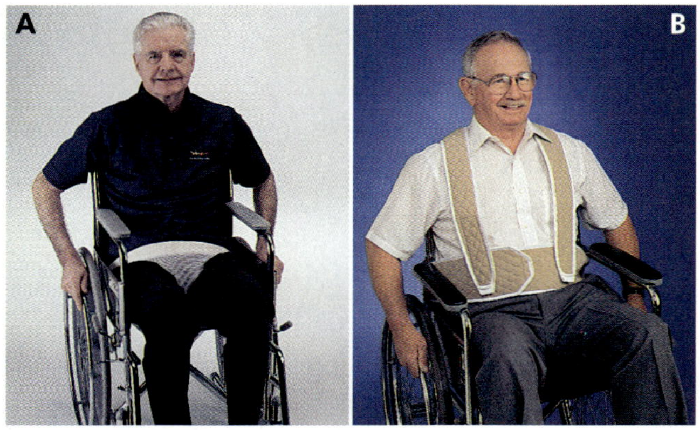

Fig. 10-49 *Restraints as postural supports.* ***A,*** *Pelvic holder.* ***B,*** *Torso support.* (Courtesy of Posey, Arcadia, CA.)

SUMMARY

Good body mechanics are used to lift, move, and transfer persons to protect yourself and them from injury. You need to keep yourself and the person in good alignment for comfort and well-being.

You have learned many ways to move, lift, transfer, and position persons. Their comfort and safety must always be protected during these activities. Be sure you know about any position restrictions ordered for a person. Also provide for privacy and protect the person from falling. Encourage the person to help with repositioning or transfers to the extent possible.

You may need to change some lifelong posture and body movement habits. As you use good body mechanics, you will feel better and work with greater efficiency. Remember to follow the rules of body mechanics in all activities.

REVIEW QUESTIONS

Circle T *if the answer is true and* F *if the answer is false.*

1 **T** **F** Body mechanics is the way body segments are aligned with one another.

2 **T** **F** Good body mechanics help protect you and your patients or residents from injury.

3 **T** **F** Base of support is the area on which an object rests.

4 **T** **F** Objects are kept away from the body when lifting, moving, or carrying them.

5 **T** **F** Face the direction you are working to prevent unnecessary twisting.

6 **T** **F** Push, slide, or pull heavy objects rather than lift them.

7 **T** **F** Consult with the nurse for any limitations or restrictions in positioning or moving a person.

8 **T** **F** The right to privacy is protected when moving, lifting, or transferring persons.

9 **T** **F** You need help to move Mrs. Lund. You should ask a co-worker to help before you begin the procedure.

10 **T** **F** A lift sheet is used to move Mrs. Lund. It should extend from her shoulders to above the knees.

11 **T** **F** You are going to turn Mrs. Lund to the side-lying position. First move her to the side of the bed.

12 **T** **F** Logrolling is rolling the person in segments.

13 **T** **F** Persons with spinal cord injuries are logrolled.

14 **T** **F** A person may dangle to gradually increase activity.

15 **T** **F** A transfer belt is part of a mechanical lift.

16 **T** **F** You are going to transfer Mrs. Lund from the bed to a chair. Move her from the direction of the weak side of her body.

17 **T** **F** Safety straps are applied only if the person is left unattended on a stretcher.

18 **T** **F** Repositioning prevents deformities and pressure on body parts.

19 **T** **F** The head of the bed is elevated 45 to 60 degrees for the supine position.

20 **T** **F** The Sims' position is a side-lying position.

Circle the best *answer.*

21 Body mechanics involves the following *except*

- **a** Good posture
- **b** Balance
- **c** The small muscles of the body
- **d** The large muscles of the body

22 The small muscles of the body are located in the

- **a** Back
- **b** Shoulders
- **c** Upper arms
- **d** Hips and thighs

23 Which will *not* reduce friction and shearing?

- **a** Sliding the person
- **b** Lifting the person
- **c** Rolling the person
- **d** Using a turning sheet

24 Mrs. Lund is to be transferred from the bed to a chair. She should

- **a** Be barefoot
- **b** Wear socks
- **c** Wear slippers
- **d** Wear nonskid shoes

25 Mrs. Lund is positioned in a chair. Which is *false?*

- **a** Her back and buttocks are against the back of the chair.
- **b** Her feet are flat on the floor or wheelchair footrests.
- **c** Her paralyzed arm rests on her lap.
- **d** The backs of her knees and calves are away from the chair.

Answers to these questions are on page 750.

The Patient/Resident Unit

11

OBJECTIVES

- Define the key terms listed in this chapter
- Identify the temperature range comfortable for most people
- Identify the temperature range required by OBRA
- Describe how to protect patients and residents from drafts
- List ways to prevent or reduce odors in the person's room
- Describe how to control common causes of noise in health care facilities
- Explain how lighting affects comfort
- Know the basic bed positions
- Describe the use of furniture and equipment found in a patient/resident unit
- Describe how a bathroom is equipped
- Explain how to maintain the person's unit
- Know the OBRA requirements for resident rooms

KEY TERMS

caster A small wheel made of rubber or plastic

patient/resident pack Personal care equipment provided by the health care facility (wash basin, emesis or kidney basin, bedpan, urinal, water pitcher and glass, soap, and soap dish)

patient/resident unit The furniture and equipment provided for the person by the health care facility

reverse Trendelenburg's position The head of the bed is raised, and the foot of the bed is lowered

semi-Fowler's position The head of the bed is raised 45 degrees, and the knee portion is raised 15 degrees; or the head of the bed is raised 30 degrees

Trendelenburg's position The head of the bed is lowered, and the foot of the bed is raised

Hospital patients and nursing facility residents spend a lot of time in their rooms. Rooms may be private, for one person. Semiprivate rooms, furnished for two people, are more common. Rooms must be comfortable, safe, and allow enough space for activities of daily living. This chapter describes the furnishings in a patient/resident unit. A **patient/resident unit** is the furniture and equipment provided for the person by the facility (Fig. 11-1). The conditions that affect comfort also are presented. So are OBRA requirements for long-term care.

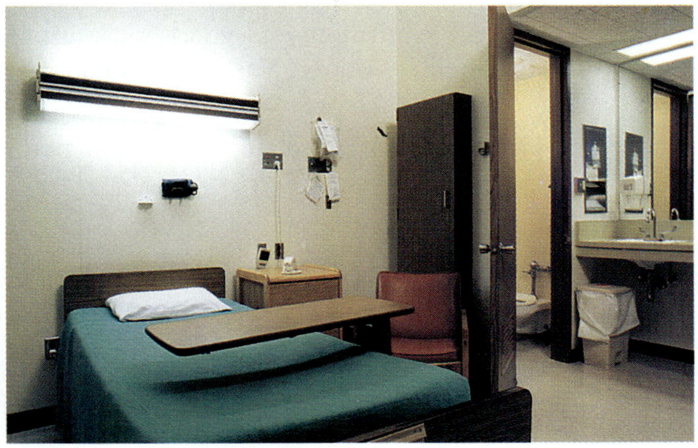

Fig. 11-1 *Furniture and equipment in a typical patient/resident unit.*

COMFORT

Age, illness, and activity affect comfort. So do factors like temperature, ventilation, noise, odors, and lighting. Those factors can be controlled to meet the person's needs.

Temperature and Ventilation

Health care facilities have heating, air conditioning, and ventilation systems. The systems maintain a comfortable temperature and provide fresh air in the rooms. A temperature range of 68° F to 74° F is usually comfortable for most healthy people. A comfortable temperature for one person may be too hot or too cold for another. Infants, the elderly, and ill persons generally need higher room temperatures for comfort. Therefore higher temperatures are usually needed in hospitals and nursing facilities. OBRA requires that nursing facilities maintain a temperature range of 71° F to 81° F.

Stale room air and lingering odors affect comfort and rest. A good ventilation system provides fresh air and moves room air. Drafts can occur as air moves. Infants, the elderly, and ill persons are sensitive to drafts and need protection from them. Adequate clothing is necessary.

The elderly may wear sweaters even in warm weather. Persons sensitive to drafts need to be well covered with blankets. Those sitting in chairs or wheelchairs may want lap robes (blankets, afghans) for warmth. Patients and residents are moved from drafty areas when possible.

Odors

Many odors occur in health facilities. Some are pleasant, like food aromas and flower scents. Others are unpleasant. Draining wounds, vomitus, and bowel movements have unpleasant smells that can embarrass the person. Body, breath, and smoking odors may offend patients, residents, visitors, and staff. Odors may be unnoticed by ill persons and the elderly who have a reduced sense of smell. Good nursing care, good ventilation, and good housekeeping practices help eliminate odors. Nursing personnel can reduce odors by

- Emptying and washing bedpans and emesis basins promptly
- Changing soiled linens promptly
- Cleaning incontinent patients or residents promptly
- Providing individuals with good personal hygiene to prevent body and breath odors
- Using room deodorizers when necessary and if allowed by the facility

Smoke odors cause special problems. Many facilities ban smoking. Patients, residents, staff, and visitors cannot smoke anywhere in the building. However, nursing facilities may let residents smoke in certain areas. If you smoke, you must follow the employer's policy. Wash your hands after handling smoking materials and before giving care. Careful attention must be given to your uniforms, hair, and breath because of clinging smoke odors.

Noise

Ill people are sensitive to noises and sounds around them. Patients and residents are often disturbed by common health care sounds. The clanging of metal bedpans, urinals, and wash basins can be annoying. So can the clatter of dishes and trays. Loud talking and laughing in hallways and at the nurses' station, loud televisions and radios, ringing telephones, and buzzing intercoms can be irritating. So is noise from equipment needing repair or oil. Wheels on stretchers, wheelchairs, carts, and other equipment must be oiled properly.

When in a strange place, people want to know the cause and meaning of new sounds. This is part of the basic need to feel safe and secure. Patients and residents may find sounds dangerous, frightening, or irritating. They may become upset, anxious, and uncomfortable. Remember, noise to one person may not be noise to another. For example, loud stereo music may please a teenager but irritate parents.

Health care facilities are designed to reduce noise. Drapes, carpeting, and acoustical tiles help absorb noise. Plastic items have replaced some metal equipment (bedpans, urinals, and wash basins). Staff can reduce noise by controlling the loudness of their voices and handling equipment carefully. Keeping equipment working properly and promptly answering telephones and intercoms also decrease noise.

Lighting

Good lighting is needed for the safety and comfort of patients, residents, and staff. Glares, shadows, and dull lighting can cause falls, headaches, and eyestrain. People usually relax and rest better in dim light. However, a bright room is more cheerful and stimulating.

Lighting is adjusted to meet the person's changing needs. Shades are pulled or drapes drawn to control natural light. The overbed light is adjusted to provide soft, medium, and bright lighting. Some facilities have ceiling lights over beds. These provide low to very bright light. Bright lighting is helpful when care is given. Light controls should be within the person's reach.

ROOM FURNITURE AND EQUIPMENT

Patient or resident rooms are furnished and equipped for the person's basic needs. There is furniture and equipment for comfort, sleep, elimination, nutrition, personal hygiene, and activity. There is also equipment for communicating with the nursing team, relatives, and friends. The right to privacy is considered when equipping the room.

OBRA requires rooms in long-term care settings to be as homelike as possible. Therefore the resident is allowed to have and use personal items. To the extent possible, residents can bring furniture and personal items from home. This promotes the person's dignity and esteem.

The Bed

Hospital beds have electrical or manual controls. Beds are raised horizontally to give care. This reduces the amount of bending or reaching needed. The lowest horizontal position lets the person get out of bed with ease (Fig. 11-2). The head of the bed can be kept flat or raised to varying degrees.

Electric beds are common. Bed positions are easily changed by hand controls. The controls are on a side panel, attached to the bed by a cable, or on a panel at the foot of the bed (Fig. 11-3). Patients and residents are taught how to use the controls. They are warned not to

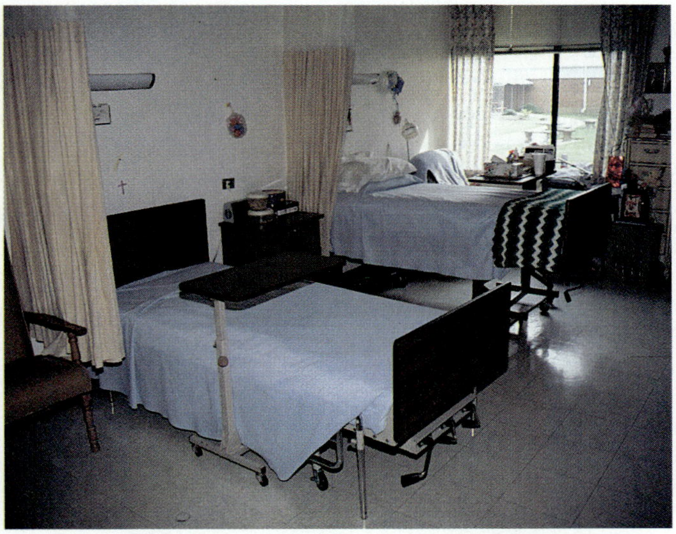

Fig. 11-2 *One bed in the highest horizontal position and the other bed in the lowest horizontal position.*

raise the bed to the high position and not to adjust the bed to harmful positions. They are told of any position limits or restrictions.

Some electric beds can be locked in certain positions. This prevents the person from raising or lowering the head or foot of the bed. Persons restricted to certain positions may need to have their beds locked. The locking feature is useful for confused persons.

Manually operated beds have cranks at the foot of the bed (Fig. 11-4). The left crank raises or lowers the head of the bed. The right crank adjusts the knee portion. The center crank raises or lowers the entire bed. The cranks are pulled up for use and kept down at all other times. Cranks in the *up* position are safety hazards. Anyone walking past may bump into them.

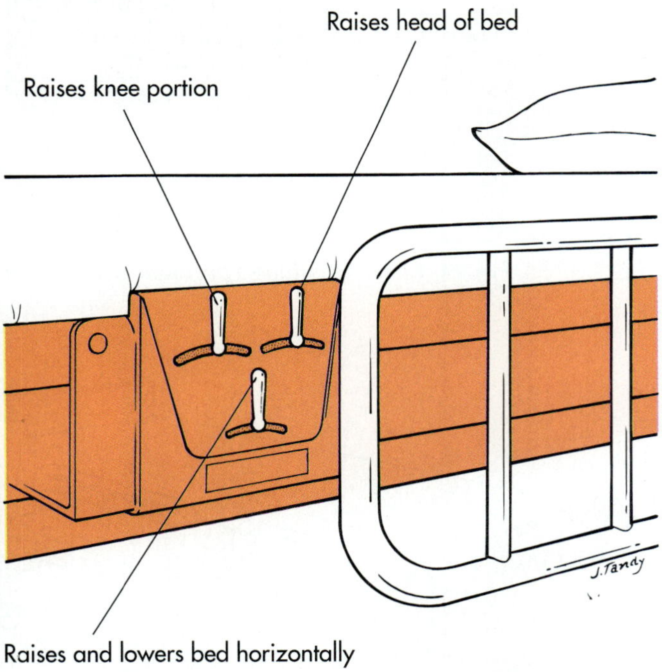

Fig. 11-3 *Controls for an electric bed.*

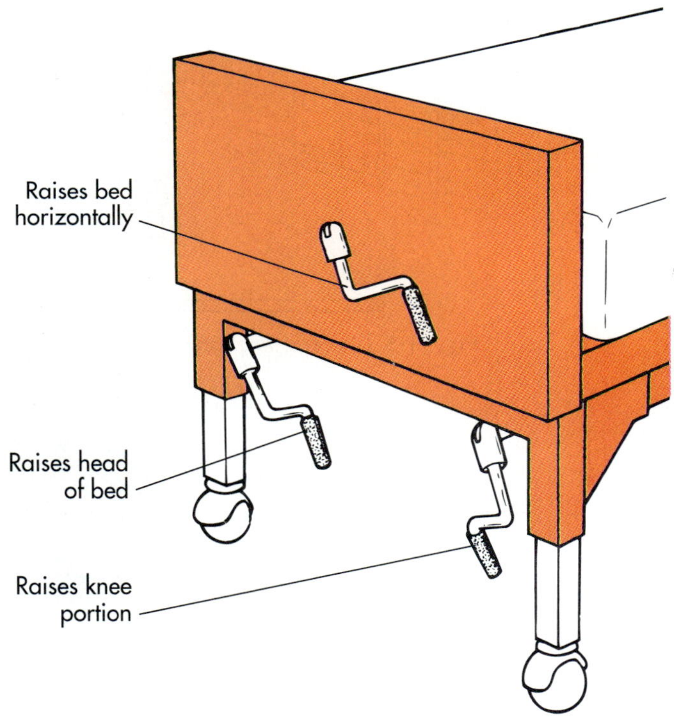

Fig. 11-4 *Manually operated hospital bed.*

Bed positions There are four basic bed positions: Fowler's, semi-Fowler's, Trendelenburg's, and reverse Trendelenburg's. **Fowler's position** is a semisitting position. The head of the bed is elevated 45 to 60 degrees (Fig. 11-5). The reasons for positioning a person in Fowler's position are described in Chapter 10.

In **semi-Fowler's position** the head of the bed is raised 45 degrees and the knee portion is raised 15 degrees (Fig. 11-6). This position is comfortable and prevents persons from sliding down in bed. However, raising the knee portion can interfere with circulation. Consult with the nurse before positioning a person in semi-Fowler's position. Many facilities define semi-Fowler's position as when the head of the bed is raised 30 degrees and the knee portion is *not* raised. You must know which definition your employer uses so you give safe care.

Trendelenburg's position involves lowering the head of the bed and raising the foot of the bed (Fig. 11-7). A doctor's order is required for this position. Blocks are placed under the legs at the foot of the bed. Some beds are made so the entire bedframe can be tilted into Trendelenburg's position.

Reverse Trendelenburg's position is the opposite of Trendelenburg's position. The head of the bed is raised and the foot of the bed is lowered (Fig. 11-8). Blocks are put under the legs at the head of the bed, or the bedframe is tilted. This position requires a doctor's order.

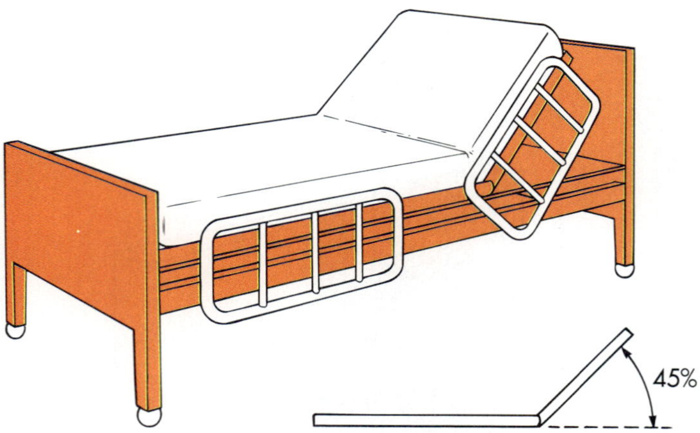

Fig. 11-5 *Fowler's position.*

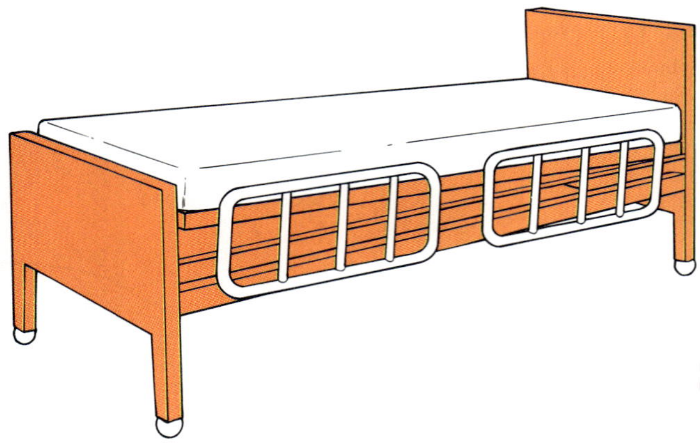

Fig. 11-7 *Trendelenburg's position.*

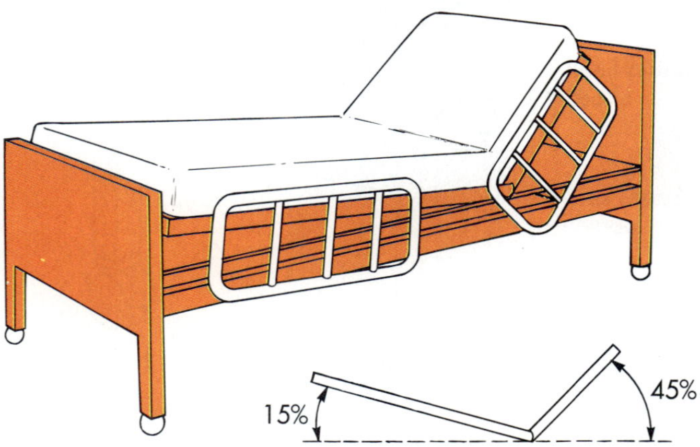

Fig. 11-6 *Semi-Fowler's position.*

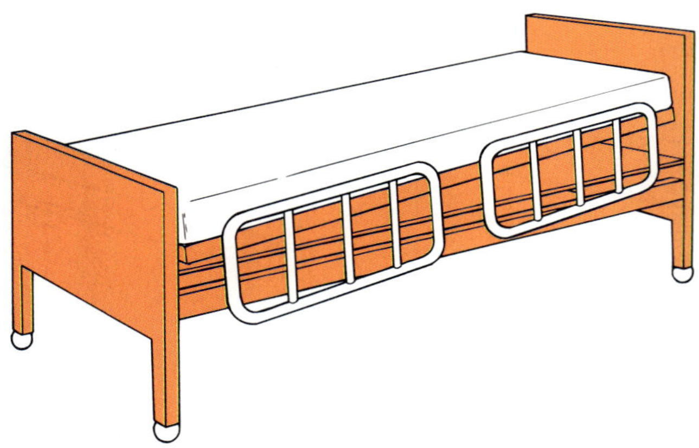

Fig. 11-8 *Reverse Trendelenburg's position.*

Safety Considerations

Bed legs have wheels or casters. A **caster** is a small wheel made of rubber or plastic that allows the bed to move easily. Each wheel or caster has a lock to prevent the bed from moving (Fig. 11-9). Bed wheels are locked when giving bedside care. They are also locked when you transfer a person to and from the bed. The person can be injured if the bed moves.

The importance of side rails on hospital beds is discussed in Chapter 8.

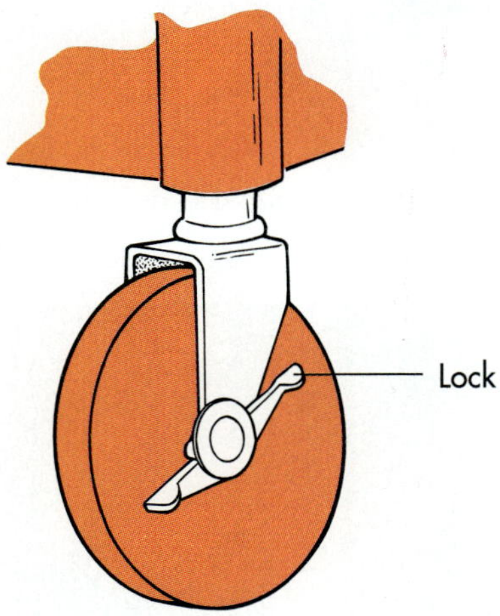

Fig. 11-9 *Lock on bed wheel.*

The Overbed Table

The overbed table (see Fig. 11-1) is positioned over the bed by sliding the base under the bed. The height is adjusted for the person in bed or in a chair. Turn the side handle or lever to raise or lower the table. The overbed table is used for meal trays and for eating, writing, reading, and other activities.

Many overbed tables have movable tops with a storage area underneath. The storage area is often used for makeup, hair care, or shaving items. Many also have a flip-up mirror.

The nursing team uses the overbed table as a work area. Only clean and sterile items are placed on the table. The table is cleaned after being used as a working surface.

The Bedside Stand

The bedside stand is next to the bed. The stand is a storage area for personal items and personal care equipment. It has 2 or 3 drawers or 1 drawer at the top and a lower cabinet with a shelf (Fig. 11-10). The top drawer can be used for money, eyeglasses, books, and other personal items. The first shelf (or second drawer) is used for the wash basin, which can hold personal care items. These include soap and soap dish, powder, lotion, deodorant, towels, washcloth, bath blanket, and a clean gown or pajamas. An emesis or kidney basin (shaped like a kidney) is often used to hold oral hygiene items. The kidney basin can be stored on the top shelf or in the top drawer. The bedpan and its cover, the urinal, and toilet paper are on the lower shelf (or third drawer).

The top of the stand is often used for tissues and the telephone. It may also be used for a radio, flowers, gifts, cards, and other items important to the person. Some stands have a rod at the side or back for towels and washcloths.

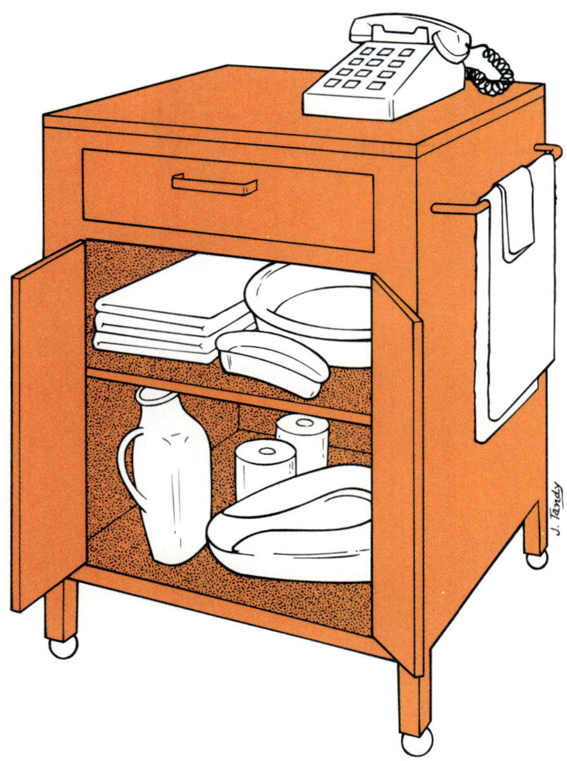

Fig. 11-10 *The bedside stand is used to store personal care equipment.*

Chairs

The patient/resident unit usually has 1 or 2 chairs. One is a straight-back chair without arms. The other is an upholstered chair with armrests. It is used by the person and visitors and is placed near the bed. Nursing facility residents may bring their own chairs from home (Fig. 11-11).

Curtains or Screens

Rooms have privacy curtains. The curtain is pulled around the bed to provide privacy for the person (Fig. 11-12). The curtain is always pulled while care is being given. If a portable screen is used (Fig. 11-13), it is placed between the two beds. Curtains and screens protect the person from being seen by others. However, they do not block sound or prevent conversations from being overheard.

Personal Care Items

Personal care items are used for hygiene and elimination. A **patient pack** is provided by the facility. It usually has a wash basin, emesis or kidney basin, bedpan, urinal, water pitcher and glass, and soap and soap dish. Powder, lotion, toothbrush, toothpaste, mouthwash, tissues, and a comb may be included. Often patients and residents bring their own oral hygiene equipment, hair care supplies, and deodorant. Some choose to use their own soap, lotion, and powder. Be sure to respect the individual's choice of personal care products.

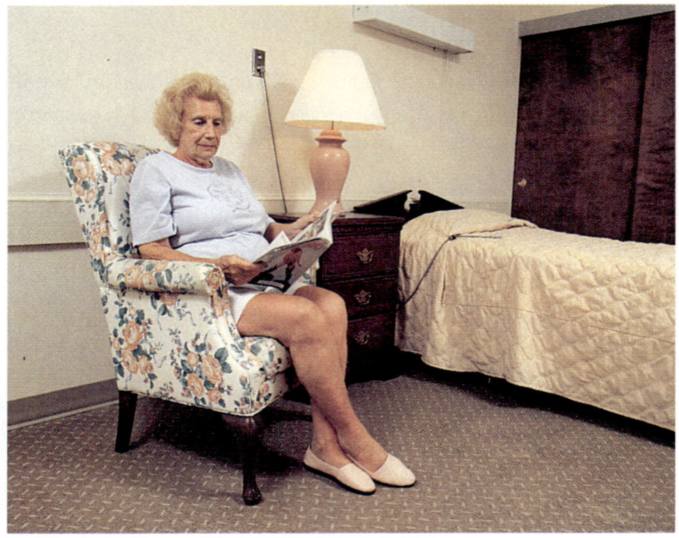

Fig. 11-11 *Resident's chair from home.*

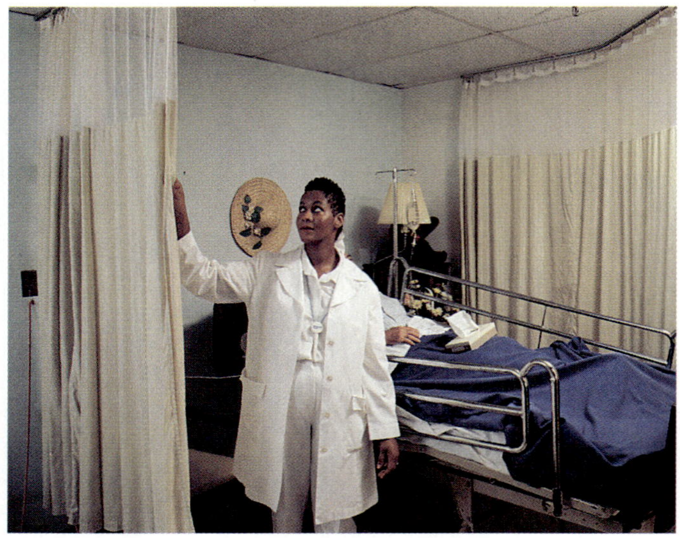

Fig. 11-12 *The privacy curtain is pulled around the person's bed while care is being given.*

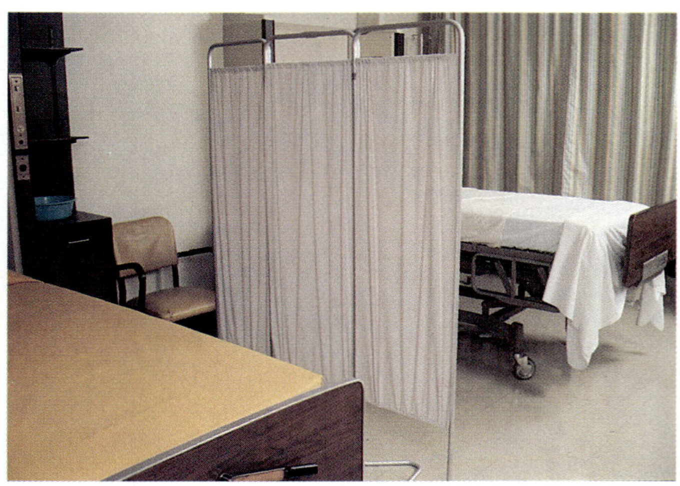

Fig. 11-13 *Portable screen between two units.*

Call System

The call system lets the person signal when help is needed. A call bell at the bedside is connected to a light above the room door and to a light panel or intercom system at the nurses' station (Fig. 11-14). The call bell is at the end of a long cord (Fig. 11-15). It is attached to the bed or chair so it is always within the person's reach and vision. The person presses a button at the end of the call bell when help is needed. The nurse or nursing assistant shuts off the call bell at the bedside when the person is given the help needed.

An intercom system lets a nursing team member talk with the person from the nurses' station. It also allows the light to be turned off from the station. Sometimes a tap bell is used in place of a call bell (Fig. 11-16). The call bell or tap bell must always be on the person's good side. Patients and residents are shown how to use the call system when admitted to the facility.

Some people cannot use the call bell. They must be checked often to make sure their needs are met.

A

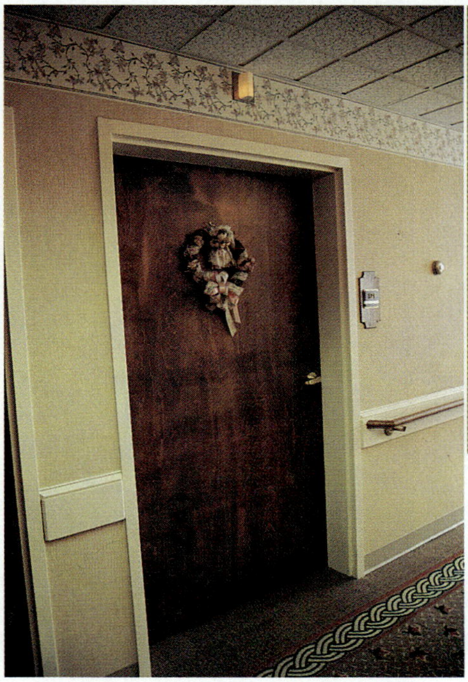

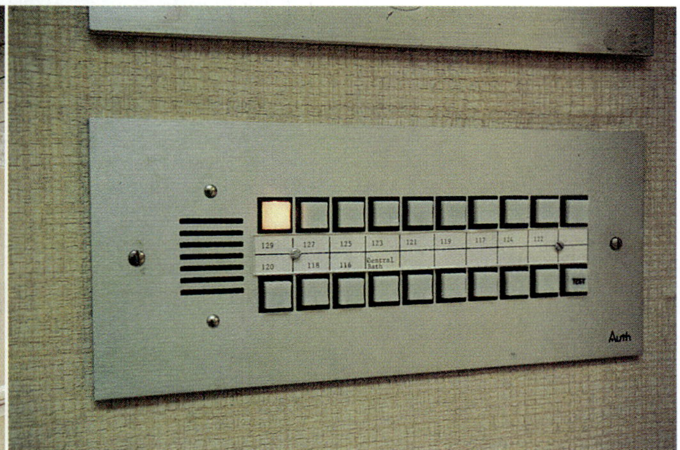

B

Fig. 11-14 *A, The light above the door of the person's room. B, Light panel or intercom system at the nurses' station.*

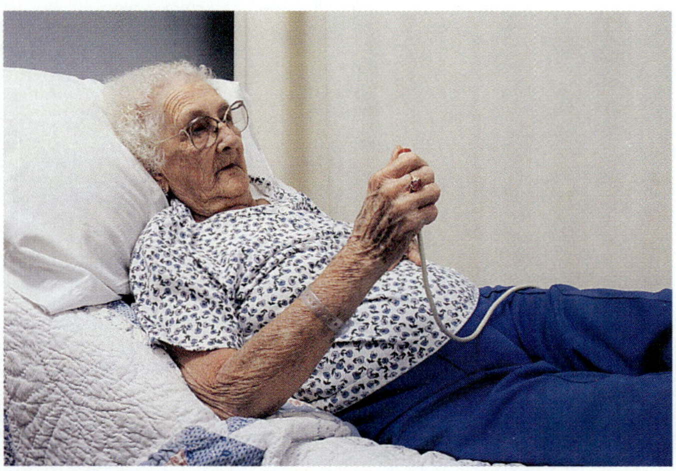

Fig. 11-15 *The person presses the button of the signal light when assistance is needed.*

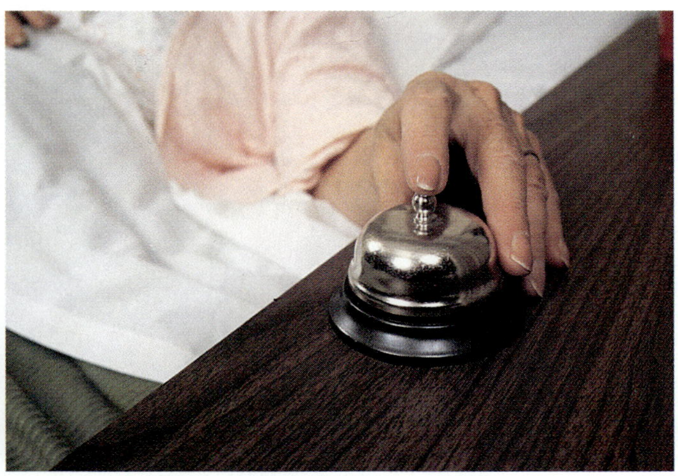

Fig. 11-16 *Tap bell.*

The Bathroom

Many facilities have a bathroom in each room. Some have a bathroom between two rooms. A toilet, sink, call system, and mirror are standard equipment (Fig. 11-17). There may also be a tub and shower. Hand rails are installed by the toilet for the person's safety. Toilets in some facilities are higher than the standard toilet. Higher toilets make transfers to and from wheelchairs easier and are helpful for persons with joint problems.

Towel racks, toilet paper, soap, a paper towel dispenser, wastebasket, and call system are in the bathroom. They are placed within easy reach of the person.

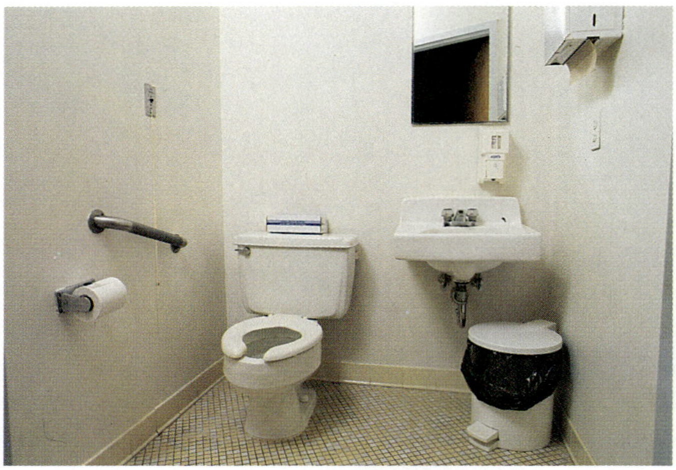

Fig. 11-17 *Bathroom in a health care facility.*

Closet and Drawer Space

Closet and drawer space are provided for the person's clothing. OBRA (see Chapter 7) requires closet space for each nursing facility resident. Such closet space must have shelves and a clothes rack. The resident must have free access to the closet and its contents (Fig. 11-18).

Items in the closet or drawers are the person's private property. You must not search the closet or drawers without the person's permission.

Sometimes people hoard items like napkins, straws, sugar, salt and pepper, and food in their drawers. Such hoarding can cause safety or health risks. Facility representatives can inspect a person's closet or drawers if hoarding is suspected. The person must be informed of the inspection and be present when it takes place.

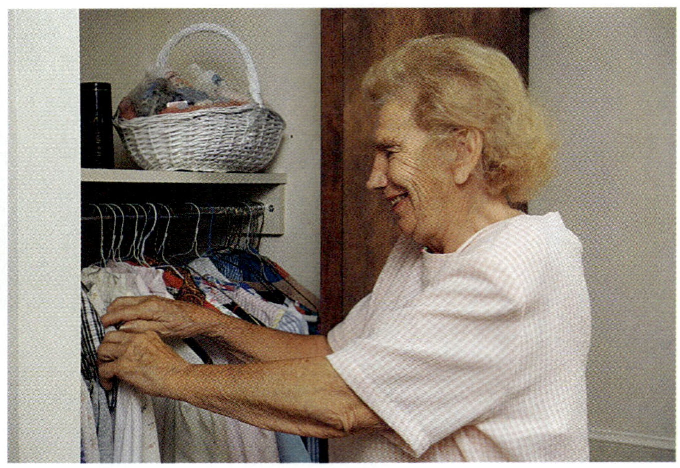

Fig. 11-18 *The resident can access items in her closet.*

Other Equipment

Many facilities furnish patient and resident units with other equipment. A television, radio, and clock are often included for comfort and relaxation. Hospital rooms have telephones. Some nursing facilities also provide telephones. Residents may bring favorite furniture and items from home.

Blood pressure equipment is often mounted on the walls. There are also wall outlets for oxygen and suction. Oxygen tanks and portable suction equipment are common in long-term care and home care settings. An IV pole (IV standard) is used to hang an intravenous infusion bottle or bag or a feeding bag. Some hospital beds have an IV pole stored in the bedframe. The IV pole may be a separate piece of equipment that is brought to the bedside when needed. Figure 11-19 shows blood pressure equipment and oxygen and suction outlets.

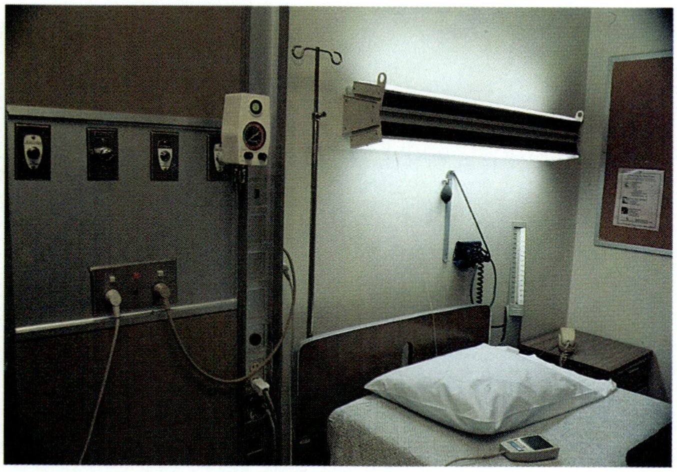

Fig. 11-19 *This room has blood pressure equipment and oxygen and suction outlets.*

General Rules

The patient or resident unit is kept clean, neat, and safe. This is a responsibility of everyone involved in the person's care. The rules in Box 11-1 are followed to maintain the person's unit.

BOX 11-1 Rules for Maintaining the Patient/Resident Unit

- Make sure the person can reach the overbed table and the bedside stand.
- Arrange personal items as the individual prefers. Make sure they are easily reached.
- Keep the call bell within the person's reach at all times.
- Make sure the person can reach the telephone, television, and light controls.
- Provide the person with enough tissues and toilet paper.
- Adjust lighting, temperature, and ventilation for the person's comfort.
- Handle equipment carefully to prevent noise.
- Explain the causes of strange noises to the person.
- Use room deodorizers if necessary.
- Empty the person's wastebasket as often as needed.
- Respect the person's belongings. An item may not be important or valuable to you yet it has great significance to the person. Even a scrap of paper can have great meaning to the person.
- Do not throw away any items belonging to the patient or resident.
- Do not move furniture or the person's belongings. Persons with poor vision rely on memory or feel for the location of items.

QUALITY OF LIFE

Nursing facility residents have left their homes. Each once had a home or apartment with furniture, appliances, a private bathroom, and many personal belongings and treasures. Now the person lives in a strange place and probably shares a room with another resident. Leaving one's home is a difficult part of growing old with poor health. Therefore it is important to make the resident's unit as homelike as possible.

The resident may bring some furniture and personal belongings. A chair, footstool, lamp, or small table are some items that may be allowed. Residents can always bring such things as family photos, religious items, and books. Some may have plants to care for.

The resident is allowed personal choice in arranging personal items. The health care team must make sure that such choices are safe and will not cause falls or other accidents. In addition, the resident's choices must not interfere with the rights of others. You may have to help the resident in choosing the best place for personal items.

Remember, the facility is now the person's home. You and other health team members must help the person feel safe, secure, and comfortable. A homelike environment is important for the person's quality of life. OBRA serves to promote quality of life. Box 11-2 lists OBRA's requirements for resident rooms.

BOX 11-2 OBRA Requirements for Resident Rooms

- Designed for 1 to 4 residents
- Direct access to an exit corridor
- Full visual privacy (privacy curtain that extends around the bed, movable screens, door)
- At least one window to the outside
- Individual closet space with racks and shelves
- Toilet facilities in the room or nearby (includes bathing facilities)
- Call system in the room and in toilet/bathing facilities
- Bed of proper height and size
- Clean, comfortable mattress with bedding appropriate to the weather and climate
- Furniture to accommodate clothing, personal items, and a chair for visitors
- Clean, and orderly room
- Odor-free room
- Room temperature between 71° and 81° F
- Acceptable noise level
- Adequate ventilation and room humidity
- Appropriate lighting
- No glares from floors, windows, and lighting
- Clean orderly drawers, shelves, and personal items
- Pest-free room
- Handrails in needed areas
- Side rails only if needed
- Clean, dry floor; pathways free of clutter and furniture
- Bed in low position and locked
- Personal supplies and items labeled and stored appropriately
- Drawers free of unwrapped food
- Items within reach for use in bed or bathroom
- Space for wheelchair or walker use
- Elevated toilet seat
- Stool and skidproof tub or shower

SUMMARY

The patient/resident unit is designed and equipped to meet basic needs. Equipment is provided for comfort, hygiene, elimination, and activity. The overbed table is used for meals. Side rails, hand rails, and the call system are for safety. Safety is also promoted by controlling temperature, ventilation, lighting, noise, and odors. Curtains or screens provide privacy and help the person feel safe and secure. A telephone lets the person talk with family and friends. The television and radio provide entertainment and relaxation.

Review Questions

Circle the best *answer.*

1 Which is a comfortable temperature range for most people?
- **a** 60° F to 66° F
- **b** 68° F to 74° F
- **c** 74° F to 80° F
- **d** 80° F to 86° F

2 Mr. Lance is protected from drafts by
- **a** Wearing enough clothing
- **b** Being covered with adequate blankets
- **c** Being moved out of a drafty area
- **d** All of the above.

3 Which does *not* prevent or reduce odors?
- **a** Placing fresh flowers in the room
- **b** Emptying bedpans promptly
- **c** Using room deodorizers
- **d** Practicing good personal hygiene

4 Which does *not* control noise?
- **a** Using plastic equipment
- **b** Handling dishes with care
- **c** Speaking softly
- **d** Talking with others in the hallway

5 Which is Fowler's position?
- **a** The head of the bed is raised 45 degrees.
- **b** The head of the bed is raised 45 degrees and the knee portion is raised 15 degrees.
- **c** The head of the bed is lowered and the foot of the bed is raised.
- **d** The head of the bed is raised and the foot of the bed is lowered.

6 The overbed table is *not* used
- **a** For eating
- **b** As a working surface
- **c** To store the urinal
- **d** To store shaving articles

Circle T *if the answer is true and* F *if the answer is false.*

7 **T** **F** Soft, dim lighting is usually relaxing and comfortable.

8 **T** **F** The curtain is pulled around Mr. Lance's bed to prevent conversations from being heard.

9 **T** **F** The call system is used by Mr. Lance to signal when help is needed.

10 **T** **F** The signal light must always be within Mr. Lance's reach except when he is in the bathroom.

11 **T** **F** The overbed table and bedside stand should be within the person's reach.

12 **T** **F** You should explain the cause of strange noises to Mr. Lance.

The answers to these questions are on page 750.

Bedmaking

12

OBJECTIVES

- Define the key terms listed in this chapter
- Describe unoccupied (open and closed), occupied, and surgical beds
- Identify when bed linens are changed
- Explain the use of plastic drawsheets and cotton drawsheets
- Identify the type of bed to make for certain situations
- Handle linens according to the rules of medical asepsis
- Perform the procedures in this chapter

KEY TERMS

drawsheet A small sheet placed over the middle of the bottom sheet; it helps keep the mattress and bottom linens clean and dry and can be used to turn and move the person in bed; the cotton drawsheet

mitered corner A way of tucking linens under the mattress to help keep them straight and smooth

plastic drawsheet A drawsheet made of plastic; it is placed between the bottom sheet and the cotton drawsheet to keep the mattress and bottom linens clean and dry

Patients and residents spend a lot of time in bed. Most residents are out of bed most of the day. Some patients and residents are up only part of the day. Others are in bed all the time. Some cannot get out of bed to use the bathroom. Meals are eaten in bed. Some persons are bathed in bed. Many other procedures are done with the person in bed.

Bedmaking is important. A clean, neat bed helps the person's comfort. Think of how nice it is getting into a freshly made bed at home. How does it feel getting into an unmade bed that does not have the sheets and blankets tucked in?

Linens are changed daily in hospitals. In nursing facilities, a complete linen change is done on the person's bath day or as needed. The bed is usually made in the morning after the person's bath. It can also be made while the person is in the shower or tub or out of the room. In nursing facilities, beds are made after breakfast. People like to have their beds made and rooms cleaned before visitors arrive.

Linens are straightened if they become loose and wrinkled during the day. Check linens for crumbs after meals and properly remove them. Also straighten linens at bedtime. You must change linens whenever they become wet, soiled, or damp. Remember to wear gloves for contact with the person's blood, body fluids, secretions, or excretions.

Beds are made in the following ways:

- An *unoccupied bed* is a closed or open bed.
- A *closed bed* is not being used. Top linens are not folded back, and the bed is ready for a new person (Fig. 12-1).
- An *open bed* is being used. Top linens are folded back so the person can get into bed. A closed bed becomes an open bed when the top linens are folded back (Fig. 12-2 on page 266).
- An *occupied bed* is made with the person in it (Fig. 12-3 on page 266).
- A *surgical bed* is made so the person can be moved from a stretcher to the bed. It may be called a post-operative bed, recovery bed, or anesthetic bed (Fig. 12-4 on page 266).

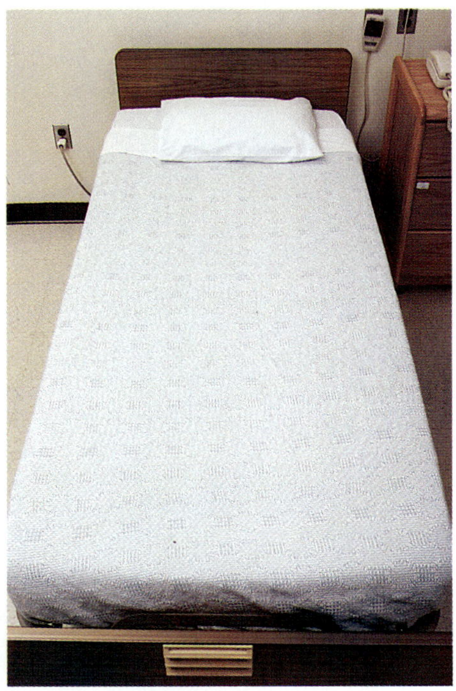

Fig. 12-1 *Closed bed.*

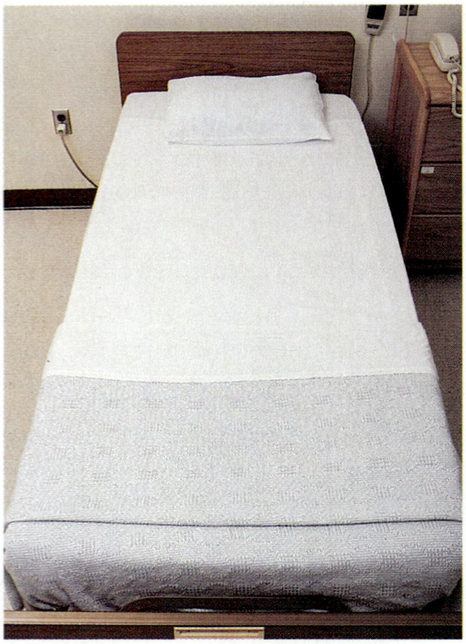

Fig. 12-2 *Open bed. Top linens are folded to the foot of the bed.*

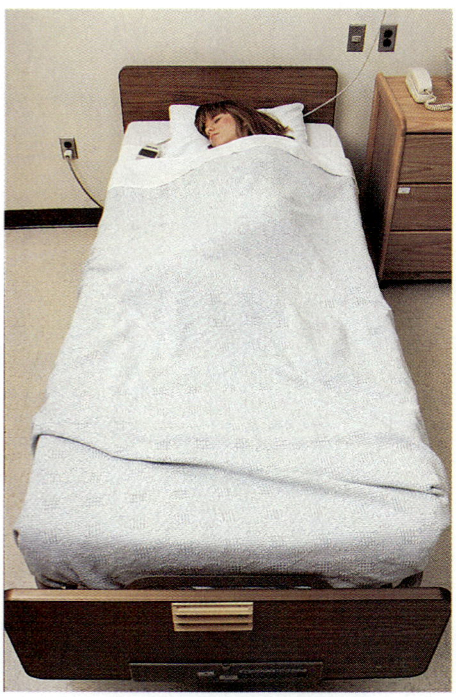

Fig. 12-3 *Occupied bed.*

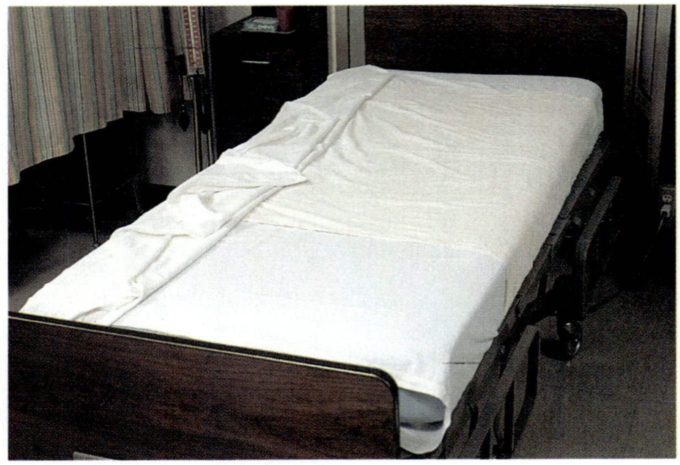

Fig. 12-4 *Surgical bed.*

LINENS

Special attention is given to the care and use of linens. The rules of medical asepsis are followed when handling linens and making beds. Your uniform is considered dirty. Therefore always hold linens away from your body and uniform (Fig. 12-5). Never shake linens in the air. Shaking them causes the spread of microbes. Clean linens are placed on a clean surface. Never put dirty linens on the floor.

Clean linens are collected in the order of use. Linens for personal care are also collected. Be sure to collect enough linens. If the person has 2 pillows, get 2 pillowcases. Extra blankets may be needed for the person's warmth. Do not bring unneeded linens to a person's room. Extra linen in a person's room is considered contaminated and cannot be used for another person.

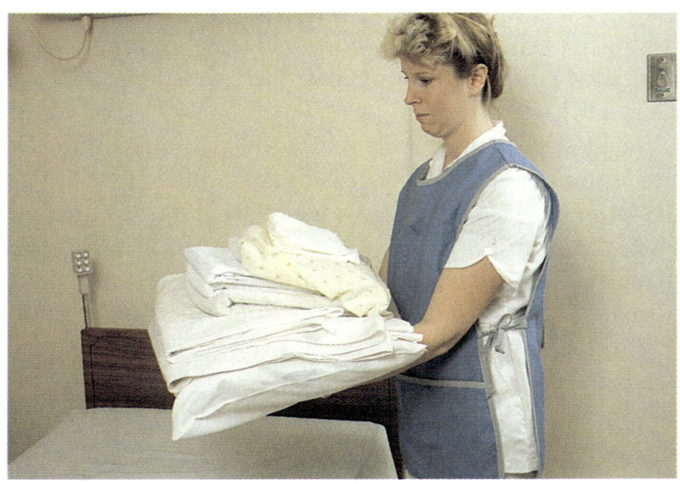

Fig. 12-5 *Linens are held away from the body and uniform.*

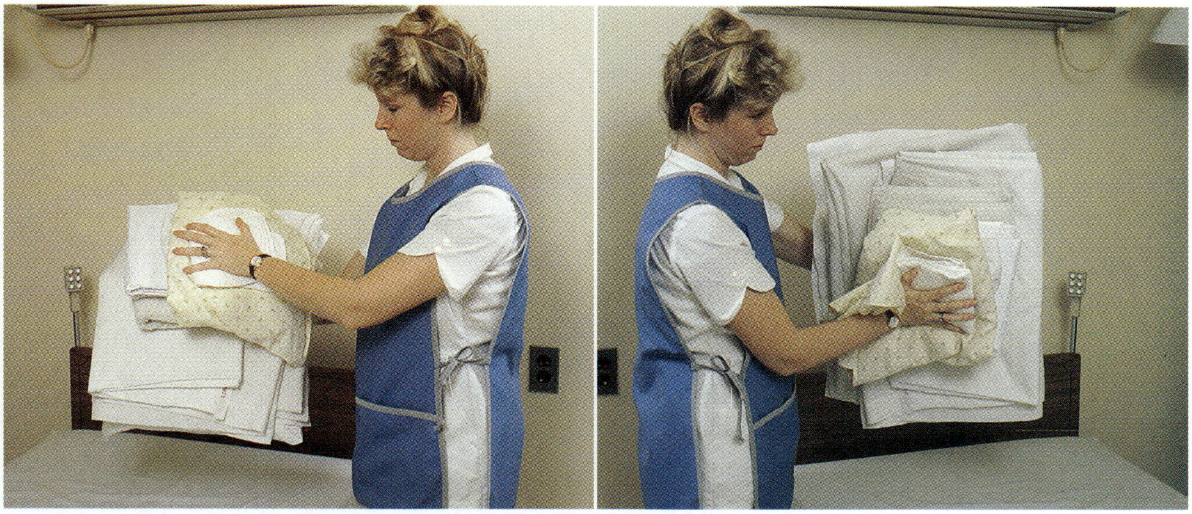

Fig. 12-6 *A, The arm is placed over the top of the stack of linens. B, The stack of linens is turned over onto the free arm.*

You should collect linens in the following order:

- Mattress pad
- Bottom sheet (flat sheet or contour sheet)
- Plastic drawsheet (optional)
- Cotton drawsheet
- Top sheet (flat sheet)
- Blanket
- Bedspread
- Pillowcase(s)
- Bath towel(s)
- Hand towel
- Washcloth
- Gown or pajamas
- Bath blanket

Use one arm to hold the linens and the other hand to pick them up. The item to be used first is at the bottom of your stack. (You picked up the mattress pad first, therefore it is at the bottom. The bath blanket is on top.) You need the mattress pad first. To get it on top, simply place your free arm over the bath blanket. Then turn the stack over to the free arm (Fig. 12-6). The arm that had been holding the linens will then be free. Place clean linens on a clean surface.

Linens are pressed and folded to prevent the spread of microbes and to make bedmaking easy. They are pressed with a center crease, which is placed in the center of the bed from the head to the foot. The linens unfold easily.

To remove dirty linens from the bed, roll the linens away from you. The side that touched the person is inside the roll. The side that has not touched the person is outside (Fig. 12-7).

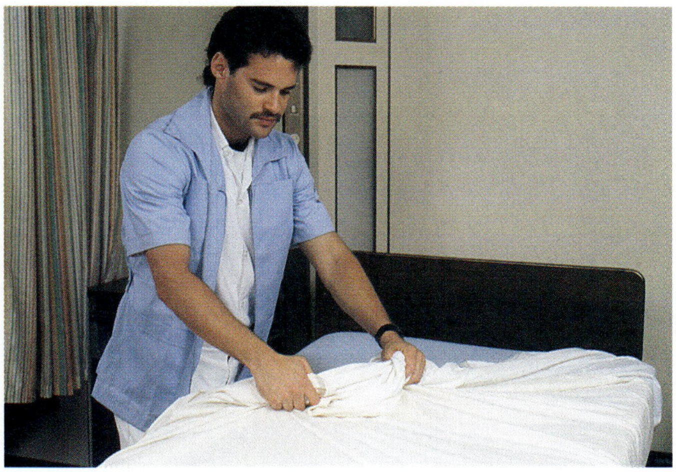

Fig. 12-7 *Roll linens away from you when removing them from the bed.*

Not all linens are changed every time the bed is made. Some are reused for an open bed. The mattress pad, plastic drawsheet, blanket, and bedspread are reused for the same person. They are reused if not soiled, wet, or very wrinkled. Some facilities use only flat sheets. The flat top sheet can be reused as the bottom sheet. If a person has been discharged, all linens are removed and a closed bed is made. Check the facility's policy about linen changes. *Remember, linens that are wet, damp, or soiled must be changed right away.*

A bed may have a plastic drawsheet and a cotton drawsheet. A **drawsheet** is a small sheet placed over the middle of the bottom sheet. It helps keep the mattress and bottom linens clean and dry. A **plastic drawsheet** protects the mattress and bottom linens from becoming damp or soiled. It is placed between the bottom sheet and cotton drawsheet. The cotton drawsheet protects the person from contact with the plastic and absorbs moisture.

Although the bottom linen and mattress are protected, discomfort and skin breakdown may occur. This is because heat is retained and it is hard to keep drawsheets tight and wrinkle free.

Clinical mattresses are covered with plastic or plastic mattress covers are used. Disposable waterproof pads are often used instead of plastic drawsheets. Plastic and cotton drawsheets are used only for certain persons. They include those with bowel or bladder control problems or those with excessive wound drainage.

A cotton drawsheet may be used without a plastic drawsheet. Plastic covered-mattresses cause some persons to perspire heavily and can increase discomfort. A cotton drawsheet helps to reduce heat retention and absorbs moisture. Cotton drawsheets are often used as lift sheets to move and position persons in bed (see Chapter 10). When used for this purpose, they are not tucked in at the sides.

The bedmaking procedures in this chapter include plastic and cotton drawsheets so you learn how to properly use them. Consult the nurse about their use. Also, know your employer's policies about using plastic and cotton drawsheets.

GENERAL RULES

Your job description will include making beds. No matter what type of bed you make, safety and medical asepsis are important. Box 12-1 lists the rules for bedmaking.

THE CLOSED BED

A closed bed is made after a person has been discharged so it is ready for a new person. The bed is made after the bed frame and mattress have been cleaned and disinfected according to facility policy.

BOX 12-1 Rules for Bedmaking

- Use good body mechanics at all times.
- Follow the rules of medical asepsis.
- Practice Standard Precautions.
- Follow the Bloodborne Pathogen Standard.
- Always wash your hands before handling clean linen and after handling dirty linen.
- Bring enough linen to the person's room.
- Never shake linens. Shaking linens causes the spread of microorganisms.
- Extra linen in a person's room is considered contaminated. Do not use it for other patients or residents. Put it with the dirty laundry so it is not used for other persons.
- Hold linens away from your uniform. Dirty and clean linen should never touch your uniform.
- Never put dirty linens on the floor or on clean linens. Follow facility policy about dirty linen.
- Linens the person lies on (bottom linens) must be tightly tucked in without wrinkles.
- A cotton drawsheet must completely cover the plastic drawsheet. A plastic drawsheet must never touch the person's body.
- Straighten and tighten loose sheets, blankets, and bedspreads whenever necessary.
- Make as much of one side of the bed as possible before going to the other side. This saves time and energy.

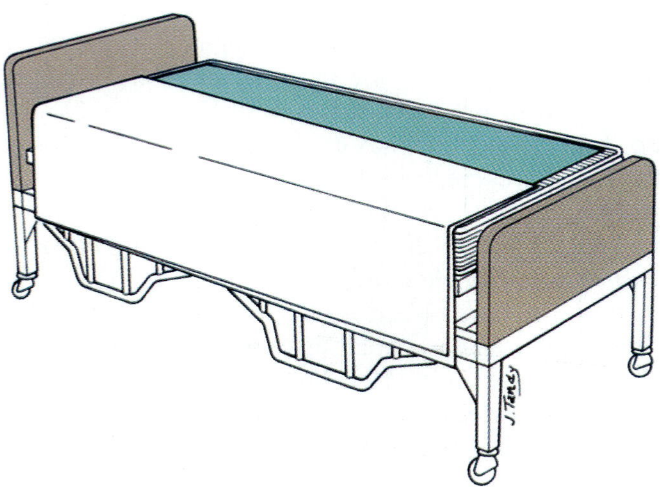

Fig. 12-8 *The bottom sheet is on the bed with the center crease in the middle. The lower edge of the sheet is even with the bottom of the mattress.*

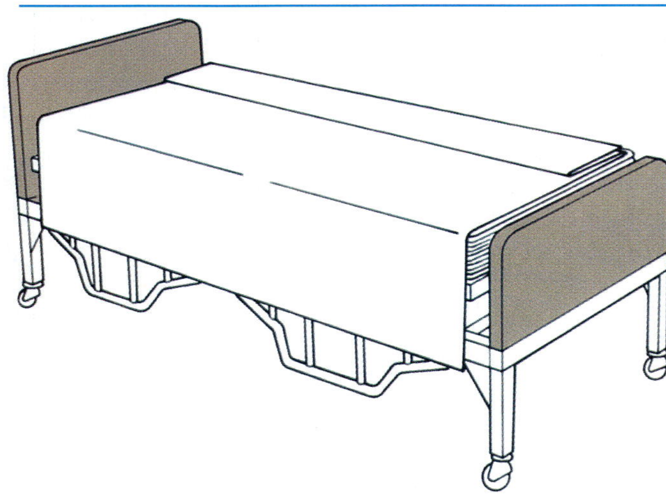

Fig. 12-9 *The bottom sheet is fanfolded to the other side of the bed.*

Text continued on page 274.

Making a Closed Bed

Pre-procedure

1 Wash your hands
2 Collect clean linen:
- Mattress pad
- Bottom sheet
- Plastic drawsheet
- Cotton drawsheet
- Top sheet
- Blanket
- Bedspread
- Two pillowcases
- Bath towel(s)
- Hand towel
- Washcloth
- Hospital gown or pajamas
- Bath blanket

3 Place linen on a clean surface.
4 Raise the bed for good body mechanics.

Procedure

5 Move the mattress to the head of the bed.
6 Put the mattress pad on the mattress. It is even with the top of the mattress.
7 Place the bottom sheet on the mattress pad (Fig. 12-8).
  - **a** Unfold it lengthwise.
  - **b** Place the center crease in the middle of the bed.
  - **c** Position the lower edge even with the bottom of the mattress.
  - **d** Place the large hem at the top and the small hem at the bottom.
  - **e** Face hem stitching downward.

8 Pick the sheet up from the side to open it. Fanfold it toward the other side of the bed (Fig. 12-9).
9 Go to the head of the bed. Tuck the top of the sheet under the mattress. You will lift the mattress slightly. Make sure the sheet is tight and smooth.
10 Make a mitered corner (Fig. 12-10 on page 271).
11 Place the plastic drawsheet on the bed about 14 inches from the top of the mattress.
12 Open the plastic drawsheet and fanfold it toward the other side of the bed.
13 Place a cotton drawsheet over the plastic drawsheet. It must cover the entire plastic drawsheet (Fig. 12-11 on page 271). Hem stitching must face down.
14 Open the cotton drawsheet and fanfold it toward the other side of the bed.
15 Tuck both drawsheets under the mattress. Or tuck each in separately.
16 Go to the other side of the bed.
17 Miter the top corner of the bottom sheet.
18 Pull the bottom sheet tight so there are no wrinkles. Tuck in the sheet.
19 Pull the drawsheets tight so there are no wrinkles. Tuck both in together or pull each tight and tuck them in separately (Fig. 12-12 on page 272).
20 Go to the other side of the bed.
21 Put the top sheet on the bed.
  - **a** Unfold it lengthwise.
  - **b** Place the center crease in the middle.
  - **c** Place the large hem at the top, even with the top of the mattress.
  - **d** Open the sheet and fanfold the extra part toward the other side.
  - **e** Face hem stitching outward.
  - **f** Do not tuck the bottom in yet.
  - **g** Never tuck top linens in on the sides.

Continued.

Making a Closed Bed

Procedure—cont'd

22 Place the blanket on the bed.
  - **a** Unfold it so the center crease is in the middle.
  - **b** Put the upper hem about 6 to 8 inches from the top of the mattress.
  - **c** Open the blanket and fanfold the extra part toward the other side.
  - **d** If steps 28 and 29 are not done, turn the top sheet down over the blanket. Hem stitching is down.

23 Place the bedspread on the bed.
  - **a** Unfold it so the center crease is in the middle.
  - **b** Place the upper hem even with the top of the mattress.
  - **c** Open the bedspread and fanfold the extra part toward the other side.
  - **d** Make sure the bedspread facing the door is even and covers all the top linens.

24 Tuck in top linens together at the foot of the bed. They should be smooth and tight. Make a mitered corner.

25 Go to the other side.

26 Straighten all top linen, working from the head of the bed to the foot.

27 Tuck in the top linens together. Make a mitered corner.

28 Turn the top hem of the bedspread under the blanket to make a cuff (Fig. 12-13 on page 272).

29 Turn the top sheet down over the spread. Hem stitching is down. (Steps 28 and 29 are not done in some facilities.)

30 Place the pillow on the bed.

31 Open the pillowcase so it is flat on the bed.

32 Put the pillowcase on the pillow as in Figure 12-14 on page 273. Fold extra pillowcase material under the pillow at the seam end of the pillowcase.

33 Place the pillow on the bed so the open end is away from the door. The seam of the pillowcase is toward the head of the bed.

Post-procedure

34 Attach the call bell to the bed.

35 Lower the bed to its lowest position.

36 Put towels, washcloth, gown or pajamas, and bath blanket in the bedside stand.

37 Wash your hands.

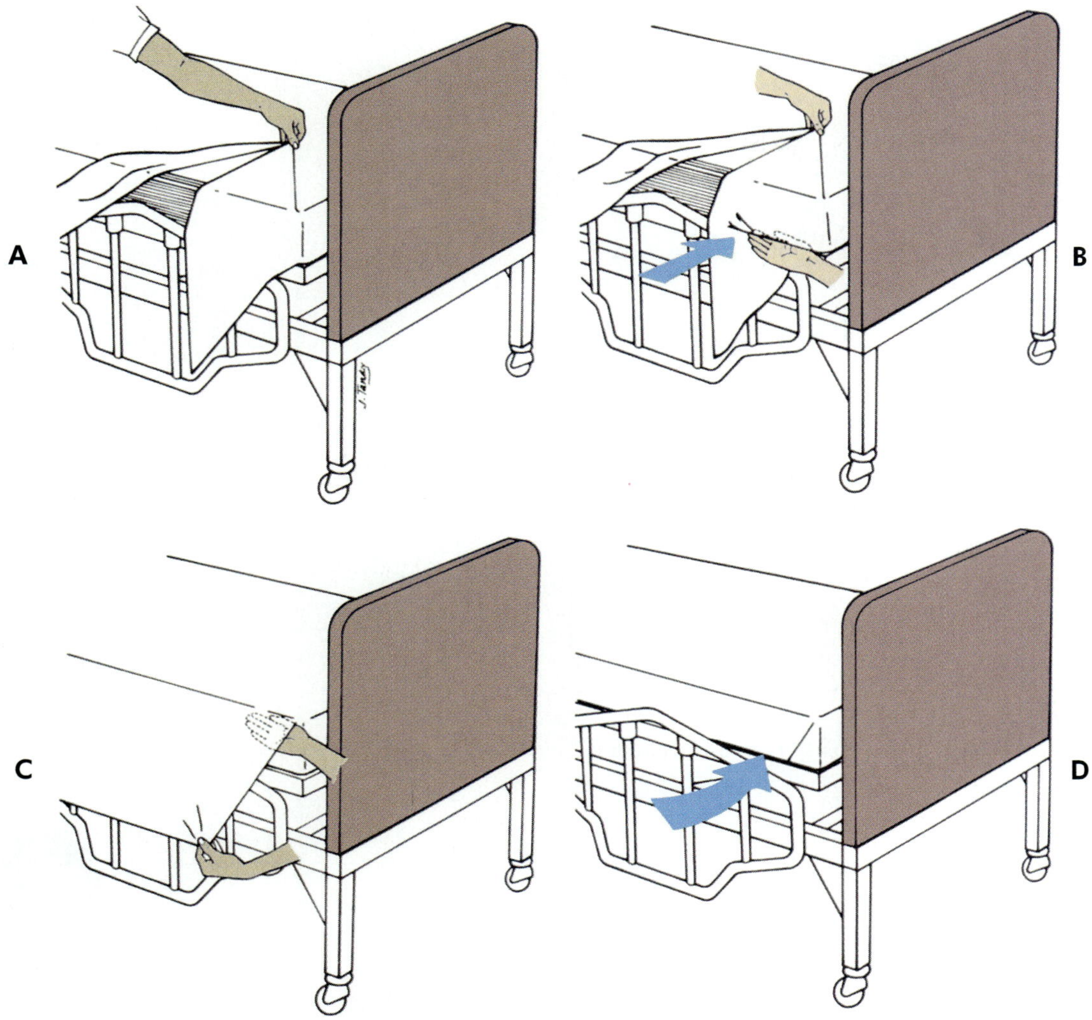

Fig. 12-10 *Making a mitered corner. A, Bottom sheet is tucked under the mattress and the side of the sheet is raised onto the mattress. B, The remaining portion of the sheet is tucked under the mattress. C, The raised portion of the sheet is brought off the mattress. D, The entire side of the sheet is tucked under the mattress.*

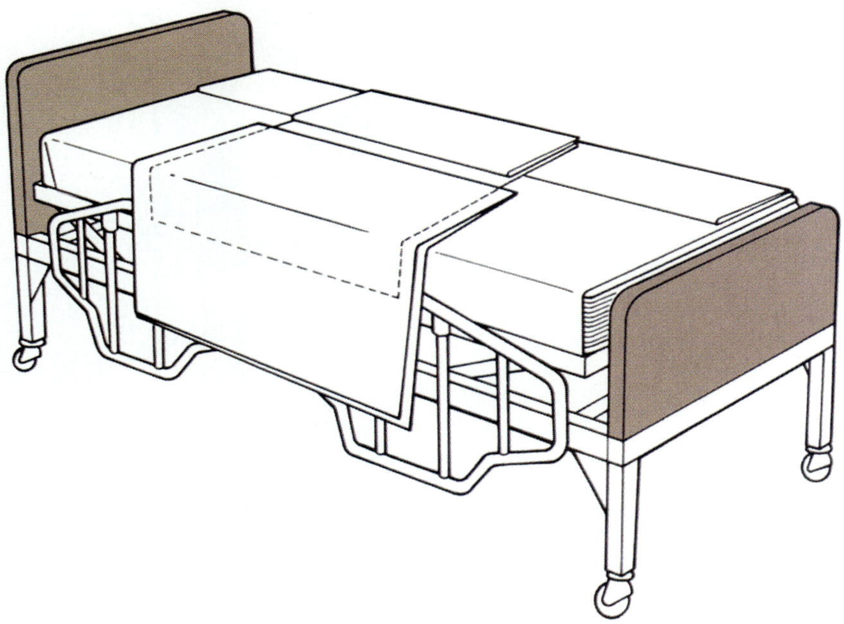

Fig. 12-11 *A cotton drawsheet over the plastic drawsheet. The cotton drawsheet completely covers the plastic drawsheet.*

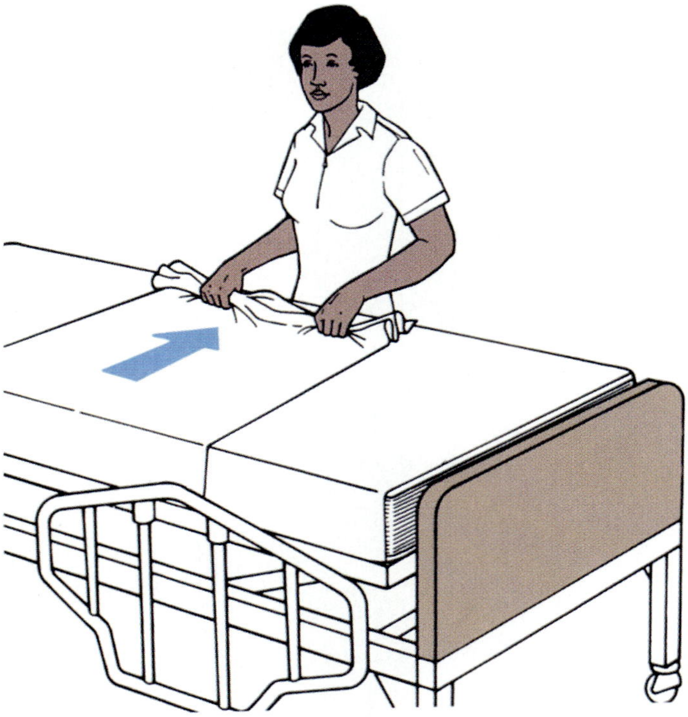

Fig. 12-12 *The drawsheet is pulled tight to remove wrinkles.*

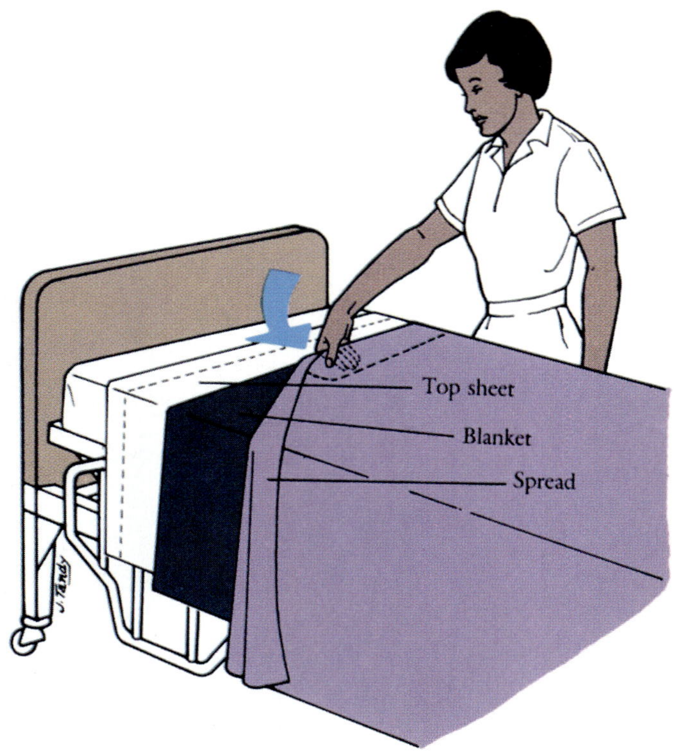

Fig. 12-13 *The top hem of the bedspread is turned under the top hem of the blanket to make a cuff.*

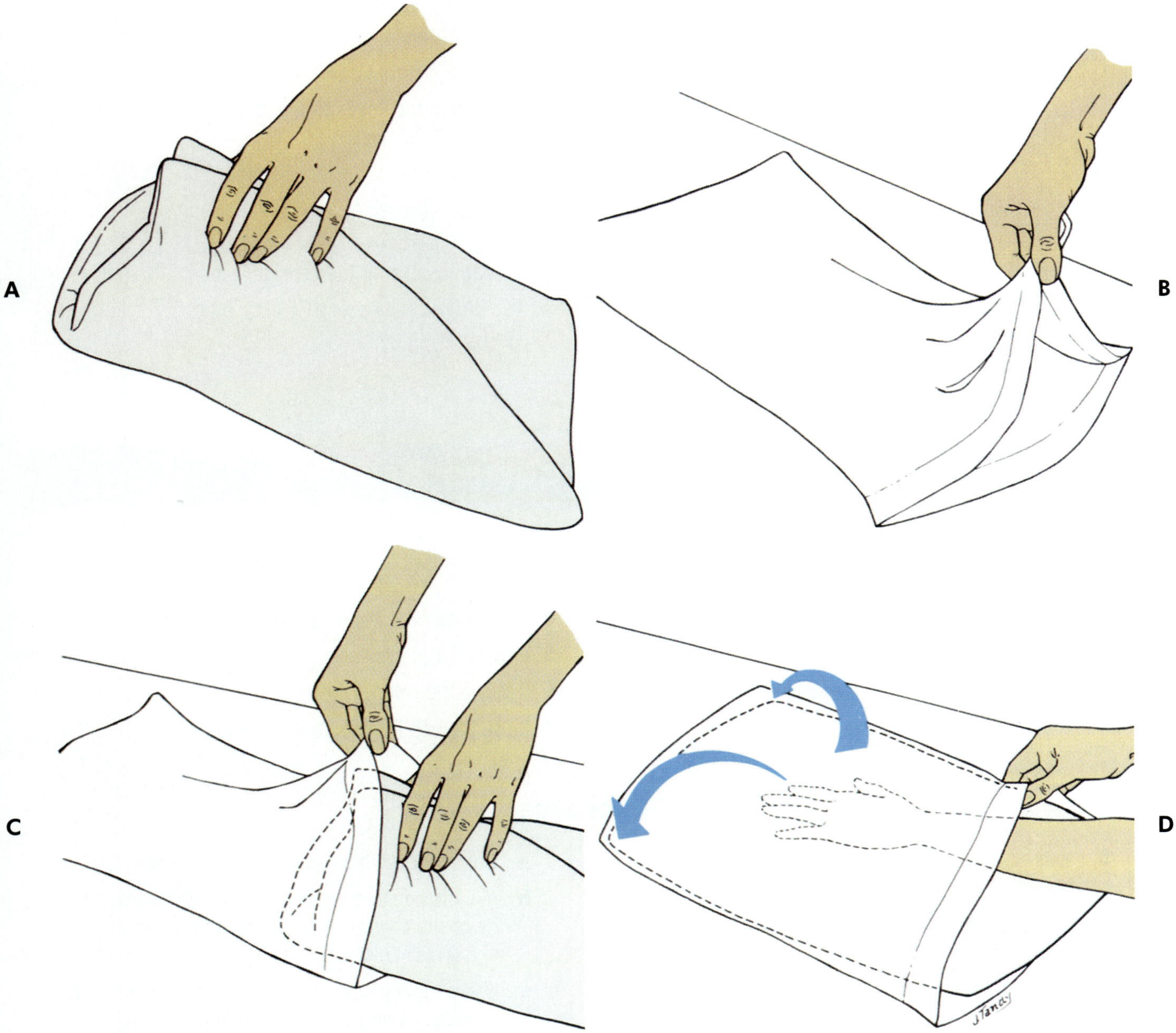

Fig. 12-14 *Putting a pillowcase on a pillow.* ***A,*** *Grasp the corners of the pillow at the seam end and form a "V" with the pillow.* ***B,*** *The pillowcase is flat on the bed; the pillowcase is opened with the free hand.* ***C,*** *The "V" end of the pillow is guided into the pillowcase.* ***D,*** *The "V" end of the pillow falls into the corners of the pillowcase.*

THE OPEN BED

The open bed is an unoccupied bed. Linens are folded back so the person can get into bed with ease. Open beds are made when persons are admitted to the facility. They are also made for persons who can be out of bed when their beds are being made. A closed bed becomes an open bed when top linens are folded back.

THE OCCUPIED BED

An occupied bed is made when a person cannot get out of bed. When making an occupied bed, you must keep the person in good body alignment. You must also be aware of restrictions or limits in the person's movement or positioning. Be sure to explain each step of the procedure to the person before it is done.

MAKING AN OPEN BED

PROCEDURE

1 Wash your hands.
2 Collect linen for a closed bed.
3 Make a closed bed.
4 Fanfold top linens to the foot of the bed (see Fig. 12-2).
5 Attach the call bell to the bed.
6 Lower the bed to its lowest position.
7 Put towels, washcloth, gown or pajamas, and bath blanket in the bedside stand.
8 Follow facility policy for dirty linen.
9 Wash your hands.

MAKING AN OCCUPIED BED

PRE-PROCEDURE

1 Explain the procedure to the person.
2 Wash your hands.
3 Collect gloves and clean linen (see *Making a Closed Bed,* page 269).
4 Place linen on a clean surface.
5 Provide for privacy.
6 Remove the call bell.
7 Raise the bed for good body mechanics.

PROCEDURE

8 Lower the head of the bed to a level appropriate for the person. It should be as flat as possible.
9 Lower the side rail near you. Make sure the far one is up and secure.
10 Put on gloves if linens are soiled with blood, body fluids, secretions, or excretions. Practice Standard Precautions and follow the Bloodborne Pathogen Standard. Remove gloves when soiled linens have been removed and before touching clean linens.
11 Loosen top linens at the foot of the bed.
12 Remove the bedspread and blanket separately. Fold them as in Figure 12-15 on page 276 if they are to be reused.
13 Cover the person with a bath blanket for warmth and privacy:
  a Unfold a bath blanket over the top sheet.
  b Ask the person to hold onto the bath blanket. If he or she cannot, tuck the top part under the person's shoulders.
  c Grasp the top sheet under the bath blanket at the shoulders. Bring the sheet down to the foot of the bed. Remove the sheet from under the blanket (Fig. 12-16 on page 276).
14 Move the mattress to the head of the bed.
15 Position the person on the side of the bed away from you. Adjust the pillow for the person's comfort. It should be on the far side of the bed.
16 Loosen bottom linens from the head to the foot of the bed.

Text continued on page 278.

PROCEDURE—CONT'D

17 Fanfold bottom linens one at a time toward the person: cotton drawsheet, plastic drawsheet, bottom sheet, and mattress pad (Fig. 12-17 on page 277). Do not fanfold the mattress pad if it will be reused.

18 Place a clean mattress pad on the bed. Unfold it lengthwise so the center crease is in the middle. Fanfold the top part toward the person. If reusing the mattress pad, straighten and smooth any wrinkles.

19 Place the bottom sheet on the mattress pad so hem stitching is away from the person. Unfold the sheet so the crease is in the middle. The small hem should be even with the bottom of the mattress. Fanfold the top part toward the person.

20 Make a mitered corner at the head of the bed. Tuck the sheet under the mattress from the head to the foot.

21 Pull the fanfolded plastic drawsheet toward you over the bottom sheet. Tuck excess material under the mattress. Do the following if you are using a clean plastic drawsheet (Fig. 12-18 on page 278):

- **a** Place the plastic drawsheet on the bed about 14 inches from the mattress top.
- **b** Fanfold the top part toward the person.
- **c** Tuck in the excess material.

22 Place the cotton drawsheet over the plastic drawsheet. It must cover the entire plastic drawsheet. Fanfold the top part toward the person. Tuck in excess material.

23 Raise the side rail. Go to the other side and lower the side rail.

24 Position the person on the side of the bed away from you. Adjust the pillow for the person's comfort.

25 Loosen bottom linens. Remove the soiled linen one piece at a time. Follow facility policy for soiled linen. Remove and discard the gloves.

26 Straighten and smooth the mattress pad.

27 Pull the clean bottom sheet toward you. Make a mitered corner at the top. Tuck the sheet under the mattress from the head to the foot of the bed.

28 Pull the drawsheets tightly toward you. Tuck both under together or tuck each in separately.

29 Position the person supine in the center of the bed. Adjust the pillow for comfort.

30 Put the top sheet on the bed. Unfold it lengthwise. Make sure the crease is in the middle, the large hem is even with the top of the mattress, and hem stitching is on the outside.

31 Ask the person to hold onto the top sheet so you can remove the bath blanket. You may have to tuck the top sheet under the person's shoulders. Remove the bath blanket.

32 Place the blanket on the bed. Unfold it so the crease is in the middle. Unfold the blanket so it covers the person. The upper hem should be 6 to 8 inches from the top of the mattress.

33 Place the bedspread on the bed. Unfold it so the center crease is in the middle and it covers the person. The top hem is even with the mattress top.

34 Turn the top hem of the bedspread under the blanket to make a cuff.

35 Bring the top sheet down over the bedspread to form a cuff.

36 Go to the foot of the bed.

37 Lift the mattress corner with one arm. Tuck all top linens under the mattress together. Be sure the linens are loose enough to allow movement of the person's feet. Make a mitered corner.

38 Raise the side rail. Go to the other side and lower the side rail.

39 Straighten and smooth top linens.

40 Tuck the top linens under the mattress as in step 37. Make a mitered corner.

41 Change the pillowcase(s).

42 Place the call bell within reach.

43 Raise or lower side rails as instructed by the nurse.

POST-PROCEDURE

44 Raise the head of the bed to a level appropriate for the person. Make sure the person is comfortable.

45 Lower the bed to its lowest position.

46 Put towels, washcloth, gown, and bath blanket in the bedside stand.

47 Unscreen the person. Thank him or her for cooperating.

48 Follow facility policy for dirty linen.

49 Wash your hands.

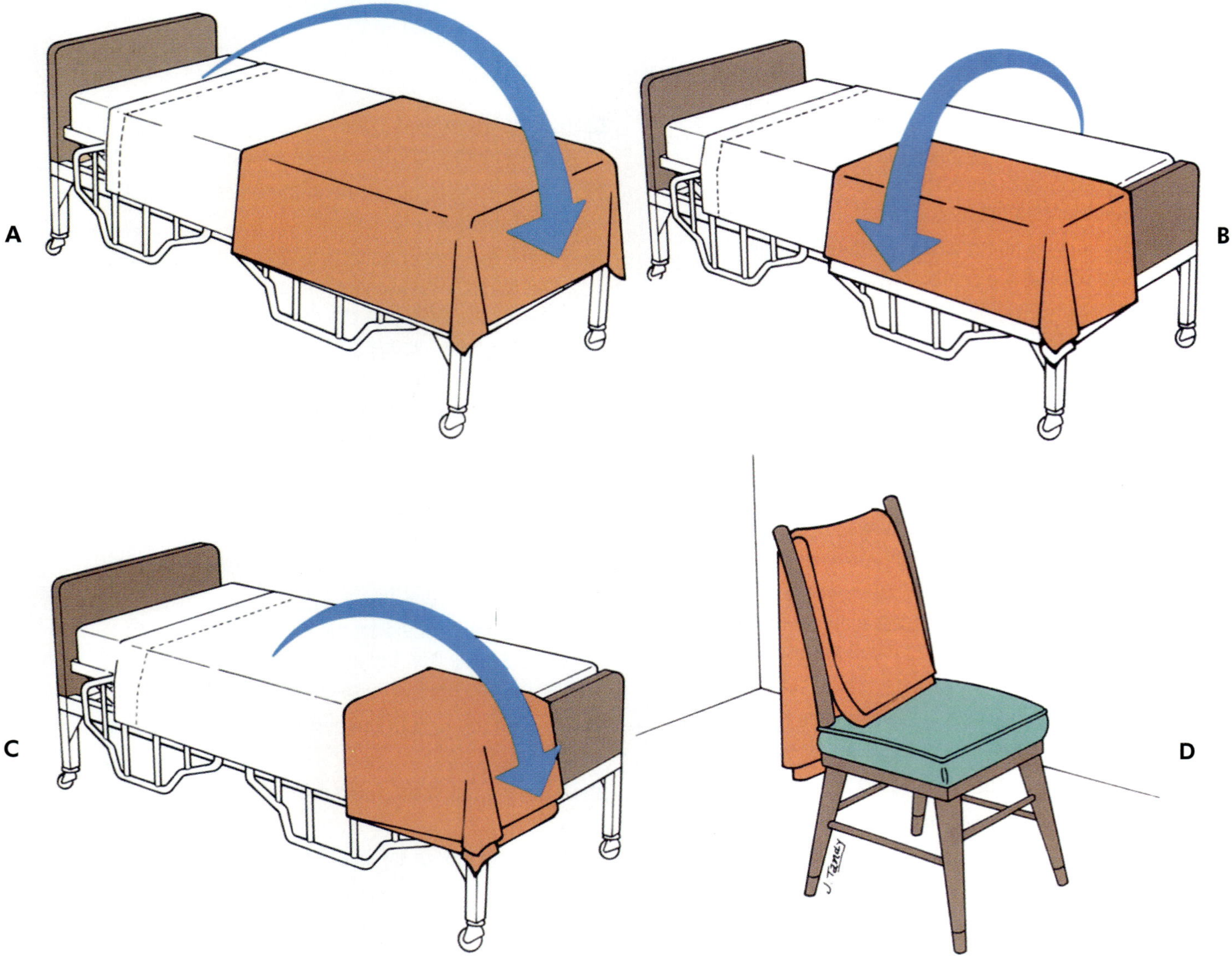

Fig. 12-15 *Folding linen for reuse.* ***A,*** *The top edge of the blanket is folded down to the bottom edge.* ***B,*** *The blanket is folded from the far side of the bed to the near side.* ***C,*** *The top edge of the blanket is folded down to the bottom edge again.* ***D,*** *The folded blanket is placed over the back of a straight chair.*

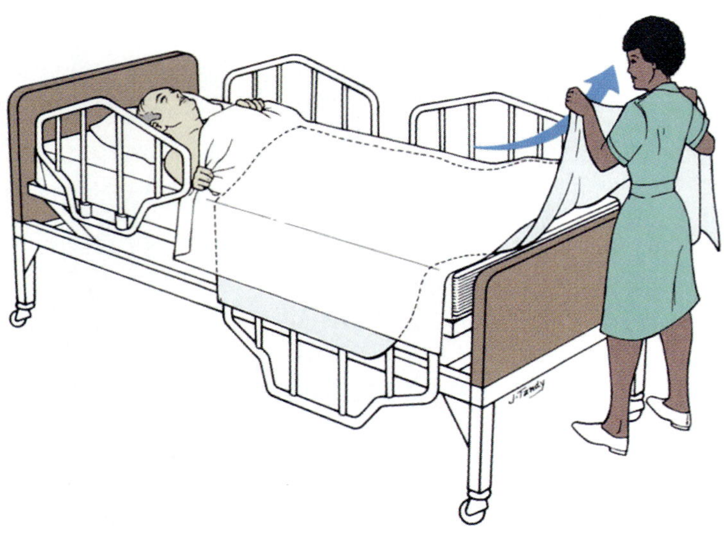

Fig. 12-16 *The person is holding onto the bath blanket. The nursing assistant at the foot of the bed is removing the top sheet from under the bath blanket.*

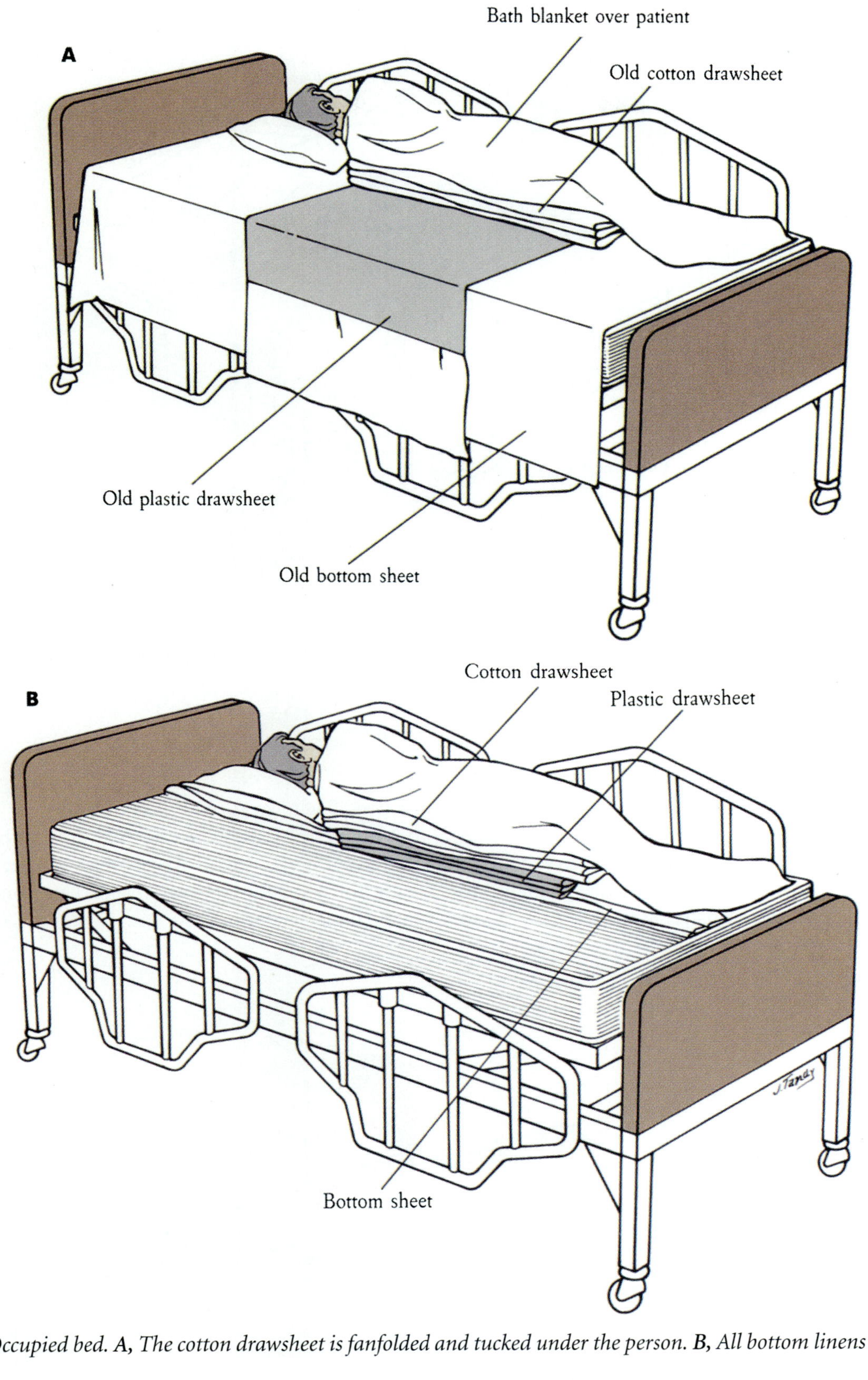

Fig. 12-17 *Occupied bed. A, The cotton drawsheet is fanfolded and tucked under the person. B, All bottom linens are tucked under the person.*

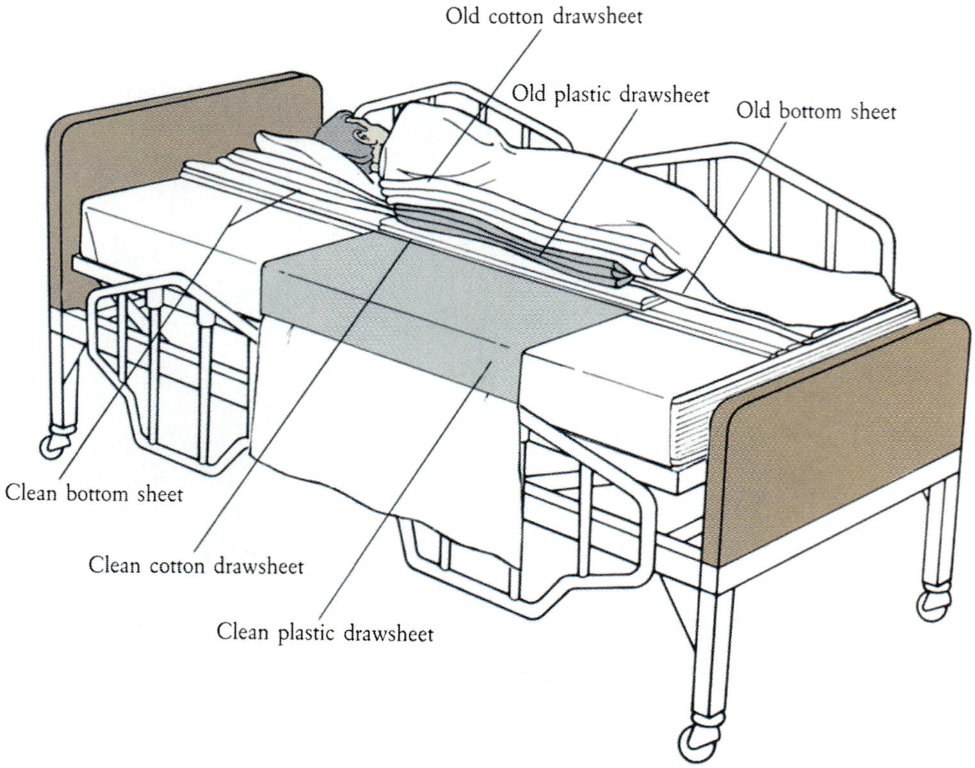

Fig. 12-18 *A clean bottom sheet and plastic drawsheet are on the bed with both fanfolded and tucked under the person. The clean cotton drawsheet is put in place in step 22.*

THE SURGICAL BED

The surgical bed (recovery bed, postoperative bed, or anesthetic bed) is a form of the open bed. Top linens are folded so the person can be transferred from a stretcher to the bed. The term *surgical bed* and its other names imply that the person has had surgery. However, this bed is also needed for persons who arrive on a stretcher. If the bed is made for a postoperative (surgical) person, a complete linen change is done.

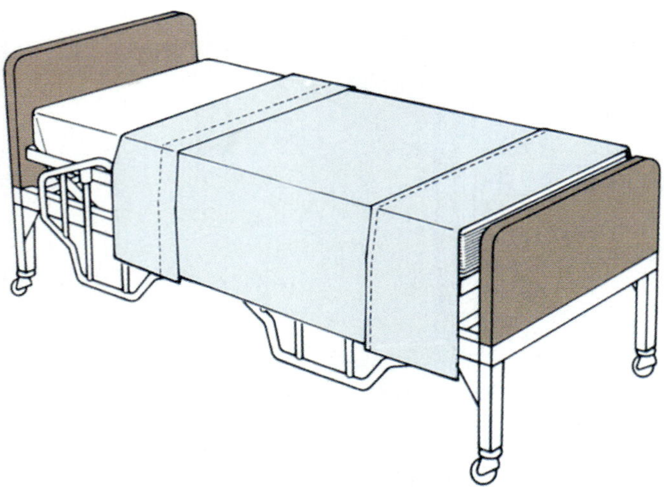

Fig. 12-19 *Surgical bed. The bottom of the top linens is folded back onto the bed. The fold is even with the edge of the mattress.*

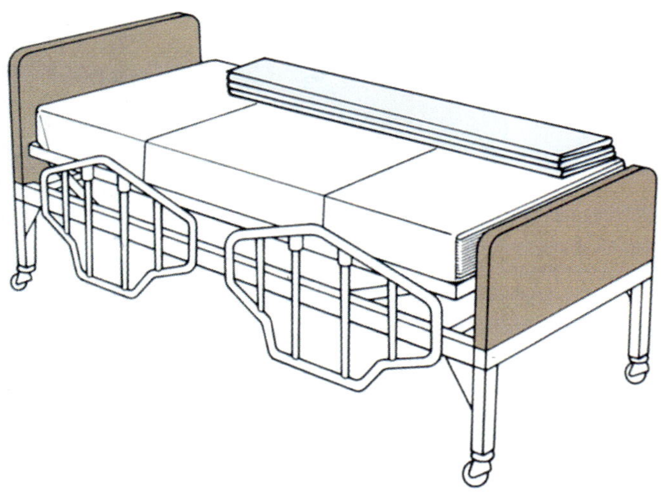

Fig. 12-20 *A surgical bed with top linens fanfolded lengthwise to the opposite side of the bed.*

MAKING A SURGICAL BED

PROCEDURE

1 Wash your hands.
2 Collect the following:
   a Clean linen (see *Making a Closed Bed,* page 269)
   b IV pole
   c Tissues
   d Kidney basin
   e Gloves
   f Other equipment as requested by the nurse
3 Place linen on a clean surface.
4 Remove the call bell.
5 Raise the bed for good body mechanics.
6 Remove all linen from the bed. Wear gloves for contact with the person's blood, body fluids, secretions, or excretions.
7 Make a closed bed (see *Making a Closed Bed,* page 269). Do not tuck the top linens under the mattress.
8 Fold all top linens at the foot of the bed back onto the bed. The fold is even with the edge of the mattress (Fig. 12-19).
9 Use one of these methods to fold top linen:
   a Fanfold linen lengthwise to the side of the bed farthest from the door (Fig. 12-20).
   b Fanfold linens from the head of the bed to the foot (Fig. 12-21).
10 Put the pillowcase(s) on the pillow(s).
11 Place the pillow(s) on a clean surface.
12 Leave the bed in its highest position.
13 Make sure both side rails are down.
14 Put the towels, washcloth, gown or pajamas, and bath blanket in the bedside stand.
15 Place the tissues and kidney basin on the bedside stand. Place the IV pole near the head of the bed.
16 Move all furniture away from the bed. Make sure there is room for the stretcher and for the staff to move about.
17 Do not attach the call bell to the bed.
18 Follow facility policy for soiled linen.
19 Wash your hands.

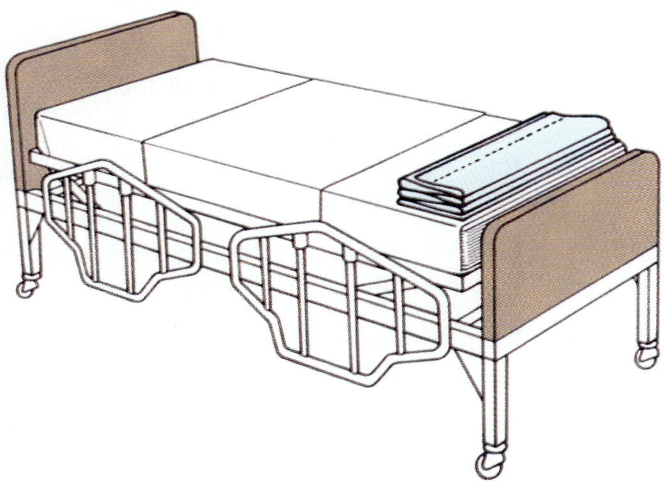

Fig. 12-21 *A surgical bed with top linens fanfolded from the head of the bed to the foot.*

QUALITY OF LIFE

The bed is the largest piece of equipment in the person's unit. The patient or resident, family, and visitors will question the quality of care and the person's quality of life if the bed is unmade or messy. The bed must be neat and well made so the person's environment is orderly and pleasant. If the person must stay in bed, you need to straighten and tighten loose linen whenever necessary.

Some residents bring their own bedspreads, pillows, blankets, or afghans from home. Be sure to use these when making the bed. Such items are the person's property. Therefore they are handled with care and respect. Make sure the items are marked with the person's name to prevent them from becoming lost or confused with property of other residents.

Allow personal choice whenever possible. The facility may use white, blue, yellow, pink, or other colored linens. If so, let the person choose which color to use. Also let the person decide how many pillows or blankets to use. If possible, the person also chooses when the bed is made. The more choices you allow, the greater the person's sense of usefulness and quality of life.

Summary

You have learned how to make hospital beds. You have also learned the principles of bedmaking and of handling linens. Facility policies and procedures or a person's condition may require changes in these procedures. However, the principles must be followed. The person's comfort and safety are the focus of bedmaking. Remember, the person spends a lot of time in bed. Therefore the bed must be neat, clean and free of wrinkles. A well-made bed promotes the person's comfort.

Be sure to handle linens properly so you do not spread microorganisms. Also follow the rules of medical asepsis, bedmaking, and good body mechanics. Standard Precautions and the Bloodborne Pathogen Standard must also be followed.

Review Questions

Circle T *if the statement is true and* F *if the statement is false.*

1 **T F** Linens are changed whenever soiled, wet, or damp.

2 **T F** An open bed is made after a person is discharged.

3 **T F** A surgical bed is only for persons who have had surgery.

4 **T F** A postoperative bed is made with the person in bed.

5 **T F** Linens are held away from your body and uniform.

6 **T F** Dirty linens can be put on the floor.

7 **T F** Extra linen in a person's room is used for another person.

8 **T F** Complete linen changes are required for closed beds and surgical beds.

9 **T F** A cotton drawsheet is always used when a plastic drawsheet is used.

10 **T F** To remove crumbs from the bed, loosen linens and shake them in the air.

11 **T F** The hem stitching of the bottom sheet is placed downward so it is away from the person.

12 **T F** The plastic drawsheet is placed 6 to 8 inches from the top of the mattress.

13 **T F** A cotton drawsheet must completely cover the plastic drawsheet.

14 **T F** The upper hem of the bedspread is even with the top of the mattress.

15 **T F** A closed bed becomes an open bed when top linens are fanfolded to the foot of the bed.

16 **T F** An occupied bed is made for an ambulatory person.

17 **T F** A person is screened when an occupied bed is made.

18 **T F** When making an occupied bed, the far side rail is up at all times.

19 **T F** After a surgical bed is made, it is left in its lowest position.

20 **T F** A cotton drawsheet is used only with a plastic drawsheet.

Answers to these questions are on page 750.

Cleanliness and Skin Care

13

OBJECTIVES

- Define the key terms listed in this chapter
- Explain the importance of cleanliness and skin care
- Describe the routine care given before and after breakfast, after lunch, and in the evening
- Explain the importance of oral hygiene and list the observations to report
- Describe the rules for bathing and the observations to make
- Identify the safety precautions for persons taking tub baths or showers
- Explain the purposes of a back massage
- Identify the purposes of perineal care
- Describe the signs, symptoms, and causes of pressure sores
- Locate the pressure points of the body in the prone, supine, lateral, Fowler's, and sitting positions
- Describe how to prevent pressure sores
- Perform the procedures described in this chapter

KEY TERMS

AM care Routine care performed before breakfast; early morning care

antiperspirant A skin care product that reduces the amount of perspiration

aspiration Breathing fluid or an object into the lungs

bedsore A decubitus ulcer; a pressure sore; a pressure ulcer

decubitus ulcer A bedsore, pressure sore, or pressure ulcer

deodorant A skin preparation that masks and controls body odors

evening care HS care or PM care

HS care Care given in the evening at bedtime; evening care or PM care

morning care Care given after breakfast; cleanliness and skin care measures are more thorough at this time

oral hygiene Measures performed to keep the mouth and teeth clean; mouth care

pericare Perineal care

perineal care Cleansing the genital and anal areas

plaque A thin film that sticks to the teeth; it contains saliva, microorganisms, and other substances

PM care HS care or evening care

pressure sore An area where the skin and underlying tissues are eroded because of a lack of blood flow; a decubitus ulcer; a bedsore; a pressure ulcer

pressure ulcer A bed sore; a decubitus ulcer; a pressure sore

tartar Hardened plaque on teeth

Cleanliness and skin care are needed for comfort, safety, and health. The skin is the body's first line of defense against disease. Intact skin prevents microbes from entering the body and causing an infection. Likewise, mucous membranes of the mouth, genital area, and anus must be kept clean and intact. Besides cleansing, hygiene practices prevent body and breath odors, promote relaxation, and increase circulation.

Culture and personal choice affect hygiene. Some people take showers. Others take tub baths. Some bathe at bedtime. Others bathe in the morning. Bathing frequency also varies. Some bathe daily or twice a day—such as before work and after work or exercise. Some people do not have water for bathing. Others cannot afford soap, deodorant, shampoo, toothpaste, or other hygiene products.

Patients and residents usually need some help with personal hygiene. Weakness from illness and the changes of aging affect the ability to practice hygiene. The need for cleanliness and skin care is affected by perspiration, vomiting, urinary and bowel elimination, drainage from wounds or body openings, bed rest, and activity. The nurse uses the nursing process to meet the person's hygiene needs. The nurse and the nursing care plan tell you how to meet the person's hygiene needs.

A review of the body structures and functions important for this chapter is contained in Box 13-1 on page 284. See Chapter 5 for more detailed information.

DAILY CARE OF THE PERSON

Personal hygiene is practiced to stay clean and comfortable. People usually have routines and habits for hygiene. For example, teeth are brushed and the face and hands washed after rising in the morning. These and other hygiene measures may be done routinely before and after meals and at bedtime.

Infants, young children, and some weak or disabled adults need help with hygiene. Routine care is given at certain times. However, you need to help with personal hygiene whenever necessary.

Before Breakfast

Routine care before breakfast is called **early morning care** or **AM care.** Night shift or day shift staff give AM care. They get patients and residents ready for breakfast or tests to be done early in the day. Personal hygiene measures performed at this time include:

- Offering bedpans or urinals or assisting persons to the bathroom
- Helping persons wash their faces and hands
- Assisting with oral hygiene

Text continued on page 285.

BOX 13-1 REVIEW OF BODY STRUCTURE AND FUNCTION

The Teeth and Gums

The teeth cut, chop, and grind food into small bits for digestion and swallowing. A tooth has three parts: the crown, neck, and root (Fig. 13-1). The crown is the outer part. It is covered by enamel. The neck is surrounded by the gums (gingivae). The root fits into the bone of the lower or upper jaw.

Cavities (dental caries) and periodontal disease *(pyorrhea)* are common problems. Poor oral hygiene allows the build of plaque and tartar. **Plaque** is a thin film that sticks to the teeth. It contains saliva, bacteria, and other substances. Plaque leads to tooth decay or cavities. When plaque hardens it is called **tartar.** Tartar builds up at the gum line near the neck of the tooth. Tartar buildup leads to periodontal disease. The gums are red, swollen, and bleed easily. As the disease progresses, bone is destroyed and teeth loosen. Loss of teeth is common.

The Skin

The skin is the largest system of the body. The skin is the body's natural covering. There are two skin layers: the epidermis and the dermis (Fig. 13-2). The *epidermis* is the outer layer; it contains living and dead cells. Dead cells constantly flake off and are replaced by living cells. Living cells also die and flake off. The epidermis has no blood vessels and few nerve endings. The *dermis* is the inner layer of the skin and is made up of connective tissue. Blood vessels, nerves, sweat and oil glands, and hair roots are found in the dermis.

Sweat glands help regulate body temperature. Sweat is secreted through the skin's pores. The body is cooled as sweat evaporates. Oil glands secrete an oily substance into the space near the hair shaft. Oil travels to the skin surface, helping to keep the hair and skin soft and shiny.

The skin is the protective covering of the body. Intact skin prevents bacteria and other substances from entering the body. It also prevents excessive amounts of water from leaving the body and protects organs from injury. Nerve endings in the skin sense both pleasant and unpleasant stimulation. Cold, pain, touch, and pressure can be sensed. The skin also helps regulate body temperature. Blood vessels dilate (widen) when temperature outside the body is high. More blood is brought to the body surface for cooling during evaporation. When blood vessels constrict (narrow), the body retains heat because less blood reaches the skin.

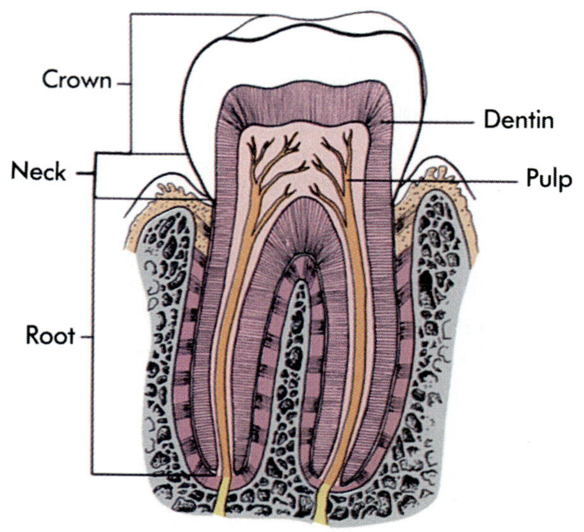

Fig. 13-1 *Parts of the tooth. (From Potter PA and Perry AG: Fundamentals of nursing, ed 3, St Louis, 1993, Mosby-Year Book.)*

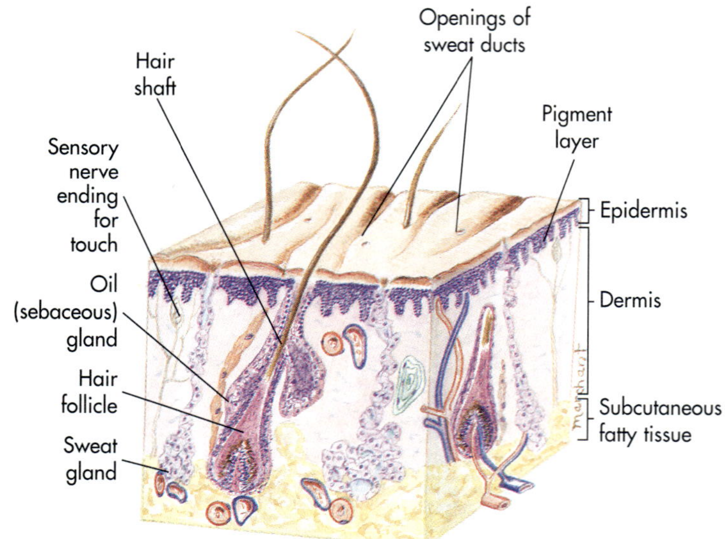

Fig. 13-2 *Structures of the skin.*

- Positioning persons in Fowler's position or in chairs for breakfast
- Straightening bed linens
- Straightening patient or resident units

After Breakfast

Morning care is given after breakfast. Cleanliness and skin care measures are more thorough at this time. Routine morning care usually involves:

- Offering bedpans or urinals or assisting persons to the bathroom
- Helping persons wash their faces and hands
- Assisting with oral hygiene
- Shaving patients and residents
- Providing showers, tub baths, or bed baths
- Giving perineal care
- Giving back massages
- Changing gowns or pajamas or assisting with dressing
- Brushing and combing hair
- Changing bed linens
- Straightening patient and resident units

Afternoon Care

Routine hygiene is performed after lunch and the evening meal. If done before visiting hours, patients and residents feel more refreshed. They can also visit with family and friends without interruption. Afternoon care involves:

- Offering bedpans or urinals or assisting persons to the bathroom
- Helping patients and residents wash their faces and hands
- Assisting with oral hygiene
- Changing gowns, pajamas, or clothing if needed
- Brushing or combing hair if needed
- Changing damp or soiled bed linens
- Straightening patient and resident units

Evening Care

Care given at bedtime is called HS **care, evening care,** or PM **care.** Hygiene measures are performed right before the person is ready for sleep. HS care promotes comfort and relaxation. It involves:

- Offering bedpans or urinals or assisting persons to the bathroom
- Helping patients and residents wash their faces and hands
- Assisting with oral hygiene
- Changing damp or soiled linens and straightening all other linens
- Changing gowns or pajamas if needed
- Helping persons in street clothes to undress and put on gowns or pajamas
- Giving back massages
- Straightening patient and resident units

ORAL HYGIENE

Oral hygiene (mouth care) keeps the mouth and teeth clean. This prevents mouth odors and infections, increases comfort, and makes food taste better. Cavities and periodontal disease (gum disease) are prevented. Illness and disease may cause a bad taste in the mouth. Some drugs and diseases cause coating of the mouth and tongue with a whitish material. Other drugs and diseases cause redness and swelling of the mouth and tongue. A dry mouth is common from some medications, supplemental oxygen, smoking, decreased fluid intake, and anxiety.

The nurse assesses the person's need for mouth care. Then the nurse decides the type of mouth care and amount of assistance needed. Oral hygiene is provided on awakening, after each meal, and at bedtime. Many people also practice oral hygiene before meals.

Equipment

A toothbrush, toothpaste, dental floss, and mouthwash are needed. The toothbrush should have soft bristles. Persons with dentures need a denture cleaner, denture cup, and denture brush or regular toothbrush. Toothettes or other applicators are used for persons with sore, tender mouths and for unconscious patients or residents. A *toothette* is a piece of spongy foam attached to a stick. Other needed items include a kidney basin, water glass, straw, tissues, and towels.

Needed items may be in the patient pack. Nursing unit supply carts have oral hygiene items. Most facility gift shops have them too. However, many people bring oral hygiene items from home.

Standard Precautions are necessary when giving oral hygiene. The Bloodborne Pathogen Standard is also followed. You have contact with the person's mucous membranes. Gums may bleed during oral care. Also, the mouth contains many microbes. Pathogens spread through sexual contact may be in the mouths of some persons.

Brushing Teeth

Many people perform oral hygiene themselves. Others need help gathering and setting up equipment. You may have to brush the teeth of persons who are very weak or who cannot use or move their arms. The following observations are reported to the nurse:

- Dry, cracked, swollen, or blistered lips
- Redness, swelling, irritation, sores, or white patches in the mouth or on the tongue
- Bleeding, swelling, or redness of the gums

Text continued on page 289.

Assisting the Person to Brush the Teeth

Pre-procedure

1. Explain the procedure to the person.
2. Wash your hands.
3. Collect the following:
   - Toothbrush
   - Toothpaste or dentifrice
   - Mouthwash
   - Dental floss
   - Water glass with cool water
   - Straw
   - Kidney basin
   - Face towel
   - Paper towels
4. Place the paper towels on the overbed table. Arrange items on top of them.
5. Identify the person. Check the ID bracelet and call the person by name.
6. Provide for privacy.
7. Raise the head so the person can brush with ease.

Procedure

8. Place the towel over the person's chest. This protects the gown and linens from spills.
9. Lower the side rail if up.
10. Place the overbed table in front of the person. Adjust table height for the person.
11. Allow the person to brush the teeth.
12. Remove the towel when the person is done.
13. Move the overbed table next to the bed. Lower it to a level appropriate for the person.

Post-procedure

14. Make sure the person is comfortable.
15. Place the call bell within reach.
16. Raise or lower side rails as instructed.
17. Clean and return items to their proper place.
18. Wipe off the overbed table with the paper towels and discard them.
19. Unscreen the person.
20. Follow facility policy for dirty linen.
21. Wash your hands.
22. Report your observations to the nurse.

Brushing the Person's Teeth

Pre-procedure

1 Explain the procedure to the person.

2 Wash your hands.

3 Collect gloves and items listed in *Assisting the Person to Brush the Teeth.*

4 Place the paper towels on the overbed table. Arrange items on top of them.

5 Identify the person. Check the ID bracelet and call the person by name.

6 Provide for privacy.

7 Raise the bed to the best level for good body mechanics.

Procedure

8 Raise the head of the bed so the person can sit comfortably. Position the person in a side-lying position on the side near you if he or she cannot sit up.

9 Lower the side rail.

10 Place the towel over the person's chest. This protects the gown and linens from spills.

11 Position the overbed table so you can reach it with ease. Adjust the height as needed.

12 Put on the gloves.

13 Apply toothpaste to the toothbrush.

14 Hold the toothbrush over the kidney basin. Pour some water over the brush.

15 Brush the person's teeth gently as shown in Figure 13-3 on page 288.

16 Let the person rinse the mouth with water. Hold the kidney basin under the person's chin (Fig. 13-4 on page 288). Repeat this step as necessary.

17 Floss the person's teeth (see *Flossing the Person's Teeth*, page 289).

18 Let the person use mouthwash. Hold the kidney basin under the chin.

Post-procedure

19 Remove the towel when done.

20 Remove and discard the gloves.

21 Make sure the person is comfortable.

22 Place the call bell within reach.

23 Lower the bed to its lowest position.

24 Raise or lower side rails as instructed by the nurse.

25 Clean and return equipment to its proper place.

26 Wipe off the overbed table with the paper towels and discard them.

27 Lower the overbed table to a level appropriate for the person.

28 Unscreen the person.

29 Follow facility policy for dirty linen.

30 Wash your hands.

31 Report your observations to the nurse.

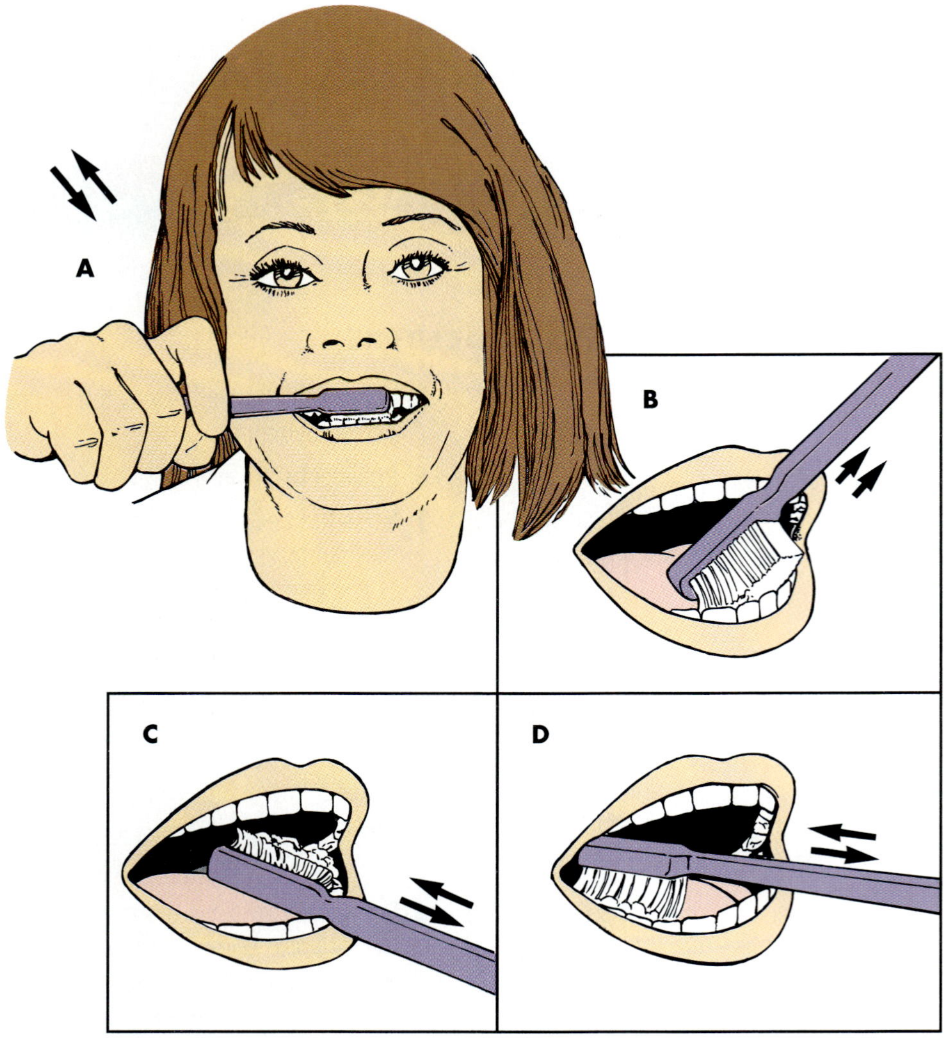

Fig. 13-3 *A, Position the brush at a 45-degree angle to the gums. Brush with short strokes. B, Position the brush at 45-degree angle against the inside of the front teeth. Brush from the gum to the crown of the tooth with short strokes. C, Hold the brush horizontally against the inner surfaces of the teeth. Brush back and forth. D, Position the brush on the biting surfaces of the teeth. Brush back and forth.*

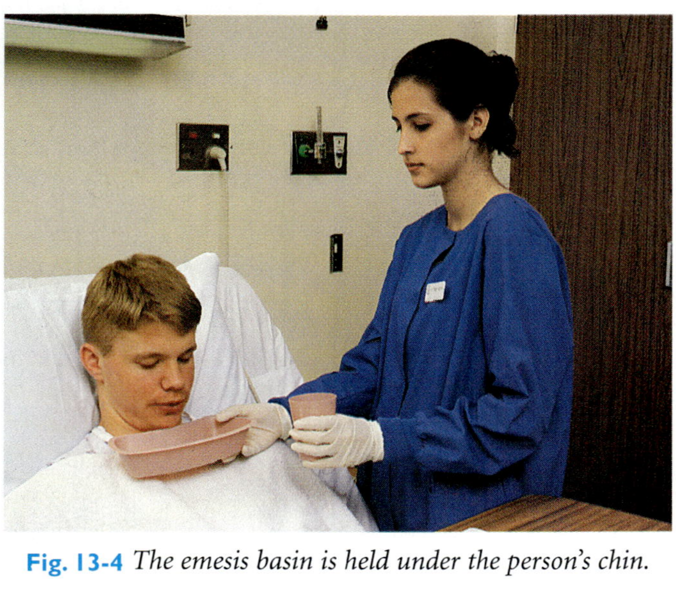

Fig. 13-4 *The emesis basin is held under the person's chin.*

Flossing

Flossing teeth removes plaque and tartar from the teeth. These substances can cause serious gum disease that leads to loosening and loss of teeth. Therefore flossing is a preventive measure. Flossing also removes food from between the teeth. It is usually done after brushing but can be done at other times. Some people floss after meals. If done only once a day, bedtime is the best time to floss.

Dental floss is waxed or unwaxed. Waxed floss does not fray as easily as the unwaxed type. Waxed floss is easier to use because it slides between the teeth. However, particles on tooth surfaces are more likely to attach to unwaxed floss. Many dentists recommend unwaxed floss, which is thinner than waxed floss.

You need to floss for persons who cannot tend to oral hygiene.

Flossing the Person's Teeth

Pre-procedure

1 Explain to the person what you are going to do.
2 Wash your hands.
3 Collect the following:
   - Kidney basin
   - Water glass with cool water
   - Dental floss
   - Face towel
   - Paper towels
   - Disposable gloves
4 Place the paper towels on the overbed table. Arrange items on top of them.
5 Identify the person. Check the ID bracelet and call the person by name.
6 Provide for privacy.
7 Raise the bed to the best level for good body mechanics.

Procedure

8 Raise the head of the bed so the person can sit comfortably. Position the person in a side-lying position near you if he or she cannot sit up.
9 Place the towel over the person's chest.
10 Position the overbed table so you can reach it with ease. Adjust the height as needed.
11 Lower the side rail.
12 Put on the gloves.
13 Break off an 18-inch piece of floss from the dispenser.
14 Hold the floss between the middle fingers of each hand (Fig. 13-5, A on page 290).
15 Stretch the floss with your thumbs.
16 Start at the upper back tooth on the right side and work around to the left side.
17 Move the floss gently up and down between the teeth (Fig. 13-5, B on page 290). Move floss up and down from the top of the crown to the gum line.
18 Move to a new section of floss after every second tooth.
19 Floss the lower teeth. Hold the floss with your index fingers (Fig. 13-5, C on page 290). Use up and down motions and go under the gums as for the upper teeth. Start on the right side and work around to the left side.
20 Let the person rinse his or her mouth. Hold the kidney basin under the chin. Repeat rinsing as necessary.

Post-procedure

21 Remove the towel when done.
22 Remove and discard the gloves.
23 Follow steps 21 through 30 for *Brushing the Person's Teeth,* page 287.

A
B
C
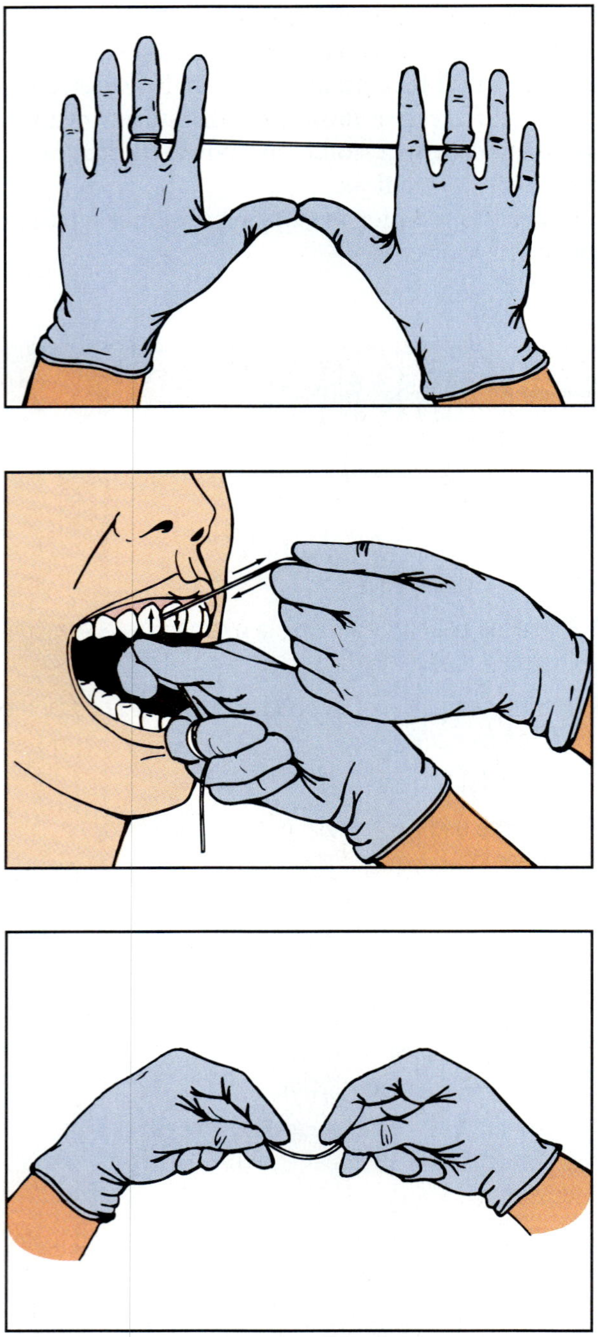

Fig. 13-5 *A, Dental floss is held between the middle fingers to floss the upper teeth. B, Floss is moved in up and down motions between the teeth. Floss is moved up and down from the crown to the gum line. C, Floss is held with the index fingers to floss the lower teeth.*

Mouth Care for the Unconscious Person

Unconscious persons need special mouth care. They cannot eat and drink, they breathe with their mouths open, and they usually receive supplemental oxygen. These factors cause mouth dryness. They also cause crusts to form on the tongue and mucous membranes. Good mouth care helps keep the mouth clean and moist. It is also important for preventing infection.

The nurse tells you what cleaning agent to use for the person. Toothettes dipped in a small amount of mouthwash, hydrogen peroxide, or a salt solution can be used. So can commercial swabs of lemon and oil. However, lemon and oil swabs have a drying effect. They should not be the only method of mouth care used. Petrolatum jelly is applied to the lips after cleaning to prevent cracking.

Unconscious persons usually cannot swallow. They must be protected from choking and aspiration. **Aspiration** is the breathing of fluid or an object into the lungs. To prevent aspiration, position the person on one side with the head turned well to the side (Fig. 13-6). In this position, excess fluid runs out of the mouth. Thus the risk of aspiration is reduced. Using only a small amount of fluid also reduces the risk of aspiration.

The person's mouth must be kept open for mouth care. A padded tongue blade is used for this purpose. (Figure 13-7 shows how to make a padded tongue blade.) Do not use your fingers to hold the mouth open. The person can bite down on them. The bite breaks the skin and creates a

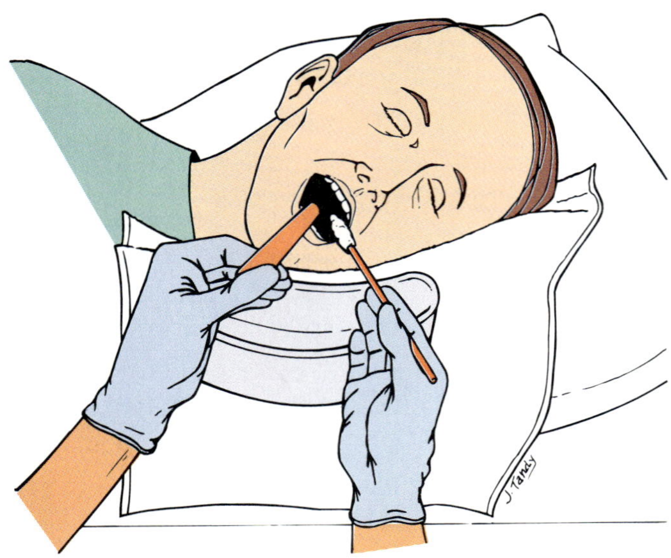

Fig. 13-6 *The head of the unconscious person is turned well to the side to prevent aspiration. A padded tongue blade is used to keep the mouth open while cleaning the mouth with applicators.*

portal of entry for microorganisms. An infection could develop.

Unconscious persons cannot speak or respond to what is happening. However, some can hear. Always assume that unconscious persons can hear. Explain what you are doing step by step. Also tell the person when you are done and when you are leaving the room.

Mouth care is usually given at least every 2 hours. The nurse assesses the person's needs and then writes a care plan. Check with the nurse and the nursing care plan. They tell you how often oral hygiene is to be done and what to use. Unconscious persons are also repositioned at least every 2 hours. Combining mouth care, skin care, and other comfort measures increases their comfort and safety. The risk of forgetting to give mouth care is reduced if oral hygiene is part of this routine care.

A

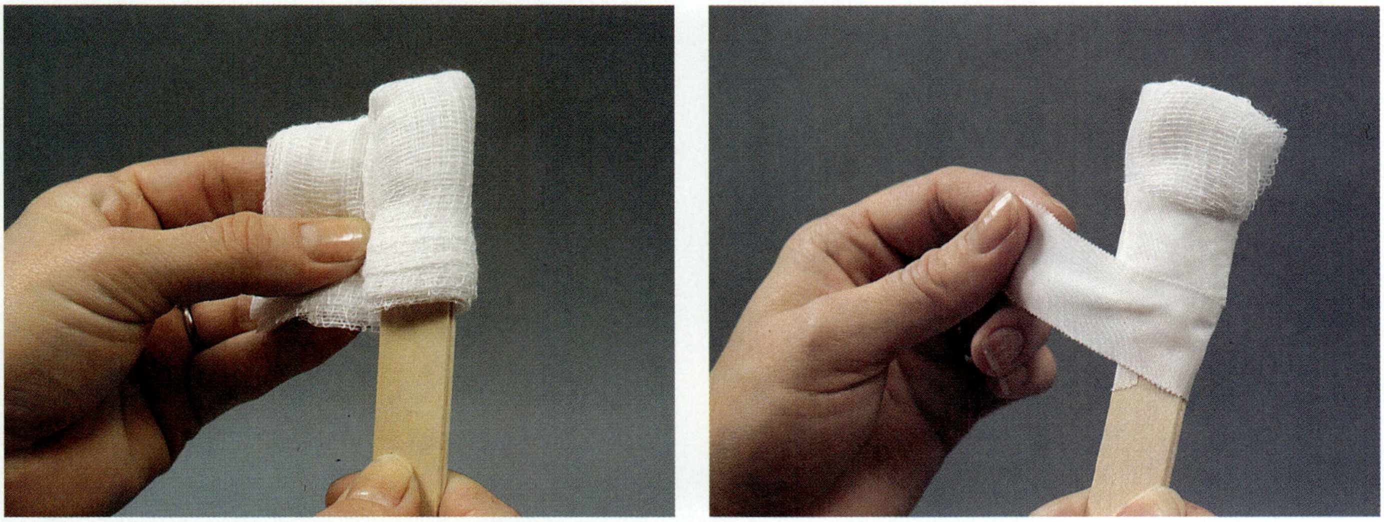

B

Fig. 13-7 *Padded tongue blade. **A**, Place two wooden tongue blades together and wrap gauze around the top half. **B**, Tape the gauze in place.*

Providing Mouth Care for an Unconscious Person

Pre-procedure

1 Wash your hands.
2 Collect the following:
   - Commercial swabs if ordered by the nurse
   - Antiseptic mouthwash or other solution
   - Toothettes or other applicators
   - Padded tongue blade
   - Water glass with cool water
   - Face towel
   - Kidney basin
   - Petrolatum jelly
   - Paper towels
   - Disposable gloves
3 Place the paper towels on the overbed table. Arrange items on top of them.
4 Identify the person. Check the ID bracelet and call the person by name.
5 Explain the procedure to the person.
6 Provide for privacy.
7 Raise the bed to the best level for good body mechanics.

Continued.

Providing Mouth Care for an Unconscious Person—cont'd

Procedure

8 Lower the side rail near you.
9 Put on the gloves.
10 Position the person in a side-lying position on the side toward you. Turn his or her head well to the side.
11 Place the towel under the person's face.
12 Place the kidney basin under the chin.
13 Position the overbed table so you can reach it. Adjust the height as needed.
14 Separate the upper and lower teeth with the padded tongue blade.
15 Clean the mouth using the toothettes or applicators moistened with mouthwash or other solution (see Fig. 13-6).
  a Clean the chewing and inner surfaces of the teeth.
  b Clean the outer surfaces of the teeth.
  c Swab the roof of the mouth, inside of the cheeks, and the lips.
  d Swab the tongue.
  e Moisten a clean applicator with water and swab the mouth to rinse.
  f Place used applicators in the kidney basin.
16 Repeat step 15 using commercial swabs if ordered by the nurse.
17 Apply petrolatum jelly to the person's lips.
18 Remove the towel.
19 Remove and discard the gloves.
20 Explain that the procedure is done and that you will reposition him or her.
21 Reposition the person.
22 Raise the side rail. Make sure both side rails are up.

Post-procedure

23 Make sure the call bell is within reach.
24 Lower the bed to its lowest position.
25 Clean and return equipment to its proper place. Discard disposable items.
26 Unscreen the person.
27 Tell the person that you are leaving the room.
28 Follow facility policy for dirty linen.
29 Wash your hands.
30 Report your observations to the nurse.

Denture Care

Dentures are cleaned for persons who cannot do so themselves. Mouth care is given and dentures are cleaned as often as natural teeth. Remember, dentures are the person's property. They are expensive. Losing or damaging dentures is negligent conduct.

Dentures are slippery when wet. They can easily break or chip if dropped onto a hard surface such as floors or sinks. You must hold them firmly. During cleaning they are held firmly over a basin of water lined with a towel. Hot water causes them to warp. Do not use hot water to clean or store dentures. If not worn, dentures are stored in a container of cool water. Dentures can dry out and warp if not stored in water.

Dentures are generally removed at bedtime. Some people choose not to wear their dentures. Others wear dentures for eating and remove them after meals. Remind patients and residents not to wrap dentures in tissues or napkins. There is the risk that they will be discarded. Dentures are stored in water when not being worn.

Many patients and residents can clean their own dentures. However, they may need help collecting cleaning items. They may also need help getting to the bathroom.

Text continued on page 295.

Denture Care

Pre-procedure

1 Explain the procedure to the person.

2 Wash your hands.

4 Collect the following:
- Denture brush or toothbrush
- Denture cup labeled with the person's name and room number
- Denture cleaner or toothpaste
- Water glass with cool water
- Straw
- Mouthwash
- Kidney basin
- Two face towels
- Gauze squares
- Disposable gloves

4 Identify the person. Check the ID bracelet and call the person by name.

5 Provide for privacy.

Procedure

6 Lower the side rail if up.

7 Place a towel over the person's chest.

8 Put on the gloves.

9 Ask the person to remove the dentures. Carefully place them in the kidney basin.

10 Remove the dentures using gauze if the person cannot do so. (The gauze lets you get a good grip on the slippery dentures.)

- a Grasp the upper denture with your thumb and index finger (Fig. 13-8 on page 294). Move the denture up and down slightly to break the seal. Gently remove the denture once the seal is broken. Place it in the kidney basin.
- b Remove the lower denture by grasping it with your thumb and index finger. Turn it slightly and lift it out of the person's mouth. Place it in the kidney basin.

11 Raise the side rail if instructed by the nurse.

12 Take the kidney basin, denture cup, brush, and denture cleaner or toothpaste to the sink.

13 Line the sink with a towel and fill it with water.

14 Rinse each denture under warm running water. Return them to the denture cup.

15 Apply denture cleaner or toothpaste to the brush.

16 Brush the dentures as in Figure 13-9 on page 294.

17 Rinse dentures under cool running water. Handle them carefully; do not drop them.

18 Place them in the denture cup. Fill it with cool water until the dentures are covered.

19 Clean the kidney basin.

20 Bring the denture cup and kidney basin to the bedside table.

21 Lower the side rail if up.

22 Position the person for oral hygiene.

23 Assist the person to rinse his or her mouth with mouthwash. Hold the kidney basin under the chin.

24 Ask the person to insert the dentures. Insert them if the person cannot.

- a Grasp the upper denture firmly with your thumb and index finger. Raise the upper lip with the other hand and insert the denture. Use your index fingers to gently press on the denture to make sure it is securely in place.
- b Grasp the lower denture securely with your thumb and index finger. Pull down slightly on the lower lip and insert the denture. Gently press down on it to make sure it is in place.

25 Put the denture cup in the top drawer of the bedside stand if the dentures are not reinserted.

26 Remove the towel.

27 Remove the gloves.

Continued.

DENTURE CARE—CONT'D

POST-PROCEDURE

28 Make sure the person is comfortable.

29 Make sure the call bell is within reach.

30 Raise or lower side rails as instructed by the nurse.

31 Unscreen the person.

32 Clean and return equipment to its proper place. Discard disposable items.

33 Follow facility policy for dirty linen.

34 Wash your hands.

35 Report your observations to the nurse.

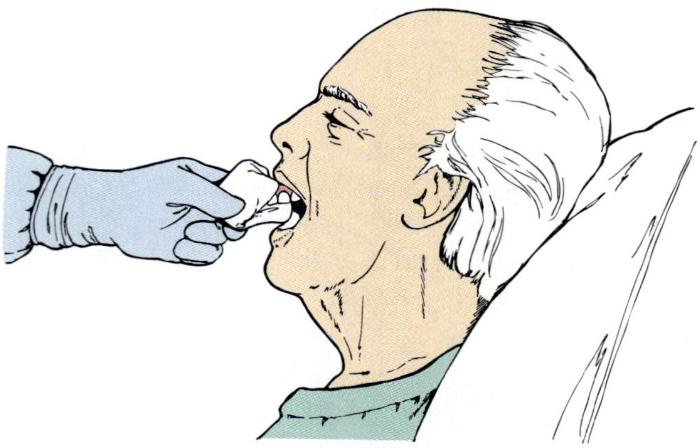

Fig. 13-8 *Remove the upper denture by grasping it with the thumb and index finger of one hand. Use a piece of gauze to grasp the slippery denture.*

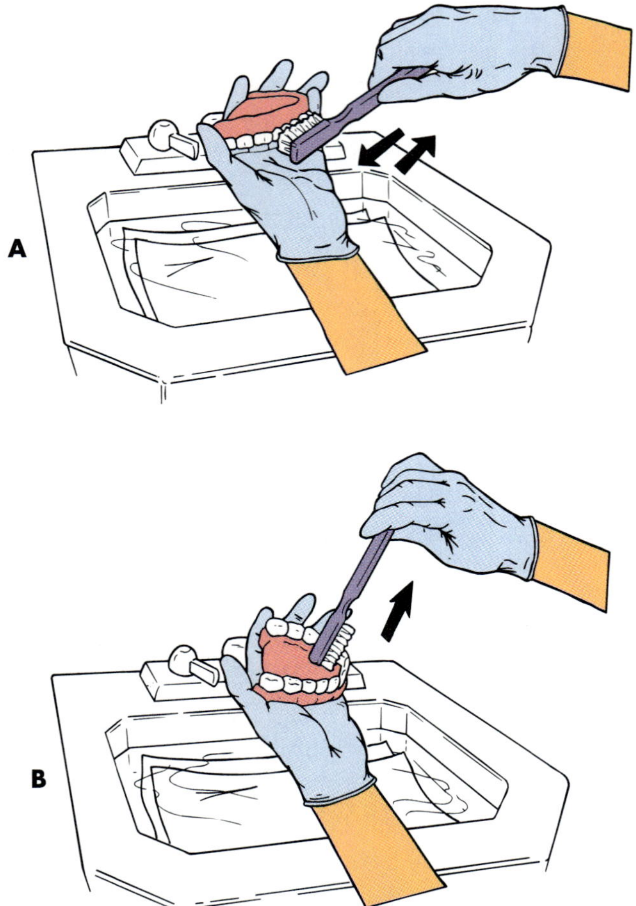

Fig. 13-9 *A, Outer surfaces of the upper denture are brushed with back-and-forth motions. Note that the denture is held over the sink, which is filled halfway with water and lined with a towel. B, Position the brush vertically to clean the inner surfaces of the denture. Use upward strokes.*

BATHING

Bathing cleans the skin and mucous membranes of the genital and anal areas. Microorganisms, dead skin, perspiration, and excess oils are removed. A bath also is refreshing and relaxing. Circulation is stimulated and body parts are exercised. Observations are made during the bath. The bath also gives you time to talk with and get to know the person.

A person may get a complete or partial bed bath, a tub bath, or a shower. The method depends on the person's condition, ability to provide self-care, and personal choice. In hospitals, bathing usually occurs after breakfast. In nursing facilities, baths and showers are given in the morning and evening. The person should be given choices in regard to time of day and frequency. A person who normally bathes at bedtime should be allowed to continue the practice if possible.

Bathing frequency is a personal matter. Some people bathe daily. Others take a complete bath only once or twice a week. Personal choice, weather, physical activity, and illness affect how often a person bathes. Illness usually increases the need for bathing because of fever and increased perspiration. Other illnesses and dry skin may require bathing every 2 or 3 days.

Age also affects bathing frequency. Dry skin occurs with aging. Bathing with soap also drys the skin. Dry skin is easily damaged. Therefore the elderly usually need a complete bath once a week. Partial baths are taken the other days. Some bathe daily but do not always use soap. Thorough rinsing is essential when soap is used. Lotions and oils help keep the skin soft.

Certain rules are followed for bed baths, showers, or tub baths. They are listed in Box 13-2.

BOX 13-2 Rules for Bathing

- Ask the nurse what type of bath a person is to have.
- Find out which skin care products to use. Allow personal choice when possible.
- Offer the bedpan or urinal or assist the person to the bathroom. Bathing usually results in the need to urinate. The person is more comfortable and relaxed if the need to urinate has been met.
- Collect equipment before beginning the procedure.
- Protect the person's privacy. Properly screen the person and close doors.
- Make sure the person is well covered for warmth and privacy.
- Reduce drafts by closing doors and windows.
- Protect the person from falling.
- Use good body mechanics at all times.
- Make sure water temperature is not too hot, particularly for elderly persons.
- Keep soap in the soap dish between latherings. This prevents the water from becoming very soapy. If a tub bath is taken, the person will not slip on the soap.
- Wash from the cleanest to the dirtiest areas.
- Encourage the person to help as much as is safely possible.
- Rinse the skin thoroughly to remove all soap.
- Pat the skin dry to avoid irritating or breaking the skin.
- Bathe the skin whenever fecal material or urine is on the skin.

Skin Care Products

There are many skin care products. Some are used for cleansing. Others protect the skin from drying or friction. The products used depend on personal choice and cost. Table 13-1 on page 296 describes the common skin care products.

Observations

When bathing a person or assisting a person to bathe, the skin is observed. The following observations are reported to the nurse:

- The color of the skin, lips, nail beds, and sclera (whites of the eyes)
- The location and description of rashes
- Dry skin
- Bruises or open skin areas
- Pale or reddened areas, particularly over bony parts
- Drainage or bleeding from wounds or body openings
- Skin temperature
- Complaints of pain or discomfort

TABLE 13-1

COMMON SKIN CARE PRODUCTS

Type	Purpose	Nursing Care Considerations
Soaps	Clean the skin Remove dirt, dead skin, skin oil, some microorganisms, and perspiration	Tend to dry and irritate the skin Dry skin is easily injured and causes itching and discomfort Skin must be rinsed well to remove all soap Not needed for every bath; plain water can clean the skin Plain water is often used for the elderly because of dry skin People with dry skin may prefer soaps containing bath oils Not used if a person has very dry skin
Bath oils	Keep the skin soft and prevent drying	Some soaps contain bath oil Liquid bath oil can be added to bath water Showers and tubs become slippery from bath oils; safety precautions are necessary to prevent falls
Creams and lotions	Protect the skin from the drying effect of air and evaporation	Do not feel greasy but leave an oily film on the skin Most are scented
Powders	Absorb moisture and prevent friction when two skin surfaces rub together	Usually applied under the breasts, under the arms, and in the groin area, and sometimes between the toes Applied to dry skin in a thin, even layer Excessive amounts cause caking and crusts that can irritate skin
Deodorants	Mask and control body odors	Applied to the axillae (under arms) Not applied to irritated skin Do not take the place of bathing
Antiperspirants	Reduce the amount of perspiration	Applied to the axillae (under arms) Not applied to irritated skin Do not take the place of bathing

The Complete Bed Bath

The *complete bed bath* involves washing the person's entire body in bed. Persons who are unconscious, paralyzed, in a cast or traction, or weak from illness or surgery generally require bed baths. Complete bed baths are given to persons who cannot bathe themselves.

Ask the nurse about the person's ability to assist with the bath. Also ask about any activity or position limits. Remember to follow Standard Precautions and the Bloodborne Pathogen Standard as needed. Consult with the nurse if you are unsure if they apply for a person.

Many people have never had a bed bath. It may be embarrassing to have another person see his or her body. The person may fear being exposed. Every person must get an explanation about how a bed bath is given and how the body is covered to protect privacy.

The following bed bath procedure is for adults. Bathing of infants is discussed in Chapter 32.

Text continued on page 301.

Giving a Complete Bed Bath

Pre-procedure

1. Identify the person. Check the ID bracelet and call the person by name.
2. Explain the procedure to the person.
3. Offer the bedpan or urinal. Provide for privacy.
4. Wash your hands.
5. Collect clean linen for a closed bed. Place linen on a clean surface.
6. Collect the following:
   - Wash basin
   - Soap dish with soap
   - Bath thermometer
   - Orange stick or nail file
   - Washcloth
   - Two bath towels and two face towels
   - Bath blanket
   - Gown, pajamas, or clothing
   - Equipment for oral hygiene
   - Body lotion
   - Talcum powder
   - Deodorant or antiperspirant
   - Brush and comb
   - Other toilet articles if requested
   - Paper towels
   - Disposable gloves

Procedure

7. Arrange items on the overbed table. Adjust the height as needed. Use the bedside stand if necessary.
8. Close doors and windows to prevent drafts.
9. Provide for privacy.
10. Raise the bed to the best level for good body mechanics.
11. Remove the call bell and lower the side rail near you.
12. Provide oral hygiene.
13. Remove top linens and cover the person with a bath blanket (see *Making an Occupied Bed,* page 274).
14. Lower the head of the bed to a level appropriate for the person. Keep it as flat as possible. Let the person have at least one pillow.
15. Place paper towels on the overbed table.
16. Raise the side rail and go fill the wash basin.
17. Fill the wash basin two-thirds full with water. Water temperature should be 110° to 115° F (43° to 46° C) for adults. These higher water temperatures are needed because the water cools rapidly.
18. Place the basin on the overbed table on top of the paper towels.
19. Lower the side rail.
20. Place a face towel over the person's chest.
21. Make a mitt with the washcloth (Fig. 13-10 on page 299). Use a mitt throughout the procedure.
22. Wash the person's eyes with water. Do not use soap. Gently wipe from the inner aspect with a corner of the mitt (Fig. 13-11 on page 299). Clean the far eye first. Repeat this step for the near eye.
23. Ask the person if you should use soap to wash the face.
24. Wash the face, ears, and neck. Rinse and dry the skin well using the towel on the chest.
25. Help the person move to the side of the bed near you.
26. Remove the gown. Do not expose the person.
27. Place a bath towel lengthwise under the far arm.
28. Support the arm with your palm under the person's elbow. His or her forearm rests on your forearm.
29. Wash the arm, shoulder, and underarm with long, firm strokes (Fig. 13-12 on page 299). Rinse and pat dry.
30. Place the basin on the towel. Put the person's hand into the water (Fig. 13-13 on page 300). Wash it well. Clean under fingernails with an orange stick or nail file.
31. Encourage the person to exercise the hand and fingers.

Continued.

GIVING A COMPLETE BED BATH—CONT'D

PROCEDURE—CONT'D

32 Remove the basin and dry the hand well. Cover the arm with the bath blanket.

33 Repeat steps 27 to 32 for the near arm.

34 Place a bath towel over the chest crosswise. Hold the towel in place and pull the bath blanket from under the towel to the waist.

35 Lift the towel slightly and wash the chest (Fig. 13-14 on page 300). Do not expose the person. Rinse and pat dry, especially under breasts.

36 Move the towel lengthwise over the chest and abdomen. Do not expose the person. Pull the bath blanket down to the pubic area.

37 Lift the towel slightly and wash the abdomen (Fig. 13-15 on page 300). Rinse and pat dry.

38 Pull the bath blanket up to the shoulders, covering both arms. Remove the towel.

39 Change the water if it is soapy or cool. Raise the side rail before you leave the bedside. Lower it when you return.

40 Uncover the far leg. Do not expose the genital area. Place a towel lengthwise under the foot and leg.

41 Bend the knee and support the leg with your arm. Wash it with long, firm strokes. Rinse and pat dry.

42 Place the basin on the towel near the foot.

43 Lift the leg slightly. Slide the basin under the foot.

44 Place the foot in the basin (Fig. 13-16 on page 300). Use an orange stick or nail file to clean under toenails if necessary.

45 Remove the basin and dry the leg. Cover the leg with the bath blanket. Remove the towel.

46 Repeat steps 40 to 45 for the near leg.

47 Change the water. Raise the side rail before leaving the bedside. Lower it when you return.

48 Turn the person onto the side away from you. Keep him or her covered with the bath blanket.

49 Uncover the back and buttocks. Do not expose the person. Place a towel lengthwise on the bed along the back.

50 Wash the back, working from the back of the neck to the lower end of the buttocks. Use long, firm, continuous strokes (Fig. 13-17 on page 300). Rinse and dry well.

51 Give a back massage. (The person may prefer to have the back massage after the bath.)

52 Turn the person onto the back.

53 Change the water for perineal care. Raise the side rail before you leave the bedside. Lower it when you return.

54 Let the person wash the genital area. Adjust the overbed table so he or she can reach the wash basin, soap, and towels with ease. Place the call bell within reach. Ask the person to signal when finished. Make sure the person understands what to do. Answer the call bell promptly. Provide perineal care if the person cannot do so (see *Perineal Care,* page 308).

55 Give a back massage if you have not already done so.

56 Apply deodorant or antiperspirant.

57 Put a clean gown, pajamas, or clothing on the person (see Chapter 14).

58 Comb and brush the hair.

59 Make the bed. Attach the call bell.

POST-PROCEDURE

60 Make sure the person is comfortable.

61 Lower the bed to its lowest position.

62 Raise or lower side rails as instructed by the nurse.

63 Empty and clean the wash basin. Return it and other supplies to their proper place.

64 Wipe off the overbed table with the paper towels and discard them.

65 Unscreen the person.

66 Follow facility policy for dirty linen.

67 Wash your hands.

68 Report your observations to the nurse (see page 295).

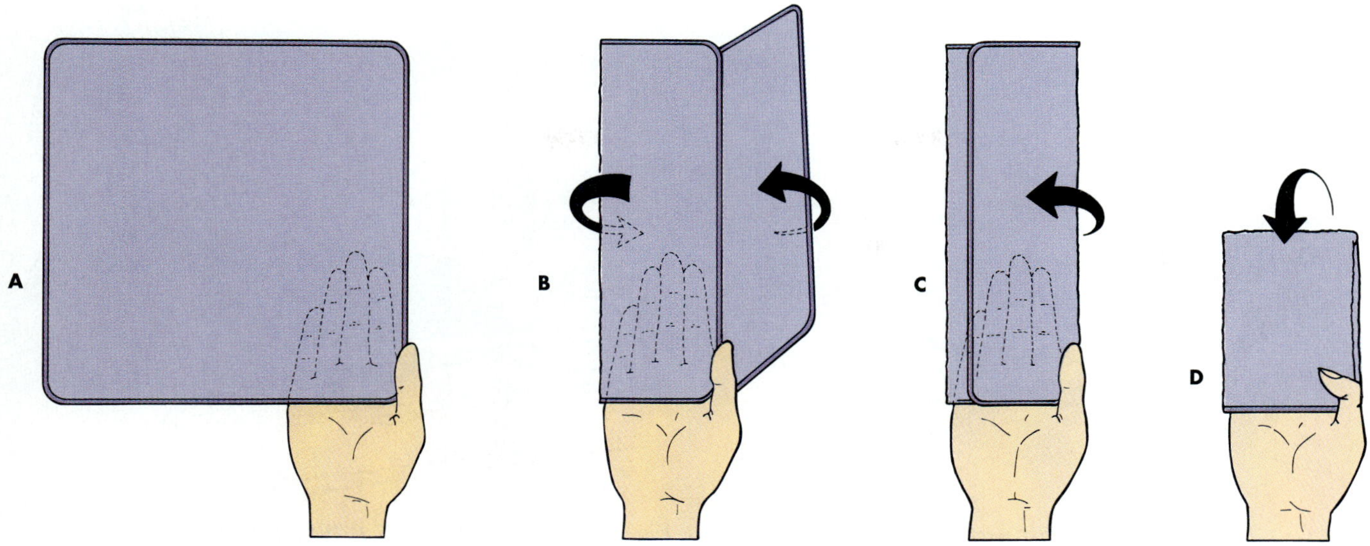

Fig. 13-10 *A, Make a mitt with a washcloth by grasping the near side of the washcloth with your thumb. B, Bring the washcloth around and behind your hand. C, Fold the side of the washcloth over your palm as you grasp it with your thumb. D, Fold the top of the washcloth down and tuck it under next to your palm.*

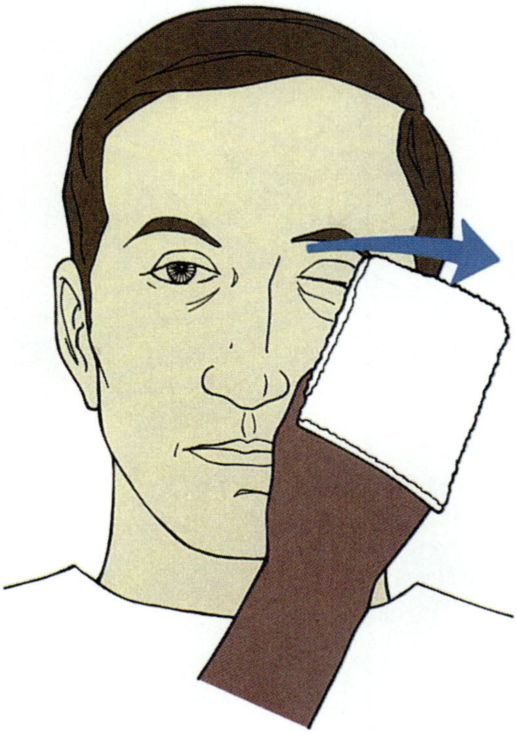

Fig. 13-11 *Wash the person's eyes with a mitted washcloth. Wipe from the inner to the outer aspect of the eye.*

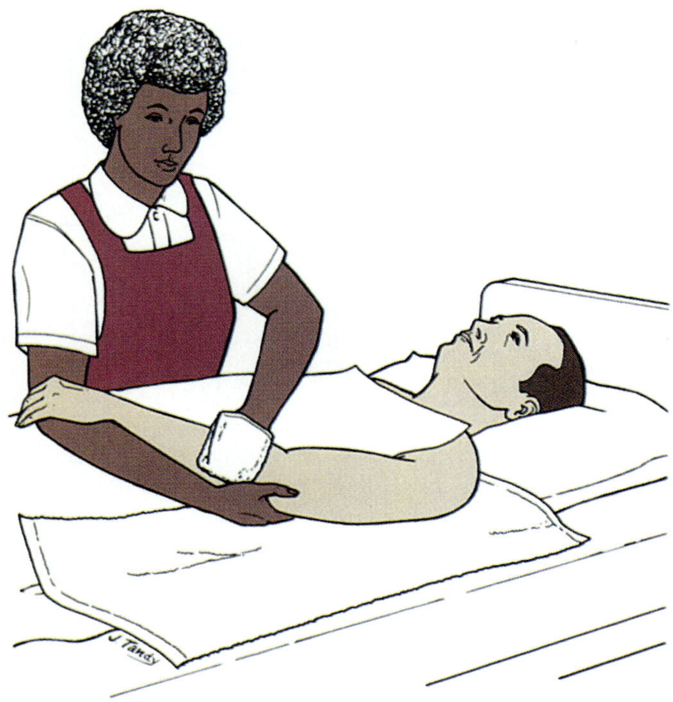

Fig. 13-12 *Wash the person's arm with firm, long strokes using a mitted washcloth.*

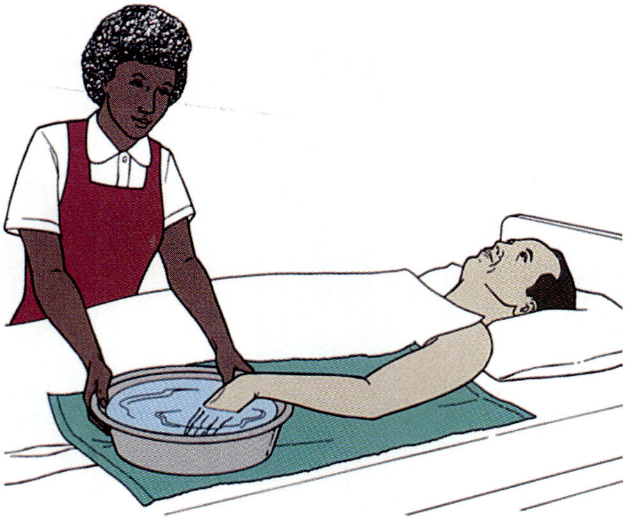

Fig. 13-13 *The person's hands are washed by placing the wash basin on the bed.*

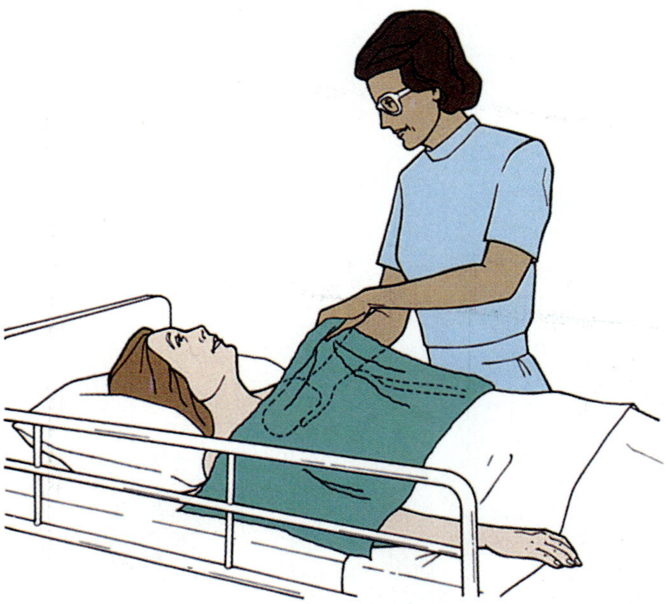

Fig. 13-14 *The person's breasts are not exposed during the bath. A bath towel is placed horizontally over the chest area. The towel is lifted slightly to reach under to wash the breasts and chest.*

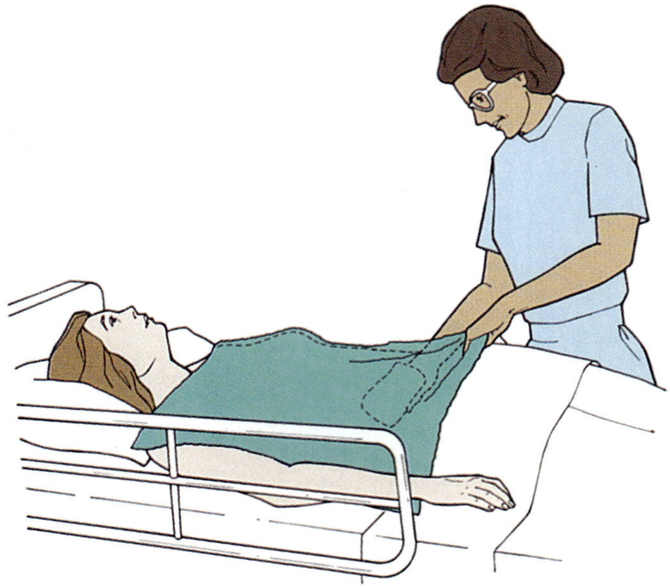

Fig. 13-15 *The bath towel is turned so that it is vertical to cover the breasts and abdomen. The towel is lifted slightly to bathe the abdomen. The bath blanket covers the pubic area.*

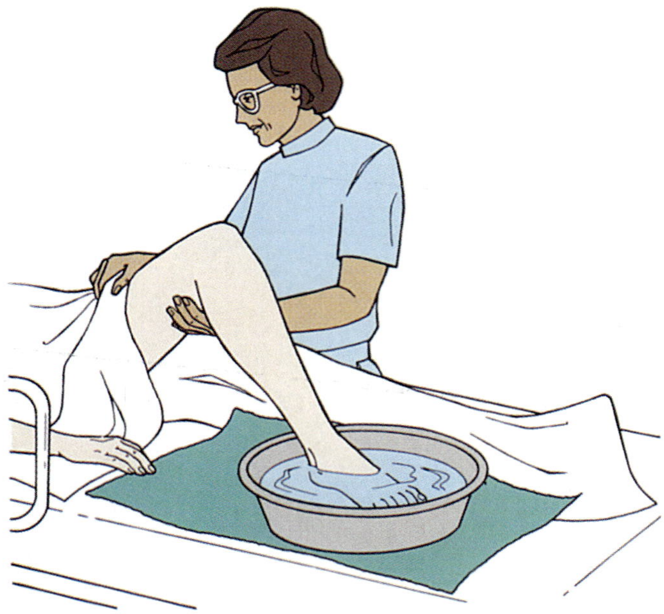

Fig. 13-16 *The foot is washed by placing it in the wash basin on the bed.*

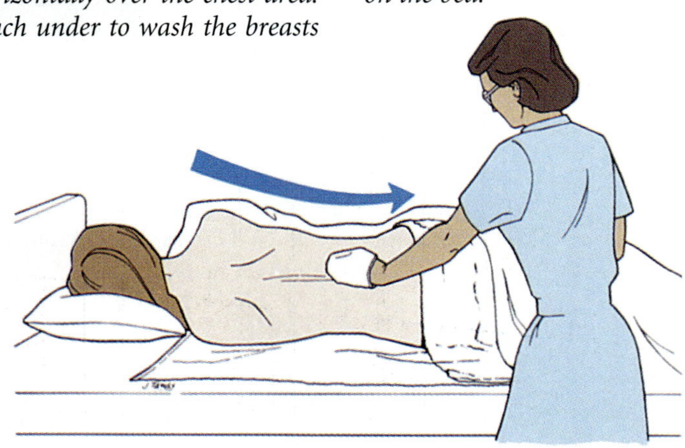

Fig. 13-17 *The back is washed with long, firm, continuous strokes. Note that the person is in a side-lying position. A towel is placed lengthwise on the bed to protect the linens from water.*

The Partial Bath

The partial bath involves bathing the face, hands, axillae (underarms), genital and rectal areas, back, and buttocks. These areas develop odors or cause discomfort if not clean. Partial bed baths are given to persons who cannot bathe themselves. Persons who are able may bathe themselves in bed or at the bathroom sink. Nursing personnel assist as needed, especially with washing the back.

The general rules for bathing apply for partial bed baths. The considerations involved in giving a complete bed bath also apply.

Giving a Partial Bath

Pre-procedure

1 Follow steps 1 through 9 in *Giving a Complete Bed Bath,* pages 297 and 298.

Procedure

2 Make sure the bed is in the lowest position.

3 Assist with oral hygiene. Adjust the height of the overbed table to an appropriate level.

4 Remove top linen. Cover the person with a bath blanket.

5 Place the paper towels on the overbed table.

6 Fill the wash basin with water. Water temperature should be 110° to 115° F (43° to 46° C) for adults.

7 Place the basin on the overbed table on top of the paper towels.

8 Raise the head of the bed so the person can bathe comfortably. Assist him or her to sit at the bedside if allowed this position.

9 Position the overbed table so the person can easily reach the basin and supplies.

10 Help the person remove the gown or pajamas.

11 Ask the person to wash the body parts that can be reached with ease (Fig. 13-18 on page 302). Explain that you will wash the back and those areas that cannot be reached.

12 Place the call bell within reach. Ask him or her to signal if help is needed or when bathing is complete.

13 Leave the room after washing your hands.

14 Return when the call light is on. Knock before entering.

15 Change the bath water.

16 Ask what was washed. Wash areas the person could not reach. The face, hands, axillae, genital and rectal areas, back, and buttocks are washed for the partial bath.

17 Give a back massage.

18 Apply deodorant or antiperspirant.

19 Help the person put on a clean gown, pajamas, or clothing (see Chapter 14).

20 Assist with hair care.

21 Assist him or her to a chair. Otherwise, turn the person onto the side away from you.

22 Make the bed.

23 Lower the bed to its lowest position.

24 Assist the person to return to bed.

Post-procedure

25 Make sure the person is comfortable.

26 Place the call bell within reach.

27 Raise or lower side rails as instructed by the nurse.

28 Empty and clean the basin. Return the basin and supplies to their proper place.

29 Wipe off the overbed table with the paper towels and discard them.

30 Unscreen the person.

31 Follow facility policy for dirty linen.

32 Wash your hands.

33 Report your observations to the nurse (see pages 295).

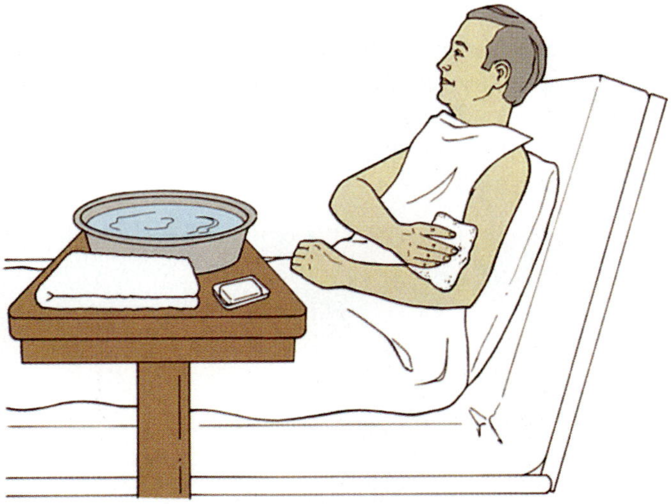

Fig. 13-18 *The person is bathing himself in bed. Necessary equipment is within his reach.*

The Tub Bath

Many people like tub baths because they are relaxing. Persons must be protected from falling when getting in and out of tubs. They must also be protected from burns caused by hot water temperatures. A tub bath can cause a person to feel faint, weak, or tired. These are greater risks for the person who has been on bed rest. A bath lasts no longer than 20 minutes. The nurse's approval is needed for a person to take a tub bath.

Some rooms have private baths. If not, you need to reserve the tub room. The tub is cleaned before use. This prevents the spread of microbes and infection. Preventing falls is also important. Safety measures to prevent falls include:

- Placing a bath mat on the bottom of the tub, unless there are nonskid strips or a nonskid surface. Tubs in private homes may not have nonskid strips or nonskid surfaces.
- Placing needed items within the person's reach. This includes the call bell.
- Draining the tub before the person gets out of the tub. If the tub is drained first, keep the person covered to protect from exposure and chilling.
- Having the person use safety bars when getting in and out of the tub.
- Avoiding the use of bath oils. They make tub surfaces slippery.

Some facilities have portable tubs. The sides are lowered and the person is transferred from the bed to the tub (Fig. 13-19). After the transfer, the sides are raised into position. The person is transported to the tub room. The portable tub is filled, and the person is bathed in the usual manner. Nursing facilities, burn units, and rehabilitation units have portable tubs.

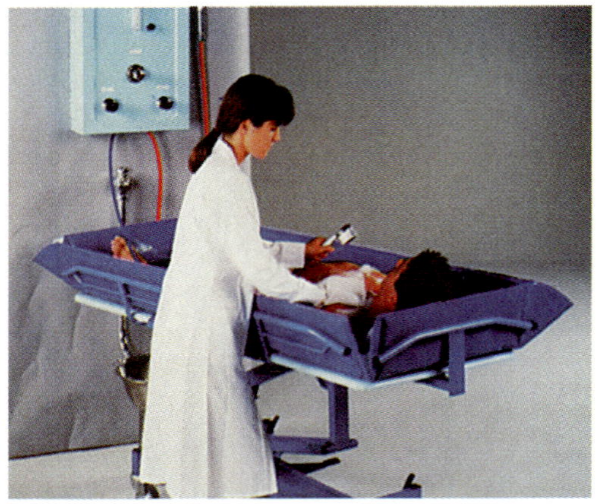

Fig. 13-19 *The person is given a bath in a portable tub.*

Assisting With a Tub Bath

Pre-procedure

1. Reserve the bathtub if necessary.
2. Identify the person. Check the ID bracelet and call the person by name.
3. Explain the procedure to the person.
4. Wash your hands.
5. Collect the following:
   - Washcloth
   - Two bath towels
   - Soap
   - Bath thermometer
   - Clean gown or pajamas
   - Deodorant or antiperspirant
   - Other toilet articles as requested
   - Robe and nonslip slippers or shoes
   - Rubber bath mat if needed
   - Disposable bath mat

Procedure

6. Place items in the bathroom in the space provided or on a chair.
7. Clean the tub if needed.
8. Place a rubber bath mat in the tub if needed.
9. Place a disposable bath mat on the floor in front of the tub.
10. Put the *occupied* sign on the bathroom door.
11. Return to the person's room. Provide for privacy.
12. Help the person sit on the side of the bed.
13. Help the person put on a robe and slippers.
14. Assist the person to the bathroom. Use a wheelchair if necessary.
15. Have the person sit on the chair by the tub.
16. Fill the tub halfway with warm water (105° F; 41° C).
17. Help the person remove slippers, robe, and gown.
18. Assist the person into the tub (Fig. 13-20 on page 304).
19. Ask the person to use the call bell when done or when help is needed.
20. Remind the person not to stay in the tub longer than 20 minutes.
21. Place a towel across the chair.
22. Leave the room and wash your hands.
23. Check the person every 5 minutes.
24. Return when he or she has signaled for you. Knock before entering.
25. Help the person out of the tub and onto the chair.
26. Help the person dry off; pat gently.
27. Assist with lotion, powder, deodorant, or antiperspirant as needed.
28. Help the person put on a clean gown or pajamas, a bathrobe, and slippers or shoes.
29. Help the person return to the room and to bed.
30. Provide a back massage.
31. Assist with hair care.

Post-procedure

32. Make sure the person is comfortable.
33. Raise or lower side rails as instructed by the nurse.
34. Clean the tub. Remove soiled linen and discard disposable items. Put the *unoccupied* sign on the door. Return supplies to their proper place.
35. Follow facility policy for dirty linen.
36. Wash your hands.
37. Report your observations to the nurse.

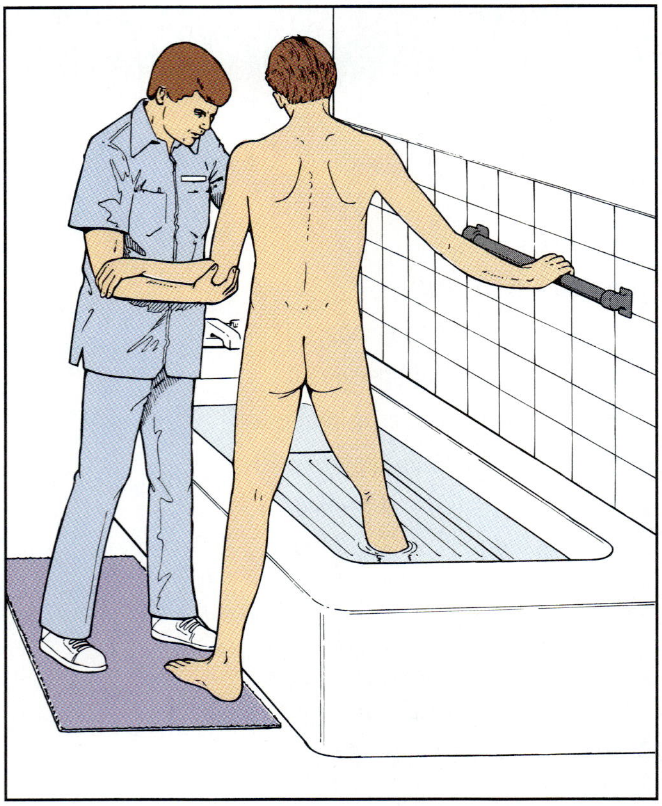

Fig. 13-20 *The nursing assistant helps the person into the tub to protect the person from falling. A bath mat is in the tub, the tub is filled halfway with water, and a floor mat is in front of the tub.*

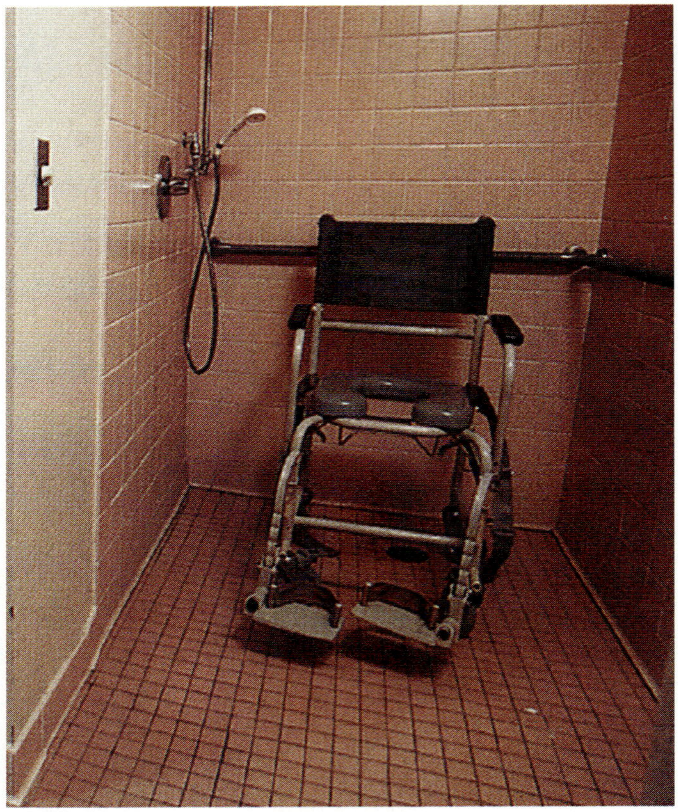

Fig. 13-21 *A shower chair has a round opening in the center of the seat.*

The Shower

A shower may be part of the bathtub or a separate stall. A shower stall has advantages. The person walks into the stall rather than stepping over the side of the tub. A weak or paralyzed person can use a shower chair. The shower chair is wheeled into the shower stall. Shower chairs are made of plastic, with wheels on the legs. Water drains through a round open area in the seat (Fig. 13-21). The wheels are locked during the shower to prevent the chair from moving. A straight-backed chair or a stool can be used in place of a shower chair. Sturdy lawn chairs have been used as shower chairs in private homes.

Persons must be protected from falling and chilling. The safety measures listed for bathing and for tub baths apply to showers. Privacy is also protected. Weak or unsteady persons are not allowed to stand in the shower. They are not left unattended. Encourage persons to use the safety bars for support when getting in and out of the shower. The safety bars are especially important if the shower is part of a tub unit. As with the tub bath, persons shower only with a nurse's approval. Your hospital or nursing facility may have additional safety rules for showers.

Spotlight On…

Toni D of Albuquerque, New Mexico, *received an unexpected compliment when a nurse, checking on her patients during rounds, asked a female patient how she was doing and if she needed anything. The patient responded, "I don't need anything right now. I've just had my bath and I feel sparkling clean." Toni then peeked around the curtains, thanked the patient, introduced herself to the nurse, and told them she had just graduated from the nursing assistant program!*

Assisting the Person to Shower

Pre-procedure

1 Reserve the shower if necessary.
2 Identify the person. Check the ID bracelet and call the person by name.
3 Explain the procedure to the person.
4 Wash your hands.
5 Collect items as for the tub bath (page 297).
6 Place items on a chair or space provided near the shower.

Procedure

7 Clean the shower if needed.
8 Place a rubber bath mat on the shower floor. Do not block the drain.
9 Place a disposable bath mat on the floor in front of the shower.
10 Place the *occupied* sign on the shower door.
11 Return to the person's room. Provide for privacy.
12 Help the person sit on the side of the bed.
13 Help the person put on a robe and slippers or shoes.
14 Assist the person to the shower room. Use a wheelchair if necessary.
15 Ask the person to use the call bell when done showering or when assistance is needed.
16 Turn the shower on. Adjust water temperature and pressure.
17 Help the person remove slippers, gown, and robe.
18 Help him or her into the shower. If using a shower chair, place it in position and lock the wheels.
19 Assist the person with washing if necessary.
20 Place a towel across the chair that is outside of the shower.
21 Wash your hands and leave the room only if the person can stand without help. Stay outside the stall if the person is weak.
22 Return to the shower room when the person has signaled. Knock before entering.
23 Turn the shower off.
24 Assist the person out of the shower and onto the chair.
25 Help the person dry off; pat gently.
26 Assist with lotion, powder, deodorant, or antiperspirant as needed.
27 Help the person put on a clean gown or pajamas, a bathrobe, and slippers or shoes.
28 Help the person return to the room and to bed.
29 Provide a back massage.
30 Assist with hair care.

Post-procedure

31 Make sure the person is comfortable.
32 Raise or lower side rails as instructed by the nurse.
33 Place the call bell within reach.
34 Clean the shower. Remove soiled linen and discard disposable items. Put the *unoccupied* sign on the door. Return supplies to their proper place.
35 Follow facility policy for dirty linen.
36 Wash your hands.
37 Report your observations to the nurse.

THE BACK MASSAGE

The back massage (back rub) relaxes muscles and stimulates circulation. The massage is normally given after the bath and with HS care. It should last 3 to 5 minutes. Observe the skin before starting the procedure. Look for breaks in the skin, bruises, reddened areas, and other signs of skin breakdown.

Lotion is used to reduce friction when giving the massage. It is warmed before being applied. Place the lotion bottle in the bath water or hold it under warm running water to warm. You can also rub some between your hands.

The prone position is best for a massage. The side-lying position is often used. Firm strokes are used, and your hands are always in contact with the person's skin. After the massage, you can apply some lotion to the elbows, knees, and heels to keep the skin soft. These bony areas are at risk for skin breakdown.

Some persons should not have back massages as described in this procedure. They may be dangerous for those with certain heart diseases, back injuries, back surgeries, skin diseases, and some lung disorders. Check with the nurse before giving back massages to persons with these conditions.

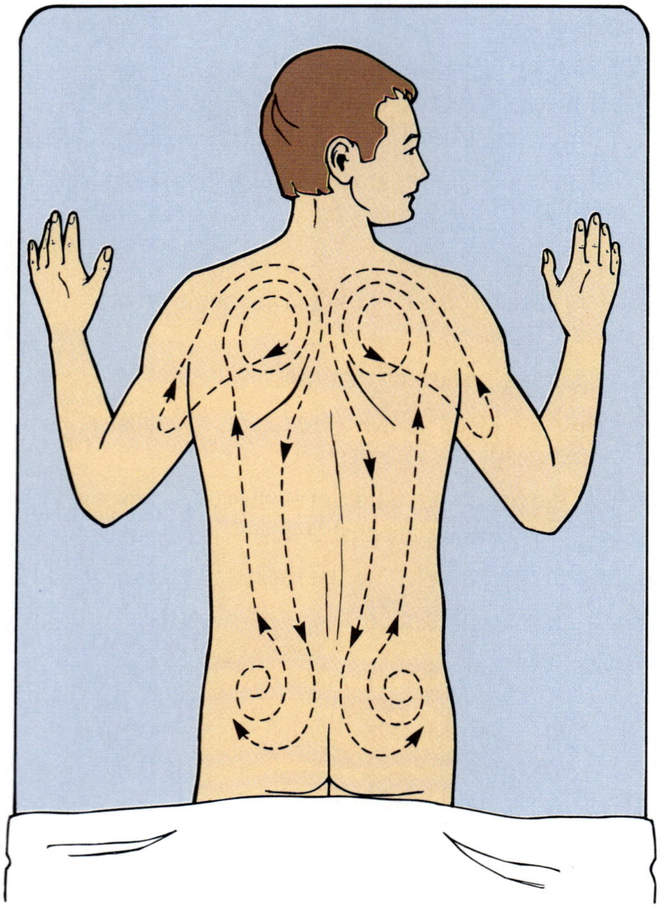

Fig. 13-22 *The person lies in the prone position for a back massage. Stroke upward from the buttocks to the shoulders, down over the upper arms, back up the upper arms, across the shoulders, and down the back to the buttocks.*

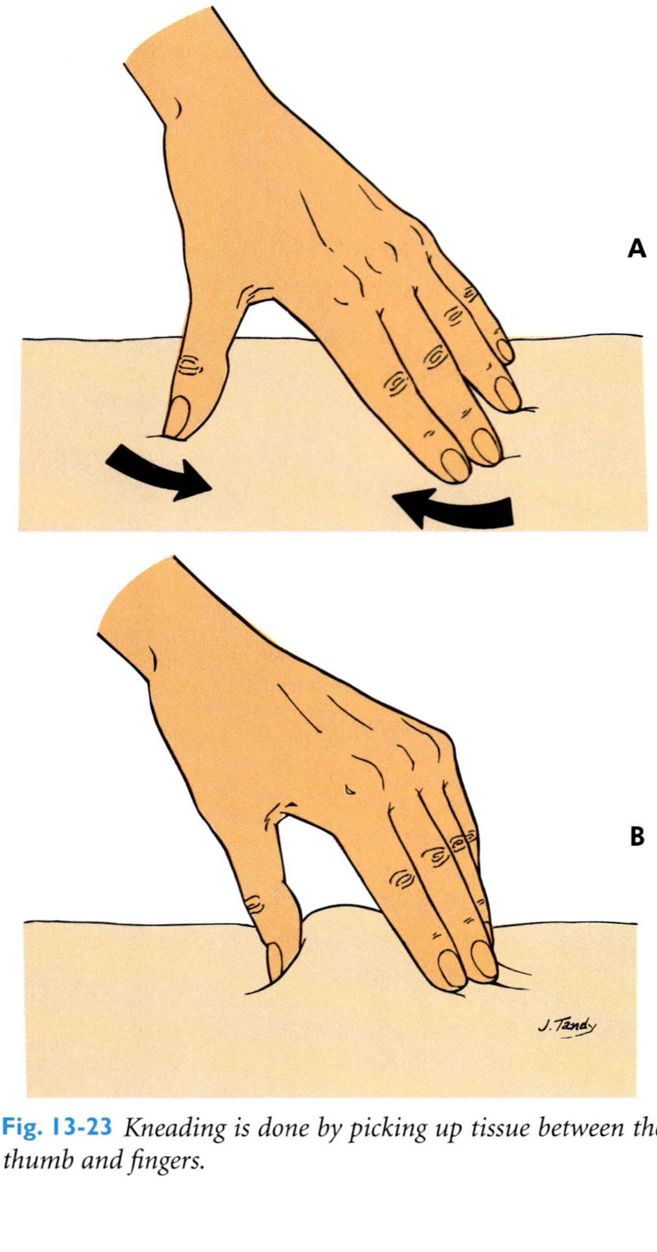

Fig. 13-23 *Kneading is done by picking up tissue between the thumb and fingers.*

Giving a Back Massage

Pre-procedure

1 Identify the person. Check the ID bracelet and call the person by name.

2 Explain the procedure to the person.

3 Wash your hands.

4 Collect the following:
- Bath blanket
- Bath towel
- Lotion

5 Provide for privacy.

6 Raise the bed to the best level for good body mechanics.

Procedure

7 Lower the side rail.

8 Position the person in the prone or side-lying position with the back toward you.

9 Expose the back, shoulders, upper arms, and buttocks. Cover the rest of the body with the bath blanket.

10 Lay the towel on the bed along the back.

11 Warm some lotion between your hands.

12 Explain that the lotion may feel cool and wet.

13 Apply lotion to the lower back area.

14 Stroke up from the buttocks to the shoulders. Then stroke down over the upper arms. Stroke up the upper arms, across the shoulders, and down the back to the buttocks (Fig. 13-22). Use firm strokes. Keep your hands in contact with the person's skin.

15 Repeat step 14 for at least 3 minutes.

16 Knead by grasping skin between your thumb and fingers (Fig. 13-23). Knead half of the back starting at the buttocks and moving up to the shoulder. Then knead down from the shoulder to the buttocks. Repeat on the other half of the back.

17 Massage bony areas. Use circular motions with the tips of your index and middle fingers.

18 Use fast movements to stimulate and slow movements to relax the person.

19 Stroke with long, firm movements to end the massage. Tell the person you are finishing.

20 Cover the person. Remove the towel and bath blanket.

Post-procedure

21 Make sure the person is comfortable.

22 Lower the bed to its lowest position.

23 Raise or lower side rails as instructed by the nurse.

24 Place the call bell within reach.

25 Return lotion to its proper place.

26 Unscreen the person.

27 Follow facility policy for dirty linen.

28 Wash your hands.

29 Report your observations to the nurse.

PERINEAL CARE

Perineal care (**pericare**) involves cleaning the genital and anal areas. These areas are warm, moist, and dark. They provide a place for microbes to grow. The genital and anal areas are cleaned to prevent infection and odors and to promote comfort.

Perineal care is done at least once a day during the bath. The procedure is also done whenever the area is contaminated with urine or feces. Persons with certain disorders need perineal care more often. It is given before and after some surgeries and after childbirth.

Patients and residents should do their own perineal care if able. Otherwise it is given by nursing staff. Many people and nursing personnel find the procedure embarrassing, especially when given to the opposite sex. People may not know the terms *perineum* and *perineal.* Most understand the following terms: *privates, private parts, crotch, genitals,* or the *area between your legs.* Be sure to use terms the person understands. The term must also be in good taste professionally.

Standard Precautions, the rules of medical asepsis, and the Bloodborne Pathogen Standard are followed. Work from the cleanest area to the dirtiest. The urethral area is the cleanest and the anal area the dirtiest. Therefore clean from the urethra to the anal area. The perineal area is very delicate and easily injured. Use warm water, not hot. Washcloths are used if the pericare is part of the bath. The nurse may have you use cotton balls or swabs at other times. The area must be rinsed thoroughly. Pat dry after rinsing to reduce moisture and promote comfort.

Text continued on page 312.

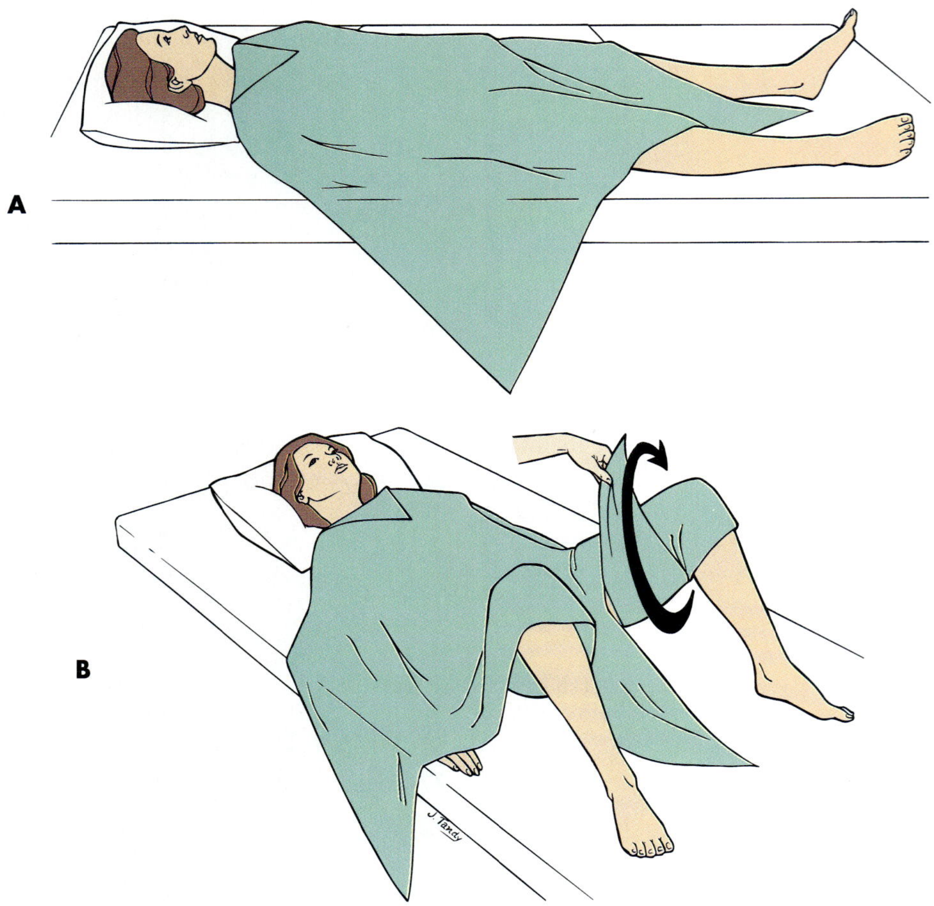

Fig. 13-24 *A, Drape the person for perineal care by positioning the bath blanket like a diamond: one corner is at the neck, there is a corner at each side, and one corner is between the person's legs.* ***B,*** *Wrap the blanket around the leg by bringing the corner around under the leg and over the top. Tuck the corner under the hip.*

Giving Female Perineal Care

Pre-procedure

1. Explain the procedure to the person.
2. Wash your hands.
3. Collect the following:
   - Soap dish with soap
   - At least four washcloths
   - Bath towel
   - Bath blanket
   - Bath thermometer
   - Waterproof pad
   - Disposable gloves
   - Paper towels
4. Arrange items on the overbed table.
5. Identify the person. Check the ID bracelet and call her by name.
6. Provide for privacy.

Procedure

7. Raise the bed to the best level for good body mechanics.
8. Lower the side rail.
9. Cover the person with a bath blanket. Move top linens to the foot of the bed.
10. Position the person on her back.
11. Position the waterproof pad under her buttocks.
12. Drape the person as in Figure 13-24.
13. Raise the side rail.
14. Fill the wash basin. Water temperature should be about 105° to 109° F (41° to 43° C).
15. Place the basin on the overbed table on top of the paper towels.
16. Lower the side rail.
17. Help the person flex her knees and spread her legs.
18. Put on the gloves.
19. Fold the corner of the bath blanket between the person's legs onto her abdomen.
20. Wet the washcloths. Squeeze out excess water from washcloths before using them.
21. Apply soap to a washcloth.
22. Separate the labia. Clean downward from front to back with one stroke (Fig. 13-25 on page 310).
23. Repeat steps 21 and 22 until the area is clean. Use a different part of the washcloth for each stroke.
24. Rinse the perineum with a clean washcloth. Separate the labia. Stroke downward from front to back. Repeat the step as necessary using a different part of the washcloth for each stroke.
25. Pat the area dry with the towel.
26. Fold the blanket back between her legs.
27. Help the person lower her legs and turn onto her side away from you.
28. Apply soap to a washcloth.
29. Clean the rectal area. Clean from the vagina to the anus with one stroke (Fig. 13-26 on page 310).
30. Repeat steps 28 and 29 until the area is clean. Use a different part of the washcloth for each stroke.
31. Rinse the rectal area with a washcloth. Stroke from the vagina to the anus. Repeat the step as necessary using a different part of the washcloth for each stroke.
32. Pat the area dry with the towel.
33. Remove and discard the gloves.

Continued.

GIVING FEMALE PERINEAL CARE—CONT'D

POST-PROCEDURE

34 Position the person so she is comfortable.

35 Return linens to their proper position and remove the bath blanket.

36 Lower the bed to its lowest position.

37 Raise or lower side rails as instructed by the nurse.

38 Place the call bell within reach.

39 Empty and clean the wash basin.

40 Return the basin and supplies to their proper place.

41 Wipe off the overbed table with the paper towels and discard them.

42 Unscreen the person.

43 Follow facility policy for dirty linen.

44 Wash your hands.

45 Report your observations to the nurse:

- Any odors
- Redness, swelling, discharge, or irritation
- Complaints of pain, burning, or other discomfort

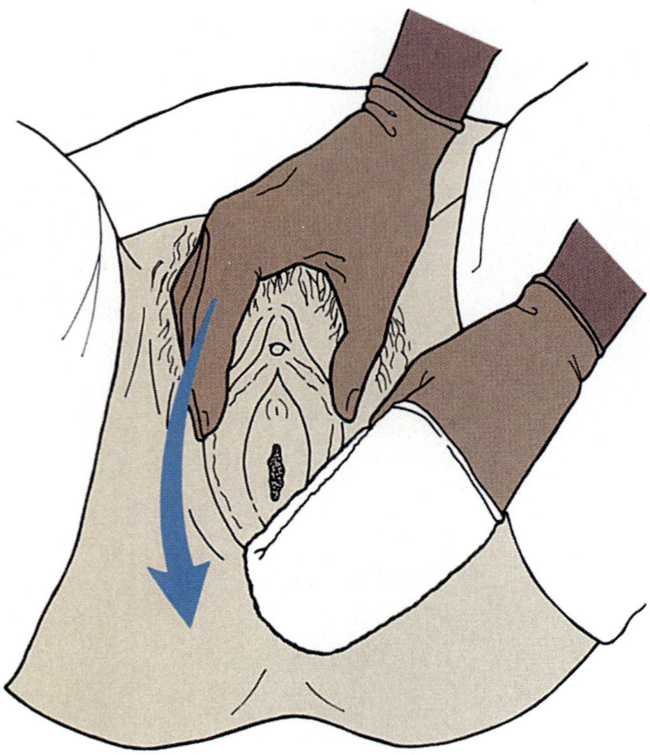

Fig. 13-25 *Perineal care is given to the female by separating the labia with one hand. The nursing assistant uses a mitted washcloth to cleanse between the labia with downward strokes.*

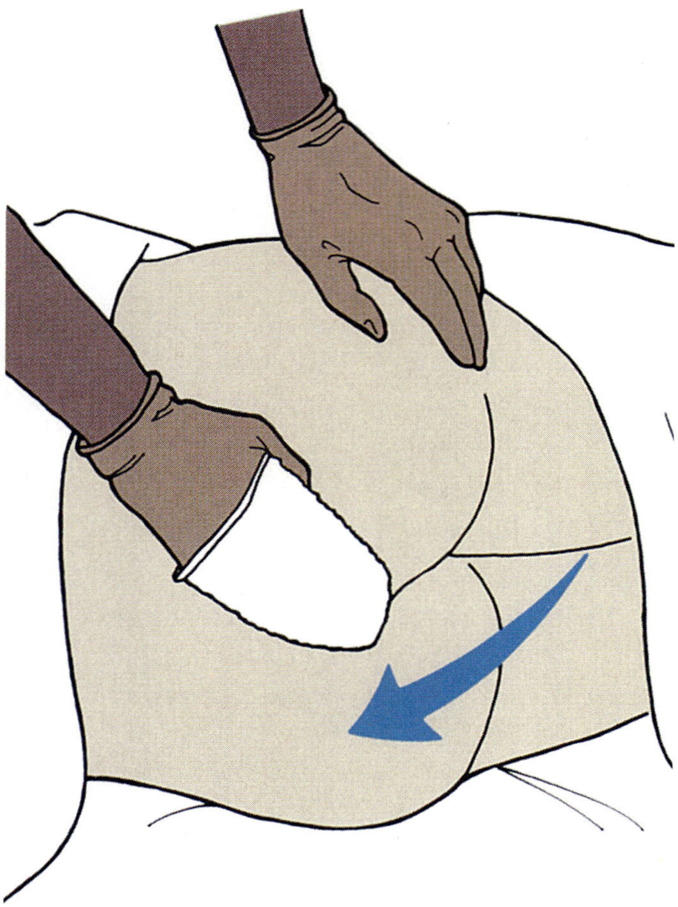

Fig. 13-26 *The rectal area is cleaned by wiping from the vagina to the anus. The side-lying position allows the anal area to be cleaned more thoroughly.*

Giving Male Perineal Care

Pre-procedure

1 Follow steps 1 through 21 in *Female Perineal Care*, p. 309.

Procedure

2 Retract the foreskin if the person is uncircumcised (Fig. 13-27).

3 Grasp the penis.

4 Clean the tip using a circular motion. Start at the urethral opening and work outward (Fig. 13-28). Repeat this step as necessary using a different part of the washcloth each time.

5 Rinse the area with another washcloth.

6 Return the foreskin to its natural position.

7 Clean the shaft of the penis with firm downward strokes. Rinse the area.

8 Help the person flex his knees and spread his legs.

9 Clean the scrotum and rinse well.

10 Pat dry the penis and scrotum.

11 Fold the bath blanket back between his legs.

12 Help him lower his legs and turn onto his side away from you.

13 Clean the rectal area (see *Female Perineal Care*). Rinse and dry well.

14 Remove and discard the gloves.

Post-procedure

15 Follow steps 34 through 45 in *Female Perineal Care.*

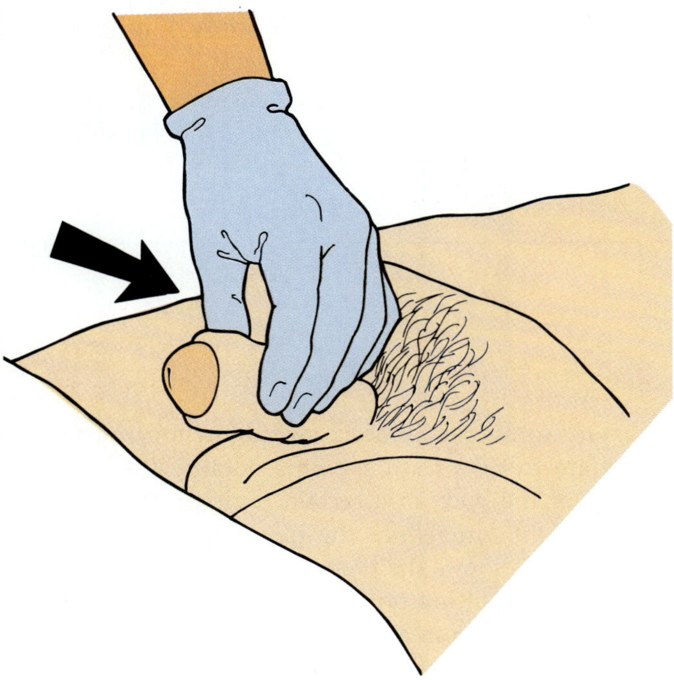

Fig. 13-27 *The foreskin of the uncircumcised male is pulled back for perineal care. It is returned to the normal position immediately after cleaning.*

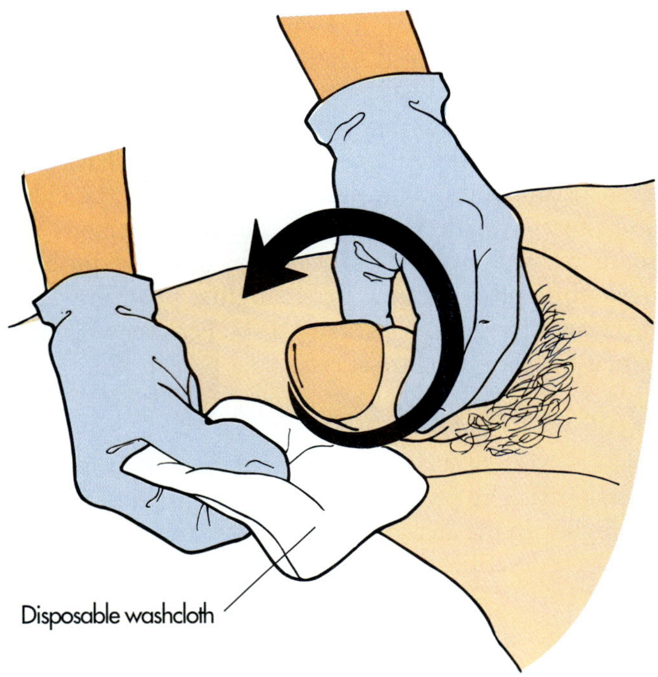

Fig. 13-28 *The penis is cleaned with circular motions starting at the urethra.*

PRESSURE SORES

Pressure sores (**decubitus ulcers** [decubiti], **bedsores, pressure ulcers**) are sores or ulcers in the skin over a bony prominence. Prominence means to stick out. Therefore a bony prominence is an area where the bone sticks out or projects out from the flat surface of the body. The shoulder blades, elbows, hip bones, sacrum, knees, ankle bone, heels, and toes are bony prominences.

Causes

Pressure, friction, and shearing are common causes of skin breakdown and pressure sores. Other factors include breaks in the skin, poor circulation to an area, moisture, dry skin, and irritation by urine and feces.

Pressure occurs when the skin over a bony prominence is squeezed between hard surfaces. The bone itself is one hard surface. The other is usually the mattress. The squeezing or pressure prevents blood flow to the skin and underlying tissues. Lack of blood flow means oxygen and nutrients cannot get to the cells. Therefore the involved skin and tissues die (Fig. 13-29).

Friction scrapes the skin. The scrape is an open area that is a portal of entry for microorganisms. The open area needs to heal. A good blood supply to the area is necessary. Infection must be prevented so healing occurs. A poor blood supply or an infection can lead to a pressure sore.

Shearing is when the skin sticks to a surface (usually the bed or chair) and deeper tissues move downward (see Fig. 10-8, page 219). This occurs when a person is sitting in a chair or in Fowler's position. Shearing occurs when the person slides down in the bed or chair. Blood vessels and tissues are damaged. Therefore blood flow to the area is reduced.

Elderly, obese, and very thin and malnourished persons are at risk for pressure sores. So are those who have problems sensing pain or pressure. This includes the elderly and those with nervous system disorders. Persons with some nervous system disorders or mobility problems have difficulty moving or changing positions. That increases their risk for pressure sores. Persons with circulatory problems also are at risk.

Signs of Pressure Sores

The first sign of a decubitus ulcer is pale skin or a reddened area. The person may complain of pain, burning, or tingling in the area. Some do not feel anything unusual. Box 13-3 describes the four stages of pressure sore development.

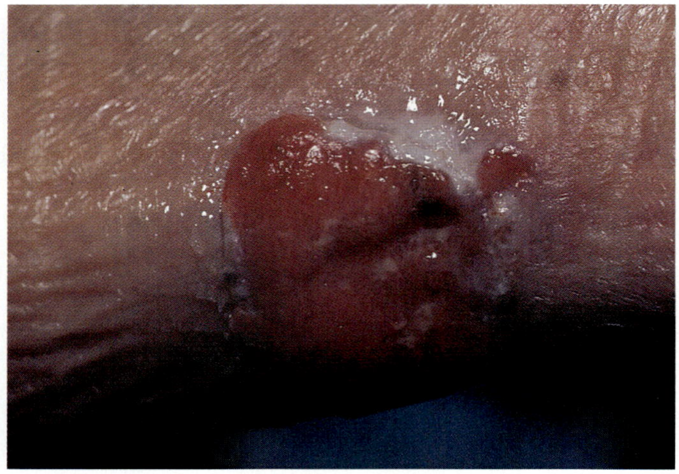

Fig. 13-29 *A pressure sore.*

BOX 13-3 STAGES OF PRESSURE SORES

Stage 1	The skin is red. The color does not return to normal when the skin is relieved of pressure (Fig. 13-30, A).
Stage 2	The skin cracks, blisters, or peels (Fig. 13-30, B). There may be a shallow crater.
Stage 3	The skin is gone and the underlying tissues are exposed (Fig. 13-30, C). The exposed tissue is damaged. There may be drainage from the area.
Stage 4	Muscle and bone are exposed and may be damaged (Fig. 13-30, D). Drainage is likely.

Sites

Pressure sores usually occur over bony areas. The bony areas are called pressure points because they bear the weight of the body in a certain position. Pressure from body weight can reduce the blood supply to the area. Figure 13-31 shows the pressure points for the bed positions and the sitting position. In obese people, pressure sores can develop in areas where skin is in contact with skin. Friction results when this occurs. Pressure sores can develop between abdominal folds, the legs, and the buttocks, and underneath the breasts.

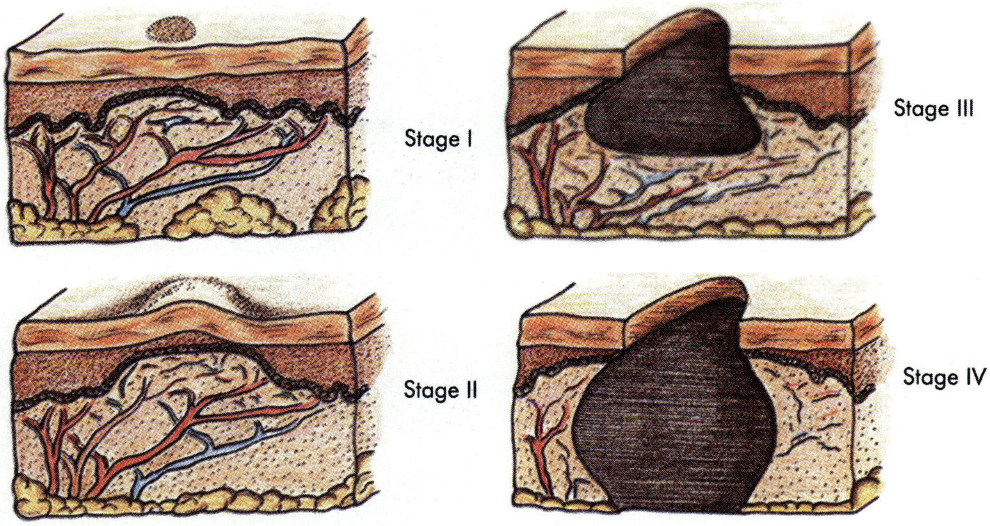

Fig. 13-30 *Stages of pressure sores. A, Stage 1. B, Stage 2. C, Stage 3. D, Stage 4.* (From Potter PA and Perry AG: Fundamentals of nursing: concepts, process, and practice, ed 3, St Louis, Mosby-Year Book.)

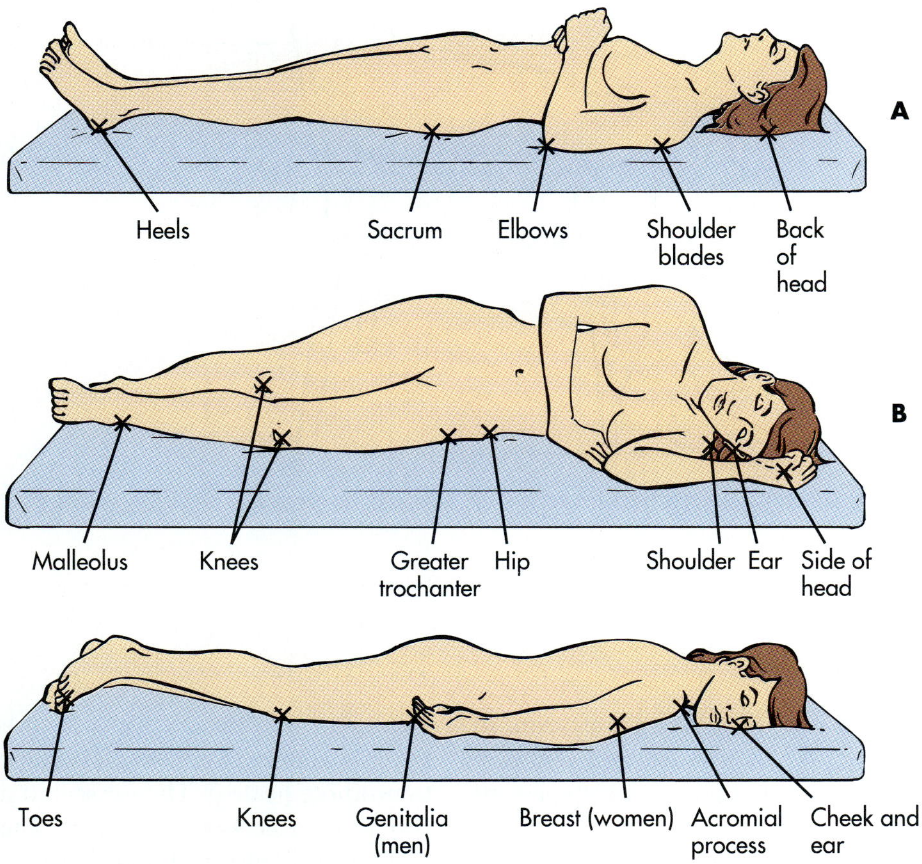

Fig. 13-31 *Pressure points. A, The supine position. B, The lateral position. C, The prone position.* *Continued.*

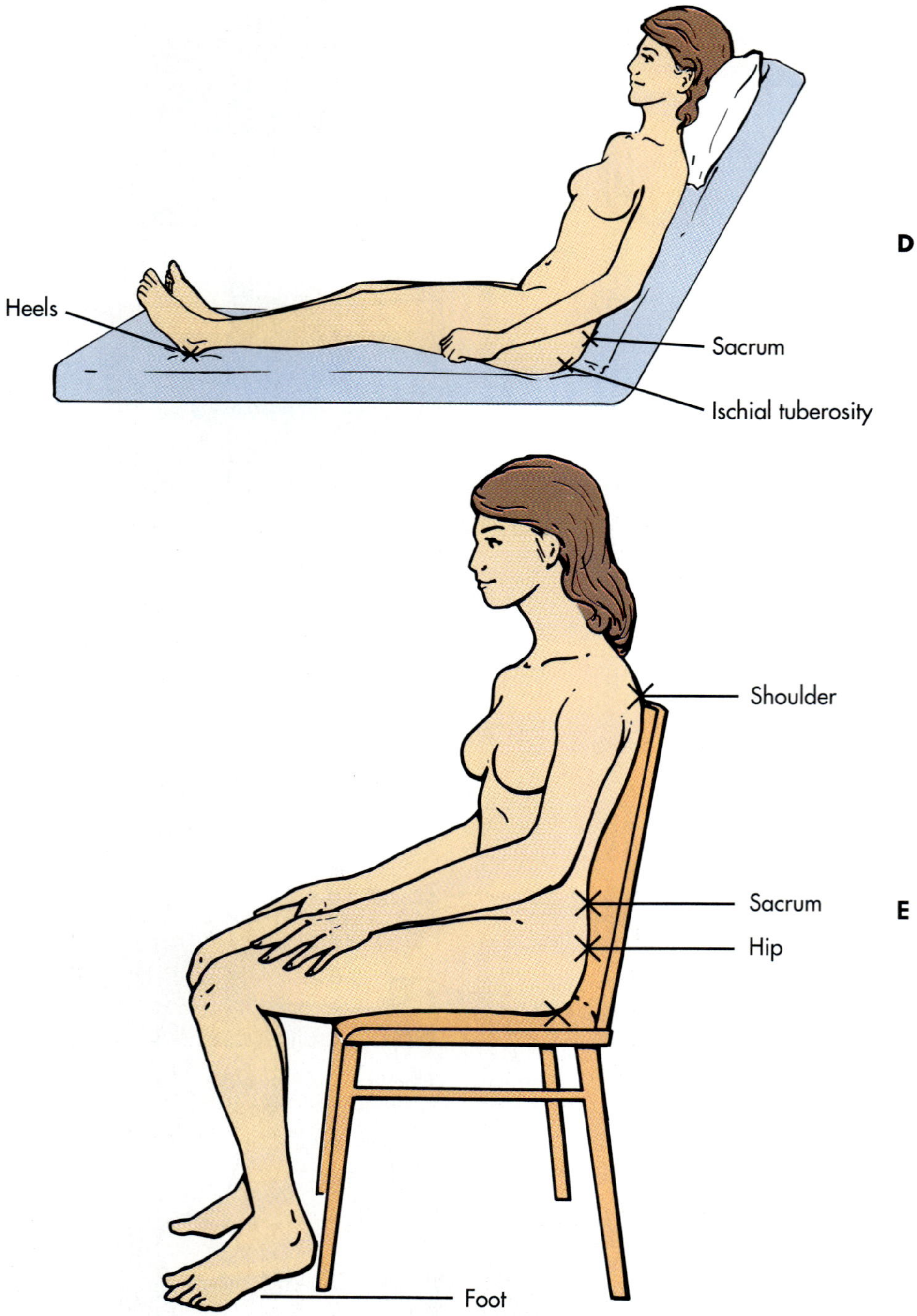

Fig. 13-31—cont'd *Pressure points. D, Fowler's position. E, The sitting position.*

Prevention

Preventing pressure sores is much easier than trying to heal them. Good nursing care, cleanliness, and skin care are essential. The measures listed in Box 13-4 help prevent skin breakdown and pressure sores.

Treatment

Treatment of pressure sores is directed by the doctor. Drugs, treatments, and special equipment may be ordered to promote healing. The nurse and nursing care plan tell you about a person's treatment. There is a lot of equipment available to treat and prevent pressure sores. Some are described in this section.

BOX 13-4 Measures to Prevent Pressure Sores

- Reposition the person at least every 2 hours or according to the schedule in the person's care plan. Some persons are repositioned every 15 minutes. Use pillows for support as instructed by the nurse.
- Prevent shearing and friction during lifting and moving procedures.
- Prevent shearing by not raising the head of the bed more than 30 degrees or as instructed by the nurse.
- Prevent friction by applying a thin layer of cornstarch to the bottom sheets.
- Provide good skin care. The skin must be clean and dry after bathing. Make sure the skin is free of moisture from urine, feces, and perspiration.
- Check incontinent persons (those without bowel or bladder control) often. Change linens and clothing as needed and provide good skin care.
- Check with the nurse before using soap on a person at risk for pressure sores. Remember, soap can dry and irritate the skin.
- Apply a moisturizer to dry areas such as the hands, elbows, legs, ankles, and heels. The nurse tells you what to use and the areas that need attention.
- Give a back massage when repositioning the person.
- Keep linens clean, dry, and free of wrinkles.
- Apply powder where skin touches skin.
- Do not irritate the skin. Avoid scrubbing or vigorous rubbing when bathing or drying the person.
- Avoid massaging over pressure points. *Never rub or massage reddened areas.*
- Use pillows and blankets to prevent skin from being in contact with skin and to reduce moisture and friction.
- Use protective devices as instructed by the nurse (see pages 315-317).
- Remind persons sitting in chairs to shift their positions every 15 minutes. This decreases pressure on bony points.
- Report any signs of skin breakdown or pressure sores immediately to the nurse.

Sheepskin Sheepskin (lamb's wool) is placed on the bottom sheet (Fig. 13-32). It protects the skin from the irritating bed linens. Friction is reduced between the skin and the bottom sheet. Air circulates between the tufts to help keep the skin dry. Sheepskin comes in many sizes for use under the shoulders, buttocks, or heels. It can also be placed in chair seats.

Bed cradle A bed cradle (Anderson frame) is a metal frame placed on the bed and over the patient or resident. Top linens are brought over the cradle to prevent pressure on the legs and feet (Fig. 13-33). Top linens are tucked in at the bottom of the mattress and mitered. They are also tucked under both sides of the mattress to protect the person from air drafts and chilling.

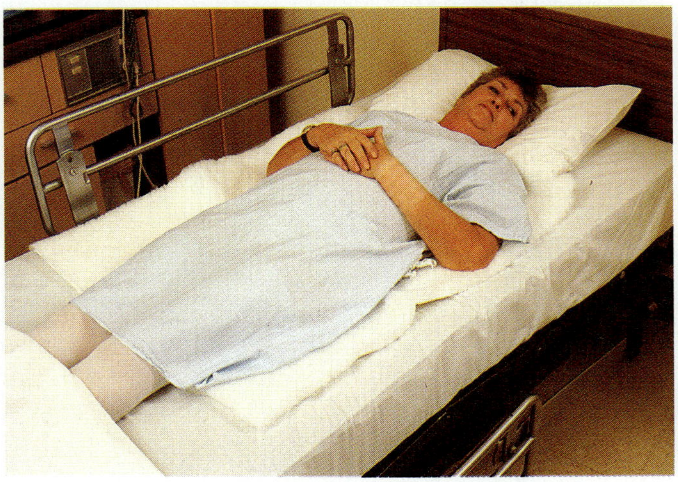

Fig. 13-32 *Sheepskin.*

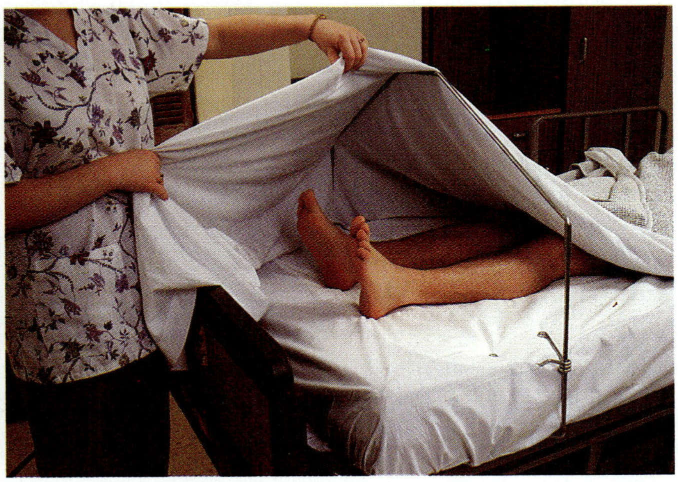

Fig. 13-33 *A bed cradle is placed on top of the bed. Linens are brought over the top of the cradle.*

A

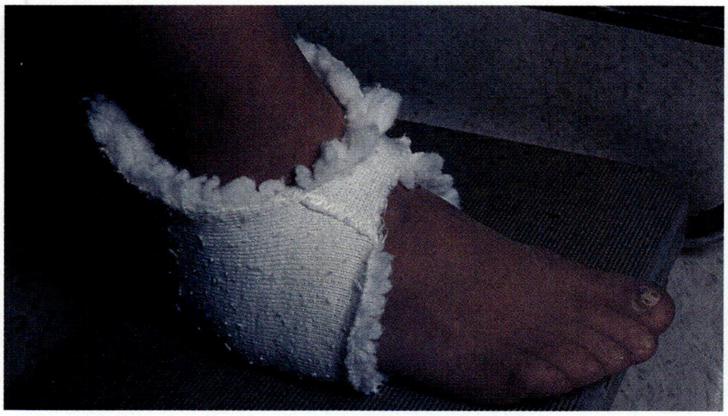

B

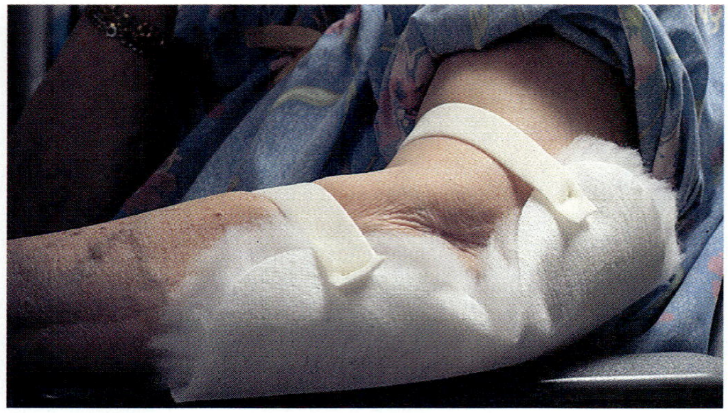

Fig. 13-34 *A, Heel protector. B, Elbow protectors.*

Heel and elbow protectors Heel and elbow protectors are made of foam rubber or sheepskin. They fit the shape of the heel or elbow (Fig. 13-34) and are secured in place with straps. Friction is prevented between the bed and the heel or elbow.

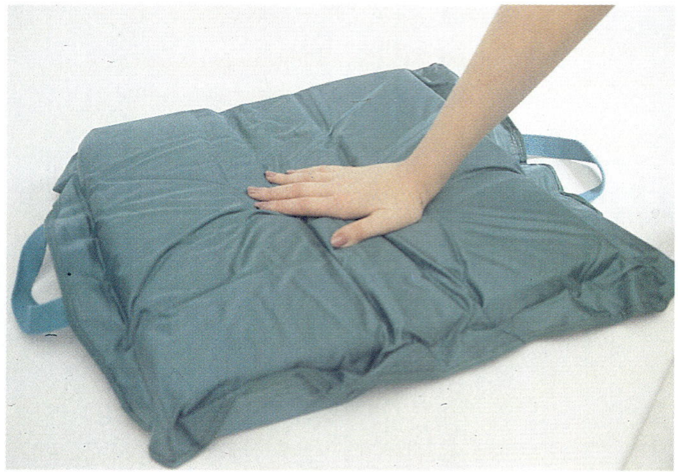

Fig. 13-35 *Flotation pad.*

Flotation pads Flotation pads or cushions (Fig. 13-35) are like water beds. They are made of a gel-like substance. The outer case is heavy plastic. They are used for chairs and wheelchairs. The pad is placed in a pillowcase so the plastic does not touch the skin.

Egg crate mattress The egg crate mattress is a foam pad that looks like an egg carton (Fig. 13-36). Peaks in the mattress distribute the person's weight more evenly. The egg crate mattress is placed on top of the regular mattress. Only a bottom sheet covers the egg crate mattress. Before the bottom sheet is put on, the egg crate mattress is put in a special cover. The cover protects against moisture and soiling.

Water bed or mattress A water bed or mattress lets the person *float* on top of the mattress (Fig. 13-37). Weight is distributed along the entire length of the body. Therefore pressure on bony points is avoided.

Alternating pressure mattress An alternating pressure mattress operates electrically. It has vertical tubelike sections (Fig. 13-38). Every other section is inflated with air. The other sections are deflated. Every 3 to 5 minutes the sections deflate or inflate automatically. Constant pressure on any area is avoided.

Only a bottom sheet is used with an alternating pressure mattress. Drawsheets and waterproof bed protectors are avoided. They add layers of material between the person and the air tubes. The air tubes should not be kinked. Pins are not used.

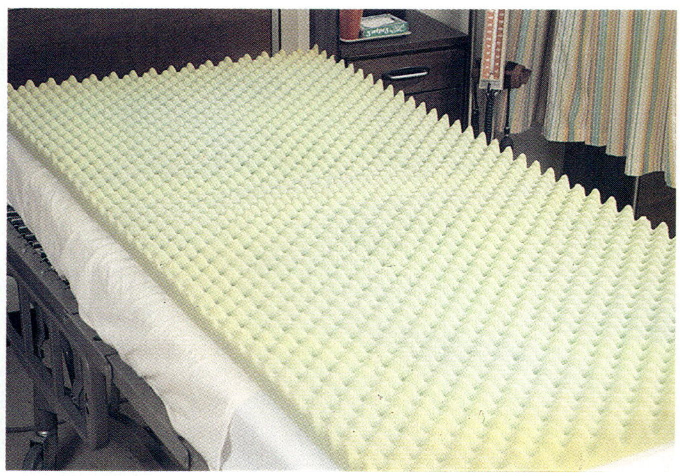

Fig. 13-36 *Egg crate mattress on the bed.*

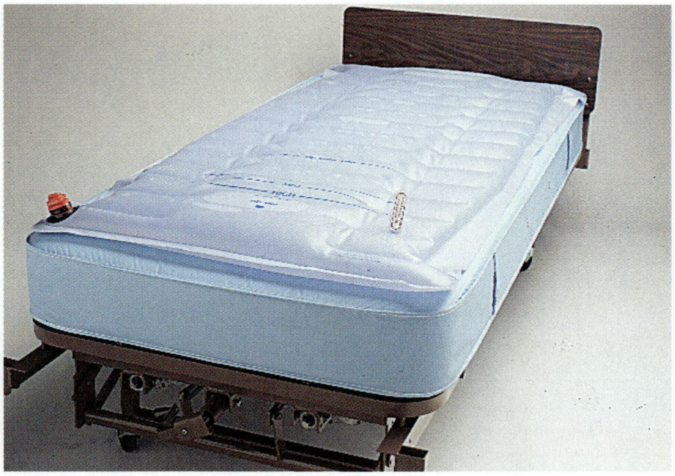

Fig. 13-37 *Water mattress. (Courtesy of Mason Medical Product Division of MRC Industries, Inc., Glendale, NY.)*

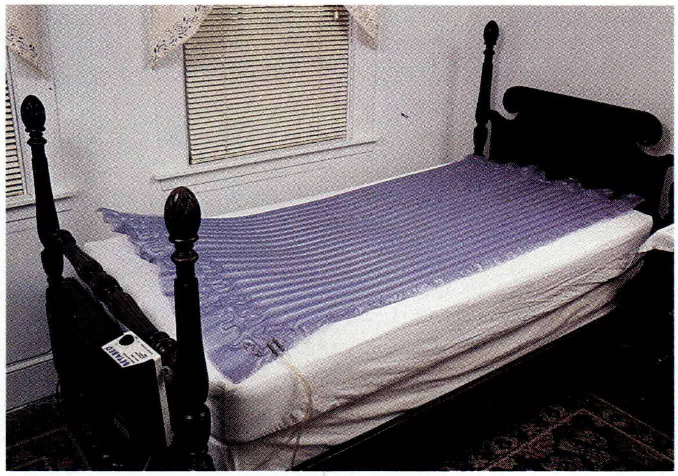

Fig. 13-38 *Alternating pressure mattress.*

Special beds There are many special beds available to prevent and treat pressure sores. Some beds have air flowing through the mattresses. The *person floats* on the mattress. Body weight is distributed evenly. There is little pressure on bony parts.

Another type of bed allows the person to be repositioned without moving. Depending on the bed, the person can be turned to the prone or supine position or titled various degrees. Body alignment does not change. Pressure points change as the position changes. There is little friction.

Some beds constantly rotate from side to side. These beds are useful for persons with spinal cord injuries.

Other equipment Trochanter rolls and footboards are also used to prevent and treat pressure sores. These are described in Chapter 19.

SUMMARY

Cleanliness and skin care are important. Physical and mental well-being are affected by good personal hygiene. Cultural and personal choice influence hygiene practices. Whenever possible, the person should make the choices.

The skin must be kept clean and intact. This promotes comfort and prevents infection. Oral hygiene, bathing, back massages, and perineal care are necessary measures. Patients and residents should do as much self-care as possible. You need to assist as necessary. Giving personal care provides a good time to get to know the person and to observe the skin.

Pressure sores result from poor nursing and skin care. They are very hard to heal. The sores can have serious effects on the person and can cause death. The person faces long nursing and medical care. Bills from such care can cause a financial burden. You must practice measures to prevent pressure sores. Should they occur, follow the nurse's directions for treating them. Remember, it is easier to prevent pressure sores than to treat and heal them.

Review Questions

Circle T *if the answer is true or* F *if the answer is false.*

1 T F Cleanliness and skin care are needed for comfort, safety, and health.

2 T F Mrs. Boyd asks for a back massage as part of HS care. It is okay to reply that a back massage is given only during morning care.

3 T F Mrs. Boyd's toothbrush has hard bristles. They are good for oral hygiene.

4 T F Unconscious persons are supine for mouth care.

5 T F Your fingers are used to keep an unconscious person's mouth open for oral hygiene.

6 T F Mrs. Boyd has a lower denture. It is washed in warm water over a hard surface.

7 T F Bath oils cleanse and soften the skin.

8 T F Powders absorb moisture and prevent friction.

9 T F Deodorants reduce the amount of perspiration.

10 T F The nurse says that Mrs. Boyd can have a tub bath. Mrs. Boyd says that she usually takes half-hour baths at home. You can allow her to take a 30-minute bath.

11 T F You can give permission for showers, but not tub baths.

12 T F Weak persons can be left alone in the shower if they are sitting.

13 T F A back massage relaxes muscles and stimulates circulation.

14 T F Perineal care helps prevent infection.

15 T F A reddened area is the first sign of a pressure sore.

16 T F Bony areas are the common sites for pressure sores.

17 T F Shearing and friction can cause pressure sores.

REVIEW QUESTIONS—CONT'D

Circle the best *answer.*

18 Oral hygiene is part of
- **a** AM care and HS care
- **b** Morning care
- **c** Care given after lunch
- **d** All of the above

19 You note the following after Mrs. Boyd's teeth are brushed. Which are reported to the nurse?
- **a** Bleeding, swelling, or redness of the gums
- **b** Irritations, sores, or white patches in the mouth or on the tongue
- **c** Lips that are dry, cracked, swollen, or blistered
- **d** All of the above

20 Which is *not* a purpose of bathing?
- **a** Increasing circulation
- **b** Promoting drying of the skin
- **c** Exercising body parts
- **d** Refreshing and relaxing the person

21 Soaps do the following *except*
- **a** Remove dirt and dead skin
- **b** Remove pigment
- **c** Remove skin oil and perspiration
- **d** Dry the skin

22 Which action is *wrong* when bathing Mrs. Boyd?
- **a** Cover her for warmth and privacy.
- **b** Rinse her skin thoroughly to remove all soaps.
- **c** Wash from the dirtiest to cleanest area.
- **d** Pat her skin dry.

23 Water for Mrs. Boyd's complete bed bath should be at least
- **a** 100° F
- **b** 105° F
- **c** 110° F
- **d** 120° F

24 You are going to give Mrs. Boyd a back massage. Which is *false?*
- **a** The massage should last about 5 minutes.
- **b** Lotion is warmed before being applied.
- **c** Your hands are always in contact with the skin.
- **d** The side-lying position is best.

25 Which will *not* prevent pressure sores?
- **a** Repositioning the person every 2 hours
- **b** Applying lotion to dry areas
- **c** Scrubbing and rubbing the skin vigorously
- **d** Keeping bed linens clean, dry, and free of wrinkles

Answers to these questions are on page 750

Personal Care and Grooming

14

OBJECTIVES

- Define the key terms listed in this chapter
- Explain the importance of hair care
- Identify the factors that affect hair care
- Explain how to care for matted and tangled hair
- Describe ways to shampoo a person
- Explain why shaving is important
- Identify the measures that are practiced when shaving a person
- Explain why nail and foot care are important
- Explain why wearing makeup is important to women
- Describe the rules for changing hospital gowns and clothing
- Perform the procedures described in this chapter

KEY TERMS

alopecia Hair loss

dandruff The excessive amount of dry, white flakes from the scalp

hirsutism Excessive body hair in women and children

pediculosis (lice) The infestation with lice

pediculosis capitis The infestation of the scalp (capitis) with lice

pediculosis corporis The infestation of the body (corporis) with lice

pediculosis pubis The infestation of the pubic (pubis) hair with lice

Cleanliness and skin care meet basic physical and safety and security needs. Clean and intact skin protects against infection. Procedures such as bathing and back massage promote circulation and exercise. They also promote comfort and relaxation. For many people, being clean is necessary for love and belonging and esteem needs.

Additional personal care and grooming measures are important to many people. Such measures include hair care, shaving, nail care, and dressing. While these are all activities of daily living, the attention given to such measures varies greatly among people. Some are only concerned with having clean hair. Others want hair styled in a certain way. Clean hands may be enough for some people. Others want nails clean, manicured, and polished. Being shaved or having a groomed beard is important to many men. Likewise, many women want their legs and underarms shaved.

These measures are less important to those who are very weak and ill. A simple bath may take much energy. Acutely ill persons usually are concerned with the basic physical needs necessary for survival. However, interest in other personal care and grooming measures usually increases as the person gains strength. Long-term care residents and disabled persons usually are interested in personal care and grooming. Although they have chronic health care problems, they generally maintain a certain level of health. Besides physical needs, they can focus on the higher-level needs of safety and security, love and belonging, esteem, and self-actualization.

HAIR CARE

Appearance and mental well-being are affected by how the hair looks and feels. Illness and disability can interfere with hair care. Patients and residents are assisted with hair care whenever necessary. Some nursing facilities have barbers and beauticians for cutting, shampooing, and styling hair.

The nurse uses the nursing process to meet the person's hair care needs. Culture, personal choice, condition of the skin and scalp, health history, and self-care ability are among the factors considered by the nurse. Certain terms may be used in the person's medical record and nursing care plan. You need to be familiar with the following:

- **Alopecia** means hair loss. Hair loss may be complete or partial. Male pattern baldness occurs with aging and is due to heredity. Thinning of hair occurs in some women with aging. Cancer treatments (radiation therapy to the head and chemotherapy) often cause alopecia in both men and women. Skin disease is another cause. Other causes include stress, poor nutrition, pregnancy, some drugs, and hormone changes. Except for hair loss from aging, the hair grows back in many cases.

- **Hirsutism** is excessive body hair in women and children. The condition is due to heredity and abnormal amounts of male hormones.
- **Dandruff** is the excessive amount of dry, white flakes from the scalp. Itching often occurs. Sometimes the eyebrows and ear canals are involved. Medicated shampoo can correct the problem.
- **Pediculosis (lice)** is the infestation with lice. Lice are parasites. The infestation causes severe itching in the affected body area from the lice bites. **Pediculosis capitis** is the infestation of the scalp (capitis) with lice. **Pediculosis pubis** is the infestation of the pubic (pubis) hair with lice. Both head and pubic lice attach their eggs to hair shafts. **Pediculosis corporis** is the infestation of the body (corporis) with lice. Lice eggs attach to clothing and furniture. Lice easily spread to other persons through clothing, furniture, bed linen, and sexual contact. Medicated shampoos, lotions, and creams are used to treat lice. Thorough bathing and washing clothing and linen in hot water are also necessary.

Brushing and Combing Hair

Brushing and combing a person's hair are part of morning care. They are also done as needed during the day. Many people want their hair styled before visitors arrive. Encourage patients and residents to do their own hair care. However, you must assist as needed. Hair care is performed for those who cannot do so. Let the person choose how hair is to be brushed, combed, and styled.

Long hair is easily matted and tangled. Daily brushing

Brushing and Combing a Person's Hair

Pre-procedure

1. Identify the person. Check the ID bracelet and call the person by name.
2. Explain the procedure to the person.
3. Collect the following:
   - Comb and brush
   - Bath towel
   - Hair care items as requested by the person
4. Arrange items on the bedside stand.
5. Wash your hands.
6. Provide for privacy.

Procedure

7. Lower the side rail.
8. Help the person to a chair or to Fowler's position if possible. The person puts on a robe and nonskid slippers if to be up.
9. Place a towel across the shoulders or across the pillow if the person is in bed.
10. Ask the person to remove eyeglasses. Put them in the glass case. Put the case inside the bedside stand.
11. Part hair into 2 sections (Fig. 14-1, A). Divide one side into 2 sections (Fig. 14-1, B).
12. Brush the hair. Start at the scalp and brush toward the hair ends (Fig. 14-2).
13. Style the hair as the person prefers.
14. Remove the towel.
15. Let the person put on the eyeglasses.

Post-procedure

16. Assist him or her to a comfortable position.
17. Raise or lower side rails as instructed by the nurse.
18. Place the call bell within reach.
19. Unscreen the person.
20. Clean and return items to their proper place.
21. Follow facility policy for dirty linen.
22. Wash your hands.

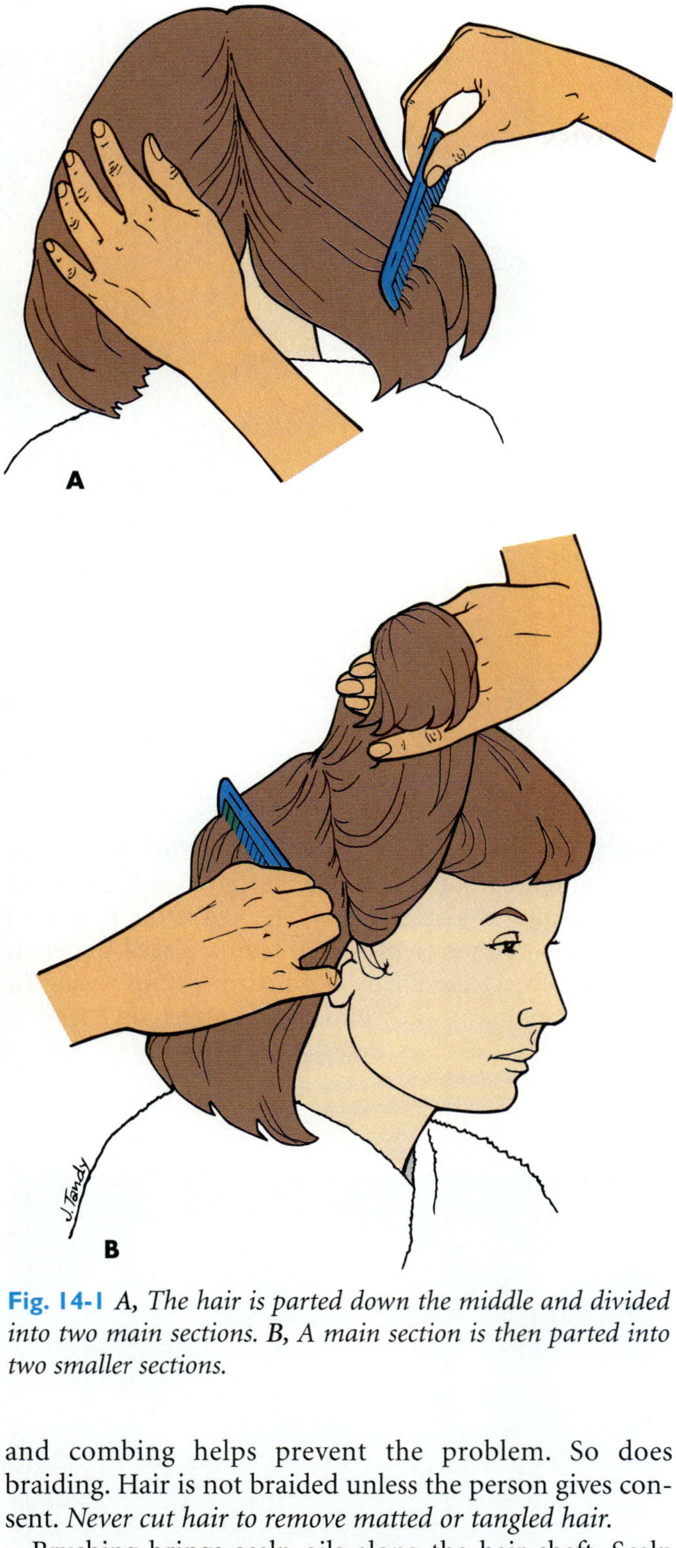

Fig. 14-1 *A, The hair is parted down the middle and divided into two main sections. **B,** A main section is then parted into two smaller sections.*

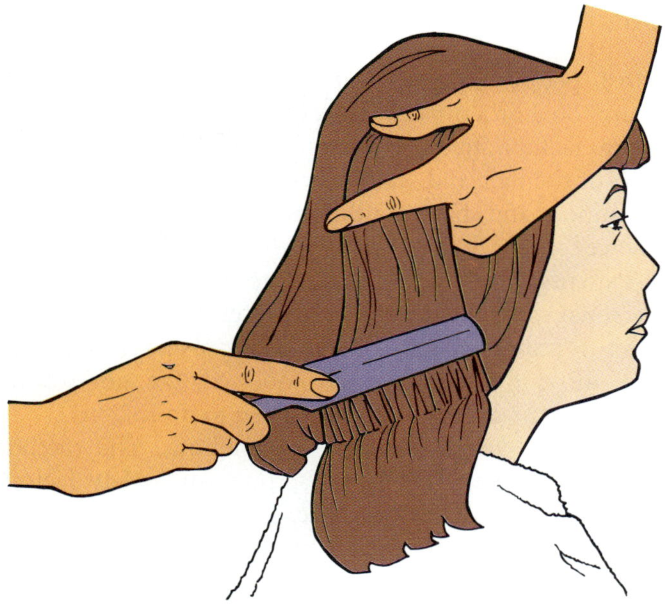

Fig. 14-2 *The hair is brushed by starting at the scalp and brushing toward the hair ends.*

and combing helps prevent the problem. So does braiding. Hair is not braided unless the person gives consent. *Never cut hair to remove matted or tangled hair.*

Brushing brings scalp oils along the hair shaft. Scalp oils help keep hair soft and shiny. Brushing and combing keep hair from tangling and matting. They also are used to style hair. When brushing and combing hair, start at the scalp. Then brush or comb to the hair ends. Be sure to consult with the nurse if the person has matted or tangled hair. Special measures may be needed. The nurse may ask you to comb or brush through the matting and tangling. This is done by taking a small section of hair near the ends and combing or brushing through to the hair ends. Working up to the scalp, small sections of hair are added. Comb or brush through each longer section to the hair ends. Finally, brush or comb from the scalp to the hair ends. *Never cut matted or tangled hair.*

Special measures are needed for curly, coarse, and dry hair. A wide-toothed comb is used for curly hair. Wetting the hair or applying a conditioner or petrolatum jelly makes combing easier. The person may have certain practices or use special hair care products. When planning for hair care, the nurse asks the patient or resident about personal preferences and routine hair care measures. These become part of the person's care plan. The person can guide you when giving hair care.

When giving hair care, a towel is placed across the shoulders to protect the person's gown or clothing. If hair care is given when the person is in bed, it is done before changing the pillowcase. If done after a linen change, place a towel across the pillow to collect falling hair.

Shampooing

Most people shampoo at least once a week. Some shampoo 2 or 3 times a week. Others shampoo every day. Many factors affect frequency. These include the condition of the hair and scalp, hairstyle, and personal choice. Shampoo and hair conditioner also involve personal choice.

Patients and residents often need help shampooing. Personal choice is followed whenever possible. However, safety is important and the nurse's approval is needed. Tell the nurse if a shampoo is requested. Do not wash a person's hair unless a nurse asks you to do so.

There are many shampooing methods. The method used depends on the person's condition, safety factors, and personal choice if possible. The nurse decides which method to use. Hair is dried and styled as quickly as possible after shampooing. Women may want hair curled or rolled up before drying. Consult with the nurse before curling or rolling up a person's hair.

Shampooing during the shower or tub bath Persons who shower can usually shampoo at the same time. Shampooing can also be done for those using shower chairs. A hand-held nozzle is used. It can also be used during a tub bath. A spray of water is directed to the hair. The person shampooing during a tub bath is likely to need some help. An extra towel, shampoo, and hair conditioner (if requested) are placed within the person's reach.

Shampooing at the sink Persons who can sit in a chair can usually be shampooed at a sink. The chair is placed so the person faces away from the sink. The person's head is tilted back over the edge of the sink. A folded towel is placed over the sink edge to protect the neck. A water pitcher or hand-held nozzle is used to wet and rinse the hair.

Shampooing a person on a stretcher The stretcher is positioned in front of a sink. A pillow is placed under the head and neck, and the head is tilted over the edge of the sink (Fig. 14-3). A water pitcher or hand-held nozzle is used to wet and rinse the hair. Safety measures include locking the stretcher wheels, using the safety straps, and raising the far side rail.

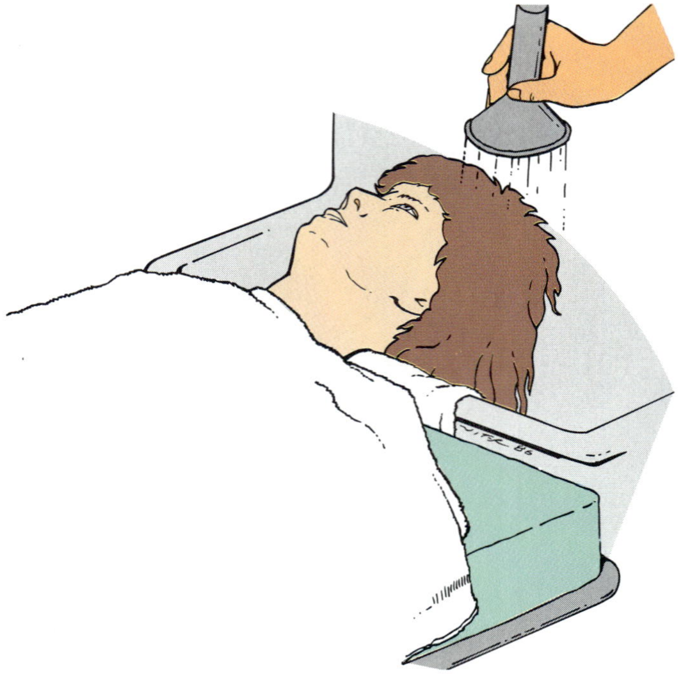

Fig. 14-3 *Shampooing while on a stretcher. The stretcher is in front of the sink.*

Shampooing a person in bed This method is for those who cannot be out of bed. The person's head and shoulders are moved to the edge of the bed if the position is allowed. A rubber or plastic trough is placed under the head to protect the linens and mattress from water. The trough also drains water into a basin placed on a chair by the bed (Fig. 14-4). A water pitcher is used to wet and rinse the hair.

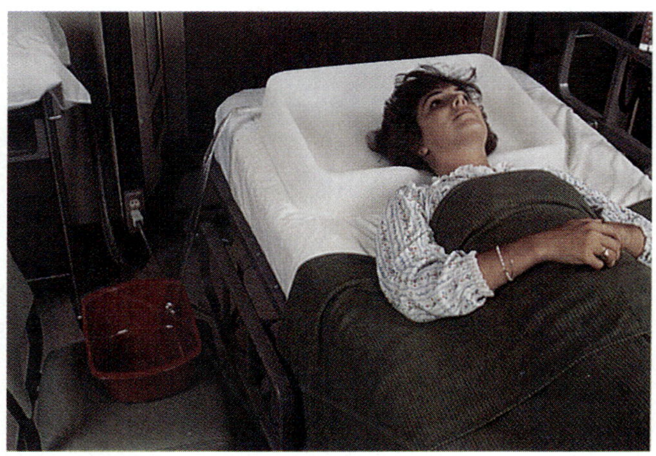

Fig. 14-4 *A trough is used when shampooing a person in bed. The trough is directed to the side of the bed so water drains into a collecting basin.*

Shampooing the Person's Hair

Pre-procedure

1 Explain the procedure to the person.

2 Wash your hands.

3 Collect the following:

- Two bath towels
- Face towel or washcloth folded lengthwise
- Shampoo
- Hair conditioner if requested
- Bath thermometer
- Pitcher or hand-held nozzle
- Equipment for the shampoo in bed (if needed)
  - *Trough
  - *Basin or pail
  - *Bath blanket
  - *Waterproof bed protector
- Comb and brush
- Hair dryer

4 Arrange items nearby.

5 Identify the person. Check the ID bracelet and call the person by name.

6 Provide for privacy.

Procedure

7 Position the person for the method you are going to use.

8 Place a bath towel across the shoulders or across the pillow under the person's head.

9 Brush and comb the hair to remove snarls and tangles.

10 Obtain water. Water temperature should be about 110° F (43° to 44° C).

11 Ask the person to hold the face towel or washcloth over the eyes.

12 Apply water until the hair is completely wet. Use the pitcher or nozzle.

13 Apply a small amount of shampoo.

14 Work up a lather with both hands. Start at the hairline and work toward the back.

15 Massage the scalp with your fingertips.

16 Rinse the hair.

17 Repeat steps 13 through 15.

18 Rinse the hair thoroughly.

19 Apply conditioner and rinse as directed on the container.

20 Wrap the person's head with a bath towel.

21 Dry his or her face with the towel or washcloth used to protect the eyes.

22 Help the person raise the head if appropriate.

23 Rub the hair and scalp with the towel. Use the second towel if the first is wet.

24 Comb the hair to remove snarls and tangles. A woman may want hair curled or rolled up.

25 Dry the hair as quickly as possible.

Post-procedure

26 Make sure the person is comfortable.

27 Place the call bell within reach.

28 Raise or lower side rails as instructed by the nurse.

29 Clean and return equipment to its proper place. Discard disposable items.

30 Follow facility policy for dirty linen.

31 Wash your hands.

BOX 14-1 RULES FOR SHAVING

- Follow Standard Precautions and the Bloodborne Pathogen Standard.
- Protect the bed linens by placing a towel under the part being shaved.
- Make sure the skin is soft before shaving.
- Encourage the person to do as much for himself or herself as safely possible.
- Hold the skin taut as necessary.
- Shave in the direction of hair growth when shaving the male face and female underarms.
- Shave upward, starting at the ankle, when shaving legs.
- Rinse the body part thoroughly.
- Apply direct pressure to any nicks or cuts.
- Report nicks and cuts to the nurse immediately.

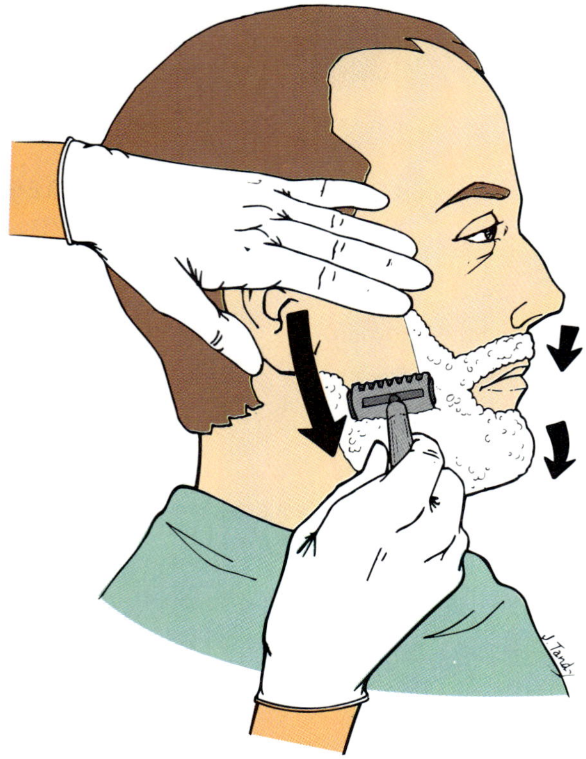

Fig. 14-5 *Shaving is done in the direction of hair growth. Longer strokes are used on the larger areas of the face. Short strokes are used around the chin and lips.*

SHAVING

A clean-shaven face is important for the comfort and well-being of many men. Likewise, many women shave their legs and underarms. Persons may prefer electric shavers or razor blades. When using an electric shaver, practice safety precautions for using electrical equipment. Razor blades can cause nicks or cuts. Standard Precautions and the Bloodborne Pathogen Standard are followed to prevent contact with the person's blood. Box 14-1 lists the measures that are followed when shaving men or the legs and underarms of women.

Shaving Men

The beard and skin are softened before shaving with a razor blade. The skin is softened by applying a warm washcloth or face towel to the face for a few minutes. Then lather the face with soap and water or a shaving cream. Be careful not to cut or irritate the skin while shaving.

Caring for Mustaches and Beards

Beards and mustaches need daily care. Food can collect in beards and mustaches. So can drainage from the mouth and nose. A beard and mustache must be kept clean. Daily washing and combing are usually enough to keep them clean. Ask the person how he wants his beard or mustache groomed. *Never trim or shave a beard or mustache without the person's consent.*

Shaving Female Legs and Underarms

Many women shave their legs and underarms. This practice varies among cultures. Personal choice is a factor. Some women shave only the lower legs. Others choose to shave to the mid-thigh while others shave the entire leg. Some women only shave their legs in the summer months when the legs are exposed.

Women's legs and underarms can be shaved during or after the tub bath or shower when the skin is soft. Shaving can also be part of the complete bed bath. Soap and water or a shaving cream are used for lather. Needed shaving items are collected with the bath items. The areas are shaved after they are washed. You may want to use the kidney basin to rinse the razor rather than using the bath water.

Shaving underarms and legs is similar to shaving the male face. You need to practice the measures in Box 14-1.

Shaving a Man

Pre-procedure

1 Explain the procedure to the person.
2 Wash your hands.
3 Collect the following:
- Wash basin
- Bath towel
- Face towel
- Washcloth
- Bath thermometer
- Razor or shaver
- Mirror
- Shaving cream or soap
- Shaving brush
- After-shave lotion
- Tissues
- Paper towel
- Disposable gloves

4 Arrange items on the overbed table.
5 Identify the person. Check the ID bracelet and call the person by name.
6 Provide for privacy.
7 Raise the bed to the best level for good body mechanics.

Procedure

8 Fill the wash basin. Water temperature should be about 115° F (46° C).
9 Place the basin on the overbed table on top of the paper towels.
10 Lower the side rail.
11 Position the person in semi-Fowler's position if allowed or on his back.
12 Adjust lighting so you can clearly see the person's face.
13 Place the bath towel over his chest.
14 Position the overbed table within easy reach and at a comfortable working height.
15 Put on the gloves.
16 Wash the person's face. Do not dry.
17 Place a washcloth or face towel in the water and wet it thoroughly. Wring it out.
18 Apply the washcloth or towel to the face to soften the beard. Remove it after 3 to 5 minutes.
19 Apply shaving cream to the face with your hands. Use a shaving brush if using soap for lather.
20 Tighten the razor blade to the razor.
21 Hold the skin taut with one hand.
22 Shave in the direction of hair growth. Use shorter strokes around the chin and lips (Fig. 14-5).
23 Rinse the razor often and wipe with tissues.
24 Apply direct pressure to any bleeding areas.
25 Wash off any remaining shaving cream or soap. Dry with a towel.
26 Apply after-shave lotion if requested.
27 Remove the towel.
28 Remove the gloves.
29 Move the overbed table to the side of the bed.

Post-procedure

30 Make sure the person is comfortable.
31 Place the call bell within reach.
32 Lower the bed to its lowest position.
33 Raise or lower side rails as instructed by the nurse.
34 Clean and return equipment and supplies to their proper place. Discard disposable items.
35 Wipe off the overbed table with the paper towels. Discard the paper towels.
36 Position the table as appropriate for the person.
37 Unscreen the person.
38 Follow facility policy for dirty linen.
39 Wash your hands.
40 Report any nicks or bleeding to the nurse.

CARE OF NAILS AND FEET

Nails and feet need special attention to prevent infection, injury, and odors. Hangnails, ingrown nails (nails that grow in at the side), and nails torn away from the skin cause breaks in the skin. These breaks are portals of entry for microbes. Long or broken nails can scratch skin or snag clothing.

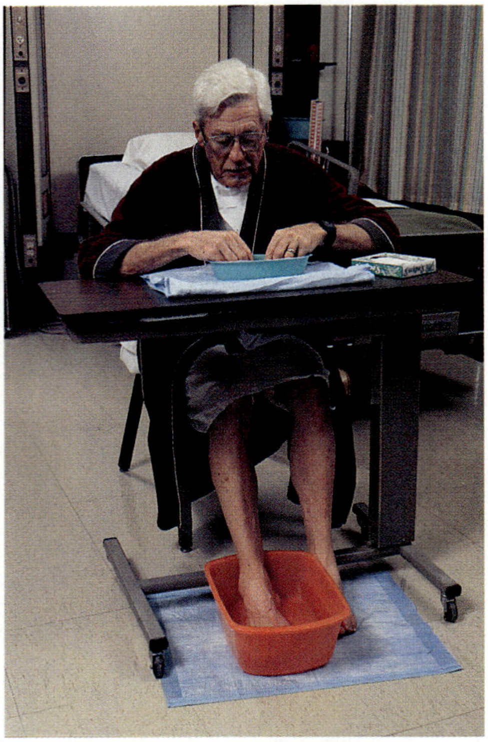

Fig. 14-6 *Nail and foot care. The feet soak in a foot basin, and the fingers soak in a kidney basin.*

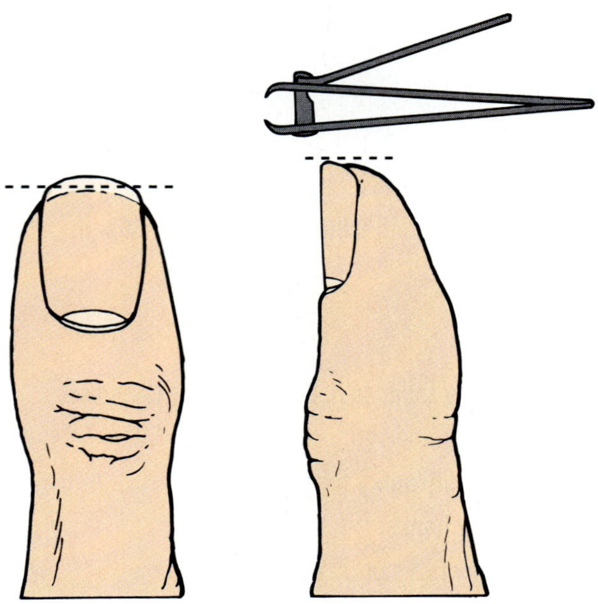

Fig. 14-7 *Fingernails are clipped straight across. A nail clipper is used.*

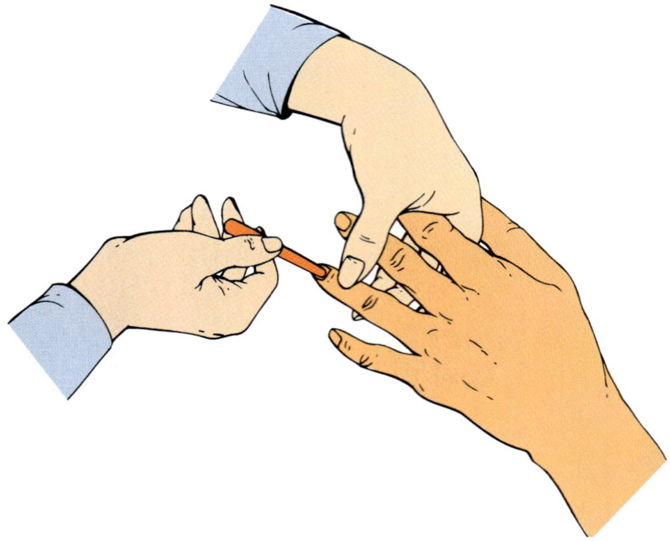

Fig. 14-8 *The cuticle is pushed back with an orange stick.*

The feet are easily infected and injured. Dirty feet, socks, or stockings harbor microbes and cause odors. Shoes and socks provide a warm, moist environment for the growth of microbes. Injuries occur from stubbing toes, stepping on sharp objects, or being stepped on by others. Blisters develop from shoes that fit poorly. Healing is prolonged in persons with poor circulation to the feet. Diabetes mellitus and vascular disease are common causes of poor circulation. Infections or foot injuries are particularly serious for the elderly and persons with circulatory disorders. Gangrene and amputation of the part are serious complications (see Chapter 28). Trimming and clipping toenails can easily result in injuries. *Therefore nursing assistants do not cut or trim toenails.*

Cleaning and trimming fingernails is easier after they have been soaked. Nail clippers are used to cut fingernails. Scissors are never used. Extreme caution is taken when clipping and trimming fingernails to prevent damage to surrounding tissues. Also, check with the nurse about the desired water temperature. The feet are easily burned. Persons with decreased sensation or circulatory problems may not feel hot temperatures.

Giving Nail and Foot Care

Pre-procedure

1 Explain the procedure to the person.
2 Wash your hands.
3 Collect the following:
- Wash basin
- Bath thermometer
- Bath towel
- Face towel
- Washcloth
- Kidney basin
- Nail clippers
- Orange stick
- Emery board or nail file
- Lotion or petrolatum jelly
- Paper towels
- Disposable bath mat

4 Arrange items on the overbed table.
5 Identify the person. Check the ID bracelet and call the person by name.
6 Provide for privacy.

Procedure

7 Help the person to a bedside chair. Place the call bell within reach.
8 Place the bath mat under the feet.
9 Fill the wash basin. Water temperature should be 105° (40° C) unless otherwise instructed by the nurse.
10 Place the basin on the bath mat. Help the person put the feet into the basin.
11 Position the overbed table in front of the person. It should be low and close to the person.
12 Fill the kidney basin. Water temperature should be 105° to 110° F (40° to 43° C).
13 Place the basin on the overbed table on top of the paper towels.
14 Place the person's fingers into the basin. Position the arms so he or she is comfortable (Fig. 14-6).
15 Let the feet and fingernails soak for 10 to 20 minutes. Rewarm the water as needed.
16 Clean under the fingernails with the orange stick.
17 Remove the kidney basin and dry the fingers thoroughly.
18 Clip fingernails straight across with the nail clippers (Fig. 14-7).
19 Shape nails with an emery board or nail file.
20 Push cuticles back with the orange stick or a washcloth (Fig. 14-8).
21 Move the overbed table to the side.
22 Scrub callused areas of the feet with a washcloth.
23 Remove the feet from the basin. Dry thoroughly.
24 Apply lotion or petrolatum jelly to the feet.

Post-procedure

25 Assist the person back to bed and to a comfortable position. Place the call bell within reach.
26 Raise or lower side rails as instructed by the nurse.
27 Clean and return equipment and supplies to their proper place. Discard disposable items.
28 Unscreen the person.
29 Follow facility policy for dirty linen.
30 Wash your hands.
31 Report your observations to the nurse:
- Reddened, irritated, or callused areas
- Breaks in the skin

APPLYING MAKEUP

Wearing makeup is important to many women. Usually makeup is worn to enhance beauty and attractiveness. For others, it is worn to mask skin blemishes. Wearing makeup is often a cultural practice. Whatever the reason it is worn, makeup can improve one's body image and sense of esteem. So can wearing a fragrance such as a perfume or cologne.

Every women has her own routine for applying makeup. Usually it is part of daily routine hygiene measures. For others, makeup is only applied for work, school, or social events. Acutely ill persons may not think about applying makeup. However, interest may increase as strength is gained. You may need to assist patients and residents with applying makeup. Sometimes you need to apply makeup for the person.

You need to follow the woman's routine. Personal choice is important. She knows what cosmetics to use, how she wants them applied, and the order of application. Be sure to give her a mirror so she can see how you are applying the makeup. Also offer to touch up makeup during afternoon and evening care. Many women reapply blush and lipstick many times during the day.

Spotlight On...

Sheila A of Davenport, Iowa, *works as a nursing assistant in a postcardiac care unit. Her nurse manager describes her as "a person who is punctual and can always be counted on. She has excellent skills related to patients' personal hygiene, always turns her patients at least every 2 hours, and goes above and beyond in the personal grooming of patients. Her caring attitude and professionalism is respected by her peers, patients, and families. Sheila has good organizational skills and never leaves her work undone. Her confidence and pride in her work cause her to often recommend improvements in the care of patients."*

CHANGING HOSPITAL GOWNS AND CLOTHING

Hospital gowns or pajamas are changed after the bath and when wet or soiled. Persons who wear regular clothing during the day change into a gown or pajamas for bed. Then they dress in the morning. Patients and residents may need help with these activities. The following rules are followed:

- Provide for privacy. Do not expose the person.
- Encourage the person to do as much as possible.
- Allow the person to choose what to wear.
- Remove clothing from the strong or *good* side first.
- Put clothing on the weak side first.

Changing Hospital Gowns

Special measures are needed for arm injuries, paralysis, or IV infusions. If there is injury or paralysis, the gown is removed from the good arm first. The weak arm is supported while removing the gown. The clean gown is put on the weak arm first and then on the good arm.

Some facilities have special gowns for persons receiving IV infusions. The gowns open along the entire sleeve and close with ties or snaps. Standard hospital gowns may be used for persons with IV infusions.

CHANGING THE GOWN OF A PERSON WITH AN IV

PRE-PROCEDURE

1 Explain the procedure to the person.
2 Wash your hands.
3 Get a clean gown.
4 Identify the person. Check the ID bracelet and call the person by name.
5 Provide for privacy.

PROCEDURE

6 Untie the back of the gown. Free parts of the gown that the person is lying on.
7 Remove the gown from the arm with no IV.
8 Gather up the sleeve of the arm with the IV. Slide it over the IV site and tubing. Remove the arm and hand from the sleeve (Fig. 14-9, A on page 332).
9 Keep the sleeve gathered. Slide your arm along the tubing to the bottle (Fig. 14-9, B on page 332).
10 Remove the bottle from the pole. Slide the bottle and tubing through the sleeve (Fig. 14-9, C on page 332). Do not pull on the tubing. Keep the bottle above the person's arm.
11 Hang the IV bottle on the pole.
12 Gather the sleeve of the clean gown that will go on the arm with the IV infusion.
13 Remove the bottle from the pole. Quickly slip the gathered sleeve over the bottle at the shoulder part of the gown (Fig. 14-9, D on page 332). Hang the bottle on the pole.
14 Slide the gathered sleeve over the tubing, hand, arm, and IV site. Then slide the sleeve onto the person's shoulder.
15 Put the other side of the gown on the person.
16 Fasten the back of the gown.

POST-PROCEDURE

17 Make sure the person is comfortable.
18 Place the call bell within reach.
19 Lower the bed to its lowest position.
20 Raise or lower side rails as instructed by the nurse.
21 Unscreen the person.
22 Follow facility policy for dirty linen.
23 Wash your hands.
24 Ask the nurse to check the IV flow rate.

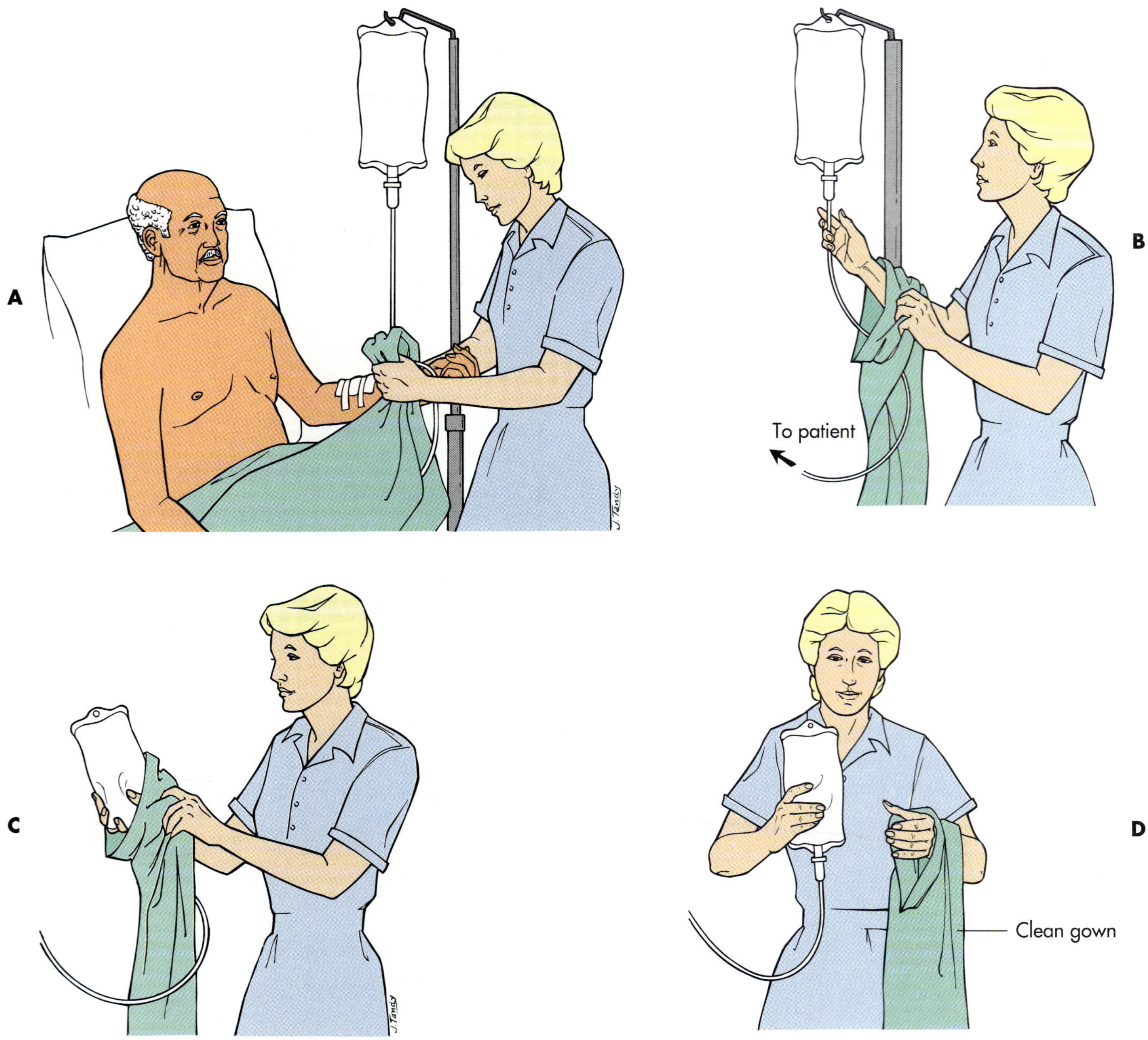

Fig. 14-9 *A, The gown is removed from the good arm. The sleeve on the arm with the IV is gathered up, slipped over the IV site and tubing, and removed from the arm and hand. B, The gathered sleeve is slipped along the IV tubing to the bag. C, The IV bag is removed from the pole and passed through the sleeve. D, The gathered sleeve of the clean gown is slipped over the IV bag at the shoulder part of the gown.*

Dressing and Undressing

Clothing changes are usually necessary on admission and discharge. Some people enter and leave the facility in a gown or pajamas. However, most wear street clothes. Nursing facility residents and persons receiving home care often wear street clothes during the day. Some persons and residents dress and undress themselves. Others need some help. The rules listed on page 333 and 338 are followed when dressing or undressing individuals.

Text continued on page 340.

Undressing a Person

Pre-procedure

1 Explain the procedure to the person.

2 Wash your hands.

3 Get a bath blanket.

4 Identify the person. Check the ID bracelet and call the person by name.

5 Provide for privacy.

6 Raise the bed to the best level for good body mechanics.

Procedure

7 Lower the side rail on the person's weak side.

8 Position him or her supine.

9 Cover the person with the bath blanket. Fanfold linens to the foot of the bed. Do not expose the person during the procedure.

10 Remove garments that open in the back.

- a Raise the person's head and shoulders. Or turn him or her onto the side away from you.
- b Undo buttons, zippers, ties, or snaps.
- c Bring the sides of the garment to the sides of the person (Fig. 14-10 on page 334). Do the following if he or she is in a side-lying position:
  1. Tuck the far side under the person.
  2. Fold the near side onto the chest (Fig. 14-11 on page 335).
- d Position the person supine.
- e Slide the garment off the shoulder on the strong side. Remove it from the arm (Fig. 14-12 on page 335).
- f Repeat step 10e for the weak side.

11 Remove garments that open in the front.

- a Undo buttons, zippers, snaps, or ties.
- b Slide the garment off the shoulder and arm on the strong side.
- c Raise the head and shoulders. Bring the garment over to the weak side (Fig. 14-13 on page 336). Lower the head and shoulders.
- d Remove the garment from the weak side.
- e Do the following if you cannot raise the person's head and shoulders:
  1. Turn the person toward you. Tuck the removed part under the person.
  2. Turn him or her onto the side away from you.
  3. Pull the side of the garment out from under the person. Make sure he or she will not lie on it when supine.
  4. Return the person to the supine position.
  5. Remove the garment from the weak side.

12 Remove pullover garments.

- a Undo any buttons, zippers, ties, or snaps.
- b Remove the garment from the strong side.
- c Raise the head and shoulders. You may need to turn him or her onto the side away from you. Bring the garment up to the person's neck (Fig. 14-14 on page 336).
- d Remove the garment from the weak side.
- e Bring the garment over the person's head.
- f Position him or her in the supine position.

13 Remove pants or slacks.

- a Remove shoes or slippers.
- b Position the person supine.
- c Undo buttons, zippers, ties, snaps, or buckles.
- d Remove the belt if one is worn.
- e Ask the person to lift the buttocks off the bed. Slide the pants down over the hips and buttocks (Fig. 14-15 on page 336). Have the person lower the hips and buttocks.
- f Do the following if the person cannot raise the hips off the bed:
  1. Turn the person toward you.
  2. Slide the pants off the hip and buttock on the strong side (Fig. 14-16 on page 337).
  3. Turn the person away from you.

Continued.

UNDRESSING A PERSON—cont'd

PROCEDURE—CONT'D

4. Slide the pants off the hip and buttock on the weak side (Fig. 14-17 on page 337).

g Slide the pants down the legs and over the feet.

14 Dress or put a clean gown or pajamas on the person.

15 Help the person get out of bed if he or she is to be up. Cover the person and remove the bath blanket if the person will not be up.

16 Lower the bed.

POST-PROCEDURE

17 Raise or lower side rails as instructed by the nurse.

18 Place the call bell within reach.

19 Unscreen the person.

20 Follow facility policy for soiled clothing.

21 Report your observations to the nurse.

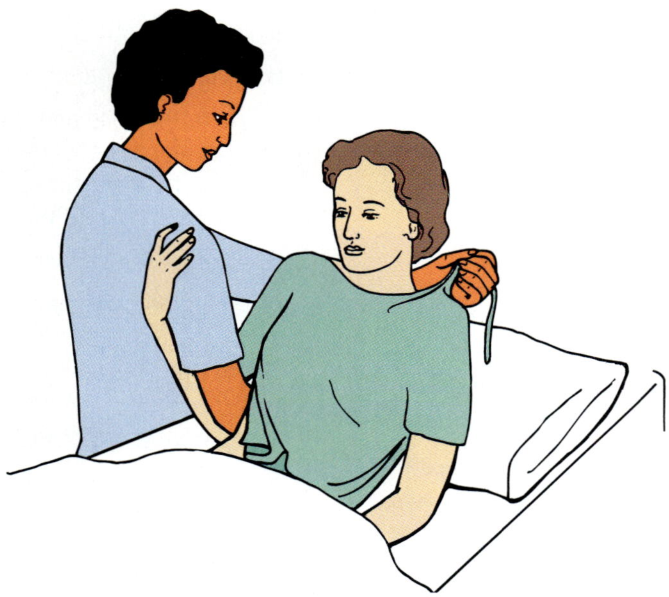

Fig. 14-10 *The sides of the garment are brought from the back to the sides of the person.*

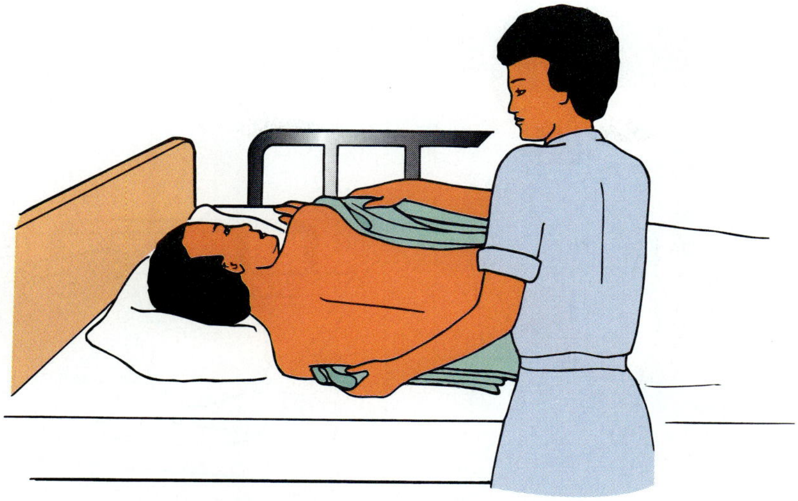

Fig. 14-11 *A garment that opens in back is removed from the person in the side-lying position. The far side of the garment is tucked under the person. The near side is folded onto the person's chest.*

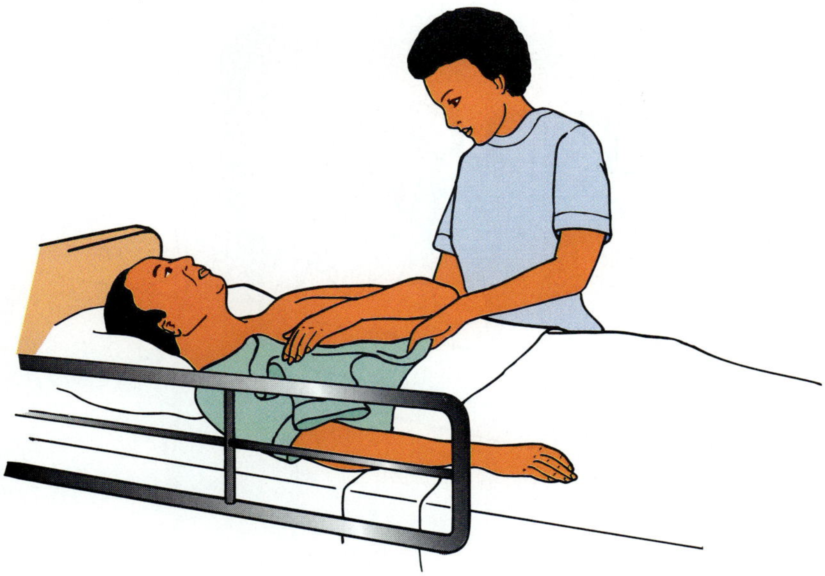

Fig. 14-12 *The garment is removed from the strong side first.*

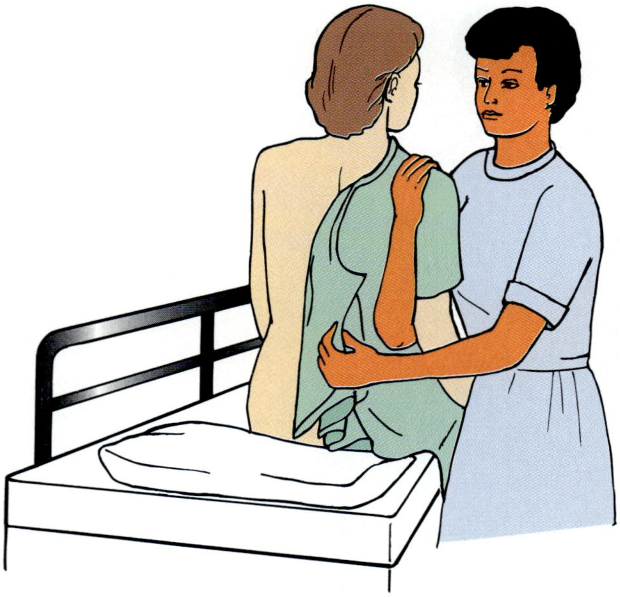

Fig. 14-13 *A front-opening garment is removed with the person's head and shoulders raised. The garment is removed from the strong side first. Then it is brought around the back to the weak side.*

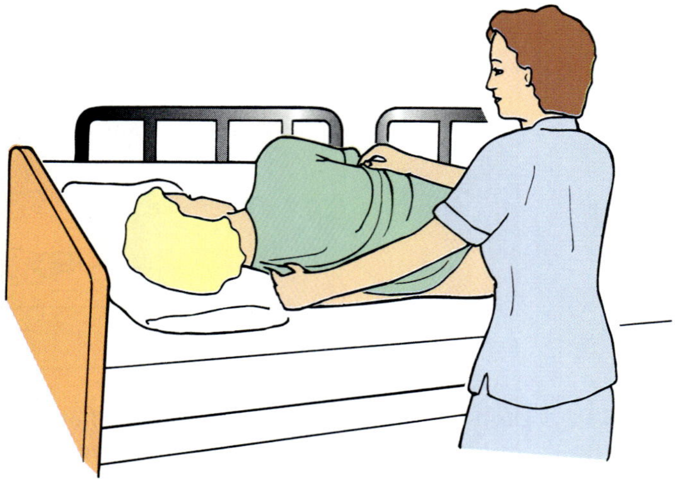

Fig. 14-14 *A pullover garment is removed from the strong side first. Then the garment is brought up to the person's neck so that it can be removed from the weak side.*

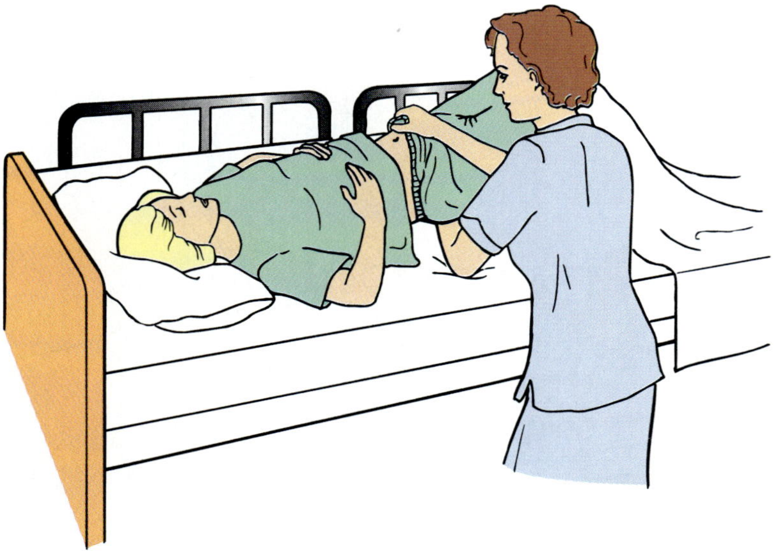

Fig. 14-15 *The person lifts the hips and buttocks so that the pants can be removed. The pants are slid down over the hips and buttocks.*

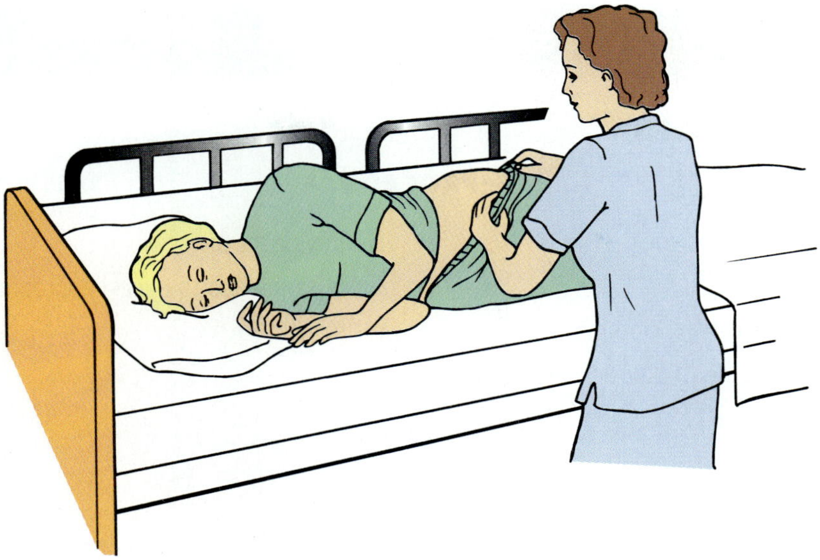

Fig. 14-16 *Pants are removed in the side-lying position. They are removed from the strong side first. They are slid over the hips and buttocks.*

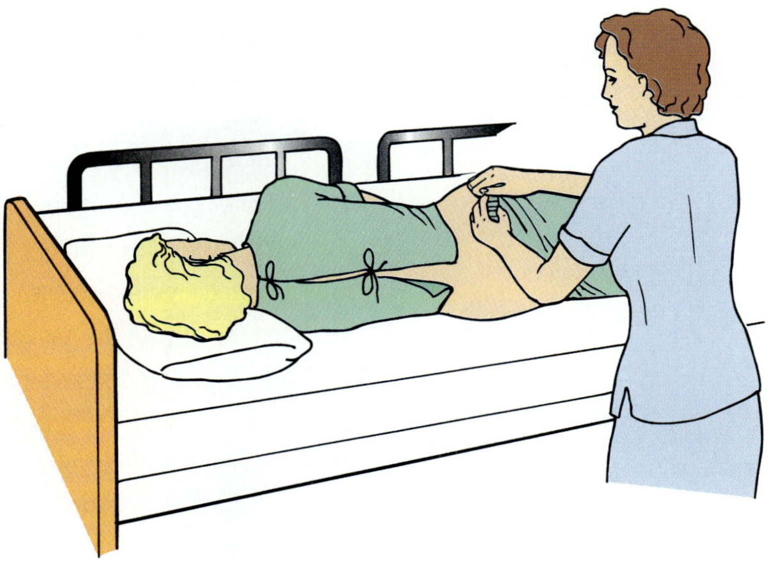

Fig. 14-17 *The person is turned onto the other side. The pants are removed from the weak side.*

DRESSING THE PERSON

PRE-PROCEDURE

1 Explain the procedure to the person.
2 Wash your hands.
3 Get a bath blanket and necessary clothing.
4 Identify the person. Check the ID bracelet and call the person by name.
5 Provide for privacy.
6 Raise the bed to a level appropriate for good body mechanics.

PROCEDURE

7 Undress the person if indicated.
8 Lower the side rail on the person's strong side.
9 Position the person supine.
10 Cover the person with the bath blanket. Fanfold linens to the foot of the bed. Do not expose the person during the procedure.
11 Put on garments that open in the back.
   - a Slide the garment onto the arm and shoulder of the weak side.
   - b Slide the garment onto the arm and shoulder of the strong side.
   - c Raise the person's head and shoulders.
   - d Bring the sides to the back if he or she is in a semisitting position.
   - e Do the following if the person is in a side-lying position:
     1. Turn the person toward you.
     2. Bring one side of the garment to the person's back (Fig. 14-18, A).
     3. Turn the person away from you.
     4. Bring the other side to the person's back (Fig. 14-18, B).
   - f Fasten buttons, snaps, ties, or zippers.
   - g Position the person in the supine position.
12 Put on garments that open in the front.
   - a Slide the garment onto the arm and shoulder on the weak side.
   - b Raise the person's head and shoulders. Bring the other side of the garment around to the back. Lower the person to the supine position. Slide the garment onto the arm and shoulder of the strong arm.
   - c Do the following if the person cannot raise the head and shoulders:
     1. Turn the person toward you.
     2. Tuck the garment under him or her.
     3. Turn the person away from you.
     4. Pull the garment out from under him or her.
     5. Turn the person back to the supine position.
     6. Slide the garment over the arm and shoulder of the strong arm.
   - d Fasten buttons, snaps, ties, or zippers.
13 Put on pullover garments.
   - a Position the person supine.
   - b Bring the neck of the garment over the head.
   - c Slide the arm and shoulder of the garment onto the person's weak side.
   - d Raise the person's head and shoulders.
   - e Bring the garment down.
   - f Slide the arm and shoulder of the garment onto the person's strong side.
   - g Do the following if the person cannot assume a semisitting position:
     1. Turn the person toward you.
     2. Tuck the garment under him or her.
     3. Turn the person away from you.
     4. Pull the garment out from under him or her.
     5. Return the person to the supine position.
     6. Slide the arm and shoulder of the garment onto the strong side.
   - h Fasten buttons, snaps, ties, or zippers.

DRESSING THE PERSON

PROCEDURE—CONT'D

14 Put on pants or slacks.

- **a** Slide the pants over the feet and up the legs.
- **b** Ask him or her to raise the hips and buttocks off the bed.
- **c** Bring the pants up over the buttocks and hips.
- **d** Ask the person to lower the hips and buttocks.
- **e** Do the following if the person cannot raise the hips and buttocks:
  - **1.** Turn person on the strong side.
  - **2.** Pull the pants over the buttock and hip on the weak side.
  - **3.** Turn the person onto the weak side.
  - **4.** Pull the pants over the buttock and hip on the strong side.
  - **5.** Return him or her to the supine position.
- **f** Fasten buttons, ties, snaps, the zipper, and the belt buckle.

15 Put socks and shoes or slippers on the person.

16 Help the person to the chair if he or she can be up. Otherwise, help the person assume a comfortable position in bed.

17 Cover the person and remove the bath blanket.

18 Lower the bed to its lowest position.

POST-PROCEDURE

19 Raise or lower side rails as instructed by the nurse.

20 Make sure the call bell is within reach.

21 Unscreen the person.

22 Follow facility policy for soiled clothing.

23 Report your observations to the nurse.

A

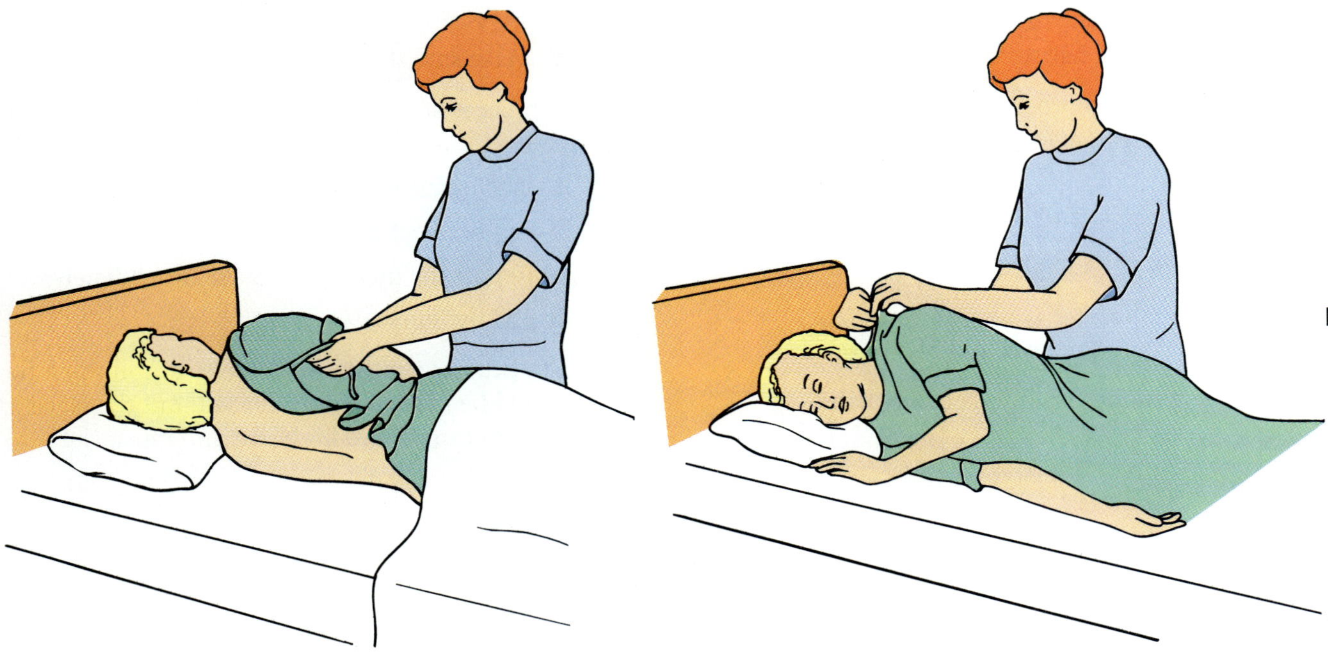

B

Fig. 14-18 *A, The side-lying position can be used to put on garments that open in the back. The person is turned toward the nursing assistant after the garment is put on the arms. The side of the garment is brought to the person's back. B, The person is then turned away from the nursing assistant. The other side of the garment is brought to the back and fastened.*

Summary

Personal care and grooming measures are important for physical comfort. They also help the person's body image and esteem needs. Being well-groomed is important to many people. Clean hair and nails and wearing clean clothes all help a person feel good mentally. Being clean shaven or having a well-groomed beard or mustache affects a man's well-being.

The person may not have energy for some procedures. The nurse tells you what care to give and when it is to be given. Personal choice is encouraged and allowed whenever possible. Personal care and grooming practices vary from person to person. Be sure to provide assistance whenever it is necessary.

Review Questions

Circle the best *answer.*

1 You read the word *alopecia* in Mr. Lee's medical record. The term means
- **a** Excessive body hair
- **b** Dry, white flakes from the scalp
- **c** An infestation of lice
- **d** Hair loss

2 Which prevents hair from matting and tangling?
- **a** Bed rest
- **b** Daily brushing and combing
- **c** Daily shampooing
- **d** Cutting long hair

3 You are going to brush a woman's hair. The hair is not matted or tangled. When brushing the hair, start at
- **a** The forehead and brush backward
- **b** The hair ends
- **c** The scalp
- **d** The back of the neck and brush forward

4 Brushing is important to keep the hair
- **a** Soft and shiny
- **b** Clean
- **c** Free from pediculosis
- **d** All of the above

5 Mr. Lee wants his hair washed. You should
- **a** Wash his hair during his shower
- **b** Wash his hair at the sink
- **c** Shampoo him in bed
- **d** Follow the nurse's instructions

6 When shaving Mr. Lee, you need to do the following *except*
- **a** Practice Standard Precautions
- **b** Follow the Bloodborne Pathogen Standard
- **c** Shave in the opposite direction of hair growth
- **d** Make sure the skin is soft before shaving

7 Mr. Lee is nicked during shaving. Your first action is to
- **a** Wash your hands
- **b** Apply direct pressure
- **c** Report the nick to the nurse immediately
- **d** Tell the nurse

8 Mr. Lee has a mustache and beard. You think he would be more comfortable without the facial hair. You can shave his beard and mustache.
- **a** True
- **b** False

REVIEW QUESTIONS—CONT'D

9 You are going to cut a person's fingernails. You should use

a Toenail clippers

b Scissors

c An emery board

d Nail clippers

10 Nursing assistants can cut and trim toenails.

a True

b False

11 Fingernails are trimmed

a Before they are soaked

b After they are soaked

c Before the toenails are trimmed

d After the toenails are trimmed

12 Makeup is applied

a As the woman prefers

b As instructed by the nurse

c After the bath

d Before the woman gets out of bed

13 Clothing is removed from the strong side first.

a True

b False

14 The person is allowed to choose what to wear.

a True

b False

Answers to these questions are on page 750.

Urinary Elimination

15

OBJECTIVES

- Define the key terms listed in this chapter
- Identify the characteristics of normal urine
- Identify the usual times for urination
- Describe the rules for maintaining normal urinary elimination
- List the observations to be made about urine
- Describe urinary incontinence and the care required
- Explain why catheters are used
- Describe the rules for caring for persons with catheters
- Describe two methods of bladder training
- Describe the rules for collecting urine specimens
- Perform the procedures described in this chapter

Key Terms

acetone Ketone bodies that appear in the urine because of the rapid breakdown of fat for energy

catheter A tube used to drain or inject fluid through a body opening

catheterization The process of inserting a catheter

diabetes mellitus A chronic disease in which the pancreas fails to secrete enough insulin; the body is prevented from using sugar for energy

dysuria Painful or difficult (dys) urination (uria)

Foley catheter A catheter that is left in the urinary bladder so urine drains continuously into a collection bag; an indwelling or retention catheter

functional incontinence The involuntary, unpredicted passage of urine from the bladder; the person does not have nervous system or urinary system diseases or injuries

glucosuria Sugar (glucose) in the urine (uria); glycosuria

glycosuria Sugar (glycos) in the urine (uria); glucosuria

hematuria Blood (hemat) in the urine (uria)

indwelling catheter A retention or Foley catheter

ketone body Acetone

micturition The process of emptying the bladder; urination or voiding

nocturia Frequent urination (uria) at night (noct)

oliguria Scant amount (olig) of urine (uria); usually less than 500 ml in 24 hours

polyuria The production of abnormally large amounts (poly) of urine (uria)

retention catheter A Foley or indwelling catheter

stress incontinence The leakage of small amounts of urine (less than 50 ml)

total incontinence The continuous loss of urine from the bladder; the passage of urine cannot be predicted

urge incontinence The involuntary passage of urine after feeling a strong need to void

urinary frequency Voiding at frequent intervals

urinary incontinence The inability to control the passage of urine from the bladder

urinary urgency The need to void immediately

urination The process of emptying the bladder; micturition or voiding

voiding Urination or micturition

Eliminating waste is a basic physical need. Body wastes are removed through the respiratory system, the digestive system, the skin, and the urinary system. The digestive system rids the body of solid wastes. The lungs rid the body of carbon dioxide. Water and other substances are contained in sweat. There are other waste products in the blood from body cells burning food for energy. The urinary system removes waste products from the blood and maintains water balance within the body. Box 15-1 on page 344 contains a review of the structure and function of the urinary system. See Chapter 5 for more detailed information.

NORMAL URINATION

The healthy adult excretes about 1500 ml (milliliters) (3 pints) of urine a day. Many factors affect the amount of urine produced. These include age, illnesses, the amount and kinds of fluid ingested, the amount of salt in the diet, and drugs. Certain substances increase urine production. Examples are coffee, tea, alcohol, and some drugs. A diet high in salt causes the body to retain water. When water is retained, less urine is produced. Urine production is also influenced by body temperature, perspiration, the external temperature, and some drugs.

Urinary frequency also depends on many factors. The amount of fluid ingested, personal habits, and available toilet facilities affect frequency. So do activity, work, and illness. People usually urinate at bedtime, after getting up, and before meals. Some people urinate every 2 to 3 hours. Others void every 8 to 12 hours. Sleep may be disturbed if large amounts of urine are produced.

MAINTAINING NORMAL URINATION

Patients or residents may need help maintaining normal elimination. Some need help getting to the bathroom. Others use bedpans, urinals, or commodes. The rules listed in Box 15-2 on page 345 are followed to maintain normal elimination in patients and residents.

What to Report to the Nurse

Before disposing of urine, it is carefully observed. Urine is normally pale yellow, straw colored, or amber. It is clear with no particles. A faint odor is normal. Urine is observed for color, clarity, odor, amount, and the presence of particles. Some foods normally affect urine color. Red-colored urine may result from red food dyes, beets, blackberries, and rhubarb. Carrots and sweet potatoes cause bright yellow urine. Certain drugs can cause changes in urine color. Asparagus causes a urine odor.

BOX 15-1 The Urinary System: Review of Body Structure and Function

The kidneys, ureters, urinary bladder, and urethra are the major urinary tract structures (Fig. 15-1). The two kidneys lie in the upper abdomen against the muscles of the back on each side of the spine. Blood passes through the two kidneys, where urine is formed. Urine consists of wastes and excess fluids filtered out of the blood. Urine flows through the two ureters to the urinary bladder, where it is stored until urination. The urethra is the tube that connects the urinary bladder to the outside of the body. Urine is eliminated from the body through the urethra. **Urination, micturition,** and **voiding** all mean the process of emptying the bladder.

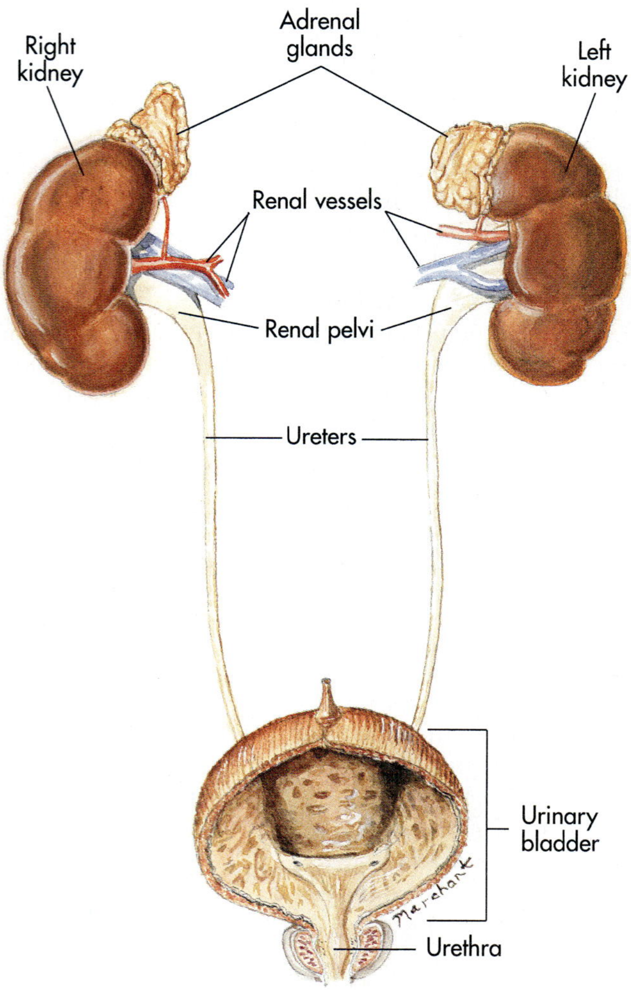

Fig. 15-1 *The urinary system.*

Urine that looks or smells abnormal is saved for the nurse to observe. Complaints of urgency, burning on urination, or dysuria are also reported. **Dysuria** means painful or difficult (dys) urination (uria). The problems described in Table 15-1 on page 345 are also reported. This information is needed for the nursing process.

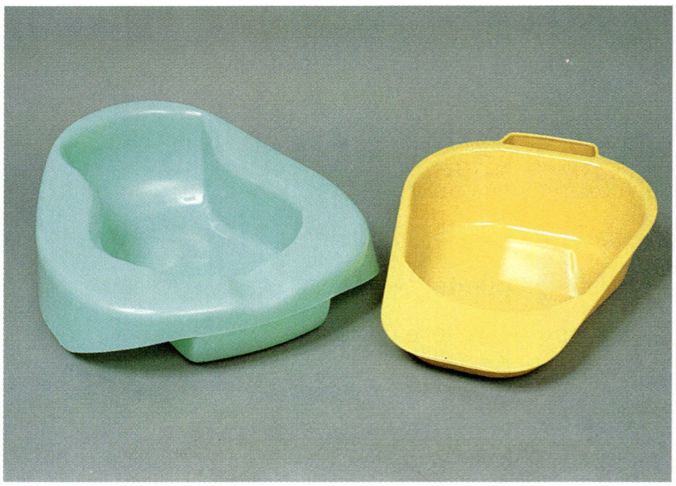

Fig. 15-2 *The regular bedpan and the fracture pan.*

Bedpans

Bedpans are used by persons who cannot be out of bed. Women use bedpans for voiding and bowel movements. Men use them only for bowel movements. Bedpans are made of plastic or stainless steel. Stainless steel bedpans tend to be cold and are warmed before use.

Fracture pans are also available (Fig. 15-2). A *fracture pan* has a thinner rim and is only about ½-inch deep at one end. The smaller end is placed under the buttocks (Fig. 15-3 on page 346). Fracture pans are used for persons with casts or those in traction.

Medical asepsis, Standard Precautions, and the Bloodborne Pathogen Standard are followed when handling bedpans and their contents. The bedpan is covered after use and is taken to the toilet or dirty utility room. After being emptied and rinsed, it is cleaned with a disinfectant. The bedpan is returned to the bedside stand with a clean cover.

Text continued on page 349.

BOX 15-2 Rules for Maintaining Normal Elimination

- Practice medical asepsis and Standard Precautions. Also follow the Bloodborne Pathogen Standard.
- Provide fluids as instructed by the nurse.
- Follow the person's normal voiding routines and habits. Check with the nurse and the nursing care plan.
- Provide the bedpan, urinal, or commode, or help the person to the bathroom as soon as the request is made. The need to void may be urgent.
- Help the person assume a normal position for voiding if possible. Women sit or squat; men stand.
- Make sure the bedpan or urinal is warm.
- Cover the person for warmth and privacy.
- Provide for privacy. Pull the curtain around the bed, close doors to the room and bathroom, and pull drapes or window shades. Portable screens or room dividers may be needed for home care patients. Leave the room if the person can be alone.
- Tell the person that running water, flushing the toilet, or playing the radio or music can mask urination sounds. This is important for persons embarrassed about voiding with others close by.
- Remain nearby if the person is weak or unsteady.
- Place the call bell and toilet tissue within reach.
- Allow the person enough time to void. Do not rush the person.
- Promote relaxation. Some people like to read when eliminating.
- Run water in a nearby sink if the person has difficulty starting the stream. You may need to place the person's fingers in some water.
- Provide perineal care as needed.
- Have the person wash his or her hands after voiding. Provide a wash basin, soap, washcloth, and towel. Assist as necessary.
- Offer the bedpan or urinal at regular intervals. Some people are embarrassed or are too weak to ask.

TABLE 15-1

Common Urinary Elimination Problems

	Definition	Causes
dysuria	Painful or difficult (dys) urination (uria)	Urinary tract infection, trauma, urinary tract obstruction
hematuria	Blood (hemat) in the urine (uria)	Kidney disease, urinary tract infection, trauma
nocturia	Frequent urination (uria) at night (noct)	Excessive fluid intake, kidney disease, disease of the prostate
oliguria	Scant amount (olig) of urine (uria), usually less than 500 ml in 24 hours	Inadequate fluid intake, shock, burns, kidney disease, heart failure
polyuria	The production of abnormally large amounts (poly) of urine (uria)	Drugs, excessive fluid intake, diabetes mellitus, hormone imbalance
urinary frequency	Voiding at frequent intervals	Excessive fluid intake, bladder infections, pressure on the bladder, drugs
urinary incontinence	Inability to control the passage of urine from the bladder	Trauma, disease, urinary tract infections, reproductive or urinary tract surgeries, aging, fecal impaction, constipation, not getting to the bathroom
urinary urgency	The need to void immediately	Urinary tract infection, fear of incontinence (see page 351), full bladder, stress

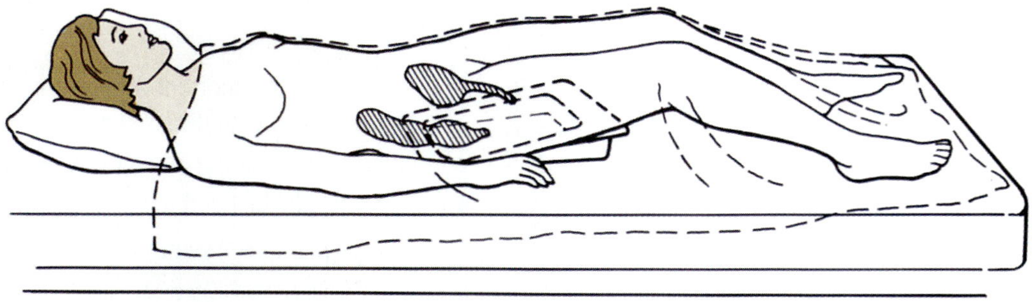

Fig. 15-3 *A person positioned on a fracture pan. The smaller end is placed under the buttocks.*

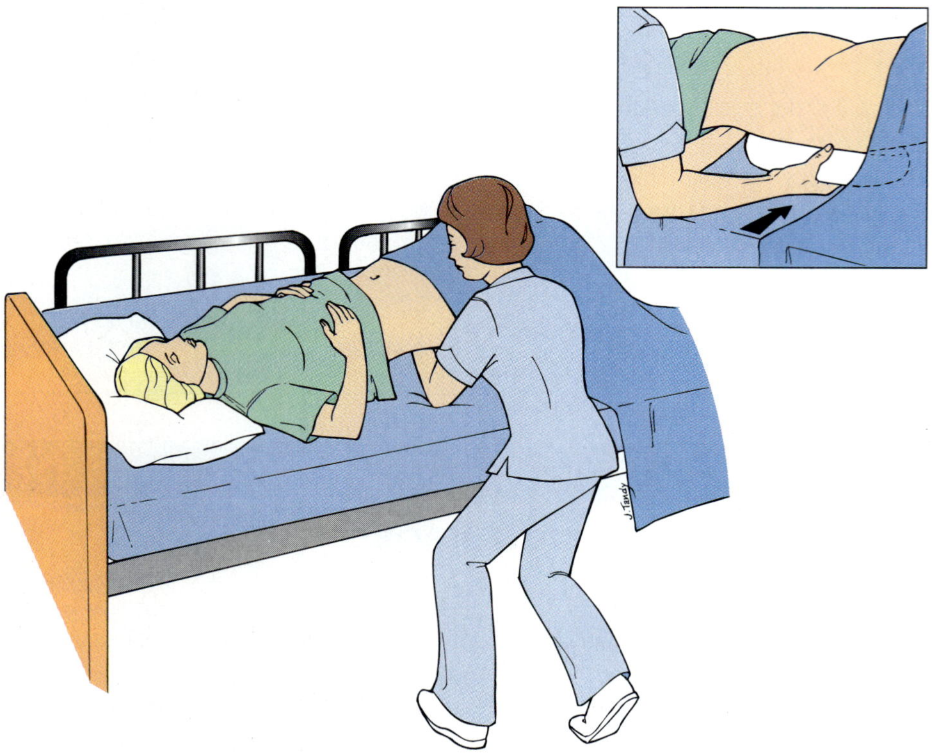

Fig. 15-4 *The person raises the buttocks off the bed with the help of the nursing assistant. The bedpan is slid under the person.*

Giving the Bedpan

Pre-procedure

1 Provide for privacy.

2 Collect the following:
- Bedpan
- Bedpan cover
- Toilet tissue
- Disposable gloves

3 Arrange equipment on the chair or bed.

4 Explain the procedure to the person.

5 Raise the bed to the best level for good body mechanics.

Procedure

6 Make sure the side rails are up.

7 Warm and dry the bedpan if necessary.

8 Lower the side rail.

9 Position the person supine. Slightly elevate the head of the bed.

10 Fold the top linens and gown out of the way. Keep the lower body covered.

11 Ask the person to flex the knees and raise the buttocks by pushing against the mattress with his or her feet.

12 Slide your hand under the lower back and help him or her raise the buttocks.

13 Slide the bedpan under the person (Fig. 15-4).

14 Do the following if the person cannot assist in getting on the bedpan:

a Turn the person onto the side away from you.

b Place the bedpan firmly against the buttocks (Fig. 15-5, A on page 348).

c Push the bedpan down and toward the person (Fig. 15-5, B).

d Hold the bedpan securely. Turn the person onto the back. Make sure the bedpan is centered under the person.

15 Return top linens to their proper position.

16 Raise the head of the bed so the person is in a sitting position.

17 Make sure the person is correctly positioned on the bedpan (Fig. 15-6 on page 348).

18 Raise the side rail.

19 Place the toilet tissue and call bell within reach.

20 Ask the person to signal when done or when help is needed.

21 Leave the room and close the door. Wash your hands.

22 Return when the person signals. Knock before entering.

23 Lower the side rail and the head of the bed.

24 Put on the gloves.

25 Ask the person to raise the buttocks. Remove the bedpan. Or hold the bedpan securely and turn him or her onto the side away from you.

26 Clean the genital area if the person cannot do so. Clean from front to back with toilet tissue. Use fresh tissue for each wipe. Provide perineal care if necessary.

27 Cover the bedpan. Take it to the bathroom or dirty utility room. Raise the side rail before leaving the bedside.

28 Measure urine if the person is on intake and output (I&O) (see Chapter 17). Collect a urine specimen if needed. Note the color, amount, and character of urine or feces.

29 Empty and rinse the bedpan. Clean it with a disinfectant.

30 Remove the gloves.

31 Return the bedpan and clean cover to the bedside stand.

32 Help the person wash the hands.

Continued.

GIVING THE BEDPAN—CONT'D

POST-PROCEDURE

33 Make sure the person is comfortable.
34 Place the call bell within reach.
35 Raise or lower side rails as instructed by the nurse.
36 Lower the bed to its lowest position.
37 Unscreen the person.
38 Follow facility policy for soiled linen.
39 Wash your hands.
40 Report your observations to the nurse.

A
B
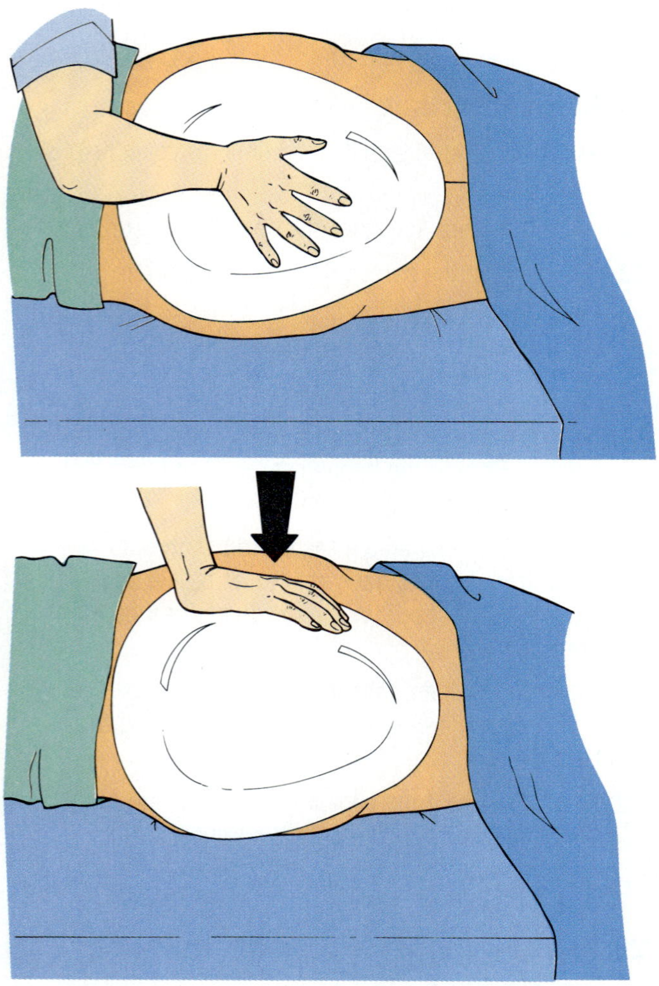

Fig. 15-5 *A, Position the person on one side and place the bedpan firmly against the buttocks. B, Push downward on the bedpan and toward the person.*

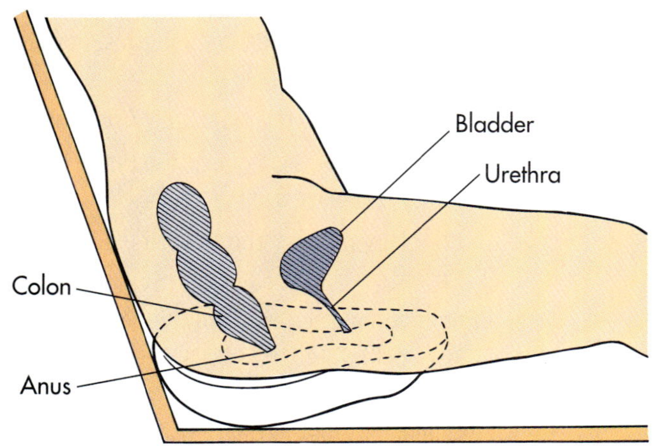

Fig. 15-6 *The person is positioned on the bedpan so the urethra and anus are directly over the opening.*

Urinals

Men use urinals to void (Fig. 15-7, A). Urinals are made of plastic or stainless steel. Plastic ones have caps at the top and hook-type handles. The hook is used to hang the urinal from the side rail within the man's reach (Fig. 15-7, B). The urinal is used while lying in bed, sitting on the edge of the bed, or standing at the bedside. The man stands if possible. Some men stand with the support of 1 or 2 workers. You may have to place and hold the urinal for some men.

Urinals are emptied promptly to prevent odors and the spread of microbes. A filled urinal can easily spill and cause safety hazards. Urinals are cleaned like bedpans.

After using urinals, many men place them on nearby tables until someone empties them. This practice is discouraged. The overbed table is used for eating and as a working surface for the nursing team. Bedside stands are also used for supplies. For these reasons, table surfaces should not be contaminated with urine. In addition, a filled urinal is an unpleasant sight and a source of odor. Men are reminded to hang urinals on the side rails. They also are reminded to signal when urinals need emptying.

There are also female urinals. However, they are not commonly used.

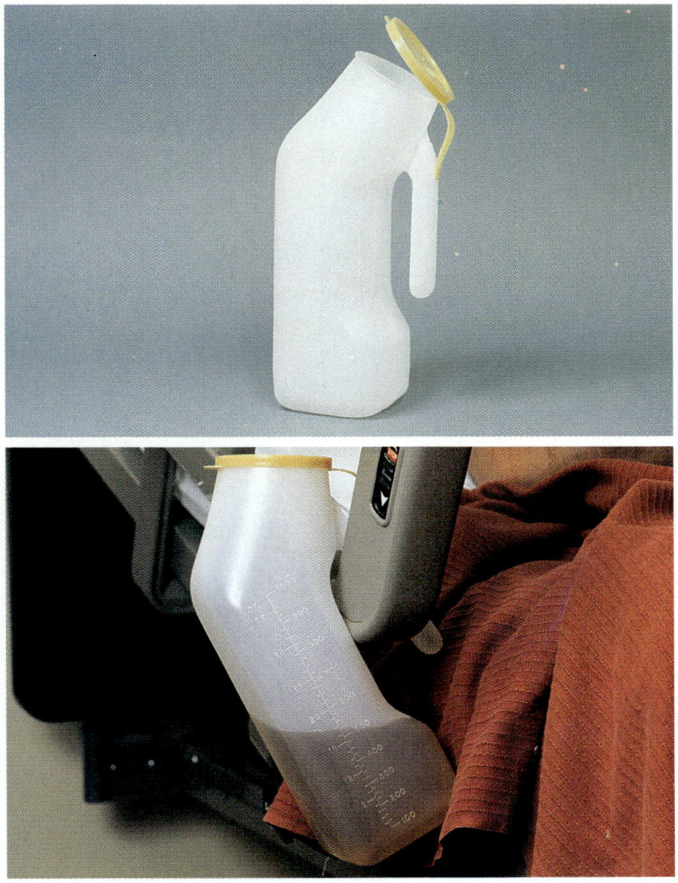

A

B

Fig. 15-7 *A, Urinal for a male. B, The urinal hangs from the side rail within the person's reach.*

Giving the Urinal

Procedure

1 Provide for privacy.

2 Determine if the man will stand or stay in bed.

3 Give him the urinal if he will stay in bed. Remind him to tilt the bottom down to prevent spills.

4 Do the following if he is going to stand:

- **a** Help him sit on the side of the bed.
- **b** Put slippers on him.
- **c** Assist him to a standing position.
- **d** Provide support if he is unsteady.
- **e** Give him the urinal.

5 Position the urinal between his legs if necessary. Position his penis in the urinal if he cannot hold the urinal. (Wear gloves for this step.)

6 Cover him to provide for privacy.

7 Place the call bell within reach. Ask him to signal when done or when he needs help.

8 Wash your hands. Leave the room and close the door.

9 Return when he signals for you. Knock before entering.

10 Put on gloves.

11 Cover the urinal. Take it to the bathroom or dirty utility room.

12 Measure urine if I&O is ordered. Collect a urine specimen if needed. Note the color, amount, and character of the urine.

Continued.

Giving the Urinal—cont'd

Procedure

13 Empty the urinal and rinse it with cold water. Clean it with a disinfectant.

14 Remove the gloves.

15 Return the urinal to the bedside stand.

16 Help the person wash his hands.

Post-procedure

17 Make sure he is comfortable.

18 Raise or lower side rails as instructed by the nurse.

19 Place the call bell within reach.

20 Unscreen him.

21 Wash your hands.

22 Report your observations to the nurse.

Commodes

A bedside commode is a portable chair or wheelchair with an opening for a bedpan or similar receptacle (Fig. 15-8). Persons unable to walk to the bathroom are often able to use commodes. The commode allows a normal position for elimination. The bedpan or receptacle is cleaned after use like the regular bedpan.

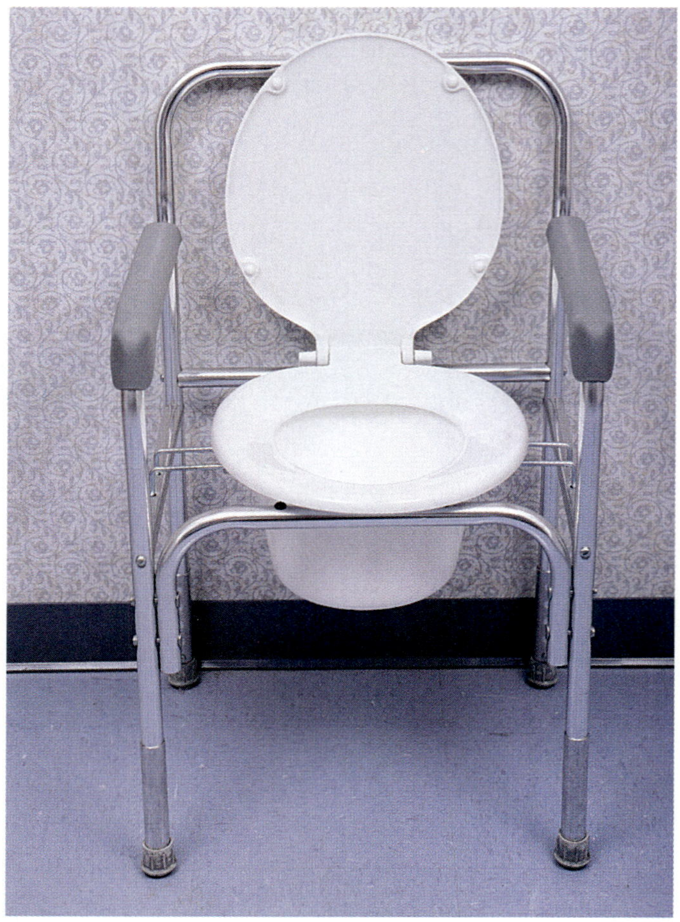

Fig. 15-8 *The bedside commode has a toilet seat with a container. The container slides out from under the toilet seat for emptying.*

HELPING THE PERSON TO THE COMMODE

PRE-PROCEDURE

1 Explain the procedure to the person.
2 Provide for privacy.
3 Collect the following:
- Commode
- Toilet tissue
- Bath blanket
- Disposable gloves

PROCEDURE

4 Bring the commode next to the bed. Remove the chair seat and lid from the container.
5 Help the person sit on the side of the bed.
6 Help him or her put on a robe and slippers.
7 Assist the person to the commode.
8 Place a bath blanket over his or her lap for warmth.
9 Place the toilet tissue and call bell within reach.
10 Ask him or her to signal when done or when help is needed.
11 Wash your hands. Leave the room and close the door.
12 Return when the person signals. Knock before entering.
13 Put on the gloves.
14 Help the person clean the genital area if indicated. Remove the gloves.
15 Help the person back to bed. Remove the robe and slippers. Raise the side rail if instructed by the nurse.
16 Put on another pair of gloves. Cover and remove the container from the commode. Clean the commode if necessary.
17 Take the container to the bathroom or dirty utility room.
18 Check urine and feces for color, amount, and character. Measure urine if I&O is ordered. Collect a specimen if one is needed.
19 Clean and disinfect the container. Remove the gloves.
20 Return the container to the commode. Return other supplies to their proper place.
21 Return the commode to its proper place.
22 Help the person wash the hands.

POST-PROCEDURE

23 Make sure he or she is comfortable and the call bell is within reach.
24 Raise or lower side rails as instructed by the nurse.
25 Unscreen the person.
26 Follow facility policy for soiled linen.
27 Wash your hands.
28 Report your observations to the nurse.

PROBLEMS WITH URINARY ELIMINATION

Illness, injury, and aging are common causes of urinary elimination problems. So are drugs and too little or too much fluid intake. Some problems are minor. Others cause great distress. (See Table 15-1 for some common problems.)

Urinary Incontinence

Urinary incontinence is the inability to control the passage of urine from the bladder. It may be temporary or permanent. There are different types of incontinence.

- **Total incontinence** is when there is continuous loss of urine from the bladder. The passage of urine cannot be predicted. Causes include nervous system disorders, injury or disease of the spinal cord, and disease or injury of urinary structures.

- **Stress incontinence** is the leakage of small amounts of urine (less than 50 ml). Often called dribbling, stress incontinence can occur with laughing, sneezing, coughing, lifting, or other physical exertion. Late pregnancy and obesity are other causes. The problem is common in women from multiple pregnancies, weak pelvic muscles, and aging.
- **Urge incontinence** is the involuntary passage of urine after feeling a strong need to void. The person cannot stop urinating and cannot get to the bathroom in time. Urinary frequency and nighttime voidings are common. This type is more common among elderly persons. Urinary tract infections, tumors, and diseases are causes.
- **Functional incontinence** is the involuntary, unpredicted passage of urine from the bladder. The person does not have any nervous system or urinary system diseases or injuries. Not being able to get to use the bathroom, bedpan, urinal, or commode is the cause. Immobility, restraints, unanswered call bells, not having a call bell within reach, and not knowing where to find the bathroom are common causes in health care settings. Difficulty removing clothes may delay urination.

Incontinence is embarrassing. Clothing becomes wet, odors develop, and the person is uncomfortable. Irritation, infection, and pressure sores can also occur.

The nurse uses the nursing process to meet the person's needs. You need to follow the nurse's instructions and the nursing care plan. Good skin care is essential. Be sure to provide dry clothing and linens. Following the rules for maintaining normal urinary elimination will prevent incontinence in some people. Others need bladder training programs (see page 359). Sometimes catheters are ordered. Some people wear garment protectors or incontinence pads (Fig. 15-9). Incontinence drawsheets can help keep the person dry. The drawsheet has two layers and a waterproof back. Fluid passes through the first layer and is absorbed by the lower layer. A variety of incontinent products are available. Many can be bought in drugstores or home care equipment stores.

Incontinence has been linked to abuse, mistreatment, and neglect of patients and residents. Caring for these persons can be very stressful. They need frequent care and may wet again just after you have given skin care and changed wet clothing and linens. You must not lose patience with these people. Their needs are great and your role is to meet their needs. If you find yourself short-tempered and impatient, discuss the problem with the nurse immediately. The nurse may need to reassign you to other patients or residents for a while. Remember, the person has the right to be free from abuse, mistreatment, or neglect. The incontinence is beyond the person's control. It is not something he or she chooses to let happen. Kindness, empathy, understanding, and patience are very important.

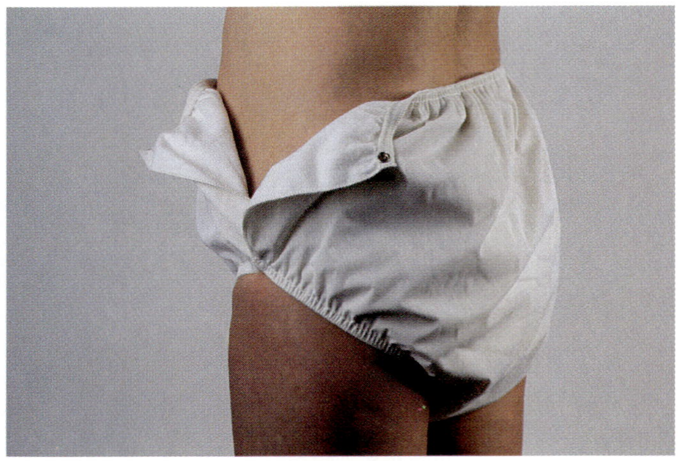

Fig. 15-9 *Garment protector (incontinence pad).*

CATHETERS

A **catheter** is a rubber or plastic tube used to drain or inject fluid through a body opening. A urinary catheter is inserted through the urethra into the bladder to drain urine. An **indwelling catheter** (**retention** or **Foley catheter**) is left in the bladder so urine drains constantly into a drainage bag. A balloon near the tip is inflated after the catheter is inserted. The balloon prevents the catheter from slipping out of the bladder (Fig. 15-10). Tubing connects the catheter to the collection bag. Catheter insertion (**catheterization**) is done by a nurse or doctor.

Catheters may be used before, during, and after surgery to keep the bladder empty. A full bladder can be accidentally injured during surgery. After surgery, a full bladder can cause pressure on nearby organs. A catheter may be used as a last resort for urinary incontinence.

You may care for persons with indwelling catheters. The rules listed in Box 15-3 promote their comfort and safety.

Text continued on page 355.

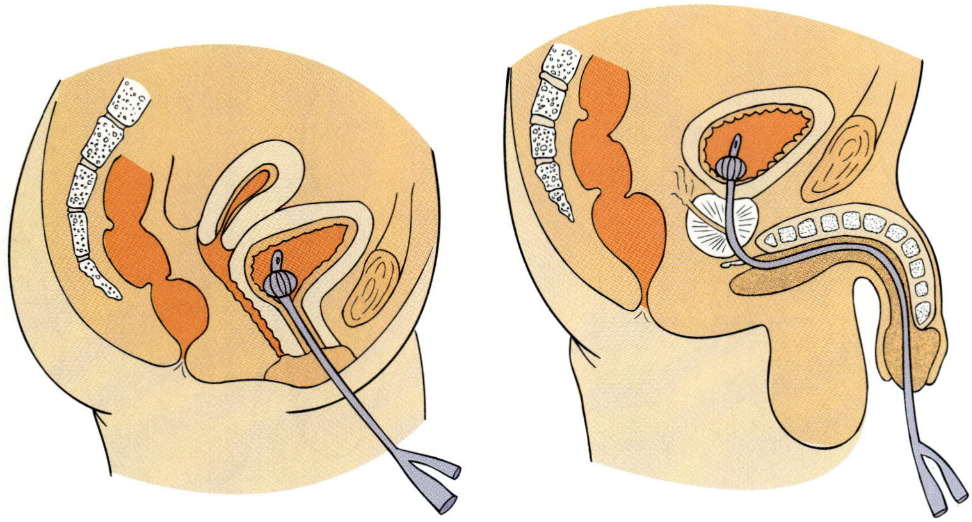

Fig. 15-10 *A, The Foley catheter in the female bladder. The inflated balloon at the top prevents the catheter from slipping out through the urethra. B, A Foley catheter with the balloon inflated in the male bladder.*

BOX 15-3 Rules for Indwelling Catheters

- Practice handwashing. Also follow the rules of medical asepsis, Standard Precautions, and the Bloodborne Pathogen Standard.
- Make sure urine flows freely through the catheter or tubing. Tubing should not have kinks. The person should not lay on the tubing.
- Keep the drainage bag below the bladder. This prevents urine from flowing backward into the bladder. Attach the drainage bag to the bed frame. *Never attach the drainage bag to the side rail.* The drainage bag would be higher than the bladder when the side rail is raised.
- Coil the drainage tubing on the bed and pin it to the bottom linen (Fig. 15-11 on page 354).
- Secure the catheter to the inner thigh as in Figure 15-11. Or secure it to the man's abdomen. This prevents excessive movement of the catheter and reduces friction at the insertion site. Tape or other devices ordered by the nurse are used to secure catheters.
- Check for leaks. Check the site where the catheter connects to the drainage bag. Report any leaks to the nurse immediately.
- Provide catheter care if ordered. Catheter care is done daily or twice a day in some facilities (see *Catheter Care,* p. 355). Some facilities consider perineal care to be sufficient. Catheter care is sometimes needed after bowel movements.
- Provide perineal care daily and after bowel movements.
- Empty the drainage bag at the end of the shift or at time intervals as directed by the nurse. Measure and record the amount of urine (see *Emptying a Urinary Drainage Bag,* p. 356). Report increases or decreases in the amount of urine.
- Use a separate measuring container for each person. This prevents the spread of microbes from one person to another.
- Do not let the drain on the drainage bag touch any surface.
- Report complaints to the nurse immediately. These include complaints of pain, burning, the need to urinate, or irritation. Also report the color, clarity, and odor of urine and the presence of particles.
- Encourage fluid intake as instructed by the nurse.

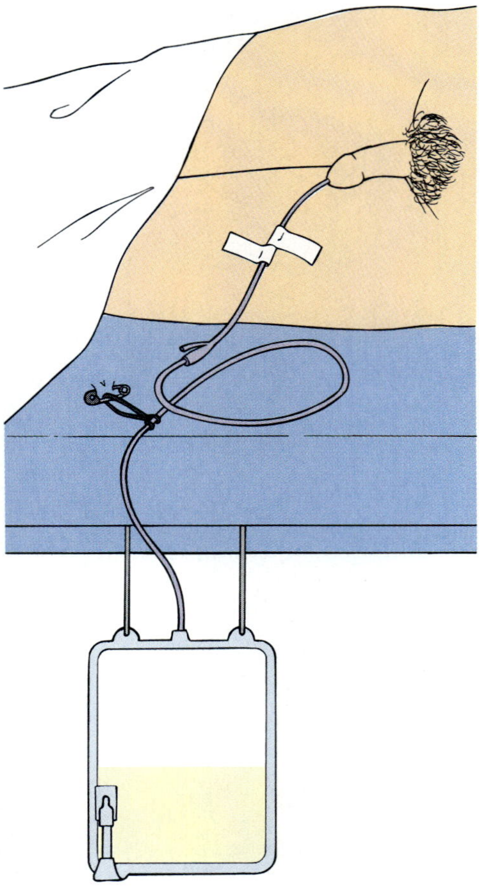

Fig. 15-11 *The drainage tubing is coiled on the bed and pinned to the bottom linens so urine flows freely. A rubber band is placed around the tubing with a clove hitch. The safety pin is passed through the loops and pinned to the linens. The catheter is taped to the inner thigh. Enough slack is left on the catheter to prevent friction at the urethra.*

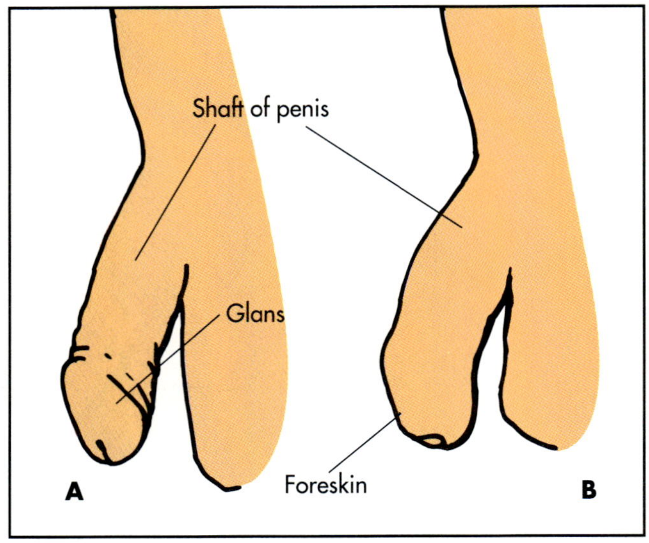

Fig. 15-12 *A, Circumcised male. B, Uncircumcised male.*

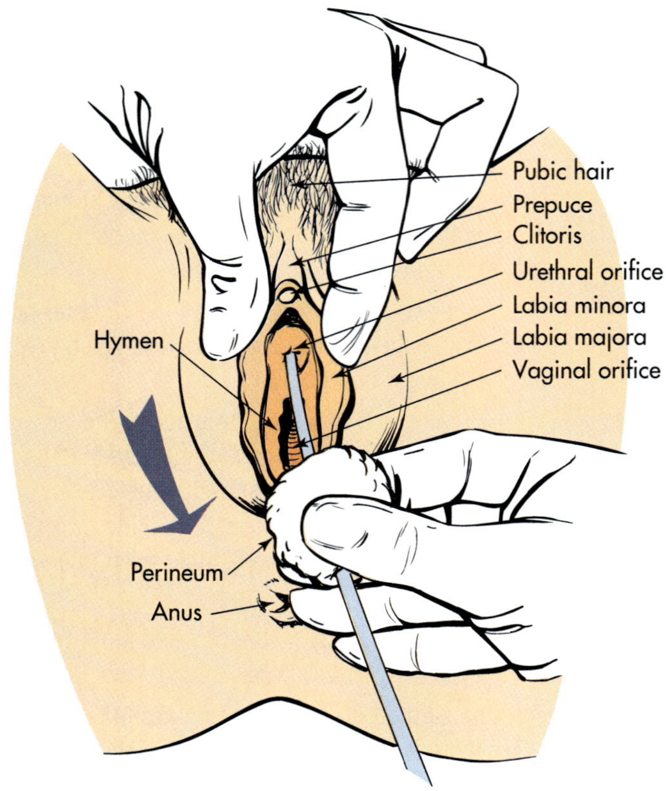

Fig. 15-13 *The catheter is cleaned beginning at the meatus. About 4 inches of the catheter is cleaned.*

Catheter Care

Facility policy or the care plan may require catheter care for a person. This involves special attention to the catheter and the insertion site. The Centers for Disease Control (CDC) suggest that perineal care daily and after bowel movements is adequate. Vaginal drainage also may require frequent perineal care. The following procedure is one way to provide catheter care. However, you must follow facility policy and the person's care plan.

CATHETER CARE

PRE-PROCEDURE

1. Explain the procedure to the person.
2. Wash your hands.
3. Collect the following:
   - Equipment for perineal care
   - Disposable gloves
   - Disposable bed protector
   - Bath blanket
4. Identify the person. Check the ID bracelet with the treatment card.
5. Provide for privacy.
6. Raise the bed to the best level for good body mechanics.

PROCEDURE

7. Lower the side rail.
8. Cover the person with a bath blanket. Fanfold top linens to the foot of the bed.
9. Drape the person for perineal care (see Fig. 13-24).
10. Fold back the bath blanket between the legs to expose the genital area.
11. Place the bed protector under the buttocks. Ask the person to flex the knees and raise the buttocks off the bed by pushing against the mattress with the feet.
12. Put on gloves. Perform perineal care (see *Female Perineal Care* or *Male Perineal Care,* pages 309-311).
13. Separate the labia (female) or retract the foreskin (uncircumcised male) as in Figure 15-12. Check for crusts, abnormal drainage, or secretions.
14. Clean the catheter from the meatus down the catheter about 4 inches (Fig. 15-13). Use soap and water and a clean washcloth. Avoid tugging or pulling on the catheter. Repeat if necessary with a clean washcloth.
15. Make sure the catheter is secured properly. Coil and secure tubing (see Fig. 15-11).
16. Remove the bed protector.
17. Remove the gloves.
18. Cover the person and remove the bath blanket.

POST-PROCEDURE

19. Make sure the person is comfortable and the call bell is within reach.
20. Lower the bed to its lowest position.
21. Raise or lower side rails as instructed by the nurse.
22. Clean and return equipment to its proper place. Discard disposable items.
23. Unscreen the person.
24. Follow facility policy for soiled linen.
25. Wash your hands.
26. Report your observations to the nurse.

Emptying a Urinary Drainage Bag

Pre-procedure

1 Collect equipment:
- Graduate (measuring container)
- Disposable gloves

2 Wash your hands.

3 Explain the procedure to the person.

4 Identify the person. Check the ID bracelet and call the person by name.

5 Provide for privacy.

Procedure

6 Put on the gloves.

7 Place the measuring container (graduate) so urine can be collected when the drain is opened.

8 Open the clamp on the bottom of the drainage bag.

9 Let all urine drain into the graduate. Do not let the drain touch the graduate (Fig. 15-14).

10 Close the clamp. Replace the clamped drain in the holder on the bag (see Fig. 15-11).

11 Measure urine.

12 Rinse the graduate and return it to its proper place.

13 Remove the gloves and wash your hands.

14 Record the time and amount on the I&O record.

Post-procedure

15 Unscreen the person.

16 Report the amount and other observations.

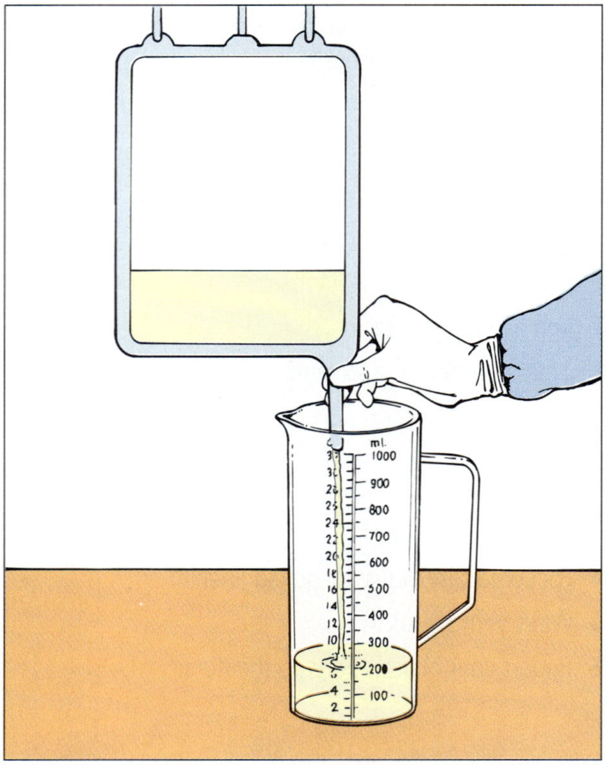

Fig. 15-14 *The clamp on the drainage bag is opened and the drain is directed into the measuring container. The drain must not touch the inside of the container.*

The Condom Catheter

Condom catheters (external catheter, urinary sheath, Texas catheter) are often used for incontinent men. A condom catheter is a soft, rubber sheath that slides over the penis. Tubing connects the condom catheter and the drainage bag. Residents and home care patients may prefer leg bags during the day (Fig. 15-15 on page 358).

A new condom catheter is applied daily. The penis is thoroughly washed with soap and water and dried before a new catheter is applied. The manufacturer's instructions are followed when applying a condom catheter. Elastic tape is used to secure the catheter in place. Elastic tape expands when the penis changes size. This allows blood flow to the penis. *Adhesive tape is never used to secure catheters. It does not expand. Blood flow to the penis will be cut off causing injury to the penis.* Medical asepsis and Standard Precautions are followed when removing or applying condom catheters. The Bloodborne Pathogen Standard is also followed if there are breaks in the skin or if the urine contains blood or is potentially infectious.

Text continued on page 359.

Applying a Condom Catheter

Pre-procedure

1 Explain the procedure to the man.
2 Wash your hands.
3 Collect the following:
- Condom catheter
- Elastic tape
- Drainage bag or leg bag
- Basin of warm water
- Soap
- Towel
- Washcloths
- Bath blanket
- Disposable gloves
- Disposable bed protector
- Paper towels

4 Arrange paper towels and equipment on the overbed table.
5 Provide for privacy.
6 Raise the bed to the best level for good body mechanics.

Procedure

7 Lower the side rail.
8 Cover the person with a bath blanket. Bring top linens to the foot of the bed.
9 Ask the person to raise his buttocks off the bed. Or turn him onto his side away from you.
10 Slide the bed protector under his buttocks.
11 Have the person lower his buttocks or turn him onto his back.
12 Bring top linens up to cover his knees and lower legs.
13 Secure the drainage bag to the bed frame or have a leg bag ready. Make sure the drain is closed.
14 Raise the bath blanket to expose the genital area.
15 Put on the gloves.
16 Remove the condom catheter.
  a Remove the tape and roll the sheath off the penis.
  b Disconnect the drainage tubing from the condom.
  c Discard the tape and condom.
17 Provide perineal care (see *Male Perineal Care*, page 311). Observe the penis for skin breakdown or irritation.
18 Remove the protective backing from the condom. This exposes the adhesive strip.
19 Hold the penis firmly. Roll the condom onto the penis. Leave a 1-inch space between the penis and the end of the catheter (Fig. 15-16 on page 358).
20 Secure the condom with elastic tape. Apply tape in a spiral (Fig. 15-17 on page 358). Tape must not go completely around the penis.
21 Connect the condom to the drainage tubing. Coil excess tubing on the bed as shown in Figure 15-11, or attach a leg bag.
22 Remove the bed protector.
23 Remove the gloves.
24 Return top linens and remove the bath blanket.

Post-procedure

25 Make sure the person is comfortable.
26 Place the call bell within reach.
27 Lower the bed to its lowest position.
28 Raise or lower side rails as instructed by the nurse.
29 Clean and return the wash basin and other equipment to their proper place.
30 Unscreen the person.
31 Take the bag, used collection bag, and disposable items to the dirty utility room. Measure and record the amount of urine in the bag. Use Standard Precautions.
32 Wash your hands.
33 Report your observations.

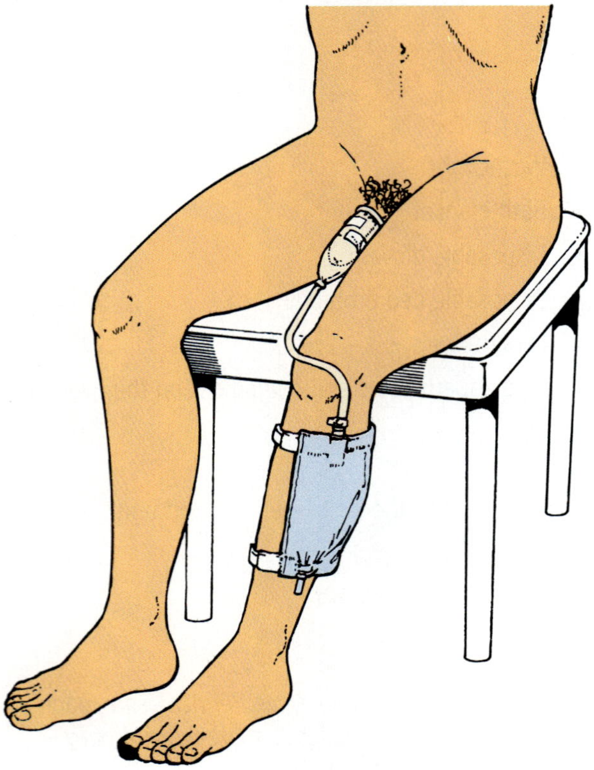

Fig. 15-15 *A condom catheter attached to a leg bag.*

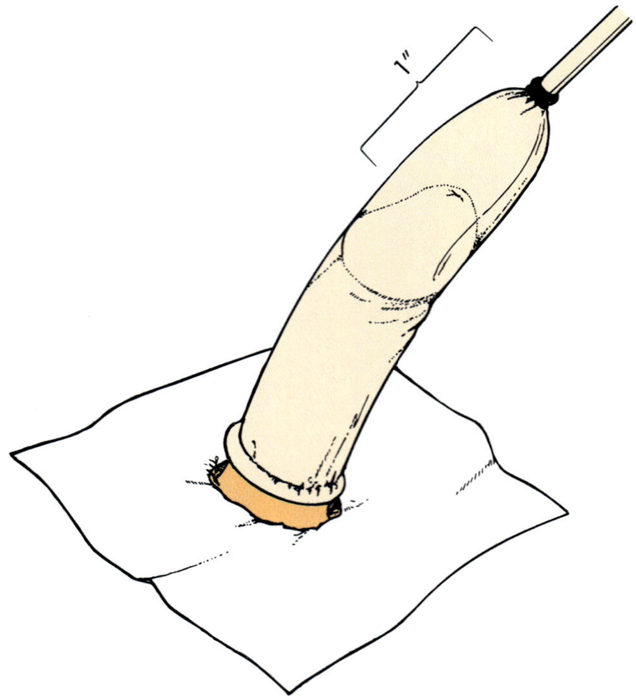

Fig. 15-16 *A condom catheter applied to the penis. There is a 1-inch space between the penis and the end of the catheter.*

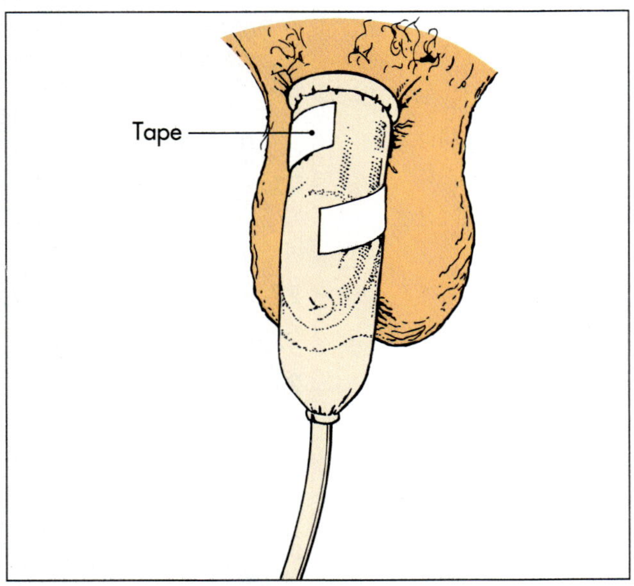

Fig. 15-17 *Tape is applied in spiral fashion to secure the condom catheter to the penis.*

BLADDER TRAINING

Bladder training programs are developed for persons with urinary incontinence. Voluntary control of urination is the goal. With the doctor's approval, the nurse develops a plan for bladder training. This becomes part of the nursing care plan. You assist in the bladder training program as directed by the nurse.

There are two basic methods for bladder training. With one, the person uses the toilet, commode, bedpan, or urinal at scheduled intervals. The person is given 15 or 20 minutes to start voiding. The rules for maintaining normal urination are followed. The normal position for urination is assumed if possible. Privacy is important.

The second method is used for those with catheters. The catheter is clamped (Fig. 15-18) to prevent urine from draining out of the bladder. Usually the catheter is clamped for 1 hour at first. Eventually it is clamped for 3 to 4 hours at a time. When the catheter is removed, the toilet, commode, bedpan, or urinal is used every 3 to 4 hours.

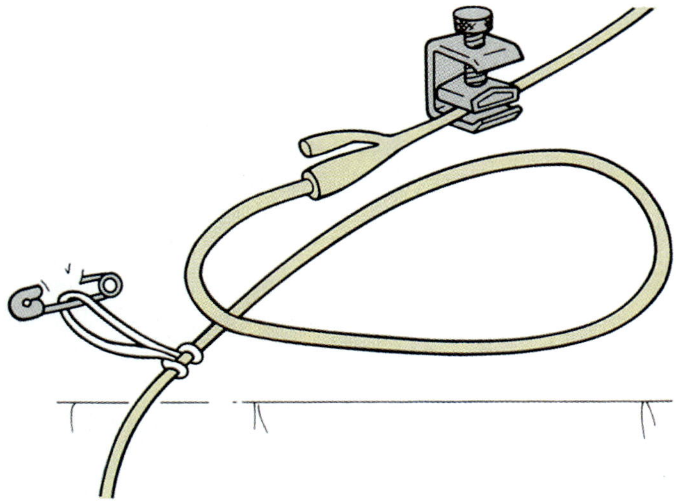

Fig. 15-18 *The catheter clamp prevents urine from draining out of the bladder. The clamp is applied directly to the catheter—not to the drainage tubing.*

COLLECTING AND TESTING URINE SPECIMENS

Urine specimens (samples) are collected for laboratory study. Urine tests are used by the doctor to make a diagnosis or to evaluate treatment. There are many types of specimens. The nurse completes a requisition slip for each specimen sent to the laboratory. The slip has the person's identifying information and the test to be done. Nursing assistants often collect urine specimens. Box 15-4 lists the rules to follow when collecting specimens.

BOX 15-4 RULES FOR COLLECTING URINE SPECIMENS

- Wash your hands before and after collecting the specimen.
- Follow the rules of medical asepsis, Standard Precautions, and the Bloodborne Pathogen Standard.
- Use a clean container for each specimen.
- Use a container appropriate for the specimen.
- Label the container accurately with the requested information. Most request the person's full name, room and bed number, date, and time the specimen was collected.
- Do not touch the inside of the container or lid.
- Collect the specimen at the time specified.
- Ask the person not to have a bowel movement while the specimen is being collected. The specimen must be free of fecal material.
- Ask the person to put toilet tissue in the toilet or wastebasket. The specimen should not contain tissue.
- Take the specimen and requisition slip to the laboratory or designated storage place. The specimen container should be in a plastic bag.

The Random Urine Specimen

The random urine specimen is collected for a urinalysis. No special preparations are needed. It also can be collected at any time. Many persons can collect the specimen themselves. Weak and very ill persons need assistance.

The Clean-Voided Specimen

The clean-voided specimen is also called a *midstream specimen* or a *clean-catch specimen.* The perineal area is cleaned before collecting the specimen. This reduces the number of microbes in the urethral area when the specimen is collected. The person starts to void into the toilet, bedpan, urinal, or commode. Then the stream is stopped and the specimen container positioned. The person voids into the container until the specimen is obtained.

Stopping the stream of urine is hard for many people. You may need to position and hold the specimen container in place after the person starts to void. Wear gloves when collecting a clean-voided specimen. Clean-voided specimen kits are obtained from the central supply area.

Collecting a Random Urine Specimen

Pre-procedure

1 Explain the procedure to the person.

2 Wash your hands.

3 Collect the following:
- Bedpan and cover, urinal, or disposable specimen pan
- Specimen container and lid
- Label
- Disposable gloves
- Plastic bag

Procedure

4 Fill out the label. Put it on the container.

5 Put the container and lid in the bathroom or dirty utility room.

6 Identify the person. Check the ID bracelet against the requisition slip.

7 Provide for privacy.

8 Ask the person to urinate in the receptacle. Remind him or her to put toilet tissue into the wastebasket or toilet. Caution the person not to put toilet tissue into the bedpan or specimen pan.

9 Put on the gloves.

10 Take the bedpan or urinal to the bathroom or dirty utility room.

11 Measure urine if I&O is ordered.

12 Pour urine into the specimen container so it is about three-fourths full. Dispose of excess urine.

13 Place the lid on the specimen container. Put the container in the plastic bag.

14 Clean the bedpan or urinal. Remove the gloves.

15 Return the bedpan or urinal to its proper place.

16 Help the person wash the hands.

Post-procedure

17 Make sure he or she is comfortable.

18 Raise or lower side rails as instructed by the nurse.

19 Place the call bell within reach.

20 Unscreen the person.

21 Take the specimen and the requisition slip to the nurses' station or laboratory.

22 Wash your hands.

23 Report your observations to the nurse.

Collecting a Clean-Voided Specimen

Pre-procedure

1 Explain the procedure to the person.
2 Wash your hands.
3 Collect the following:
- Clean-voided specimen kit
- Disposable gloves
- Bedpan, urinal, or commode if the person cannot use the bathroom
- Plastic bag

Procedure

4 Label the container with the requested information.
5 Identify the person. Check the ID bracelet with the requisition slip.
6 Provide for privacy.
7 Let the person complete the procedure if able. Place the call bell within reach.
8 Assist as necessary.
9 Offer the bedpan or assist him or her to the bathroom or commode. The person wears a robe and slippers if he or she is to be up.
10 Open the kit. Remove the specimen container and towelettes. Put on the gloves.
11 Clean the penis or perineal area with towelettes or other specified solution (see *Male Perineal Care* or *Female Perineal Care,* pages 309-311).
12 Keep the woman's labia separated until the specimen is collected. For the uncircumcised male, keep the foreskin retracted until the specimen is collected.
13 Collect the specimen.
a Ask the person to urinate into the receptacle.
b Ask him or her to stop the stream.
c Hold the specimen container under the person.
d Ask him or her to start urinating again.
e Ask the person to stop the stream when urine has been collected.
f Let him or her finish urinating.
14 Put the lid on the container immediately. Do not touch the inside of the lid. Put the container in the plastic bag.
15 Help the person clean the perineal area. Return foreskin to its natural position.
16 Clean the bedpan or commode. Remove the gloves.
17 Return equipment to its proper place. Discard disposable items.
18 Help the person wash the hands.

Post-procedure

19 Make sure the person is comfortable.
20 Raise or lower side rails as instructed by the nurse.
21 Place the call bell within reach.
22 Unscreen the person.
23 Take the requisition slip and the specimen to the nurses' station or laboratory.
24 Wash your hands.
25 Report your observations to the nurse.

The 24-Hour Urine Specimen

All urine voided during a 24-hour period is collected for a 24-hour urine specimen. Urine is chilled on ice or refrigerated during the collection period. This prevents the growth of microorganisms. A preservative is added to the collection container for some tests.

The person voids to begin the test; this voiding is discarded. *All* voidings during the next 24 hours are collected. The procedure and test period must be clearly understood by the person and everyone involved in the person's care. The rules for collecting urine specimens are followed.

COLLECTING A 24-HOUR URINE SPECIMEN

PRE-PROCEDURE

1 Review the procedure with the nurse.
2 Explain the procedure to the person.
3 Wash your hands.
4 Collect the following:
- Urine container for a 24-hour collection
- Preservative from the laboratory if needed
- Bucket with ice if needed
- Two 24-hour urine specimen labels
- Funnel
- Bedpan, urinal, commode, or specimen pan
- Disposable gloves
- Measuring containers

PROCEDURE

5 Label the specimen container.
6 Identify the person. Check the ID bracelet with the requisition slip.
7 Arrange equipment in the person's bathroom or dirty utility room.
8 Place one 24-hour specimen label in the appropriate place in the bathroom or dirty utility room. Place the other near the bed.
9 Offer the bedpan or urinal, or assist the person to the bathroom or bedside commode. The person wears a robe and slippers when up.
10 Ask the person to void.
11 Discard the specimen (wear gloves for this step) and note the time. This begins the 24-hour collection period.
12 Clean the bedpan, urinal, commode, or specimen pan.
13 Remove the gloves.
14 Mark the time the test began and the time it will end on the room and bathroom labels. Also mark the specimen container.
15 Ask the person to use the bedpan, urinal, commode, or specimen pan when voiding during the next 24 hours. Tell the person to signal when urine needs to be emptied. Remind him or her not to have a bowel movement at the same time and not to put toilet tissue in the receptacle.
16 Measure all urine if I&O is ordered. Use a clean measuring container each time.
17 Pour urine into the specimen container using the funnel. Do not spill any urine. The test is restarted if urine is spilled or discarded.
18 Add ice to the bucket as necessary.
19 Ask the person to void at the end of the 24-hour period. Pour the urine into the specimen container.
20 Thank the person for cooperating.

POST-PROCEDURE

21 Make sure he or she is comfortable.
22 Place the call bell within reach.
23 Raise or lower side rails as instructed by the nurse.
24 Wash your hands.
25 Take the specimen and requisition slip to the laboratory.
26 Remove the labels from the room and bathroom. Clean and return equipment to its proper place. Discard disposable items.
27 Report your observations to the nurse.

The Double-Voided Specimen

Fresh-fractional urine specimen is another term for a double-voided specimen. The person voids twice. The first time is to empty the bladder of "stale" urine. In 30 minutes the person voids again. "Fresh" urine has collected in the bladder since the first voiding. The second voiding is usually a very small or "fractional" amount of urine.

Fresh-fractional specimens are used to test urine for glucose and ketones (see page 365).

Collecting a Double-Voided Specimen

Pre-procedure

1. Explain the procedure to the person.
2. Wash your hands.
3. Collect the following:
   - Bedpan, urinal, commode, or disposable specimen pan
   - Two specimen containers
   - Urine testing equipment
   - Disposable gloves
4. Identify the person. Check the ID bracelet with the treatment card.
5. Provide for privacy.

Procedure

6. Offer the bedpan or urinal, or assist the person to the bathroom or commode. A robe and slippers are worn when up.
7. Ask the person to urinate.
8. Put on the gloves.
9. Take the receptacle to the bathroom or dirty utility room.
10. Measure urine if I&O is ordered. Pour some urine into the specimen container.
11. Test the specimen as ordered in case a second specimen cannot be obtained. Discard the urine.
12. Clean the receptacle. Remove the gloves.
13. Return the receptacle to its proper place.
14. Help the person wash the hands.
15. Ask the person to drink an 8-ounce glass of water.
16. Make sure the person is comfortable, the side rails are up if needed, and the call bell is within reach. Unscreen the person.
17. Wash your hands.
18. Return to the room in 20 to 30 minutes.
19. Repeat steps 5 through 17.
20. Report the results of the second test and any other observations to the nurse.

Collecting a Specimen from an Infant or Child

Specimens may be needed from infants and children who have not been toilet trained. A collection bag is applied over the urethra. Two workers may be needed to apply the bag if the baby or child is agitated.

Collecting a Urine Specimen from an Infant or Child

Pre-procedure

1 Explain the procedure to the child.
2 Wash your hands.
3 Collect the following:
- Disposable collection bag
- Wash basin
- Sterile cotton balls
- Bath towel
- Two diapers
- Specimen container
- Disposable gloves
- Plastic bag

4 Identify the child. Check the ID bracelet with the requisition slip.
5 Provide for privacy.

Procedure

6 Put on the gloves.
7 Remove the diaper and dispose of it properly.
8 Clean the perineal area. Use a sterile cotton ball for each stroke. Rinse and dry the area.
9 Position the child on the back. Flex the child's knees and separate the legs.
10 Remove the adhesive backing from the collection bag.
11 Apply the bag to the perineum. Do not cover the anus (Fig. 15-19).
12 Diaper the child. Remove the gloves.
13 Raise the head of the crib if allowed. This helps urine to collect in the bottom of the bag.
14 Unscreen the child.
15 Return to the room periodically. Open the diaper to see if the child has urinated. Provide for privacy if the child has urinated.
16 Put on gloves and remove the diaper.
17 Remove the collection bag gently.
18 Press the adhesive surfaces of the bag together. Or transfer urine to the specimen container through the drainage tab.
19 Clean the perineal area, rinse, and dry well.
20 Diaper the child and remove the gloves.

Post-procedure

21 Make sure the child is comfortable. Raise the side rail.
22 Unscreen the child.
23 Write the requested information on the specimen container. Place the container in the plastic bag.
24 Clean and return equipment to its proper place. Discard disposable items.
25 Take the requisition slip and the specimen to the nurses' station or laboratory.
26 Wash your hands.
27 Report your observations to the nurse.

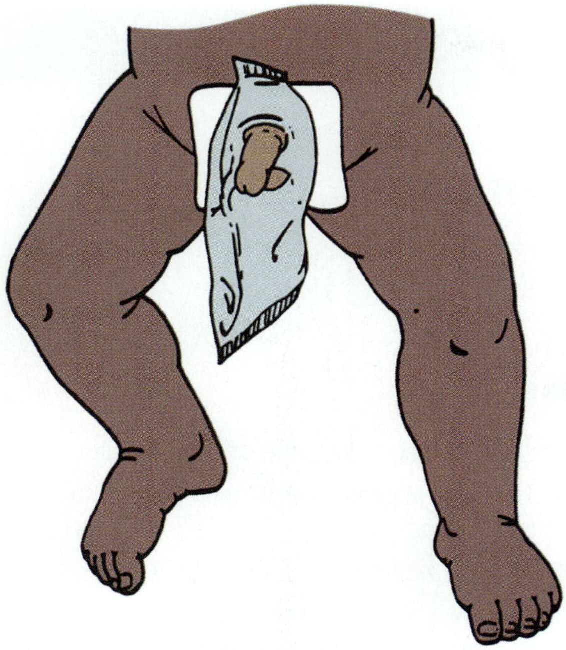

Fig. 15-19 *A disposable collection bag is applied to the perineal area of the infant. Urine collects in the bag for a specimen.*

Testing Urine

Diabetes mellitus is a chronic disease in which the pancreas fails to secrete enough insulin. Insufficient amounts of insulin prevent the body from using sugar for energy. Sugar builds up in the blood if it cannot be used. Some sugar appears in the urine. **Glucosuria** or **glycosuria** means sugar (glucos, glycos) in the urine (uria).

Simple blood tests have replaced urine tests for sugar. These tests are done by nurses. Sometimes nursing assistants are taught how to do them. Persons with diabetes are also taught how to do the tests. Blood glucose (blood sugar) testing is more accurate than urine testing. However, urine testing for sugar is still ordered for some persons.

The diabetic person may also have **acetone (ketone bodies, ketones)** in the urine. These appear in urine because of the rapid breakdown of fat for energy. Fat is used for energy if the body cannot use sugar because of the lack of insulin. Urine is also tested for ketones.

The doctor orders the type and frequency of urine tests. They are usually done four times a day: 30 minutes before each meal (ac) and at bedtime (HS). The doctor uses the test results to regulate the amount of medication given. They are also used to regulate the person's diet. You must be accurate when testing urine. The results are promptly reported to the nurse. Double-voided specimens are best for testing urine for sugar and ketones.

There are different types of tests. They involve dipping a reagent strip into the urine. The strip changes color when it reacts with the urine. The strip is compared to the color chart on the bottle (Fig. 15-20). The nurse gives you specific instructions for the urine test ordered. Be sure to read the manufacturer's instructions before you begin.

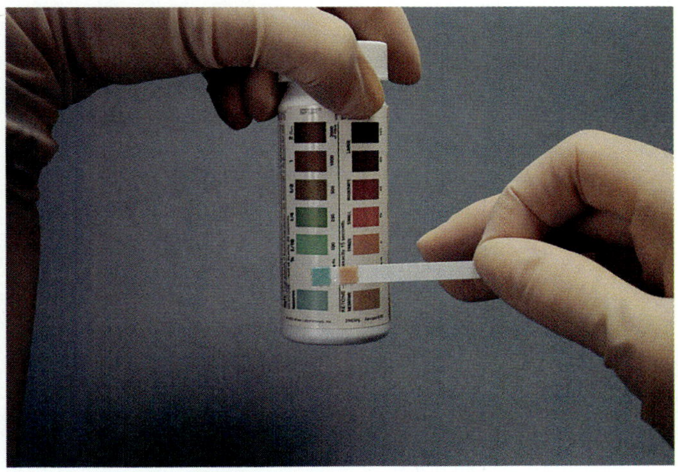

Fig. 15-20 *Reagent strip for sugar and ketones.*

Testing Urine for Sugar and Ketones

Pre-procedure

1. Explain the procedure to the person.
2. Wash your hands.
3. Identify the person. Check the ID bracelet with the treatment card.

Procedure

4. Collect the following:
    - **a** Double-voided specimen (see *Collecting a Double-Voided Specimen,* page 363)
    - **b** Reagent strip as ordered
    - **c** Wristwatch
    - **d** Disposable gloves
5. Put on the gloves.
6. Remove a strip from the bottle. Put the cap on the bottle immediately. Make sure it is tight.
7. Dip the 2 test areas of the strip into the specimen.
8. Remove the strip. The manufacturer's instructions tell you how long to keep the strip in the urine.
9. Tap the strip gently against the container to remove excess urine.
10. Wait the required amount of time as specified in the manufacturer's instructions.
    - **a** Compare the strip with the color chart on the bottle for ketones. Read the results.
    - **b** Compare the strip with the color chart for glucose. Read the results.
11. Discard disposable items and the specimen.

Post-procedure

12. Clean equipment. Remove the gloves.
13. Return equipment to its proper place.
14. Wash your hands.
15. Report the results and other observations to the nurse.

Straining Urine

Stones (calculi) can develop in the urinary system. They may be in the kidneys, ureters, or bladder. Stones may be as small as a pinhead or as large as an orange. Stones that cause severe pain and damage to the urinary system may require surgical removal. A stone may exit the body with the urine. Therefore all of the person's urine is strained. If a stone is passed, it is sent to the laboratory to be examined.

STRAINING URINE

PRE-PROCEDURE

1. Explain the procedure to the person. Also explain that the urinal, bedpan, commode, or specimen pan is used for voiding.
2. Wash your hands.
3. Collect the following:
   - Disposable strainer or 4 × 4 gauze
   - Specimen container
   - Urinal, bedpan, commode, or specimen pan
   - Two labels stating that all urine is strained
   - Disposable gloves
4. Identify the person. Check the ID bracelet with the treatment card.

PROCEDURE

5. Arrange items in the person's bathroom.
6. Place one label in the bathroom. Place the other near the bed.
7. Offer the bedpan or urinal. Or assist the person to the bedside commode or bathroom. The person wears a robe and slippers when up. Provide for privacy.
8. Tell the person to signal after voiding.
9. Put on the gloves.
10. Place the strainer or gauze into the specimen container.
11. Pour urine into the specimen container. Urine passes through the strainer or gauze (Fig. 15-21).
12. Place the strainer or gauze in the container if any crystals, stones, or particles appear.
13. Discard the urine.
14. Help the person clean the perineal area if necessary.
15. Help the person wash the hands.
16. Remove the gloves.
17. Make sure the person is comfortable.
18. Raise or lower side rails as instructed by the nurse.
19. Place the call bell within reach.
20. Unscreen the person.
21. Label the specimen container with the requested information. Put the container in the plastic bag.
22. Clean and return items to their place.
23. Take the specimen to the nurses' station or laboratory. Make sure you have a requisition slip if you are taking the specimen to the laboratory.
24. Wash your hands.
25. Report your observations to the nurse.

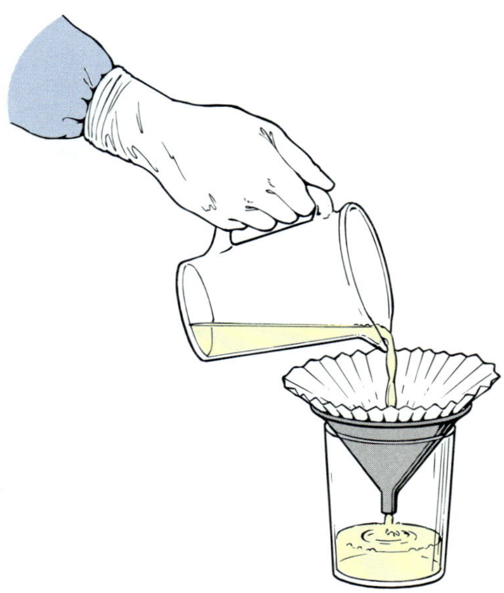

Fig. 15-21 *A disposable strainer is placed in a specimen container. Urine is poured through the strainer into the specimen container.*

Summary

You are responsible for helping patients and residents maintain normal urination. You also assist with bladder training and collect specimens. You must follow the rules of medical asepsis, Standard Precautions, cleanliness, and skin care. The Bloodborne Pathogen Standard is also followed if the urine contains blood or is potentially infectious. Your observations of the person's urine are valuable to doctors and nurses. They use them to plan and evaluate the person's treatment and progress.

Position and privacy are important for urinary elimination. Voiding is a private function. Voiding is easier and more comfortable if the person can urinate in a normal position and in private. However, some people are so weak and disabled that they cannot be left alone to use the bathroom, commode, bedpan, or urinal.

You must do all you can to protect the person's privacy. Pull privacy curtains and close doors, shades, and drapes. If you must stay in the room, position yourself so the person has as much privacy as possible. You may need to stand just outside the bathroom door. Or it may be safe to stand on the other side of the privacy curtain. The nurse will help you with ways to protect the person's privacy. Playing music is useful to mask the sounds of elimination. This may help the person who does not have total privacy.

Review Questions

Circle the best *answer.*

1 Which mean urination?
- **a** Glucosuria and dysuria
- **b** Acetone and ketone bodies
- **c** Micturition and voiding
- **d** Catheter and urinal

2 Which is *false?*
- **a** Urine is normally clear and yellow or amber in color.
- **b** Urine normally has an ammonia odor.
- **c** People normally urinate before going to bed and on rising.
- **d** A person normally voids about 1500 ml a day.

3 Which is *not* a rule for maintaining normal elimination?
- **a** Help the person assume a normal position for urination.
- **b** Provide for privacy.
- **c** Help the person to the bathroom or commode, or provide the bedpan or urinal as soon as requested.
- **d** Always stay with the person who is on a bedpan.

4 The best position for using a bedpan is
- **a** Fowler's position
- **b** The supine position
- **c** The prone position
- **d** The side-lying position

5 After a man uses the urinal, you should ask him to
- **a** Cover the urinal
- **b** Use the call bell
- **c** Put the urinal on the overbed table
- **d** Empty the urinal

6 Urinary incontinence
- **a** Is always permanent
- **b** Requires good skin care
- **c** Is treated with an indwelling catheter
- **d** All of the above

7 A person has a catheter. Which is *incorrect?*
- **a** Keep the drainage bag above the level of the bladder.
- **b** Make sure the drainage tubing is free of kinks.
- **c** Coil the drainage tubing on the bed.
- **d** Tape the catheter to the inner thigh.

Review Questions—cont'd

8 A person has a catheter. Which is *false?*

a Leaks at the connection site are taped.
b The rules of medical asepsis are followed.
c The drainage bag is emptied at the end of each shift.
d Complaints of pain, burning, the need to urinate, or irritation are reported immediately.

9 Mr. Powers has a condom catheter. Elastic tape is applied

a Completely around the penis
b To the inner thigh
c To the abdomen
d In a spiral fashion

10 The goal of bladder training is to

a Remove the catheter
b Allow the person to walk to the bathroom
c Gain voluntary control of urination
d All of the above

11 When collecting a urine specimen, you should

a Label the container with the requested information
b Use the correct container
c Collect the specimen at the time specified
d All of the above

12 The perineum is cleaned immediately before collecting a

a Random specimen
b Clean-voided specimen
c 24-hour urine specimen
d Double-voided specimen

13 A 24-hour urine specimen involves

a Collecting all urine voided by a person during a 24-hour period
b Collecting a random specimen every hour for 24 hours
c A catheterization
d Testing the urine for sugar and acetone

14 Urine is tested for sugar and ketones

a At bedtime
b 30 minutes after meals and at bedtime
c 30 minutes before meals and at bedtime
d Before breakfast

15 Which specimen is best for sugar and ketone testing?

a A random specimen
b A clean-voided specimen
c A 24-hour urine specimen
d A double-voided specimen

16 You are instructed to strain Mr. Power's urine. You know that straining urine is done to find

a Hematuria
b Stones
c Nocturia
d Urgency

Answers to these questions are on page 750.

Bowel Elimination

16

OBJECTIVES

- Define the key terms listed in this chapter
- Describe normal stools and the normal pattern and frequency of bowel movements
- List the observations about defecation that are reported to the nurse
- Identify the factors that affect bowel elimination
- Describe common bowel elimination problems
- Describe the measures that promote comfort and safety during defecation
- Describe bowel training
- Explain why enemas are given
- Know the common enema solutions
- Describe the rules for administering enemas
- Explain the purpose of rectal tubes
- Insert a rectal tube
- Describe how to care for a person with a colostomy or ileostomy
- Perform the procedures described in this chapter

KEY TERMS

anal incontinence The inability to control the passage of feces and gas through the anus

chyme Partially digested food and fluid that pass from the stomach into the small intestine

colostomy An artificial opening between the colon and abdominal wall

constipation The passage of a hard, dry stool

defecation The process of excreting feces from the rectum through the anus; a bowel movement

diarrhea The frequent passage of liquid stools

enema The introduction of fluid into the rectum and lower colon

fecal impaction The prolonged retention and accumulation of feces in the rectum

feces The semisolid mass of waste products in the colon

flatulence The excessive formation of gas in the stomach and intestines

flatus Gas or air in the stomach or intestines

ileostomy An artificial opening between the ileum (small intestine) and the abdominal wall

ostomy The surgical creation of an artificial opening

peristalsis The alternating contraction and relaxation of intestinal muscles

stoma An opening; see colostomy and ileostomy

stool Feces that have been excreted

suppository A cone-shaped solid medication that is inserted into a body opening; it melts at body temperature

Like urinary elimination, bowel elimination is a basic physical need. Many factors affect bowel elimination. They include privacy, personal habits, age, diet, exercise and activity, fluids, and drugs. Problems easily occur. Promoting normal bowel elimination is important. You will assist patients and residents in meeting their elimination needs.

Box 16-1 on page 372 contains a review of the structure and function of the gastrointestinal system.

NORMAL BOWEL MOVEMENTS

The frequency of bowel movements varies from person to person. Some have a bowel movement every day. Others have one every 2 to 3 days. Some people have 2 or 3 bowel movements a day. The elimination pattern also involves the time of day. Many people defecate after breakfast, others in the evening.

Stools are normally brown in color. Bleeding in the stomach and small intestine causes black or tarry stools. Bleeding in the lower colon and rectum causes red-colored stools. So do beets. A diet high in green vegetables can cause green stools. Diseases and infection can also cause clay- or white-, pale-, orange-, or green-colored stools.

Feces are normally soft, formed, moist, and shaped like the rectum. Feces that move rapidly through the intestine are watery and unformed. This is called **diarrhea.** Stools that move slowly through the intestines are harder than normal. **Constipation** is the excretion of a hard, dry stool.

Feces have a characteristic odor. The odor is from bacterial action in the intestines. Certain foods and drugs also cause odors.

What to Report to the Nurse

The nurse uses your observations for the nursing process. Therefore stools are carefully observed before disposal. Abnormal stools are observed by the nurse. You need to observe stools and report the following to the nurse:

- Color
- Amount
- Consistency
- Odor
- Shape
- Size
- Frequency of defecation
- Any complaints of pain

BOX 16-1 The Gastrointestinal System: Review of Body Structure and Function

Bowel elimination is the excretion of wastes from the gastrointestinal system. Foods and fluids are normally taken in through the mouth and are partially digested in the stomach. The partially digested foods and fluids are called **chyme.** Chyme passes from the stomach into the small intestine. Further digestion and absorption of nutrients occur as the chyme passes through the small bowel. Chyme eventually enters the large intestine (large bowel or colon) where fluid is absorbed. There the chyme becomes less fluid and more solid in consistency. **Feces** refers to the semisolid mass of waste products in the colon.

Feces move through the intestines by peristalsis. **Peristalsis** is the alternating contraction and relaxation of intestinal muscles. The feces move through the large intestine to the rectum. Feces are stored in the rectum until excreted from the body (Fig. 16-1). **Defecation (bowel movement)** is the process of excreting feces from the rectum through the anus. The term **stool** refers to feces that have been excreted.

See Chapter 5, pages 106-108, for more detailed information.

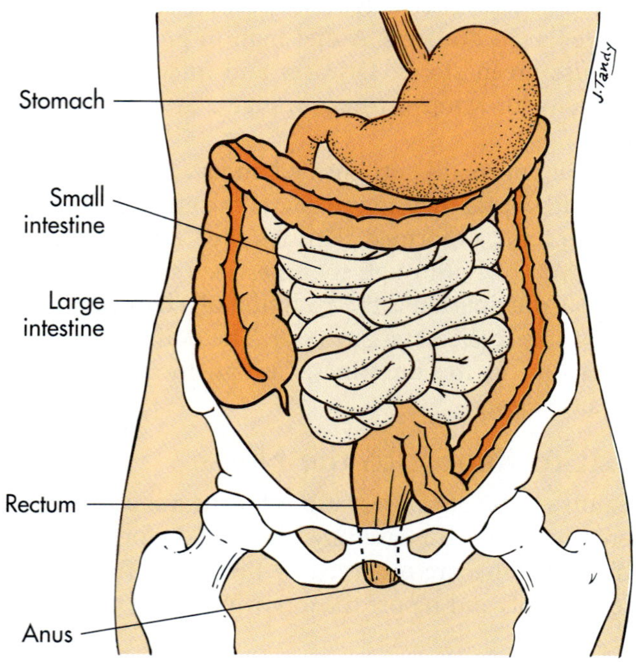

Fig. 16-1 *The gastrointestinal system.*

FACTORS AFFECTING BOWEL ELIMINATION

Normal, regular defecation is affected by many factors. The following factors affect the frequency, consistency, color, and odor of stools. The nurse considers these factors when using the nursing process to meet the person's elimination needs. Normal, regular elimination is the goal.

Privacy

Like voiding, bowel elimination is a private act. Lack of privacy prevents many people from defecating despite having the urge. Bowel movement odors and sounds can be embarrassing. Would you like to use a bedpan or commode for a bowel movement in a semiprivate room? Many people ignore the urge to defecate to avoid having a bowel movement in the presence of others. Constipation can easily result.

Personal Habits

Many people have habits and routines to promote bowel elimination. These may include drinking a hot beverage (coffee, tea, water), reading a book or newspaper, or taking a walk. These activities may relax the person. Defecation is easier when a person is relaxed rather than tense.

Time of day is another factor. Many people routinely have a bowel movement after breakfast. Habits and routines also relate to privacy and toilet access.

Age

Infants and toddlers do not have voluntary control of bowel movements. Defecation occurs whenever feces enter the rectum. Bowel training is learned between 2 and 3 years of age. Aging causes changes in the gastrointestinal system. Feces pass through the intestine at a slower rate. This results in constipation. Body changes from aging cause some elderly persons to lose control over defecation. Older persons are also at risk for intestinal tumors and disorders.

Diet

A well-balanced diet is important for normal bowel elimination. A certain amount of bulk is needed. High-fiber foods are not completely digested. They leave a residue that provides needed bulk. A diet low in fiber reduces the frequency of defecation, resulting in constipation. Fruits, vegetables, and whole grain cereals and breads are high in fiber.

Certain foods can cause diarrhea or constipation. Milk causes constipation in some people and diarrhea in others. Other milk products and chocolate can cause similar reactions. Spicy foods can irritate the intestines. Frequent stools or diarrhea can result.

Gas-forming foods stimulate peristalsis. Increased peristalsis results in defecation. Gas-forming foods include onions, beans, cabbage, cauliflower, radishes, and cucumbers.

Fluids

Feces contain water. Water is absorbed as feces move through the large intestine. Stool consistency depends on how much water is absorbed. The amount of fluid ingested, urine output, and vomiting affect the amount of water absorbed by the large intestine. Feces become hard and dry when large amounts of water are absorbed or when fluid intake is poor. Hard, dry feces move through the intestines at a slower rate. Constipation can occur.

Activity

Exercise and activity maintain muscle tone and stimulate peristalsis. Irregular elimination and constipation often occur from inactivity and bed rest. Inactivity may result from disease, surgery, injury, and aging.

Medications

Medications can prevent constipation or control diarrhea. Other drugs have the side effects of diarrhea or constipation. Drugs for pain relief often cause constipation. Antibiotics, used to fight or prevent infection, often cause diarrhea. Diarrhea occurs when the antibiotics kill normal flora in the large intestine. Normal flora is necessary for the formation of stool.

COMMON PROBLEMS

Many factors affect normal bowel elimination. Common problems include constipation, fecal impaction, diarrhea, anal incontinence, and flatulence.

Constipation

Constipation is the passage of a hard, dry stool. The person usually strains to have a bowel movement. Stools may be large or marble-sized. Large stools cause pain as they pass through the anus. Constipation occurs when feces move through the intestine slowly. This allows more time for water absorption. Common causes include a low-fiber diet, ignoring the urge to defecate, decreased fluid intake, inactivity, drugs, aging, and certain diseases. Dietary changes, fluids, activity, enemas, and medications may be ordered to prevent or relieve constipation.

Fecal Impaction

A **fecal impaction** is the prolonged retention and accumulation of feces in the rectum. Feces are hard or putty-like in consistency. Fecal impaction results if constipation is not relieved. The person cannot defecate, and more water is absorbed from the already hardened feces. Liquid seeping from the anus is a sign of fecal impaction. Liquid feces pass around the hardened fecal mass in the rectum.

The person with a fecal impaction tries many times to have a bowel movement. Abdominal discomfort, cramping, and rectal pain are common. The nurse checks for an impaction by doing a digital examination. This is done by inserting a gloved finger into the rectum (Fig. 16-2) and

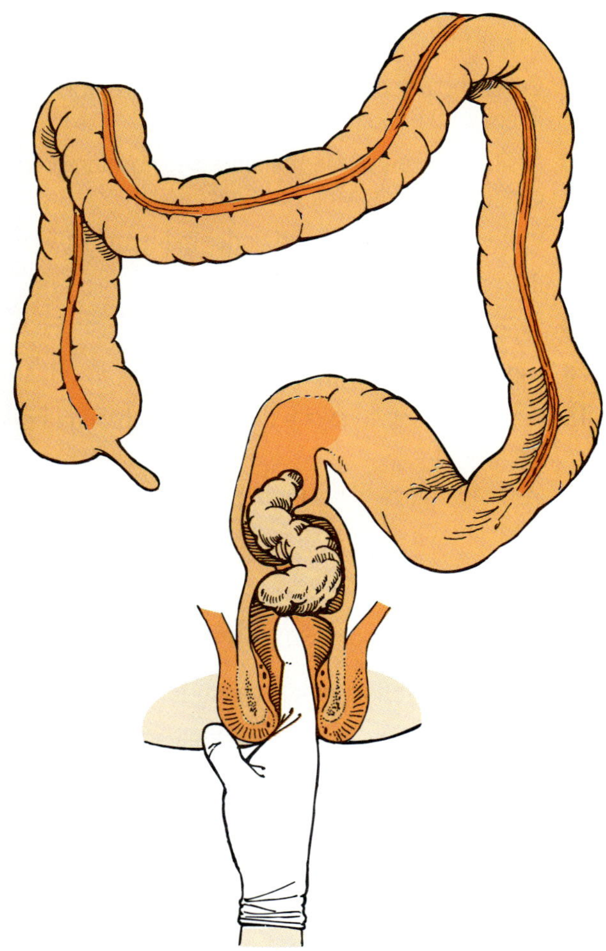

Fig. 16-2 *An index finger is used to check for a fecal impaction.*

Checking for a Fecal Impaction

Pre-procedure

1 Discuss the procedure and its need with the nurse. Make sure facility policy allows you to perform this procedure.
2 Explain the procedure to the person.
3 Wash your hands.
4 Collect the following:
   - Bedpan and bedpan cover
   - Bath blanket
   - Toilet tissue
   - Disposable gloves
   - Lubricant
   - Waterproof pad
   - Basin of warm water
   - Soap
   - Washcloth
   - Bath towel
5 Identify the person. Check the ID bracelet and call the person by name.
6 Provide for privacy.
7 Raise the bed to the best level for body mechanics. Make sure the far side rail is up.

Procedure

8 Lower the side rail near you.
9 Cover the person with a bath blanket. Fanfold top linens to the foot of the bed.
10 Position the person in the left Sims' position or in a comfortable side-lying position.
11 Place the waterproof pad under the buttocks.
12 Put on the gloves.
13 Expose the anal area.
14 Lubricate your gloved index finger.
15 Ask the person to take a deep breath through his or her mouth.
16 Insert the gloved finger while the person is taking a deep breath.
17 Check for a fecal mass.
18 Withdraw your finger.
19 Help the person onto the bedpan or to the bathroom if needed. Remember to lower the bed if the person will use the bathroom. The person also wears a robe and slippers when up. Be sure to provide for privacy and follow the *Giving the Bedpan* procedure on page 347.
20 Remove and discard the gloves. Wash your hands.
21 Put on clean gloves.
22 Wash the person's anal area with soap and water. Pat dry.
23 Remove the waterproof pad.

Post-procedure

24 Help the person assume a comfortable position.
25 Return top linens and remove the bath blanket.
26 Place the call bell within the person's reach.
27 Lower the bed to its lowest position.
28 Raise or lower side rails as instructed by the nurse.
29 Unscreen the person.
30 Clean and return equipment to its proper place. Discard disposable items.
31 Follow facility policy for soiled linen.
32 Remove the gloves and wash your hands.
33 Report your observations to the nurse.

feeling for a hard mass. The mass may be felt in the lower rectum. Sometimes it is higher in the colon and out of reach. The digital examination often produces the urge to defecate. The doctor may order medications and enemas to remove the impaction.

The nurse may have to remove the fecal mass with a lubricated, gloved finger. This is called *digital removal of an impaction.* A doctor's order is required in many facilities. The nurse inserts a finger into the rectum and hooks a finger around a piece of feces. Then the finger and stool are removed. The stool is dropped into the bedpan. The nurse repeats the process until the impaction is removed. The procedure is uncomfortable and embarrassing for most people.

Checking for and removing impactions can be very dangerous. The vagus nerve in the rectum can be stimulated. This nerve also affects the heart. Stimulation of the vagus nerve slows the heart rate. The heart rate can slow to dangerous levels in some persons. Some facilities allow nursing assistants to check for and remove impactions. Therefore the procedures are included in this book. However, you must discuss the procedure and its need with the nurse. *You must have the nurse's approval before checking for or removing an impaction. You must be very careful and gentle. Rectal bleeding can occur with both procedures. Standard Precautions and the Bloodborne Pathogen Standard must be followed.*

Diarrhea

Diarrhea is the frequent passage of liquid stools. Feces move through the intestines rapidly. This reduces the time for fluid absorption. There is an urgent need to defecate.

Removing a Fecal Impaction

Procedure

1. Follow steps 1 through 14 in *Checking for a Fecal Impaction.*
2. Ask the person to take a deep breath through the mouth.
3. Insert your lubricated, gloved index finger.
4. Hook your index finger around a small piece of feces.
5. Remove your finger and the feces.
6. Drop the stool into the bedpan.
7. Clean your finger with toilet tissue and reapply lubricant as needed.
8. Repeat steps 2 through 7 until you no longer feel feces.
9. Wipe the anal area with toilet tissue.
10. Cover the person with the bath blanket.
11. Cover the bedpan.
12. Remove and discard the gloves. Then put on a clean pair of gloves.
13. Raise the side rail and take the bedpan to the bathroom.
14. Empty, clean, and disinfect the bedpan.
15. Return the bedpan to the bedside stand.
16. Remove and discard the gloves.
17. Fill the wash basin with warm water.
18. Return to the bedside and lower the side rail near you.
19. Put on a clean pair of gloves.
20. Wash the buttocks and give perineal care.
21. Remove the waterproof pad.

Post-procedure

22. Help the person assume a comfortable position.
23. Return top linens and remove the bath blanket.
24. Place the call bell within the person's reach.
25. Lower the bed to its lowest position.
26. Raise or lower side rails as instructed by the nurse.
27. Unscreen the person.
28. Clean and return equipment to its proper place. Discard disposable items.
29. Follow facility policy for soiled linen.
30. Remove the gloves and wash your hands.
31. Report your observations to the nurse.

Some people cannot control elimination until getting to a bathroom. Abdominal cramping, nausea, and vomiting may also occur.

Causes of diarrhea include infections, certain drugs, irritating foods, and microorganisms in food and water. Medical treatment involves reducing peristalsis by diet or medications. Nursing measures include promptly assisting the person to the bathroom or providing the bedpan or commode. Stools require prompt disposal to reduce odors and prevent the spread of microorganisms. Good skin care is essential. Liquid feces are very irritating to the skin. Frequent wiping of the anal area with toilet tissue is also irritating. Pressure sores may develop if cleanliness and good skin care are not practiced.

Fluid lost through diarrhea must be replaced. This is especially important for infants, children, and the elderly. The nurse uses the nursing process to meet the person's fluid needs. The doctor may order intravenous fluids in severe cases.

Anal Incontinence

Anal incontinence (fecal incontinence) is the inability to control the passage of feces and gas through the anus. Infants and toddlers normally have anal incontinence until toilet trained. Diseases or injuries to the nervous system may cause anal incontinence. Persons with mental health problems or cognitive disorders (Chapters 29 and 30) may not recognize the need or act of defecating. Anal incontinence also can result from unanswered call bells when the person needs to use the bedpan, commode, or bathroom.

Good skin care is required. A bowel training program may be developed. Providing the bedpan or commode after meals or every 2 to 3 hours may be helpful. Waterproof pads or incontinent pants are used to keep linens and clothes clean. Consider the psychological impact of anal incontinence on the person. Frustration, embarrassment, anger, and humiliation are some emotions experienced.

Flatulence

Gas and air are normally found in the stomach and intestines. They are expelled through the mouth (belching, eructating) and anus. Gas and air passed through the anus is called **flatus. Flatulence** is the excessive formation of gas or air in the stomach and intestines. Common causes are

- Swallowing air while eating and drinking. This includes chewing gum, eating fast, drinking through a straw, and drinking carbonated beverages. Tense or anxious people may swallow large amounts of air when drinking.
- Bacterial action in the intestines
- Gas-forming foods (onions, beans, cabbage, cauliflower, radishes, and cucumbers)
- Constipation
- Bowel and abdominal surgeries
- Drugs that decrease peristalsis

If flatulence is not expelled, the intestines distend. That is, they swell or enlarge from the pressure of the gases. There may be abdominal cramping or pain, shortness of breath, and a swollen abdomen. "Bloating" is a common complaint. Ambulation (walking) and positioning in the left side-lying position often produce flatus. Doctors may prescribe enemas, medications, or rectal tubes for relief of flatulence.

COMFORT AND SAFETY DURING ELIMINATION

Certain measures help promote normal bowel elimination. The nurse uses the nursing process to meet the person's elimination needs. The nursing care plan may include measures that involve diet, fluids, and exercise. The actions listed in Box 16-2 are routinely practiced to promote comfort and safety during bowel elimination.

BOWEL TRAINING

Bowel training has two goals. One is to gain control of bowel movements. The other is to develop a regular pattern of elimination. Fecal impaction, constipation, and anal incontinence are prevented.

The urge to defecate is usually felt after a meal, particularly breakfast. Use of the toilet, commode, or bedpan is encouraged at this time. Other factors that promote elimination are included in the nursing care plan and bowel training program. These include diet, fluids, activity, and privacy. The nurse provides instructions about a person's bowel training program.

The doctor may order a suppository to stimulate defecation. A **suppository** is a cone-shaped, solid medication that is inserted into a body opening. It melts at body temperature. The rectal suppository is inserted into the rectum by the nurse (Fig. 16-3). A bowel movement occurs about 30 minutes later. Enemas are sometimes ordered.

ENEMAS

An **enema** is the introduction of fluid into the rectum and lower colon. Enemas are ordered by doctors. They are given to remove feces and to relieve constipation or fecal impaction. They are also ordered to clean the bowel of

BOX 16-2 MEASURES TO PROMOTE COMFORT AND SAFETY DURING BOWEL ELIMINATION

- Provide the bedpan or help the person to the toilet or commode as soon as requested.
- Provide for privacy. Ask visitors to leave the room. Close doors, pull curtains around the bed, and pull window curtains or shades. Remember, defecation is a private act. Leave the room if the person can be left alone.
- Make sure the bedpan is warm.
- Position the person in a normal sitting or squatting position.
- Make sure the person is covered for warmth and privacy.
- Allow enough time for defecation.
- Place the call bell and toilet tissue within the person's reach.
- Stay nearby if the person is weak or unsteady.
- Provide perineal care.
- Dispose of feces promptly. This reduces odors and prevents the spread of microorganisms.
- Let the person wash the hands after defecating and wiping with toilet tissue.
- Offer the bedpan after meals if the person has the problem of incontinence.
- Practice Standard Precautions and follow the Bloodborne Pathogen Standard if contact with stool is possible.

B

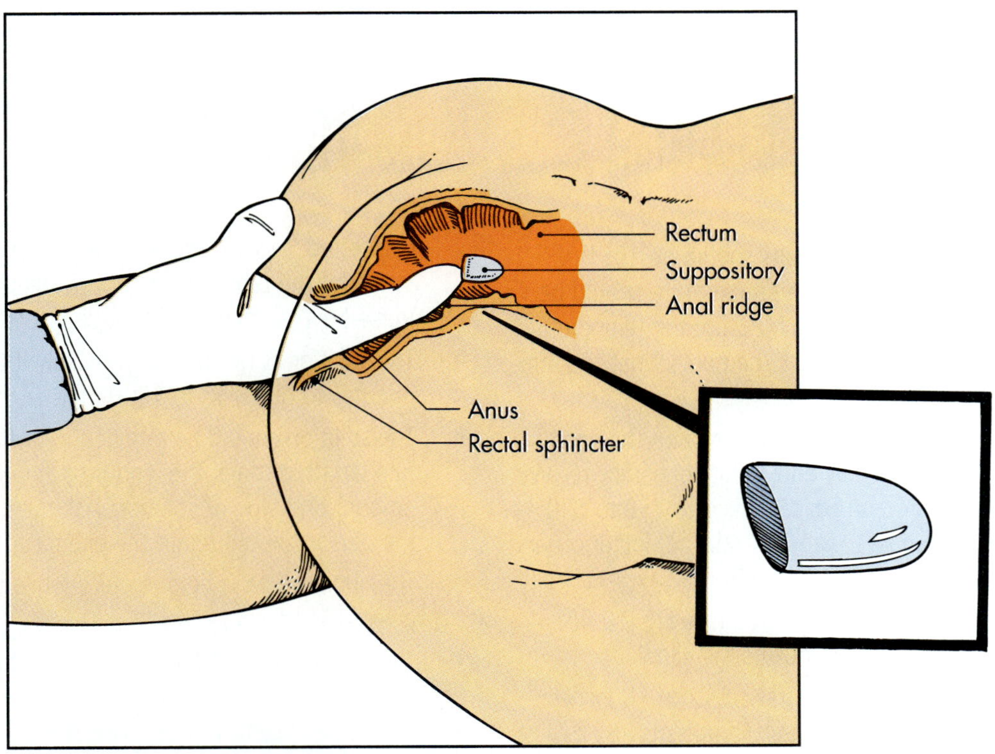

A

Fig. 16-3 *A, A rectal suppository. B, The nurse inserts a suppository into the rectum.*

feces before certain surgeries, x-ray procedures, or childbirth. Sometimes enemas are ordered to relieve flatulence and intestinal distention. Bowel training programs can involve enemas.

Enema Solutions

The enema solution is ordered by the doctor. A *tap-water* solution is obtained from a faucet. A *soapsuds* enema (SSE) is prepared by adding 5 ml of liquid soap to 1000 ml of tap water. A *saline* enema is a solution of salt and water. It is prepared by adding 2 teaspoons of table salt to 1000 ml of tap water. These solutions are generally used for cleansing enemas. Cleansing enemas are given to remove feces from the rectum and colon.

Oil is used for oil-retention enemas. They are given for constipation or fecal impactions. The oil is retained in the rectum for 30 to 60 minutes to soften feces and lubricate the rectum. This allows feces to pass with ease. Mineral oil, olive oil, or a commercial oil-retention enema are used.

Commercial enemas are often ordered for constipation. They are also ordered when complete cleansing of the bowel is not indicated. The enema contains about 120 ml (4 ounces) of solution. It causes defecation by irritating and distending the rectum.

Other enema solutions may be ordered. Consult with the nurse and use the facility procedure manual to safely prepare and give uncommon enemas.

Equipment

Disposable enema kits are used. The kit (Fig. 16-4) has a plastic enema bag, tubing, a clamp for the tubing, and a waterproof pad. The enema bag holds the solution. Most kits have packets of castile soap for soapsuds enemas. Most tubes are prelubricated. If not, a lubricant is needed. A bath thermometer is used to measure the temperature of the solution. Some solutions are obtained from central supply. If a commercial enema is ordered, you need the enema and a waterproof pad. A bedpan is usually needed for an enema. Enema procedures also require gloves. Standard Precautions and the Bloodborne Pathogen Standard are followed.

Rules for Giving Enemas

Enemas are usually safe procedures. Many people give themselves enemas at home. However, enemas are dangerous for elderly persons and those with certain heart and kidney diseases. Give an enema only after receiving clear instructions and after reviewing the procedure with the nurse.

Comfort and safety measures are practiced when giving an enema. The rules in Box 16-3 also must be followed.

BOX 16-3 GIVING ENEMAS: COMFORT AND SAFETY MEASURES

- Solution temperature for adults should be 105° to 109° F (40.5° to 43° C). The temperature should be 98.6° F (37° C) for children. Measure the temperature with a bath thermometer. Ask the nurse what the temperature should be for the person.
- The amount of solution given depends on the enema's purpose and the person's age. Adults generally receive 500 to 1000 ml. Young children receive 250 to 500 ml. Infants receive less than 250 ml. The doctor orders the amount of solution to be given.
- The left Sims' position is preferred (see Fig. 10-45). A comfortable left side-lying position is allowed.
- For adults, the enema bag is raised 12 to 18 inches above the level of the mattress. For infants, the bag is raised no more than 3 inches. Ask the nurse how high to raise the bag for the person.
- The lubricated enema tubing is inserted only 2 to 4 inches into the adult's rectum. For infants, the tubing is inserted 1 to 1½ inches. The intestine can be injured if the tube is inserted any deeper. Ask the nurse how far to insert the tubing for the person.
- The solution is given slowly. Usually it takes 10 to 15 minutes to give 750 to 1000 ml.
- The solution should be retained in the bowel for a certain length of time. The length of time depends on the amount and type of solution. Ask the nurse how long the person should retain the enema solution.
- The enema tube is held in place while the solution is given.
- The bathroom must be vacant when the person has the urge to defecate. Make sure that the bathroom will not be used by another person.
- The nurse observes the enema results.
- Standard Precautions are used and the Bloodborne Pathogen Standard is followed.

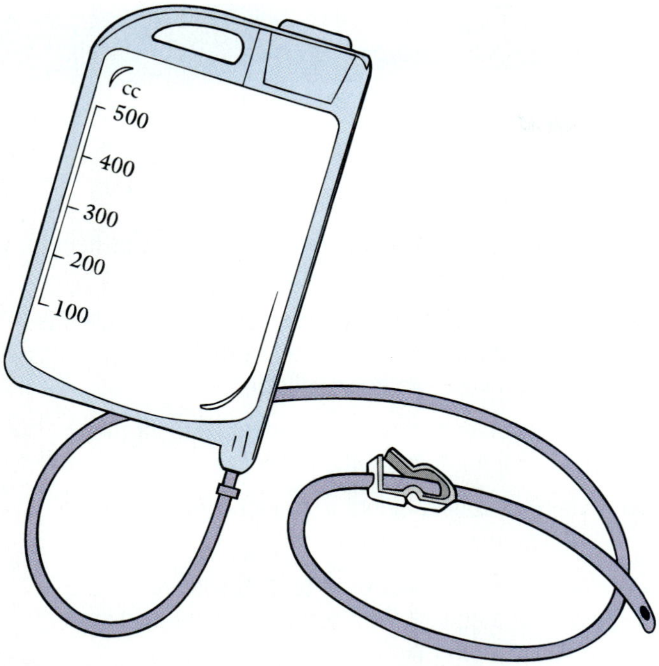

Fig. 16-4 *An enema kit contains a plastic enema bag, tubing, and a clamp.*

The Cleansing Enema

Cleansing enemas clean the bowel of feces and flatus. They are sometimes given before surgery, x-ray procedures, and childbirth. The doctor orders a soapsuds, tap-water, or saline enema. The doctor may order *enemas until clear.* This means that enemas are given until the return solution is clear and free of fecal material. Ask the nurse how many enemas can be given. Facility policy may allow repeating enemas only 2 or 3 times.

Tap-water enemas can be dangerous. The large intestine may absorb some of the water into the bloodstream. This creates a fluid imbalance in the body. Repeated enemas increase the risk of excessive fluid absorption. Soapsuds enemas are very irritating to the bowel's mucous lining. Damage to the bowel can result with repeated enemas. Using more than 5 ml of castile soap or using stronger soaps can also damage the bowel. The saline enema solution is similar to body fluid. However, some of the salt solution may be absorbed. This too can cause a fluid imbalance. When there is excess salt in the body, the body retains water.

Text continued on page 382.

Giving a Cleansing Enema

Pre-procedure

1. Explain the procedure to the person.
2. Wash your hands.
3. Collect the following:
   - Bedpan or bedside commode
   - Disposable enema kit (enema bag, tubing, clamp, and waterproof bed protector)
   - Bath thermometer
   - Waterproof bed protector
   - Water-soluble lubricant
   - Disposable gloves
   - Material for enema solution: 5 ml castile soap or 2 teaspoons of salt
   - Toilet tissue
   - Bath blanket
   - IV pole
   - Large measuring container
   - Robe and slippers
   - Specimen container if needed
   - Paper towels
4. Identify the person. Check the ID bracelet with the treatment card.
5. Provide for privacy.
6. Raise the bed to the best level for good body mechanics.

Procedure

7. Lower the side rail.
8. Cover the person with a bath blanket. Fanfold top linens to the foot of the bed.
9. Position the IV pole so the enema bag will be 12 to 18 inches above the mattress.
10. Raise the side rail.

Continued.

GIVING A CLEANSING ENEMA—CONT'D

PROCEDURE—CONT'D

11 Prepare the enema:
- **a** Close the clamp on the tubing.
- **b** Adjust water flow until it is lukewarm.
- **c** Fill the measuring container to the 1000 ml mark or as otherwise ordered.
- **d** Measure water temperature. It should be 105° F (40.5° C).
- **e** Prepare the enema solution:
  - **1.** Saline enema: add 2 teaspoons of salt
  - **2.** Soapsuds enema: add 5 ml of castile soap
  - **3.** Tap-water enema: add nothing to the water
- **f** Stir the solution with the bath thermometer. Scoop off any suds (SSE).
- **g** Pour the solution into the enema bag.
- **h** Seal the top of the bag.
- **i** Hang the bag on the IV pole.

12 Lower the side rail.

13 Position the person in the left Sims' position or in a comfortable left side-lying position.

14 Place a waterproof pad under the buttocks.

15 Put on the gloves.

16 Expose the anal area.

17 Place the bedpan behind the person.

18 Position the enema tubing in the bedpan. Open the clamp. Let solution flow through the tubing to remove air. Clamp the tubing.

19 Lubricate the tubing with the lubricant. Lubricate 2 to 4 inches from the tip.

20 Separate the buttocks to see the anus.

21 Ask the person to take a deep breath through the mouth.

22 Insert the tubing gently 2 to 4 inches into the rectum when the person is exhaling (Fig. 16-5). Stop if there are complaints of pain or if you feel resistance.

23 Check how much solution is in the enema bag.

24 Unclamp the tubing and administer the solution slowly (Fig. 16-6).

25 Ask the person to take slow deep breaths. This helps the person relax while the enema is given.

26 Clamp the tubing if the person needs to defecate, has abdominal cramping, or starts to expel solution. Unclamp when symptoms subside.

27 Give the amount of solution ordered. Stop if the person cannot tolerate the procedure.

28 Clamp the tubing before it is empty. This prevents air from entering the bowel.

29 Hold several thicknesses of toilet tissue around the tubing and against the anus. Remove the tubing.

30 Discard the soiled toilet tissue into the bedpan.

31 Wrap the tubing tip with paper towels and place it inside the enema bag.

32 Help the person onto the bedpan. Raise the head of the bed. Or assist the person to the bathroom or commode. The person wears a robe and slippers when up. The bed is in the lowest position.

33 Place the call bell and toilet tissue within reach. Remind the person not to flush the toilet.

34 Discard disposable items.

35 Remove the gloves and wash your hands.

36 Leave the room if the person can be left alone.

37 Return when the person signals. Knock before entering.

38 Observe enema results for amount, color, consistency, and odor.

39 Put on the gloves.

40 Obtain a stool specimen if ordered.

41 Provide perineal care as needed.

42 Remove the bed protector.

43 Empty, clean, and disinfect the bedpan or commode. Flush the toilet after the nurse observes the results. Return items to their proper place. Remove the gloves and wash your hands.

44 Help the person wash the hands. Wear gloves for this step if necessary.

45 Return top linens and remove the bath blanket.

POST-PROCEDURE

46 Make sure the person is comfortable and the call bell is within reach.

47 Lower the bed to its lowest position.

48 Raise or lower side rails as instructed by the nurse. Unscreen the person.

49 Follow facility policy for soiled linen.

50 Wash your hands.

51 Report your observations.

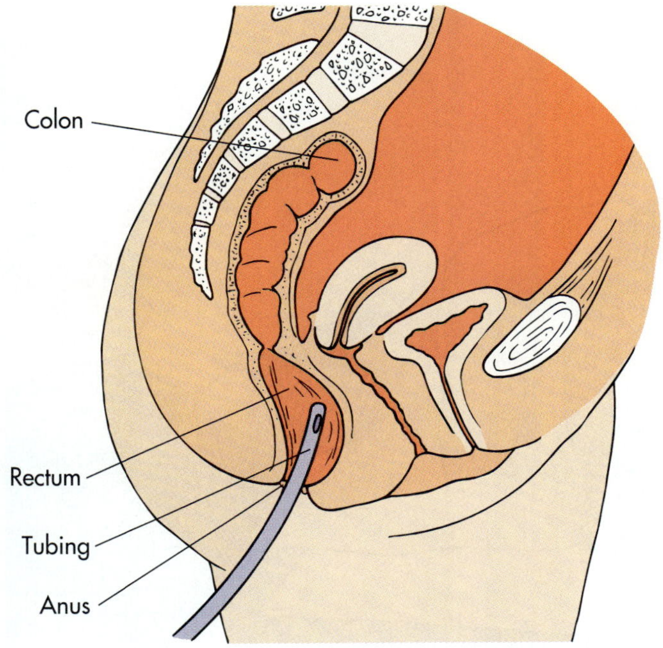

Fig. 16-5 *The enema tubing is inserted 2 to 4 inches into the rectum.*

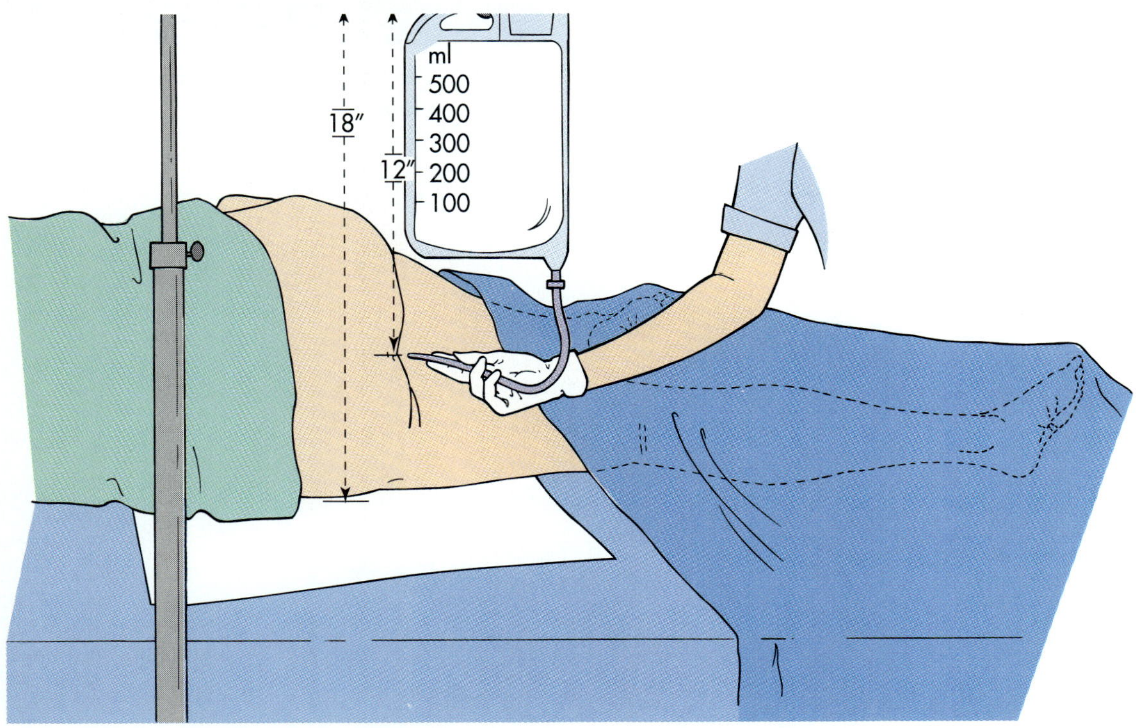

Fig. 16-6 *An enema is given with the person in the left Sims' position. For adults, the IV pole is positioned so that the enema bag is 12 inches above the anus and 18 inches above the mattress.*

The Commercial Enema

The commercial enema is ready to be given (Fig. 16-7). The solution is usually given at room temperature. However, the nurse may have you warm the enema in a basin of warm water. The left Sims' or a left side-lying position is often used. Some nursing theories suggest using the knee-chest position (see Fig. 22-2, C, page 507). The knee-chest position lets more solution flow into the colon. The nurse tells you how to position the person.

The plastic bottle is squeezed and rolled up from the bottom to give the solution. Squeezing and rolling are done until all the solution has been given. Do not release pressure on the bottle. If pressure is released, solution is drawn from the rectum back into the bottle. Encourage the person to retain the solution until the urge to defecate is felt. Remaining in the left Sims' or side-lying position helps retain the enema longer.

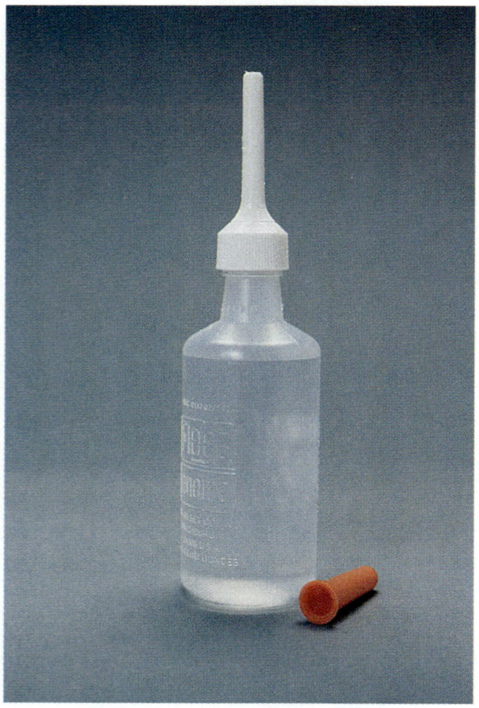

Fig. 16-7 *A commercial enema.*

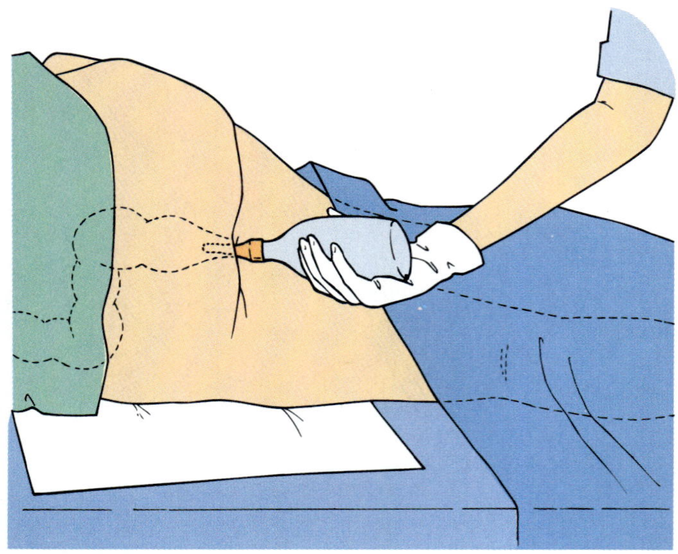

Fig. 16-8 *The tip of the commercial enema is inserted 2 inches into the rectum.*

Giving a Commercial Enema

Pre-procedure

1 Explain the procedure to the person.
2 Wash your hands.
3 Collect the following:
- Commercial enema
- Bedpan, commode, or specimen pan
- Waterproof bed protector
- Toilet tissue
- Disposable gloves
- Robe and slippers
- Specimen container if needed
- Bath blanket

4 Identify the person. Check the ID bracelet with the treatment card.
5 Provide for privacy.
6 Raise the bed to the best level for good body mechanics.

Procedure

7 Lower the side rail.
8 Cover the person with a bath blanket. Fanfold top linens to the foot of the bed.
9 Position the person in the left Sims' or a comfortable left side-lying position.
10 Place the bed protector under the buttocks.
11 Put on the gloves.
12 Expose the anal area.
13 Position the bedpan near the person.
14 Remove the cap from the enema.
15 Separate the buttocks to see the anus.
16 Ask the person to take a deep breath through the mouth.
17 Insert the enema tip 2 inches into the rectum when the person is exhaling (Fig. 16-8). Insert the tip gently.
18 Squeeze and roll the bottle gently. Do not release pressure on the bottle until all solution has been given.
19 Remove the tip from the rectum. Put the bottle into the box, tip first.
20 Help the person onto the bedpan. Raise the head of the bed. Assist the person to the bathroom or commode if appropriate. The person wears a robe and slippers when up, and the bed is in the lowest position.
21 Place the call bell and toilet tissue within reach. Remind the person not to flush the toilet.
22 Discard used disposable items. Remove the gloves and wash your hands.
23 Leave the room if the person can be left alone.
24 Return when the person signals. Knock before entering.
25 Observe enema results for amount, color, consistency, and odor.
26 Put on gloves.
27 Obtain a stool specimen if ordered.
28 Help the person clean the perineal area if indicated.
29 Remove the bed protector.
30 Empty, clean, and disinfect the bedpan or commode. Flush the toilet after the nurse observes the results. Return equipment to its proper place. Remove the gloves and wash your hands.
31 Help the person wash the hands. Wear gloves for this step if necessary.
32 Cover the person. Remove the bath blanket.

Post-procedure

33 Make sure the person is comfortable and the call bell is within reach.
34 Lower the bed to its lowest position.
35 Raise or lower side rails as instructed by the nurse.
36 Unscreen the person.
37 Follow facility policy for soiled linen.
38 Wash your hands.
39 Report your observations to the nurse.

The Oil-Retention Enema

Commercial oil-retention enemas are given like other commercial enemas. However, the solution is retained in the rectum so feces soften. The enema is retained for a specified length of time, usually 30 to 60 minutes. Oil-retention enemas are ordered to relieve constipation or fecal impaction.

Giving an Oil-Retention Enema

Pre-procedure

1 Explain the procedure to the person.
2 Wash your hands.
3 Collect the following:
- Commercial oil-retention enema
- Waterproof bed protector
- Disposable gloves
- Bath blanket

4 Identify the person. Check the ID bracelet with the treatment card.
5 Provide for privacy.
6 Raise the bed to the best level for good body mechanics.

Procedure

7 Lower the side rail.
8 Cover the person with a bath blanket. Fanfold top linens to the foot of the bed.
9 Position the person in the left Sims' or left side-lying position.
10 Place a bed protector under the buttocks.
11 Put on the gloves.
12 Expose the anal area.
13 Remove the cap from the enema.
14 Separate the buttocks to see the anus.
15 Ask the person to take a deep breath through the mouth.
16 Insert the tip 2 inches into the rectum when the person is exhaling. Insert the tip gently.
17 Squeeze and roll the bottle slowly and gently. Do not release pressure until all solution has been given.
18 Remove the tip from the rectum. Put the bottle in the box, tip first.
19 Cover the person. Leave him or her in the Sims' or side-lying position.
20 Encourage him or her to retain the enema for the time ordered.
21 Place additional waterproof protectors on the bed if indicated.
22 Lower the bed to its lowest position.
23 Raise or lower side rails as instructed by the nurse.

Post-procedure

24 Make sure the person is comfortable. Place the call bell within reach.
25 Unscreen the person.
26 Discard used disposable items.
27 Remove the gloves and wash your hands.
28 Check the person often.
29 Report your observations to the nurse.

RECTAL TUBES

A rectal tube is inserted into the rectum to relieve flatulence and intestinal distention. Flatus passes from the body without effort or straining. The disposable kit contains a tube and flatus bag (Fig. 16-9). The bag collects feces that may be expelled along with flatus. If a flatus bag is not included, place the open end of the tube in a folded waterproof pad.

The rectal tube is removed after 20 to 30 minutes. This helps prevent rectal irritation. The nurse tells you when to insert the tube and how long to leave it in place.

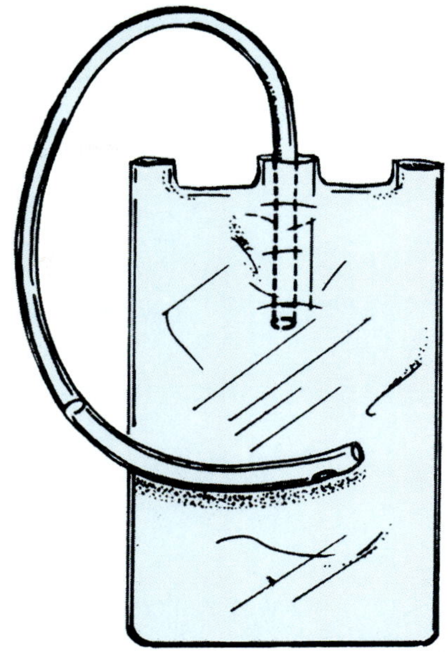

Fig. 16-9 *A disposable rectal tube and flatus bag.*

INSERTING A RECTAL TUBE

PRE-PROCEDURE

1. Explain the procedure to the person.
2. Wash your hands.
3. Collect the following:
   - Disposable rectal tube with flatus bag
   - Water-soluble lubricant
   - Adhesive tape
   - Disposable gloves
   - Waterproof bed protector
4. Identify the person. Check the ID bracelet with the treatment card.
5. Provide for privacy.
6. Raise the bed to the best level for good body mechanics.

PROCEDURE

7. Lower the side rail.
8. Position the person in the left Sims' or left side-lying position.
9. Place the waterproof bed protector under the buttocks.
10. Put on the gloves.
11. Expose the anal area.
12. Lubricate 2 to 4 inches up from the tip of the tube.
13. Separate the buttocks to see the anus.
14. Ask the person to take a deep breath through the mouth.
15. Insert the tube gently 2 to 4 inches into the rectum when the person is exhaling. Stop if there are complaints of pain or if you feel resistance.
16. Tape the rectal tube to the buttocks.
17. Position the flatus bag so it rests on the bed protector (Fig. 16-10 on page 386).
18. Cover the person.
19. Leave the tube in place for 20 minutes.
20. Lower the bed to its lowest position. Place the call bell within reach. Raise or lower side rails as instructed by the nurse.
21. Remove the gloves and wash your hands.

Continued.

INSERTING A RECTAL TUBE—CONT'D

PROCEDURE—CONT'D

22 Leave the room. Check the person often.

23 Return to the room in 20 minutes. Knock before entering the room.

24 Put on gloves and remove the tube. Wipe the rectal area.

25 Wrap the rectal tube and flatus bag in the bed protector. Remove the bed protector.

26 Ask the person about the amount of gas expelled.

POST-PROCEDURE

27 Make sure he or she is comfortable. Place the call bell within reach.

28 Unscreen the person.

29 Discard disposable items. Follow facility policy for soiled linen.

30 Remove the gloves and wash your hands.

31 Report your observations to the nurse.

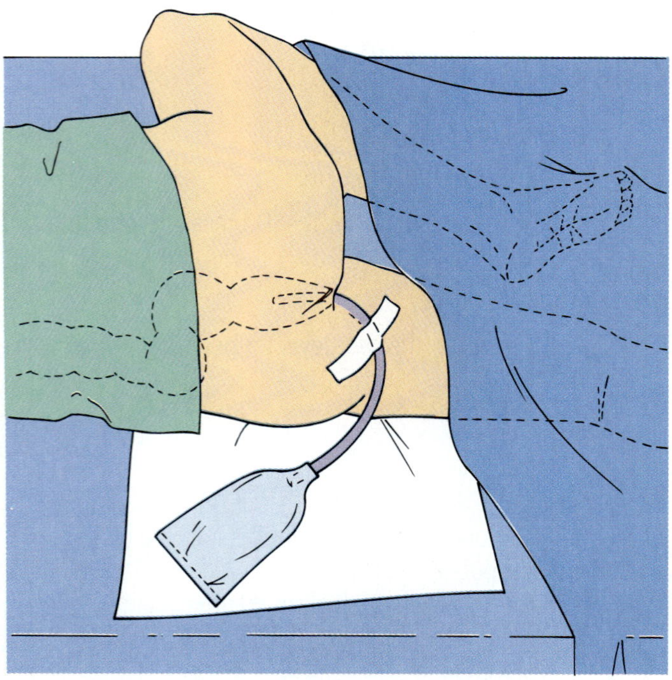

Fig. 16-10 *After being inserted, the rectal tube is taped to the buttocks and the flatus bag rests on the bed. The tube is inserted 2 to 4 inches into the rectum.*

THE PERSON WITH AN OSTOMY

Sometimes surgical removal of part of the intestines is necessary. Cancer, diseases of the bowel, and trauma (such as stab or bullet wounds) are common reasons for intestinal surgery. An ostomy may be necessary. An **ostomy** is the surgical creation of an artificial opening. The opening is called a **stoma.** The nurse may need your assistance with postoperative care. You may care for a person who has had an ostomy for a long time.

Colostomy

A **colostomy** is the surgical creation of an artificial opening between the colon and abdominal wall. Part of the colon is brought out onto the abdominal wall and a stoma made. Feces and flatus pass through the stoma rather than the anus. Colostomies may be permanent or temporary. If permanent, the diseased part of the colon is removed. A temporary colostomy gives the diseased or injured bowel time to heal. After healing, surgery is done to reconnect the bowel.

The colostomy site depends on what part of the colon is diseased or injured. Figure 16-11 shows common colostomy sites. Stool consistency depends on the colostomy site. Stools can be liquid to formed. The more colon remaining to absorb water, the more solid and formed the stool. If the colostomy is near the beginning of the colon, stools are liquid. A colostomy near the end of the large intestine results in formed stools.

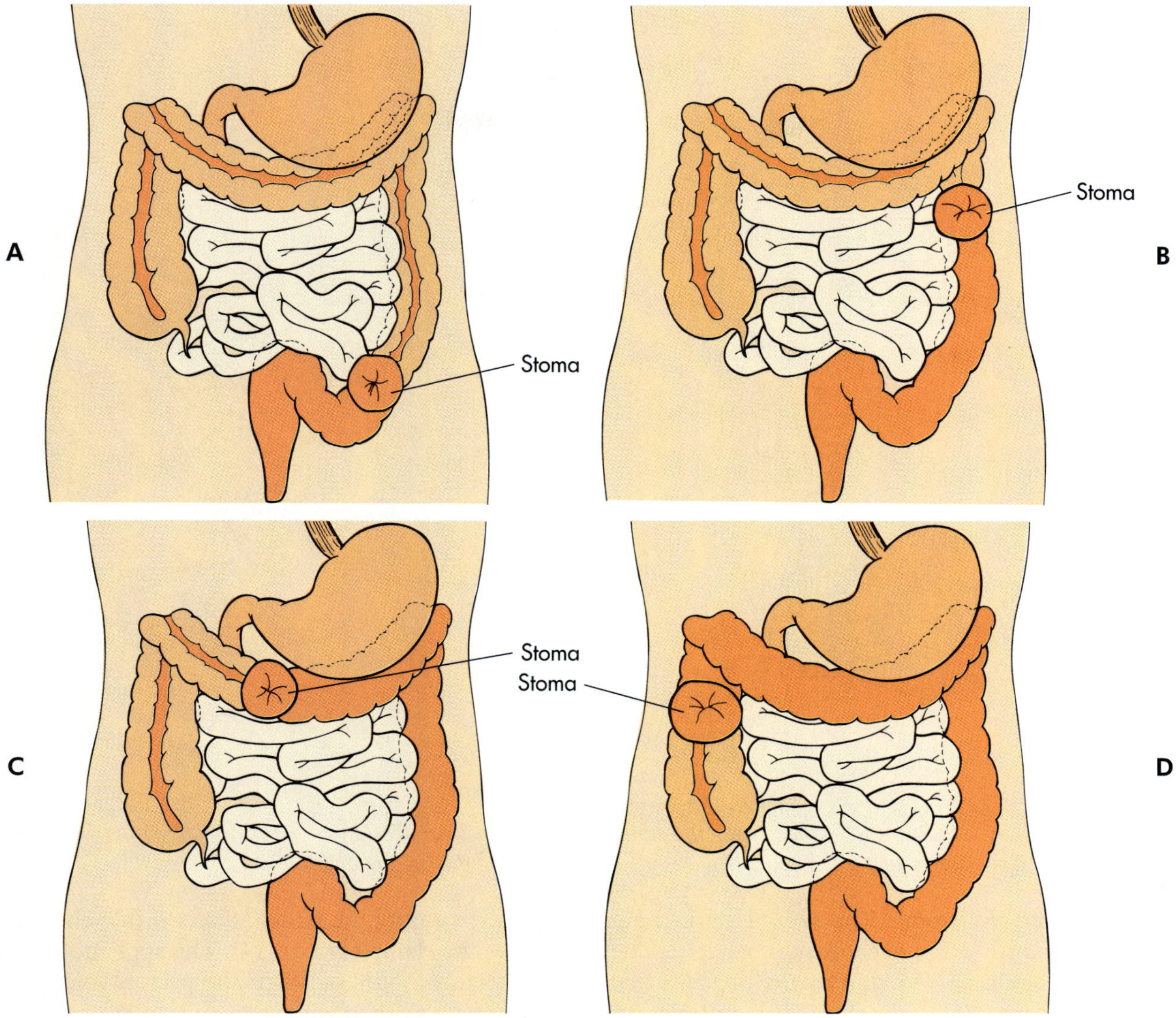

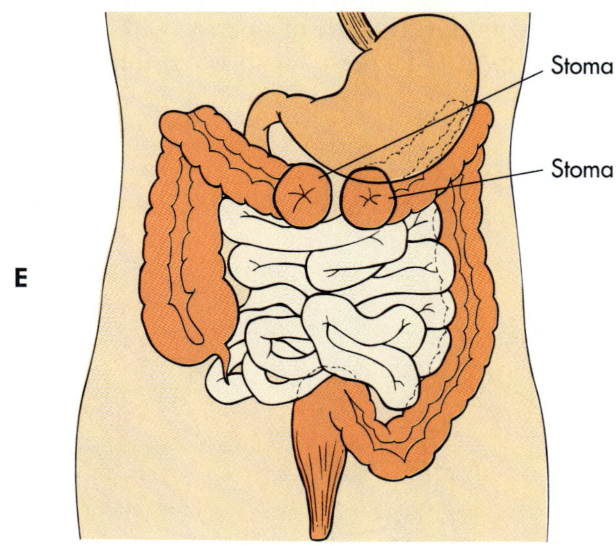

Fig. 16-11 *Colostomy sites with the shaded area indicating the part of the bowel that has been surgically removed.* ***A,*** *Sigmoid colostomy.* ***B,*** *Descending colostomy.* ***C,*** *Transverse colostomy.* ***D,*** *Ascending colostomy.* ***E,*** *Double-barrel colostomy. Two stomas are created: one allows for the excretion of fecal material. The other allows medication to be introduced to help the bowel heal. This type of colostomy is usually temporary.*

The person wears an appliance. The appliance is a disposable plastic pouch (or bag) applied over the stoma. It collects feces expelled through the stoma. Many pouches have a drain at the bottom. When soiled, the drain is opened and the pouch emptied. The pouch is changed every 3 to 5 days. Some people change the pouch whenever soiling occurs. The pouch has an adhesive backing that is applied to the skin. The pouch can also be secured to an ostomy belt (Fig. 16-12 on page 388). Many people manage their colostomies without help. If so, they are allowed to do so in the health care facility.

Feces are irritating to the skin. Skin care prevents skin

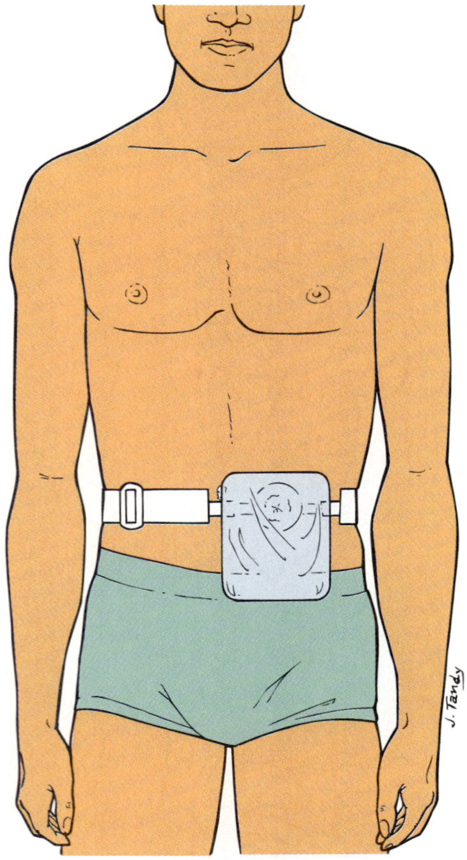

Fig. 16-12 *A colostomy appliance is in place over the stoma and is secured with a colostomy belt.*

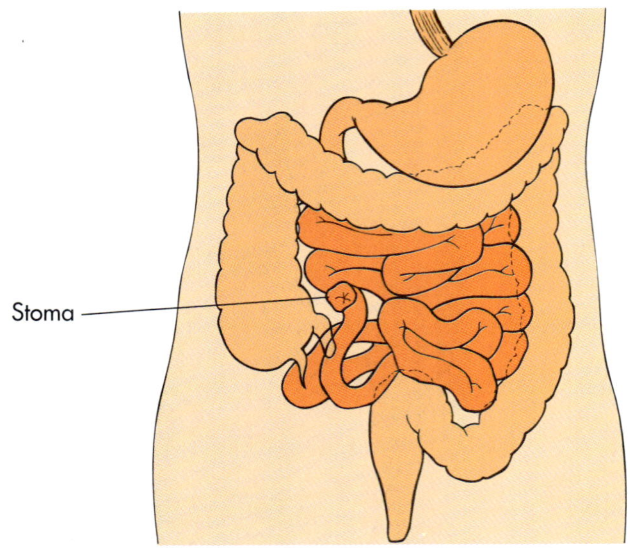

Fig. 16-13 *An ileostomy. The entire large intestine is surgically removed during the operation.*

breakdown around the stoma. The skin is washed and dried when the pouch is removed. A skin barrier is then applied around the stoma. The skin barrier prevents feces from coming in contact with the skin. Then a new pouch is applied.

Odors should be prevented. Good hygiene is essential. The pouch is emptied or a new one applied when soiling occurs. Avoiding gas-forming foods also control odors. Special deodorants can be put into the pouch. The nurse tells you which one to use.

Ileostomy

An **ileostomy** is the surgical creation of an artificial opening between the ileum (small intestine) and the abdominal wall. Part of the ileum is brought out onto the abdominal wall and a stoma made. The entire large intestine is removed (Fig. 16-13). Liquid feces drain constantly from an ileostomy. Water is not absorbed because the colon has been removed. Feces in the small intestine contain digestive juices and are very irritating to the skin. The ileostomy appliance must fit well so feces do not touch the skin. The appliance is sealed to the skin and is removed every 2 to 4 days. Good skin care is essential.

There are disposable and reusable ileostomy appliances. The appliance is clamped at the end so feces collect in the pouch. To empty the pouch, direct it into the toilet and remove the clamp (Fig. 16-14). The appliance is emptied every 4 to 6 hours or when the person voids. Reusable pouches are washed with soap and water and allowed to dry and air out. The care of a person with an ileostomy is similar to that of a person with a colostomy.

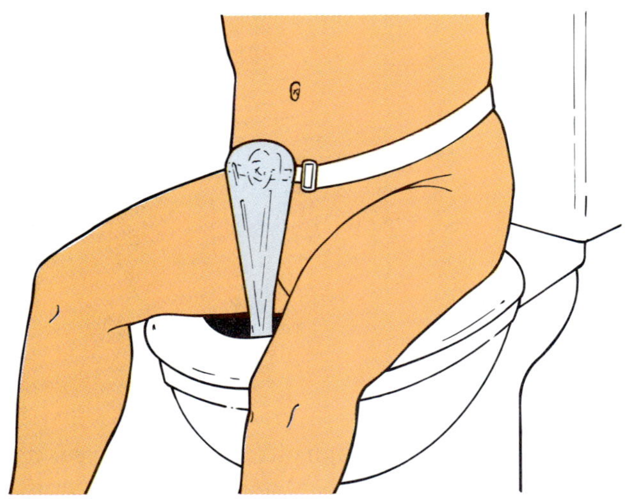

Fig. 16-14 *An ileostomy appliance is emptied by directing it into the toilet and unclamping the end.*

CARING FOR A PERSON WITH A COLOSTOMY

PRE-PROCEDURE

1 Explain the procedure to the person.
2 Wash your hands.
3 Collect the following:
- Bedpan with cover
- Waterproof bed protectors
- Bath blanket
- Toilet tissue
- Clean colostomy pouch
- Clean ostomy belt (if used)
- Wash basin
- Bath thermometer
- Prescribed soap or cleansing agent
- Skin barrier as ordered
- Deodorant for the pouch
- Disposable pouch
- Paper towels
- Disposable gloves

4 Identify the person. Check the ID bracelet and call the person by name.
5 Provide for privacy.
6 Raise the bed to the best level for good body mechanics.

PROCEDURE

7 Lower the side rail.
8 Cover the person with a bath blanket. Fanfold linens to the foot of the bed.
9 Place the waterproof pad under the buttocks.
10 Put on the gloves.
11 Disconnect the pouch from the belt if one is worn. Remove the colostomy belt.
12 Remove the pouch gently. Place it in the bedpan.
13 Wipe around the stoma with toilet tissue to remove mucus or feces. Place soiled tissue in the bedpan.
14 Cover the bedpan and take it to the bathroom.
15 Empty the pouch and bedpan into the toilet. Note the color, amount, consistency, and odor of feces. Put the pouch in the disposable bag.
16 Remove the gloves and wash your hands. Put on clean gloves.
17 Fill the wash basin. Water temperature should be 115° F (46.1° C). Place the basin on the overbed table on top of the paper towels.
18 Clean the skin around the stoma with water. Rinse and pat dry. Use soap or other cleansing agent if ordered.
19 Apply the skin barrier.
20 Put a clean colostomy belt on the person if a belt is worn.
21 Add deodorant to the new pouch.
22 Remove adhesive backing on the pouch.
23 Center the pouch over the stoma. Make sure it is sealed to the skin. Apply gentle pressure to the adhesive surface from the stoma outward.
24 Connect the belt to the pouch (if a belt is worn).
25 Remove the bed protector.
26 Cover the person. Remove the bath blanket.

POST-PROCEDURE

27 Make sure the person is comfortable.
28 Raise or lower side rails as instructed by the nurse.
29 Lower the bed to its lowest position. Place the call bell within reach. Unscreen the person.
30 Clean the bedpan, wash basin, and other equipment. Place used disposable equipment in the bag.
31 Return equipment to its proper place.
32 Discard the disposable bag according to facility policy. Follow facility policy for soiled linen.
33 Remove the gloves and wash your hands.
34 Report your observations to the nurse.

Caring for a Person with an Ileostomy

Pre-procedure

1 Explain the procedure to the person.
2 Wash your hands.
3 Collect the following:
   - Prescribed solvent
   - Medicine dropper
   - Clean appliance
   - Clean belt
   - Clamp for the appliance
   - Gauze dressing
   - Disposable washcloths
   - Towels
   - Cotton balls
   - Prescribed soap or cleansing agent
   - Skin barrier as ordered
   - Soft brush
   - Deodorant
   - Disposable gloves
   - Robe and slippers
4 Arrange items in the bathroom.
5 Identify the person. Check the ID bracelet and call the person by name.
6 Provide for privacy.

Procedure

7 Help the person put on a robe and slippers.
8 Assist the person to the bathroom.
9 Help him or her sit on the toilet.
10 Put on the gloves.
11 Direct the pouch into the toilet (see Fig. 16-14). Remove the clamp.
12 Let the pouch empty into the toilet. Wipe the end with toilet tissue. Discard tissue into the toilet. Observe feces for amount, color, consistency, and odor.
13 Disconnect the pouch from the belt. Remove the belt.
14 Apply a few drops of solvent to the skin around the pouch. (Use the medicine dropper.) The appliance will loosen and can be gently removed.
15 Cover the stoma with a gauze dressing to absorb drainage.
16 Wet the skin around the stoma with a cotton ball soaked with solvent.
17 Clean the skin around the stoma with warm water. Rinse and pat dry. Use soap or cleansing agent only if ordered.
18 Prepare the skin barrier around the stoma.
19 Remove the gauze dressing from the stoma.
20 Apply the skin barrier around the stoma.
21 Add deodorant to the pouch.
22 Apply the pouch. Be sure the bottom is clamped.
23 Put a clean belt on the person. Connect the belt to the appliance.
24 Remove the gloves and wash your hands.
25 Help the person wash the hands.
26 Assist the person back to bed or to a chair. Raise or lower side rails as instructed by the nurse.

Post-procedure

27 Make sure he or she is comfortable. Place the call bell within reach. Unscreen the person.
28 Put on another pair of gloves.
29 Clean the used appliance with soap and water using the soft brush. Wash the belt. Allow both items to dry. Clean equipment.
30 Clean and return equipment to its proper place. Discard disposable items.
31 Remove the gloves. Wash your hands.
32 Report your observations to the nurse.

STOOL SPECIMENS

When internal bleeding is suspected, feces are checked for blood. Stools are also studied for fat, microorganisms, worms, and other abnormal contents. The rules for collecting urine specimens (see Chapter 15, page 359) apply when collecting stool specimens. Standard Precautions are necessary and the Bloodborne Pathogen Standard is followed.

Specimens must not be contaminated with urine. Some tests require a warm stool. The specimen is taken to the laboratory immediately if a warm stool is needed.

COLLECTING A STOOL SPECIMEN

PRE-PROCEDURE

1 Explain the procedure to the person.
2 Wash your hands.
3 Collect the following:
   - Bedpan and cover (another bedpan may be needed if the person needs to urinate) or bedside commode
   - Urinal
   - Specimen pan if the bathroom or commode is used
   - Specimen container and lid
   - Tongue blade
   - Disposable bag
   - Disposable gloves
   - Toilet tissue
   - Laboratory requisition slip
   - Plastic bag

PROCEDURE

4 Label the container with the requested information.
5 Identify the person. Check the ID bracelet with the requisition slip.
6 Provide for privacy.
7 Offer the bedpan or urinal for voiding.
8 Assist the person onto the bedpan or to the toilet or commode. Place the specimen pan under the toilet seat (Fig. 16-15 on page 392). The person wears a robe and slippers when up.
9 Ask the person not to put toilet tissue in the bedpan, commode, or specimen pan. Provide a disposable bag for toilet tissue.
10 Place the call bell and toilet tissue within reach. Raise or lower side rails as instructed by the nurse.
11 Wash your hands and leave the room.
12 Return when the person signals. Knock before entering.
13 Lower the side rail near you.
14 Put on the gloves. Provide perineal care if necessary.
15 Use a tongue blade to take about 2 tablespoons of feces from the bedpan, commode, or specimen pan to the specimen container (Fig. 16-16 on page 392).
16 Put the lid on the specimen container. Do not touch the inside of the lid or container. Place the container in the plastic bag.
17 Place the tongue blade in the bag.
18 Empty, clean, and disinfect the bedpan, commode container, or specimen pan. Remove the gloves and wash your hands.
19 Return equipment to its proper place.
20 Help the person wash the hands.

POST-PROCEDURE

21 Make sure the person is comfortable. Place the call bell within reach.
22 Make sure the bed is in its lowest position. Raise or lower side rails as instructed by the nurse.
23 Unscreen the person.
24 Take the specimen and requisition slip to the laboratory.
25 Wash your hands.
26 Report your observations to the nurse.

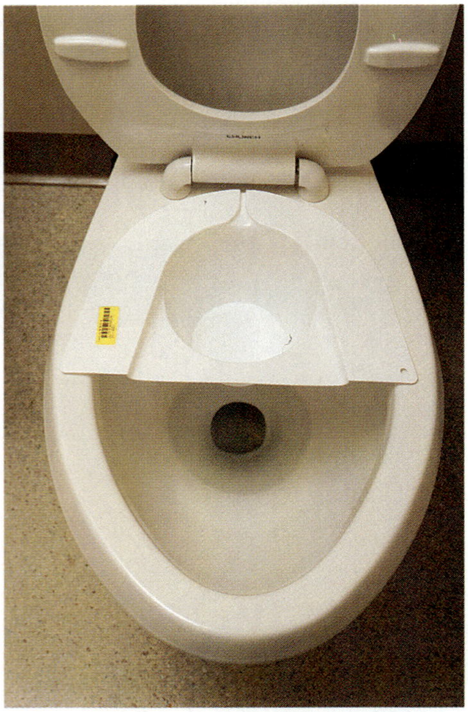

Fig. 16-15 *A specimen pan is placed in the toilet for a stool specimen.*

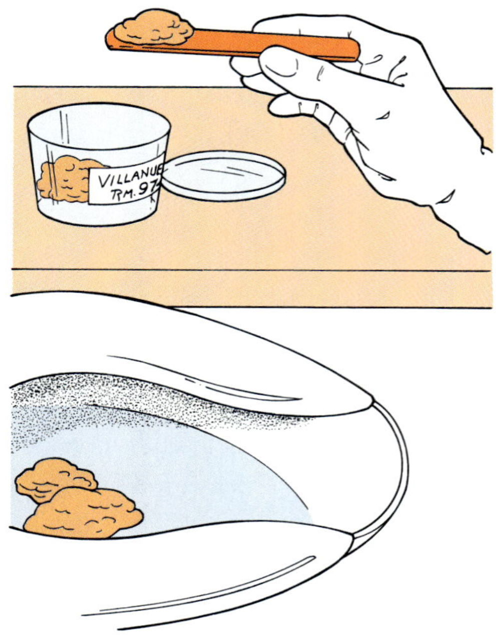

Fig. 16-16 *A tongue blade is used to transfer a small amount of stool from the bedpan to the specimen container.*

Testing Stools for Blood

Blood can appear in stools for many reasons. Ulcers, colon cancer, and hemorrhoids are common causes. Often blood is visible. Blood can usually be seen if bleeding is low in the gastrointestinal tract. Stools are black and tarry if there is bleeding in the stomach or upper GI tract.

Sometimes bleeding occurs in very small amounts. It is difficult to detect such bleeding by just observing the stools. Therefore stools are often tested for the presence of *occult blood.* Occult means hidden or unseen. The test is commonly done to screen for colon cancer.

There are many types of tests. You need to follow the manufacturer's instructions for the test ordered. Be sure to follow Standard Precautions and the Bloodborne Pathogen Standard. The nurse tells you when to collect the specimen. Many factors can affect the test results. One is eating red meat. Therefore the person cannot eat red meat for 3 days prior to the test. Bleeding from hemorrhoids can also affect the test results.

Testing a Stool Specimen for Blood

Pre-procedure

1 Explain the procedure to the person.

2 Wash your hands.

Procedure

3 Collect a stool specimen (see *Collecting a Stool Specimen).*

4 Collect the following:
- Paper towel
- Hemoccult test kit (includes developer)
- Tongue blades
- Disposable gloves

5 Put on the gloves.

6 Open the test kit.

7 Use a tongue blade to obtain a small amount of stool.

8 Apply a thin smear of stool on box **A** on the test paper (Fig. 16-17, A on page 394).

9 Use another tongue blade to obtain some feces from another part of the specimen.

10 Apply a thin smear of stool on box **B** on the test paper (Fig. 16-17, B on page 394).

11 Close the test packet.

12 Turn the test packet to the other side. Open the flap. Apply developer to boxes **A** and **B** according to the manufacturer's instructions (Fig. 16-17, C on page 394).

13 Wait the amount of time specified in the manufacturer's instructions. Time can vary from 10 to 60 seconds.

14 Note and record the color changes (Fig. 16-17, D on page 394). Follow the manufacturer's instructions.

15 Dispose of the test packet.

16 Discard the tongue blade.

17 Dispose of the specimen.

18 Remove the gloves and wash your hands.

19 Report the test results and your observations to the nurse.

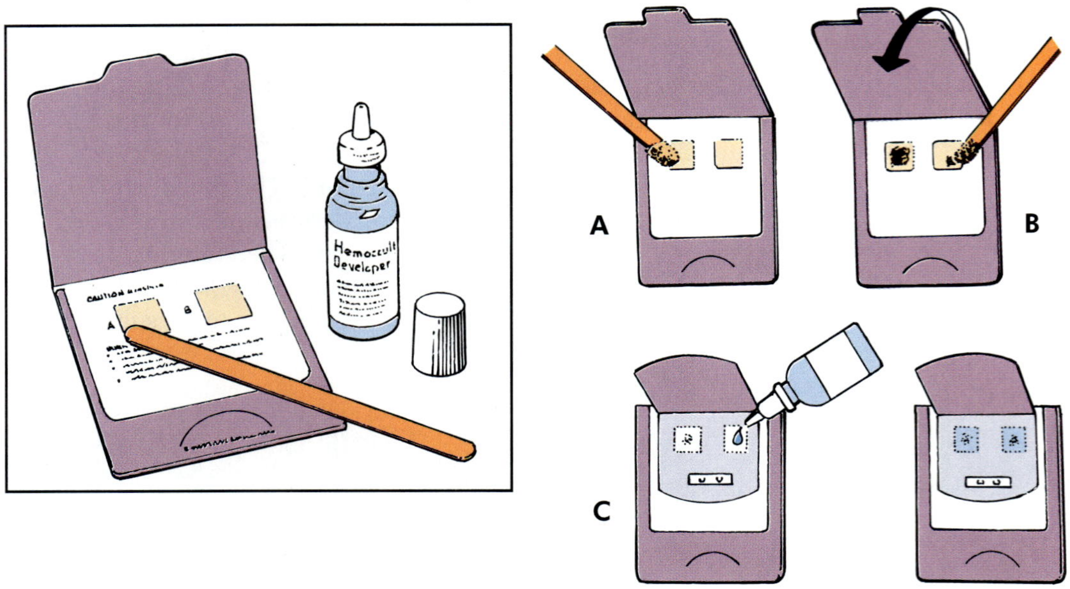

Fig. 16-17 *Testing for occult blood.* ***A,*** *Stool is smeared on box A.* ***B,*** *Stool is smeared on box B.* ***C,*** *Developer is applied to boxes A and B.* ***D,*** *Color changes are noted.*

SUMMARY

Your responsibilities in assisting persons with bowel elimination are similar to those for urinary elimination. The act of defecation is private. Bowel control is important to people. So are the hygiene practices that follow bowel movements. Physical and mental well-being are affected by normal bowel function. The personal routines related to defecation also affect well-being.

Normal bowel elimination is not always possible. Constipation, fecal impaction, diarrhea, anal incontinence, and flatulence are common problems. The doctor may order enemas, rectal tubes, medications, or dietary changes to relieve the problem. The nurse may direct you to give an enema or insert a rectal tube. The instructions and procedure must be thoroughly understood. Sometimes ileostomies or colostomies are necessary to treat bowel problems.

When assisting the person with bowel elimination, always consider the person's need for privacy and bowel control. You must do all you can to protect the person's right to privacy. The person's dignity and psychological well-being are just as important as the physical act of defecation. In addition, the rules of medical asepsis, Standard Precautions, cleanliness, skin care, and safety must be followed. The Bloodborne Pathogen Standard is also important.

REVIEW QUESTIONS

Circle the best *answer.*

1 Which is *false?*

a A person must have a bowel movement every day.

b Stools are normally brown, soft, and formed.

c Diarrhea occurs when feces move through the intestines rapidly.

d Constipation results when feces move through the large intestine slowly.

2 Bowel elimination is affected by

a Privacy and age

b Medications and diet

c Fluid intake and activity

d All of the above

3 The prolonged retention and accumulation of feces in the rectum is called

a Constipation

b Fecal impaction

c Diarrhea

d Anal incontinence

4 Which will *not* promote comfort and safety in relation to bowel elimination?

a Asking visitors to leave the room

b Helping the person assume a sitting position

c Offering the bedpan after meals

d Telling the person that you will return very soon

5 Bowel training is aimed at

a Gaining control of bowel movements and developing a regular pattern of elimination

b Colostomy or ileostomy control

c Preventing fecal impaction, constipation, and anal incontinence

d All of the above

6 Which is *not* used for a cleansing enema?

a Soap suds

b Saline

c Oil

d Tap water

7 Which is *false?*

a Enema solutions should be 105° F (40.5° C).

b The left Sims' position is used for an enema.

c The enema bag is held 12 inches above the anus.

d The enema solution is administered rapidly.

8 In adults, the enema tube is inserted

a 1 to 2 inches

b 2 to 4 inches

c 4 to 6 inches

d 6 to 8 inches

9 The oil-retention enema is retained for

a 10 to 15 minutes

b 15 to 30 minutes

c 30 to 60 minutes

d 60 to 90 minutes

10 Rectal tubes are left in place no longer than

a 20 to 30 minutes

b 10 to 20 minutes

c 10 to 15 minutes

d 5 to 10 minutes

11 Which statement about colostomies and ileostomies is *false?*

a Good skin care around the stoma is essential.

b Odors can be controlled with deodorant.

c The person will have to wear an appliance.

d Fecal material is always liquid in consistency.

12 A person wears an ileostomy pouch. It is usually emptied

a Every 4 to 6 hours

b Every morning

c Every 2 to 3 days

d When the doctor gives the order to do so

Answers to these questions are on page 751.

Foods and Fluids

11

OBJECTIVES

- Define the key terms listed in this chapter
- Explain the purpose and use of the Food Guide Pyramid
- Explain the importance of protein, carbohydrates, and fats
- Identify major sources of proteins, carbohydrates, and fats
- Describe the functions of vitamins and minerals
- Identify the dietary sources of vitamins and minerals
- Describe factors that affect eating and nutrition
- Describe the special diets
- Describe normal adult fluid requirements and the common causes of dehydration
- Explain your responsibilities when forced fluids, restricted fluids, and NPO are ordered
- Explain the purpose of intake and output records
- Identify foods that are counted as fluid intake
- Describe between-meal nourishments, tube feedings, intravenous therapy, and hyperalimentation
- Explain how to promote quality of life when meeting food and fluid needs
- Perform the procedures described in this chapter

KEY TERMS

anorexia Loss of appetite

calorie The amount of energy produced from the burning of food by the body

dehydration A decrease in the amount of water in body tissues

dysphagia Difficulty or discomfort (dys) in swallowing (phagia)

edema The swelling of body tissues with water

gastrostomy A surgically created opening (stomy) in the stomach (gastro) that allows feeding

gavage Tube feeding

graduate A calibrated container used to measure fluid

intake The amount of fluid taken in by the body

intravenous therapy Fluid administered through a needle within a vein; IV, IV therapy, and IV infusion

nutrient A substance that is ingested, digested, absorbed, and used by the body

nutrition The many processes involved in the ingestion, digestion, absorption, and use of foods and fluids by the body

output The amount of fluid lost by the body

The need for food and water is a basic physical need necessary for life and health. The amount and quality of foods and fluids in the diet are important. They affect a person's current and future physical and mental well-being. A poor diet and poor eating habits increase a person's risk for infection and chronic diseases. Healing problems and abnormal body functions are also related to poor diet and eating habits. Poor physical and mental functioning increase a person's risk for accidents and injuries. Besides survival, eating and drinking provide pleasure. They are a part of social activities with family and friends.

Many factors affect dietary practices. They include culture, finances, and personal choice. Dietary practices also include selecting, preparing, and serving food. The nurse considers these factors when using the nursing process to meet the person's nutritional needs.

BASIC NUTRITION

Nutrition is the many processes involved in the ingestion, digestion, absorption, and use of foods and fluids by the body (Box 17-1 on page 398). Good nutrition is needed for growth, healing, and maintaining body functions. It starts with properly selecting foods and fluids. They must provide a well-balanced diet and correct calorie intake. A diet high in fat and calories causes weight gain and obesity. Weight loss occurs when not enough calories are consumed.

Foods and fluids contain nutrients. A **nutrient** is a substance that is ingested, digested, absorbed, and used by the body. Many nutrients are needed for body functions. Nutrients are grouped into fats, proteins, carbohydrates, vitamins, and minerals.

Fats, proteins, and carbohydrates provide the body with fuel for energy. The amount of energy provided by a nutrient is measured in calories. A **calorie** is the amount of energy produced from the burning of food by the body.

- 1 gram of fat supplies the body with 9 calories
- 1 gram of protein provides 4 calories
- 1 gram of carbohydrate supplies 4 calories

Energy is needed for all body functions—even sitting in a chair. The amount of calories a person needs depends on many factors. They include age, activity, climate, state of health, amount of sleep, and sex (male or female). Men usually need more calories than women.

Food Guide Pyramid

Good nutrition was previously based on the four basic food groups: milk and dairy products; meats and fish; fruits and vegetables; and breads and cereals. In 1992 the U.S. Dept. of Agriculture (USDA) released its *Food Guide Pyramid.* The pyramid replaces the four basic food groups.

BOX 17-1 Digestive System: Review of Body Structure and Function

The digestive system breaks down food physically and chemically so it can be absorbed for use by the cells. This process is called *digestion.* The digestive system is also called the *gastrointestinal system (GI system).* The digestive system consists of the *alimentary canal (GI tract)* and the accessory organs of digestion (Fig. 17-1). The alimentary canal is a long tube extending from the mouth to the anus. Its major parts are the mouth, pharynx, esophagus, stomach, small intestine, and large intestine. The accessory organs of digestion are the teeth, tongue, salivary glands, liver, gallbladder, and pancreas.

Digestion begins in the *mouth (oral cavity).* The oral cavity receives food and prepares it for digestion. Using chewing motions, the *teeth* cut, chop, and grind food into smaller particles for digestion and swallowing. The *tongue* aids in chewing and swallowing. *Taste buds* on the tongue contain nerve endings. Taste buds allow sensing of sweet, sour, bitter, and salty tastes. *Salivary glands* in the mouth secrete *saliva.* Saliva moistens food particles for easier swallowing and begins the digestion of food. During swallowing, the tongue pushes food into the pharynx.

The *pharynx* (throat) is a muscular tube. The act of swallowing is continued as the pharynx contracts. Contraction of the pharynx pushes food into the *esophagus.* The esophagus is a muscular tube about 10 inches long. It extends from the pharynx to the stomach. Involuntary muscle contractions called *peristalsis* move food down the esophagus into the stomach.

The *stomach* is a muscular, pouchlike sac in the upper left portion of the abdominal cavity. Strong stomach muscles stir and churn food to break it up into even smaller particles. The stomach is lined with a mucous membrane containing glands that secrete *gastric juices.* Food is mixed and churned with the gastric juices to form a semiliquid substance called *chyme.* Through peristalsis, the chyme is pushed from the stomach into the small intestine.

The *small intestine* is about 20 feet long and has three parts. The first part is the *duodenum.* In the duodenum, more digestive juices are added to the chyme. One is called *bile.* Bile is a greenish liquid produced by the *liver* and stored in the *gallbladder.* Juices from the *pancreas* and small intestine are also added to the chyme. The digestive juices chemically break down food so it can be absorbed.

Peristalsis moves the chyme through the two remaining portions of the small intestine: the *jejunum* and the *ileum.* Tiny projections called *villi* line the small intestine. Villi absorb the digested food into the capillaries. Most of the absorption of food takes place in the jejunum and ileum. Chyme eventually enters the large intestine. More fluid is absorbed. The solid waste that remains is eventually eliminated through the anus.

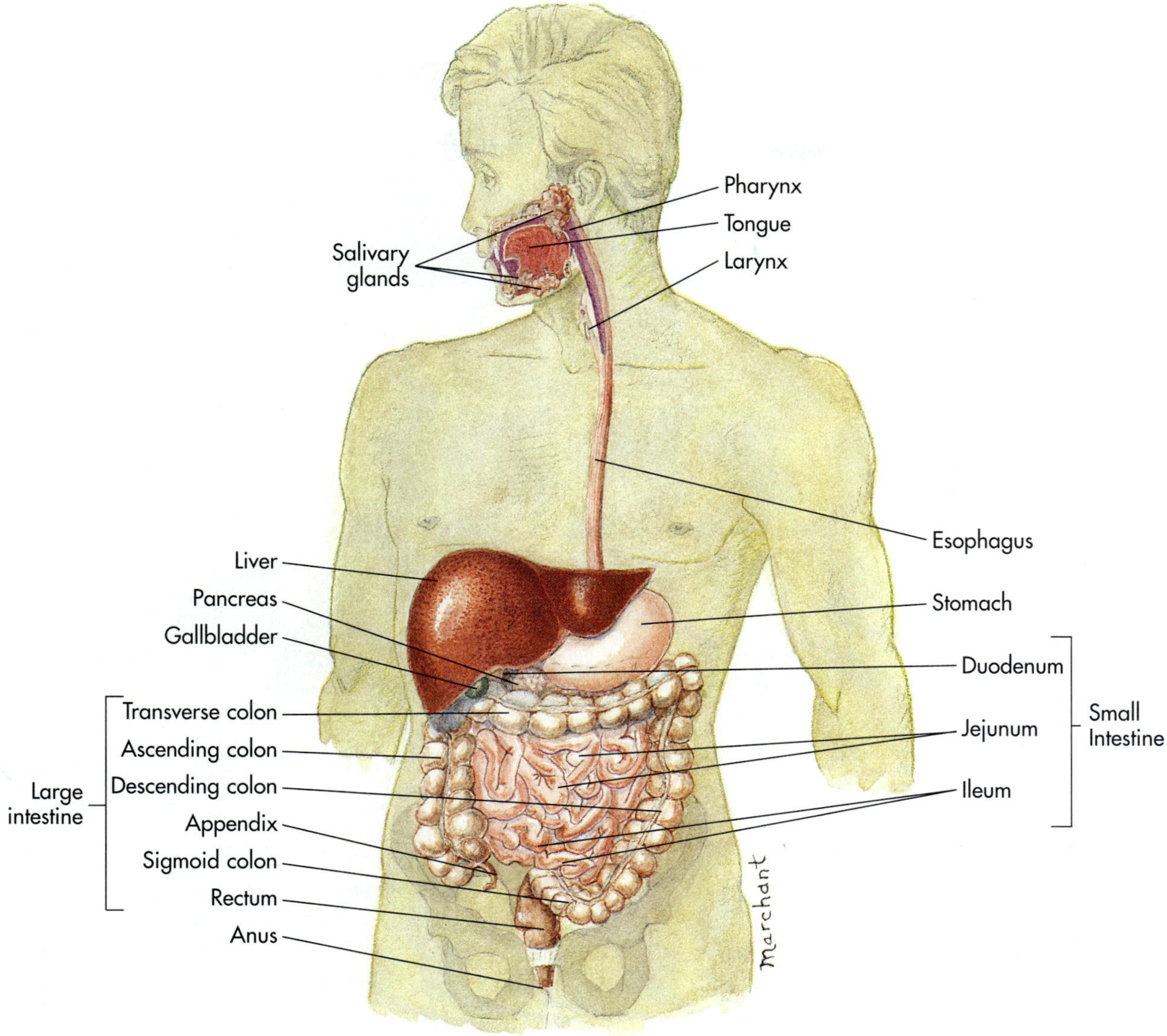

Fig. 17-1 *Structures of the digestive system.*

The purpose of the Food Guide Pyramid is to make wise food choices (Fig. 17-2 on page 400). The pyramid has 6 food groups:

- Bread, cereal, rice, and pasta
- Vegetables
- Fruits
- Milk, yogurt, and cheese
- Meat, poultry, fish, dry beans, eggs, and nuts
- Fats, oils, and sweets

The pyramid suggests eating more foods at the bottom level (level 1) and lesser amounts at each level moving to the top (level 4). The Food Guide Pyramid encourages a low-fat diet. More bread, cereal, rice, and pasta (level 1) and more vegetables and fruits (level 2) should be eaten. There should be moderate amounts from the milk, yogurt, and cheese group and from the meat, poultry, fish, beans, eggs, and nut group (level 3). Fats, oils, and sweets (level 4) should be used sparingly.

Foods from each of the five food groups in levels 1, 2, and 3 are needed daily. Those foods contain varying amounts of the essential nutrients. No one food or food group contains every nutrient needed by the body.

Note the small circles and triangles in the pyramid (see Fig. 17-2). The circles are for fat and the triangles for sugar. Some sugar and fat naturally occur in all foods. They appear in all levels of the pyramid. There are fewer fats and sugars at levels 1 and 2. Therefore the bread, vegetable, and fruit groups are low in sugar and fat. More servings are allowed from these groups than the others. The result is a low-fat diet. Level 4 foods contain more fat and calories than do foods at level 1. As you move up the Food Guide Pyramid, the amount of fat and calories increases.

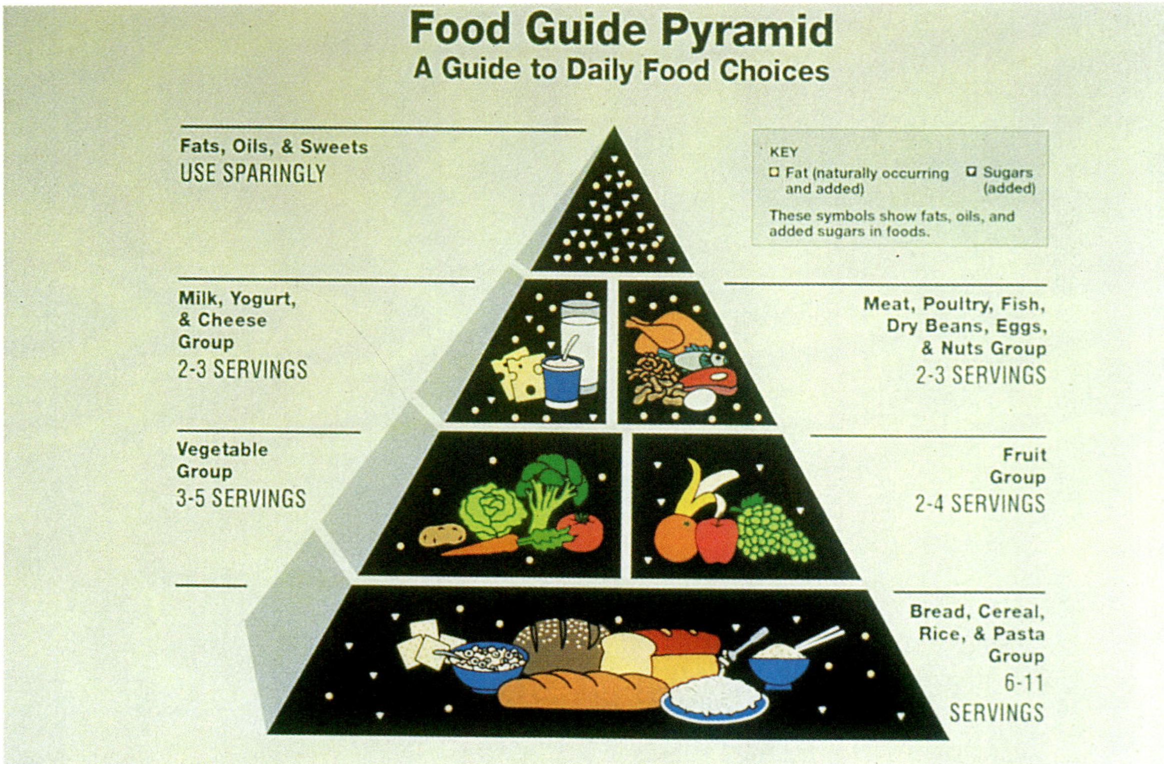

Fig. 17-2 *Food Guide Pyramid. (Courtesy U.S. Dept. of Agriculture, Washington, D.C.)*

The pyramid is for everyone over 2 years of age. Better health is the goal. Many diseases are related to diet and the kinds of food eaten. They include heart disease, high blood pressure, stroke, diabetes, and certain cancers. The risk for such diseases can be reduced by following the Dietary Guidelines for Americans. Box 17-2 lists the guidelines developed by the U.S. Dept. of Agriculture and the U.S. Dept. of Health and Human Services.

BOX 17-2 Dietary Guidelines for Americans

- Eat a variety of foods.
- Maintain a healthy weight.
- Choose a diet low in fat, saturated fat, and cholesterol.
- Choose a diet with plenty of vegetables, fruits, and grain products.
- Use sugars only in moderation.
- Use salt and sodium only in moderation.
- If you drink alcoholic beverages, do so in moderation.

BOX 17-3 FOOD GUIDE PYRAMID SERVING SIZES

Bread, Cereals, Rice, and Pasta Group

- 1 slice of bread = 1 serving
- 1 ounce of ready-to-eat cereal = 1 serving
- 1/2 cup of cooked cereal, rice, or pasta = 1 serving

Vegetable Group

- 1 cup raw leafy vegetables = 1 serving
- 1/2 cup other cooked or chopped raw vegetables = 1 serving
- 3/4 cup vegetable juice = 1 serving

Fruit Group

- 1 medium apple, orange, or banana = 1 serving
- 1/2 cup chopped, cooked, or canned fruit = 1 serving
- 3/4 cup fruit juice = 1 serving

Milk, Cheese, and Yogurt Group

- 1 cup of milk or yogurt = 1 serving
- 1/2 to 1 ounce cheese = 1 serving
- 2 ounces process cheese = 1 serving

Meat, Poultry, Fish, Dry Beans, Eggs, and Nuts Group

- 2 to 3 ounces cooked lean meat, poultry, or fish = 1 serving
- 1/2 cup cooked dry beans = 1 serving
- 1 egg = 1 serving
- 2 tablespoons peanut butter = 1 serving

Fats, Oils, and Sweets Group

- Use sparingly

Breads, cereals, rice, and pasta group The bread group forms the base of the pyramid. More servings are allowed from this group than any other group or level. The USDA recommends 6 to 11 servings a day (Box 17-3). All foods in the bread group come from grain (wheat, oats, rice, etc.). Protein, carbohydrates, iron, thiamin, niacin, and riboflavin are the main nutrients in this group. There are small amounts of fats and sugars.

Foods such as pie, cake, cookies, pastries, doughnuts, and muffins are made from grains. However, they are also made with fats and sugars. They are high-fat food choices depending on the amount of fat and sugar added.

Vegetable group The USDA recommends 3 to 5 servings a day from the vegetable group (see Box 17-3). Vegetables provide fiber, vitamins A and C, carbohydrates, and minerals. They are naturally low in fat. A variety of vegetables should be eaten: dark green and yellow vegetables, tomatoes, potatoes, and vegetable juices.

Naturally low in fat, vegetables can become high in fat during food preparation. French fries are very high in fat compared to a baked or boiled potato. Butter, oil, mayonnaise, salad dressing, sour cream, and sauces are often added to vegetables. These toppings are high in fat. Small amounts of low-fat toppings help keep vegetables low in fat.

Fruit group Fruits naturally contain some sugar and are low in fat. The USDA recommends 2 to 4 servings of fruit daily (see Box 17-3). Fruits provide carbohydrates, vitamins A and C, potassium, and other minerals. This group includes all fruits and fruit juices. Fresh fruits and juices are best. Frozen or canned fruits should be unsweetened. Often they are sweetened or syrupy and therefore higher in sugar and calories.

Milk, yogurt, and cheese group Milk and milk products are high in protein, carbohydrates, fat, calcium, and riboflavin. The USDA recommends 2 to 3 daily servings from the milk group—milk, cheese, and yogurt (see Box 17-3). Children and breast-feeding mothers need 3 servings a day.

Skim milk is lower in fat than whole milk. One cup of skim milk has only a trace of fat; 1 cup of whole milk has 8 grams of fat. There are about 86 calories in 1 cup of skim milk and 150 calories in 1 cup of whole milk (72 of the calories in 1 cup of whole milk come from fat). Besides skim milk, low-fat food choices from this group include cheeses made with skim milk, low or nonfat yogurts, and ice milk rather than ice cream.

Meat, poultry, fish, dry beans, eggs, and nuts group Meat, poultry, fish, dry beans, eggs, and nuts make up the meat group. The foods in this group are higher in fat than those in the milk, fruit, vegetable, and bread groups. The USDA recommends 2 to 3 servings a day (see Box 17-3). Protein, fat, iron, and thiamin are the main nutrients found in this group.

Serving size is very important when planning a well balanced diet. This is especially important for meat, poultry, and fish because they contain many calories. Many factors affect serving size including culture, appetite, personal choice, and the recipe used. A quarter pound hamburger, a 12-ounce T-bone steak, a 10 ounce lobster tail, and a quarter of a chicken are some servings advertised by restaurants. *One serving* in this group is 2 to 3 ounces of boned meat, fish, or poultry. A 12 ounce steak is 4 to 6 servings from this group!

Remember, foods in this group are higher in fat than foods in the other groups (except the fats, oils, and sweets group). The more fat, the greater the calories. Wise food choices can lower fat intake from this group. Fish and shellfish are low in fat. Chicken and turkey have less fat than veal, beef, pork, and lamb. Skinless chicken and turkey are even lower in fat. Veal is lower in fat than beef. Lean cuts of beef and pork should be used. Egg yolks have more fat than egg whites. Low-fat egg substitutes can be used for cooking and baking.

Food preparation is also important. Fat should be trimmed from meat and poultry. Poultry should be skinned. Roasting, broiling, and baking are better than frying. Gravies and sauces also add fat.

Nuts and peanut butter are higher in fat than the other foods in this group. They should be used wisely. As shown in Fig. 17-3, 1 serving of peanut butter (two tablespoons) equals 1 serving of meat (2 to 3 ounces)! Peas and cooked dry beans are very low in fat. They should be used often.

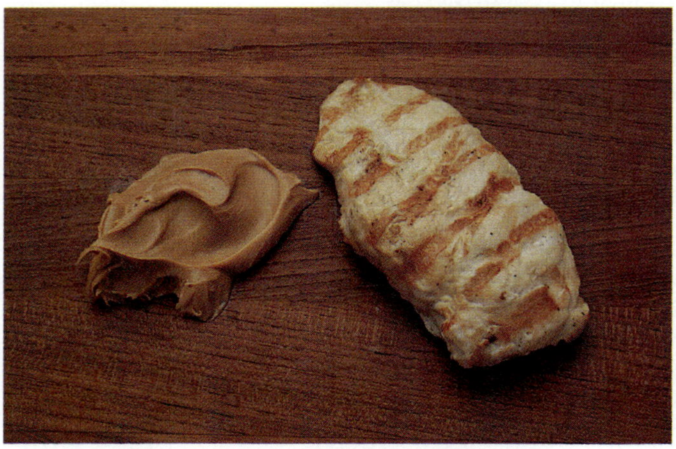

Fig. 17-3 *Two tablespoons of peanut butter (one serving) equals this 3-ounce chicken breast (one serving).*

Fats, oils, and sweets group This group is at the very top of the pyramid. The USDA recommends that they be used sparingly. There are no recommended servings or serving sizes. They should be used as little as possible. There is little nutritional value in fats, oils, and sweets (foods with added sugar). However, they are very high in calories. Foods in this group include

- Cooking oils
- Shortening
- Butter, margarine
- Salad dressing
- Soft drinks
- All candy
- Sour cream
- Cream cheese
- Frosting
- Chocolate
- Cookies
- Cake
- Pie
- Ice cream
- Many desserts
- Jellies and jams
- Syrups
- Alcohol (beer, wine, champagne, whiskey, vodka, gin, Scotch)

Some foods are high in fat, some in added sugar, and some in both. Butter and oil are high in fat. Soft drinks, jellies, jams, and syrups are high in added sugar. So are coffee and cereal if sugar is added at the table. Chocolate and ice cream are high in both fat and added sugar.

Alcohol is also included in this group. Beer, wine, champagne, whiskey, vodka, gin, and scotch are common alcoholic drinks. If used at all, alcohol use should be moderate.

Many low-fat or nonfat foods can be bought. Food labels are used to determine fat content (see Chapter 35).

Nutrients

No one food or food group has every essential nutrient needed by the body. A well balanced diet consists of servings from the five food groups in levels 1, 2, and 3 of the Food Guide Pyramid. It ensures an adequate intake of the essential nutrients.

Protein Protein is the most important nutrient—it is needed for tissue growth and repair. Protein sources include meat, fish, poultry, eggs, milk and milk products, cereals, beans, peas, and nuts. Foods high in protein are costly. Therefore persons with low incomes often lack protein in their diets.

Each body cell is made of protein. When protein intake is excessive, some is excreted in the urine. Some protein changes into body fat and some into carbohydrates.

Carbohydrates Carbohydrates provide energy. They also provide fiber for bowel elimination. Carbohydrates are found in fruits, vegetables, breads, cereals, and sugar. These foods are rather inexpensive. Diets rarely lack carbohydrates.

Carbohydrates are broken down into sugars during digestion. The sugars are then absorbed into the bloodstream. The fiber in carbohydrate foods is not digested. It provides the bulky part of chyme for elimination. When carbohydrate intake is excessive, some of the nutrient is stored in the liver. The rest changes into body fat.

Fats Fats provide energy and serve many other functions. They add flavor to food and help the body use certain vitamins. Fats also conserve body heat and protect organs from injury. Fat sources include the fat in meats, lard, butter, shortenings, salad and vegetable oils, milk, cheese, egg yolks, and nuts. These sources are more expensive than sources of carbohydrates. Dietary fat not needed by the body is stored as body fat (adipose tissue).

Vitamins Although they do not provide calories, vitamins are essential nutrients. They are ingested through food. Vitamins A, D, E, and K can be stored by the body. Vitamin C and the B complex vitamins are not stored. They must be ingested daily. Each vitamin is needed for certain body functions. The lack of a specific vitamin results in signs and symptoms of a particular disease. Table 17-1 on page 404 lists the sources and major functions of common vitamins.

Minerals A well-balanced diet also supplies needed amounts of minerals. Minerals are used for many body processes. They are needed for bone and tooth formation, nerve and muscle function, fluid balance, and other body processes. Table 17-2 on page 404 lists the major functions and dietary sources of common minerals.

Table 17-1

Major Functions and Sources of Common Vitamins

	Major Functions	Sources
Vitamin A	Growth; vision; healthy hair, skin, and mucous membranes; resistance to infection	Liver, spinach, green leafy and yellow vegetables, yellow fruits, fish liver oils, egg yolk, butter, cream, whole milk
Vitamin B_1 (thiamin)	Muscle tone; nerve function; digestion; appetite; normal elimination; utilization of carbohydrates	Pork, fish, poultry, eggs, liver, breads, pastas, cereals, oatmeal, potatoes, peas, beans, soybeans, peanuts
Vitamin B_2 (riboflavin)	Growth; healthy eyes; protein and carbohydrate metabolism; healthy skin and mucous membranes	Milk and milk products, liver, green leafy vegetables, eggs, breads, cereals
Vitamin B_3 (niacin)	Protein, fat, and carbohydrate metabolism; nervous system function; appetite; digestive system function	Meat, pork, liver, fish, peanuts, breads and cereals, green vegetables, dairy products
Vitamin B_{12}	Formation of red blood cells; protein metabolism; nervous system functioning	Liver, meats, poultry, fish, eggs, milk, cheese
Folic acid	Formation of red blood cells; functioning of the intestines; protein metabolism	Liver, meats, fish, poultry, green leafy vegetables, whole grains
Vitamin C (ascorbic acid)	Formation of substances that hold tissues together; healthy blood vessels, skin, gums, bones, and teeth; wound healing; prevention of bleeding; resistance to infection	Citrus fruits, tomatoes, potatoes, cabbage, strawberries, green vegetables, melons
Vitamin D	Absorption and metabolism of calcium and phosphorus; healthy bones	Fish liver oils, milk, butter, liver, exposure to sunlight
Vitamin E	Normal reproduction; formation of red blood cells; muscle function	Vegetable oils, milk, eggs, meats, cereals, green leafy vegetables
Vitamin K	Blood clotting	Liver, green leafy vegetables, egg yolk, cheese

Table 17-2

Major Functions and Sources of Common Minerals

	Major Functions	Sources
Calcium	Formation of teeth and bones, blood clotting, muscle contraction, heart function, nerve function	Milk and milk products, green leafy vegetables, whole grains, egg yolks, dried peas and beans, nuts
Phosphorus	Formation of bones and teeth; utilization of proteins, fats, and carbohydrates; nerve and muscle function	Meat, fish, poultry, milk and milk products, nuts, egg yolks, dried peas and beans
Iron	Allows red blood cells to carry oxygen	Liver, meat, eggs, green leafy vegetables, breads and cereals, dried peas and beans, nuts
Iodine	Thyroid gland function, growth, and metabolism	Iodized salt, seafood, and shellfish
Sodium	Fluid balance; nerve and muscle function	Almost all foods
Potassium	Nerve function, muscle contraction, heart function	Fruits, vegetables, cereals, meats, dried peas and beans

FACTORS THAT AFFECT EATING AND NUTRITION

Many factors affect nutrition and eating habits. Some begin during infancy and continue throughout life. Others develop later.

Culture

Dietary practices are greatly influenced by culture (Box 17-4). Foods available in the region of an ethnic group also affect diet. Rice and tea are common in the diets of Chinese, Japanese, Korean, and other peoples of the Far East. Hispanic people eat a lot of tacos, tamales, and burritos. Italians are known for food such as spaghetti, lasagna, and other pastas. Scandinavians eat a lot of fish. Americans enjoy foods from the meat group, fast foods, and processed foods (canned and frozen foods).

Culture also influences food preparation. Frying, baking, smoking, or roasting food or eating raw food are cultural practices. The use of sauces and spices is also related to culture.

BOX 17-4 Top Ten Countries of Origin of Immigrants to the United States*: Food Practices

Country	Food Practices
Mexico	Rice and beans provide proteins.
Vietnam	None reported.
Philippines	Rice is preferred with every meal.
Former Soviet Union	None reported.
Dominican Republic	None reported.
Mainland China	The diet is low in fat. Excessive amounts of soy sauce and dried and preserved foods cause a high sodium intake. Herbs are used to treat symptoms, wounds, and disease. The ginseng root is widely used. Raw vegetables and meats are usually not eaten. Hot and warm beverages are preferred.
India	Beef is not eaten.
El Salvador	Some believe that being thin is unhealthy and weight control does not mean good nutrition.
Poland	The diet tends to be higher in starch and fat. Potatoes, rye, and wheat products are common.
United Kingdom	Organ meats are common in England.

Information based on data gathered through 1992 by the U.S. Department of Immigration and Naturalization Services.
From Geissler EM: *Pocket guide to cultural assessment,* St Louis, 1994, Mosby–Year Book.

Religion

Many religious beliefs involve dietary practices. Selecting, preparing, and eating food are often regulated by religious practices. Some religions have days of fasting. During a fast, all or certain foods are avoided. Members of a religious group may follow all, some, or none of the dietary practices of their faith. You need to respect the person's religious practices. Box 17-5 lists the dietary practices of the major religious groups.

Finances

Cost is a major factor in food selection. People with limited incomes, like the elderly, usually buy the cheaper carbohydrate foods. Therefore their diets often lack protein and certain vitamins and minerals.

BOX 17-5 Religion and Dietary Practices

Adventist (Seventh Day Adventist)

- Coffee, tea, and alcohol are not allowed.
- Beverages with caffeine (colas) are not allowed.
- Some groups forbid the eating of meat.

Baptist

- Some groups forbid coffee, tea, and alcohol.

Christian Scientist

- Alcohol and coffee are not allowed.

Church of Jesus Christ of Latter Day Saints (Mormon)

- Alcohol and hot drinks, such as coffee and tea, are not allowed.
- Meat is not forbidden, but members are encouraged to eat meat infrequently.

Greek Orthodox Church

- Wednesdays, Fridays, and Lent are days of fasting.
- Meat and dairy products are usually avoided during days of fast.

Islam (Muslim or Moslem)

- All pork and pork products are forbidden.
- Alcohol is not allowed except for medical reasons.

Judaism (Jewish faith)

- Foods must be kosher (prepared according to Jewish law).
- Meat of kosher animals (cows, goats, and sheep) can be eaten.
- Chickens, ducks, and geese are kosher fowls.
- Kosher fish have scales and fins, such as tuna, sardines, carp, and salmon.
- Shellfish cannot be eaten.
- Milk, milk products, and eggs from kosher animals and fowl are acceptable.
- Milk and milk products cannot be eaten with or immediately after eating meat.
- Milk and milk products can be eaten 6 hours after eating meat.
- Milk and milk products can be a part of the same meal with meat—they are served separately and before the meat.
- Kosher foods cannot be prepared with utensils used to prepare nonkosher foods.
- Breads, cakes, cookies, noodles, and alcoholic beverages are not consumed during Passover.

Roman Catholic

- Fasting is required for 1 hour before receiving Holy Communion.
- Fasting from meat is required on Ash Wednesday and Good Friday—some may continue to fast from meat on Fridays

Appetite

Appetite relates to the desire for food. Hunger is an unpleasant feeling caused by the lack of food. When hungry, a person seeks food and eats until the appetite is satisfied. Aromas and thoughts of food can also stimulate the appetite. Loss of appetite (anorexia) can also occur. The many causes of anorexia include illness, medications, unpleasant thoughts or sights, anxiety, and fear.

Personal Choice

The like or dislike of certain foods is an individual matter. Food preferences begin in childhood. They are affected by the kinds of food served in the home. As a child grows older, new foods are introduced through school and social events. Many people decide if they do or do not like a certain food by the way it looks, the way it is prepared, its smell, or the recipe ingredients. Usually food preferences expand with age and with new social experiences.

Body reactions affect food choices. People usually avoid foods that cause allergic reactions, nausea, vomiting, diarrhea, indigestion, or headaches.

Personal choice is allowed in hospitals and nursing facilities to the extent possible. The doctor orders a diet for the person. Each day the person receives a menu for breakfast, lunch, and dinner. The person chooses from the various foods on the menu (Fig. 17-4). Special requests are often met.

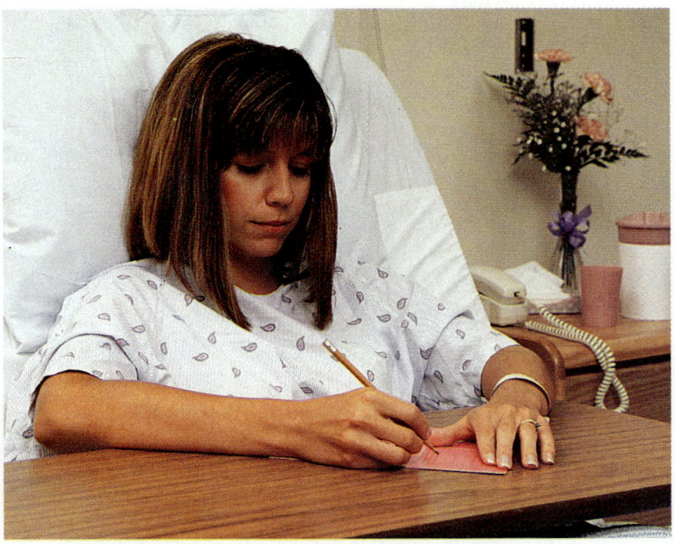

Fig. 17-4 *The person chooses foods from a menu. This protects the right to personal choice.*

Illness

Appetite usually decreases during illness and recovery from injuries. However, nutritional needs increase at these times. The body must fight infection, heal tissue, and replace lost blood cells. Nutrients lost through vomiting and diarrhea must be replaced. Some diseases and drugs cause a sore mouth, which makes eating painful. Loss of teeth affects chewing, especially protein foods.

SPECIAL DIETS

Doctors often order special diets. Special diets are ordered for a nutritional deficiency or a disease, to eliminate or decrease certain substances in the diet, or for weight control. The doctor, nurses, and dietician work together to meet the person's nutritional needs. They consider the need for dietary changes, personal choice, religion, culture, and eating problems.

Many persons do not need special diets. *Regular diet, general diet, and house diet* mean that there are no dietary limits, restrictions, or modifications. A variety of foods from the lower three levels of the Food Guide Pyramid are on the menu. Special diets are ordered for persons before and after surgery and for those with diabetes. Persons with diseases of the heart, kidneys, gallbladder, liver, stomach, or intestines may receive special diets. Allergies, obesity, and other disorders also require special diets. Table 17-3 on page 408 describes the common special diets.

The sodium-restricted diet and diabetic diet are often ordered. You will care for persons in hospitals, nursing facilities, or private homes who need these diets. They are described in greater detail.

The Sodium-Restricted Diet

The average amount of sodium in the daily diet is 3000 to 7000 mg. The body needs only half this amount daily. Healthy people excrete excess sodium in the urine. Heart and kidney diseases cause the body to retain the extra sodium.

Sodium-restricted diets are ordered for people with heart disease. They may also be ordered for those with liver diseases, kidney disease, certain complications of pregnancy, and when certain medications are being taken. Sodium causes the body to retain water. If there is too much sodium, the body retains more water. Body tissues swell with water, and there are excess amounts of fluid in the blood vessels. The increased fluid in the tissues and bloodstream forces the heart to work harder. In other words, the work load of the heart increases. With heart disease, the extra work load can cause serious complications or death. Restricting the amount of sodium in the diet decreases the amount of sodium in the body. The body retains less water. Less water in the tissues and blood vessels reduces the amount of work for the heart.

Text continued on page 410.

TABLE 17-3

SPECIAL DIETS

Diet	Description	Use	Foods Allowed
Clear-liquid	Clear liquids that do not leave a residue; nonirritating and nongas-forming	Postoperatively, acute illness, infection, and nausea and vomiting	Water, tea, and coffee (without milk or cream); carbonated beverages; gelatin; clear fruit juices (apple, grape, and cranberry); fat-free clear broth; hard candy, sugar, and popsicles
Full-liquid	Foods that are liquid at room temperature or that melt at body temperature	Advance from clear-liquid diet postoperatively; for stomach irritation, fever, and nausea and vomiting	All foods allowed on a clear-liquid diet; custard, eggnog; strained soups; strained fruit and vegetable juices; milk; creamed cereals; plain ice cream and sherbet
Soft	Semisolid foods that are easily digested	Advance from full-liquid diet; chewing difficulties, gastrointestinal disorders, and infections	All liquids; eggs (not fried); broiled, baked, or roasted meat, fish, or poultry that is chopped or shredded; mild cheeses (American, Swiss, cheddar, cream, and cottage); strained fruit juices; refined bread (no crust) and crackers; cooked cereal; cooked or pureed vegetables; cooked or canned fruit without skin or seeds; pudding; plain cakes
Low-residue	Food that leaves a small amount of residue in the colon	Diseases of the colon and diarrhea	Coffee, tea, milk, carbonated beverages, strained fruit juices; refined bread and crackers; creamed and refined cereal; rice; cottage and cream cheese; eggs (not fried); plain puddings and cakes; gelatin; custard; sherbet and ice cream; strained vegetable juices; canned or cooked fruit without skin or seeds; potatoes (not fried); strained cooked vegetables; plain pasta; *no raw fruits and vegetables*
High-fiber	Foods that increase the amount of residue in the colon to stimulate peristalsis	Constipation and colon disorders	All fruits and vegetables; whole wheat bread; whole grain cereals; fried foods; whole grain rice; milk, cream, butter, and cheese; meats
Bland	Foods that are mechanically and chemically nonirritating and low in roughage; foods served at moderate temperatures; no strong spices or condiments	Ulcers, gallbladder disorders, and some intestinal disorders; postoperatively following abdominal surgery	Lean meats; white bread; creamed and refined cereals; cream or cottage cheese; gelatin, plain puddings, cakes, and cookies; eggs (not fried); butter and cream; canned fruits and vegetables without skin and seeds; strained fruit juices; potatoes (not fried); pastas and rice; strained or soft cooked carrots, peas, beets, spinach, squash, and asparagus tips; creamed soups from allowed vegetables; no fried foods are allowed

TABLE 17-3

SPECIAL DIETS—CONT'D

Diet	Description	Use	Foods Allowed
High-calorie	Calorie intake is increased to about 4000; includes three full meals and between-meal snacks	Weight gain and some thyroid imbalances	Dietary increases in all foods
Low-calorie	The number of calories is reduced below the minimum daily requirements	Weight reduction	Foods low in fats and carbohydrates and lean meats; avoid butter, cream, rice, gravies, salad oils, noodles, cakes, pastries, carbonated and alcoholic beverages, candy, potato chips, and similar foods
High-iron	Foods that are high in iron	Anemia; following blood loss; for women during the reproductive years	Liver and other organ meats; lean meats; egg yolks; shellfish; dried fruits; dried beans; green leafy vegetables; lima beans; peanut butter; enriched breads and cereals
Low-fat (low-cholesterol)	Foods low in fat and foods prepared without adding fat	Heart disease, gallbladder disease, disorders of fat digestion, and liver disease	Skim milk or buttermilk; cottage cheese (no other cheeses are allowed); gelatin; sherbet; fruit; lean meat, poultry, and fish (baked, broiled, or roasted); fat-free broth; soups made with skim milk; margarine; rice, pasta, breads, and cereals; vegetables; potatoes
High-protein	Aid and promote tissue healing	For burns, high fever, infection, and some liver diseases	Meat, milk, eggs, cheese, fish, poultry; breads and cereals; green leafy vegetables
Sodium-restricted	A certain amount of sodium is allowed; sodium restriction ranges from mild to severe	Heart disease, fluid retention, and some kidney diseases	Fruits and vegetables and unsalted butter are allowed; adding salt at the table is not allowed; highly salted foods and foods high in sodium are not allowed; the use of salt during cooking may be restricted
Diabetic	The amount of carbohydrates and number of calories are regulated; protein and fat are also regulated	Diabetes mellitus	Determined by nutritional and energy requirements

There are three common levels of sodium-restricted diets. They range from mild to severe. The doctor orders the amount of restriction for the person. People on sodium-restricted diets need to learn how to calculate the amount of sodium in the diet. They also need to know which foods are high and which are low in sodium. A nurse or dietician teaches individuals and families about the diet. Many low-salt or salt-free foods can be bought. Food labels are used to determine salt content (see Chapter 35).

- 2000 mg to 3000 mg sodium diet. Called the low-salt diet, this diet is commonly ordered. Sodium restriction is mild. All high-sodium foods are omitted (Box 17-6). A minimum amount of salt is used for cooking. Salt is not added to foods at the table.
- 1000 mg sodium diet. Sodium restriction is moderate. Food is cooked without salt. Foods high in sodium are omitted. Vegetables high in sodium are restricted in amount. Salt-free products, such as salt-free bread, are used. Diet planning is necessary.
- 500 mg sodium diet. Sodium restriction is severe. Restrictions for the mild and moderate sodium diets are followed. In addition, vegetables high in sodium are omitted. Milk is limited to 1 cup per day, and only 1 egg per day is allowed. Meat is limited to 4 ounces per day. Diet planning is essential.

The Diabetic Diet

The diabetic diet is ordered for people with diabetes mellitus. Diabetes mellitus is a chronic disease from a deficiency of insulin (see Chapter 28). Insulin is produced and secreted by the pancreas. It allows the body to use sugar. If there is not enough insulin, sugar builds up in the bloodstream rather than being used by cells for energy. Diabetes is usually treated with insulin or medications, diet, and exercise.

Carbohydrates are broken down into sugar during digestion. The amount of carbohydrates is controlled with the diabetic diet. Only the amount of carbohydrates needed is ingested. The diabetic diet involves the correct amount and kind of food for the person. The doctor determines the amount of carbohydrate, fat, protein, and calories a person should have. The person's age, sex, activity, and weight are considered.

The calories and nutrients allowed are divided among 3 meals and between-meal nourishments. The person must eat only what is allowed and all that is allowed. This is important so the person does not get too many or too few carbohydrates. The American Diabetes Association has food lists that have equal amounts of nutrients and calories. There are 6 food lists called *exchanges:* milk, vegetables, fruits, bread, meat foods, and fat. The exchanges allow variety in menu planning. For example, a person does not want grapefruit. The exchange list is checked for other fruits. The person sees that one small orange equals one-half grapefruit. Therefore the person knows how much to eat. The nurse and dietician help the person and family learn how to use the exchange lists.

You must serve the person's meal on time. The diabetic must eat at regular times to maintain a certain blood sugar level. You need to check the tray to determine what has been eaten. If all food has not been eaten, a between-meal nourishment is needed. The nourishment makes up for what was not eaten at the regular meal. The amount of insulin given also depends on the person's daily food intake.

OBRA DIETARY REQUIREMENTS

OBRA requires that persons receive a well-balanced diet. The diet must be nourishing and taste good. The nutritional and special dietary needs of each person must be met.

Food flavor and appearance are important. OBRA requires that appetizing food be served. That is, food should have an appealing aroma and be attractive. Food should also be well seasoned. It must not be too salty or too sweet. Temperature is important. OBRA requires that hot food be served hot and cold food served cold. Facilities have special food servers to keep food at the correct temperature. Food should be served promptly in dining rooms. Persons who eat in their rooms need to have trays served promptly. Otherwise, hot food will cool and cold food will warm. Survey teams (see Chapter 7) actually taste food and measure its temperature to make sure the facility is meeting OBRA requirements.

OBRA also requires that food be prepared to meet the person's individual needs. Some persons need food cut, ground, or chopped. Others have special diets ordered by the doctor. Survey teams check to make sure the person is getting the diet ordered.

Each person must receive at least 3 meals per day and be offered a bedtime snack. The facility must also provide any special eating equipment and utensils that are needed (Fig. 17-5 on page 412). Hands, wrists, and arms may be affected by disease or injury. Special equipment may be needed so the person can eat independently. You must make sure needed equipment is used by the person.

BOX 17-6 High-Sodium Foods

Bread, Cereal, Rice, and Pasta Group

- Saltines
- Baking powder biscuits
- Muffins
- Bisquick
- Pretzels
- Salted crackers
- Quick breads (corn bread, nut bread)
- Pancakes
- Waffles
- Instant cooked cereal
- Processed bran cereals
- Rice
- Noodle mixes
- Corn chips and other salted snacks

Vegetable Group

- Sauerkraut
- Tomato juice
- V-8 juice
- Vegetables in creams or sauces
- Frozen vegetables processed with salt or sodium
- Bloody Mary mixes
- Potato chips
- French fries
- Instant potatoes
- Pickles
- Relishes

Fruit Group

- No restrictions

Milk, Yogurt, and Cheese Group

- Buttermilk
- Cheese
- Commercial dips made with sour cream

Meat, Poultry, Fish, Dry Beans, Eggs, and Nuts Group

- Bacon
- Ham
- Sausage
- Salt pork
- Hot dogs
- Luncheon meats
- Corned or chopped beef
- Organ meats
- Shellfish
- Sardines
- Herring
- Anchovies
- Caviar
- Kosher meats
- Canned tuna
- Canned salmon
- Mackerel
- Salted nuts or seeds
- Peanut butter

Fats, Oils, and Sweets

- Salad dressings
- Mayonnaise
- Baked desserts

Other

- Mineral water
- Club soda
- Canned soups
- Bouillon cubes
- Dried soup mixes
- Olives
- Salted popcorn
- Frozen or canned dinners
- Salt
- Baking powder
- Baking soda
- Celery, onion, garlic, and other seasoning salts
- Meat tenderizers
- Worcestershire sauce
- Soy sauce
- Mustard
- Catsup
- Horseradish
- Sauces: chili, tomato, steak, barbecue

Modified from Lewis SM, Collier IC: *Medical-surgical nursing: assessment and management of clinical problems,* ed 3, St Louis, 1992, Mosby–Year Book.

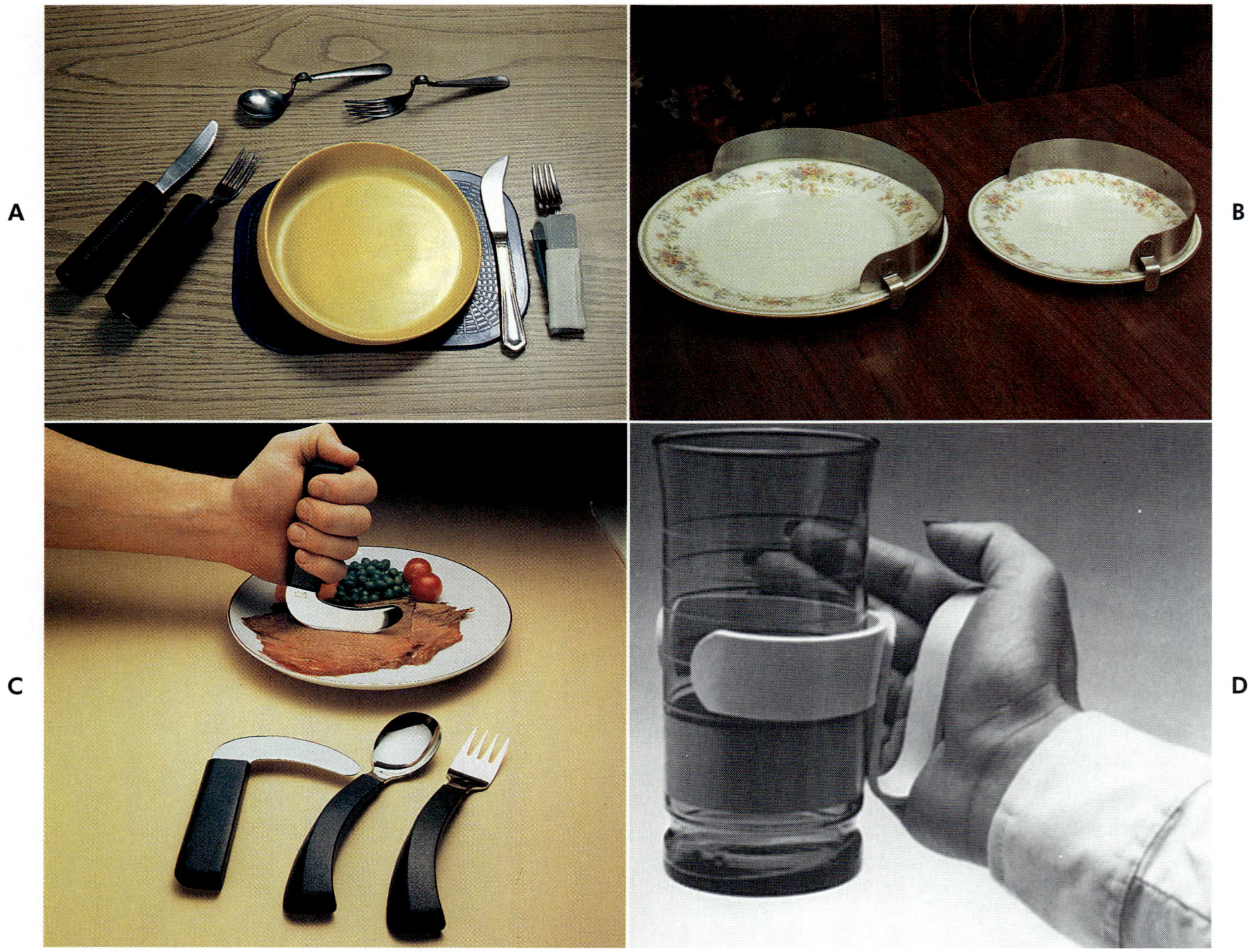

Fig. 17-5 *Eating utensils for persons with special needs. A, Note the curved fork, which fits over the hand. The rounded plate helps keep food on the plate. Special grips and swivel handles are helpful for some persons. B, Plate guards help keep food on the plate. C, Knives with rounded blades are rocked back and forth to cut food. The person does not need to have a fork in one hand and a knife in the other. D, Glass or cup holder.* (Courtesy BISSELL Healthcare Corp.; Fred Sammons, Inc.)

FLUID BALANCE

After oxygen, water is the most important physical need for survival. Death can result from an inadequate water intake or from excessive fluid loss. Water enters the body through fluids and foods. Water is lost through the urine and feces, through the skin as perspiration, and through the lungs with expiration. Fluid balance must be maintained for health. There must be a balance between the amount of fluid taken in and the amount lost.

The amount of fluid taken in (**intake**) and the amount lost (**output**) must be equal. If fluid intake exceeds fluid output, body tissues swell with water. This is called **edema.** Edema is common in people with heart and kidney diseases. **Dehydration** is a decrease in the amount of water in the tissues. It results when fluid output exceeds intake. Inadequate fluid intake, vomiting, diarrhea, bleeding, excessive sweating, and increased urine production are common causes of dehydration.

Normal Requirements

An adult needs 1500 ml of water daily to survive. Approximately 2000 to 2500 ml of fluid per day is required to maintain a normal fluid balance. The water requirement increases with high weather temperatures, exercise, fever, and illness. Excessive fluid losses also increase the water requirement.

Minimum daily water requirements vary with age. Infants and young children have more body water. They need more fluids than do adults. Excessive fluid losses cannot be tolerated and will quickly cause death in an infant or child.

Special Orders

The doctor may order the amount of fluid a person can have during a 24-hour period. This is done to maintain fluid balance. *Force fluid, restrict fluids, and nothing by mouth* may be ordered.

- **Force fluids** means having the person drink increased amounts of fluid. The force fluids order may be general or for a specific amount. A FORCE FLUIDS sign is placed by the bed. Records are kept of the intake. A variety of allowed fluids are provided. They must be within the person's reach and served at the correct temperature. You must frequently offer fluids to persons who have force fluids orders but who cannot feed themselves.
- **Restrict fluids** means restricting fluids to a certain amount. Water is offered in small amounts and in small containers. The water pitcher is removed from the room or kept out of sight. A RESTRICT FLUIDS sign is posted by the bed and accurate intake records are kept. The person needs frequent oral hygiene. Oral hygiene helps keep mucous membranes of the mouth moist.
- **Nothing by mouth** means the person cannot eat or drink anything. *NPO* is the abbreviation for the Latin term *nils per os,* which means nothing by mouth. Persons are usually NPO before and after surgery, before some laboratory tests and x-ray procedures, and in the treatment of certain illnesses. An *NPO* sign is posted by the bed. The water pitcher and glass are removed. Frequent oral hygiene is allowed, but the person cannot swallow any fluid. The person is kept NPO starting at midnight before scheduled surgery, laboratory tests, or x-ray procedures.

Intake and Output Records

The doctor or nurse may want a person's fluid intake and output measured. This involves keeping intake and output (I&O) records. I&O records are used to evaluate fluid balance and kidney function. They are also used to determine and evaluate medical treatment. I&O records are kept when forcing fluids or restricting fluid intake.

To measure fluid intake, all liquid ingested by the person through the mouth is measured. Fluids given in IV therapy and tube feedings are also measured. The obvious fluids are measured: water, milk, coffee, tea, juices, soups, and soft drinks. So are soft and semisolid foods such as ice cream, sherbet, custard, pudding, creamed cereals, gelatin, and popsicles. Output to be measured includes urine, vomitus, diarrhea, and wound drainage.

Measuring Intake and Output

Intake and output are measured in milliliters (ml) or in cubic centimeters (cc). These metric system measurements are equal in amount. One ounce equals 30 ml. A pint is about 500 ml. There are about 1000 ml in a quart. You need to know the fluid capacity of bowls, dishes, cups, pitchers, glasses, and other containers used to serve fluids. Most I&O records have tables for use in measuring intake (Fig. 17-6 on page 414).

A **graduate** is used to measure fluids. A graduate is a measuring container similar to but larger than a measuring cup. The graduate is calibrated to measure amounts. Some graduates are marked in ounces and in milliliters or cubic centimeters (Fig. 17-7 on page 415). A graduate is used to measure leftover fluids, urine, vomitus, and drainage from suction (see Chapter 24). Plastic urinals and emesis basins are often calibrated.

An I&O record is usually kept at the bedside. Whenever fluid is ingested or output is measured, the amount is recorded in the appropriate column (see Fig. 17-7). The amounts are totaled at the end of the shift. The nurse charts the total amount for the shift in the person's record. The person's I&O are also communicated to the next shift during the end-of-shift report. The nurse records any intake through IV therapy or tube feedings.

The purpose of measuring intake and output is explained to the person. How the person can participate is also explained. Some persons measure and record their own intake. Family members may be involved. The urinal, commode, bedpan, or specimen pan is used for voiding. The toilet is not used. The person is reminded not to put toilet tissue into the receptacle.

Medical asepsis, Standard Precautions, and the Bloodborne Pathogen Standard are followed when measuring output.

DAILY INTAKE AND OUTPUT RECORD
(Bedside record)

Intake | Output

11-7

Time	Oral	IV			Time	Urine	Emesis	Drainage	

Total: ______ Total: ______

7-3

Time	Oral	IV			Time	Urine	Emesis	Drainage	

Total: ______ Total: ______

3-11

Time	Oral	IV			Time	Urine	Emesis	Drainage	

Total: ______ Total: ______

Water glass	= 150 ml	Milk carton	= 240 ml
Coffee pot	= 200 ml	Large paper cup (like for eggnog, shakes, etc.)	= 240 ml
Ice cream	= 60 ml	Jello per serving	= 120 ml
Coffee cup	= 120 ml		
Soup bowl	= 180 ml		

Fig. 17-6 *An intake and output (I and O) record.*

MEASURING INTAKE AND OUTPUT

PROCEDURE

1 Explain the procedure to the person.
2 Collect the following:
   - Intake and output (I&O) record
   - 2 I&O labels
   - Graduate (see Fig. 17-7)
   - Disposable gloves
3 Place the I&O record at the bedside.
4 Place one label in the bathroom. Place the other by the bed.
5 Measure intake as follows:
   - **a** Pour liquid remaining in a container into the graduate.
   - **b** Measure the amount at eye level.
   - **c** Check the amount of the serving on the I&O record.
   - **d** Subtract the remaining amount from the full serving amount.
   - **e** Repeat steps 5a through 5d for each liquid.
   - **f** Add the amounts from 5e together. Record the time and amount on the I&O record.
6 Measure output as follows. (Wear gloves for this step.)
   - **a** Pour the fluid into the graduate.
   - **b** Measure the amount at eye level.
   - **c** Record the time and amount on the I&O record.
   - **d** Rinse and return the graduate to its proper place.
   - **e** Clean and rinse the bedpan, urinal, emesis basin, or other drainage container. Return it to its proper place.
7 Remove the gloves and wash your hands.
8 Report your observations to the nurse.

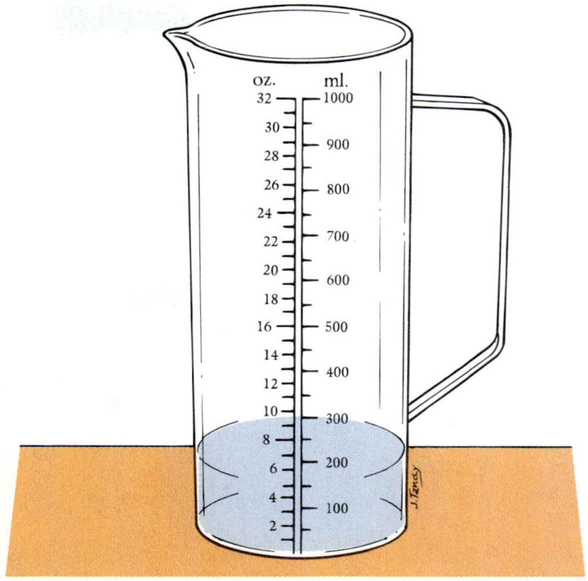

Fig. 17-7 *A graduate (measuring container) calibrated in milliliters. The graduate contains 150 ml.*

ASSISTING THE PERSON WITH FOODS AND FLUIDS

Weakness and illness can affect a person's appetite and ability to eat. Odors, unpleasant equipment, an uncomfortable position, the need for oral hygiene, and the need to void are some factors that affect appetite. Nursing staff can control these factors by getting the person ready for meals. Be sure to practice Standard Precautions and follow the Bloodborne Pathogen Standard.

Serving Meal Trays

In hospitals, food is usually served in the person's room. However, some persons eat in dining rooms, the cafeteria, or lounge areas. Nursing facility residents usually eat in dining rooms. Food is served in containers that keep hot and cold foods at the correct temperature. You will serve meal trays after preparing persons for meals. Having persons already prepared for eating means trays can be served promptly. The prompt serving of trays keeps food at the desired temperature.

Getting the Person Ready for Meals

Pre-procedure

1 Explain the procedure to the person.
2 Wash your hands.
3 Collect the following:
   - Items for oral hygiene
   - Bedpan or urinal
   - Wash basin
   - Soap
   - Washcloth
   - Towel
   - Robe and slippers
   - Disposable gloves
4 Provide for privacy.

Procedure

5 Assist the person with oral hygiene. Be sure dentures are in place. (Wear gloves for this step).
6 Offer the bedpan or urinal. Assist the person to the bathroom or bedside commode if he or she can be up. The person wears a robe and slippers when up.
7 Help the person wash the hands.
8 Do one of the following:
   a For persons who will eat in bed: Raise the head of the bed to a comfortable sitting position. Position the overbed table in front of the person. Make sure it is clean.
   b For persons who can sit in a chair: Help the person to a chair if he or she can be up. Position the overbed table in front of the person. Place the call bell within reach.
   c For persons who will eat in dining rooms: Assist the person to the dining room.
9 Clean and return items to their proper place. (Wear gloves if contact with body fluids or substances is possible.)
10 Straighten the room. Eliminate unpleasant noise, odors, or equipment.
11 Unscreen the person.
12 Wash your hands.

Serving Meal Trays

Procedure

1 Wash your hands.
2 Make sure the tray is complete. Check items on the tray with the dietary card.
3 Identify the person. Check the ID bracelet with the dietary card.
4 Have the person in a sitting position if possible.
5 Place the tray on the overbed table within the person's reach. Adjust table height as necessary.
6 Remove food covers. Open milk cartons and cereal boxes, cut meat, and butter bread if indicated (Fig. 17-8).
7 Place the napkin and silverware within reach.
8 Measure and record intake if ordered. Note the amount and type of foods eaten.
9 Remove the tray.
10 Assist the person with oral hygiene. (Wear gloves for this step.)
11 Clean any spills and change soiled linen.
12 Help the person return to bed if indicated.

Post-procedure

13 Make sure the person is comfortable and the call bell is within reach. Raise or lower side rails as instructed by the nurse.
14 Wash your hands.
15 Report your observations to the nurse.

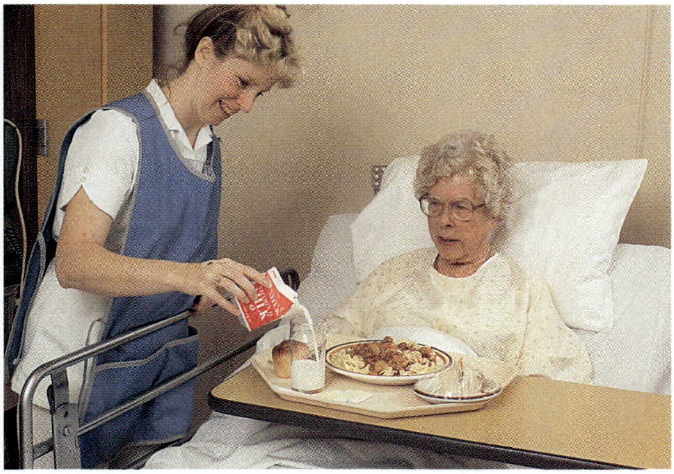

Fig. 17-8 *The nursing assistant opens cartons and other containers for the person.*

Feeding the Person

Some persons cannot feed themselves. Weakness, paralysis, casts, and other physical limitations may make self-feeding impossible. These persons must be fed. When feeding a person, you should be in a comfortable position. You also need to provide a relaxed mood so that the person does not feel rushed. Many people say a prayer before eating. Be sure to provide time and privacy for a prayer. This shows care and respect for the person. The person is asked about the order in which to offer foods and fluids. Spoons are used. They are less likely to cause injury than forks. The spoon should be only one-third full. The portion is easily chewed and swallowed.

Persons who cannot feed themselves may be angry, humiliated, and embarrassed at being dependent on others. Some may be depressed or resentful, or may refuse to eat. These persons are allowed to feed themselves as much as possible. However, they should not exceed activity limits ordered by the doctor. Be supportive and encouraging.

Visually impaired persons are often keenly aware of food aromas. They may even be able to identify some foods served. Be sure to tell the person what foods and fluids are on the tray. When feeding someone who is visually impaired, always tell the person what you are offering. If the person does not need to be fed, identify foods and fluids and their location on the tray. Use the numbers on a clock to identify the location of foods (Fig. 17-9).

Meals provide social contact. You should engage the person in pleasant conversation. However, give the person enough time to chew and swallow. Also, sit so that you face the person. Sitting is relaxing and shows that you have time for the person. Standing communicates nonverbally that you do not have time and that you are in a hurry. By facing the person, you can see how well the person is eating. You can also see if the person has problems swallowing.

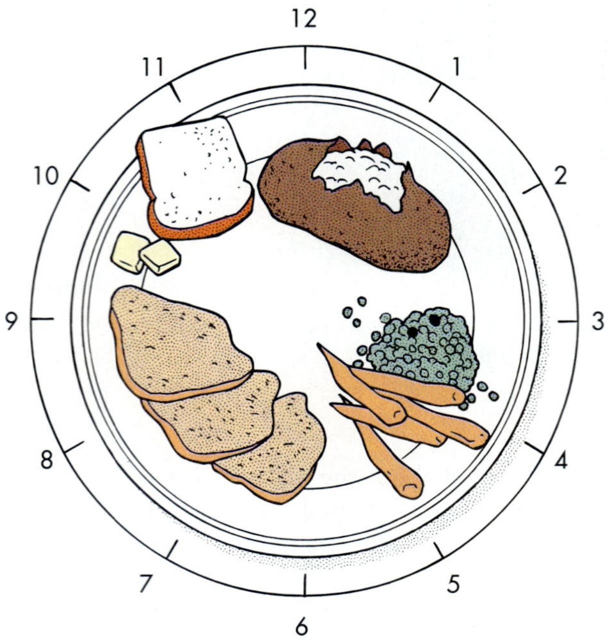

Fig. 17-9 *The numbers on a clock are used to help a visually impaired person locate food on the tray.*

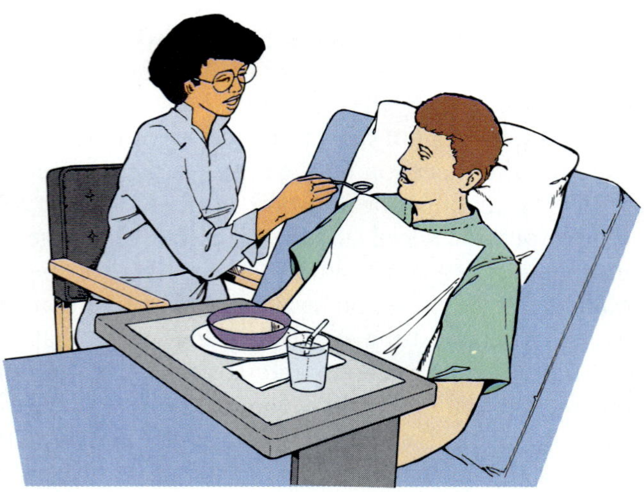

Fig. 17-10 *A spoon is used to feed the person. The spoon is no more than one-third full.*

FEEDING A PERSON

PROCEDURE

1. Explain the procedure to the person.
2. Wash your hands.
3. Position the person in a comfortable sitting position.
4. Bring the tray into the room. Place it on the overbed table.
5. Identify the person. Check the ID bracelet with the dietary card.
6. Drape a napkin across the person's chest and underneath the chin.
7. Prepare the food for eating.
8. Tell the person what foods are on the tray.
9. Serve foods in the order the person prefers. Alternate between solid and liquid foods. Use a spoon for safety as in Figure 17-10. Allow enough time for chewing. Do not rush the person.
10. Use straws for liquids if the person cannot drink out of a glass or cup. Have one straw for each liquid. Provide a short straw for weak persons.
11. Converse with the person in a pleasant manner.
12. Encourage him or her to eat as much as possible.
13. Wipe the person's mouth with a napkin.
14. Note how much and which foods were eaten.
15. Measure and record intake if ordered.
16. Remove the tray.
17. Provide oral hygiene. (Wear gloves for this step.)

POST-PROCEDURE

18. Make sure the person is comfortable and the call bell is within reach. Raise or lower side rails as instructed by the nurse.
19. Wash your hands.
20. Report your observations to the nurse:
    - The amount and kind of food eaten
    - Complaints of nausea or **dysphagia**—difficulty or discomfort (dys) in swallowing (phagia)

Between-Meal Nourishments

Many special diets involve between-meal nourishments. Commonly served nourishments are crackers, milk, juice, a milkshake, cake, wafers, a sandwich, gelatin, and custard. Nourishments are served as soon as they arrive on the nursing unit. Needed eating utensils, a straw, and a napkin are provided. The same considerations and procedures described for serving meal trays and feeding persons are followed.

Providing Drinking Water

Patients and residents need fresh drinking water. Fresh water is usually provided during the day and evening and whenever the water pitcher is empty. Before passing water you need to know about any special orders. Some persons are NPO, on restricted fluids, or not allowed ice. The rules of medical asepsis are practiced when passing drinking water.

PROVIDING FRESH DRINKING WATER

PRE-PROCEDURE

1 Get a list of persons who have special fluid orders (NPO, fluid restriction, or no ice). The list is obtained from the nurse.

2 Wash your hands.

3 Collect the following:
- Cart
- Ice chest filled with ice cubes and a cover for the chest
- Scoop
- Disposable cups
- Straws
- Paper towels
- Large water pitcher filled with cold water (optional, depending on facility procedure)

4 Arrange items on the cart on top of the paper towels.

PROCEDURE

5 Move the cart until you are just outside a person's room. Check the list to see if the person has special orders.

6 Check the ID bracelet and call the person by name.

7 Take the water pitcher from the overbed table. Empty it into the sink in the bathroom.

8 Fill the pitcher half full with water. Get water from the tap or pitcher on the cart.

9 Fill the water pitcher with ice if it is allowed. Use the scoop for the ice (Fig. 17-11 on page 420).

10 Place the pitcher, disposable cup, and straw on the overbed table. Make sure the person can easily reach the items.

11 Fill the disposable cup with fresh water.

12 Repeat steps 5 through 11 for each person.

13 Return the equipment to the utility room. Clean and return equipment to its proper place.

14 Wash your hands.

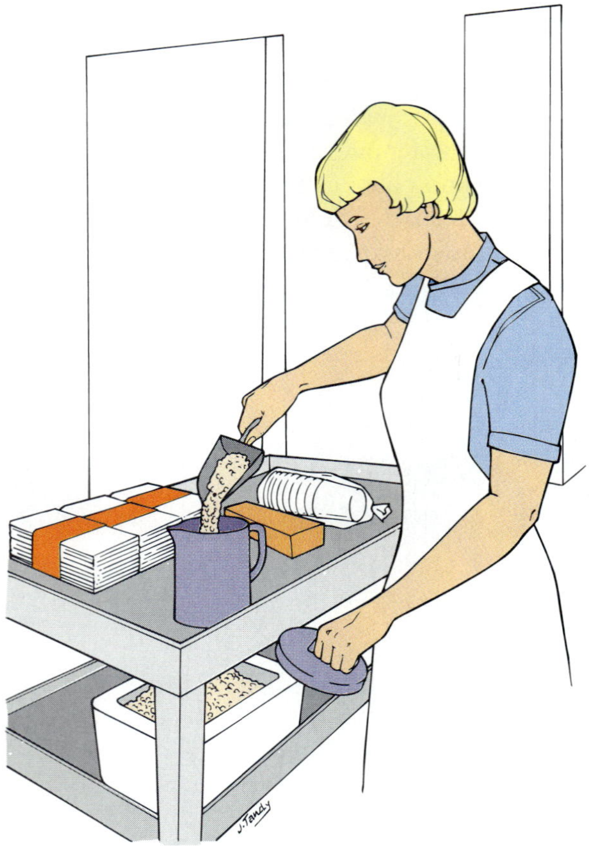

Fig. 17-11 *The rules of medical asepsis are followed when passing drinking water. The scoop does not touch any part of the water pitcher when ice is being added.*

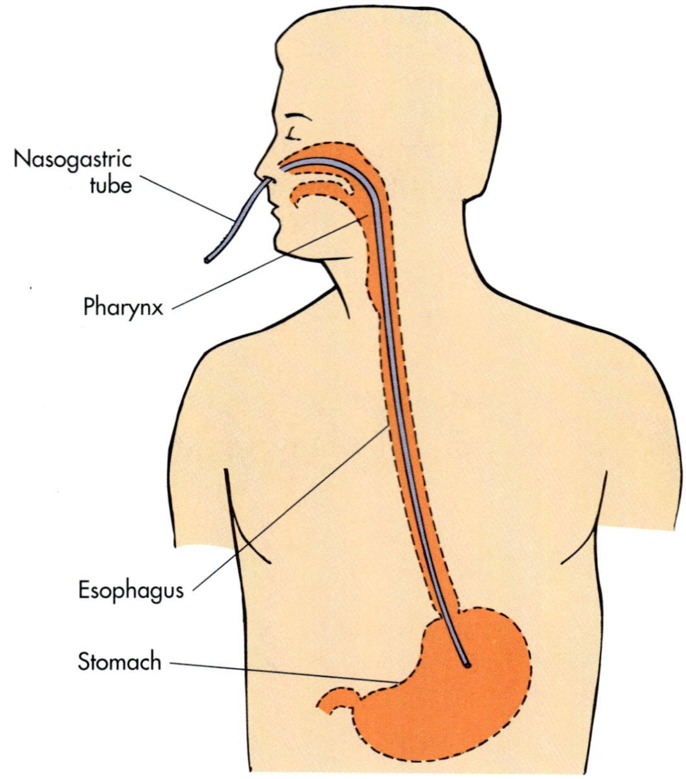

Fig. 17-12 *A nasogastric tube is inserted through the nose into the stomach.*

Other Methods of Maintaining Food and Fluid Needs

Many people cannot eat or drink because of illness, surgery, or injury. Other methods must be used to meet their food and fluid needs. These methods are ordered by the doctor. The nurse carries out the order.

Tube feedings The doctor may order a tube feeding. The nurse inserts a nasogastric (NG) tube through the nose into the stomach (Fig. 17-12). Commercial or blended fluids are passed through the tube into the stomach. The feeding can be given at scheduled intervals using a syringe (Fig. 17-13). Electronic feeding pumps are often used for continuous feedings (Fig. 17-14). **Gavage** is another term for a tube feeding.

A person may have a gastrostomy. A **gastrostomy** is an opening (stomy) in the stomach (gastro). The opening is created surgically. A tube is inserted into the opening (Fig. 17-15). Commercial or blended foods are passed through the tube into the stomach.

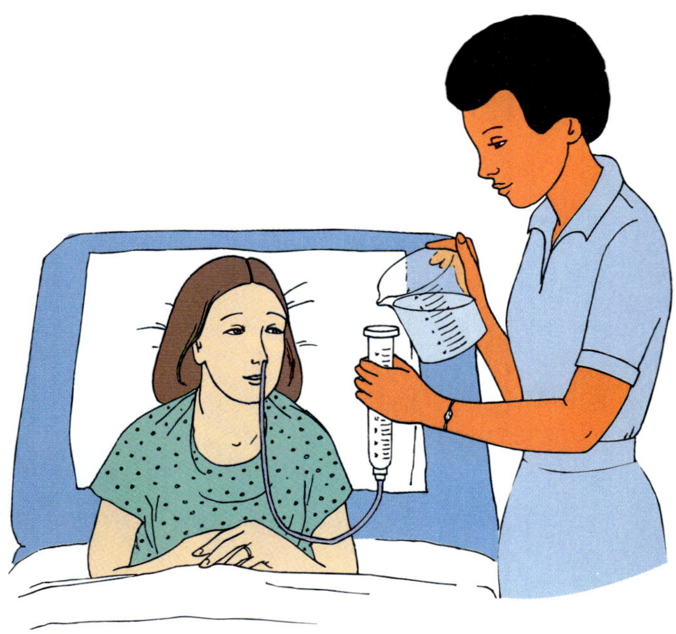

Fig. 17-13 *The nurse gives a tube feeding. A syringe is attached to the end of the NG tube. The blended fluid is poured into the syringe.*

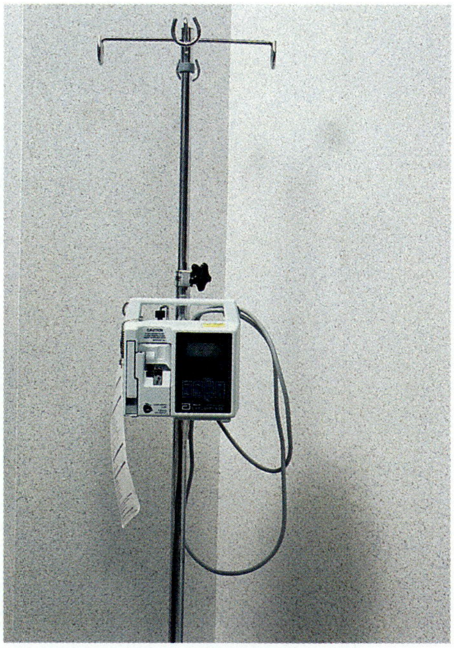

Fig. 17-14 *An electronic feeding pump.*

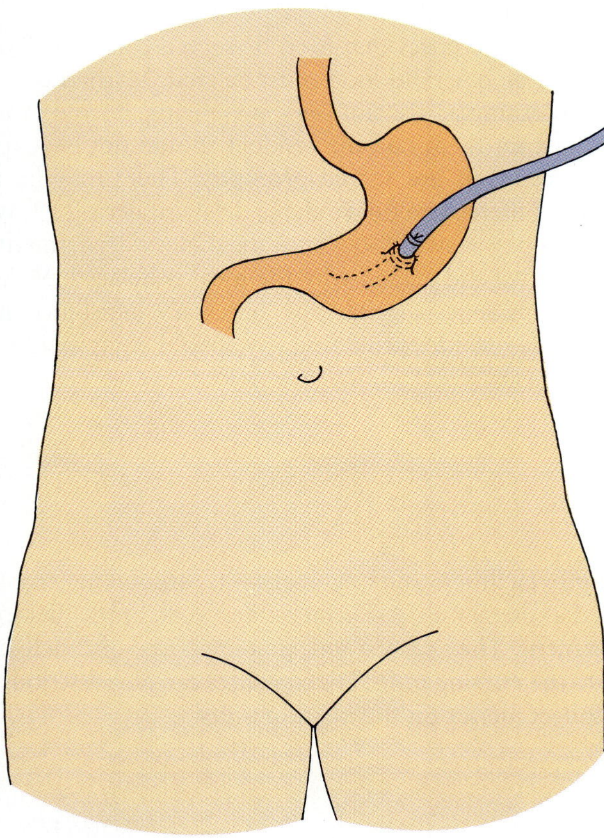

Fig. 17-15 *A gastrostomy tube.*

A gastrostomy is used when food cannot pass normally from the mouth into the esophagus and then into the stomach. Cancer of the head, neck, or esophagus may require a gastrostomy. The person with a gastrostomy cannot eat or drink fluids. The gastrostomy may be temporary or permanent.

The nurse is responsible for giving tube feedings. The person is sitting or in Fowler's position for the feeding. These positions promote flow of the fluid through the tube. They also prevent aspiration. The person remains sitting, in Fowler's position, or in semi-Fowler's position for at least 30 minutes after the feeding. This promotes movement of the feeding fluid through the gastrointestinal system and prevents aspiration.

Intravenous therapy Many persons receive fluid through a needle inserted in a vein. The fluid may contain sugar, minerals, and vitamins. **IV, IV therapy,** and **IV infusion** are often used in referring to **intravenous therapy.** The fluid is in a plastic bag. Clear IV tubing connects the container to the needle in a vein (Fig. 17-16). The amount of fluid given (infused) per hour is ordered by the doctor.

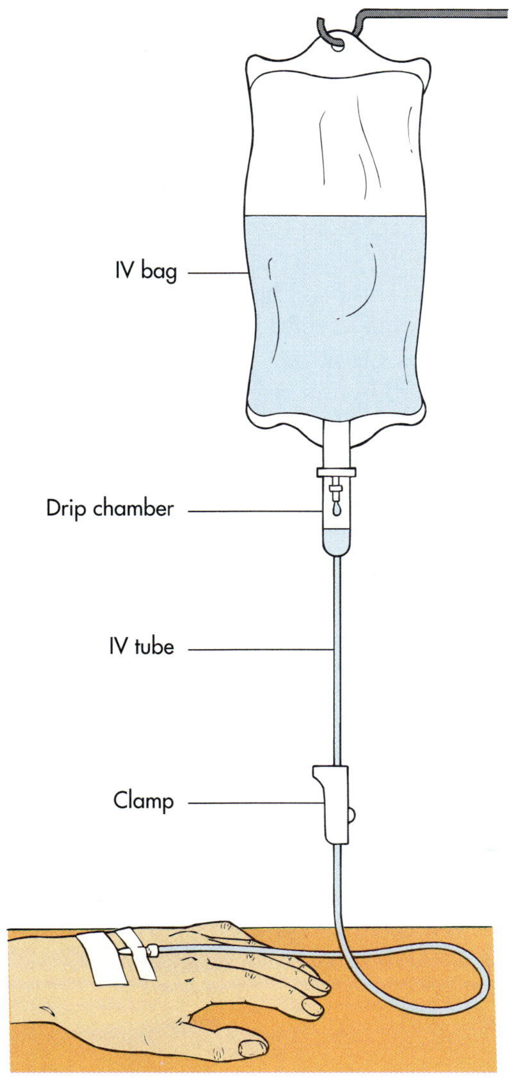

Fig. 17-16 *Intravenous therapy. The needle is inserted into a vein in the arm or hand. The needle is attached to the bag by tubing.*

The nurse makes sure the ordered amount is given. This is done by controlling the number of drops (flow rate) per minute. *Nursing assistants are never responsible for IV therapy or for regulating the flow rate.* Your role in caring for the person with an IV infusion is further discussed in Chapter 24.

IV therapy does not provide fat and protein. It provides fluids and sugar for energy. IV therapy is not used for long-term nutritional therapy.

Hyperalimentation

Hyperalimentation is the intravenous administration of a solution highly concentrated with proteins, carbohydrates, vitamins, and minerals. Fat can also be added. The solution is far more nutritious than a regular IV solution. Hyperalimentation is used for seriously ill and injured persons. *Nursing assistants are never responsible for administering or regulating hyperalimentation solutions.*

QUALITY OF LIFE

The right to personal choice is important when meeting food and fluids needs. Everyone has a lifetime of food likes and dislikes. These do not change when a person enters a health care facility. Food preferences may be based on certain religious or cultural practices. The dietician works with the person in planning healthy meals that include personal choices. The person may tell you that he or she likes or wants certain foods. You need to share this information with the nurse.

Sometimes family and friends bring the person food from home. This can help the person's need for love and belonging. Sometimes the dietary department cannot provide for all of the person's food preferences. Patients and residents are usually very pleased when family and friends bring favorite foods. Certain foods and food traditions are part of holidays. Holidays are more meaningful when lifelong family traditions are shared. Many families and friends bring food as holiday gifts. The nurse needs to know when food is brought to the person. The food must not interfere with special diets.

Some nursing facilities have dining areas where residents can dine with guests. There the resident can have a family meal with a spouse, children, grandchildren, relatives, or friends. The dietary department provides the meal or it may be brought by the family. Holidays, birthdays, anniversaries, and other special events can be celebrated (Fig. 17-17).

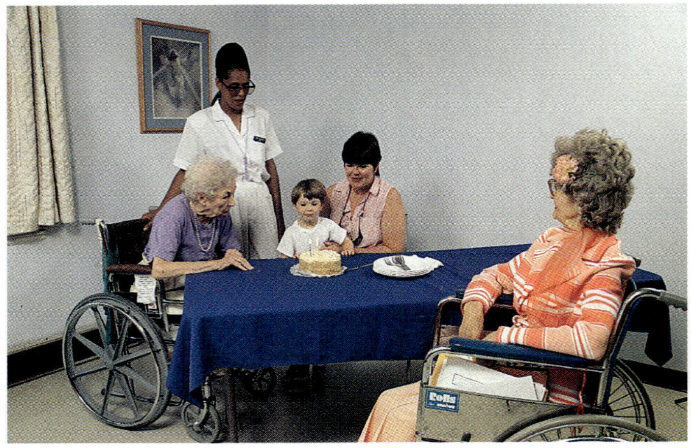

Fig. 17-17 *A grandchild's birthday is celebrated in the nursing facility.*

OBRA also requires that food be served correctly. Hot food must be hot, cold food must be cold. Mashed potatoes, for example, are not very appetizing if cold. You would not eat them and the resident should not have to. Make sure meals are served promptly. There may be a time when there is an unavoidable delay in serving a tray. If so, get a new tray of food from the dietary department. Be sure to tell the person why the meal is delayed. Make sure the resident is given any necessary assistance in eating. This includes providing any special equipment or eating utensils.

CROSS-TRAINING OPPORTUNITIES

In some facilities, nursing assistants are being cross-trained as dietary aides. Dietary aides work in the dietary department. They serve food, prepare trays, and deliver trays to the nursing units. Dietary aides can also distribute and collect menus on the nursing units.

Summary

Food and fluids are needed for health and survival. A well-balanced diet contains foods from the five groups in the lower three levels of the Food Guide Pyramid. The diet provides the necessary amounts of proteins, carbohydrates, fats, vitamins, and minerals. Eating habits vary among individuals. They are affected by many factors, including culture and religion. You must consider the factors that affect a person's eating habits or abilities. Also try to make the meal as pleasant as possible for the person.

Fluid balance is essential for health and life. Fluid intake must equal fluid output. Fluid is lost through the urine, feces, skin, and lungs. You assist doctors and nurses in evaluating a person's fluid balance by keeping accurate I&O records when directed to do so.

Patients and residents depend on nursing staff to meet some or all of their food and fluid needs. Even persons who are up and about rely on the nursing team to serve meal trays. They also need nourishments and fresh drinking water. Some persons need to be fed. Remember that meals provide pleasure and time for socializing. The person enjoys the meal even more if he or she is refreshed and in a comfortable position.

Review Questions

Circle the best *answer.*

1 Nutrition is
- **a** Fats, proteins, carbohydrates, vitamins, and minerals
- **b** The many processes involved in the ingestion, digestion, absorption, and use of food and fluids by the body
- **c** The Food Guide Pyramid
- **d** The balance between fluids taken in and lost by the body

2 The Food Guide Pyramid has
- **a** Three food groups
- **b** Four food groups
- **c** Five food groups
- **d** Six food groups

3 The Food Guide Pyramid encourages
- **a** A low-fat diet
- **b** A high-fat diet
- **c** A low-fiber diet
- **d** A low-salt diet

4 How many daily servings of breads, cereals, rice, and pasta are recommended?
- **a** 6 to 11
- **b** 3 to 5
- **c** 2 to 4
- **d** 2 to 3

5 How many daily servings of the meat group are recommended?
- **a** 6 to 11
- **b** 3 to 5
- **c** 2 to 4
- **d** 2 to 3

6 Which food groups contain the most fat?
- **a** Breads, cereal, rice, and pasta
- **b** Fruits
- **c** Milk, yogurt, and cheese
- **d** Meat, poultry, fish, dry beans, eggs, and nuts

7 Fats, oils, and sweets
- **a** Should be used in moderate amounts
- **b** Are low in calories
- **c** Should be used sparingly
- **d** Have great nutritional value

8 Protein is needed for
- **a** Tissue growth and repair
- **b** Energy and the fiber for bowel elimination
- **c** Body heat and the protection of organs from injury
- **d** Improving the taste of food

REVIEW QUESTIONS—CONT'D

9 Which foods provide the *most* protein?
- **a** Butter and cream
- **b** Tomatoes and potatoes
- **c** Meats and fish
- **d** Corn and lettuce

10 Eating and nutrition are affected by
- **a** Culture and religious practices
- **b** Personal preferences and how food is prepared
- **c** The amount of money available for food
- **d** All of the above

11 Sodium-restricted diets are usually ordered for the following persons *except* those with
- **a** Diabetes mellitus
- **b** Heart disease
- **c** Kidney disease
- **d** Liver disease

12 Mr. Bonner is on a sodium-restricted diet. He asks for some salt for his chicken. You should bring him the salt.
- **a** True
- **b** False

13 The diabetic diet controls the amount of
- **a** Water
- **b** Sodium
- **c** Carbohydrates
- **d** Nutrients

14 Diet planning for the diabetic diet involves
- **a** Calculating the amount of sodium
- **b** Exchange lists
- **c** Measuring fluid intake
- **d** Giving insulin with meals

15 Fluids are lost from the body through the
- **a** Urine and feces
- **b** Skin and lungs
- **c** Vomitus
- **d** All of the above

16 Mr. Bonner is on I&O. His fluid intake and output should be equal.
- **a** True
- **b** False

17 Adult fluid requirements for normal fluid balance are about
- **a** 1000 to 1500 ml daily
- **b** 1500 to 2000 ml daily
- **c** 2000 to 2500 ml daily
- **d** 2500 to 3000 ml daily

18 A person is NPO. You should
- **a** Provide a variety of fluids
- **b** Offer fluids in small amounts and small containers
- **c** Remove the water pitcher and glass
- **d** Prevent the person from having oral hygiene

19 Which are *not* counted as liquid foods?
- **a** Coffee, tea, juices, and soft drinks
- **b** Butter, spaghetti sauce, and melted cheese
- **c** Ice cream, sherbet, custard, and pudding
- **d** Jello, popsicles, soup, and creamed cereals

20 Which statement about feeding a person is *false?*
- **a** Ask if he or she wants to pray before eating.
- **b** A fork is used to feed the person.
- **c** The person is asked the order in which foods should be served.
- **d** Engage the person in a pleasant conversation.

21 Which is *false?*
- **a** Between-meal nourishments must be served promptly.
- **b** You are never responsible for IV therapy.
- **c** You are never responsible for hyperalimentation.
- **d** You can insert an NG tube and give a tube feeding.

22 OBRA requires that
- **a** Hot foods be served hot; cold foods be served cold
- **b** Foods smell good
- **c** Foods taste good
- **d** All of the above

Answers to these questions are on page 751.

Measurement of Vital Signs

18

OBJECTIVES

- Define the key terms listed in this chapter
- Explain why vital signs are measured
- List the factors affecting vital signs
- Identify the normal ranges of oral, rectal, axillary, and tympanic temperatures
- Know when to take oral, rectal, axillary, and tympanic temperatures
- Identify the sites for taking a pulse
- Know the normal pulse ranges for different age groups
- Describe normal respirations
- Describe the factors affecting blood pressure
- Know the normal ranges for adult blood pressures
- Describe the differences between mercury and aneroid sphygmomanometers
- Describe the practices that are followed when measuring blood pressure
- Perform the procedures described in this chapter

KEY TERMS

apical-radial pulse Taking the apical and radial pulses at the same time

apnea The lack or absence of (a) breathing (pnea)

blood pressure The amount of force exerted against the walls of an artery by the blood

body temperature The amount of heat in the body that is a balance between the amount of heat produced and the amount lost by the body

bradycardia A slow (brady) heart rate (cardia); the rate is less than 60 beats per minute

bradypnea Slow (brady) breathing (pnea); the respiratory rate is less than 10 respirations per minute

Cheyne-Stokes A pattern of breathing in which respirations gradually increase in rate and depth and then become shallow and slow; breathing may stop for 10 to 20 seconds

diastole The period of heart muscle relaxation

diastolic pressure The pressure in the arteries when the heart is at rest

dyspnea Difficult, labored, or painful (dys) breathing (pnea)

hypertension Persistent blood pressure measurements above the normal systolic (140 mm Hg) or diastolic (90 mm Hg) pressures

hyperventilation Respirations that are rapid and deeper than normal

hypotension A condition in which the systolic blood pressure is below 90 mm Hg and the diastolic pressure is below 60 mm Hg

hypoventilation Respirations that are slow, shallow, and sometimes irregular

pulse The beat of the heart felt at an artery as a wave of blood passes through the artery

pulse deficit The difference between the apical and radial pulse rates

pulse rate The number of heartbeats or pulses felt in 1 minute

respiration The act of breathing air into (inhalation) and out of (exhalation) the lungs

sphygmomanometer The instrument used to measure blood pressure

stethoscope An instrument used to listen to the sounds produced by the heart, lungs, and other body organs

systole The period of heart muscle contraction

systolic pressure The amount of force it takes to pump blood out of the heart into the arterial circulation

tachycardia A rapid (tachy) heart rate (cardia); the heart rate is over 100 beats per minute

tachypnea Rapid (tachy) breathing (pnea); the respiratory rate is usually greater than 24 respirations per minute

vital signs Temperature, pulse, respirations, and blood pressure

Vital signs reflect the function of three body processes essential for life: regulation of body temperature, breathing, and heart function. The four **vital signs** of body function are temperature, pulse, respirations, and blood pressure.

Nursing assistants often measure vital signs. Accuracy is absolutely essential. You must be accurate in measuring, reporting, and recording vital signs.

MEASURING AND REPORTING VITAL SIGNS

A person's temperature, pulse, and respirations (TPR) and blood pressure (BP) vary within certain limits during any 24-hour period. Many factors affect vital signs. They include sleep, activity, eating, weather, noise, exercise, medications, fear, anxiety, and illness.

Vital signs are measured to detect changes in normal body function. They also tell how a person is responding to treatment. Life-threatening situations can be recognized. Vital signs are an important part of the assessment step of the nursing process. Vital signs are always measured:

- During physical examinations
- When a person is admitted to a health care facility
- Several times a day for hospital patients
- Before and after surgery
- Before and after complex procedures or diagnostic tests
- After some nursing procedures or measures, such as ambulation
- When medications are taken that affect the respiratory or circulatory systems
- Whenever the person complains of pain, fainting, shortness of breath, rapid heart rate, or not feeling well

Nursing facility residents do not have vital signs measured as often as hospital patients. The nurse tells you when to obtain vital signs. Unless otherwise ordered, vital signs are taken with the person lying or sitting. The person should be at rest when vital signs are measured.

Vital signs show even minor changes in a person's condition. They must be measured accurately. If unsure of your measurements, promptly ask the nurse to take them again. Vital signs must also be accurately reported and recorded. Any vital sign that is changed from a previous measurement is reported to the nurse immediately. Vital signs that are above or below the normal range are also reported immediately.

Many facilities have *temp boards* or *TPR books.* These

are divided into columns. Patient or resident names are written down the left side of the page. The other columns are for times of day (such as 0800, 1200, 1600, 2000). Vital signs are recorded on the line in the column appropriate for the person and time. In some facilities, changed or abnormal vital signs are circled in red. Besides recording them, verbally report changed or abnormal vital signs to the nurse right away. The nurse or doctor compares the current measurements with previous ones.

BODY TEMPERATURE

Body temperature is the amount of heat in the body. It is a balance between the amount of heat produced and the amount lost by the body. Heat is produced as food is used for energy. It is lost through the skin, breathing, urine, and feces. Body temperature remains fairly stable. It is lower in the morning and higher in the afternoon and evening. Factors affecting body temperature include age, weather, exercise, pregnancy, the menstrual cycle, emotions, stress, and illness.

Normal Body Temperature

The Fahrenheit (F) and Centigrade or Celsius (C) scales are used to measure temperature. Common sites for measuring body temperature are the mouth, rectum, axilla (underarm), and ear (tympanic). Normal body temperature depends on the site.

- Oral—98.6° F (37° C)
- Rectal—99.6° F (37.5° C)
- Axillary—axillary temperature is 97.6° F (36.5° C)
- Tympanic—98.6° F (37° C)

A person may have a temperature higher or lower than these measurements. That temperature may be normal for that person.

Body temperature usually stays within a normal range. Normal ranges of body temperature for healthy adults are:

- Oral—97.6° to 99.6° F (36.5° to 37.5° C)
- Rectal—98.6° to 100.6° F (37.0° to 38.1° C)
- Axillary (underarm)—96.6° to 98.6° F (36.0° to 37.0° C)
- Tympanic (ear)—98.6° F (37° C)

Thermometers are used to measure temperature. Glass and disposable thermometers are common in homes. So are tympanic thermometers. Electronic and tympanic thermometers are common in hospitals and nursing facilities.

> ## *Spotlight On...*
>
> ***Heather R of Atlanta, Georgia,*** *completed the nursing course at the Atlanta Job Corps Center. She then entered a work experience program in a doctor's office. During her work experience she was cross-trained to perform electrocardiograms, blood glucose tests, and venous punctures. After completing her work experience, Heather's interest is working as a home health aide.*

Glass Thermometers

The glass thermometer (clinical thermometer) is a hollow glass tube with a mercury-filled bulb. When heated by the body, the mercury expands and rises in the tube. The mercury contracts and moves down the tube when cooled.

There are three types of glass thermometers. Each has a different bulb or tip (Fig. 18-1). Long- or slender-tip thermometers are used for oral and axillary temperatures. So are thermometers with stubby and pear-shaped tips. Rectal thermometers have stubby tips that are color coded in red. Glass thermometers have a Fahrenheit or Centigrade scale. Some have both scales.

Glass thermometers can be reused after disinfection. However, they have the following disadvantages:

- They take a long time to register—3 to 10 minutes depending on the site used. Oral temperatures take 2 to 3 minutes, rectal temperatures take at least 2 minutes, and axillary temperatures take 5 to 10 minutes.
- They break easily.
- When used orally, there is the danger of the person biting down on the thermometer and causing it to break. The broken glass can cut the mucous membranes of the mouth. Any swallowed mercury can cause mercury poisoning.
- Broken rectal thermometers can injure the rectum and colon.

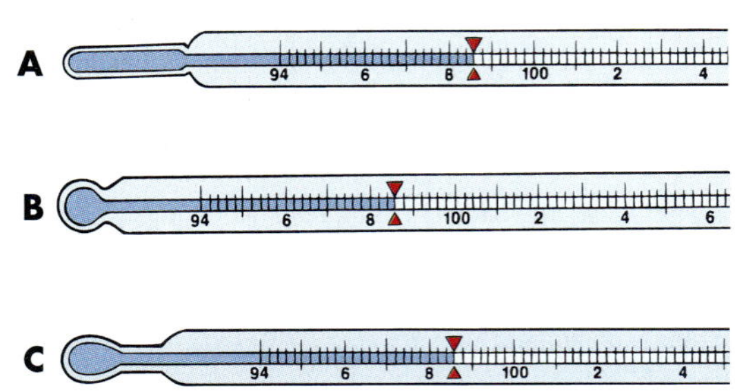

Fig. 18-1 *Types of glass thermometers.* ***A,*** *The long or slender tip.* ***B,*** *The stubby tip (rectal thermometer).* ***C,*** *The pear-shaped tip.*

How to read a glass thermometer Fahrenheit thermometers have long and short lines. Every other long line is marked in an even degree from 94° to 108° F. The short lines indicate 0.2 (two tenths) of a degree (Fig. 18-2, A).

Centigrade thermometers also have long and short lines. Each long line represents 1 degree, from 34° to 42° C. Each short line represents 0.1 (one tenth) of a degree (Fig. 18-2, B). Table 18-1 shows equivalent values for Fahrenheit and Centigrade scales.

TABLE 18-1

FAHRENHEIT AND CENTIGRADE EQUIVALENTS

Fahrenheit	Centigrade
95.0	35.0
95.9	35.5
96.8	36.0
97.7	36.5
98.6	37.0
99.5	37.5
100.4	38.0
101.3	38.5
102.2	39.0
103.1	39.5
104.0	40.0
104.9	40.5
105.8	41.0
106.7	41.5
107.6	42.0
108.5	42.5
109.4	43.0
110.3	43.5

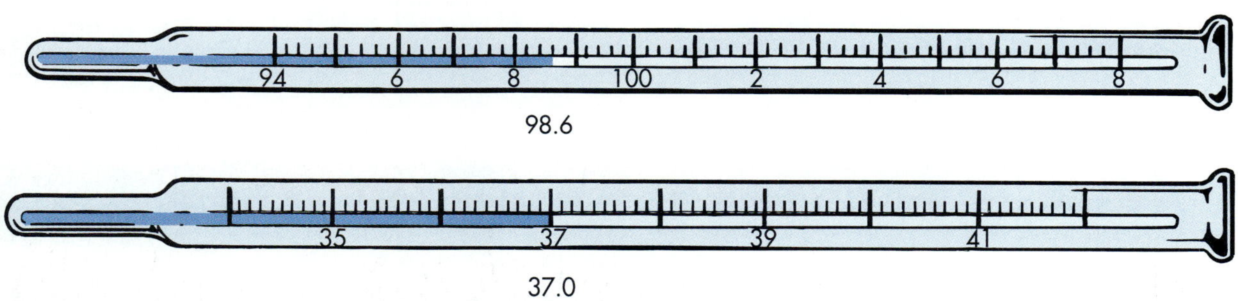

Fig. 18-2 *A, Fahrenheit thermometer. The mercury level is at 98.6° F. B, Centigrade thermometer. The mercury level is at 37.0° C.*

HOW TO READ A GLASS THERMOMETER

PROCEDURE

1. Make sure you have good lighting.
2. Hold the thermometer at the stem with your thumb and fingertips (Fig. 18-3 on page 430).
3. Bring the thermometer to eye level (Fig. 18-4 on page 430).
4. Rotate the thermometer until you can see both the numbers and the long and short lines.
5. Note that each long line measures 1° and each small line measures 0.1° on a Centigrade thermometer. Each small line on a Fahrenheit thermometer represents 0.2° (see Fig. 18-2).
6. Turn the thermometer back and forth slowly until the silver (or red) mercury line is seen.
7. Read the thermometer to the nearest degree (long line). Read the nearest tenth of a degree (short line)—an even number if you are using a Fahrenheit thermometer.
8. Record the person's name and temperature.

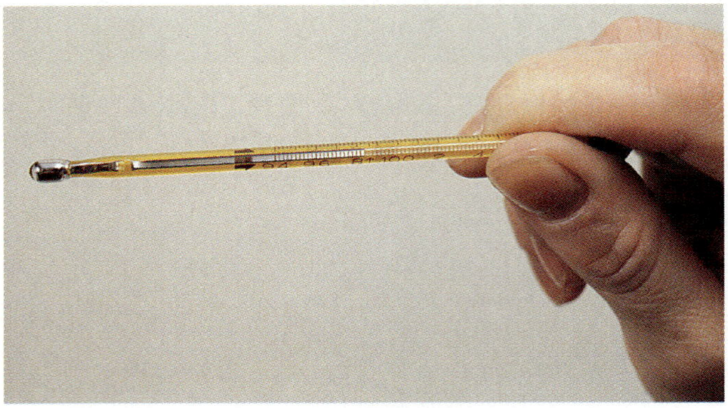

Fig. 18-3 *The thermometer is held at the stem with the thumb and fingertips.*

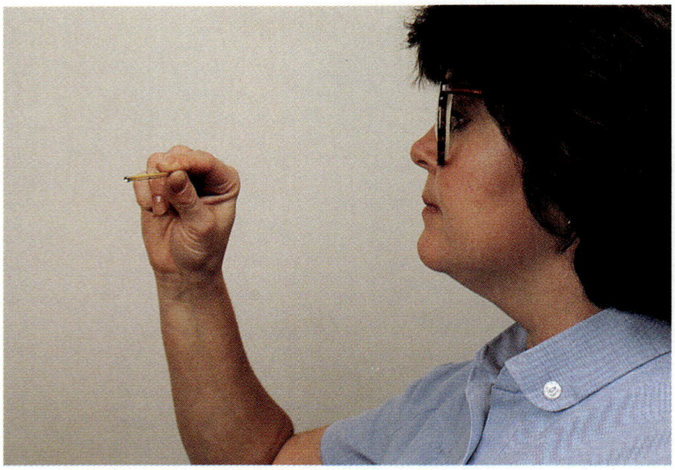

Fig. 18-4 *The thermometer is read at eye level.*

Using a glass thermometer The thermometer is inserted into the mouth, rectum, or axilla. Each area has many microorganisms. Therefore each person has a thermometer. This prevents the spread of microbes and infection. Thermometers are disinfected after use. They are often stored in a disinfectant solution between uses. Before being used again, a thermometer is rinsed under cold running water and wiped with a tissue to remove the disinfectant.

After being used, the glass thermometer is cleaned. Cleaning methods vary among facilities. The thermometer is usually first wiped with a tissue to remove mucus or feces. Then it is washed in warm soapy water. Hot water is not used. It causes the mercury to expand so much that the thermometer could break. After cleaning, thermometers are rinsed under cold running water. They are stored in a case or a container filled with disinfectant solution.

Many facilities use plastic covers for thermometers (Fig. 18-5). A cover is used once and then discarded. The thermometer is inserted into a cover and the temperature is taken. The cover is removed to read the thermometer. The thermometer never touches the person.

Before taking a temperature, you must shake the thermometer down to move the mercury into the bulb. The thermometer is checked for breaks or chips, which could cause the person injury.

How to Use a Glass Thermometer

Procedure

1. Collect a thermometer and tissues.
2. Wash your hands.
3. Hold the thermometer at the stem.
4. Rinse the thermometer under cold running water if it was soaking in a disinfectant. Dry it from the stem to the bulb end with tissues.
5. Shake down the thermometer. The mercury must be below the lines and numbers.
   a. Hold the thermometer at the stem.
   b. Stand away from walls, tables, or other hard surfaces to avoid breaking the thermometer.
   c. Flex and snap your wrist until the mercury is shaken down (Fig. 18-6).
6. Insert the thermometer into a plastic cover (if used).
7. Take the person's temperature. (See procedures for taking oral, rectal, and axillary temperatures with glass thermometers.)
8. Remove the thermometer.
9. Remove and discard the plastic cover if used. If a cover was not used, wipe the thermometer with tissues from the stem to the bulb end.
10. Read the thermometer and record the temperature.
11. Shake down the thermometer after use.
12. Clean the thermometer according to facility policy.

A

B

C

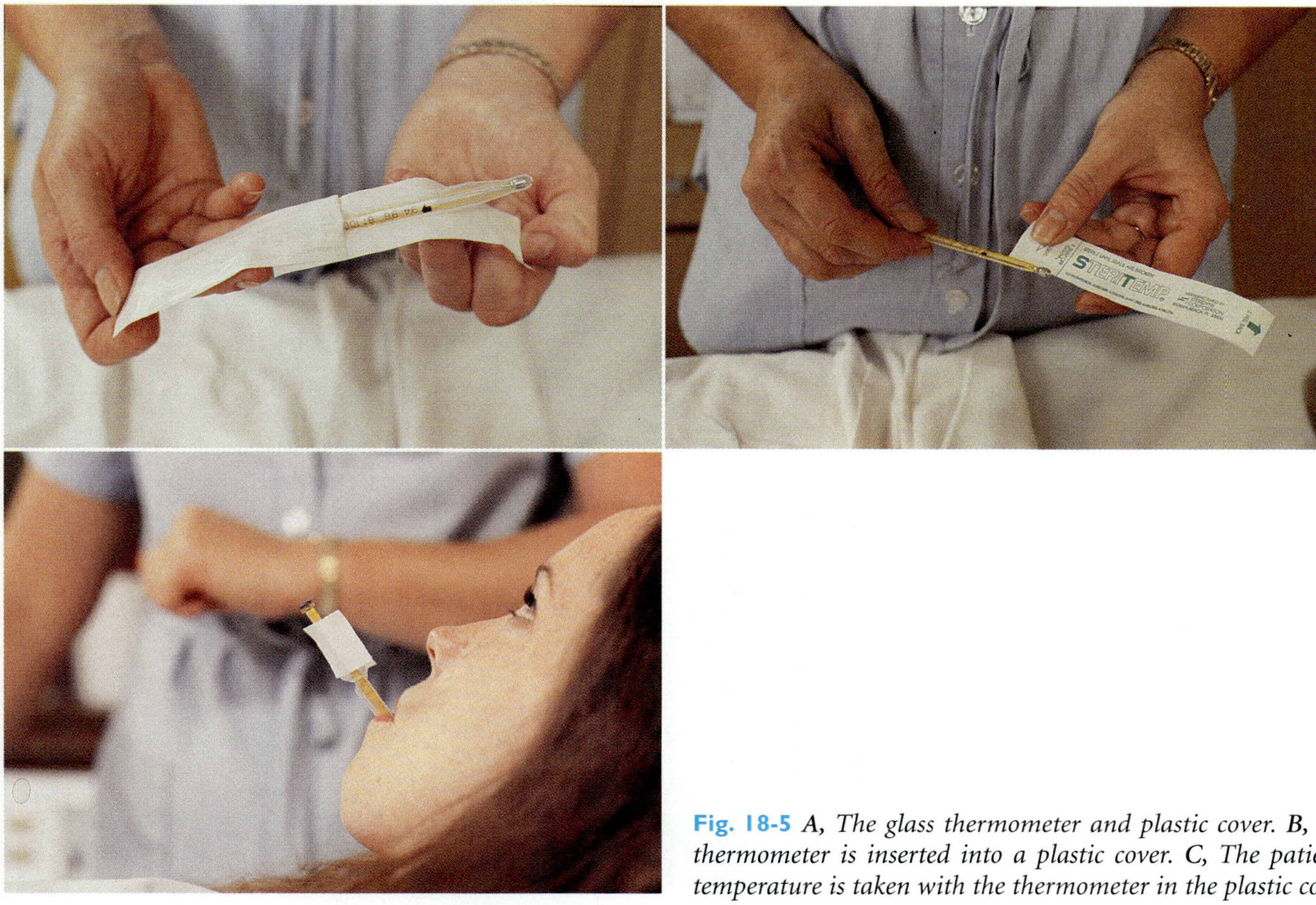

Fig. 18-5 *A, The glass thermometer and plastic cover. B, The thermometer is inserted into a plastic cover. C, The patient's temperature is taken with the thermometer in the plastic cover.*

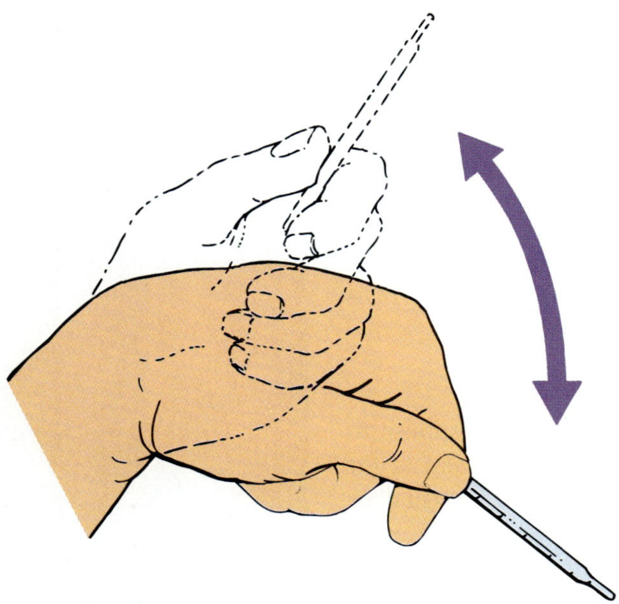

Fig. 18-6 *The wrist is snapped to shake down the thermometer.*

Electronic Thermometers

Electronic thermometers are portable and battery operated (Fig. 18-7). They measure temperatures in 2 to 60 seconds. The temperature is displayed on the front of the instrument. The hand-held unit is kept in a battery charger when not in use.

Electronic thermometers have oral and rectal probes. A disposable cover (sheath) covers the probe. Disposable probe covers are used once and then are discarded.

Electronic thermometers are expensive. However, they have several advantages.

- Disposable probe covers help prevent the spread of infection.
- The temperature is measured rapidly.
- The temperature display is easy to read.

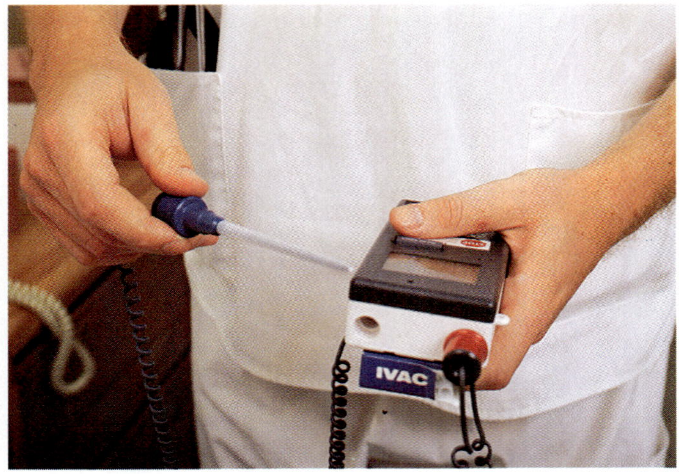

Fig. 18-7 *An electronic thermometer.*

Disposable Oral Thermometers

Disposable oral thermometers (Fig. 18-8) have small chemical dots. The dots change color when heated by the body. Each dot must be heated to a certain temperature before it changes color. These thermometers are used only once. They measure temperatures in 45 to 60 seconds.

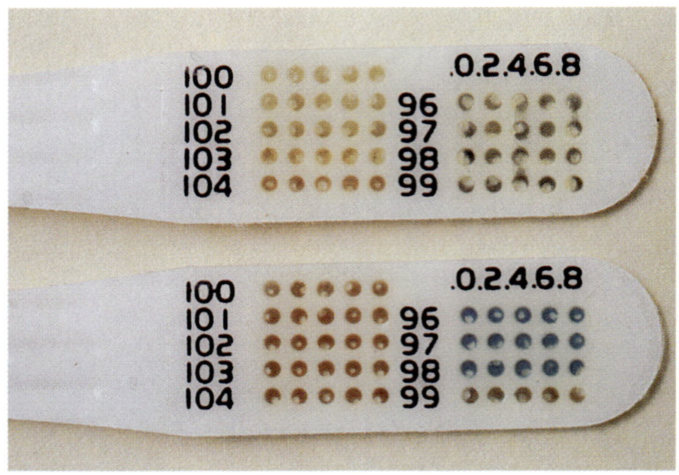

Fig. 18-8 *A, Disposable oral thermometer with chemical dots. B, The dots change color when the temperature is taken.*

Tympanic Thermometers

Tympanic thermometers measure temperature at the tympanic membrane in the ear (Fig. 18-9). They are the newest and fastest way to measure body temperature. The covered probe is inserted into the ear. The temperature is measured in 1 to 3 seconds. Like electronic thermometers, tympanic thermometers are battery operated and use disposable probe covers.

Tympanic thermometers have many advantages. They are comfortable for the person. They are not invasive like rectal thermometers. They are useful for children because of their speed and comfort. Infection control is another advantage. There are fewer microbes in the ear than in the mouth or rectum. Therefore the risk of spreading infection is reduced. Tympanic thermometers are available in drugstores for home use. They are not used if there is drainage from the ear.

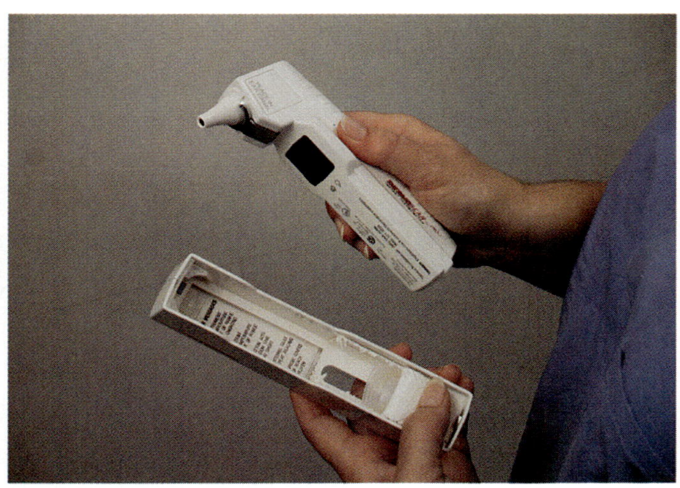

Fig. 18-9 *Tympanic thermometer.* (Courtesy of Thermoscan, Inc., San Diego, Calif.)

Temperature-Sensitive Tape

Temperature-sensitive tape changes color in response to body heat. The tape is applied to the forehead or abdomen. It indicates if the temperature is normal or above normal. Exact body temperature is not measured. The color change takes about 15 seconds.

Taking Oral Temperatures

Oral temperatures are usually taken on older children and adults. Drinking, eating, smoking, and chewing gum affect measurements. If the person has engaged in these activities, wait at least 15 minutes before taking an oral temperature. The glass thermometer remains in place 2 to 3 minutes or as required by facility policy. Temperatures are not taken orally if the person:

- Is an infant or a child younger than 4 or 5 years of age
- Is unconscious
- Has had surgery or an injury to the face, neck, nose, or mouth
- Is receiving oxygen
- Breathes through the mouth
- Has a nasogastric tube in place
- Is delirious, restless, confused, or disoriented
- Is paralyzed on one side of the body
- Has a sore mouth
- Has a history of convulsive disorders

Taking an Oral Temperature with a Glass Thermometer

Pre-procedure

1 Explain the procedure to the person. Ask him or her not to eat, drink, smoke, or chew gum for at least 15 minutes.

2 Collect the following:
- Oral thermometer and holder
- Tissues
- Plastic covers if used
- Disposable gloves

3 Wash your hands.

4 Identify the person. Check the ID bracelet and call the person by name.

5 Provide for privacy.

Procedure

6 Put on the gloves.

7 Rinse the thermometer in cold water if it was soaking in a disinfectant solution. Dry it with tissues.

8 Check the thermometer for breaks or chips.

9 Shake down the thermometer.

10 Place a plastic cover on the thermometer.

11 Ask the person to moisten his or her lips.

12 Place the bulb end of the thermometer under the person's tongue (Fig. 18-10 on page 434).

13 Ask the person to close his or her lips around the thermometer to hold it in place.

14 Leave the thermometer in place for 2 to 3 minutes or as required by facility policy.

15 Remove the thermometer by grasping the stem.

16 Use tissues to remove the plastic cover. Wipe the thermometer with a tissue from the stem to the bulb end if no cover was used.

17 Read the thermometer.

18 Record the person's name and temperature on your note pad.

19 Shake down the thermometer.

20 Clean the thermometer according to facility policy.

Post-procedure

21 Make sure the person is comfortable and the call bell is within reach.

22 Unscreen the person.

23 Remove the gloves and wash your hands.

24 Report any abnormal temperature to the nurse. Record the measurement in the proper place.

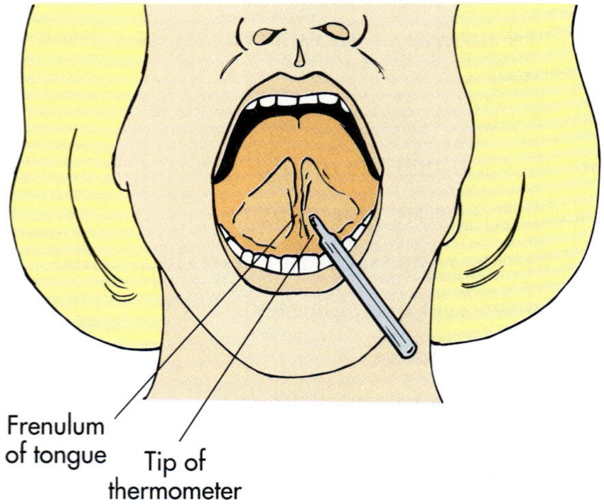

Fig. 18-10 *The thermometer is positioned at the base of the tongue next to the frenulum.*

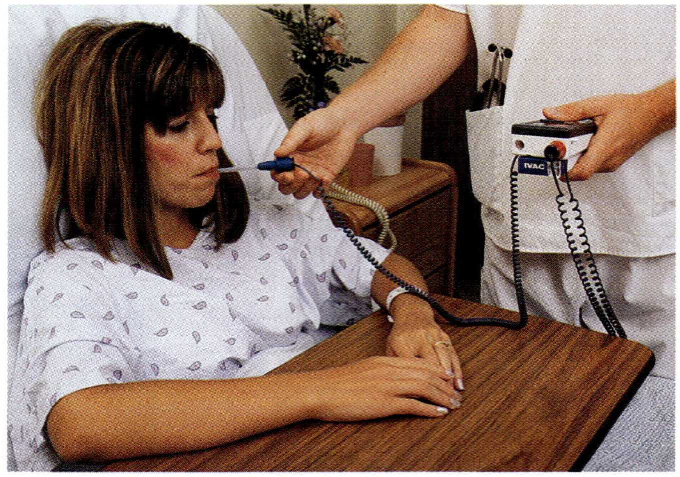

Fig. 18-11 *The covered probe of the electronic thermometer is inserted under the tongue.*

Taking an Oral Temperature with an Electronic Thermometer

Pre-procedure

1. Explain the procedure to the person. Ask him or her not to eat, drink, smoke, or chew gum for at least 15 minutes.
2. Collect the following:
   - Electronic thermometer
   - Oral probe (usually blue)
   - Disposable probe covers
   - Disposable gloves
3. Plug the oral probe into the thermometer.
4. Wash your hands.
5. Identify the person. Check the ID bracelet and call the person by name.
6. Provide for privacy.

Procedure

7. Put on gloves if contact with body fluid or body substances is likely.
8. Insert the probe into a probe cover.
9. Ask the person to open the mouth and raise the tongue.
10. Place the covered probe at the base of the tongue on either side (Fig. 18-11).
11. Ask the person to lower the tongue and close the mouth.
12. Hold the probe in place.
13. Read the temperature on the display. A tone or a flashing or steady light means the temperature has been measured.
14. Remove the probe from the person's mouth. Press the eject button to discard the cover.
15. Record the person's name and temperature on your note pad.
16. Return the probe to the holder.

Post-procedure

17. Make sure the person is comfortable and the call bell is within reach.
18. Unscreen the person.
19. Remove the gloves and wash your hands.
20. Return the thermometer to the charging unit.
21. Wash your hands.
22. Report any abnormal temperature to the nurse. Record the measurement in the proper place.

Taking an Oral Temperature with a Disposable Thermometer

Pre-procedure

1. Explain the procedure to the person. Ask him or her not to eat, drink, smoke, or chew gum for at least 15 minutes.
2. Get a disposable thermometer and disposable gloves.
3. Wash your hands.
4. Identify the person. Check the ID bracelet and call the person by name.
5. Provide for privacy.

Procedure

6. Put on the gloves.
7. Remove the wrapper from the thermometer.
8. Ask the person to open the mouth and raise the tongue.
9. Place the thermometer at the base of the tongue on either side.
10. Ask the person to lower the tongue and close the mouth.
11. Leave the thermometer in place for 45 seconds.
12. Remove the thermometer and read the last colored dot.
13. Record the person's name and temperature on your note pad.

Post-procedure

14. Make sure the person is comfortable and the call bell is within reach.
15. Unscreen the person.
16. Remove the gloves and wash your hands.
17. Report any abnormal temperature to the nurse. Record the measurement in the proper place.

Taking Rectal Temperatures

The rectal temperature is an accurate and reliable measurement of body temperature. This route is used when oral temperatures cannot be taken (see above). Rectal temperatures are not taken if the person has diarrhea, a rectal disorder or injury, heart disease, or has had rectal surgery.

The rectal thermometer is lubricated for easy insertion and to prevent tissue injury. The thermometer is held in place so it is not lost into the rectum or broken. A glass thermometer remains in the rectum for 2 minutes or as required by facility policy.

Privacy is important when taking rectal temperatures. The buttocks and anus are exposed. Many people are embarrassed by the procedure.

Taking a Rectal Temperature with a Glass Thermometer

Pre-procedure

1 Explain the procedure to the person.

2 Collect the following:
- Rectal thermometer and holder
- Toilet tissue
- Plastic covers if used
- Disposable gloves
- Water-soluble lubricant

3 Wash your hands.

4 Identify the person. Check the ID bracelet and call the person by name.

5 Provide for privacy.

Procedure

6 Rinse the thermometer in cold water if it was soaking in a disinfectant solution. Dry it with tissues.

7 Check the thermometer for breaks or chips.

8 Shake down the thermometer.

9 Place a plastic cover on the thermometer.

10 Position the person in Sims' position.

11 Put on the gloves.

12 Put a small amount of lubricant on a tissue. Lubricate the bulb end of the thermometer.

13 Fold back top linens to expose the anal area.

14 Raise the upper buttock to expose the anus (Fig. 18-12).

15 Insert the thermometer 1 inch into the rectum.

16 Hold it in place for 2 minutes or as required by facility policy (Fig. 18-13).

17 Remove the thermometer.

18 Remove the plastic cover. Wipe the thermometer with tissues from the stem to the bulb end if no cover was used.

19 Place the used toilet tissue on a paper towel or several thicknesses of toilet tissue. Place the thermometer on clean toilet tissue.

20 Wipe the anal area to remove excess lubricant and any feces. Cover the person.

21 Make sure the person is comfortable and the call bell is within reach.

22 Dispose of tissue.

23 Read the thermometer. Record the person's name and temperature on your note pad. Write *R* to indicate a rectal temperature.

24 Shake down the thermometer.

25 Clean the thermometer according to facility policy.

Post-procedure

26 Remove the gloves and wash your hands.

27 Unscreen the person.

28 Report any abnormal temperature. Record the measurement with an *R* in the proper place.

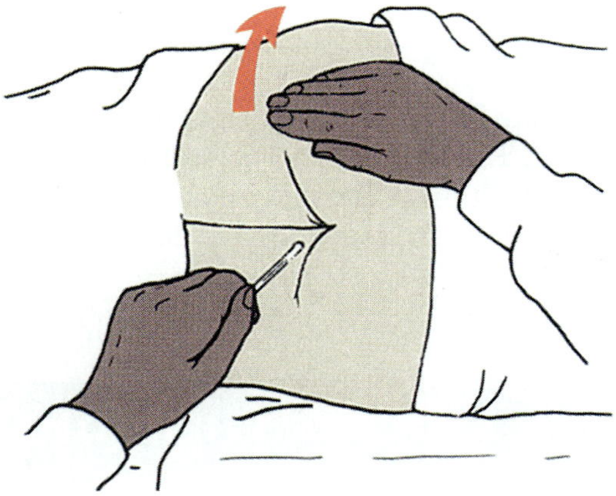

Fig. 18-12 *The rectal temperature is taken with the patient in Sims' position. The buttock is raised to expose the anus.*

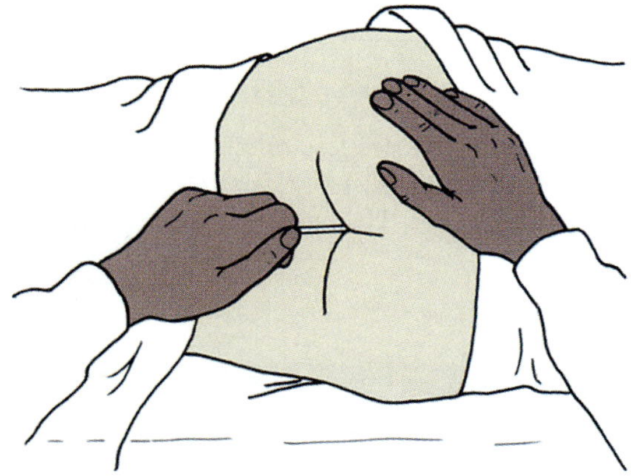

Fig. 18-13 *The rectal thermometer is held in place during the measurement.*

Taking a Rectal Temperature with an Electronic Thermometer

Pre-procedure

1 Explain the procedure to the person.

2 Collect the following:
- Electronic thermometer
- Rectal probe (usually red)
- Disposable probe covers
- Toilet tissue
- Water-soluble lubricant
- Disposable gloves

3 Plug the rectal probe into the thermometer.

4 Wash your hands.

5 Identify the person. Check the ID bracelet and call the person by name.

6 Provide for privacy.

Procedure

7 Position the person in Sims' position.

8 Put on the gloves.

9 Put a small amount of lubricant on some toilet tissue.

10 Insert the probe into a probe cover.

11 Lubricate the end of the covered probe using the lubricant on the toilet tissue.

12 Fold back top linens to expose the anal area.

13 Raise the upper buttock to expose the anus.

14 Insert the probe one-half inch into the rectum.

15 Hold the probe in place until you hear a tone or see a flashing or steady light.

16 Read the temperature on the display.

17 Remove the probe from the rectum.

18 Press the eject button to discard the probe cover. Return the probe to the holder.

19 Wipe the anal area with toilet tissue to remove excess lubricant and any feces. Cover the person.

20 Dispose of toilet tissue.

21 Remove the gloves and wash your hands.

22 Record the person's name and temperature with an *R* (for rectal temperature) on your note pad.

Post-procedure

23 Make sure the person is comfortable and the call bell is within reach.

24 Unscreen the person.

25 Return the thermometer to the charging unit.

26 Wash your hands.

27 Report any abnormal temperature. Record the measurement with an *R* in the proper place.

Taking Axillary Temperatures

Axillary temperatures are less reliable than oral, rectal, or tympanic temperatures. They are used when the other routes cannot be used. The axilla must be dry for the measurement. This site is not used right after the axilla has been bathed. The thermometer is held in place to maintain proper position. A glass thermometer is held in place for 5 to 10 minutes or as required by facility policy.

Taking an Axillary Temperature with a Glass Thermometer

Pre-procedure

1. Explain the procedure to the person.
2. Collect the following:
   - Oral glass thermometer and holder
   - Plastic covers if used
   - Tissues
   - Towel
3. Wash your hands.
4. Identify the person. Check the ID bracelet and call the person by name.
5. Provide for privacy.

Procedure

6. Rinse the thermometer in cold water if it was soaking in a disinfectant solution. Dry it with tissues.
7. Check the thermometer for breaks or chips.
8. Shake down the thermometer.
9. Place a plastic cover on the thermometer.
10. Help the person remove an arm from the gown. Do not expose the person.
11. Dry the axilla with the towel.
12. Place the bulb end of the thermometer in the center of the axilla.
13. Ask the person to place the arm over the chest to hold the thermometer in place (Fig. 18-14). Hold it and the arm in place if he or she cannot help or if the person is an infant or child (Fig. 18-15).
14. Leave the thermometer in place for 5 to 10 minutes or as required by facility policy.
15. Remove the thermometer from the plastic cover. Wipe it with tissues from the stem to the bulb end if no cover was used.
16. Read the thermometer.
17. Record the person's name and temperature with an *A* (for axillary temperature) on your note pad.
18. Help the person put the gown back on.
19. Make sure the person is comfortable and the call bell is within reach.
20. Shake down the thermometer.
21. Rinse and wash the thermometer. Place it in the holder with disinfectant or in a plastic cover.

Post-procedure

22. Unscreen the person.
23. Follow facility policy for soiled linen.
24. Wash your hands.
25. Report any abnormal temperature. Record the measurement with an *A* in the proper place.

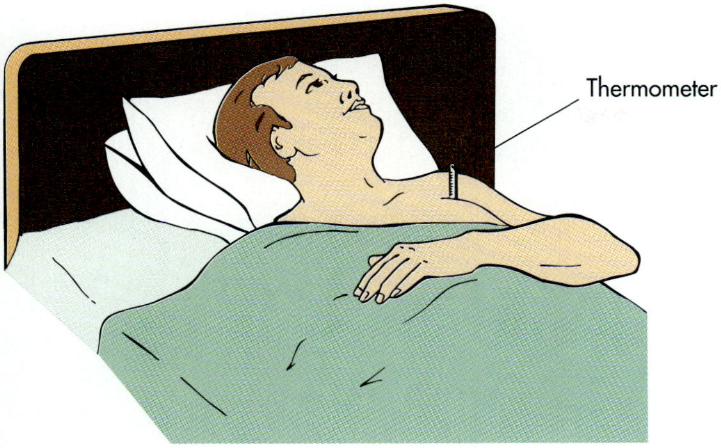

Fig. 18-14 *The thermometer is held in place in the axilla by bringing the patient's arm over the chest.*

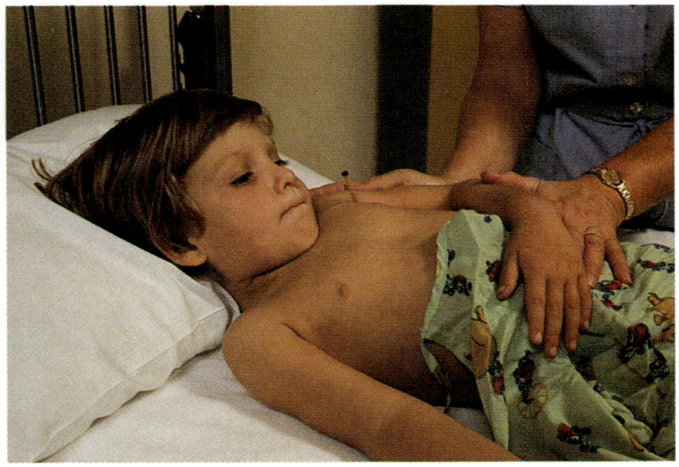

Fig. 18-15 *Axillary temperature taken on a child. The nursing assistant holds the thermometer and the child's arm in place.*

Taking an Axillary Temperature with an Electronic Thermometer

Pre-procedure

1. Explain the procedure to the person.
2. Collect the following:
   - Electronic thermometer
   - Oral probe (usually blue)
   - Disposable probe covers
   - Towel
3. Plug the oral probe into the thermometer.
4. Wash your hands.
5. Identify the person. Check the ID bracelet and call the person by name.
6. Provide for privacy.

Procedure

7. Help the person remove an arm from the gown. Do not expose the person.
8. Dry the axilla with the towel.
9. Insert the probe into a probe cover.
10. Place the covered probe in the axilla. Place the person's arm over the chest. Hold the probe in place until you hear a tone or see a steady or flashing light.
11. Remove the probe. Read the temperature on the display.
12. Record the person's name and temperature with an *A* (for axillary temperature) on your note pad.
13. Press the eject button and discard the probe cover. Return the probe to the holder.
14. Help the person put the gown back on.

Post-procedure

15. Make sure the person is comfortable and the call bell is within reach.
16. Unscreen the person.
17. Follow facility policy for soiled linen.
18. Return the thermometer to the charging unit.
19. Wash your hands.
20. Report any abnormal temperature. Record the measurement with an *A* in the proper place.

Taking Tympanic Temperatures

Tympanic temperatures are quick and easy to take. The probe is gently inserted into the ear canal. Do not shove the probe into the ear or insert the probe deeply. Like electronic thermometers, tympanic thermometers must be kept charged.

Taking a Tympanic Temperature

Pre-procedure

1 Explain the procedure to the person.
2 Get the tympanic thermometer and a probe cover.
3 Wash your hands.
4 Identify the person. Check the ID bracelet and call the person by name.
5 Provide for privacy.

Procedure

6 Ask the person to turn his or her head so the ear is in front of you.
7 Insert the probe gently. Pull back on the ear to straighten the ear canal (Fig. 18-16).
8 Start the thermometer.
9 Read the thermometer when you hear a tone or see a flashing light.
10 Remove the probe from the ear.
11 Record the person's name and temperature on your note pad. Note that a tympanic temperature was taken.
12 Press the ejection button and discard the probe.

Post-procedure

13 Make sure the person is comfortable and the call bell is within reach.
14 Unscreen the person.
15 Return the thermometer to the charging unit.
16 Wash your hands.
17 Report any abnormal temperature. Record the measurement in the proper place. Note that a tympanic temperature was taken.

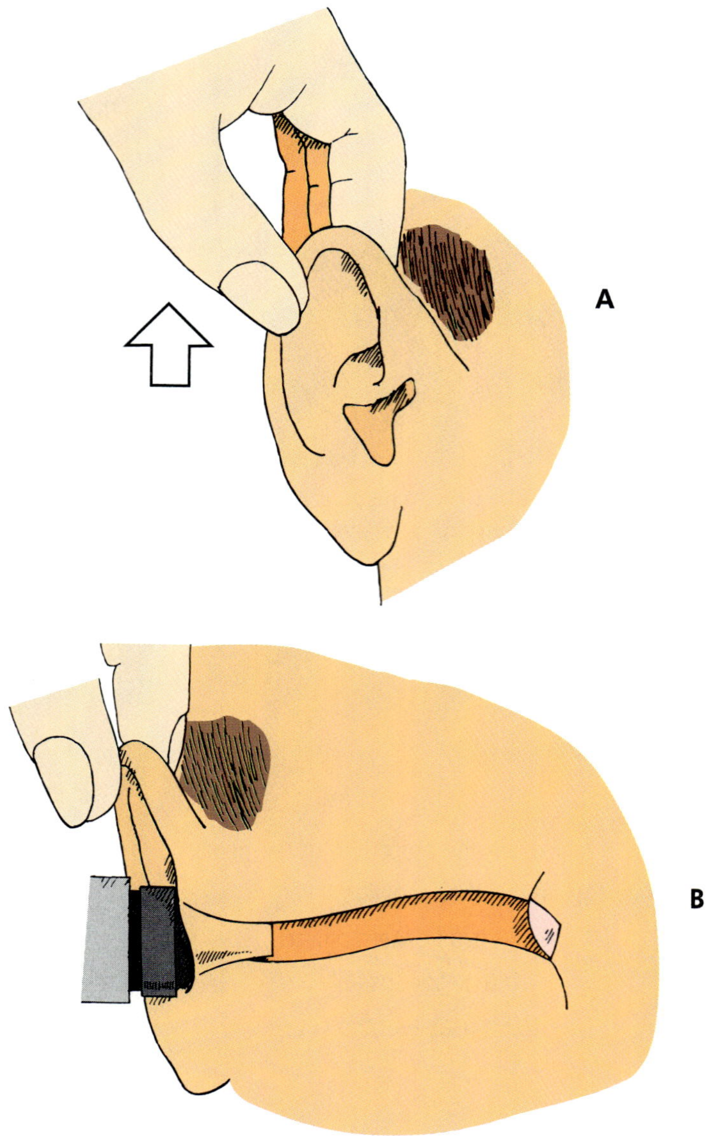

Fig. 18-16 ***A,*** *The ear is pulled back and,* ***B,*** *the tympanic thermometer probe is inserted into the ear canal.*

PULSE

Arteries carry blood from the heart to all parts of the body (Box 18-1). The **pulse** is defined as the beat of the heart felt at an artery as a wave of blood passes through the artery. A pulse can be felt every time the heart beats.

BOX 18-1 REVIEW: STRUCTURE AND FUNCTION OF THE HEART AND BLOOD VESSELS

The heart is a muscle. It pumps blood through the blood vessels to the tissues and cells. The heart lies in the middle to lower part of the chest cavity toward the left side (Fig. 18-17).

The heart has four chambers (see Fig. 5-17). Upper chambers receive blood and are called the *atria.* The *right atrium* receives blood from body tissues. The *left atrium* receives blood from the lungs. Lower chambers are called ventricles. Ventricles pump blood. The *right ventricle* pumps blood to the lungs for oxygen. The *left ventricle* pumps blood to all parts of the body.

There are two phases of heart action. During *diastole,* the resting phase, heart chambers fill with blood. During *systole,* the working phase, the heart contracts. Blood is pumped through the blood vessels when the heart contracts.

Blood flows to body tissues and cells through the blood vessels. *Arteries* carry blood away from the heart. Arterial blood is rich in oxygen. The *aorta* is the largest artery. The aorta receives blood directly from the left ventricle. The aorta branches into other arteries that carry blood to all parts of the body (Fig. 18-18). *Veins* return blood to the heart.

See Chapter 5 for more detailed information.

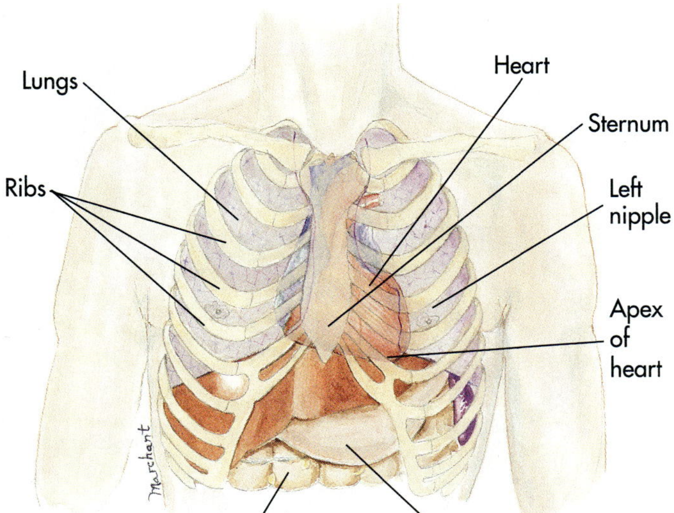

Fig. 18-17 *Location of the heart.*

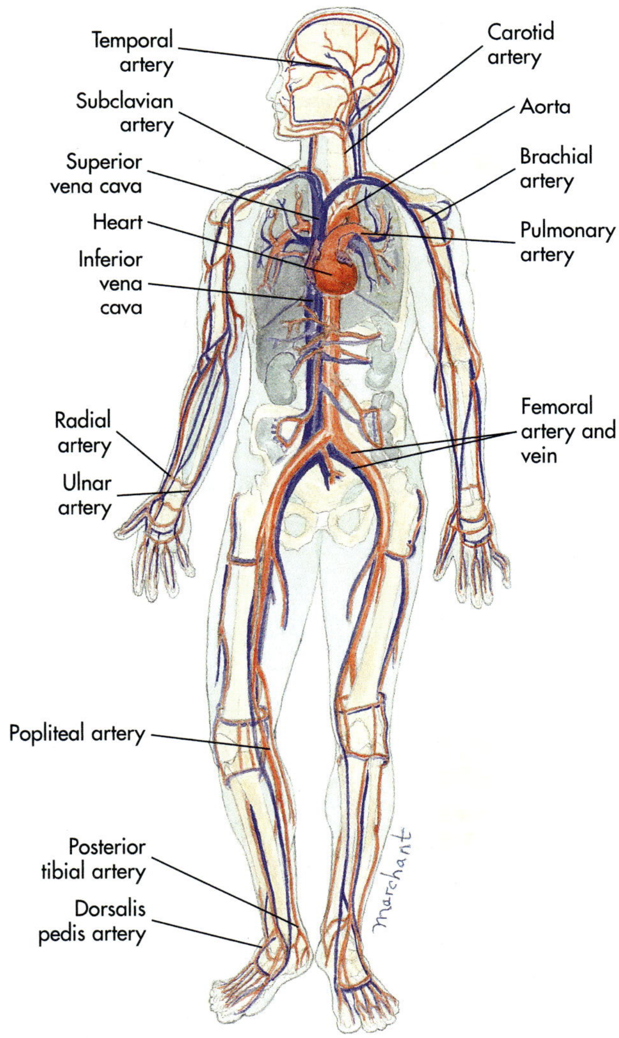

Fig. 18-18 *The arterial system.*

Sites for Taking a Pulse

The pulse can be taken at a number of sites (Fig. 18-19). Pulses are easy to feel at these sites. The arteries are close to the body's surface and lie over a bone. The radial site is used most often because it is easy to reach and find. The radial pulse can be taken without disturbing or exposing the person.

The temporal, carotid, brachial, radial, femoral, popliteal, and dorsalis pedis (pedal) arteries are found on both sides of the body. The apical pulse is felt over the apex (top) of the heart. It is taken with a stethoscope. The carotid pulse is taken during cardiopulmonary resuscitation (CPR) and other emergencies (see Chapter 33).

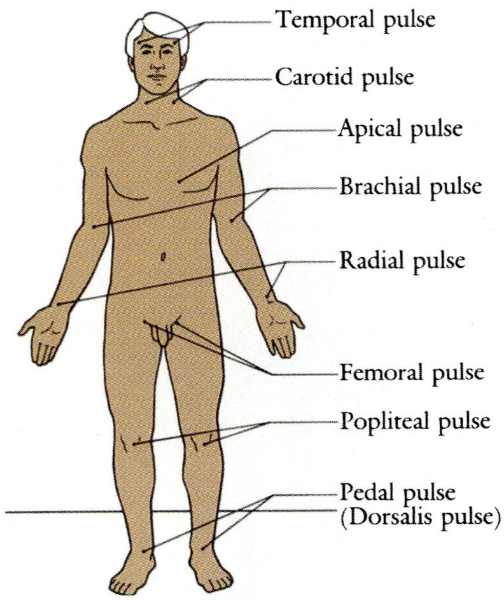

Fig. 18-19 *The pulse sites.*

Using a Stethoscope

A **stethoscope** is an instrument used to listen to the sounds produced by the heart, lungs, and other body organs. The stethoscope amplifies the sounds so they can be heard easily. The parts of a stethoscope are shown in Figure 18-20. The earpieces should fit snugly to block out external noises. However, they should not cause pain or ear discomfort.

Stethoscopes are shared by doctors and the nursing team. Stethoscopes are in contact with many persons and workers. Therefore infection control is important. The earpieces and diaphragm are cleaned before and after use. Cleaning prevents the spread of microorganisms.

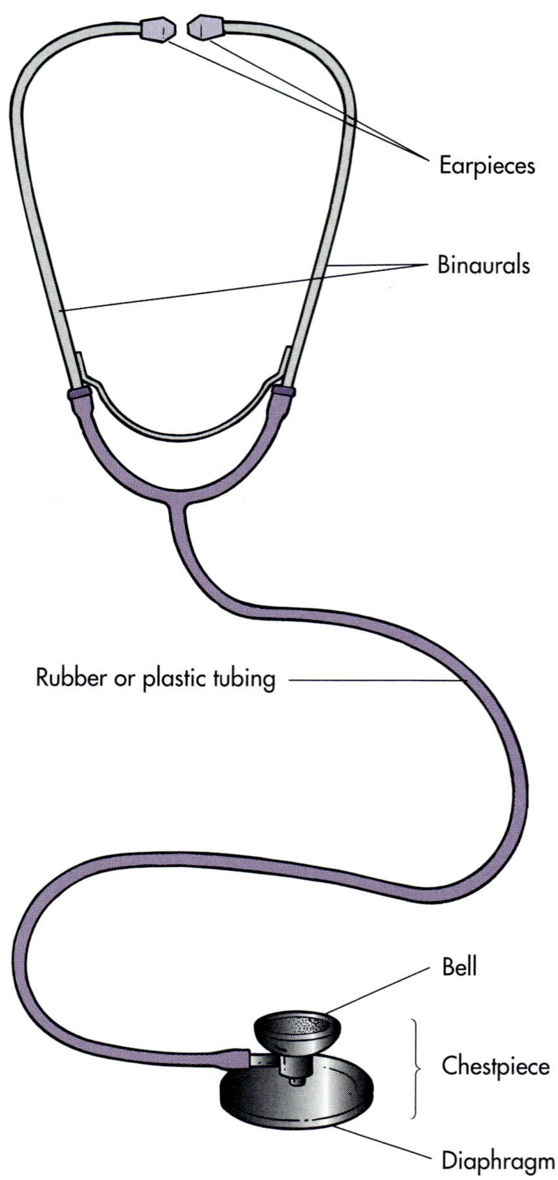

Fig. 18-20 *Parts of a stethoscope.*

How to Use a Stethoscope

Procedure

1. Collect the following:
   - Stethoscope with diaphragm
   - Alcohol wipes
2. Wash your hands.
3. Wipe the earpieces and diaphragm with alcohol wipes.
4. Warm the diaphragm in your hand (Fig. 18-21).
5. Place the earpiece tips in your ears so the bend of the tips points forward.
6. Place the diaphragm over the artery. Hold it in place as in Figure 18-22.
7. Do not let anything touch the tubing.
8. Ask the person to be silent during the procedure.
9. Wipe the earpiece tips and diaphragm with alcohol wipes when the procedure is completed.
10. Return the stethoscope to its proper place.

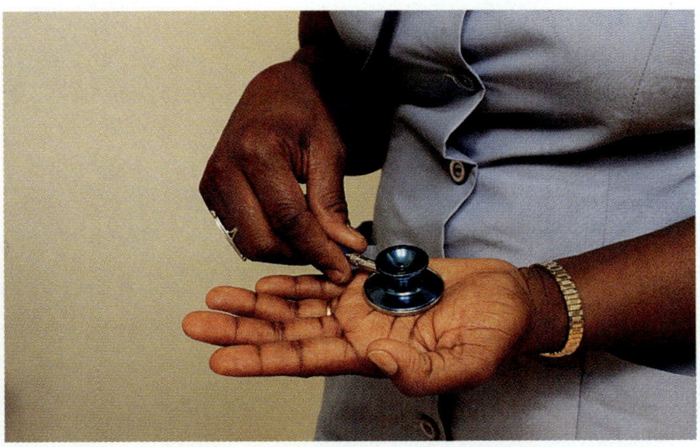

Fig. 18-21 *The diaphragm of the stethoscope is warmed in the palm of the hand.*

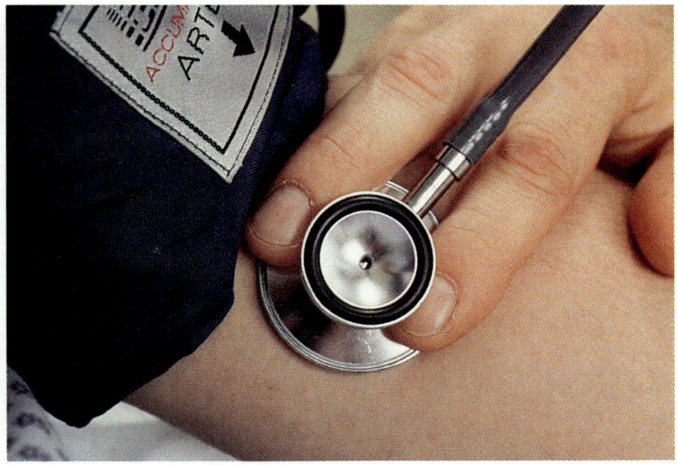

Fig. 18-22 *The stethoscope is held in place with the fingertips of the index and middle fingers.*

Pulse Rate

The **pulse rate** is the number of heartbeats or pulses felt in 1 minute. The rate varies for different age groups (Table 18-2). The pulse rate is influenced by many factors. They include elevated body temperature (fever), exercise, fear, anger, anxiety, excitement, heat, position, and pain. These and other factors cause the heart to beat faster. Some medications also increase the pulse rate. Other drugs slow down the pulse.

The adult pulse rate is between 60 and 100 beats per minute. A rate of less than 60 or greater than 100 is considered abnormal. **Tachycardia** is a rapid (tachy) heart rate (cardia). The heart rate is over 100 beats per minute. **Bradycardia** is a slow (brady) heart rate (cardia). The rate is less than 60 beats per minute. Abnormal rates are reported to the nurse immediately.

Table 18-2

Pulse Ranges for Different Ages

Age	Pulse rates per minute
Birth to 4 weeks	80-180
4 weeks to 1 year	80-160
1 to 2 years	80-130
2 to 6 years	80-120
6 to 12 years	70-110
12 years and older	60-100

Rhythm and Force of the Pulse

When taking a pulse, give attention to its rhythm and force. The rhythm should be regular. That is, a pulse should be felt in a pattern. The same time interval should occur between beats (Fig. 18-23, A). An irregular pulse occurs when the beats are unevenly spaced or beats are skipped (Fig. 18-23, B). The force of the pulse relates to its strength. A forceful pulse is easy to feel and is described as strong, full, or bounding. Pulses that are hard to feel are described as weak, thready, or feeble.

Electronic blood pressure equipment (see page 451) can also count pulses. The pulse rate is displayed along with the blood pressure. However, no information is given about the rhythm and force of the pulse. If electronic blood pressure equipment is used, you still need to feel the pulse to determine rhythm and force.

A

B

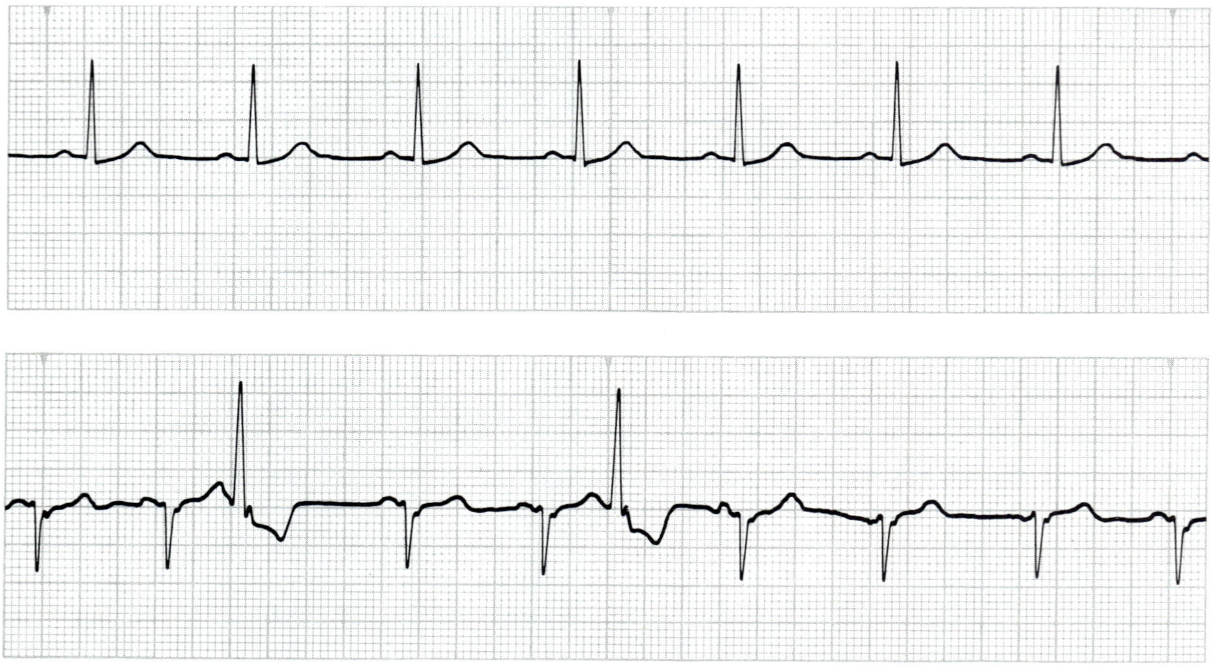

Fig. 18-23 *A, The electrocardiogram shows a regular pulse. The beats occur at regular intervals. B, The beats in this electrocardiogram occur at irregular intervals.* (From Huszar RJ: Basic dysrhythmias: interpretation and management, St Louis, 1988, Mosby-Year Book.)

Taking a Radial Pulse

The radial pulse is used for routine vital signs. The pulse is felt by placing the first three fingers of one hand against the radial artery. The radial artery is on the thumb side of the wrist (Fig. 18-24). Do not use your thumb to take a pulse; it has a pulse of its own. The pulse in your thumb could be mistaken for the person's pulse. The pulse is counted for 30 seconds. The number is multiplied by 2 to obtain the number of beats per minute. If the pulse is irregular, it is counted for 1 full minute.

Some facilities require that all radial pulses be taken for 1 full minute. You need to follow your facility's policy.

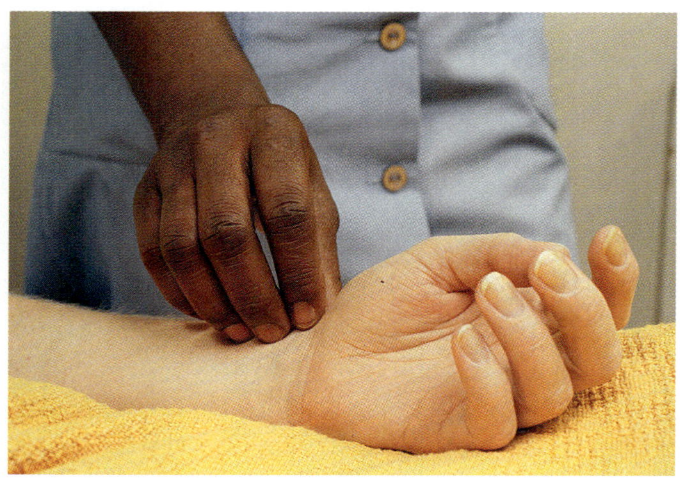

Fig. 18-24 *The middle three fingers are used to locate the radial pulse on the thumb side of the wrist.*

Taking a Radial Pulse

Pre-procedure

1. Wash your hands.
2. Identify the person. Check the ID bracelet and call the person by name.
3. Explain the procedure to the person.
4. Provide for privacy.

Procedure

5. Have the person sit or lie down.
6. Locate the radial pulse with your 3 middle fingers (see Fig. 18-24).
7. Note if the pulse is strong or weak, and regular or irregular.
8. Count the pulse for 30 seconds. Multiply the number of beats by 2. Or count the pulse for 1 full minute if required by facility policy.
9. Count the pulse for 1 full minute if it is irregular.
10. Record the person's name and pulse on your note pad. Make a note about the strength of the pulse and if it was regular or irregular.

Post-procedure

11. Make sure the person is comfortable and the call bell is within reach.
12. Unscreen the person.
13. Wash your hands.
14. Report the following to the nurse:
    - A pulse rate of less than 60 or greater than 100 beats per minute is reported immediately
    - Whether the pulse is regular or irregular
    - The pulse rate
    - The strength of the pulse (strong, full, or bounding; or weak, thready, or feeble)
15. Record the pulse rate in the proper place.

Taking an Apical Pulse

The apical pulse is taken with a stethoscope. This method is used on infants and children up to about 3 years of age. Apical pulses are also taken on adults who have heart disease or who take medications that affect the heart. The apical pulse is on the left side of the chest slightly below the nipple (Fig. 18-25). The apical pulse is counted for 1 full minute.

The heartbeat normally sounds like a *lub-dub*. Each *lub-dub* is counted as 1 beat. Do not count the *lub* as 1 beat and the *dub* as another.

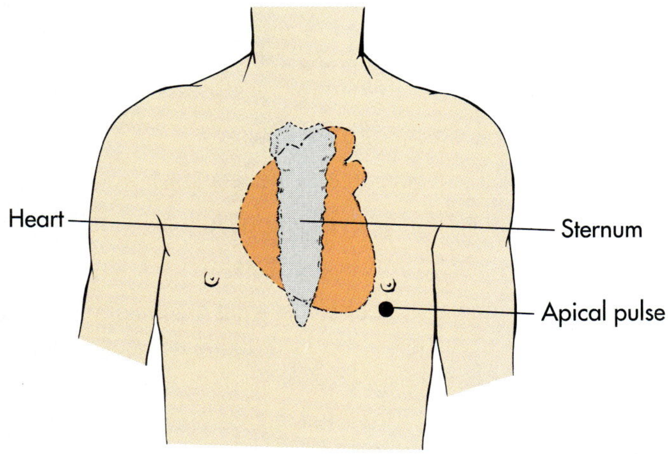

Fig. 18-25 *The apical pulse is located 2 to 3 inches to the left of the sternum (breastbone) and below the left nipple.*

Taking an Apical Pulse

Pre-procedure

1. Collect the following:
   - Stethoscope with diaphragm
   - Alcohol wipes
2. Wash your hands.
3. Identify the person. Check the ID bracelet and call the person by name.
4. Explain the procedure to the person.
5. Provide for privacy.

Procedure

6. Wipe the earpieces and diaphragm with alcohol wipes.
7. Have the person sit or lie down.
8. Expose the nipple area of the left chest.
9. Warm the diaphragm in your palm.
10. Place the earpieces in your ears.
11. Locate the apical pulse. Place the diaphragm 2 to 3 inches to the left of the breastbone and below the left nipple (see Fig. 18-25).
12. Count the pulse for 1 full minute. Note if it is regular or irregular.
13. Cover the person. Remove the earpieces.
14. Record the person's name and pulse on your note pad. Note whether the pulse was regular or irregular.
15. Make sure the person is comfortable and the call bell is within reach.
16. Unscreen the person.
17. Clean the earpieces and diaphragm of the stethoscope with alcohol wipes.
18. Return the stethoscope to its proper place.

Post-procedure

19. Wash your hands.
20. Report the following to the nurse:
    - A pulse rate of less than 60 or greater than 100 beats per minute is reported immediately
    - Whether the pulse was regular or irregular
    - The pulse rate
    - Any unusual heart sounds
21. Record the pulse rate in the proper place with an *Ap* for an apical pulse.

Taking an Apical-Radial Pulse

The apical and radial pulse rates should be equal. Sometimes heart contractions are not strong enough to create pulses in the radial artery. This may occur in people with heart disease. The radial pulse may be less than the apical pulse. To see if there is a difference between the apical and radial rates, the pulses are taken at the same time by two workers. This is called an **apical-radial pulse.** The **pulse deficit** is the difference between the apical and radial pulse rates. To obtain the pulse deficit, subtract the radial rate from the apical rate. The apical pulse rate is never less than the radial pulse rate.

Taking an Apical-Radial Pulse

Pre-procedure

1 Ask a nurse or another nursing assistant to help you.

2 Collect the following:
- Stethoscope with diaphragm
- Alcohol wipes

3 Wash your hands.

4 Identify the person. Check the ID bracelet and call the person by name.

5 Explain the procedure to the person.

6 Provide for privacy.

Procedure

7 Wipe the earpieces and diaphragm with the alcohol wipes.

8 Have the person sit or lie down.

9 Warm the diaphragm in your palm.

10 Expose the left nipple area of the chest.

11 Place the earpieces in your ears.

12 Find the apical pulse. Have your helper find the radial pulse (Fig. 18-26).

13 Give the signal to begin counting.

14 Count the pulse for 1 full minute.

15 Give the signal to stop counting.

16 Cover the person. Remove the earpieces.

17 Record the person's name and the apical and radial pulses on your note pad. Subtract the radial pulse from the apical pulse for the pulse deficit. Note whether the pulse was regular or irregular.

18 Make sure the person is comfortable and the call bell is within reach.

19 Unscreen the person.

20 Clean the earpieces and diaphragm with alcohol wipes.

21 Return the stethoscope to its proper place.

Post-procedure

22 Wash your hands.

23 Report the following to the nurse:
- An apical pulse rate of less than 60 or greater than 100 beats per minute is reported immediately
- The apical and radial pulse rates
- The pulse deficit
- Whether the pulse was regular or irregular
- Any unusual heart sounds

24 Record the pulses in the proper place. Indicate that an apical-radial pulse was taken.

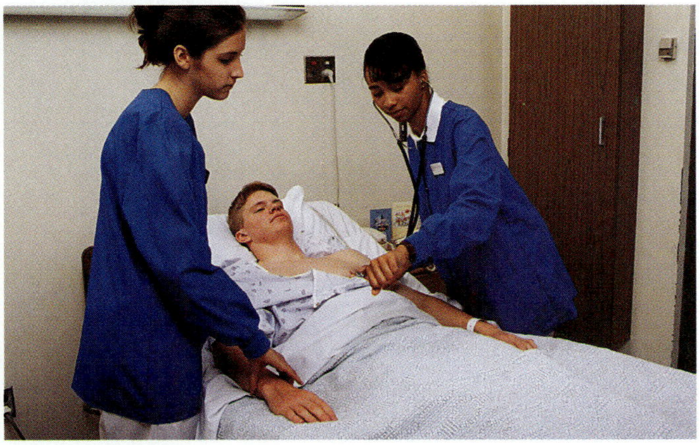

Fig. 18-26 *Two workers take an apical-radial pulse. One worker takes the apical pulse, and the other takes the radial pulse.*

RESPIRATIONS

Respiration is the act of breathing air into the lungs (inhalation) and out of the lungs (exhalation). Oxygen is taken into the lungs during inhalation. Carbon dioxide is moved out of the lungs during exhalation. Each respiration involves one inhalation and one exhalation. The chest rises during inhalation and falls during exhalation. The respiratory system is reviewed in Box 18-2.

The healthy adult has 10 to 20 respirations per minute. Infants and children normally breathe faster than adults. The respiratory rate is affected by many of the factors that affect body temperature and pulse. Heart and respiratory diseases usually cause an increased number of respirations per minute.

Abnormal Respirations

Normal respirations occur between 10 and 20 times per minute in the adult. They are quiet, effortless, and regular. Both sides of the chest rise and fall equally. You should know the following abnormal respiratory patterns:

- **Tachypnea**—rapid (tachy) breathing (pnea); the respiratory rate is usually greater than 24 respirations per minute
- **Bradypnea**—slow (brady) breathing (pnea); the respiratory rate is less than 10 respirations per minute
- **Apnea**—the lack or absence (a) of breathing (pnea)
- **Hypoventilation**—respirations that are slow (hypo), shallow, and sometimes irregular
- **Hyperventilation**—respirations that are rapid (hyper) and deeper than normal
- **Dyspnea**—difficult, labored, or painful (dys) breathing (pnea)
- **Cheyne-Stokes**—a breathing pattern in which respirations gradually increase in rate and depth and then become shallow and slow; breathing may stop (apnea) for 10 to 20 seconds

BOX 18-2 THE RESPIRATORY SYSTEM: REVIEW OF STRUCTURE AND FUNCTION

Oxygen is needed for survival. Every cell needs oxygen. The respiratory system brings oxygen into the lungs and eliminates carbon dioxide. The process of supplying the cells with oxygen and removing carbon dioxide from them is called *respiration.* Respiration involves *inhalation* (breathing in) and *exhalation* (breathing out). The terms *inspiration* (breathing in) and *expiration* (breathing out) are also used. The respiratory system is shown in Figure 18-27.

Air enters the body through the *nose.* The air then passes into the *pharynx* (throat), a tube-shaped passageway for both air and food. Air passes from the pharynx into the *larynx* (the voice box). Air passes from the larynx into the *trachea* (the windpipe). The trachea divides at its lower end into the *right bronchus* and *left bronchus.* Each bronchus enters a lung. On entering the lungs, the bronchi further divide several times into smaller branches called *bronchioles.* Eventually the bronchioles subdivide and end in tiny one-celled air sacs called *alveoli.* They are supplied by capillaries. Oxygen and carbon dioxide are exchanged between the alveoli and capillaries. Blood in the capillaries picks up oxygen from the alveoli. Then the blood is returned to the left side of the heart and pumped to the rest of the body. Alveoli pick up carbon dioxide from the capillaries for exhalation.

Each lung is divided into lobes. The right lung has three lobes, the left lung has two. The lungs are separated from the abdominal cavity by a muscle called the *diaphragm.* A bony framework consisting of the ribs, sternum, and vertebrae protects the lungs.

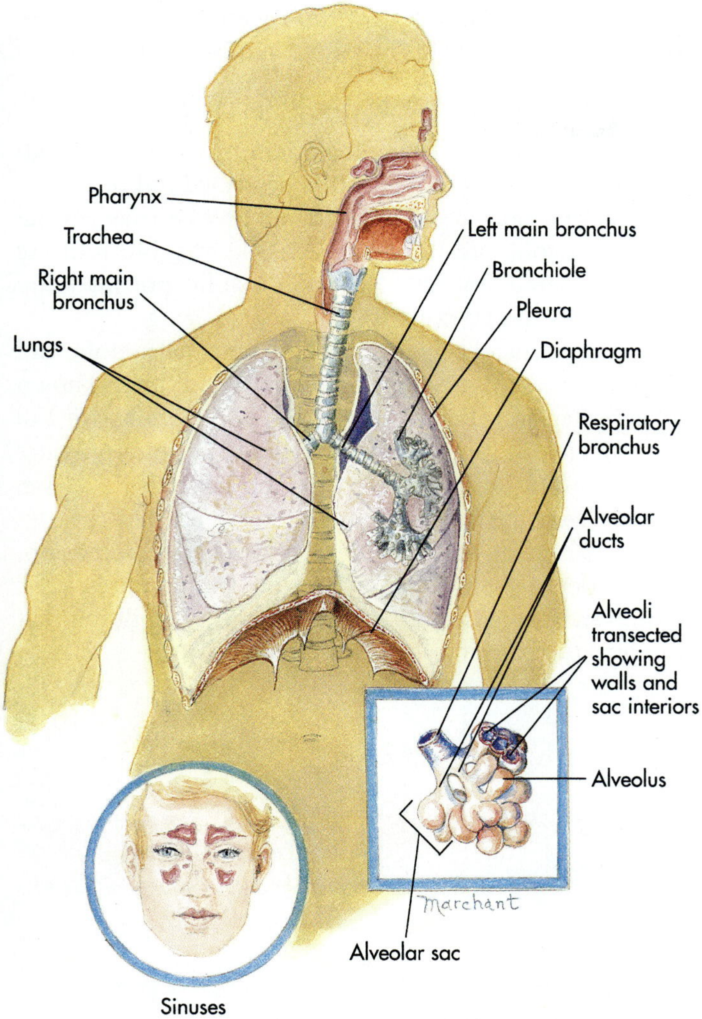

Fig. 18-27 *The respiratory system.*

Counting Respirations

Respirations are counted when the person is at rest. The person is positioned so you can see the chest rise and fall. The depth and rate of breathing can be voluntarily controlled to a certain extent. People tend to change breathing patterns when they know their respirations are being counted. Therefore the person should be unaware that the respirations are being counted.

Respirations are counted right after taking a pulse. The fingers or stethoscope stay over the pulse site. The person assumes that the pulse is still being taken. Respirations are counted by watching the rise and fall of the chest. They are counted for 30 seconds. The number is multiplied by 2 for the total number of respirations in 1 minute. If an abnormal pattern is noted, the respirations are counted for 1 full minute.

Counting Respirations

Procedure

1. Continue to hold the wrist after taking the radial pulse. Keep the stethoscope in place if you took an apical pulse.
2. Do not tell the person you are counting respirations.
3. Begin counting when the chest rises. Count each rise and fall of the chest as 1 respiration.
4. Observe if respirations are regular and if both sides of the chest rise equally. Also note the depth of respirations and if the person has any pain or difficulty in breathing.
5. Count respirations for 30 seconds. Multiply the number by 2. Count an infant's respirations for 1 minute.
6. Count an adult's respirations for 1 full minute if they are abnormal or irregular.
7. Record the person's name, respiratory rate, and other observations on your note pad.

Post-Procedure

8. Make sure the person is comfortable and the call bell is within reach.
9. Wash your hands.
10. Report the following to the nurse:
    - The respiratory rate
    - Equality and depth of respirations
    - If the respirations were regular or irregular
    - If the person experienced pain or difficulty in breathing
    - Any respiratory noises
    - Any abnormal respiratory patterns
11. Record the respiratory rate in the proper place.

BLOOD PRESSURE

Blood pressure is the amount of force exerted against the walls of an artery by the blood. Blood pressure is controlled by:

- The force of heart contractions
- The amount of blood pumped with each heartbeat
- How easily the blood flows through the blood vessels

The period of heart muscle contraction is called **systole.** The period of heart muscle relaxation is called **diastole.**

Both the systolic and diastolic pressures are measured. The **systolic pressure** is the higher pressure. It represents the amount of force needed to pump blood out of the heart into the arterial circulation. The **diastolic pressure** is the lower pressure. It reflects the pressure in the arteries when the heart is at rest. Blood pressure is measured in millimeters (mm) of mercury (Hg). The systolic pressure is recorded over the diastolic pressure. The average adult has a systolic pressure of 120 mm Hg and a diastolic pressure of 80 mm Hg. This is written as 120/80 mm Hg.

Factors Affecting Blood Pressure

Blood pressure can change from minute to minute. Such changes are related to the factors described in Box 18-3.

Because it can vary so easily, blood pressure has normal ranges. Systolic pressures between 100 and 140 mm Hg are considered normal. Normal diastolic pressures are between 60 and 90 mm Hg.

Persistent measurements above the normal systolic and diastolic pressures are abnormal. This condition is known as **hypertension.** Report any systolic pressure above 140 mm Hg to the nurse immediately. A diastolic pressure above 90 mm Hg also is reported immediately. Likewise, systolic pressures below 90 mm Hg and diastolic pressures below 60 mm Hg are reported. This is called **hypotension.** Some people normally have low blood pressures. However, hypotension is a sign of a serious condition that can lead to death if it is not corrected.

BOX 18-3 Factors Affecting Blood Pressure

- **Age**—blood pressure increases as a person grows older. It is lowest in infancy and childhood and highest in adulthood. Blood pressure continues to increase with aging.
- **Sex** (male or female)—women usually have lower blood pressures than men. Blood pressures rise in women after menopause.
- **Blood volume**—is the amount of blood in the system. Severe bleeding lowers the blood volume. Therefore the blood pressure lowers. The rapid administration of IV fluids increases the blood volume. The blood pressure rises.
- **Stress**—includes anxiety, fear, and emotions. Heart rate and blood pressure increase as part of the body's response to stress.
- **Pain**—generally increases blood pressure. However, severe pain can cause shock. Blood pressure is seriously low in the state of shock (see Chapter 33).
- **Exercise**—increases heart rate and blood pressure. Blood pressure should not be measured right after exercise.
- **Weight**—blood pressure is higher in overweight persons. The blood pressure lowers with weight loss.
- **Race**—black persons generally have higher blood pressures than white persons.
- **Diet**—a high-sodium diet increases the amount of water in the body. The extra fluid volume increases blood pressure (see Chapter 17).
- **Medications**—drugs can be given to raise or lower blood pressure. Other drugs have the side effects of high or low blood pressure.
- **Position**—blood pressure is generally lower when lying down and higher in the standing position. Sudden changes in position can cause sudden changes in blood pressure. A person who stands suddenly may have a sudden drop in blood pressure. Dizziness and fainting can occur.
- **Smoking**—increases blood pressure. Nicotine in cigarettes causes blood vessels to narrow. The heart must work harder to pump blood through narrowed vessels.
- **Alcohol**—excessive alcohol intake can raise blood pressure.

Equipment

A stethoscope and a sphygmomanometer are used to measure blood pressure. The **sphygmomanometer** consists of a cuff and a measuring device. There are three types of sphygmomanometers: aneroid, mercury, and electronic. The aneroid type has a round dial and a needle that points to the calibrations (Fig. 18-28, A). The aneroid manometer is small and easy to carry. The mercury manometer is more accurate than the aneroid type. The mercury type has a column of mercury within a calibrated tube (Fig. 18-28, B). Many facilities have wall-mounted mercury sphygmomanometers in patient and resident rooms.

The blood pressure cuff is wrapped around the upper arm. Tubing connects the cuff to the manometer. Another tube connects the cuff to a small handheld bulb. A valve on the bulb is turned to allow inflation of the cuff as the bulb is squeezed. The inflated cuff causes pressure over the brachial artery. The valve is turned in the opposite direction for cuff deflation. Blood pressure is measured as the cuff is deflated.

Sounds are produced as blood flows through the arteries. The stethoscope is used to listen to the sounds in the brachial artery as the cuff is deflated. Stethoscopes are not needed with electronic sphygmomanometers.

There are many types of electronic sphygmomanometers (Fig. 18-29). The systolic and diastolic blood pressures are displayed on the front of the instrument. The pulse is usually displayed also. The cuff automatically inflates and deflates on some models. Others have automatic deflation only. If electronic blood pressure equipment is used where you work, you need to learn how to use the equipment. Ask the nurse to show you what to do. The manufacturer's instructions are also helpful. Electronic devices are available for home use.

A

B

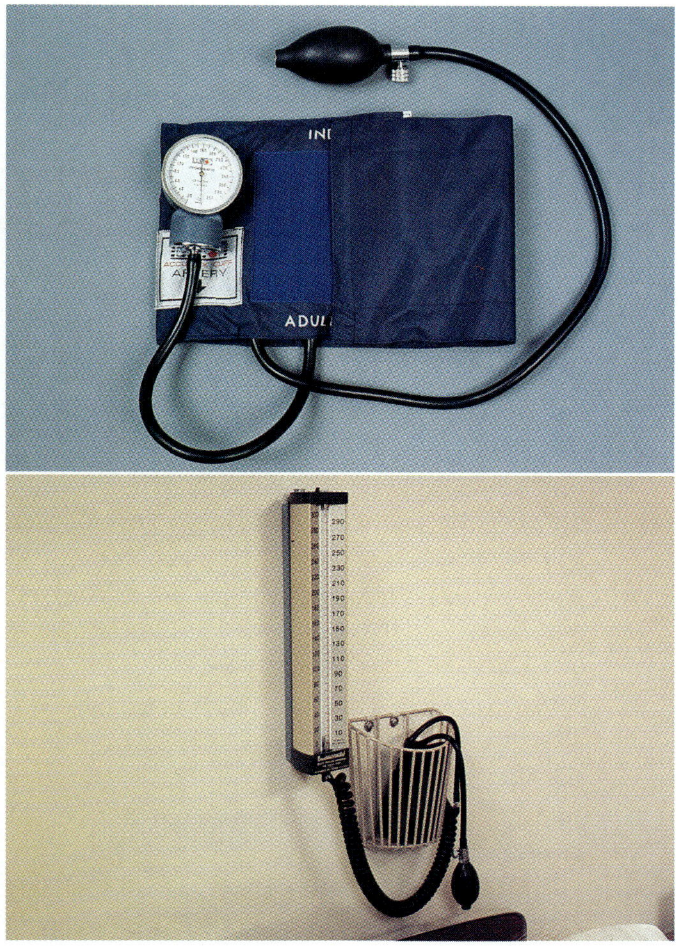

Fig. 18-28 *A, Aneroid manometer and cuff. B, Mercury manometer and cuff.*

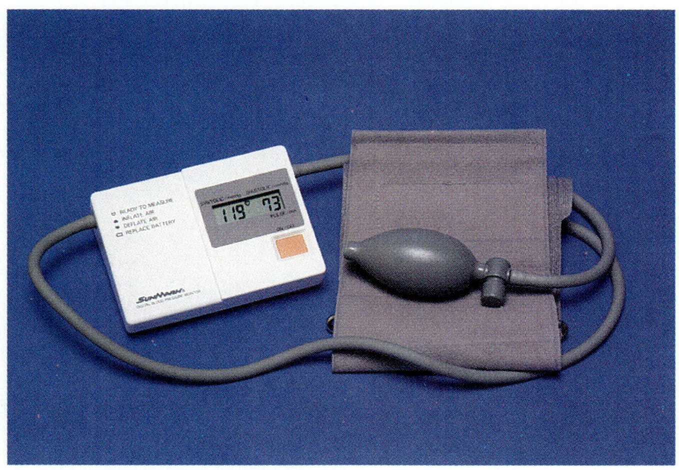

Fig. 18-29 *Electronic sphygmomanometer.*

Measuring Blood Pressure

Blood pressure is normally measured in the brachial artery. Box 18-4 lists the guidelines for measuring blood pressure.

BOX 18-4 GUIDELINES FOR MEASURING BLOOD PRESSURE

- Blood pressure is not taken on an arm with an IV infusion or a cast, or on an injured arm. If a person has had breast surgery, blood pressure is not taken on that side.
- Let the person rest for 10 to 20 minutes before measuring the blood pressure. Do not measure blood pressure right after exercise.
- Blood pressure is measured with the person sitting or lying. Sometimes the doctor orders measurement of blood pressure in the standing position.
- The cuff is applied to the bare upper arm. Clothing can affect the measurement. Do not apply the cuff over clothing.
- The cuff should be snug. Loose cuffs can cause inaccurate readings.
- The diaphragm of the stethoscope is placed firmly over the artery. The entire diaphragm must be in contact with the skin.
- The room should be quiet so the blood pressure can be heard. Talking, television, radio, and sounds from the hallway can affect an accurate measurement.
- The sphygmomanometer must be clearly visible.
- The radial artery is located, and the cuff is inflated. When the radial pulse is no longer felt, the cuff is inflated an additional 30 mm Hg. This prevents cuff inflation to an unnecessarily high pressure, which is painful to the person.
- The systolic and diastolic pressures are measured. The point at which the radial pulse is no longer felt is where you should expect to hear the first blood pressure sound. The first sound is the systolic pressure. The point where the sound disappears is the diastolic pressure.
- If you are not sure of an accurate measurement, take the blood pressure again. Wait 30 to 60 seconds before repeating the measurement.
- Notify the nurse immediately if you cannot hear the blood pressure.

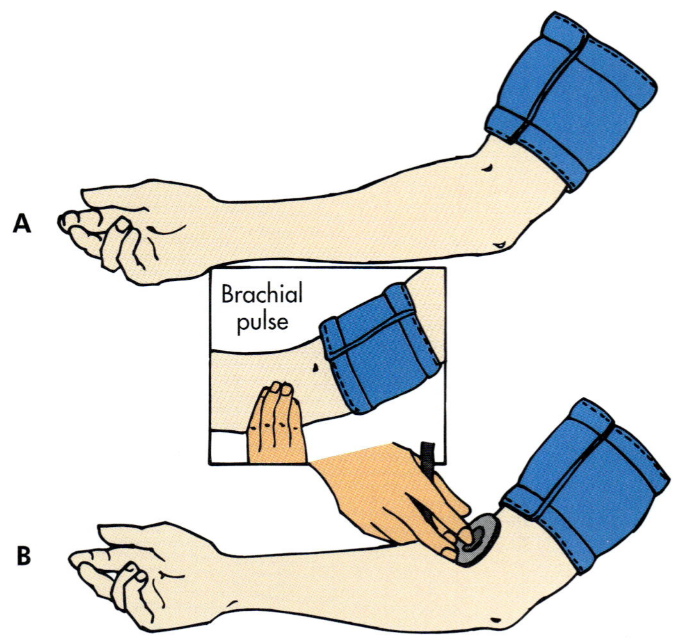

Fig. 18-30 *A, The cuff is over the brachial artery. B, The diaphragm of the stethoscope is over the brachial artery.*

Measuring Blood Pressure

Pre-procedure

1 Collect the following:
- Sphygmomanometer (blood pressure cuff)
- Stethoscope
- Alcohol wipes

2 Wash your hands.

3 Identify the person. Check the ID bracelet and call the person by name.

4 Explain the procedure to the person.

5 Provide for privacy.

Procedure

6 Wipe the stethoscope earpieces and diaphragm with alcohol wipes.

7 Have the person sit or lie down.

8 Position the person's arm so it is level with the heart. The palm should be up.

9 Stand no more than 3 feet away from the sphygmomanometer. A mercury model should be vertical, on a flat surface, and at eye level. The aneroid type should be directly in front of you.

10 Expose the upper arm.

11 Squeeze the cuff to expel any remaining air. Close the valve on the bulb.

12 Find the brachial artery at the inner aspect of the elbow.

13 Place the arrow on the cuff over the brachial artery (Fig. 18-30, A). Wrap the cuff around the upper arm at least 1 inch above the elbow. It should be even and snug.

14 Place the stethoscope earpieces in your ears.

15 Locate the radial artery. Inflate the cuff until you can no longer feel the pulse. Inflate the cuff 30 mm Hg beyond the point at which you last felt the pulse.

16 Position the diaphragm over the brachial artery (Fig. 18-30, B).

17 Deflate the cuff at an even rate of 2 to 4 millimeters per second. Turn the valve counterclockwise to deflate the cuff.

18 Note the point on the scale where you hear the first sound. This is the systolic reading. It should be near the point where the radial pulse disappeared.

19 Continue to deflate the cuff. Note the point where the sound disappears for the diastolic reading.

20 Deflate the cuff completely. Remove it from the person's arm. Remove the stethoscope.

21 Record the person's name and blood pressure on your note pad.

22 Return the cuff to the case or wall holder.

Post-procedure

23 Make sure the person is comfortable and the call bell is within reach.

24 Unscreen the person.

25 Clean the earpieces and diaphragm with alcohol wipes.

26 Return the equipment to its proper place.

27 Wash your hands.

28 Report the blood pressure. Record it in the proper place.

SUMMARY

Temperature, pulse, respirations, and blood pressure are used for the nursing process. They give valuable information about a person's state of health or illness. Vital signs can vary within certain normal ranges. Changes above or below the normal range signal a disorder or serious illness. Vital signs can change in response to the slightest change in body functions. Therefore they are a part of routine physical examinations and are taken several times a day for hospital patients.

Measuring vital signs is an important part of your job. Measurements must be accurate. Abnormal measurements are immediately reported to the nurse. They could signal serious threats to the person's life. Clear and accurate recording of vital signs is equally important. Doctors and nurses use them to decide on treatment and to evaluate care.

REVIEW QUESTIONS

Circle the best *answer.*

1 Which statement is *false?*

- **a** The vital signs are temperature, pulse, respirations, and blood pressure.
- **b** Vital signs detect changes in body function.
- **c** Vital signs change only during illness.
- **d** Sleep, exercise, medications, emotions, and noise affect vital signs.

2 Which temperature should you report immediately?

- **a** An oral temperature of 98.4° F
- **b** A rectal temperature of 101.6° F
- **c** An axillary temperature of 97.6° F
- **d** An oral temperature of 99.0° F

3 Electronic thermometers measure temperatures in

- **a** 2 to 60 seconds
- **b** 45 seconds
- **c** 2 to 3 minutes
- **d** 8 to 9 minutes

4 A rectal temperature is *not* taken when the person

- **a** Is unconscious
- **b** Is an infant
- **c** Has a nasogastric tube
- **d** Has had rectal surgery

5 Which gives the least accurate measurement of body temperature?

- **a** Oral temperature
- **b** Rectal temperature
- **c** Axillary temperature
- **d** Tympanic temperature

6 Which is usually used to take a pulse?

- **a** The radial pulse
- **b** The apical-radial pulse
- **c** The apical pulse
- **d** The brachial pulse

7 Which is reported to the nurse immediately?

- **a** An adult has a pulse of 120 beats per minute
- **b** An infant has a pulse of 130 beats per minute
- **c** An adult has a pulse of 80 beats per minute
- **d** All of the above

8 Which statement about apical-radial pulses is true?

- **a** The pulse can be taken by one person.
- **b** The radial pulse can be greater than the apical pulse.
- **c** The apical pulse can be greater than the radial pulse.
- **d** The apical and radial pulses are always equal.

REVIEW QUESTIONS—CONT'D

9 Normal respirations are
- **a** Between 10 and 20 per minute
- **b** Quiet and effortless
- **c** Regular with both sides of the chest rising and falling equally
- **d** All of the above

10 Difficult, painful, or labored breathing is known as
- **a** Tachypnea
- **b** Bradypnea
- **c** Apnea
- **d** Dyspnea

11 Respirations are usually counted
- **a** After taking the temperature
- **b** After taking the pulse
- **c** Before taking the pulse
- **d** After taking the blood pressure

12 Which blood pressure is normal?
- **a** 88/54 mm Hg
- **b** 210/100 mm Hg
- **c** 130/82 mm Hg
- **d** 152/90 mm Hg

13 When taking a blood pressure, you should do the following *except*
- **a** Take the blood pressure in the arm with an IV infusion
- **b** Apply the cuff to a bare upper arm
- **c** Turn off the television and radio
- **d** Locate the brachial artery

14 Which is the systolic blood pressure?
- **a** The point at which the pulse is no longer felt
- **b** The point where the first sound is heard
- **c** The point where the last sound is heard
- **d** The point 30 mm Hg above where the pulse was felt

Answers to these questions are on page 751.

Exercise and Activity

19

OBJECTIVES

- Define the key terms listed in this chapter
- Describe bed rest
- Identify the complications of bed rest
- Explain how to prevent muscle atrophy and contractures
- Describe the devices used to support and maintain the body in alignment
- Explain why a trapeze is used
- Describe range-of-motion exercises
- Perform range-of-motion exercises
- Help a person walk
- Explain how to help a falling person
- Describe four walking aids
- Explain why recreational activities are important for the elderly

Key Terms

abduction Moving a body part away from the body

adduction Moving a body part toward the body

atrophy A decrease in size or a wasting away of tissue

contracture The abnormal shortening of a muscle

dorsiflexion Bending backward

extension Straightening of a body part

external rotation Turning the joint outward

flexion Bending a body part

footdrop Plantar flexion

hyperextension Excessive straightening of a body part

internal rotation Turning the joint inward

plantar flexion The foot is bent; footdrop

pronation Turning downward

range of motion The movement of a joint to the extent possible without causing pain

supination Turning upward

Being active is important for physical and mental well-being. Ideally, we can move about and function without help. However, illnesses, surgery, injuries, and pain cause weakness and some degree of activity limitation. Some people are weak from chronic illnesses. Others are confined to bed for a long time. Some have permanent paralysis. Some disorders are progressive, causing decreases in activity. Examples include multiple sclerosis, Parkinson's disease, arthritis, and nervous system and muscular disorders (see Chapter 28). Inactivity, whether minor or severe, affects the normal function of every body system. Mental well-being is also affected.

The nursing process is used to promote exercise and activity in all persons to the degree possible. The nurse assesses and plans for the person's need. The nursing care plan includes the person's activity level and what exercises to perform. To assist in promoting exercise and activity, you need to understand

- Bed rest
- How to prevent complications from bed rest
- How to help persons exercise

BED REST

Bed rest may be ordered by the doctor because of a person's health problem. It may also be a nursing measure because of a person's apparent helplessness. Generally bed rest is ordered to

- Reduce physical activity
- Reduce pain
- Encourage rest
- Regain strength
- Promote healing

Bed rest has many meanings. The person may be allowed to perform activities of daily living (ADL). Bathing, oral hygiene, hair care, and feeding may be allowed. *Strict* or *absolute* bed rest means everything is done for the person. The person is not allowed to perform any activities of daily living. You must know what activities are allowed for each person on bed rest. The nurse provides this information.

Complications of Bed Rest

Bed rest and lack of exercise and activity can cause serious complications. Every body system is affected. Pressure sores, constipation, and fecal impaction can result. Blood clots, urinary tract infections, renal calculi (renal stones), and pneumonia (infection of the lung) can occur. Contractures and muscle atrophy are other complications.

A **contracture** is the abnormal shortening of a muscle. The contracted muscle is fixed into position, is deformed, and cannot be stretched (Fig. 19-1). The person is permanently deformed and disabled. Contractures must be prevented. **Atrophy** is the decrease in size or the wasting away of tissue. Muscle atrophy is a decrease in size or a wasting away of muscle (Fig. 19-2). These complications must be prevented to maintain normal body movement.

Preventing the Complications of Bed Rest

Complications from bed rest are prevented by good nursing care. Positioning in good body alignment and range-of-motion exercises are important preventive measures. These are part of the person's care plan.

Positioning

Body alignment and positioning were discussed in Chapter 10. Supportive devices are often used to support and maintain the person in a certain position.

- **Bed boards** are placed under the mattress. They keep the person in alignment because sagging of the mattress is prevented (Fig. 19-3). They are usually made of plywood and have a covering of canvas or other material. There are two sections: one for the head of the bed and one for the foot. The two sections allow the head of the bed to be raised.
- **Footboards** are placed at the foot of mattresses (Fig. 19-4). They prevent **plantar flexion (footdrop).** In plantar flexion the foot (plantar) is bent (flexion).

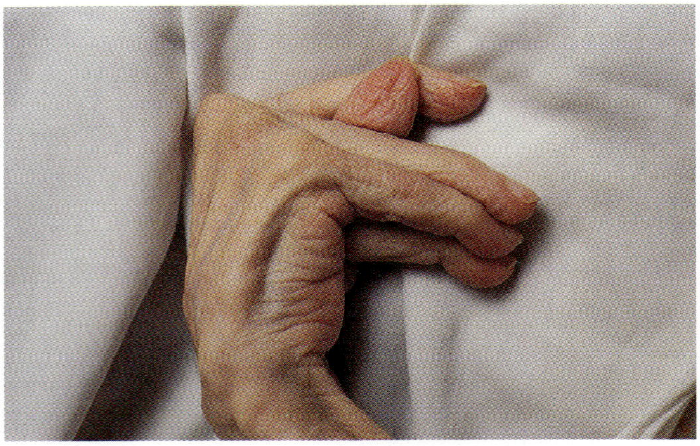

Fig. 19-1 *A contracture.*

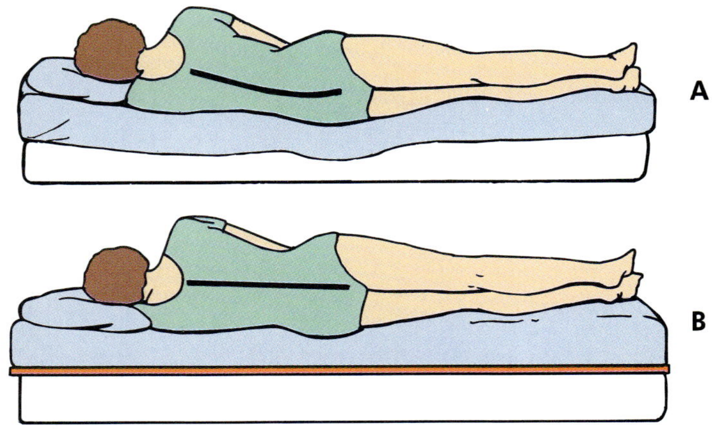

Fig. 19-3 *A, Mattress sagging without bed boards. B, Bed boards are placed under the mattress. No sagging occurs.*

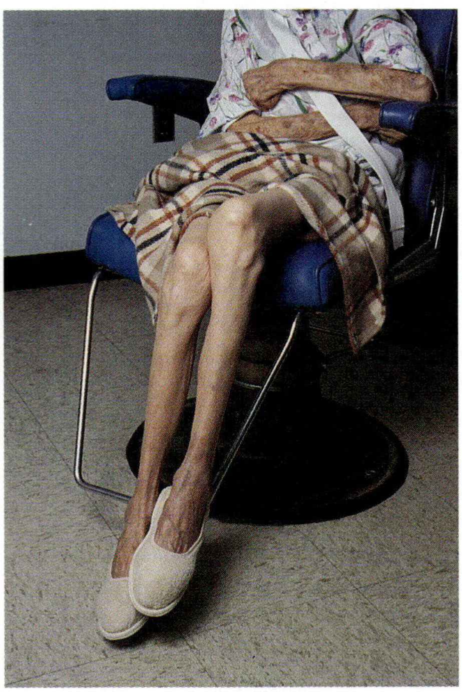

Fig. 19-2 *Muscle atrophy.*

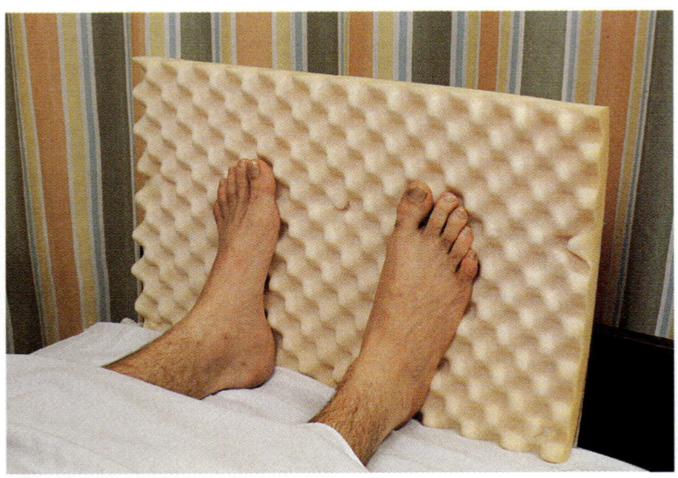

Fig. 19-4 *Footboard. Feet are flush with the board to keep them in normal alignment.*

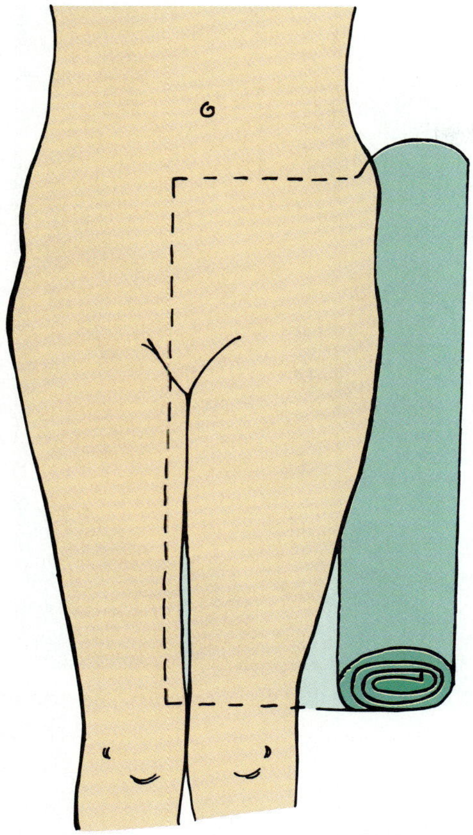

Fig. 19-5 *Trochanter roll made from a bath blanket. It extends from the hip to the knee.*

The footboard is placed so the soles of the feet are flush against it. The feet are in good alignment as when standing. The footboard can be used as a bed cradle to keep top linens off the feet.

- **Trochanter rolls** (Fig. 19-5) prevent the hips and legs from turning outward (external rotation). They are made from bath blankets. A blanket is folded to the desired length and rolled up. The loose end is placed under the person from the hip to the knee. Then the roll is tucked alongside the body. Pillows or sandbags can be used to keep the hips and knees in alignment.
- **Hip abduction wedges** keep the hips abducted (Fig. 19-6). The wedge is positioned between the person's legs. These are common after hip replacement surgery.
- **Hand rolls or hand grips** prevent contractures of the thumb, fingers, and wrist. Commercial hand rolls are common (Fig. 19-7 on page 460). Rolled-up washcloths (see Fig. 8-25, page 170), foam rubber sponges, rubber balls, and finger cushions (Fig. 19-8 on page 460) can be used.
- **Bed cradles** keep the weight of top linens off the feet (see Fig. 13-33, page 315). The weight of top linens can cause footdrop and pressure sores.

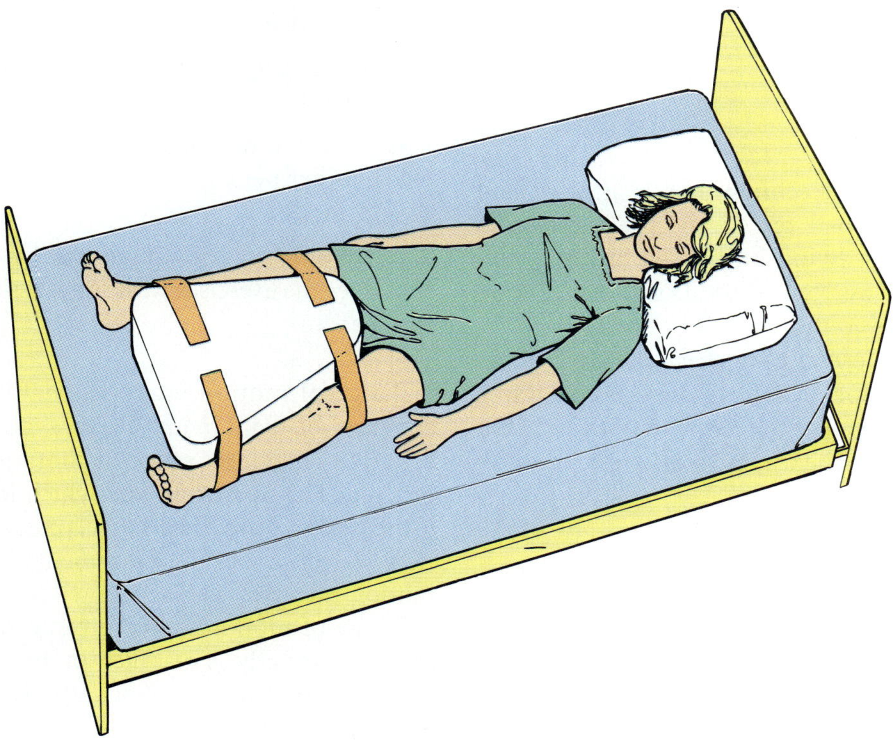

Fig. 19-6 *Hip abduction wedge.*

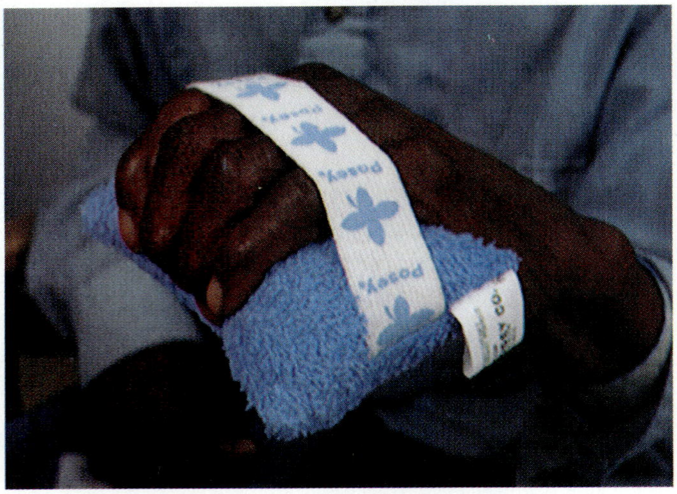

Fig. 19-7 *Hand roll.* (*Courtesy of Posey Co, Arcadia, Calif.*)

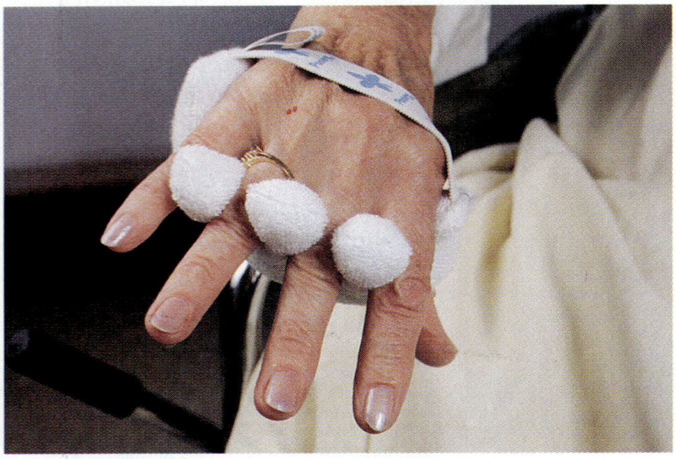

Fig. 19-8 *Finger cushion* (*Courtesy of Posey Co, Arcadia, Calif.*)

Exercise

Exercise helps prevent contractures, muscle atrophy, and other complications of bed rest. Some exercise occurs with activities of daily living and when turning and moving in bed without assistance. Additional exercises are needed for muscles and joints.

A trapeze is used for exercises to strengthen arm muscles. The trapeze is suspended from an overbed frame (Fig. 19-9). The person grasps the bar with both hands to lift the trunk off the bed. The trapeze is also used to move up and turn in bed.

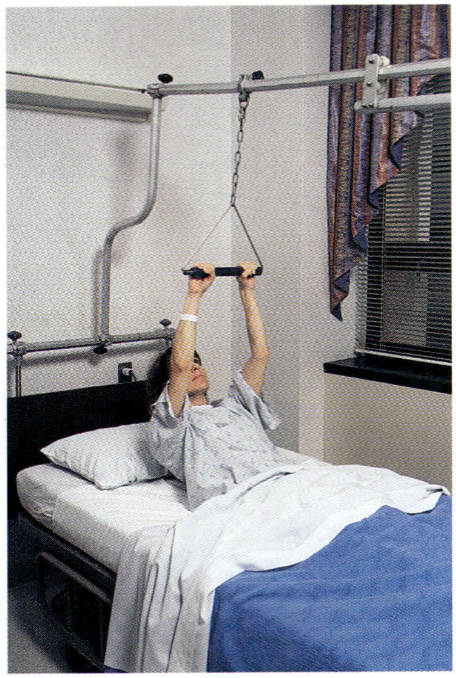

Fig. 19-9 *Trapeze is used to strengthen the arm muscles.*

Range-of-motion exercises The movement of a joint to the extent possible without causing pain is the **range of motion (ROM)** of that joint. Range-of-motion exercises involve exercising the joints through their complete range of motion. The exercises are usually done at least twice a day. Range-of-motion exercises may be active, passive, or active-assistive.

- *Active* range-of-motion exercises are done by the person.
- *Passive* range-of-motion exercises involve having another person move the joints through their range of motion.
- *Active-assistive* range of motion is when the person does the exercises with some assistance from another person.

Range-of-motion exercises naturally occur during activities of daily living. Persons on bed rest have little activity. Therefore range-of-motion exercises may be ordered. The nurse tells you which joints to exercise and if the exercises are to be active, passive, or active-assistive. Box 19-1 describes the movements involved in range-of-motion exercises.

Range-of-motion exercises can cause injury if not performed properly. The rules in Box 19-2 are practiced when performing or assisting with range-of-motion exercises.

Text continued on page 466.

BOX 19-1 JOINT MOVEMENTS

Abduction—moving a body part away from the body
Adduction—moving a body part toward the body
Extension—straightening a body part
Flexion—bending a body part
Hyperextension—excessive straightening of a body part
Dorsiflexion—bending backward
Rotation—turning the joint
Internal rotation—turning the joint inward
External rotation—turning the joint outward
Pronation—turning downward
Supination—turning upward

BOX 19-2 RULES FOR PERFORMING RANGE-OF-MOTION EXERCISES

- Exercise only the joints the nurse tells you to exercise.
- Expose only the body part being exercised.
- Use good body mechanics.
- Support the extremity being exercised.
- Move the joint slowly, smoothly, and gently.
- Do not force a joint beyond its present range of motion or to the point of pain.
- Perform range-of-motion exercises to the neck only if allowed by facility policy. In some facilities neck exercises are done only by physical therapists or occupational therapists. This is because of the danger of neck injuries.

PERFORMING RANGE-OF-MOTION EXERCISES

PRE-PROCEDURE

1. Identify the person. Check the ID bracelet and call the person by name.
2. Explain the procedure to the person.
3. Wash your hands.
4. Obtain a bath blanket.
5. Provide for privacy.
6. Raise the bed to the best level for good body mechanics.

PROCEDURE

7. Lower the side rails.
8. Position the person supine and in good alignment.
9. Cover the person with a bath blanket. Fanfold top linens to the foot of the bed.
10. Exercise the neck (Fig. 19-10 on page 464):
    - **a** Place your hands over the person's ears to support the head.
    - **b** Flexion—bring the head forward so the chin touches the chest.
    - **c** Extension—straighten the head.
    - **d** Hyperextension—bring the head backward until the chin is pointing up.
    - **e** Rotation—turn the head from side to side.
    - **f** Lateral flexion—move the head to the right and to the left.
    - **g** Repeat flexion, extension, hyperextension, rotation, and lateral flexion 5 times.

Continued.

PROCEDURE—CONT'D

11 Exercise the shoulder (Fig. 19-11 on page 464):
- **a** Grasp the wrist with one hand and the elbow with the other.
- **b** Flexion—raise the arm straight in front and over the head.
- **c** Extension—bring the arm down to the side.
- **d** Hyperextension—move the arm behind the body. (This can be done if the person is standing or sitting in a straight-backed chair.)
- **e** Abduction—move the straight arm away from the side of the body.
- **f** Adduction—move the straight arm to the side of the body.
- **g** Internal rotation—bend the elbow and place it at the same level as the shoulder. Move the forearm down toward the body.
- **h** External rotation—move the forearm toward the head.
- **I** Repeat flexion, extension, hyperextension, abduction, adduction, and internal and external rotation 5 times.

12 Exercise the elbow (Fig. 19-12 on page 464):
- **a** Grasp the person's wrist with one hand and the elbow with the other.
- **b** Flexion—bend the arm so the same-side shoulder is touched.
- **c** Extension—straighten the arm.
- **d** Repeat flexion and extension 5 times.

13 Exercise the forearm (Fig. 19-13 on page 464):
- **a** Pronation—turn the hand so the palm is down.
- **b** Supination—turn the hand so the palm is up.
- **c** Repeat pronation and supination 5 times.

14 Exercise the wrist (Fig. 19-14 on page 465):
- **a** Hold the wrist with both of your hands.
- **b** Flexion—bend the hand down.
- **c** Extension—straighten the hand.
- **d** Hyperextension—bend the hand back.
- **e** Radial flexion—turn the hand toward the thumb.
- **f** Ulnar flexion—turn the hand toward the little finger.
- **g** Repeat flexion, extension, hyperextension, and radial and ulnar flexion 5 times.

15 Exercise the thumb (Fig. 19-15 on page 465):
- **a** Hold the person's hand with one hand and the thumb with your other hand.
- **b** Abduction—move the thumb out from the inner part of the index finger.
- **c** Adduction—move the thumb back next to the index finger.
- **d** Opposition—touch each fingertip with the thumb.
- **e** Flexion—bend the thumb into the hand.
- **f** Extension—move the thumb out to the side of the fingers.
- **g** Repeat flexion, extension, abduction, adduction, and opposition 5 times.

16 Exercise the fingers (Fig. 19-16 on page 465):
- **a** Abduction—spread the fingers and the thumb apart.
- **b** Adduction—bring the fingers and thumb together.
- **c** Extension—straighten the fingers so the fingers, hand, and arm are straight.
- **d** Flexion—make a fist.
- **e** Repeat abduction, adduction, extension, and flexion 5 times.

17 Exercise the hip (Fig. 19-17 on page 465):
- **a** Place one hand under the knee and the other under the ankle to support the leg.
- **b** Flexion—raise the leg.
- **c** Extension—straighten the leg.
- **d** Abduction—move the leg away from the body.
- **e** Adduction—move the leg toward the other leg.
- **f** Internal rotation—turn the leg inward.
- **g** External rotation—turn the leg outward.
- **h** Repeat flexion, extension, abduction, adduction, and inward and outward rotation 5 times.

18 Exercise the knee (Fig. 19-18 on page 465):
- **a** Place one hand under the knee and the other under the ankle to support the leg.
- **b** Flexion—bend the leg.
- **c** Extension—straighten the leg.
- **d** Repeat flexion and extension of the knee 5 times.

PROCEDURE—CONT'D

19 Exercise the ankle (Fig. 19-19 on page 465):
- **a** Place one hand under the foot and the other under the ankle to support the part.
- **b** Dorsiflexion—pull the foot forward and push down on the heel at the same time.
- **c** Plantar flexion—turn the foot down or point the toes.
- **d** Repeat dorsiflexion and plantar flexion 5 times.

20 Exercise the foot (Fig. 19-20 on page 465):
- **a** Pronation—turn the outside of the foot up and the inside down.
- **b** Supination—turn the inside of the foot up and the outside down.
- **c** Repeat pronation and supination 5 to 6 times.

21 Exercise the toes (Fig. 19-21 on page 465):
- **a** Flexion—curl the toes.
- **b** Extension—straighten the toes.
- **c** Abduction—spread the toes apart.
- **d** Adduction—pull the toes together.
- **e** Repeat flexion, extension, abduction, and adduction 5 times.

22 Cover the leg and raise the side rail.

23 Go to the other side. Lower the side rail.

24 Repeat steps 11 through 21.

POST-PROCEDURE

25 Make sure the person is comfortable.

26 Cover the person. Remove the bath blanket.

27 Raise or lower side rails as instructed by the nurse.

28 Lower the bed to its lowest level.

29 Place the call bell within reach.

30 Unscreen the person.

31 Return the bath blanket to its proper place.

32 Wash your hands.

33 Report the following to the nurse:
- The time the exercises were performed
- The joints exercised
- The number of times the exercises were performed on each joint
- Any complaints of pain or signs of stiffness or spasm
- The degree to which the person participated in the exercises

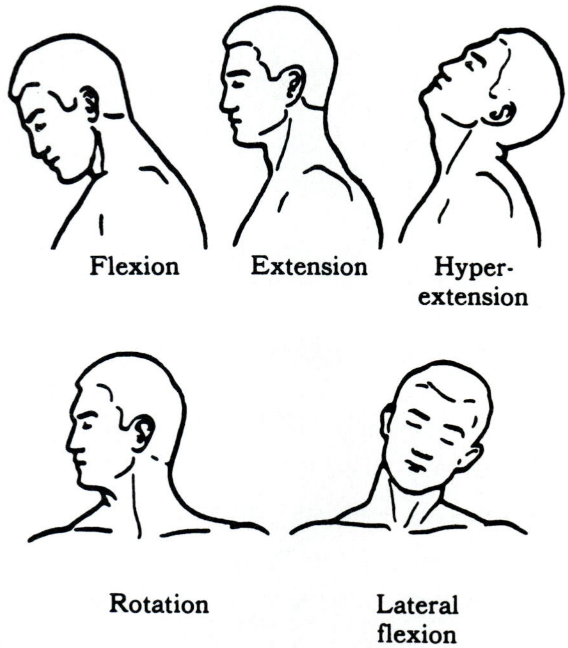

Fig. 19-10 *Range-of-motion exercises for the neck. (Figs. 19-10 through 19-21 from Phipps WJ, Long BC, Woods NF: Medical-surgical nursing: concepts and practice, ed 5, St Louis, 1995, Mosby–Year Book.)*

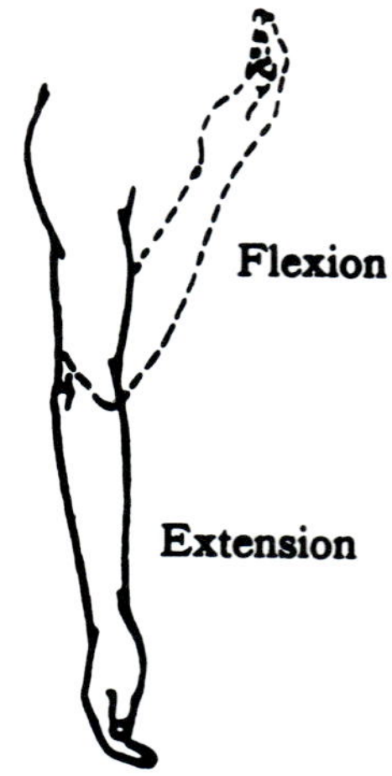

Fig. 19-12 *Range-of-motion exercises for the elbow.*

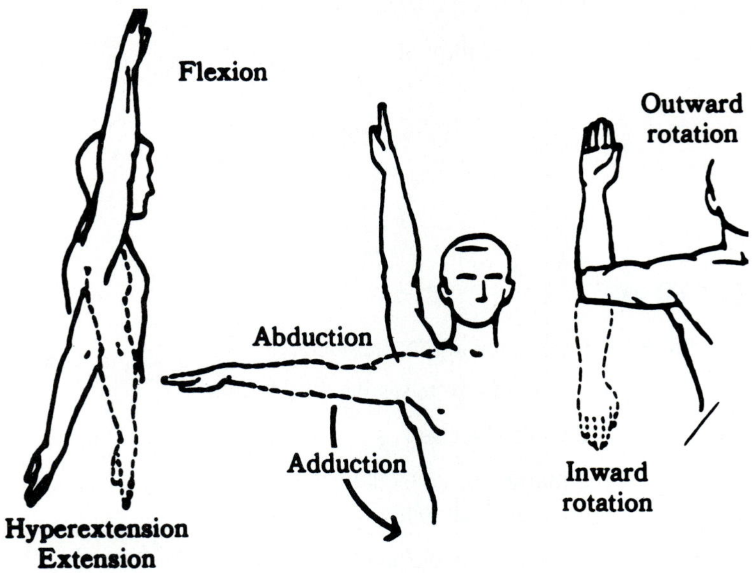

Fig. 19-11 *Range-of-motion exercises for the shoulder.*

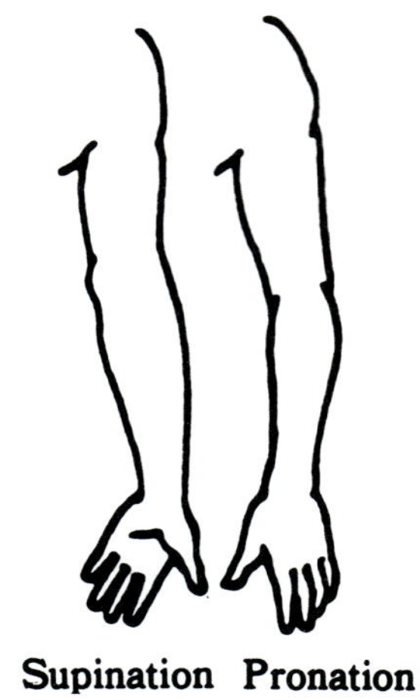

Fig. 19-13 *Range-of-motion exercises for the forearm.*

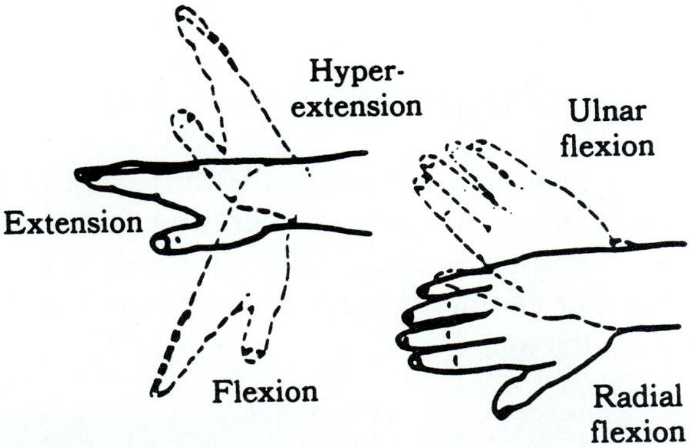

Fig. 19-14 *Range-of-motion exercises for the wrist.*

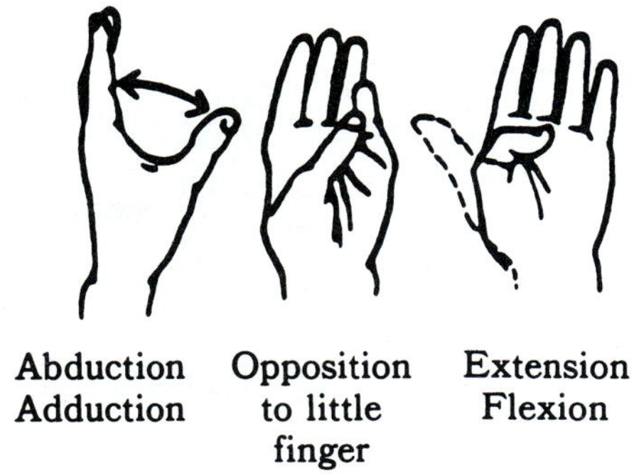

Fig. 19-15 *Range-of-motion exercises for the thumb.*

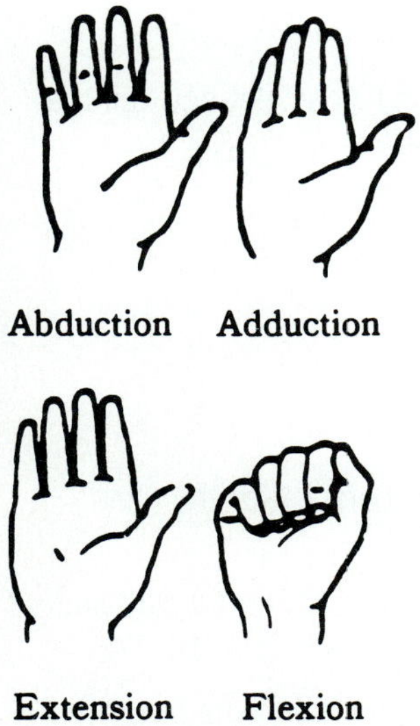

Fig. 19-16 *Range-of-motion exercises for the fingers.*

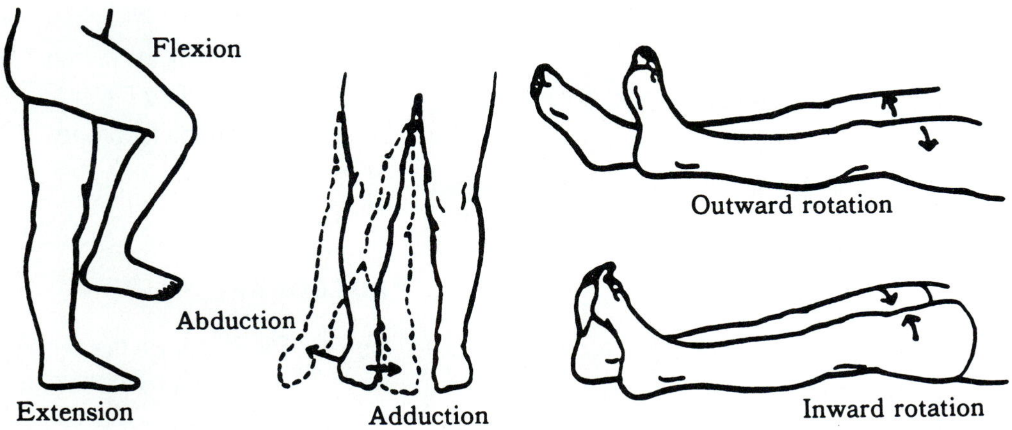

Fig. 19-17 *Range-of-motion exercises for the hip.*

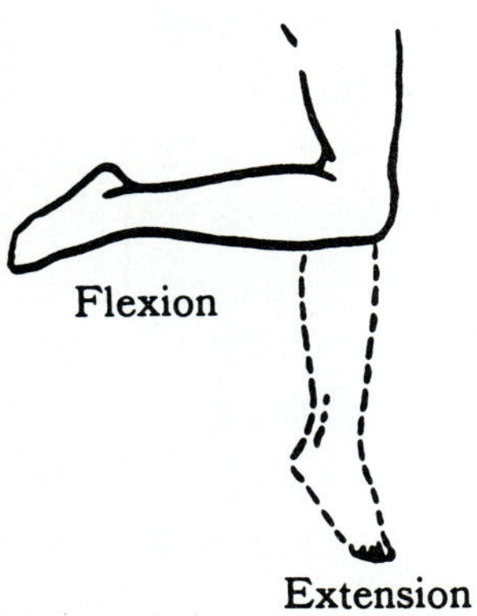

Fig. 19-18 *Range-of-motion exercises for the knee.*

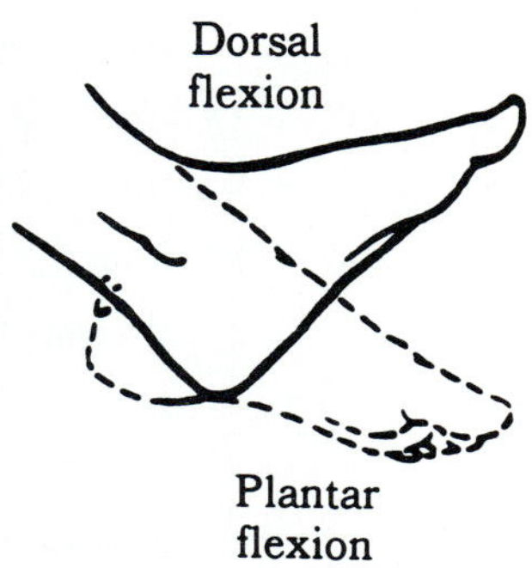

Fig. 19-19 *Range-of-motion exercises for the ankle.*

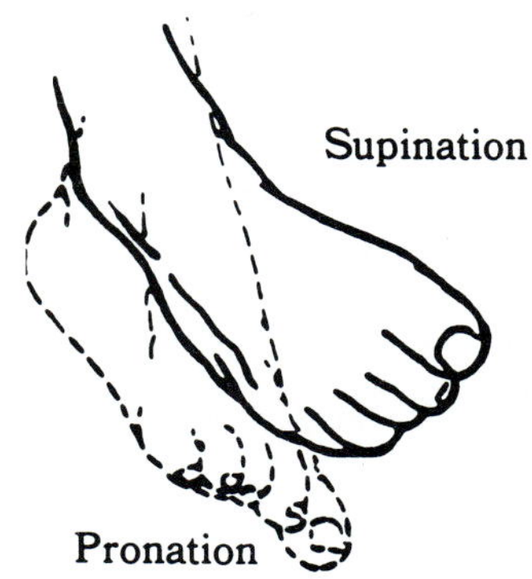

Fig. 19-20 *Range-of-motion exercises for the foot.*

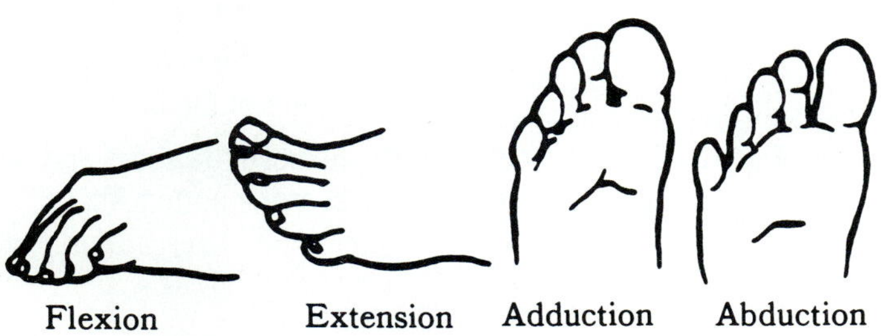

Fig. 19-21 *Range-of-motion exercises for the toes.*

AMBULATION

For most persons on bed rest, activity is increased slowly and in steps. First the person dangles (sits on the side of the bed). The next step is to sit in a bedside chair. Walking about in the room and then in the hallway are the next steps. **Ambulation,** the act of walking, is not a problem if complications have been prevented. Contractures and muscle atrophy are prevented by proper positioning and exercise.

Persons may be weak and unsteady from bed rest, surgery, or injury. You need to help these persons walk. Use a gait (transfer or safety) belt if the person is weak or unsteady. For additional support, the person uses hand rails along the wall.

HELPING THE PERSON TO WALK

PRE-PROCEDURE

1 Explain the procedure to the person.
2 Wash your hands.
3 Collect the following:
- Robe and shoes
- Paper or sheet to protect bottom linens
- Transfer (gait or safety) belt

4 Identify the person. Check the ID bracelet and call the person by name.
5 Provide for privacy.

PROCEDURE

6 Move furniture if necessary for moving space for you and the person.
7 Lower the bed to its lowest position. Lock the bed wheels.
8 Fanfold top linens to the foot of the bed.
9 Place the paper or sheet under the person's feet. This protects the bottom sheet from the shoes. Put the shoes on the person.
10 Help the person to dangle. (See *Helping the Person to Sit on the Side of the Bed,* page 234.)
11 Help the person put on the robe.
12 Apply the transfer belt. (See *Applying a Transfer [Gait] Belt,* page 236.)
13 Help the person stand:
- a Stand facing the person.
- b Grasp the transfer belt at each side.
- c Brace your knees against the person's knees. Block his or her feet with your feet (see Fig. 10-29, page 239).
- d Pull the person up into a standing position as you straighten your knees (see Fig. 10-30, page 240).

14 Stand at the person's side while he or she gains balance. Do not let go of the transfer belt. Grasp the belt at the side and back.
15 Encourage the person to stand erect with the head up and back straight.
16 Assist the person to walk. Walk at his or her side and provide support with the transfer belt (Fig. 19-22).
17 Encourage the person to walk normally. The heel of the foot strikes the floor first. Discourage shuffling, sliding, or walking on tiptoes.
18 Walk the required distance if the person can tolerate the activity. Do not rush the person.
19 Help the person return to bed:
- a Have the person stand at the side of the bed.
- b Pivot him or her a quarter turn. The backs of the knees should touch the bed.
- c Grasp the sides of the transfer belt.
- d Lower the person onto the bed as you bend your knees. Remove the transfer belt and robe.
- e Help the person lie down. (See *Helping the Person to Sit on the Side of the Bed,* page 234.)

20 Lower the head of the bed. Help the person to the center of the bed.
21 Remove the shoes and remove the paper or sheet over the bottom sheet.

POST-PROCEDURE

22 Make sure the person is comfortable. Cover the person.

23 Place the call bell within reach.

24 Raise or lower side rails as instructed by the nurse.

25 Return the robe and shoes to their proper place.

26 Return furniture to its proper location.

27 Unscreen the person.

28 Wash your hands.

29 Report the following to the nurse:
- How well the person tolerated the activity
- The distance walked

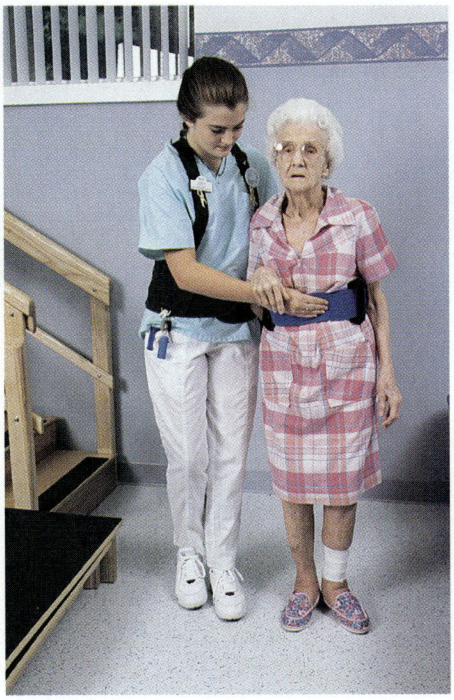

Fig. 19-22 *The nursing assistant walks at the person's side. A transfer (safety) belt is used for the person's safety.*

The Falling Person

Patients and residents may start to fall when standing or walking. They may be weak, lightheaded, or dizzy. Fainting may occur. Falling may be due to slipping or sliding on spills, waxed floors, throw rugs, or improper shoes (see Chapter 8). When a person is falling, there is a tendency to try to prevent the fall. However, trying to prevent a fall could cause greater harm. You could injure yourself and the person as you twist and strain to stop the fall. Balance is lost as a person is falling. If you try to prevent the fall, you could lose your balance. Thus both you and the person could fall or cause the other person to fall. Head, hip, and knee injuries are common from falls.

If a person starts to fall, ease him or her to the floor. This lets you control the direction of the fall. You can also protect the person's head.

HELPING THE FALLING PERSON

PROCEDURE

1 Stand with your feet apart. Keep your back straight.

2 Bring the person close to your body as quickly as possible. Use the gait belt if one is worn. If not, wrap your arms around the person's waist. You can also hold the person under the arms (Fig. 19-23, A on page 468).

3 Move your leg so the person's buttocks rest on it (Fig. 19-23, B). Move the leg near the person.

4 Lower the person to the floor. Let him or her slide down your leg to the floor (Fig. 19-23, C). Bend at your hips and knees as you lower the person.

5 Call a nurse to check the person.

6 Help the nurse return the person to bed. Get other workers to help if necessary.

7 Report the following to the nurse:
- How the fall occurred
- How far the person walked
- How activity was tolerated before the fall
- Any complaints before the fall
- The amount of assistance needed by the person while walking

8 Complete an incident report.

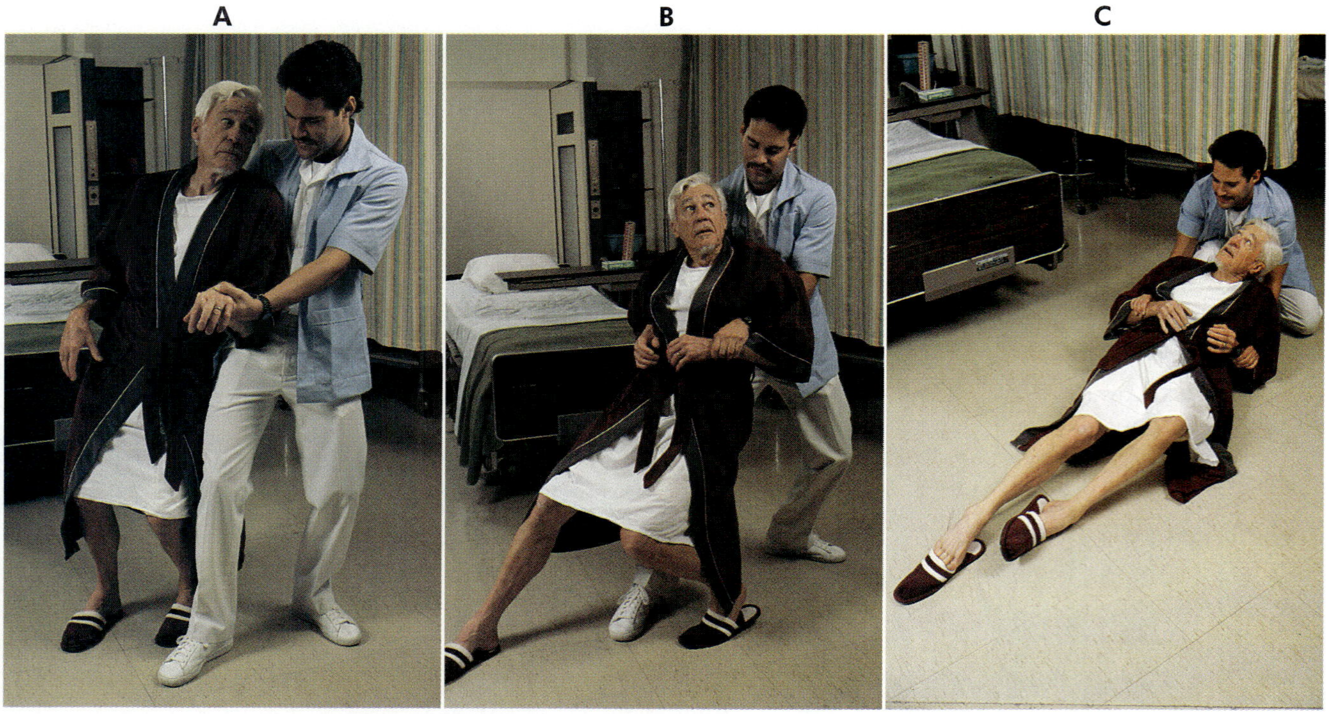

Fig. 19-23 *A, The falling person is supported under the arms. B, The person's buttocks are on the orderly's leg. C, The person is eased to the floor on the orderly's leg.*

Walking Aids

Walking aids support the body. They are ordered by the doctor. The type ordered depends on the person's physical condition, the amount of support needed, and the type of disability. The physical therapist or nurse teaches the person to use the walking aid. Its use may be temporary or permanent.

Crutches Crutches (Fig. 19-24) are used when the person cannot use one leg or when one or both legs need to gain strength. Some persons with permanent leg weakness are able to use crutches.

Safety is important. The person on crutches is at risk of falling. Though crutches provide support, certain safety measures are followed.

- The crutches must fit. A nurse or physical therapist measures and fits the person with crutches. An improper fit increases the risk of falling and further injury. Back pain, nerve damage, and injuries to the underarms and palms are other risks.
- Crutch tips must be attached to the crutches. They must not be worn down or wet.
- Crutches are checked for flaws. Check wooden crutches for cracks and aluminum crutches for bends. All bolts on both types must be tight.
- Street shoes are worn. They must be flat and have nonskid soles.

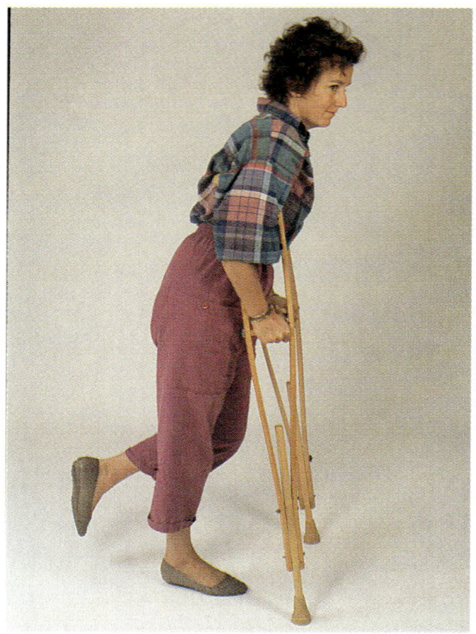

Fig. 19-24 *A person using crutches.*

- Clothes must fit well. Loose clothing may get caught between the crutches and underarms. Loose clothing can also hang forward and block the person's view of the feet and crutch tips.
- Safety rules to prevent falls must be followed (see Chapter 8).

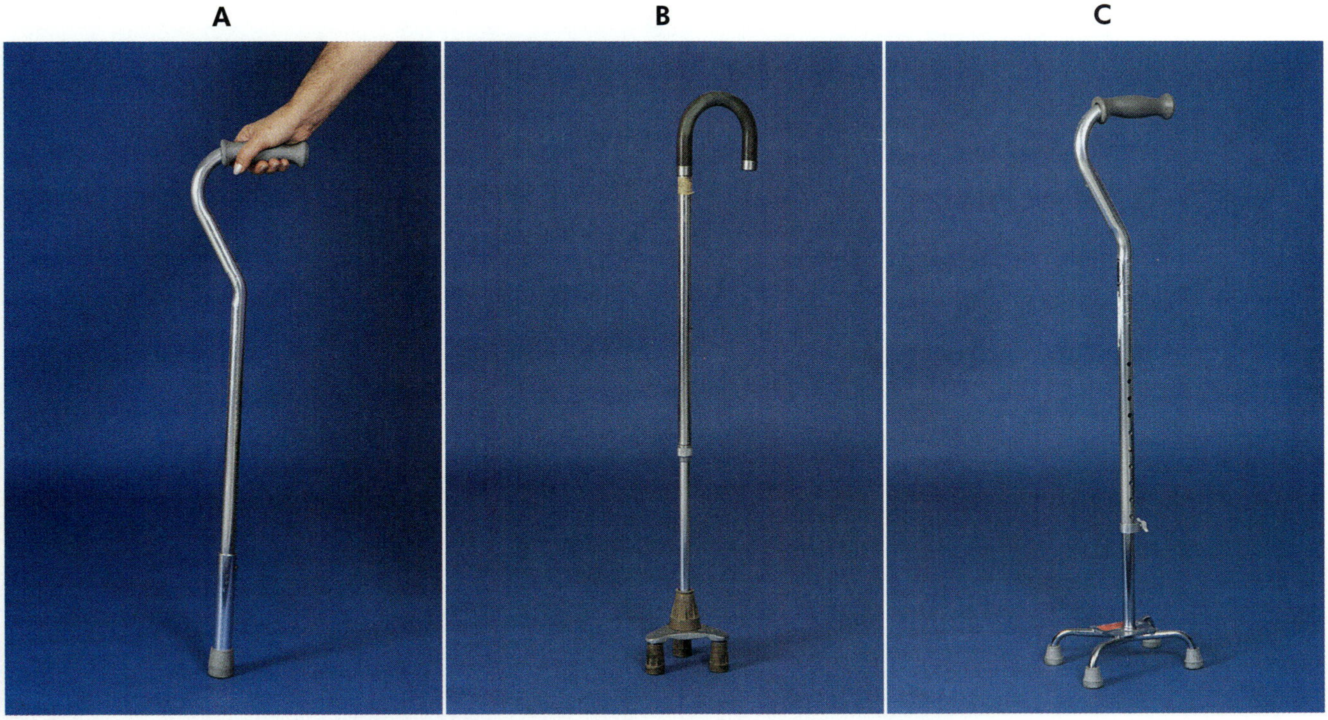

Fig. 19-25 *A, Single-tipped cane. B, Tri-pod cane. C, Four-point (quad) cane.*

Canes Canes are used when there is weakness on one side of the body. They help provide balance and support. There are single-tipped, three-point, and four-point (quad) canes (Fig. 19-25). A cane is held on the *strong side* of the body. (If the left leg is weak, the cane is held in the right hand.) Three-point and four-point canes give more support than single-tipped canes. However, they are harder to move.

The cane tip is about 6 to 10 inches to the side of the foot and about 6 inches in front of the foot. The grip is level with the hip (Fig. 19-26). The person walks as follows:

Step A: The cane is moved forward about 12 inches (Fig. 19-27, A on page 470).

Step B: The weak leg (opposite the cane) is moved forward even with the cane (Fig. 19-27, B).

Step C: The strong leg is brought forward and ahead of the cane and the weak leg (Fig. 19-27, C).

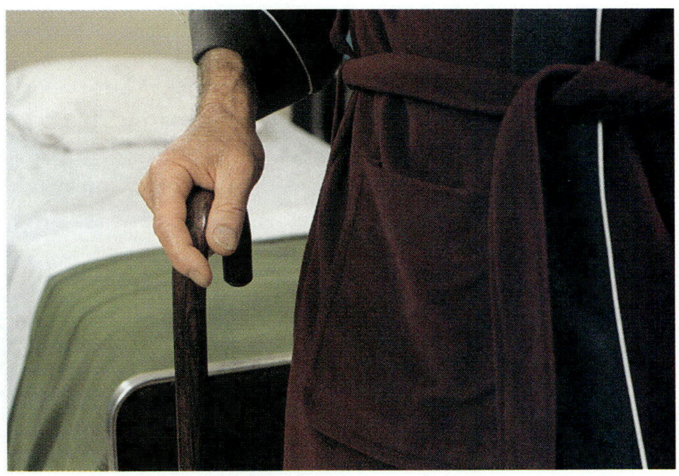

Fig. 19-26 *The cane grip is held level with the hip.*

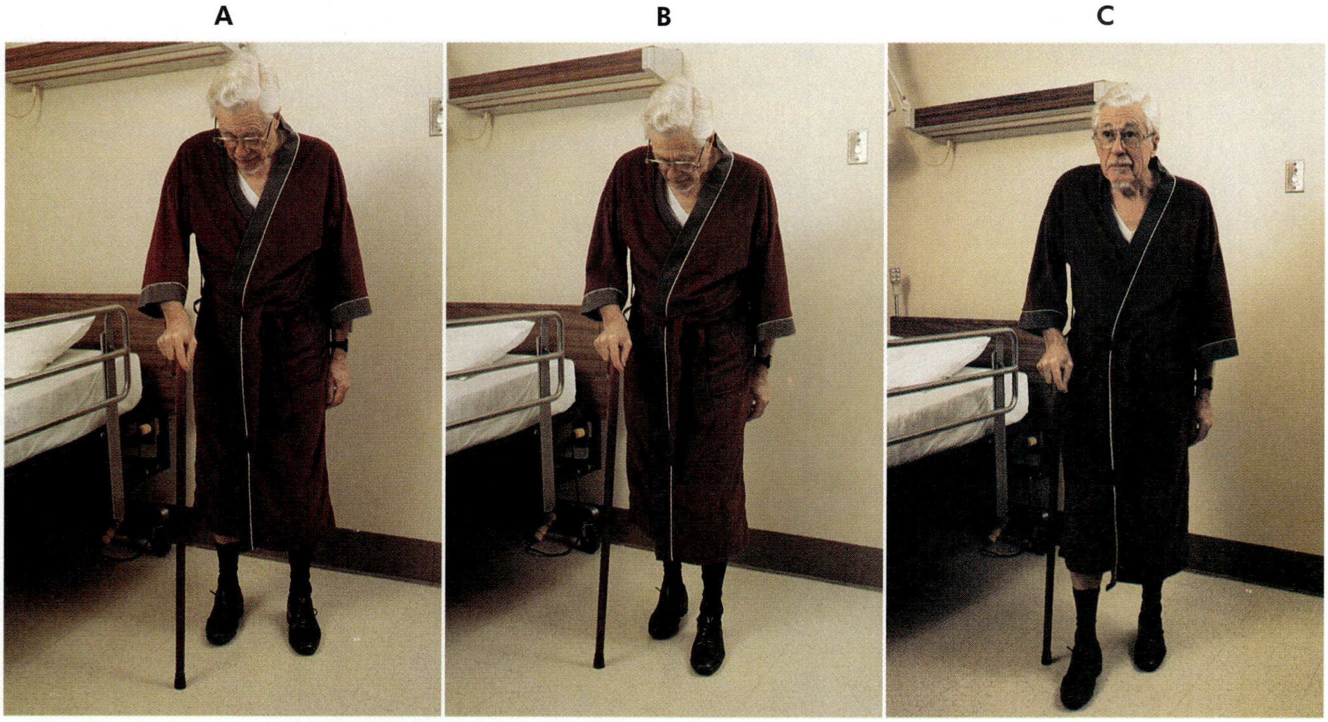

Fig. 19-27 *Walking with a cane. A, The cane is moved forward about 1 foot. B, The leg opposite the cane (weak leg) is brought forward even with the cane. C, The leg on the cane side (strong leg) is moved ahead of the cane and the weak leg.*

Walkers A walker is a four-point walking aid (Fig. 19-28). It gives more support than a cane. Many people feel safer and more secure with a walker than with a cane. There are many kinds of walkers. The standard walker is picked up and moved about 6 inches in front of the person. The person then moves the right foot and then the left foot up to the walker (Fig. 19-29).

Baskets, pouches, and trays can be attached to walkers (Fig. 19-30). The attachment is used to carry needed items. The person is more independent and does not have to rely on others. The attachment also keeps the hands free to grip the walker.

Braces Braces support weak body parts. They are also used to prevent or correct deformities or to prevent the movement of a joint. Metal, plastic, or leather are used for braces. A brace is applied over the ankle, knee, or back (Fig. 19-31). An ankle-foot orthosis (AFO) is positioned in the shoe (Fig. 19-32). Then the foot is inserted. The device is secured in place with a Velcro strap. Bony points under braces are protected. Otherwise skin breakdown can occur.

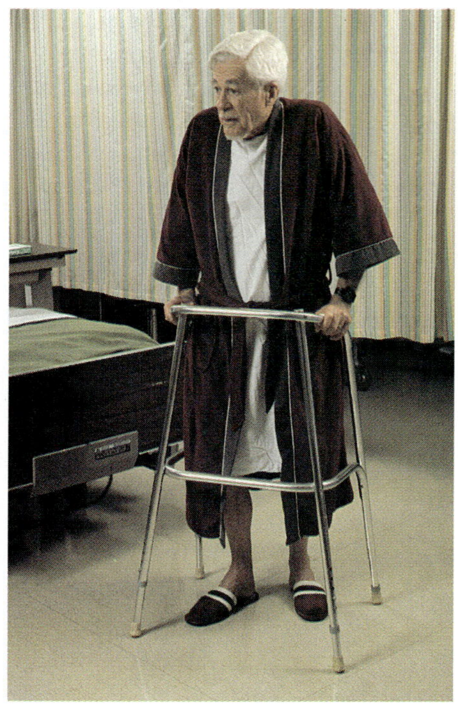

Fig. 19-28 *A walker.*

A

B

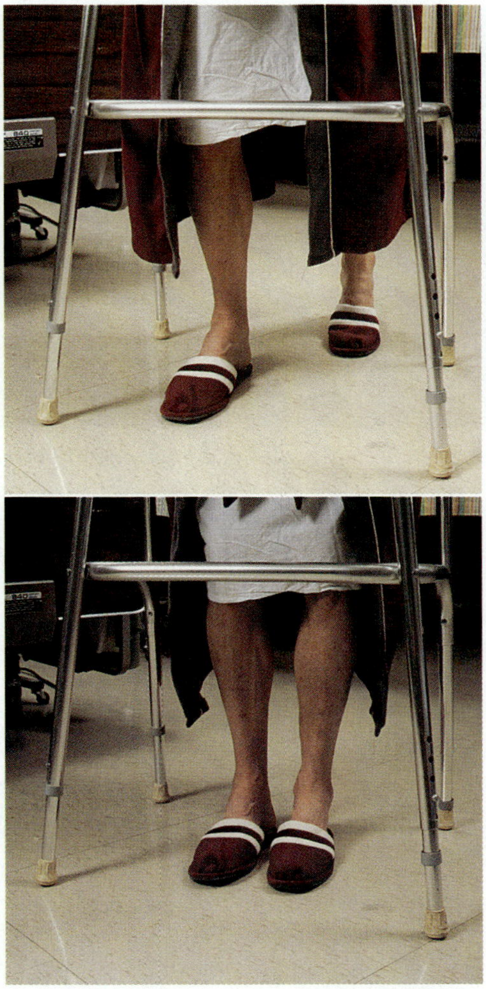

Fig. 19-29 *Walking with a walker. A, The walker is moved about 6 inches in front of the person. B, Both feet are moved up to the walker.*

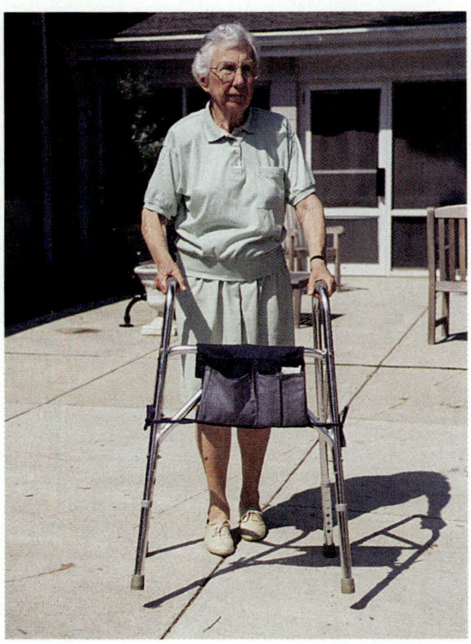

Fig. 19-30 *The pouch is a walker attachment.*

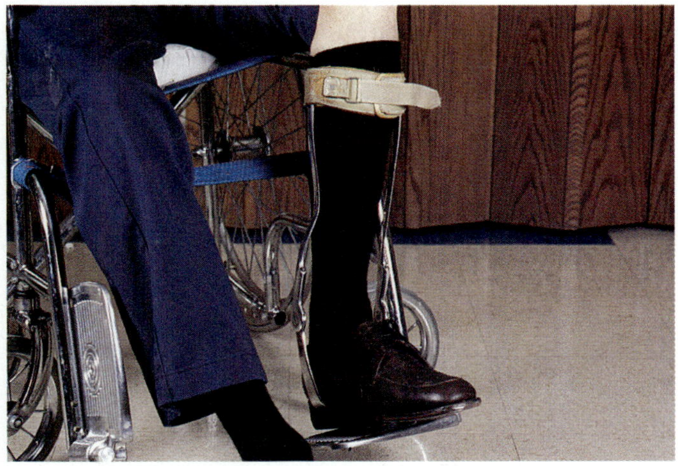

Fig. 19-31 *Leg brace.*

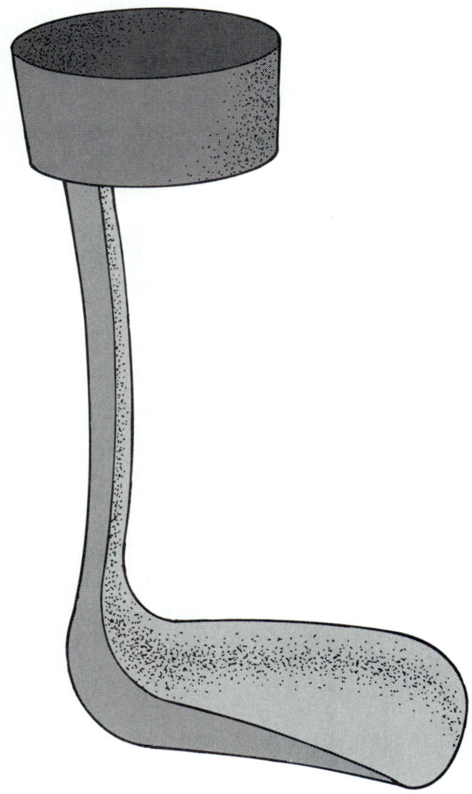

Fig. 19-32 *Ankle-foot orthosis (AFO).*

RECREATIONAL ACTIVITIES

OBRA requires activity programs for nursing facility residents. Recreational activities are important for the physical and mental well-being of elderly persons. Joints and muscles are exercised, and circulation is stimulated. Recreational activities also provide social opportunities and are mentally stimulating (Fig. 19-33).

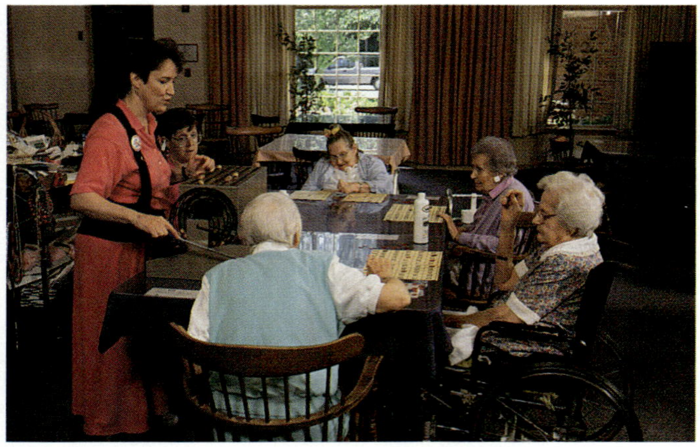

Fig. 19-33 *Recreational activities are important for the elderly.*

The activities must meet the interests and physical, mental, and psychosocial needs of each resident. Bingo, movies, dances, exercise groups, shopping trips, museum trips, concerts, and guest speakers are often arranged by nursing facilities. Some facilities have fashion shows, gourmet meal nights, family cookouts, and gardening activities. Grade school, high school, and college music groups often perform in nursing facilities.

The right to personal choice is protected. The resident chooses which activities to take part in. OBRA requires that activities promote physical, intellectual, social, and emotional well-being. Well-being is promoted when the resident attends activities of personal choice. The resident must not be forced to take part in an activity that has no interest to him or her.

Residents may need help getting to an activity. Some also need help in participating. You must provide assistance as necessary.

SUMMARY

Exercise and activity are necessary for physical and mental well-being. Complications from a lack of activity or exercise can occur from bed rest. You will position and exercise persons. Exercises prevent the complications of bed rest, especially muscle atrophy and contractures. Muscle atrophy makes walking difficult. A contracture causes loss of function and movement of the body part. A leg contracture may make normal walking impossible. Supportive devices and range-of-motion exercises also help prevent muscle atrophy and contractures.

Most persons eventually ambulate after illness, surgery, or injury. Many may need some assistance with walking at first. Some people need walking aids on a permanent or temporary basis. Doctors may prescribe crutches, canes, walkers, or braces.

Review Questions

Circle the best answer.

1 Mr. Parker is on bed rest. Which statement is *false?*

a No activities of daily living are allowed.
b Bed rest helps reduce pain and promote healing.
c Complications of bed rest include pressure sores, constipation, and blood clots.
d Contractures and muscle atrophy can occur.

2 Which helps to prevent plantar flexion?

a Bed boards
b A footboard
c Trochanter rolls
d Hand rolls

3 Which prevents the hip from turning outward?

a Bed boards
b A footboard
c Trochanter roll
d All of the above

4 A trapeze can be used to

a Lift the trunk off the bed
b Move up or turn in bed
c Strengthen arm muscles
d All of the above

5 Passive range-of-motion exercises are performed by

a The person
b A health team member
c The person with the assistance of another
d The person with the use of a trapeze

6 ROM exercises are ordered for Mr. Parker. You should do the following *except*

a Support the extremity being exercised
b Move the joint slowly, smoothly, and gently
c Force the joint through full range of motion
d Exercise only the joints indicated by the nurse

7 Flexion involves

a Bending the body part
b Straightening the body part
c Moving the body part toward the body
d Moving the body part away from the body

8 Which statement about ambulation is *false?*

a A transfer belt is used if the person is weak or unsteady.
b The person is allowed to shuffle or slide when beginning to walk after bed rest.
c Walking aids may be needed permanently or temporarily.
d Crutches, canes, walkers, and braces are common walking aids.

9 You are getting a person ready to crutch walk. You should do the following *except*

a Check the crutch tips
b Have the person wear street shoes
c Get any pair of crutches from physical therapy
d Tighten the bolts on the crutches

10 A single-tipped cane is used

a At waist level
b On the strong side
c On the weak side
d On either side

Circle T *if the answer is true and* F *if the answer is false.*

11 **T** **F** A single-tipped cane and a four-point cane give equal support.

12 **T** **F** When using a cane, the feet are moved first.

13 **T** **F** Mr. Parker uses a walker. First he moves the walker in front of him. Then he moves his right and left feet forward.

14 **T** **F** Mr. Parker starts to fall. You should try to prevent the fall.

15 **T** **F** A person has a brace. Bony areas need protection from skin breakdown.

16 **T** **F** Recreational activities exercise only muscles and joints.

Answers to these questions are on page 751.

Comfort, Rest, and Sleep

20

OBJECTIVES

- Define the key terms listed in this chapter
- Explain why comfort, rest, and sleep are important
- Describe four types of pain
- Explain why pain is a personal experience
- Describe the factors that affect pain
- List the signs and symptoms of pain
- Explain how you help the nurse assess pain
- List the nursing measures that relieve pain
- Explain why basic needs must be met before a person can rest
- Describe the nursing measures that promote rest
- Identify when rest is needed
- Describe the factors that affect sleep
- Describe the common sleep disorders
- Explain the importance of sleep
- Explain circadian rhythm and how it affects sleep
- Describe the stages of sleep
- Know the sleep requirements for each age group
- List the nursing measures that promote sleep
- List the OBRA requirements for comfort, rest, and sleep
- Describe the nursing measures that promote the resident's quality of life and comfort, rest, and sleep

KEY TERMS

acute pain Pain that is felt suddenly from injury, disease, trauma, or surgery; it generally lasts less than 6 months

chronic pain Pain lasting longer than 6 months; it may be constant or occur off and on

comfort A state of well-being; the person has no physical or emotional pain and is calm and at peace

discomfort To ache, hurt, or be sore; pain

distraction To change the person's center of attention

enuresis Urinary incontinence in bed at night

guided imagery Creating and focusing on an image

insomnia A chronic condition in which the person cannot sleep or stay asleep throughout the night

NREM sleep The stage of sleep when there is no rapid eye movement; nonREM sleep

pain Discomfort

phantom pain Pain felt in a body part that is no longer there

radiating pain Pain felt at the site of tissue damage and in nearby areas

relaxation To be free from mental or physical stress

REM sleep The stage of sleep when there is rapid eye movement

rest To be calm, at ease, and relaxed; to be free of anxiety and stress

sleep A state of unconsciousness, reduced voluntary muscle activity, and lowered metabolism

Comfort, rest, and sleep are needed for well-being. The total person—the physical, emotional, social, and spiritual—is affected by comfort, rest, and sleep problems. People need to be comfortable and free of pain. Discomfort and pain can be physical or emotional. Whatever the cause, discomfort and pain affect rest and sleep. Rest and sleep are needed for health and healing. The ill and injured need more rest and sleep than healthy persons.

Nursing plays a major role in promoting comfort, rest, and sleep. You will study about pain in this chapter. You will also learn how to promote comfort, rest, and sleep.

COMFORT

Comfort is a state of well-being. There is no physical or emotional pain. The person is calm and at peace. **Discomfort** or **pain** means to ache, hurt, or be sore. Discomfort is unpleasant. Comfort and discomfort are subjective (see page 478). That is, you cannot see, hear, touch, or smell the person's comfort or discomfort. You must rely on what the person tells you. Complaints are reported to the nurse. The information is used for the nursing process.

Pain is personal. It differs for each person. What *hurts* to one person may *ache* to another. What one person calls *sore,* another may call *aching.* Pain is subjective. If a person complains of pain or discomfort, the person *has* pain or discomfort. You must believe the person. Remember, you cannot see, hear, feel, or smell the pain.

Pain is a warning from the body. It means there is damage to body tissues. Pain often causes the person to seek health care.

Types of Pain

There are different types of pain. The doctor uses the type of pain when diagnosing. The type of pain also is used in the nursing process.

- **Acute pain** is felt suddenly from injury, disease, trauma, or surgery. There is tissue damage. It lasts a short time, usually less than 6 months. Acute pain decreases with healing.
- **Chronic pain** lasts longer than 6 months. Pain may be constant or occur off and on. There is no longer tissue damage. Chronic pain remains long after healing. Arthritis and cancer are common causes of chronic pain.

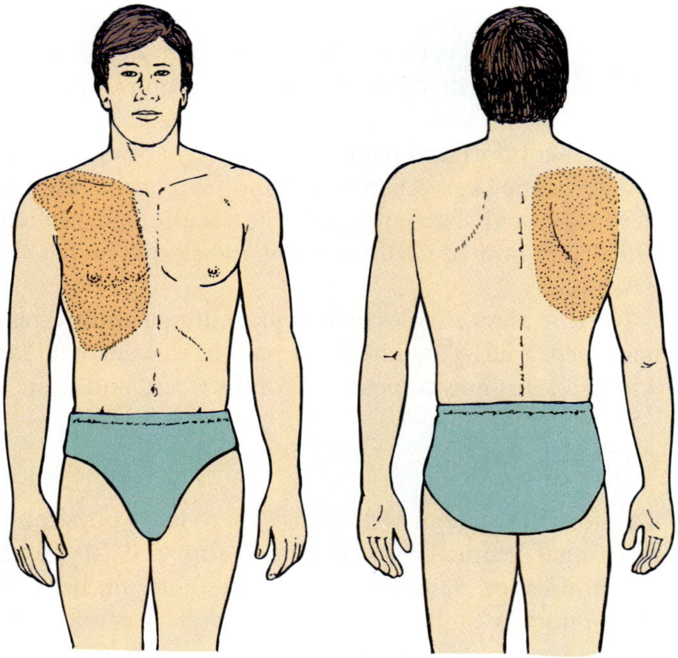

Fig. 20-1 *Gallbladder pain radiates to the right upper abdomen, the back, and the right shoulder.*

- **Radiating pain** is felt at the site of tissue damage and in nearby areas. Pain from a heart attack can be felt in the left chest, left jaw, left shoulder, and left arm. Pain from a diseased gallbladder may be felt in the right upper abdomen, the back, and the right shoulder (Fig. 20-1).
- **Phantom pain** is felt in a body part that is no longer there. A person with an amputated leg may still sense leg pain (see page 612).

Factors Affecting Pain

A person may handle pain well one time and poorly the next time. Many factors affect reactions to pain.

Past experience We learn from past experiences. They help us know what to do or what to expect at other times. Whether its going to school, driving a car, taking a test, shopping, having a baby, or caring for children, the past prepares us for similar events at another time. We also learn from the past experiences shared by family and friends.

A person may have had pain before. The severity of pain, its cause, how long it lasted, and if there was relief all affect the person's current response to pain. Knowing what to expect can help or hinder how the person handles pain.

Some have never had pain. When pain is felt, the person may be very afraid and anxious. Fear and anxiety affect pain.

Anxiety Anxiety relates to feelings of fear, dread, worry, and concern. The person feels uneasy and tense. The person may feel troubled or threatened or sense danger. Something is wrong but the person may not know what or why.

Pain and anxiety are related. Pain can cause anxiety. Anxiety increases how much pain the person feels. Lessening anxiety helps reduce pain. For example, the nurse explains to Mr. Smith that he will have pain after surgery. The nurse also explains that medication will be given for the pain. Mr. Smith knows the cause of the pain and what to expect. This helps reduce his anxiety and, therefore, the amount of pain felt.

Rest and sleep Rest and sleep restore energy. Body demands are reduced and the body repairs itself. Lack of needed rest and sleep affects how a person thinks and copes with daily life demands. Ill and injured persons need more sleep than usual. Many also have pain. Lack of rest and sleep can affect how the person deals with pain. Pain seems worse when the person is tired or restless. Also, the person usually pays more attention to pain when tired and unable to rest or sleep.

Attention The more a person thinks about the pain, the worse it can seem. The pain may be so severe that it is all the person thinks about. However, even mild pain can seem worse if the person thinks about it all the time. Pain often seems worse at night. Activity is less, it is quiet, there are no visitors, the radio or television is off, others are asleep. This applies to home, hospitals, or nursing facilities. Being unable to sleep also allows the person to think about the pain.

Personal and family duties How a person deals with pain often relates to personal and family obligations. Pain may be ignored if children must be cared for. Some people go to work when having pain. Others deny pain because they fear a serious illness. The illness can interfere with earning money, going to school, or caring for children, a spouse, or ill parents.

The value or meaning of pain To admit pain is a sign of weakness for some people. It also may mean a serious illness and the need for painful procedures and treatments. Therefore pain is ignored or denied. Sometimes pain results in pleasure. The pain of childbirth is one example.

For some persons, pain means not having to work or assume daily routines. Pain can be used to avoid certain people or things. Pain is useful for the person. Some people like being doted on and pampered by others when in pain. Such attention is wanted and valued by the person.

Support from others Pain is often easier to deal with when family and friends offer comfort and support. The pain of childbirth is made easier when a loving father gives support and encouragement. A child can bear pain much better when comforted by a caring mother, father, or family member. The use of touch by an important person in the individual's life is very comforting. Just being nearby also helps.

Some people do not have caring family or friends. They must deal with the pain alone. Being alone can increase anxiety. It also gives the person more time to think about the pain. Facing pain alone is hard for everyone, especially children and the elderly.

Age Children may not understand pain. They know it is a bad feeling. They have had fewer experiences with pain and do not know what to expect. They also have fewer ways of dealing with the pain. Adults can take some pain medications bought in stores. They also know that heat or cold applications help to relieve pain. They can take measures to distract their attention away from the pain. Music, working, reading, and hobbies are distracting for some adults. Children do not know how to help relieve their own pain. They must rely on adults for help.

Babies, infants, toddlers, and preschool children have difficulty alerting adults to pain. Babies and infants cry, fuss, and are restless. Such behaviors also mean hunger and the need for a diaper change. Toddlers and preschool children may not have the words to express pain. Adults must be alert for behaviors and situations that signal pain.

Elderly persons may have decreased pain sensations. They may not feel pain as greatly as younger people (see Chapter 7). The need for pain medication may be less. The elderly may not feel pain or it may not feel severe. This places them at greater risk for undetected disease or injury. Remember, pain occurs when there is tissue damage. Therefore, pain alerts the person to illness or injury. If pain is not felt, the person does not know to seek health care.

Some elderly persons have many health problems that cause pain. New pain may not be felt because of chronic pain in nearby body parts. Elderly persons may also ignore or deny new pain. They may think it is related to an existing health problem. Like other adults, the elderly may deny or ignore pain because of what it may mean.

Some elderly persons have cognitive impairments. That is, thinking and reasoning are affected. Some cannot verbally communicate pain. Nursing staff must be alert to signs of pain in all persons. This is especially important for the elderly with cognitive impairments and for young children.

Culture Culture affects how a person responds to pain (Box 20-1 on page 478). In some cultures the person in pain is stoic. To be stoic means to show no reaction to joy, sorrow, pleasure, or pain. Strong verbal and nonverbal reactions to pain are seen in other cultures.

BOX 20-1 TOP TEN COUNTRIES OF ORIGIN OF IMMIGRANTS TO THE UNITED STATES:* PAIN REACTIONS

Country	Pain Reactions
Mexico	Emotional self-restraint and stoic inhibition of strong feelings and emotional expression are seen. Expression of pain may be a self-help relief mechanism. Pain relief might be refused as a means for atonement. During labor the loud verbal repetition of "Aye, yie, yie" requires long, slow breaths, thus becoming a culturally and medically appropriate method of pain relief.
Vietnam	Pain may be severe before relief is requested.
Philippines	People may appear stoic, believing that pain is the will of God and that God will give them the strength to bear it.
Former Soviet Union	People are communicative about pain. Some prefer injections for pain relief.
Dominican Republic	None reported.
Mainland China	Strong negative feelings, such as anger and pain, are often suppressed. A display of emotion is considered a weakness of character. Because it is considered impolite to accept something the first time it is offered, pain relief interventions must be offered more than once.
India	The person has a quiet acceptance of pain and will accept some relief measures.
El Salvador	None reported.
Poland	Tolerance of pain is valued. Pain may be expressed by facial grimaces or by crying out.
United Kingdom	None reported.

*Information based on data gathered through 1992 by the U.S. Department of Immigration and Naturalization Services.
From Geissler EM: *Pocket guide to cultural assessment,* St Louis, 1994, Mosby–Year Book.

Signs and Symptoms

Remember, pain is subjective. You cannot see, hear, feel, or smell pain. You must rely on what the person tells you. Be sure to promptly report to the nurse any information you collect about pain. Use the person's exact words when you report and record. The nurse needs the following information when assessing the person's pain.

- **Location.** Where is the pain? Ask the person to point to the area of pain (Fig. 20-2). Remember, pain can radiate. Ask the person if the pain is anywhere else and to point to those areas.
- **Onset and duration.** When did the pain start? How long has the pain lasted?
- **Intensity.** Does the person complain of mild, moderate, or severe pain? Ask the person to rate the pain on a scale of 1 to 10, with 10 being the most severe.
- **Description.** Ask the person to describe the pain. Box 20-2 lists some words used to describe pain. Make notes of the words used by the person and report them to the nurse. Use the person's own words when reporting.
- **Factors causing pain.** These are called *precipitating* factors. To precipitate means to cause. Such factors include moving or turning in bed, coughing or deep breathing, and exercise. Ask what the person was doing both before and when the pain started.
- **Vital signs.** What are the person's pulse, respirations, and blood pressure? Increases in these vital signs often occur with pain.
- **Other signs and symptoms.** Does the person have other symptoms: dizziness, nausea, vomiting, weakness, numbness or tingling, or others? Box 20-3 lists the signs and symptoms that often occur with pain.

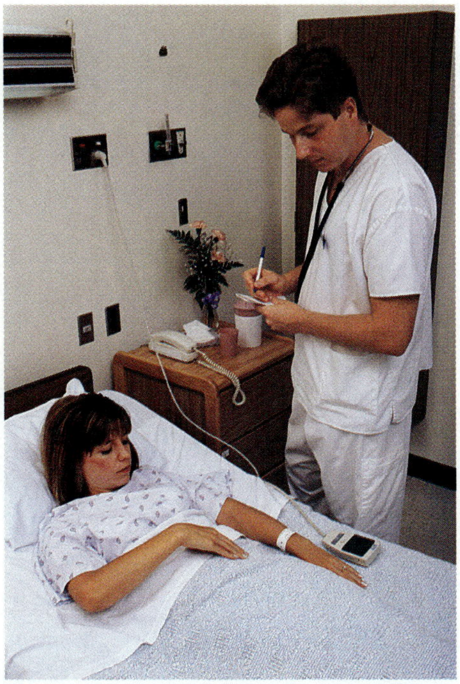

Fig. 20-2 *The person points to the area of pain so the nursing assistant knows its exact location.*

BOX 20-2 Words Used to Describe Pain

- Aching
- Burning
- Cramping
- Crushing
- Dull
- Gnawing
- Knifelike
- Piercing
- Pressure
- Sharp
- Sore
- Squeezing
- Stabbing
- Throbbing
- Viselike

BOX 20-3 Signs and Symptoms of Pain

Body responses

- Increased pulse, respirations, and blood pressure
- Sweating (diaphoresis)
- Nausea
- Vomiting
- Pale skin (pallor)

Behaviors

- Changes in speech: slow or rapid; loud or quiet
- Crying
- Gasping
- Grimacing
- Groaning
- Grunting
- Holding the affected body part (splinting)
- Irritability
- Maintaining one position; refusing to move
- Moaning
- Quietness
- Restlessness
- Rubbing
- Screaming

Nursing Measures

The nurse uses the nursing process to promote comfort and relieve pain. Box 20-4 lists the nursing measures that may be part of the person's care plan. You have learned how to perform most of these measures in earlier chapters (Fig. 20-3). You have also learned why they are important for comfort.

Other measures may be used to control pain. These include distraction, relaxation, and guided imagery. The nurse may ask you to assist with these measures. You will be given instruction or guidance to perform them properly.

Distraction means to change the person's center of attention. The person's attention is moved away from the pain. Listening to music, playing games, singing, praying, watching television, and needlework are some ways to distract attention.

Relaxation means to be free from mental or physical stress. This state reduces pain and anxiety. The nurse teaches the person relaxation techniques. The person is taught to breathe deeply and slowly and to contract and relax muscle groups. The person must be in a comfortable position in a quiet room. Box 20-5 is an example of how the nurse teaches the person relaxation.

Guided imagery is creating and focusing on an image. The person is asked to create a pleasant scene. The nurse notes this on the care plan so nursing team members use

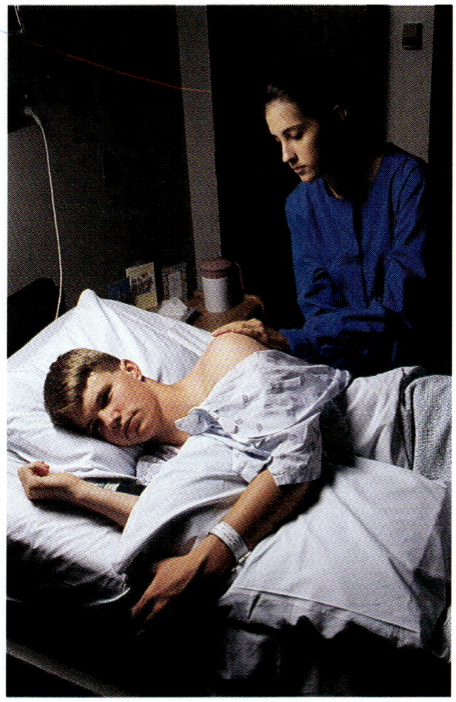

Fig. 20-3 *The nursing assistant implements nursing measures to relieve pain. The person is positioned in good body alignment with pillows used for support. The room is darkened. Blankets provide warmth. A back massage is given to provide touch and promote relaxation.*

BOX 20-4 Nursing Measures to Promote Comfort and Relieve Pain

- Position the person in good body alignment; use pillows for support.
- Make sure bed linens are tight and wrinkle-free.
- Make sure the person is not lying on drainage tubes.
- Offer the bedpan or urinal or assist the person to the bathroom or commode.
- Provide blankets for warmth and to prevent chilling.
- Use correct lifting, moving, and turning procedures.
- Wait one-half hour after pain medication has been given before giving care or performing procedures.
- Give a back massage.
- Provide soft music to distract the person.
- Use touch to provide comfort.
- Allow family members and friends at the bedside as requested by the person.
- Avoid sudden or jarring movements of the bed.
- Handle the person gently.
- Practice safety measures if the person is receiving strong pain medication or sedatives:
  - *Keep the bed in the low position.
  - *Raise side rails as directed.
  - *Check on the person every 10 to 15 minutes.
  - *Provide assistance when the person is up.
- Apply warm or cold applications as directed by the nurse.
- Provide a calm, quiet, darkened environment.

BOX 20-5 Relaxation Taught by the Nurse

Let's begin by finding as comfortable a position as possible. Arms at your side . . . legs uncrossed. . . . Move until you feel at ease. . . . Take a deep breath. Feel your stomach and chest slowly rise. . . . Relax. . . . Now breathe out slowly . . . slowly . . . and relax.

Count to 4, inhaling on 1 and 2, exhaling on 3 and 4. . . . Continue to breathe slowly. . . . Your body is beginning to relax. . . . Think "relax". . . . Feel the parts of your body. . . . Notice any tension in your muscles. . . . Continue to breathe slowly . . . and relax.

Concentrate on your face . . . your jaws . . . your neck. . . . Notice any tightness. . . . Breathe in warmth and relaxation. . . . Concentrate on any tension in your hands. . . . Notice how it feels. . . . Now make a fist—a tight fist! As you begin to exhale, relax your fist. . . . Good! Notice how your hand feels . . . Think "relax". . . . Your hand feels warm . . . heavy or light. . . . Just relax more . . . and more. Now focus on your forearms. . . . Notice any tension. . . . Relax your arms. . . . Feel your body relaxing. . . . Let the feelings of relaxation spread from your fingers and hands through the muscles of your arms.

From Potter PA, Perry AG: *Fundamentals of nursing: concepts, process and practice*, St Louis, 1993, Mosby–Year Book.

BOX 20-6 Guided Imagery

Imagine yourself lying on a cool bed of grass with sounds of rushing water from a nearby stream. It's a balmy day. You turn to see a patch of blue wildflowers in bloom and can smell their fragrance.

From Potter PA and Perry AG: *Fundamentals of nursing: concepts, process and practice*, St Louis, 1993, Mosby–Year Book.

the same image with the person. The nurse uses a calm, soft voice when helping the person focus on the image. Soft music, a blanket for warmth, and a darkened room may help. The nurse coaches the person to focus on the image and then to practice relaxation exercises. Box 20-6 is an example of how the nurse assists the person with guided imagery.

The doctor may order medications to control or relieve pain. The nurse gives these medications. Such medications can cause drowsiness, dizziness, and coordination problems. Therefore the person must be protected from injury. The nurse will alert you to any needed safety measures.

REST AND SLEEP

Comfort, rest, and sleep are related (Fig. 20-4). To rest, a person must be free of pain or discomfort. A person must be at rest before sleep occurs. Rest and sleep restore energy and well-being. Illness and injury increase the need for rest and sleep. The body needs more energy for healing and repair. When ill or injured, more energy than normal is needed to perform daily activities. Pain interferes with rest and sleep. Health care environments, routines, and procedures can too.

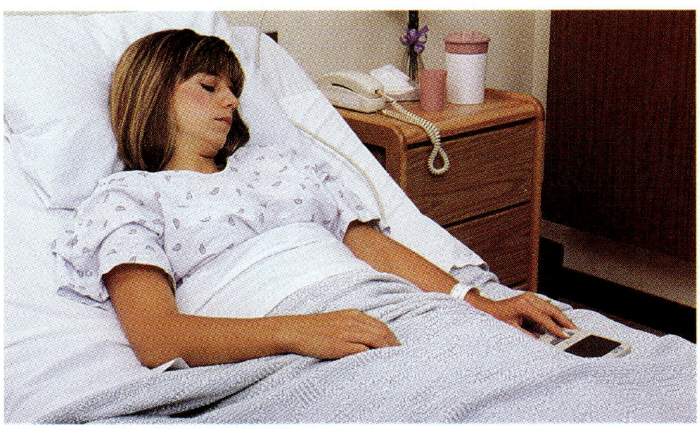

Fig. 20-4 *Comfort is needed to rest. Rest precedes sleep.*

Rest

Rest means being calm, at ease, and relaxed. The person is free of anxiety and stress. Rest may involve physical inactivity. Or the person may do things that he or she finds calming and relaxing. Reading, music, television, needlework, prayer, gardening, baking, golf, walking, and carpentry are among the activities some people find to be restful (Fig. 20-5).

Basic needs must be met for a person to rest. Thirst, hunger, the need to eliminate, and pain or discomfort can affect rest. You can promote rest by meeting physical needs. The person must also be in a comfortable position and in good body alignment. A quiet environment promotes rest. So does a bed that is clean, dry, and wrinkle-free. Some find it easier to rest in a clean, neat, and uncluttered room.

Safety and security needs must be met. The person must feel safe from falling or being injured in some other way. Having the call bell within reach helps the person feel secure. The person knows that help can be called if needed. Understanding the purpose of treatments and therapies also helps the person feel safe. So does knowing how procedures are done. That is why you always explain the procedure before it is performed.

Many persons have certain rituals or routines before resting. These may include going to the bathroom, brushing teeth, washing the face and hands, praying, having a snack or beverage, locking doors, or making sure children or loved ones are safe at home. Rest may involve being warm. The person may want a favorite blanket or afghan. Routines and rituals are followed whenever possible.

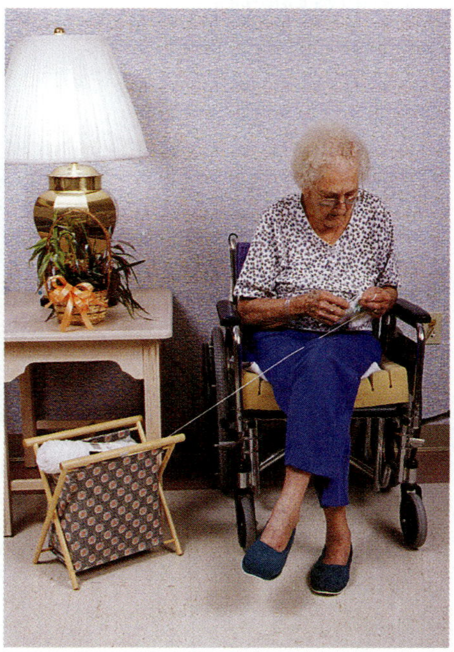

Fig. 20-5 *Needle work is relaxing for this lady.*

The need for love and belonging is also important for rest. Visits or telephone calls from family and friends may help the person relax. The person knows that others care and are concerned. Reading cards and letters may also help the person relax and rest (Fig. 20-6).

Esteem needs relate to feeling good about oneself. A person may find hospital gowns embarrassing. Others fear being exposed. Many persons rest better wearing their own gowns or pajamas. Personal appearance also affects esteem. Hair care, being clean and free of body odors, and other hygiene and grooming measures all help people feel good about themselves. If esteem needs are met, the person may rest easier.

Some people are refreshed after resting for 15 or 20 minutes. Others need more time. Hospital routines usually allow time for rest in the afternoon. Nursing facilities often have rest periods in the afternoon after lunch and before afternoon activities.

Ill or injured persons need to rest more often. They may need to rest during or after a procedure. For example, a bath may tire Mr. Smith. Then you need to allow him to rest before making the bed. Getting dressed may tire him. Some people may need a few hours to complete oral hygiene, bathing, grooming, and dressing. Others need to rest after meals. Needed rest is important. Do not push the person beyond his or her limits. Allow rest periods as they are needed. Do not rush the person.

Distraction, relaxation, and guided imagery also promote rest. So does a back massage. You must also plan and organize care so that the person can rest without interruptions.

The doctor may order bed rest for a person. Bed rest, its complications, and how to prevent complications are presented in Chapter 19.

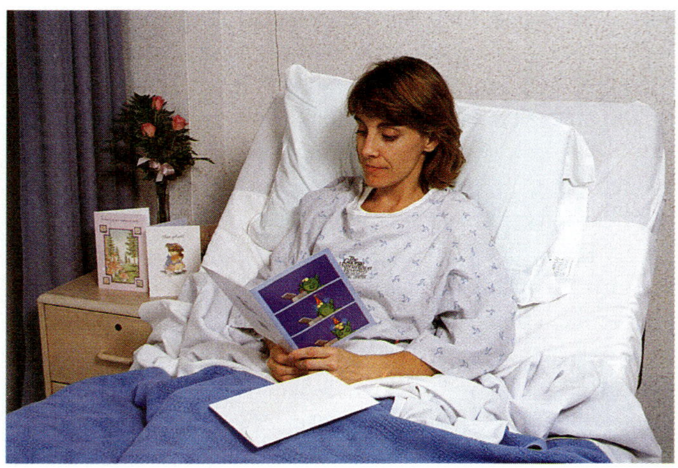

Fig. 20-6 *The person is reading cards and letters received from family and friends.*

Sleep

Sleep is a state of unconsciousness, reduced voluntary muscle activity, and lowered metabolism. An unconscious person is unaware of the environment and cannot respond to people and things in the environment. As you know, people can be awakened from sleep. Alarm clocks, voices, and crying babies or children easily awaken sleeping persons. The unconsciousness is temporary. Voluntary muscles are skeletal muscles. During sleep, there are no voluntary arm or leg movements. Metabolism is the burning of food and energy for use by the body. Less energy is needed during sleep. Thus metabolism is reduced during sleep.

Sleep is a basic need. It allows the mind and body to rest. The body saves energy. Body functions slow. Vital signs fall. That is, blood pressure, temperature, pulse, and respirations are less than when awake. Tissue healing and repair occur during sleep. Sleep is also restorative. It lowers stress, tension, and anxiety. It refreshes and renews the person. That is, the person regains energy and mental alertness. The person thinks and functions better after needed sleep.

Circadian rhythm Sleep is a natural state. It occurs regularly. Sleep is part of circadian rhythm. Circadian comes from the Latin words *circa* meaning *about* and *dies* meaning *day.* **Circadian rhythm** is a pattern based on a 24-hour cycle. It is a daily rhythm called the *day-night cycle* or *body rhythm.* Functioning is affected by circadian rhythm. Some people function better in the morning. They are more alert and active; they think and react better. Others function better in the evening.

Circadian rhythm includes a sleep-wake cycle. The person's *biological clock* signals the time for sleep and the time to wake up. You have usual times for going to sleep and waking up. You may awaken before the alarm clock goes off. That is all part of your biological clock. Health care facilities often interfere with a person's circadian rhythm and the sleep-wake cycle. Sleep problems easily occur.

Many people work evening and night shifts. They include health care workers, police officers, fire fighters, fast food workers, and factory workers. Their bodies must adjust to changes in the sleep-wake cycle.

Sleep cycle There are two phases of sleep. Nonrapid eye movement is **NREM sleep** or **nonREM sleep.** NREM sleep has four stages. Sleep goes from light to deep as the person moves through the four stages.

The rapid eye movement phase is called **REM sleep.** The person is hard to arouse. Mental restoration occurs during REM sleep. Events and problems of the previous day are thought to be reviewed during REM sleep. The person prepares for the next day.

Box 20-7 on page 484 shows the stages of NREM and REM sleep. There are usually 4 to 6 cycles of NREM and REM sleep during the 7 to 8 hours of sleep each night. Stage 1 of NREM is usually not repeated (Fig. 20-7).

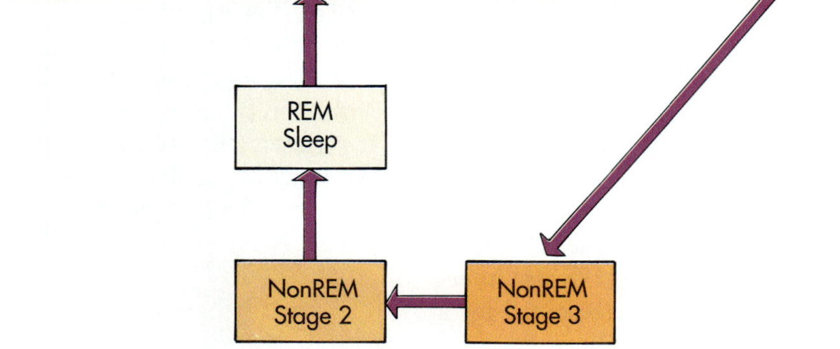

Fig. 20-7 *Adult sleep cycle.*

BOX 20-7 Sleep Cycle

Stage 1: NREM sleep
- Lightest sleep level
- Lasts a few minutes
- Gradual fall in vital signs
- Gradual lowering of metabolism
- Person feels drowsy and relaxed
- Person easily aroused
- Daydreaming feeling after being aroused

Stage 2: NREM sleep
- Sound sleep
- Relaxation increases
- Still easy to arouse
- Lasts 10 to 20 minutes
- Body functions continue to slow

Stage 3: NREM sleep
- First stages of deep sleep
- Hard to arouse the person
- Person rarely moves
- Muscles relax completely
- Vital signs fall
- Lasts 15 to 30 minutes

Stage 4: NREM sleep
- Deepest stage of sleep
- Hard to arouse the person
- Body rests and is restored
- Vital signs much lower than when awake
- Lasts about 15 to 30 minutes
- Sleepwalking and **enuresis** (urinary incontinence in bed at night) may occur

REM sleep
- Vivid, full-color dreaming
- Usually starts 50 to 90 minutes after sleep has begun
- Rapid eye movements
- Blood pressure, pulse, and respirations may fluctuate
- Voluntary muscles are relaxed
- Mental restoration occurs
- Hard to arouse the person
- Lasts about 20 minutes

Modified from Potter PA and Perry AG: *Fundamentals of nursing: concepts, process and practice,* St Louis, 1993, Mosby–Year Book.

Sleep requirements The amount of sleep needed varies for each age group. The amount needed decreases with age (Table 20-1). Infants need more sleep than toddlers. Toddlers need more than preschool children. School-age children need more than teenagers. The elderly need less sleep than middle-age adults.

Factors affecting sleep Several factors affect the amount and quality of sleep. Quality relates to how well the person slept and if needed amounts of NREM and REM sleep were obtained.

- **Illness.** Illness increases the need for sleep. However, the signs and symptoms of illness can interfere with sleep. They include pain, nausea, vomiting, coughing, difficulty breathing, diarrhea, frequent voiding, and itching. Treatments and therapies can also interfere with sleep. The person may be awakened for a

TABLE 20-1 Average Sleep Requirements

Age Group	Hours Per Day
Newborns (birth to 4 weeks)	14 to 18
Infants (4 weeks to 1 year)	12 to 14
Toddlers (1 to 3 years)	11 to 12
Preschoolers (3 to 6 years)	11 to 12
Middle and late childhood (6 to 12 years)	10 to 11
Adolescents (12 to 18 years)	8 to 9
Young adults (18 to 40 years)	7 to 8
Middle-age adults (40 to 65 years)	7
Older adults (65 years and older)	5 to 7

treatment or a medication. Dressing changes may be needed. Vital signs may need to be taken. Traction or a cast can cause uncomfortable positions (see Fig. 28-13). The emotional effects of illness can affect sleep. These include fear, anxiety, and worry.

- **Nutrition.** Weight loss or gain affect sleep. The need for sleep increases with weight gain. It decreases with weight loss. Some foods affect sleep. Those with caffeine (chocolate, coffee, tea, and colas) prevent sleep. The protein L-tryptophan tends to help sleep. It is found in milk, cheese, and beef (Fig. 20-8).
- **Exercise.** Exercise is good for the body. It improves health and fitness. Exercise requires energy. The person usually feels good after exercising. Eventually the person tires. Being tired helps the person sleep well at night. Exercising right before bedtime interferes with sleep. Exercise causes the release of substances into the bloodstream that stimulate the body. Therefore a person should exercise no more than 2 hours before bedtime.
- **Environment.** People adjust to their usual sleeping environments. They get used to such things as the bed, pillows, noises in the home or neighborhood, lighting, and sleeping partner. Any change in the usual environment can affect the amount and quality of sleep.
- **Drugs and other substances.** Some drugs promote sleep. These are commonly called *sleeping pills.* Drugs given for anxiety, depression, and pain may cause the person to sleep. However, these drugs and sleeping pills reduce the length of REM sleep. Remember, mental restoration occurs during REM sleep. Behavior problems and sleep deprivation can occur. Alcohol is a drug. Alcohol tends to cause drowsiness and sleep. However, it interferes with REM sleep. Those under the influence of alcohol may awaken during sleep. Difficulty returning to sleep is common. Some drugs contain caffeine. As stated earlier, caffeine is a stimulant and prevents sleep. Besides drugs, it is found in coffee, tea, chocolate, and colas. The side effects of some drugs can disrupt sleep. These include frequent voiding and nightmares.

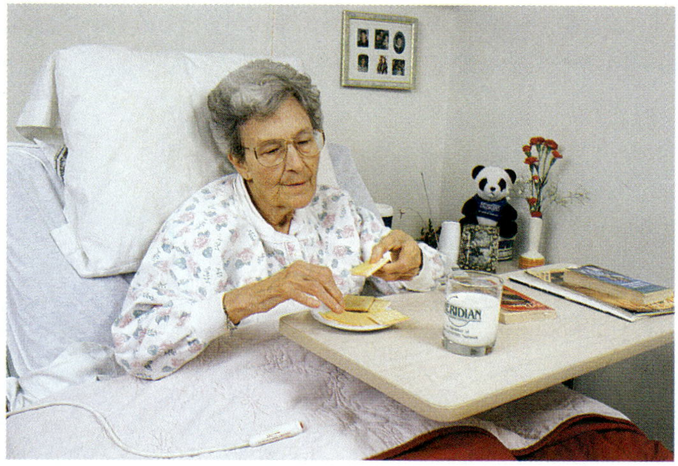

Fig. 20-8 *A bedtime snack of milk, cheese, and crackers helps to promote sleep.*

- **Lifestyle changes.** Lifestyle relates to a person's daily routines and way of living. Work, school, play, and social events are all part of lifestyle. Lifestyle changes can affect sleep. Travel, vacation, and social events often affect usual bedtimes and when the person awakens. Children usually stay up later during school holidays. They may sleep later, too. If work hours change, the person needs to change sleep hours. Such changes affect normal sleep-wake cycles and the circadian rhythm.
- **Emotional problems.** Fear, worry, and anxiety affect sleep. These may be due to work, personal, or family problems. Loss of a close family member or friend is another cause. Money problems are stressful. People may have difficulty falling asleep or they awaken often. Difficulty getting back to sleep may occur.

Sleep disorders Difficulty sleeping one night is not a sleep disorder. Sleep disorders involve repeated problems. The quantity and quality of sleep are affected. Sleep disorders affect lifestyle. Box 20-8 on page 486 lists the signs and symptoms that may be observed.

BOX 20-8 Signs and Symptoms of Sleep Disorders

- Hand tremors
- Slowed responses to questions, conversations, or situations
- Reduced word memory; difficulty finding the right word
- Decreased reasoning and judgment
- Irregular pulse
- Red, puffy eyes
- Dark circles under the eyes
- Moodiness; mood swings
- Disorientation
- Irritability
- Fatigue
- Sleepiness
- Agitation
- Restlessness
- Decreased attention
- Hallucinations
- Coordination problems
- Slurred speech

Insomnia **Insomnia** is a chronic condition in which the person cannot sleep or stay asleep throughout the night. There are three forms of insomnia:

- Being unable to fall asleep
- Being unable to stay asleep
- Early awakening and being unable to fall back asleep

Emotional problems are common causes of insomnia. The fear of dying during sleep is another cause. Some people are afraid of falling asleep and not waking up. This may occur after recent heart disease or after being told of a terminal illness. The fear of not being able to sleep is another cause. The physical and emotional discomforts of illness can also cause insomnia.

The nurse plans measures to promote sleep (page 473). However, the emotional or physical problems causing the insomnia also must be treated.

Sleep deprivation When a person experiences sleep deprivation, the amount and quality of sleep are decreased. Sleep is interrupted. NREM and REM sleep stages are not completed. Illness and hospital care are common causes of sleep deprivation. Patients in intensive care units (ICUs) are at great risk. ICU lights are on much of the time, there are many care measures, and there are many sounds from the equipment needed for treatment and care. Factors that affect sleep can also lead to sleep deprivation. Sleep deprivation results in many of the signs and symptoms listed in Box 20-8.

Sleepwalking The person who sleepwalks leaves the bed and walks about. The person is not aware of sleepwalking and has no memory of the event on awakening. Children sleepwalk more than adults. The event may last 3 to 4 minutes or longer.

Stress, fatigue, and some medications can cause sleepwalking. The person must be protected from injury. The risk of falling is great. Intravenous infusions, catheters, nasogastric tubes, and other tubings are also sources of injury. The tubes or catheters can be pulled out of the body when the person gets out of bed. Sleepwalkers must be guided back to bed. They startle easily so you must gently awaken them.

Promoting sleep The nurse assesses the person to see if there is a problem with sleep. Your observations are important. Be sure to report any of the signs and symptoms listed in Box 20-8. The nurse plans measures to promote sleep. Several of the measures listed in Box 20-9 may be chosen. Be sure to check the care plan so that you give the correct care. Also report your observations so the nurse can evaluate whether the goal of a regular sleep pattern has been met.

BOX 20-9 Nursing Measures to Promote Sleep

- Organize care to allow for uninterrupted rest.
- Avoid physical activity before bedtime.
- Encourage the person to avoid tending to business or family matters before bedtime.
- Let bedtime be flexible: bedtime should be when the person is tired and fatigued, not because it is a certain time.
- Provide a comfortable room temperature.
- Allow the person to take a warm bath or shower.
- Provide a bedtime snack (milk).
- Avoid caffeine (coffee, tea, colas, chocolate).
- Avoid alcoholic beverages.
- Have the person void before going to bed; change diapers.
- Follow bedtime rituals.
- Make sure the person wears loose-fitting nightwear.
- Provide adequate warmth (blankets, socks) for those who tend to be cold.
- Reduce noise.
- Darken the room by closing shades, blinds, and the privacy curtain; shut off or dim lights.
- Dim lights in hallways and the nursing unit.
- Make sure linens are clean, dry, and wrinkle-free.
- Position the person in good alignment.
- Support body parts as ordered.
- Make sure the person is in a comfortable position.
- Give a back massage.
- Implement measures to relieve pain.
- Allow the person to read; read to children.
- Allow the person to listen to music.
- Allow the person to watch television.
- Assist with relaxation exercises as ordered.
- Sit and talk with patients or residents.

OBRA AND QUALITY OF LIFE

OBRA requires that residents be given care that promotes well-being. Comfort, rest, and sleep are necessary for physical, emotional, and mental well-being. OBRA requires that resident rooms be designed and equipped to provide for comfort. The following room requirements under OBRA promote quality of life and comfort, rest, and sleep:

- No more than 4 residents in a room
- Suspended curtain that extends around the bed for privacy
- A bed of proper height and size for the resident
- Clean, comfortable mattress
- Linens appropriate to the weather and climate
- Clean and orderly room
- Odor-free room
- Room temperature between 71 and 81 degrees F
- Acceptable noise level
- Adequate ventilation and room humidity
- Appropriate lighting

The right to personal choice is also important. Residents may have very specific rituals and routines before bedtime. They are to be allowed if safe. The person may perform personal hygiene measures in a certain order. Some residents like to check on friends in the facility before going to bed. Some may be given the responsibility of turning off lights at bedtime. A bedtime snack may be important. Watching certain television shows in bed may be a bedtime routine. Others may read the Bible, pray, or say a rosary before going to sleep. Whatever the routine or ritual, it is important to the resident.

The resident is involved in planning care. The person should be allowed to choose when to take a nap or go to sleep. The person also has the right to choose what measures are helpful in promoting comfort, rest, and sleep. You must follow the care plan and the resident's wishes.

Remember, the elderly need less sleep than younger persons. A 9:00 PM (2100) bedtime and a 6:00 AM (0600) wake time may not suit some residents. For weak and ill residents, an early bedtime may be needed. Again, personal choice is important.

SUMMARY

Comfort, rest, and sleep affect the well-being of the total person. If in pain, a person cannot rest well. If the person cannot rest, sleep does not occur. Problems result when a person does not get enough rest and sleep. The quality of sleep is also important.

Illness and injury commonly result in pain. Pain is a personal experience. It differs for different people. The degree of pain felt depends on the person and the amount of tissue damage. Remember, you cannot see, feel, smell, or hear the person's pain. If the person complains of pain, you must report the pain to the nurse. Be sure to report its location, onset and duration, and intensity. You also need to provide the person's description of the pain and any factors causing the pain.

The nurse uses the nursing process to relieve the person's pain. Pain and factors affecting the pain are assessed. A nursing diagnosis is made and goals set. Nursing measures are planned and implemented by the nursing team. The nurse also evaluates the pain to see if the measures relieved the pain.

Rest and sleep restore energy and well-being. Ill and injured persons need more rest and sleep than healthy persons. Many factors interfere with sleep. These include pain, the health care environment, and the many routines and procedures performed by the health care team.

The person at rest is calm, at ease, and relaxed. Basic needs must be met for rest to occur. You must assist in meeting physical needs, safety and security needs, the need for love and belonging, and esteem needs. Ill and injured persons need more rest than when healthy. They should be allowed to rest whenever it is needed. Health care routines and schedules may need changing to allow for rest.

Sleep is a natural state during which the mind and body rest. Tissues heal and the body repairs itself. Energy and mental alertness are regained for functioning and clear thinking. Sleep is part of circadian rhythm. Problems occur if the person's sleep-wake cycle is affected.

The amount of sleep needed depends on the person's age. Younger persons need more sleep than older persons. The amount and quality of sleep can be affected by many factors. They include illness, nutrition, exercise, environment, drugs and other substances, lifestyle changes, and emotional problems. Sleep deprivation results when the amount and quality of sleep and NREM and REM sleep are affected. As with pain, the nurse uses the nursing process to promote sleep and prevent sleep disorders.

Comfort, rest, and sleep are important for quality of life and well-being. OBRA has certain requirements that promote the resident's comfort, rest, and sleep. They relate to the bed, mattress, room temperature, noise level, lighting, linens, odors, and the number of residents in each room. The right to personal choice and being involved in planning care are other ways to promote the resident's comfort, rest, and sleep.

REVIEW QUESTIONS

Circle the best *answer.*

1 These statements are about pain. Which is *false?*
- **a** Pain is objective. It can be seen, heard, smelled, or felt.
- **b** Pain is a warning from the body. It means there is damage to tissues.
- **c** Pain is personal. It is different for each person.
- **d** Pain is used to make diagnoses.

2 A person complains of pain in the left chest, up into the left jaw, and down to the left shoulder and left arm. This is
- **a** Acute pain
- **b** Chronic pain
- **c** Radiating pain
- **d** Phantom pain

3 Which of these factors affect how a person deals with pain?
- **a** Past experience, anxiety, and age
- **b** Rest, sleep, and attention
- **c** Family duties, support from others, and the meaning of pain
- **d** All of the above

4 Elderly persons may not report acute pain because
- **a** Pain sensations may be decreased
- **b** Chronic pain in the same area may mask new pain
- **c** The pain is being denied or ignored
- **d** All of the above

5 Mr. Smith complains of pain. You should do the following *except*
- **a** Ask him to point to where the pain is felt
- **b** Ask him when the pain started
- **c** Ask him to describe the pain
- **d** Ask to look at the pain

6 You take Mr. Smith's vital signs after he complains of pain. You should expect the following changes *except*
- **a** Increased temperature
- **b** Increased pulse rate
- **c** Increased respiratory rate
- **d** Increased blood pressure

7 The nurse decides to give Mr. Smith some pain medication ordered by the doctor. A procedure is also scheduled for this time. You should
- **a** Perform the procedure before the medication is given
- **b** Perform the procedure right after the medication is given
- **c** Wait one-half hour to let the medication take effect
- **d** Omit the procedure for the day

8 Mr. Smith must be protected from injury after the medication has been given. You should do the following *except*
- **a** Keep the bed in the high position
- **b** Raise side rails as directed
- **c** Check on him every 10 to 15 minutes
- **d** Provide assistance if he needs to get up

9 These measures to relieve pain are part of Mr. Smith's care plan. Which should you question the nurse about?
- **a** Provide blankets as needed.
- **b** Keep the room well lighted.
- **c** Provide soft music.
- **d** Give a back massage.

10 These statements are about rest and sleep. Which is *false?*
- **a** Rest and sleep restore energy and well-being.
- **b** Pain interferes with rest and sleep.
- **c** Ill and injured persons need more rest and sleep than healthy persons.
- **d** Sleep occurs even if the person is in pain and cannot rest.

REVIEW QUESTIONS—CONT'D

11 A person at rest is

- **a** In a state of well-being. The person has no physical or emotional pain.
- **b** Calm, at ease, relaxed. The person is free of anxiety and stress.
- **c** In a state of unconsciousness. The person does not move the voluntary muscles of the arms and legs.
- **d** All of the above

12 For rest to occur, Mr. Smith's basic needs must be met. Which of these basic needs must be met *first* for rest to occur?

- **a** Physical needs
- **b** The need for safety and security
- **c** The need for love and belonging
- **d** Esteem needs

13 Mr. Smith performs certain routines and rituals before he rests. Which basic need is being met?

- **a** Physical needs
- **b** The need for safety and security
- **c** The need for love and belonging
- **d** Esteem needs

14 Mr. Smith's care plan has the following nursing measures. Which will *not* help him rest or sleep?

- **a** Have patient urinate before rest or sleep.
- **b** Assist patient to assume a comfortable position.
- **c** Assist patient to ambulate before rest or sleep.
- **d** Allow him to choose sleep attire.

15 Mr. Smith tires very easily. His morning care includes a bath, hair care, and getting dressed. His bed is made after he is dressed. When should he rest?

- **a** After morning care is completed.
- **b** After his bath and before hair care.
- **c** After you make the bed.
- **d** Whenever he needs to.

16 These statements are about sleep. Which is *false?*

- **a** Tissue healing and repair occur during sleep.
- **b** Voluntary muscle activity increases during sleep.
- **c** Sleep refreshes and renews the person.
- **d** All of the above.

17 Circadian rhythm

- **a** Includes a sleep-wake cycle
- **b** Involves a 24-hour cycle
- **c** Is also called body rhythm
- **d** All of the above

18 Mr. Smith was kept awake several nights when he first entered the hospital. Which is *true?*

- **a** His circadian rhythm may be affected.
- **b** NREM and REM sleep are affected.
- **c** His biological clock will still tell him when to sleep and wake up.
- **d** His functioning will not be affected.

19 Sleepwalking and bed-wetting are most likely to occur during

- **a** Stage 2 of NREM sleep
- **b** Stage 3 of NREM sleep
- **c** Stage 4 of NREM sleep
- **d** REM sleep

20 Mr. Smith has fallen asleep. Full-color dreaming occurs during

- **a** Stage 2 of NREM sleep
- **b** Stage 3 of NREM sleep
- **c** Stage 4 of NREM sleep
- **d** REM sleep

21 Mr. Smith is 35 years old. When healthy, he probably needs about

- **a** 12 to 14 hours of sleep per day
- **b** 8 to 9 hours of sleep per day
- **c** 7 to 8 hours of sleep per day
- **d** About 6 hours of sleep per day

22 Illness interferes with sleep because

- **a** Signs and symptoms of illness can keep a person awake
- **b** Treatments or medications may need to be given
- **c** The emotional effects of illness can keep a person awake
- **d** All of the above

REVIEW QUESTIONS—CONT'D

23 Mr. Smith asks for a snack. He said a friend brought him a chocolate chip cheesecake and some beef summer sausage. He asks for milk with his snack. Which foods will prevent sleep?

a Chocolate

b Cheese

c Milk

d Beef

24 Mr. Smith awakens about 0100. Later he complains of difficulty falling back asleep. The nurse gives him a medication ordered for sleep. You know that the drug

a Contains caffeine

b Interferes with REM sleep

c Causes frequent voiding

d All of the above

25 Alcohol affects sleep because

a It interferes with REM sleep

b Causes the person to awaken during sleep

c Causes the person to have difficulty returning to sleep

d All of the above

26 Mr. Smith has difficulty sleeping and he awakens several times during the night. You report that he has difficulty answering your questions and that he seems moody. You note that his pulse is irregular and that his eyes are red and puffy. He is showing signs of

a Insomnia

b Sleep deprivation

c Enuresis

d Distraction

27 These measures are part of Mr. Smith's care plan. Which should you question?

a Let Mr. Smith choose his bedtime.

b Provide a bedtime snack of hot tea and a cheese sandwich.

c Make sure his cast is properly supported.

d Follow his bedtime rituals.

28 Mr. Smith's mother is a resident of a nursing facility. One night he tells you about her and her care. He says there are 6 ladies in the same room. You know that

a OBRA allows no more than 4 residents in a room

b He is not thinking clearly from lack of sleep

c OBRA does not have a requirement about the number of people in the room

d He is probably disoriented

29 OBRA requires that Mr. Smith's mother have

a A bed of the proper height and size for her

b A clean, comfortable mattress

c Blankets when the weather is cold or when she asks for them

d All of the above

30 Mr. Smith says that his mother likes to go to bed about 10:00 PM. She likes to watch the news and then a late-night talk show. He says the facility is very good about letting her do those things. Under OBRA she has the right to plan her care and to make choices for herself.

a True

b False

Answers to these questions are on page 751.

Admissions, Transfers, and Discharges

21

OBJECTIVES

- Describe what occurs in the admitting office
- Prepare the person's room
- Explain how to admit a person to the nursing unit
- Measure height and weight
- Know how to handle the person's clothing and valuables
- Explain why a person may be transferred to another nursing unit
- Explain how a person is prepared for discharge
- Admit, transfer, and discharge a person

KEY TERMS

admission Official entry of a person into a facility or nursing unit

discharge Official departure of a person from a facility or nursing unit

transfer Moving a person from one room, nursing unit, or facility to another

Admission to a health care facility causes anxiety and fear. Persons and families may worry about the need for treatment or surgery and its outcome. They may be afraid of finding serious health problems. The fear of pain is very common. People admitted to nursing facilities have fears of never returning home. Many people are unfamiliar with health care facilities. They worry about where to go, what to expect, and the strange sights and sounds. Similar concerns occur with transfers to other nursing units. Discharge usually brings relief and happiness. However, the person may need home care.

Admission, transfer, and discharge are critical events. Patients, residents, and families need to feel comfortable and secure. You must be courteous, kind, and respectful.

ADMISSIONS

Except in emergencies, the admission process starts in the admitting office. **Admission** is the official entry of a person into a facility or nursing unit. Admitting staff or a nurse obtains identifying information. This includes the person's full name, age, date of birth, doctor's name, social security number, and religion. The information is recorded on the admission record. The person is given an identification number and an identification bracelet. A general consent for treatment is signed at this time.

Admitting office staff notify the nursing unit that a new patient or resident is being admitted. The nursing staff is told the person's room and bed number. Someone from the admitting office brings the person to the nursing unit. Some facilities let the person walk to the nursing unit if able. Most require transport by wheelchair or stretcher.

Preparing the Room

The room must be ready for the new patient or resident. This is usually your responsibility. Figure 21-1 shows a room prepared for a person's arrival.

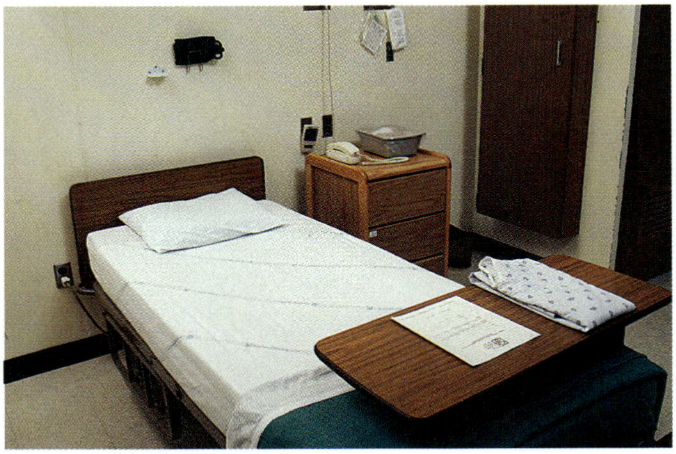

Fig. 21-1 *The room is ready for a person to be admitted.*

Preparing the Person's Room

Procedure

1. Know which room and bed to prepare. Find out if the person is arriving by wheelchair or stretcher.
2. Wash your hands.
3. Collect the following:
   - Patient pack (contains bath basin, pitcher, cup, and personal care items)
   - Admission checklist
   - Urine specimen container (if a urine specimen is ordered)
   - Sphygmomanometer
   - Stethoscope
   - Gown or pajamas
   - IV pole if needed
4. Open the bed.
5. Lower the bed if the person is walking or arriving by wheelchair. Raise the bed to its highest level for a person arriving by stretcher.
6. Attach the call bell to the bed linens.
7. Place the sphygmomanometer, stethoscope, and admission checklist on the overbed table.
8. Place the gown or pajamas on the bed.
9. Place the patient pack and specimen container on the bedside stand or overbed table.
10. Make sure a bedpan, kidney basin, and urinal (for a male) are in the bedside stand. Get missing equipment.
11. Wash your hands.

Admitting the Person

A nurse usually greets and admits the person. It may be your responsibility if the person has no serious discomfort or distress. The admission record is used to find out the person's name. When you greet the person, call him or her by name. Introduce yourself by name and title to the person and to family members who may be present (Fig. 21-2).

Admission procedures involve:

- Completing an admission checklist
- Weighing and measuring the person
- Obtaining a urine specimen if one is ordered
- Orienting the person to the room, nursing unit, and the facility

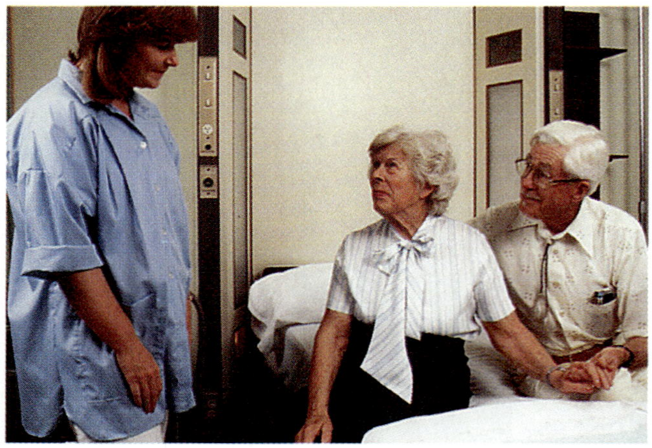

Fig. 21-2 *The nursing assistant introduces herself to the person and family member.*

Admitting the Person—Admission Checklist

Procedure

1. Wash your hands.
2. Prepare the room.
3. Greet the person by name. Ask if he or she prefers a certain name.
4. Introduce yourself to the person and relatives or friends who may be present. Explain that you are a nursing assistant and that you assist the nurses in giving care.
5. Introduce the roommate.
6. Call for a nurse immediately if the person complains of any severe pain or appears to be in distress.
7. Proceed if the person's condition does not present an immediate or serious problem.
8. Provide for privacy. Ask family members or friends to leave the room. Tell them how much time you need and where they can wait comfortably. (Allow a family member or friend to stay if the person prefers.)
9. Have the person put on a gown or pajamas. Assist as needed.
10. Make sure the person is comfortable. He or she should be in bed or in a chair as directed by the nurse.
11. Hang clothes in the closet. Put personal items in the drawers and bedside stand.
12. Obtain information for the admission checklist (Fig. 21-3 on page 496).
13. Complete a clothing and valuables list.
14. Explain any ordered activity limits.
15. Obtain a urine specimen if instructed by the nurse (see Chapter 15).
16. Take the specimen to the nurses' desk. Clean equipment and wash your hands.
17. Orient the person to the area:
    - **a** Give names of the nurses.
    - **b** Identify items in the bedside stand. Explain the purpose of each item.
    - **c** Show how the call bell is used.
    - **d** Show how to operate the bed and television controls.
    - **e** Explain how to make telephone calls. Place the phone within reach.
    - **f** Explain visiting hours and policies.
    - **g** Describe the location of the nurses' station, lounge, chapel, dining room, gift shop, and other important areas.
    - **h** Explain other services: newspaper, library, activities, educational programs, religious services, and others.
    - **i** Identify other staff: workers from x-ray, laboratory, housekeeping, dietary, and physical therapy, as well as students and others.
    - **j** Explain when meals and nourishments are served.
18. Fill the water pitcher if oral fluids are allowed.
19. Place the call bell within reach. Place other controls and needed items within reach.
20. Keep the bed in its lowest position.
21. Raise or lower side rails as instructed by the nurse.
22. Unscreen the person.
23. Clean used equipment. Discard used disposable items. Wash your hands.
24. Provide a denture container if needed. Label it with the person's name and room number.
25. Label personal property and personal care equipment for the nursing facility resident. Items are labeled with the person's name.
26. Wash your hands.
27. Report your observations to the nurse.

NURSES' ADMISSION RECORD

(To be completed by the nurse admitting the patient)

LAST NAME	FIRST NAME	MIDDLE NAME	ROOM NO.	BED NO.	ADMISSION NO.
ATTENDING PHYSICIAN			DATE		TIME A.M. P.M.
ADMITTING DIAGNOSIS					

Take and record temperature, pulse and respiration once daily during first 48 hours.

Date ________ T. ______ P. ______ R. ______ B.P. ___ /______ | Date ________ T. ______ P. ______ R. ______ B.P. ___ /______

FIRST 24 HOURS | SECOND 24 HOURS

CONDITION ON ADMISSION

Ambulatory	☐	Feeds self	☐	Admitted by ambulance	☐	Alert	☐
Semi-ambulatory	☐	Requires help w/feeding	☐	From hospital	☐	Forgetful	☐
Chair-ridden	☐	Continent	☐	From home	☐	Confused	☐
Bed ridden	☐	Incontinent	☐	From nursing home	☐	____________	☐

Patient wears: Dentures ☐ Glasses ☐ Hearing aid ☐ Other ______________________ SPECIFY

Has prosthesis of: Breast ☐ Leg ☐ Arm ☐ Other ______________________ SPECIFY

General physical appearance ____

General condition of skin ____

Indicate on diagram below all body marks such as, old or recent scars, bruises or discolorations (regardless of how slight), lacerations, decubitus ulcers and other ulcerations or questionable markings considered other than normal:

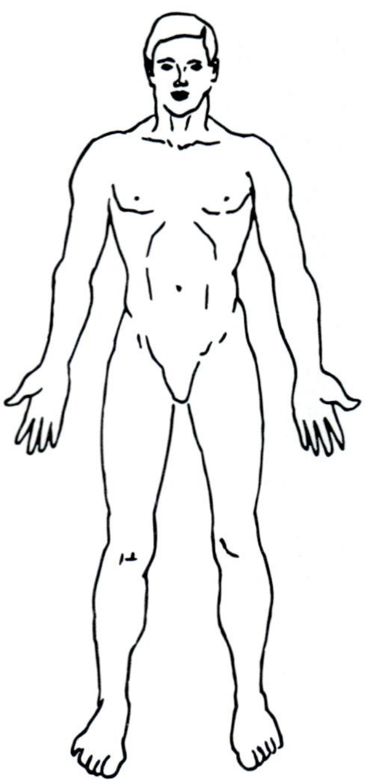

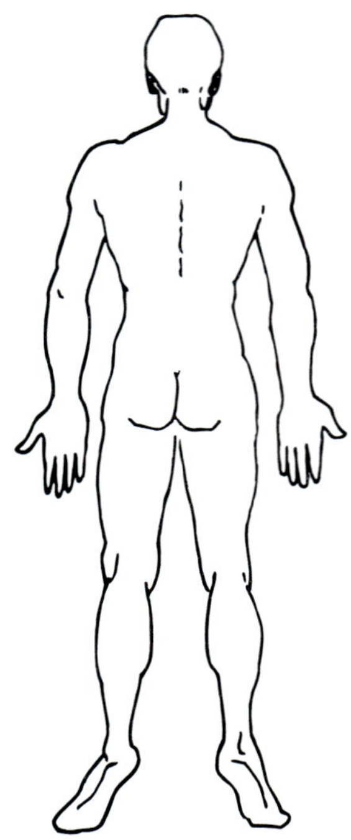

Signed ______________________________ ADMITTING NURSE

Form 3006 BRIGGS, Des Moines, Iowa 50306 PRINTED IN U.S.A. **NURSES' ADMISSION RECORD**

Fig. 21-3 *An admission checklist. (Reprinted with permission of Briggs Healthcare Products, Des Moines, Iowa.)*

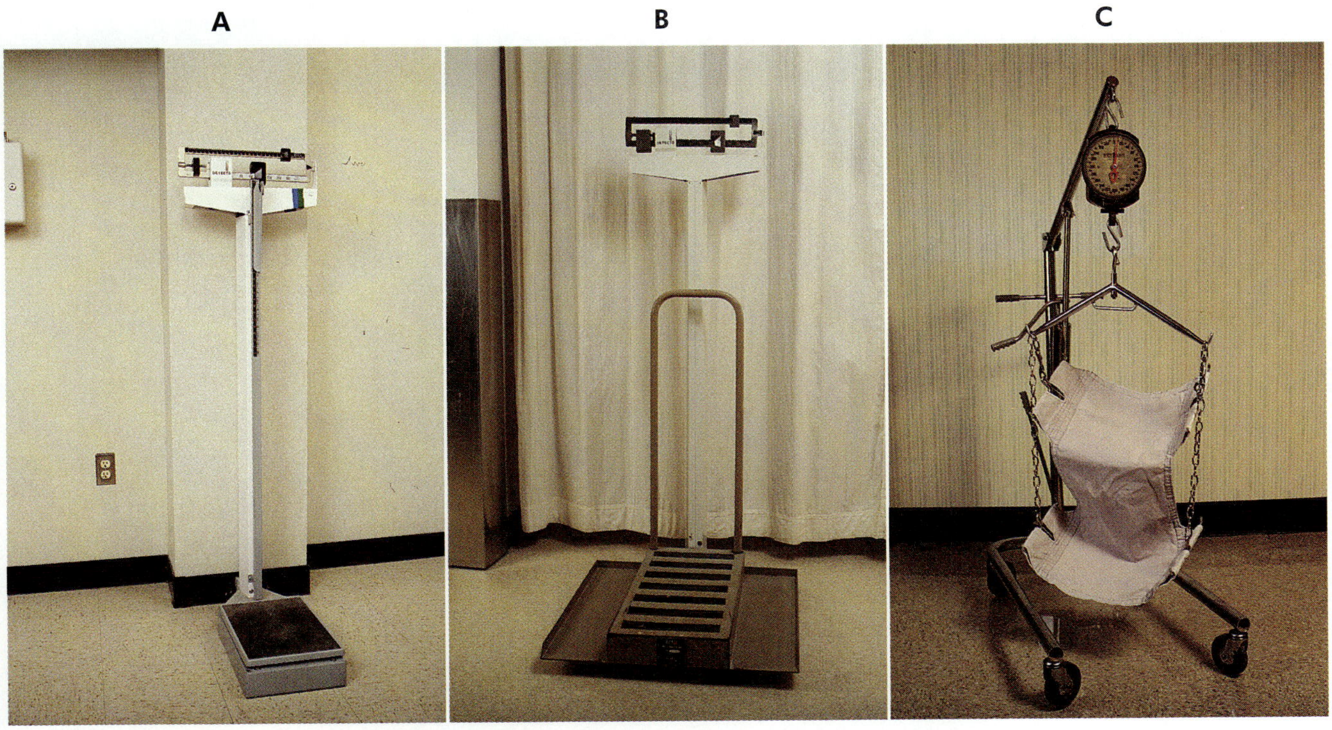

Fig. 21-4 *A, Standing scale. B, Chair scale. C, Lift scale.*

Measuring height and weight Height and weight are measured on admission. The person only wears a gown or pajamas. Clothes add weight. Shoes or slippers also add weight and add to the height measurement. The person urinates before being weighed. A full bladder affects the weight measurement. If a urine specimen is needed, collect it at this time.

Standing, chair, and lift scales are used (Fig. 21-4). Chair and lift scales are used for persons who cannot stand. The manufacturer's instructions are followed when using a chair or lift scale.

Clothing and valuables A list is made of the person's clothing and valuables. Valuables (including money and jewelry) must be kept in a safe place. Often they are sent home with the family. A clothing list is completed by the staff member admitting the person. Each item is identified and described. The staff member and person each sign the completed list. It may be signed by the person's legal representative. In nursing facilities, clothing also is labeled with the person's name.

A valuables envelope is used for money and jewelry. Each piece of jewelry is listed and described on the envelope. When describing jewelry, describe what you see. For example, a ring is described as having a white stone with six prongs in a yellow setting. Do not assume that the stone is a diamond in a gold setting. Each jewelry item is placed in the envelope while the person watches. Money is counted with the person. Then it is put in the envelope. The envelope is sealed and signed like the clothing checklist. The envelope is given to the nurse. The nurse takes it to the safe or sends it home with the family.

Some valuables are kept at the bedside. They include dentures, eyeglasses, contact lenses, watches, and radios. Valuables kept at the bedside are listed in the person's record. Some persons keep money for newspapers and gift cart items. The amount of money kept by the person is noted in the person's record.

MEASURING HEIGHT AND WEIGHT

PRE-PROCEDURE

1 Explain the procedure to the person.
2 Ask the person to urinate.
3 Wash your hands.
4 Collect the following:
   - Portable balance scale
   - Paper towels
5 Identify the person. Check the ID bracelet and call the person by name.
6 Provide for privacy.

PROCEDURE

7 Place the paper towels on the scale platform.
8 Raise the height rod.
9 Have the person remove the robe and slippers. Assist as needed.
10 Help the person stand on the scale platform. Arms are at the sides.
11 Move the weights until the balance pointer is in the middle (Fig. 21-5).
12 Record the weight on your note pad.
13 Ask the person to stand very straight.
14 Lower the height rod until it rests on the person's head (Fig. 21-6).
15 Record the height on your note pad.
16 Help the person put on the robe and slippers if he or she will be up. Help the person back to bed if necessary. Make sure he or she is comfortable.

POST-PROCEDURE

17 Place the call bell within reach.
18 Unscreen the person.
19 Discard the paper towels. Return the scale to its storage area.
20 Wash your hands.
21 Report and record the measurements.

A

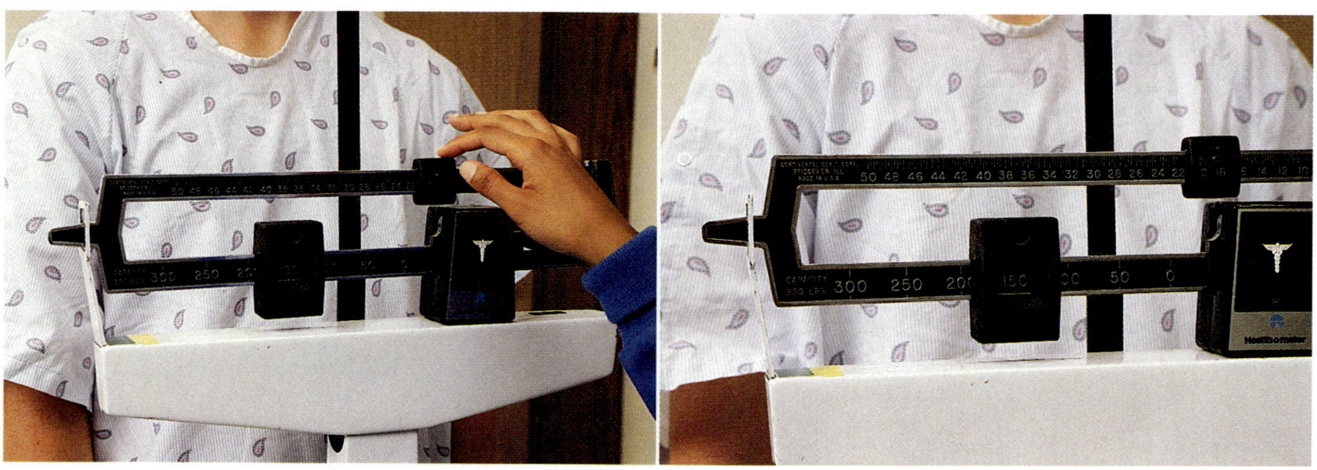

B

Fig. 21-5 *A, The person is weighed. B, The weight is read when the balance pointer is in the middle.*

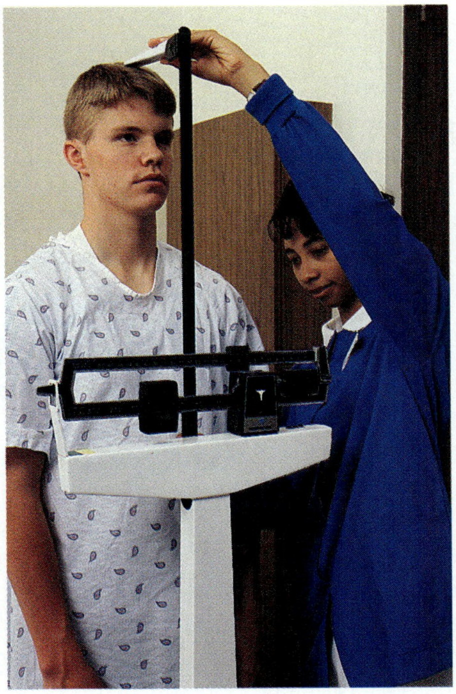

Fig. 21-6 *Height is measured.*

TRANSFERS

A **transfer** is moving a person from one room, nursing unit, or facility to another. Transfers are usually related to changes in condition. The person may or may not welcome the transfer. Reasons for the transfer are explained by the doctor or nurse. The nurse also notifies the family and business office. You may assist in the transfer or carry out the entire procedure. The person is usually transported by wheelchair or stretcher. Sometimes the bed is used.

TRANSFERRING THE PERSON TO ANOTHER NURSING UNIT

PROCEDURE

1 Ask the nurse where the person is going. Find out if the bed, a wheelchair, or a stretcher will be used.

2 Get a stretcher or wheelchair, bath blanket, and a utility cart if needed.

3 Wash your hands.

4 Identify the person. Check the ID bracelet with the transfer slip.

5 Explain the procedure to the person.

6 Collect the person's belongings and bedside equipment. Place them on the utility cart for transport.

7 Assist the person to the wheelchair or stretcher. Cover the person with a bath blanket.

8 Transport the person to the assigned place.

9 Introduce the person to the receiving nurse.

10 Help transfer the person from the wheelchair or stretcher into bed. Help position the person.

11 Bring the person's belongings and equipment to the new room. Help put them away.

12 Report the following to the receiving nurse:
- How the person tolerated the transfer
- That a nurse will bring the person's chart, care plan, Kardex, and medications

13 Return the wheelchair or stretcher and the utility cart to the storage area.

14 Wash your hands.

15 Report the following to the nurse:
- The time of transfer
- Where the person was taken
- How the person was transferred (bed, wheelchair, or stretcher)
- How the person tolerated the transfer
- Who received the person
- Any other observations

16 Strip the bed, clean the unit, and make a closed bed. (This may be done by housekeeping staff.)

17 Wash your hands.

Discharging the Person

Procedure

1. Make sure the person is to be discharged. Find out if transportation arrangements have been made.
2. Explain the procedure to the person.
3. Wash your hands.
4. Identify the person. Check the ID bracelet with the discharge slip.
5. Provide for privacy.
6. Help the person dress as needed.
7. Help the person pack. Check all drawers and closets to make sure all items are collected.
8. Check off the clothing list. Ask the person to sign the form indicating that all clothing has been returned.
9. Tell the nurse that the person is ready for the final visit. The nurse
   - a Gives prescriptions written by the physician
   - b Provides discharge instructions
   - c Gets valuables from the safe
10. Get a wheelchair and a utility cart for the person's belongings. Ask a co-worker to help you.
11. Bring the wheelchair to the bedside and lock the wheels. Lock the bed wheels. Lower the bed to its lowest position.
12. Assist the person into the wheelchair.
13. Unlock the wheels.
14. Take the person to the exit area. Lock the wheels of the wheelchair (Fig. 21-7).
15. Help the person out of the wheelchair and into the car. Help put the belongings into the car.
16. Return the wheelchair and cart to the storage area.
17. Wash your hands.
18. Report the following to the nurse:
    - The time of discharge
    - How the person was transported
    - Who accompanied the person
    - The person's destination
    - Any other observations
19. Strip the bed, clean the unit, and make a closed bed. (This may be done by housekeeping staff.)
20. Wash your hands.

DISCHARGES

Discharge is usually planned a few days in advance. **Discharge** is the official departure of a person from a facility or nursing unit. This is a happy time if the person is going home. Some people are discharged to another hospital or to a nursing facility. Some need home care. They may have other fears and concerns. The doctor, nurse, dietician, social worker, and other health team members plan the person's discharge. They teach the person and family about diet, exercise, and needed medications. They also teach about dressing changes and treatments. A doctor's appointment may be arranged.

You will often help persons pack belongings and change into street clothes. You also transport persons out of the facility. The nurse tells you when to start the discharge procedure. The doctor must write a discharge order before the person is allowed to leave. The nurse tells you when the person can leave and how to transport him or her. Usually a wheelchair is used. Some facilities let the person walk. Occasionally a person or resident leaves by ambulance. The ambulance attendants bring the stretcher to the room.

Financial arrangements are made on admission or before discharge. Before leaving the facility, the person or family makes arrangements for payment at the business office.

A person may want to leave the facility without the doctor's permission. You must notify the nurse immediately if the person expresses the wish or intent to leave. This situation is handled by the nurse.

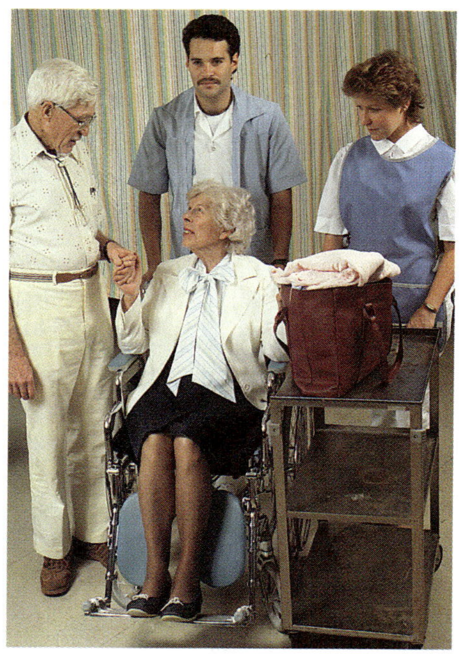

Fig. 21-7 *The person is taken to the exit by wheelchair. The person's possessions are brought along at this time.*

SUMMARY

Admission to a health care facility is often a frightening time for the person and family. Transfers can also cause fear and apprehension. This is particularly true when the transfer is due to a change in the person's condition. Discharge is a happy and pleasant time. However, it may cause worries and concerns if more care and treatment are required. You can help the person and family cope with these events. You need to be polite, courteous, caring, efficient, and competent. The person's property and valuables must be handled with care and respect. They are kept in a safe place and protected from loss or damage. Always treat the person and family the way you would like to be treated.

REVIEW QUESTIONS

Circle T *if the answer is true and* F *if the answer is false.*

1 **T** **F** The person's identifying information is obtained on arrival to the nursing unit.

2 **T** **F** A new patient or resident is usually transported to the nursing unit by wheelchair or stretcher.

3 **T** **F** The bed is opened when preparing the room for the person.

4 **T** **F** The person is greeted by name when being admitted to the nursing unit.

5 **T** **F** A patient complains of pain. The complaint is reported after the admission checklist is completed.

6 **T** **F** A urine specimen may be needed on admission.

7 **T** **F** You are not responsible for orienting a resident to the new environment.

8 **T** **F** The person wears a robe and slippers when being weighed and measured.

9 **T** **F** A list is made of the person's clothing and valuables during the admission process.

10 **T** **F** A person's condition may require a transfer to another nursing unit.

11 **T** **F** A doctor's order is required for discharge from the health care facility.

12 **T** **F** You provide the person with instructions about diet and medications.

Answers to these questions are on page 751.

Assisting with the Physical Examination

22

OBJECTIVES

- Define the key terms listed in this chapter
- Explain your responsibilities before, after, and during a physical examination
- Identify the equipment used during a physical examination
- Describe how to prepare a person for an examination
- Describe four examination positions and how to drape the person for each position
- Prepare a person for an examination
- Explain the rules for assisting with a physical examination
- Describe the differences between the examination of an infant or child and an adult

Key Terms

dorsal recumbent position The supine or back-lying examination position; the legs are together

horizontal recumbent position The dorsal recumbent position

knee-chest position The person kneels and rests the body on the knees and chest; the head is turned to one side, the arms are above the head or flexed at the elbows, the back is straight, and the body is flexed about 90 degrees at the hips

laryngeal mirror An instrument used to examine the mouth, teeth, and throat

lithotomy position The person is in a back-lying position, the hips are brought down to the edge of the examination table, the knees are flexed, the hips are externally rotated, and the feet are supported in stirrups

nasal speculum An instrument used to examine the inside of the nose

ophthalmoscope A lighted instrument used to examine the internal structures of the eye

otoscope A lighted instrument used to examine the external ear and the eardrum (tympanic membrane)

percussion hammer An instrument used to tap body parts to test reflexes

tuning fork An instrument used to test hearing

vaginal speculum An instrument used to open the vagina so that it and the cervix can be examined

Physical examinations are usually done by doctors. Many nurses also perform them. They are done for many reasons. Routine health examinations are done to promote health. Preemployment physicals are done to determine fitness for work. Physical examinations are also used to diagnose and treat disease. You may be asked to assist a doctor or nurse with a physical examination.

RESPONSIBILITIES OF THE NURSING ASSISTANT

Your responsibilities depend on the policies and procedures of the facility. The examiner's preferences also affect what you are expected to do. You may do some or all of the following:

- Collect linens for draping the person and for the procedure.
- Collect equipment to be used for the examination.
- Prepare the room for the examination.
- Make sure there is enough lighting.
- Measure vital signs, height, and weight.
- Position and drape the person for the examination.
- Hand equipment and instruments to the examiner.
- Label specimen containers.
- Dispose of soiled linen and discard used disposable supplies.
- Clean reusable equipment after the examination.
- Help the person dress or assume a comfortable position after the examination.

EQUIPMENT

Some equipment and supplies used in a physical examination are used for nursing care. You may recognize some of the instruments. Some were probably used when you were examined. You need to know the instruments in Figure 22-1 on page 504.

- **Ophthalmoscope**—a lighted instrument used to examine the internal structures of the eye.
- **Otoscope**—used to examine the external ear and the eardrum (tympanic membrane). The otoscope is a lighted instrument. Some scopes have interchangeable parts. Some can be changed into an ophthalmoscope or otoscope.
- **Percussion hammer**—used to tap body parts to test reflexes.

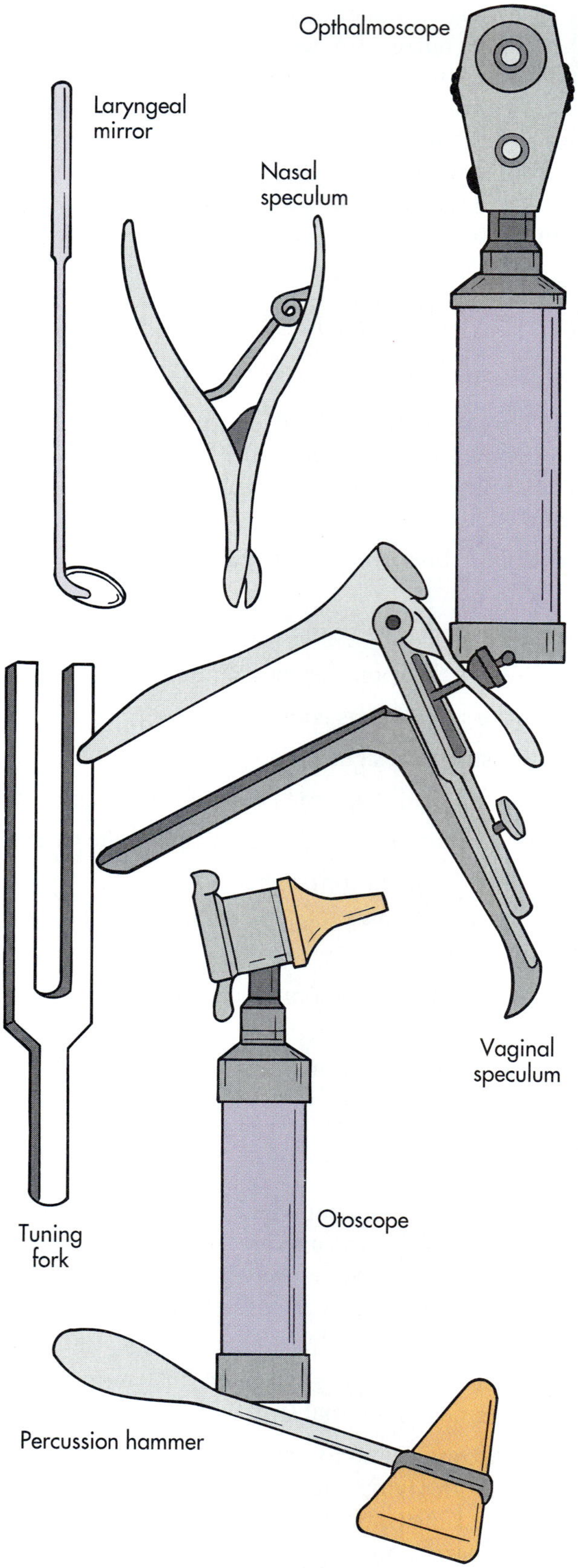

Fig. 22-1 *Instruments used for a physical examination.*

- **Vaginal speculum**—used to open the vagina so it and the cervix can be examined.
- **Nasal speculum**—used to examine the inside of the nose.
- **Tuning fork**—vibrated to test hearing.
- **Laryngeal mirror**—used to examine the mouth, teeth, and throat.

Many facilities have examination trays in the central supply department. If not, needed items are collected. Items listed in *Preparing the Person for an Examination* on page 491 are usually used for an examination. They are arranged on a tray or table for the examiner.

PREPARING THE PERSON

The physical examination causes anxiety for many people. They are concerned about possible findings. Other factors can add to their anxiety. These include discomfort, embarrassment, the fear of exposure, and unfamiliarity with the procedure. You need to be sensitive to the person's feelings and concerns. The person is prepared physically and psychologically for the examination. The nurse explains the purpose of the examination and what to expect. This could be your responsibility, depending on the situation and the employer.

Usually all clothes are removed for a complete physical examination. The person is covered with a drape. It may be a disposable paper drape, a bath blanket, a sheet, or a drawsheet. Sometimes a hospital gown is worn. It reduces the feeling of nakedness and the fear of exposure. Explain to the person that there is little exposure during the examination. The person needs to understand that some exposure is necessary to examine the body. However, only the body part being examined is exposed. You must screen the person and close the door to the room. This further protects the person's right to privacy.

The person urinates before the examination. The bladder must be empty so the examiner can feel the abdominal organs. A full bladder can change the normal position and shape of organs. It can also cause discomfort, especially when the abdominal organs are felt. If a urine specimen is needed, it is obtained at this time. Explain how to collect the specimen, and label the container properly (see Chapter 15).

Warmth is a major concern during the examination. The person is protected from chilling, especially if ill, elderly, or a child. An extra bath blanket should be nearby. Also take measures to prevent drafts.

The examiner may want height, weight, and vital signs measured. These are obtained before the exam starts. They are recorded on the examination form. The person is then positioned and draped for the examination.

PREPARING THE PERSON FOR AN EXAMINATION

PROCEDURE

1 Explain the procedure to the person.

2 Wash your hands.

3 Assemble the following items on a tray at the bedside or in the examination room:
   - Flashlight
   - Sphygmomanometer
   - Stethoscope
   - Thermometer
   - Tongue depressors (blades)
   - Laryngeal mirror
   - Ophthalmoscope
   - Otoscope
   - Nasal speculum
   - Percussion (reflex) hammer
   - Tuning fork
   - Tape measure
   - Disposable gloves
   - Water-soluble lubricant
   - Vaginal speculum
   - Cotton-tipped applicators
   - Specimen containers and labels
   - Disposable bag
   - Emesis basin
   - Towel
   - Bath blanket
   - Tissues
   - Drape (sheet, bath blanket, drawsheet, or disposable drape)
   - Paper towels
   - Cotton balls
   - Waterproof bed protector
   - Eye chart (Snellen chart)
   - Slides
   - Gown
   - Alcohol wipes
   - Wastebasket
   - Container for soiled instruments
   - Marking pencils or pens

4 Identify the person. Check the ID bracelet and call the person by name.

5 Provide for privacy.

6 Ask the person to put on the gown. Instruct him or her to remove all clothes. Assist as necessary.

7 Ask the person to urinate. If the person is not ambulatory, offer the bedpan or urinal. Provide for privacy.

8 Transport the person to the examination room. Help the person get on the examination table. Have him or her use a stool if necessary. Omit this step if the examination will be done in the person's room.

9 Position the person as directed. Raise the bed to its highest level. Raise the side rails if the person is in bed.

10 Drape the person. Untie the gown.

11 Place a bed protector under the buttocks.

12 Arrange for adequate lighting.

13 Put the call bell on for the nurse or examiner. Do not leave the person unattended.

Positioning and Draping

The person may have to assume a special position for the examination. Some examination positions (Fig. 22-2) are uncomfortable and embarrassing. The examiner tells you how to position the person. Be sure to help the person assume and maintain the position. But first explain the following to the person:

- The need for the position
- How the position is assumed
- How the body is draped
- How long the person can expect to stay in the position

The **dorsal recumbent (horizontal recumbent)** or supine position is used to examine the abdomen, anterior chest, and breasts. The person is supine with the legs together. If the perineal area is to be examined, the knees are flexed and hips externally rotated (see Fig. 22-2, A). The person is draped as for perineal care (see *Female Perineal Care*, page 309).

The **lithotomy position** (Fig. 22-2, B) is used to examine the vagina. The person lies on her back, and her hips are brought to the edge of the examination table. The knees are flexed, and the hips are externally rotated. The feet are supported in stirrups. The person is draped as for the dorsal recumbent position. Some facilities provide socks to cover the feet and calves.

The **knee-chest position** (Fig. 22-2, C) is used to examine the rectum. Sometimes it is used to examine the vagina. The person kneels on the bed or examination table. Then the person rests his or her body on the knees and chest. The head is turned to one side, and the arms are above the head or flexed at the elbows. The back is straight and the body is flexed about 90 degrees at the hips. The person wears a gown and sometimes socks. The drape is applied in a diamond shape to cover the back, buttocks, and thighs.

The **Sims' position** (Fig. 22-2, D) is sometimes used to examine the rectum or vagina (see Fig. 10-45, page 249). The drape is applied in a diamond shape. The corner near the examiner is folded back to expose the rectum or vagina.

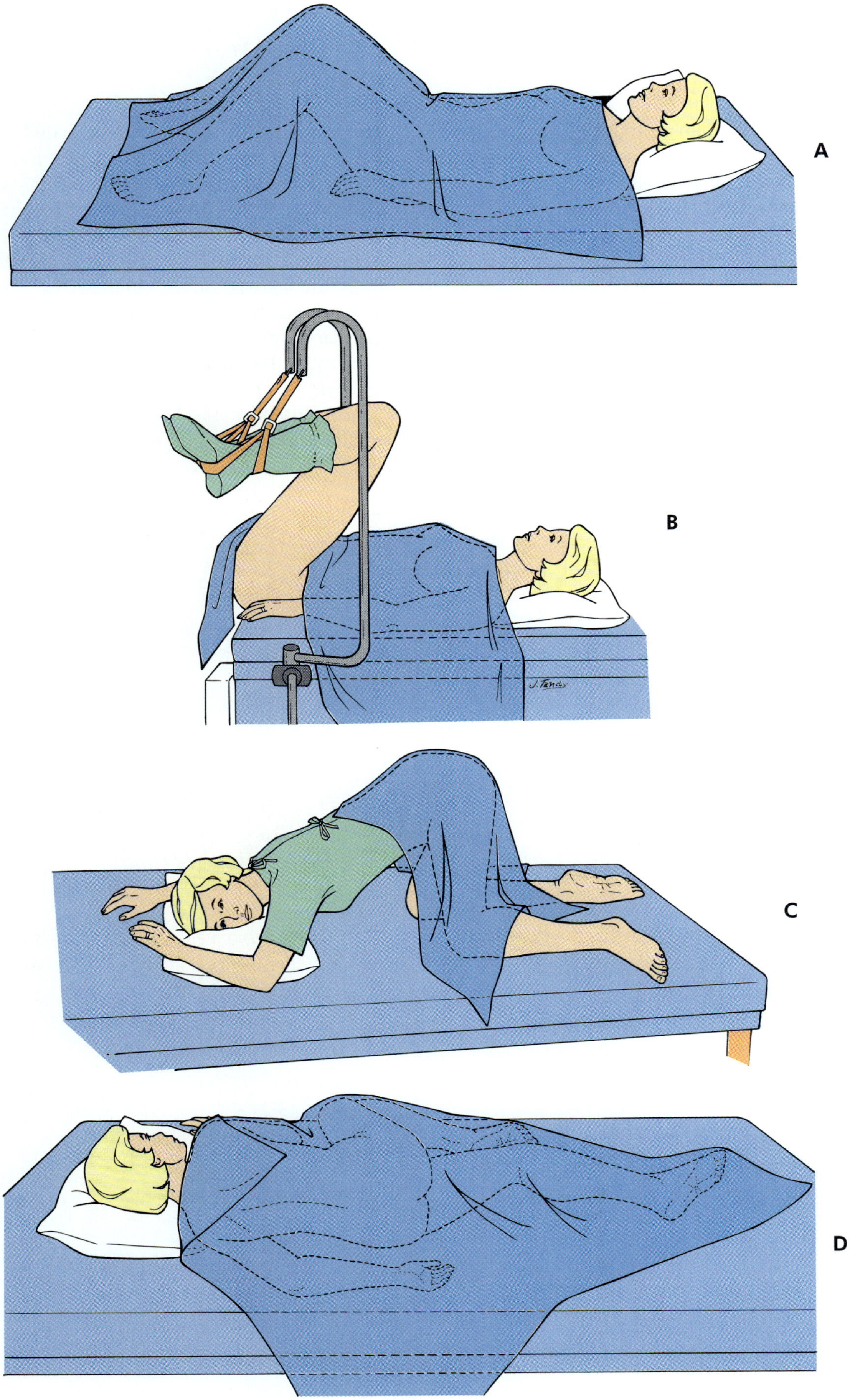

Fig. 22-2 *Positioning and draping for the physical examination.* ***A,*** *Dorsal recumbent position.* ***B,*** *Lithotomy position.* ***C,*** *Knee-chest position.* ***D,*** *Sims' position.*

ASSISTING WITH THE EXAMINATION

You may be asked to prepare, position, and drape the person. You may also be asked to assist the doctor or nurse during the examination. When assisting with the examination, the rules in Box 22-1 are followed.

After the Examination

After the examination the person is taken back to the room. In a clinic, the person gets dressed in the exam room. Assistance is given as needed. Lubricant is used for the vaginal or rectal examination. The area is wiped or cleaned before the person dresses or returns to the room.

Used disposable items are put in a bag or waste container. Examples are bed protectors, paper drapes, tongue blades, applicators, and cotton balls. These supplies are replaced so the tray is ready for the next examination. Reusable items are cleaned according to facility policy and returned to the tray. This includes the otoscope and ophthalmoscope tips, speculum, and stethoscope. The examination table is covered with a clean drawsheet or paper. All specimens are labeled and sent to the laboratory with a requisition slip. The person's unit or examination room should be neat and orderly after the examination. Follow facility policy for soiled linens.

EXAMINATION OF AN INFANT OR CHILD

The examination of an infant or child is like an adult examination. However, a parent is present. The parent may be asked to hold or restrain the infant or child during some parts of the procedure. Restraint may be necessary if the infant or child is uncooperative. Restraining may frighten an infant. The child may also fear separation from the parent. Some children fear being physically harmed during the examination. A calm, comforting manner helps both the child or infant and the parent. Remember, the parent may be anxious too. The equipment needed is like that used for the adult examination. Toys are used to assess development. Vaginal speculums are not used.

BOX 22-1 Rules for Assisting with the Physical Examination

- Wash your hands before and after the examination.
- Provide for privacy throughout the examination. This is done by screening, closing doors, and draping. Expose only the body part being examined.
- Assist the person in assuming positions as directed by the examiner.
- Place instruments and equipment in a convenient location for the examiner.
- Stay in the room during the examination of a female person (unless you are a male). When a woman is examined by a man, another female is in attendance. This is for the legal protection of the woman and the male examiner. A female attendant also adds to the psychological comfort of the woman.
- Protect the person from falling.
- Anticipate the examiner's need for equipment.
- Place paper or paper towels on the floor if the person is asked to stand.
- Practice medical asepsis and Standard Precautions. Also follow the Bloodborne Pathogen Standard.

SUMMARY

Physical examinations are frightening to many people. Many fear exposure or a serious diagnosis. Examinations may cause discomfort, especially for the ill, injured, or elderly. You may be asked to prepare persons for examinations. Collecting and arranging examination supplies and equipment are sometimes done by nursing assistants. You may also be asked to assist with the procedure. Feelings, fears, and sources of discomfort during the examination must be considered. This is essential for the person's physical and psychological comfort. In addition, you must function efficiently and competently. This allows the examination to be performed smoothly and in a reasonable length of time.

REVIEW QUESTIONS

Circle the best *answer.*

1 The otoscope is used to

- **a** Examine the internal structures of the eye
- **b** Examine the external ear and the eardrum
- **c** Test reflexes
- **d** Open the vagina

2 You are preparing Mrs. Porter for an examination. You should do the following *except*

- **a** Have her urinate
- **b** Ask her to undress
- **c** Drape her
- **d** Go tell the nurse when Mrs. Porter is ready

3 Which part of Mrs. Porter's examination can you do?

- **a** Examine her eyes and ears
- **b** Inspect her mouth, teeth, and throat
- **c** Measure her height, weight, and vital signs
- **d** Observe her perineum and rectum

4 Mrs. Porter is supine. Her hips are flexed and externally rotated. Her feet are supported in stirrups. She is in the

- **a** Dorsal recumbent position
- **b** Lithotomy position
- **c** Knee-chest position
- **d** Sims' position

5 Mary Adams is a nursing assistant. She is to assist with Mrs. Porter's examination. Which is *false?*

- **a** Handwashing is done before and after the examination.
- **b** Instruments are placed near the examiner.
- **c** The nursing assistant leaves the room when Mrs. Porter is examined.
- **d** Her privacy is protected by screening, closing the door, and proper draping.

6 An infant is being examined. Which is *true?*

- **a** Restraints are applied.
- **b** Equipment is needed as for the adult examination.
- **c** The temperature is measured orally.
- **d** The parent stays for the examination.

Answers to these questions are on page 752.

Heat and Cold Applications

23

OBJECTIVES

- Define the key terms listed in this chapter
- Identify the purposes, effects, and complications of heat applications
- Identify the persons at risk for complications from heat applications
- Explain the differences between moist and dry heat applications
- Describe the rules for the application of heat
- Identify the purposes, effects, and complications of cold applications
- Identify the persons at risk for complications from cold applications
- Explain the differences between moist and dry cold applications
- Describe the rules for the application of cold
- Perform the procedures described in this chapter

KEY TERMS

closed wound A wound in which the skin is intact; tissues below the skin are injured

constrict To narrow

cyanosis Bluish discoloration of the skin

dilate To expand or open wider

open wound A wound in which the skin is broken

wound An injury to tissues

Heat and cold applications are often ordered for wound care. A **wound** is an injury to tissues. With **open wounds,** the skin is broken. Incisions, cuts, and pressure sores are examples of open wounds. With **closed wounds,** the skin is intact. Tissues below the skin are injured. Sprains are common closed wounds. Heat and cold applications are ordered by doctors to:

- Promote healing
- Promote comfort
- Reduce tissue swelling

Heat and cold have opposite effects on body function. Severe injuries and changes in body function can occur if safety precautions are not taken. The risks are great. Therefore heat and cold applications are complex and more advanced nursing functions.

In many facilities, only nurses apply heat and cold. Some facilities let nursing assistants apply heat and cold under the direction of a nurse. You are advised to perform these procedures only if you thoroughly understand their purposes, effects, and complications. Review the procedure with a nurse first. A nurse should closely supervise your work and the effects of the procedure on the person.

HEAT APPLICATIONS

Heat applications are usually small and can be applied to almost any body part. *Local heat application* means heat is applied to a body part. They are often used for musculoskeletal injuries or problems (sprains, arthritis). Heat applications are used to:

- Relieve pain
- Relax muscles
- Promote healing
- Reduce tissue swelling
- Decrease joint stiffness

Effects

When heat is applied to the skin, blood vessels in the area dilate. **Dilate** means to expand or open wider (Fig. 23-1). More blood flows through the vessels. More oxygen and nutrients are available to the tissues for healing. Toxic (poisonous) substances and waste products are removed faster. Excess fluid is removed from the area more rapidly. The skin feels warm and appears reddened. These effects are from increased blood flow.

Complications

High temperatures can cause burns. Pain, excessive redness, and blisters are danger signs. These are reported to the nurse immediately. You must also observe for pale skin. When heat is applied for a long time, blood vessels tend to **constrict,** or narrow (see Fig. 23-1). Blood flow decreases when vessels constrict. Decreased blood flow reduces the amount of blood available to tissues. Decreased blood supply causes tissue damage and gives the skin a pale color.

Certain persons are at great risk for complications. They are infants, very young children, fair-skinned people, and the elderly. Their skin is very delicate and fragile, and is easily burned. Persons who have difficulty sensing (feeling) heat or pain are also at risk. Many factors can interfere with sensation. They include circulatory disorders, central nervous system damage, aging, and loss of consciousness. Confused persons or those receiving strong pain medications may also have decreased sensation.

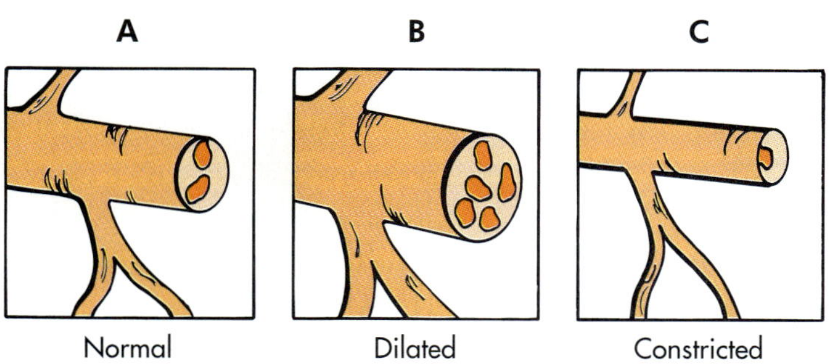

Fig. 23-1 *A, Blood vessel under normal conditions. B, Dilated blood vessel. C, Constricted blood vessel.*

Persons with metal implants are also at risk. Metal conducts heat. Deep tissues can be burned. Pacemakers and hip and knee replacements are often made of metal. Heat is not applied in the area of the implant.

Heat is not applied to the abdomen of a pregnant woman. The heat can affect fetal growth.

Moist and Dry Applications

Moist or dry applications are ordered. A *moist heat application* means that water is in contact with the skin. Water conducts heat. Therefore the effects from moist heat are greater and occur faster than from dry heat applications. Heat penetrates deeper with a moist application. To prevent injury, temperatures of moist heat applications are lower than those of dry heat applications.

Water is not in contact with the skin with *dry heat applications.* Dry heat has advantages.

- The application stays at the desired temperature longer.
- Heat is not lost through evaporation as with moist applications.
- The risk of burns is less. Dry heat does not penetrate as deeply as moist heat. Also, water, which conducts heat, is not involved.

Because water is not used, higher temperatures are needed with dry heat to achieve the desired effect. Therefore burns are still a risk.

Patients and residents must be protected from injury during local heat applications. Those who cannot protect themselves need extra attention. The rules listed in Box 23-1 are practiced to prevent burns and other complications.

Hot Compresses and Packs

Hot compresses and packs are moist heat applications. They consist of a washcloth, small towel, or gauze dressing. A compress is applied to a small area. Packs are applied to large areas. There are sterile and nonsterile compresses. Sterile applications are used for open wounds. The nurse applies sterile hot compresses or packs.

Box 23-1 Rules for Applying Heat

- Know how to operate equipment used in the procedure.
- Measure the temperature of moist heat applications. Use a bath thermometer.
- Follow facility policies for the safe temperature ranges of heat applications.
- Know the temperature ranges for warm, hot, and very hot applications. The following are guidelines:
  - *Warm*—98° to 105° F (37° to 40° C)
  - *Hot*—105° to 115° F (40° to 46° C)
  - *Very hot*—above 115° F (above 46° C)
- Do not apply *very hot* (above 115° F or 46° C) applications. Tissue damage can occur. The nurse applies *very hot* applications.
- Ask the nurse what the temperature of the application should be. Lower temperatures are used for those at risk.
- Know the precise location for the heat application. Ask the nurse to show you the site.
- Cover dry heat applications before applying them. Flannel covers are usually used.
- Observe the skin for signs of complications. Immediately report the following to the nurse:
  - Pain, numbness, or burning
  - Excessive redness
  - Blisters
  - Pale, white, or gray skin
  - Cyanosis
  - Shivering
- Do not let the person increase the temperature of the application.
- Ask the nurse how long to leave the application in place. Carefully watch the time. Heat is never applied longer than 30 minutes.
- Follow the rules of electrical safety when using electrical appliances to apply heat.
- Expose only the body part where the heat is to be applied. Provide for privacy through proper draping and screening.
- Place the call bell within the person's reach.

Applying Hot Compresses

Pre-procedure

1 Explain the procedure to the person.
2 Wash your hands.
3 Collect the following:
- Basin
- Bath thermometer
- Small towel, washcloth, or gauze squares
- Plastic wrap or aquathermia pad
- Ties, tape, or rolled gauze
- Bath towel
- Waterproof bed protector

4 Identify the person. Check the ID bracelet with the treatment card.
5 Provide for privacy.

Procedure

6 Place the protector under the body part.
7 Fill the basin one-half to two-thirds full with hot water. Water temperature should be 105° to 115° F (40.5° to 46.1° C).
8 Place the compress in the water.
9 Wring out the compress (Fig. 23-2).
10 Apply the compress to the area. Note the time.
11 Cover the compress quickly. Do one of the following as directed by the nurse:
  a Cover it with plastic wrap and then with a bath towel (Fig 23-2). Secure the towel in place with ties, tape, or rolled gauze.
  b Cover it with an aquathermia pad (see *Applying an Aquathermia Pad,* page 520).
12 Place the call bell within reach. Raise or lower side rails as instructed by the nurse.
13 Check the area every 5 minutes. Check for redness and complaints of pain, discomfort, or numbness. Remove the compress if any occur. Tell the nurse immediately.
14 Change the compress if cooling occurs.
15 Remove the compress after 20 minutes or as directed by the nurse. Pat the area dry with a towel. (Lower the side rails for this step.)

Post-procedure

16 Make sure the person is comfortable and unscreened.
17 Raise or lower side rails as instructed by the nurse.
18 Place the call bell within reach.
19 Clean equipment. Discard disposable items.
20 Follow facility policy for soiled linen.
21 Wash your hands.
22 Report the following to the nurse:
- The time, site, and length of the application
- Observations of the skin
- The person's response

Nonsterile applications are used for closed wounds. The compress or pack is placed in a basin of hot water. After it is wrung out, it is applied to the body part. The application is left in place for 20 minutes and then removed. Sometimes an aquathermia pad (page 519) is applied over the compress or pack. This maintains the temperature of the compress or pack.

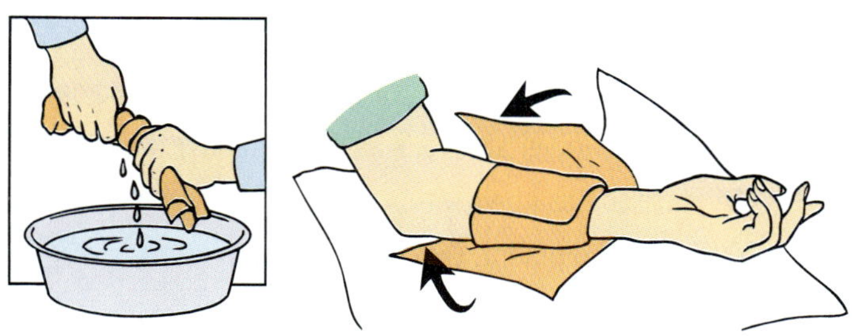

Fig. 23-2 *A hot compress is covered with plastic and a bath towel. These keep the compress warm.*

Commercial Compresses

Commercial compresses are premoistened and packaged in foil. An ultraviolet light is used to heat the wrapped compress for 10 minutes or as instructed by the manufacturer. The ultraviolet light is kept in the clean utility room, treatment room, medication room, or the person's room.

Commercial compresses are sterile. Sometimes doctors order them for nonsterile compresses. Nurses may decide they are needed in certain situations. Commercial compresses are costly and are used only when necessary.

Applying a Commercial Compress

Pre-procedure

1 Explain the procedure to the person.
2 Wash your hands.
3 Collect the following:
   - Commercial compress
   - Ultraviolet light
   - Towel
   - Ties, tape, or rolled gauze
   - Waterproof bed protector
   - Aquathermia pad (if ordered)
4 Follow the manufacturer's instructions for heating the compress. The instructions may involve placing the compress under an ultraviolet light for 10 minutes.
5 Identify the person. Check the ID bracelet with the treatment card.
6 Provide for privacy.

Procedure

7 Place the bed protector under the body part.
8 Open the foil-wrapped compress.
9 Apply the compress quickly with the foil wrap.
10 Cover it with the towel.
11 Secure the towel in place with ties, tape, or rolled gauze.
12 Apply the aquathermia pad (if ordered). See *Applying an Aquathermia Pad,* page 520.
13 Place the call bell within reach. Raise or lower side rails as instructed by the nurse.
14 Check the area every 5 minutes. Check for redness and complaints of pain, discomfort, or numbness. Remove the compress if any occur. Tell the nurse immediately.
15 Change the compress if cooling occurs.
16 Remove the compress after 20 minutes or as directed by the nurse. Pat the area dry with the towel. (Lower the side rail for this step.)

Post-procedure

17 Make sure the person is comfortable and unscreened.
18 Raise or lower side rails as instructed by the nurse.
19 Place the call bell within reach.
20 Clean equipment. Discard disposable items.
21 Follow facility policy for soiled linen.
22 Wash your hands.
23 Report the following to the nurse:
   - The time, site, and length of the application
   - Observations of the skin
   - The person's response

Hot Soaks

A hot soak involves putting the body part into water. This is usually used for smaller parts, such as a hand, lower arm, foot, or lower leg (Fig. 23-3). Sometimes large areas are soaked, such as the torso or an entire arm or leg. A tub is used for a large area. The soak lasts 15 to 20 minutes. The person's comfort and body alignment are maintained during the hot soak.

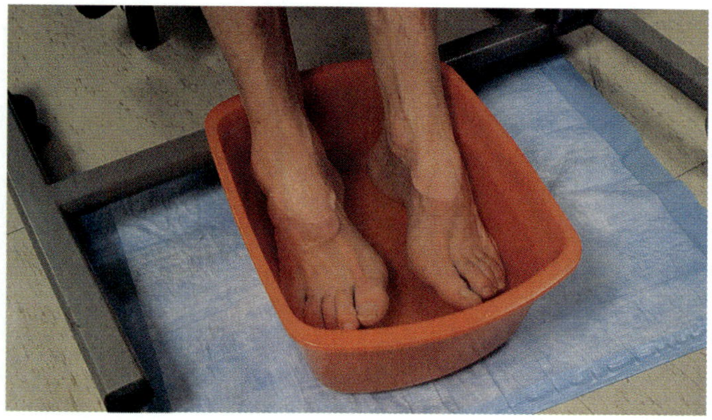

Fig. 23-3 *The hot soak.*

The Hot Soak

Pre-procedure

1 Explain the procedure to the person.

2 Wash your hands.

3 Collect the following:
- Water basin or an arm or foot bath
- Bath thermometer
- Bath blanket
- Waterproof pads

4 Identify the person. Check the ID bracelet with the treatment card.

5 Provide for privacy.

Procedure

6 Position the person for the treatment. Place the call bell within reach.

7 Place a waterproof pad under the area.

8 Fill the container one-half full with hot water. Measure water temperature. It should be 105° to 110° F (40.5° to 43.3° C) or as specified by facility policy.

9 Expose the area. Avoid unnecessary exposure.

10 Place the part into the water. Pad the edge of the container with a towel. Note the time.

11 Cover the person with a bath blanket for extra warmth.

12 Check the area every 5 minutes. Check for redness and complaints of pain, numbness, or discomfort. Remove the part from the soak if any of these occur. Wrap the part in a towel and tell the nurse immediately.

13 Check water temperature every 5 minutes. Change water as necessary. Wrap the part in a towel while changing the water.

14 Remove the part from the water in 15 to 20 minutes. Pat dry with a towel.

Post-procedure

15 Make sure the person is comfortable and unscreened.

16 Place the call bell within reach.

17 Raise or lower side rails as instructed by the nurse.

18 Clean and return equipment to its proper place. Discard disposable items.

19 Follow facility policy for soiled linen.

20 Wash your hands.

21 Report the following to the nurse:
- The time, site, and length of the application
- Observations of the skin
- The person's response

The Sitz Bath

The sitz bath (hip bath) involves immersing the pelvic area in warm or hot water for 20 minutes. (*Sitz* means seat in German.) Sitz baths are used to clean perineal or anal wounds, promote healing, relieve pain and soreness, increase circulation, or stimulate voiding. They are common after rectal or female pelvic surgery, for hemorrhoids, and after childbirth.

The disposable plastic sitz bath fits onto the toilet seat (Fig. 23-4). It can be used in the home or health facility. A sitz tub is a built-in fixture with a deep seat. The person sits in the seat that is filled with water (Fig. 23-5). A portable sitz chair is similar. The person sits with the knees flexed to keep the legs out of the water.

The sitz bath increases blood flow to the pelvic area. Therefore less blood flows to other body parts. As a result, the person may become weak or feel faint. The relaxing effect of the treatment may cause drowsiness. The person is carefully observed for signs of weakness, faintness, or fatigue. Also take precautions to keep the person safe from injury. This includes checking the person often, keeping the call bell within the person's reach, and taking measures to prevent chilling and burns.

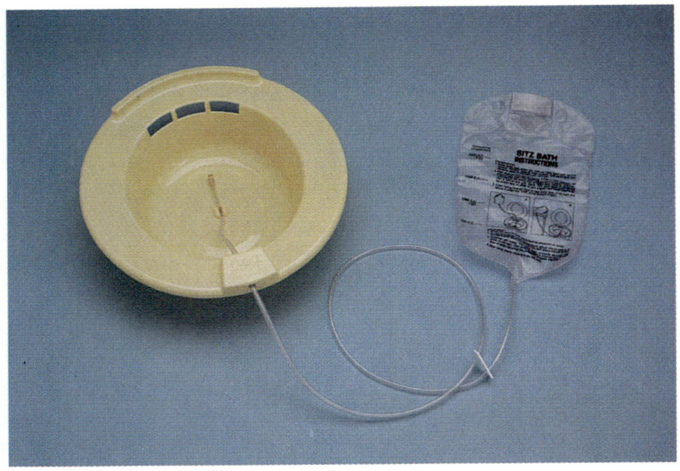

Fig. 23-4 *The disposable sitz bath.*

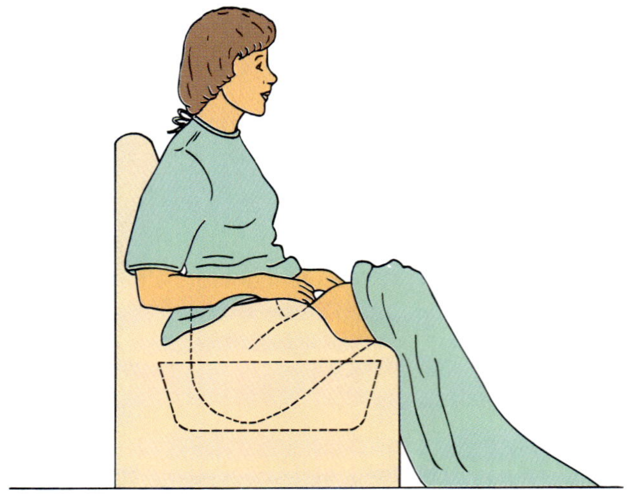

Fig. 23-5 *The built-in sitz bath.*

Assisting the Person to Take a Sitz Bath

Pre-procedure

1 Explain the procedure to the person.
2 Wash your hands.
3 Collect the following:
   - Portable or disposable sitz bath
   - Wheelchair if the built-in sitz bath is used
   - Bath thermometer
   - Large water container
   - Two bath blankets
   - Footstool if the person is short
   - Bath towels
   - Clean gown
   - Disinfectant solution
4 Identify the person. Check the ID bracelet with the treatment card.
5 Provide for privacy.

Procedure

6 Do one of the following:
   a Position the portable sitz bath at the bedside.
   b Place the disposable sitz bath on the toilet seat.
   c Transport the person by wheelchair to the sitz bath room.
7 Fill the sitz bath two-thirds full with water. Follow facility policy for water temperature. Generally the temperature is
   a 100° to 104° F (37.7° to 40° C) to clean the perineum
   b 105° to 110° F (40.5° to 43.3° C) to increase circulation
8 Lock the wheels of the portable sitz bath.
9 Use bath towels to pad the metal parts that will be in contact with the person.
10 Raise the gown and secure it above the waist.
11 Help the person sit in the sitz bath.
12 Place one bath blanket around the person's shoulders. Place another over the legs for warmth.
13 Provide a footstool if the edge of the sitz bath causes pressure under the knees.
14 Make sure the call bell is within reach and the person is comfortable.
15 Stay with a person who is weak or unsteady.
16 Check the person every 5 minutes for complaints of weakness, faintness, and drowsiness. Check for a rapid pulse. If any of these occur, get assistance to help the person back to bed.
17 Help the person out of the sitz bath after 20 minutes or as directed by the nurse.
18 Assist the person with drying and dressing.
19 Assist the person back to bed.

Post-procedure

20 Make sure he or she is comfortable and unscreened.
21 Place the call bell within reach.
22 Raise or lower side rails as instructed by the nurse.
23 Clean the sitz bath with disinfectant solution.
24 Return reusable items to their proper place.
25 Follow facility policy for soiled linen.
26 Wash your hands.
27 Report the following to the nurse:
   - The time the sitz bath started and ended
   - The person's response
   - The water temperature
   - Any other observations

Heat Lamps

A heat lamp applies dry heat. An infrared or a gooseneck lamp (Fig. 23-6) is used. The gooseneck is flexible. The lamp can be placed at various distances from the body part. First it is checked for breakage. Bulb wattage is also checked. The distance between the lamp and the body part is determined by the bulb wattage. The lamp is warmed up before the treatment starts. It is not covered with bed linens. Heat from the lamp could burn the linens and start a fire.

APPLYING A HEAT LAMP

PRE-PROCEDURE

1 Explain the procedure to the person.

2 Wash your hands.

3 Collect the following:
- Gooseneck lamp or infrared lamp
- Bath blanket
- Yardstick or tape measure

4 Identify the person. Check the ID bracelet with the treatment card.

5 Provide for privacy.

PROCEDURE

6 Plug in the lamp and allow it to warm up.

7 Cover the person with a bath blanket. Fanfold top linens to the foot of the bed.

8 Expose the body part.

9 Position the lamp a safe distance from the person. Follow facility policy. The following are offered as guidelines:
- **a** 25 watt bulb—14 inches
- **b** 40 watt bulb—18 inches
- **c** 60 watt bulb or small infrared lamp—18 to 24 inches
- **d** Large infrared lamp—24 to 30 inches

10 Note the time of application.

11 Measure the distance from the lamp to the person. Use the tape measure or yardstick (Fig. 23-7).

12 Cover body parts not being treated.

13 Check the person every 5 minutes. Check for redness or blistering of the skin. Ask about pain, burning, or decreased sensation. Stop the treatment if complications occur. Tell the nurse immediately.

14 Remove the lamp after 20 minutes or as directed by the nurse.

15 Return top linens to their proper position. Remove the bath blanket.

POST-PROCEDURE

16 Make sure the person is comfortable and unscreened.

17 Place the call bell within reach.

18 Raise or lower side rails as instructed by the nurse.

19 Clean the lamp according to facility policy. Return it and other supplies to their proper place.

20 Wash your hands.

21 Report the following to the nurse:
- The time the treatment started and ended
- The site of application
- Bulb wattage and the distance between the bulb and the person
- The person's response
- Any other observations

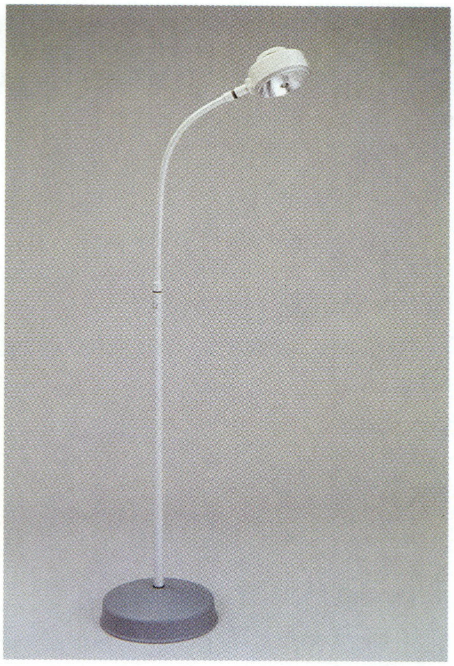

Fig. 23-6 *Gooseneck lamp. (Courtesy of Welch Allyn, Skaneateles Falls, North Carolina)*

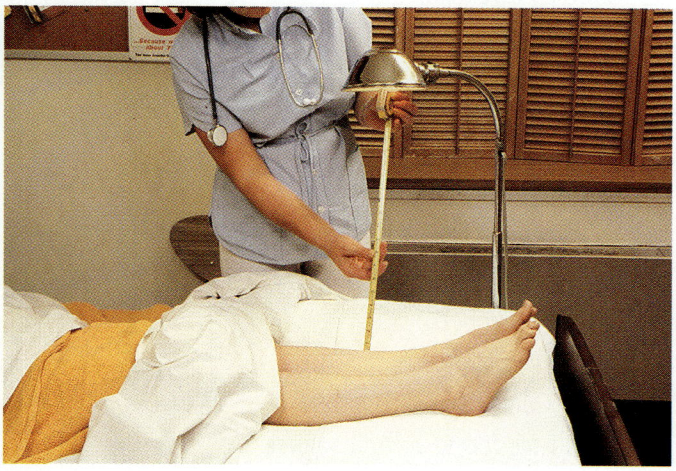

Fig. 23-7 *The distance between the heat lamp and the person is measured.*

The Aquathermia Pad

The aquathermia pad (Aqua-K, K-Pad) is an electric device used for dry heat. It is different from heating pads. Heating pads have electric coils made of wire. Tubes inside the aquathermia pad are filled with distilled water. A bedside heating unit is also filled with distilled water. The heated water flows to the pad through a connecting hose (Fig. 23-8). Another hose returns water to the heating unit. The water is reheated and circulated back into the pad.

The heating unit is kept level with the pad and connecting hoses. Water must flow freely. Hoses must be free of kinks and air bubbles. The temperature is set at 105° F (40.5° C) with a key provided by the manufacturer. After setting the temperature, the key is removed. This prevents anyone from changing the temperature. The temperature is often preset in the central supply department. The key is kept in that department.

The aquathermia pad is an electrical device. Measures are taken to prevent equipment-related accidents.

- Check the cord for fraying.
- Use a three-pronged plug to ground the device.
- Keep the cord out of the way of traffic.
- Place the heating unit on an even, uncluttered surface. This prevents it from being knocked over or knocked off of the surface.
- Secure the pad in place with ties, tape, or rolled gauze. Do not use pins. They can puncture the pad and cause leaking.
- Use a flannel cover to insulate the pad. It also absorbs perspiration at the application site.
- Do not place the pad under the person or under a body part. Weight from the body or extremity exerts pressure against the pad and mattress. This prevents the escape of heat. Burns can result if heat cannot escape.

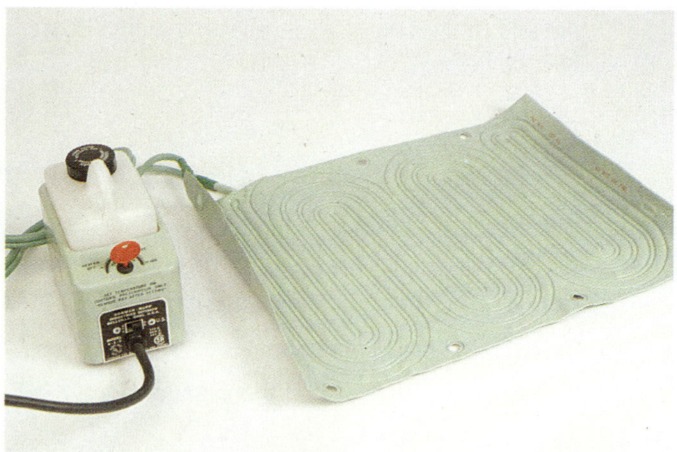

Fig. 23-8 *The aquathermia pad and heating unit.*

Applying an Aquathermia Pad

Pre-procedure

1 Explain the procedure to the person.

2 Wash your hands.

3 Collect the following:
- Aquathermia pad and heating unit
- Distilled water
- Flannel cover
- Ties, tape, or rolled gauze

4 Identify the person. Check the ID bracelet with the treatment card.

5 Provide for privacy.

Procedure

6 Fill the heating unit two-thirds full with distilled water.

7 Remove any air bubbles. Place the pad and tubing below the heating unit. Then tilt the unit from side to side.

8 Set the temperature as instructed by the nurse (usually 105° F or 40.5° C). Remove the key (give the key to the nurse when you complete the procedure).

9 Place the pad in the flannel cover.

10 Plug in the unit. Let water warm to the desired temperature.

11 Set the heating unit on the bedside stand. Keep the pad and connecting hoses level with the unit. Hoses must be free of kinks.

12 Apply the pad to the part. Note the time.

13 Secure the pad in place with ties, tape, or rolled gauze. Do not use pins.

14 Unscreen the person. Make sure the call bell is within reach.

15 Raise or lower side rails as instructed by the nurse.

16 Check the skin for redness, swelling, and blisters. Ask about pain, discomfort, or decreased sensation. Remove the pad if any occur. Tell the nurse immediately.

17 Remove the pad at the specified time. (Lower the side rail for this step.)

Post-procedure

18 Make sure the person is comfortable and unscreened.

19 Raise or lower side rails as instructed by the nurse.

20 Place the call bell within reach.

21 Clean and return equipment to its proper place.

22 Wash your hands.

23 Report the following to the nurse:
- The time of application and when it was removed
- The site of the application
- The temperature of the aquathermia pad
- The person's response
- Any other observations

Disposable Hot Packs

Disposable hot packs are dry heat applications. The pack contains chemicals. When activated, the chemicals react to cause heat. The package instructions tell how to activate the pack. Usually striking, squeezing, or kneading actions are used.

Some packs have protective outer coverings. If not, the pack is placed in a flannel cover. The pack is used once and then discarded.

Applying a Disposable Hot Pack

Pre-procedure

1. Explain the procedure to the person.
2. Wash your hands.
3. Collect the following:
   - Disposable hot pack
   - Flannel cover
   - Ties, tape, or rolled gauze
4. Identify the person. Check the ID bracelet with the treatment card.
5. Provide for privacy.

Procedure

6. Squeeze, knead, or strike the hot pack (see package directions). This causes a chemical reaction, which releases heat.
7. Cover the pack with the flannel cover.
8. Apply the hot pack to the part. Secure it in place with ties, tape, or rolled gauze. Note the time.
9. Place the call bell within reach. Raise or lower side rails as instructed by the nurse.
10. Check the skin every 5 minutes. Check for redness and for complaints of pain, discomfort, or numbness. Remove the pack if any occur. Notify the nurse immediately.
11. Remove the pack after 20 minutes or as directed by the nurse. (Lower the side rail for this step.)
12. Discard the pack and other disposable items. Place the flannel cover with the soiled linen.

Post-procedure

13. Make sure the person is comfortable and unscreened.
14. Raise or lower side rails as instructed by the nurse.
15. Place the call bell within reach.
16. Wash your hands.
17. Report the following to the nurse:
    - The time, site, and length of the application
    - Observations of the skin
    - The person's response

COLD APPLICATIONS

Cold applications are often used in the treatment of sprains and fractures. These are common sports injuries. They also occur from falls and other accidents. Cold applications reduce pain and prevent swelling. They also decrease circulation and bleeding. Cold cools the body when fever is present. Remember, heat and cold have opposite effects on body function.

Effects

When cold is applied to the skin, blood vessels constrict (see Fig. 23-1, C). Decreased blood flow results. Less oxygen and nutrients are carried to the tissues. Tissue metabolism also decreases. As a result, fewer toxic substances and waste products are produced. Cold applications are useful right after injury. The decreased circulation reduces the amount of bleeding. The amount of fluid accumulation in tissues is also reduced. Cold has a numbing effect on the skin. This helps reduce or relieve pain in the part. The skin appears pale and feels cool in the area of the cold because of decreased blood flow.

Complications

Complications can occur from local cold applications. They include pain, burns and blisters, and **cyanosis** (bluish discoloration of the skin). Burns and blisters tend to occur from intense cold. They also occur when dry cold applications are in direct contact with the skin. When cold is applied for a long time, blood vessels tend to dilate. Blood flow increases. Therefore the prolonged application of cold has the same effects as local heat applications.

Certain people are at greater risk for complications from local cold applications. They are infants, young children, the elderly, and fair-skinned persons. Persons with mental or sensory impairments are also at risk.

Moist and Dry Applications

Cold applications can be moist or dry. The ice bag and ice collar are dry cold applications. The cold compress and cold sponge bath are moist applications. Moist cold applications penetrate deeper than dry ones. Therefore temperatures of moist applications are not as cold as dry applications.

Patients and residents must be protected from injuries caused by cold applications. The rules for cold applications are listed in Box 23-2.

BOX 23-2 RULES FOR APPLYING COLD

- Know how to operate equipment used in the procedure.
- Measure the temperature of moist cold applications. Use a bath thermometer.
- Follow facility policies for the safe temperature ranges of cold applications.
- Know the different temperature ranges for cool, cold, and very cold applications. The following ranges are guidelines:
  Very cold—59° F and below (15° C and below)
  Cold—59° to 65° F (15° to 18 ° C)
  Cool—65° to 80° F (18° to 27° C)
- Do not apply *very cold* applications. These can damage tissue. The nurse applies *very cold* applications.
- Ask the nurse what the temperature of the application should be. Higher temperatures are used for those at risk.
- Know the precise location for the cold application. Ask the nurse to show you the site.
- Cover dry cold applications before applying them. Flannel covers are usually used.
- Report the following to the nurse immediately:
  *Complaints of numbness, pain, or burning
  *Blisters
  *Burns
  *Pale, white, or gray skin
  *Cyanosis
  *Shivering
- Do not let the person lower the temperature of the application.
- Ask the nurse how long to leave the application in place. Carefully watch the time. Cold is never applied longer than 30 minutes.
- Expose only the body part where the cold is to be applied. Provide for privacy through proper draping and screening.
- Place the call bell within the person's reach.

Ice Bags and Ice Collars

An ice bag and ice collar are dry cold applications. Ice collars are applied to the neck. The bag or collar is filled with crushed ice. Crushed ice is better than ice cubes. The smaller pieces of ice allow easier molding of the bag to the body part. Also, there is less air space between crushed ice for more even cooling. The ice bag or collar is placed in a flannel cover. If the cover becomes moist, it is removed and a dry one applied. Ice bags and ice collars are left in place no longer than 30 minutes. If the bag or collar is to be reapplied, wait 1 hour. This gives tissues time to recover from the cold.

Some facilities use commercial ice bags. They are filled with a special solution and are kept frozen until needed. Commercial ice bags can be refrozen for reuse. Flannel covers are also needed with ice collars or commercial ice bags.

Applying an Ice Bag or Collar

Pre-procedure

1 Explain the procedure to the person.

2 Wash your hands.

3 Collect the following:

- Ice bag or collar
- Crushed ice
- Flannel cover
- Paper towels

Procedure

4 Fill the ice bag with water. Put in the stopper. Turn the bag upside down to check for leaks.

5 Empty the bag.

6 Fill the bag one-half to two-thirds full with crushed ice or ice chips (Fig. 23-9 on page 524).

7 Remove excess air. Bend, twist, or squeeze the bag, or press it against a firm surface.

8 Place the cap or stopper on securely.

9 Dry the bag with the paper towels.

10 Place the bag in the flannel cover.

11 Identify the person. Check the ID bracelet with the treatment card.

12 Provide for privacy.

13 Apply the ice bag to the part.

14 Place the call bell within reach. Raise or lower side rails as instructed by the nurse.

15 Check the skin every 10 minutes. Check for blisters; pale, white, or gray skin; cyanosis; and shivering. Ask about numbness, pain, or burning. Remove the bag if any occur. Tell the nurse immediately.

16 Remove the bag after 30 minutes or as directed by the nurse. (Lower the side rail for this step.)

Post-procedure

17 Make sure the person is comfortable and unscreened.

18 Place the call bell within reach.

19 Raise or lower side rails as instructed by the nurse.

20 Clean equipment. Place the flannel cover with the soiled linen.

21 Wash your hands.

22 Report the following to the nurse:

- The time, site, and length of the application
- Your observations of the skin
- The person's response

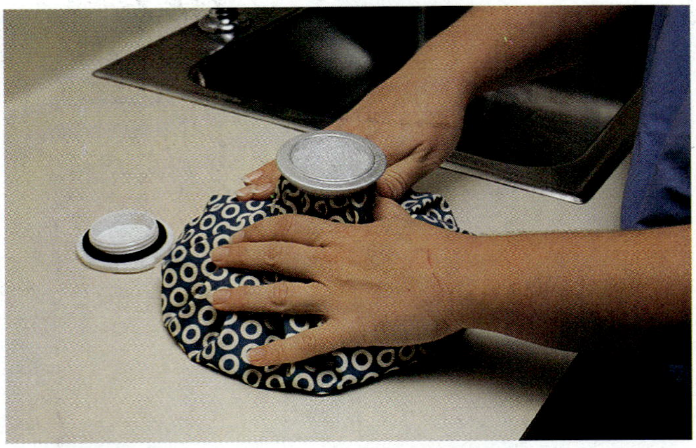

Fig. 23-9 *The ice bag is filled one-half to two-thirds full with ice.*

Disposable Cold Packs

Disposable cold packs are dry cold applications. They are used once and then discarded. They come in various sizes to fit different body parts. Some have an outer covering so the pack can be applied directly to the skin. Use a flannel cover if there is no outer covering. A cold pack is left in place no longer than 30 minutes.

APPLYING DISPOSABLE COLD PACKS

PRE-PROCEDURE

1 Explain the procedure to the person.
2 Wash your hands.
3 Collect the following:
- Disposable cold pack
- Flannel cover
- Ties, tape, or rolled gauze

4 Identify the person. Check the ID bracelet with the treatment card.
5 Provide for privacy.

PROCEDURE

6 Squeeze, knead, or strike the cold pack as directed by the manufacturer. This causes a chemical reaction, which releases cold.
7 Cover the pack with the flannel cover.
8 Apply the cold pack to the part. Secure it in place with ties, tape, or rolled gauze. Note the time.
9 Place the call bell within reach. Raise or lower side rails as instructed by the nurse.
10 Check the skin every 10 minutes. Check for blisters; pale, white, or gray skin; cyanosis; and shivering. Ask about pain, numbness, or burning. Remove the pack if any occur. Tell the nurse immediately.
11 Remove the pack after 30 minutes or as directed by the nurse. (Lower the side rails for this step.)

POST-PROCEDURE

12 Make sure the person is comfortable and unscreened.
13 Place the call bell within reach.
14 Raise or lower side rails as instructed by the nurse.
15 Discard the pack and other disposable items. Place the flannel cover with the soiled linen.
16 Wash your hands.
17 Report the following to the nurse:
- The time, site, and length of the application
- Your observations of the skin
- The person's response

Cold Compresses

Applying a cold compress is like applying a hot compress. The cold compress is a moist application. It may be sterile or nonsterile. As with hot compresses, the nurse applies sterile cold compresses. Sterile compresses are ordered for open wounds. Moist cold compresses are left in place no longer than 20 minutes.

Applying Cold Compresses

Pre-procedure

1 Explain the procedure to the person.
2 Wash your hands.
3 Collect the following:
   - Large basin with ice
   - Small basin with cold water
   - Gauze squares, washcloths, or small towels
   - Waterproof pad
   - Bath towel
4 Identify the person. Check the ID bracelet with the treatment card.
5 Provide for privacy.

Procedure

6 Place the small basin with cold water into the large basin with ice.
7 Place the compresses into the cold water.
8 Place a bed protector under the affected body part. Expose the area.
9 Wring out a compress so water is not dripping.
10 Apply the compress to the part. Note the time.
11 Check the area every 5 minutes. Check for blisters; pale, white, or gray skin; cyanosis; or shivering. Ask about numbness, pain, or burning. Remove the compress if any occur. Tell the nurse immediately.
12 Change the compress when it warms. Usually compresses are changed every 5 minutes.
13 Remove the compress after 20 minutes or as directed by the nurse.
14 Pat dry the area with the bath towel.

Post-procedure

15 Make sure the person is comfortable and unscreened.
16 Raise or lower side rails as instructed by the nurse.
17 Place the call bell within reach.
18 Clean equipment.
19 Follow facility policy for soiled linen.
20 Wash your hands.
21 Report the following to the nurse:
   - The time, site, and length of the application
   - Observations of the skin
   - The person's response

Cool Sponge Baths

The cool sponge bath (tepid sponge bath) is used to reduce body temperature when there is a high fever. A doctor's order is required in many facilities. The order may include adding alcohol to the water. Alcohol evaporates quickly, causing rapid cooling. Alcohol also dries the skin. Therefore alcohol is not often ordered.

At first the cool sponge bath causes vasoconstriction, chilling, and shivering. These reactions increase body temperature. As the body adjusts to the cold, body temperature decreases. The bath lasts for 25 to 30 minutes to allow time for the body to adjust.

Vital signs are taken before, during, and after the procedure. They are taken every 15 minutes during the procedure. Ice bags or moist cold compresses may be used to help lower body temperature. They are applied to the forehead, axillae (underarms), and groin. The nurse may also want them placed on each side of the neck.

Giving a Cool Sponge Bath

Pre-procedure

1 Explain the procedure to the person.

2 Wash your hands.

3 Collect the following:
- Bath basin
- Bath thermometer
- Equal amounts of 70% alcohol and water, if alcohol is ordered
- Six ice bags or disposable ice packs with flannel covers (if ordered)
- Bath blanket
- Two or more bath towels
- Two or more washcloths
- Thermometer for body temperature
- Sphygmomanometer and stethoscope
- Ice chips

4 Identify the person. Check the ID bracelet with the treatment card.

5 Provide for privacy.

Procedure

6 Measure and record vital signs. Note the time.

7 Raise the bed to a level appropriate for good body mechanics. Lower the side rail.

8 Cover the person with a bath blanket. Remove top linens.

9 Remove the gown without exposing the person. Raise the side rail.

10 Prepare the ice bags or packs for application. Place them in the flannel covers.

11 Lower the side rail. Move the person to the side of the bed near you.

12 Apply the ice bags or packs to the forehead, axillae, and groin. Place one on each side of the neck if requested by the nurse (Fig. 23-10). Apply cold applications only if ordered.

13 Raise the side rail.

14 Fill the basin two-thirds full with cool water. Water (and alcohol if added) temperature should be about 98° F (37° C) or as directed by the nurse. Add ice chips to cool the water if necessary.

15 Place the washcloths in the water. Alternate washcloths during the procedure. Make sure no ice chips stick to them.

16 Lower the side rail.

17 Place a bath towel under the far arm.

18 Sponge the arm for 5 minutes with long, slow, gentle strokes. Pat dry; do not rub dry.

19 Repeat steps 17 and 18 for the near arm.

20 Measure and record vital signs. Note the time.

PROCEDURE—CONT'D

21 Stop sponging and notify the nurse if one or more of the following occur:
- Body temperature is normal or slightly above normal.
- Shivering.
- Cyanosis.
- Other signs and symptoms of cold. Check the skin under the ice bags. Notify the nurse of signs of complications.

22 Place the bath towel lengthwise over the chest and abdomen. Fanfold the bath blanket to the pubic area.

23 Sponge the chest and abdomen for 3 to 5 minutes. Pat the area dry, cover the person with the bath blanket, and remove the towel.

24 Place a towel under the far leg.

25 Sponge the leg with long, slow, gentle strokes for 5 minutes. Pat the leg dry, cover, and remove the bath blanket.

26 Repeat steps 23 and 24 for the near leg.

27 Measure and record vital signs. Note the time. Follow the guidelines in step 21.

28 Help the person turn away from you.

29 Place a bath towel on the bed along the length of the person's back and buttocks.

30 Sponge the back and buttocks with long, slow, gentle strokes for 5 minutes. Pat dry and remove the towel.

31 Position the person supine. Cover the person with the bath blanket.

32 Remove the ice packs.

33 Measure and record vital signs. Note the time.

34 Put a clean gown on the person. Make the bed. Change damp or soiled linen.

POST-PROCEDURE

35 Make sure the person is comfortable.

36 Raise or lower side rails as instructed by the nurse.

37 Lower the bed to its lowest position.

38 Place the call bell within reach.

39 Unscreen the person.

40 Clean and return equipment to its proper place.

41 Remove soiled linen and disposable items.

42 Measure vital signs 15 minutes after the procedure.

43 Wash your hands.

44 Report the following to the nurse:
- The time the procedure was started and completed
- All vital sign measurements
- How the person tolerated the procedure
- Condition of the skin under the cold applications
- Other signs and symptoms

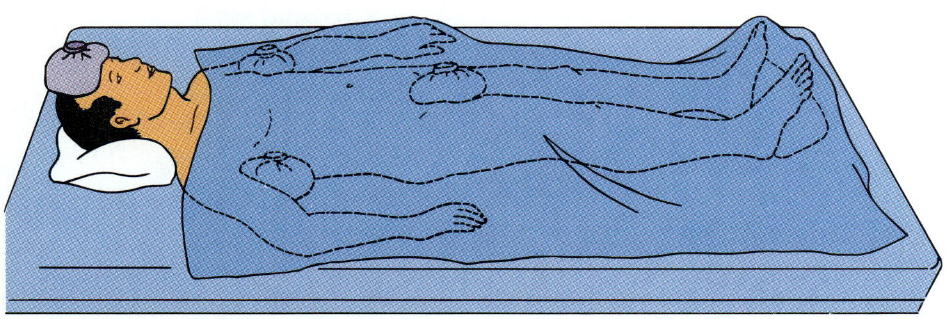

Fig. 23-10 *Ice bags are applied to the forehead, axillae, and groin to help cool the body during the sponge bath. Ice bags may also be applied on each side of the neck if requested by the nurse. A hot water bottle is applied to the feet to prevent chilling.*

Summary

Heat and cold applications are often ordered by doctors. They have opposite effects on blood flow. However, both are used for healing, comfort, and tissue swelling. Extreme care is taken to use the right temperature. Heat and cold must be applied properly. Close observation of the person is necessary. Complications can easily and quickly occur if safety precautions are not taken. Of all the complications, burns are the most serious.

Your facility may allow the application of heat and cold only by RNs or LPNs. If you are allowed to apply heat and cold, extreme caution must be taken. The dangers to the person are severe. Therefore greater knowledge and judgment are required. The purpose and steps of the procedure are reviewed with the nurse. Also ask the nurse to closely supervise the procedure and its effects on the person. The person's safety is the most important consideration.

The person's quality of life is important. Make sure the environment is safe and comfortable. Heat and cold applications take between 20 and 30 minutes. The person is not free to move about during this time. Encourage the person to use the toilet, commode, urinal, or bedpan before the procedure. Also make sure the room is free of unpleasant equipment or odors. Needed items must be within the person's reach. These include the call bell, water, books or magazines, needlework, telephone, television controls, and other items requested by the person. Be sure to check the person often. You are responsible for the person's safety.

Review Questions

Circle the best *answer.*

1 Jane Connor has arthritis in her knees and ankles. Local heat applications were ordered for these areas. Local heat has the following effects *except*

- **a** Pain relief
- **b** Muscle relaxation
- **c** Healing
- **d** Decreased blood flow

2 Which complication of heat is the greatest threat to Jane Connor?

- **a** Infection
- **b** Burns
- **c** Chilling
- **d** Pressure sores

3 Who has the greatest risk of complications from local heat applications?

- **a** A 10-year-old boy
- **b** A teenager
- **c** A 40-year-old woman
- **d** An elderly person

4 These statements are about moist heat applications. Which is *false?*

- **a** Water is in contact with the skin.
- **b** The effects of moist heat are less than with a dry heat application.
- **c** Heat penetrates deeper than with a dry heat application.
- **d** The temperature of the application is lower than a dry heat application.

5 The temperature of a hot application is usually between

- **a** 65° and 80° F
- **b** 93° and 98° F
- **c** 98° and 105° F
- **d** 105° and 115° F

6 An extremity is in a basin of hot water. This is a

- **a** Hot compress
- **b** Hot pack
- **c** Hot soak
- **d** Sitz bath

REVIEW QUESTIONS—CONT'D

7 These statements are about sitz baths. Which is *false?*

- **a** The pelvic area is immersed in warm or hot water for 20 minutes.
- **b** Weakness and fainting can occur.
- **c** The sitz bath lasts 25 to 30 minutes.
- **d** They can be used to clean the perineum, relieve pain, increase circulation, or stimulate voiding.

8 You are applying a heat lamp. You should do the following *except*

- **a** Cover the lamp with bed linens
- **b** Let the lamp warm up before starting the procedure
- **c** Check the bulb wattage
- **d** Measure the distance between the bulb and the person's body

9 Jane Connor is using an aquathermia pad. Which is *false?*

- **a** The aquathermia pad is a dry heat application.
- **b** The temperature is usually set at 105° F.
- **c** Electrical safety precautions must be practiced.
- **d** Pins secure the aquathermia pad in place.

10 Jane Connor sprained her wrist. Local cold applications were ordered to

- **a** Reduce pain, prevent swelling, and decrease circulation
- **b** Dilate blood vessels
- **c** Prevent the spread of microorganisms
- **d** All of the above

11 Which is *not* a complication of local cold applications?

- **a** Pain
- **b** Burns and blisters
- **c** Cyanosis
- **d** Infection

12 A dry cold application is ordered for Jane Connor's wrist. Which is a dry cold application?

- **a** The ice bag
- **b** The cold compress
- **c** The cold sponge bath
- **d** All of the above

13 Before applying an ice bag

- **a** The bag is placed in a freezer
- **b** The temperature of the bag is measured
- **c** The bag is placed in a flannel cover
- **d** The person is asked to void

14 Moist cold compresses are left in place no longer than

- **a** 20 minutes
- **b** 30 minutes
- **c** 45 minutes
- **d** 60 minutes

15 The cool sponge bath is ordered to

- **a** Reduce swelling
- **b** Relieve pain
- **c** Decrease circulation
- **d** Lower body temperature

16 The cool sponge bath should last

- **a** 15 to 20 minutes
- **b** 25 to 30 minutes
- **c** 45 to 50 minutes
- **d** 60 minutes or longer

Answers to these questions are on page 752.

Special Procedures and Treatments

24

OBJECTIVES

- Define the key terms listed in this chapter
- Describe how to give safe care to a person with an IV infusion
- Identify common routes and reasons for suctioning
- Describe the rules related to suctioning
- Explain the purpose of oxygen therapy
- Describe the sources and devices used to administer oxygen
- Describe the rules for oxygen therapy
- Collect a sputum specimen
- Give a vaginal irrigation

Key Terms

douche Vaginal irrigation

face mask A device used to administer oxygen; it covers the nose and mouth

nasal cannula A two-pronged device used to administer oxygen; the prongs are inserted into the nostrils

sputum Mucus secreted by the lungs, bronchi, and trachea during respiratory illnesses or disorders

suction The process of withdrawing or sucking up fluids

vaginal irrigation The introduction of a fluid into the vagina and the immediate return of the fluid; douche

Intravenous (IV) therapy, suctioning, and oxygen therapy involve complex principles. *You are not responsible for these therapies and treatments.* Risks to patients and residents are great. However, you need to understand their use and purpose. You also need to know how to safely care for persons receiving these therapies.

You may be asked to collect a sputum specimen or give a vaginal irrigation. These procedures are performed only if you have had the necessary instruction. You must understand the purpose, the procedure, and the possible complications. The procedure is first reviewed with the nurse. The nurse closely supervises the procedure and its effect on the person.

INTRAVENOUS THERAPY

An intravenous (IV) infusion is the administration of fluid through a needle within a vein. *You are never responsible for IV therapy.* However, you may care for persons receiving IV infusions. You must give safe care. Therefore you must understand the basic purposes of IV therapy and needed safety measures.

Purposes

Doctors order IV infusions. The doctor orders the amount and type of IV solution to be given. IVs are ordered for one or more of the following reasons:

- To provide needed fluids when the person cannot take fluids by mouth
- To replace minerals and vitamins lost because of illness or injury
- To provide sugar for energy
- To administer medications and blood

Safety Measures

RNs start and maintain IV infusions. The RN inserts a needle or catheter into a vein (Fig. 24-1) and connects IV tubing from the IV bag to the needle (Fig. 24-2 on page 532). RNs also regulate the flow rate (the number of drops per minute). They change the bags, tubing, and dressings at insertion sites. These are changed when necessary. Blood or medications ordered by the doctor are also given by RNs.

You need to know two parts of the IV infusion (see Fig. 24-2). One is the drip chamber. Fluid drips from the bag into the drip chamber. You can tell if the fluid is flowing by looking at the chamber. If no fluid is dripping, tell the nurse immediately. The second part is the clamp on the tubing. The RN uses the clamp to regulate the flow rate. *Never change the position of the clamp.*

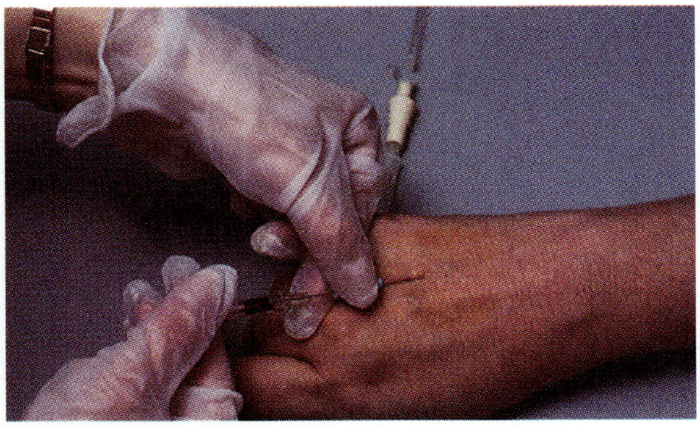

Fig. 24-1 *The nurse starts an IV by inserting a needle or catheter into a vein.* (From Potter PA, Perry AG: *Fundamentals of nursing: concepts, process, and practice,* ed 3, St Louis, 1993, Mosby—Year Book.)

Electronic pumps are often used to control the flow rate (Fig. 24-3). The nurse sets the flow rate. An alarm sounds if a problem occurs with the flow rate. Tell the nurse immediately if you hear the alarm. Never adjust any of the controls on electronic pumps.

You are never responsible for starting, maintaining, or discontinuing an IV infusion. Nor do you regulate the flow rate or change IV bags, tubing, or dressings. Nursing assistants never administer blood or medications. You may assist persons with IVs to meet personal hygiene and activity needs. The safety measures in Box 24-1 are important. Complications can occur from IV therapy. Report any of the signs and symptoms listed in Box 24-2 to the nurse immediately.

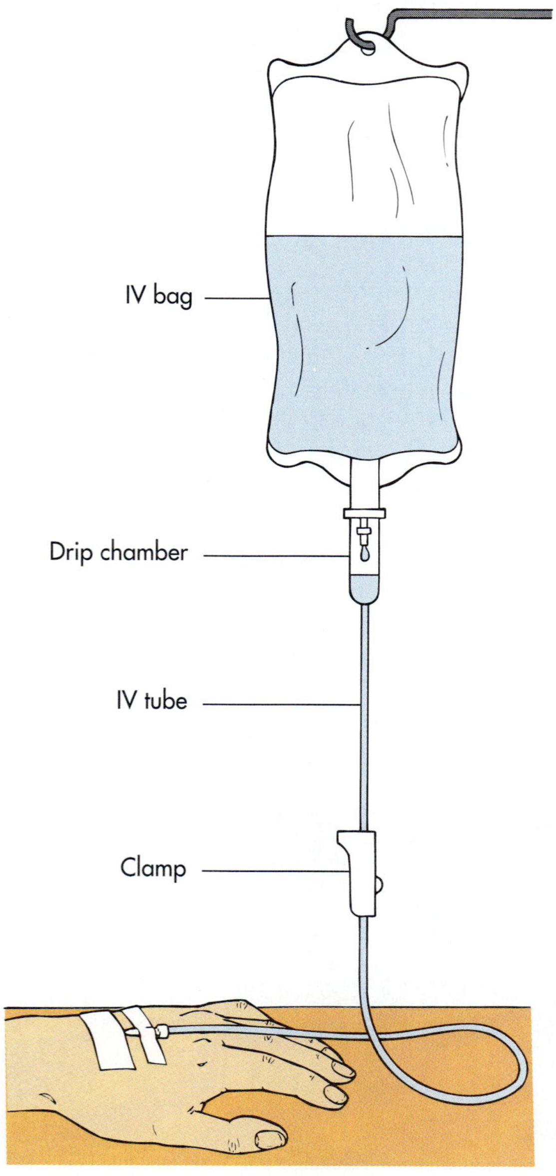

Fig. 24-2 *Tubing from the IV bag is connected to the needle.*

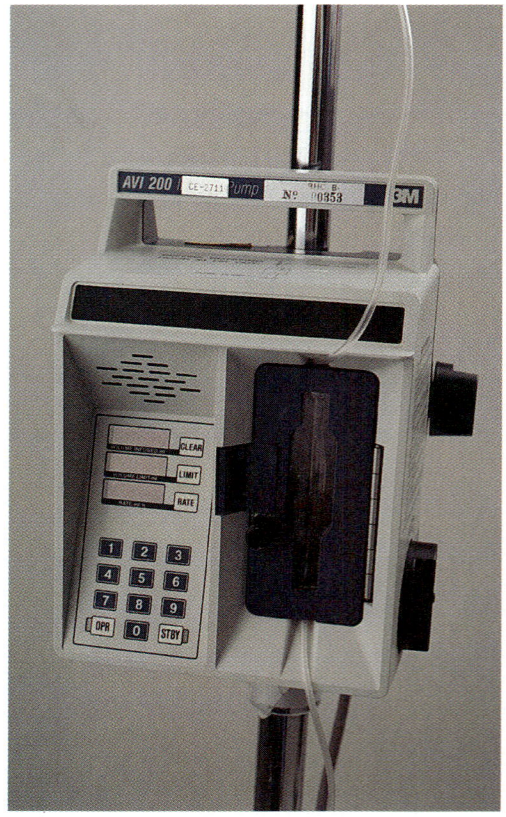

Fig. 24-3 *Electronic pump controls the IV flow rate.*

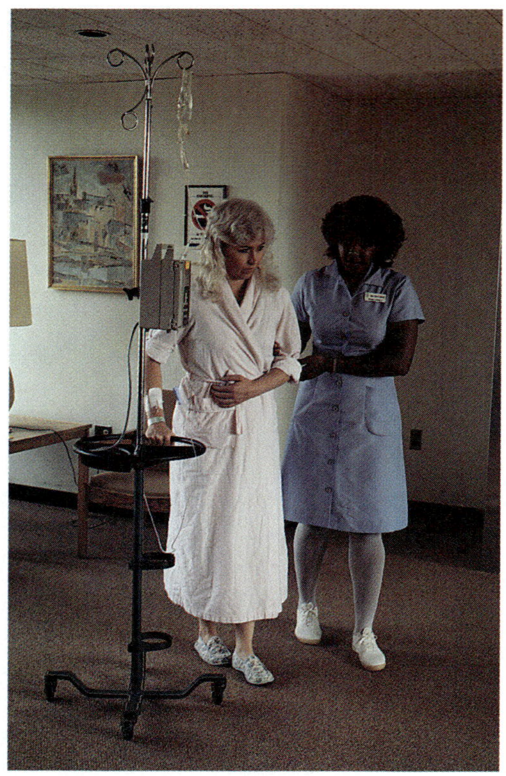

Fig. 24-4 *A person ambulating with an IV.*

BOX 24-1 SAFETY MEASURES FOR IV THERAPY

- Do not move the needle or catheter. The position of the IV needle or catheter must be maintained when assisting a person. If the needle or catheter is moved, it may come out of the vein. Then fluid flows into the tissues (infiltration), or the flow stops.
- Follow the safety measures for restraints if a restraint is used (see Chapter 8). Sometimes the nurse splints or restrains the extremity to prevent movement of the part. This helps prevent the needle or catheter from moving.
- Be careful not to move the needle or catheter when changing a gown (see *Changing the Gown of a Person with an IV,* page 331).
- Protect the IV bag, tubing, and needle or catheter when ambulating the person. Portable IV standards are rolled along next to the person (Fig. 24-4).
- Assist the person with turning and repositioning. The IV bag is moved to the side of the bed on which the person is lying. Always allow enough slack in the tubing. The needle will dislodge if pressure is exerted by the tubing.
- Notify the nurse immediately if there is bleeding from the insertion site. Be sure to follow Standard Precautions and the Bloodborne Pathogen Standard.
- Notify the nurse immediately of any of the signs and symptoms listed in Box 24-2.

SUCTIONING

Injury and illness often cause secretions to collect in body parts. Common areas are the upper airway, stomach, and surgical wounds. The secretions are removed for the person's recovery and well-being. Suction is a method ordered by the doctor to remove excess secretions. **Suction** is the process of withdrawing or sucking up fluid (secretions). A tube is connected to a wall suction outlet, a suction machine, or a disposable suction system (Fig. 24-5 on page 534). The other end is inserted into the body part. The secretions are withdrawn through the tube (or catheter) into a collecting container.

You are not responsible for inserting tubes or suctioning persons. However, you may care for a person who needs suctioning. Some states allow nursing assistants to suction persons who have long-standing tracheostomies (a surgically created opening into the trachea). If your state allows you to perform this function, special education and training are necessary.

BOX 24-2 SIGNS AND SYMPTOMS OF COMPLICATIONS OF IV THERAPY

- Bleeding
- Puffiness or swelling
- Pale or reddened skin
- Complaints of pain
- Skin at or near the site is hot or cold
- Fever
- Itching
- Drop in blood pressure
- Tachycardia (pulse rate greater than 100 beats per minute)
- Cyanosis
- Loss of consciousness
- Difficulty breathing (dyspnea)

A

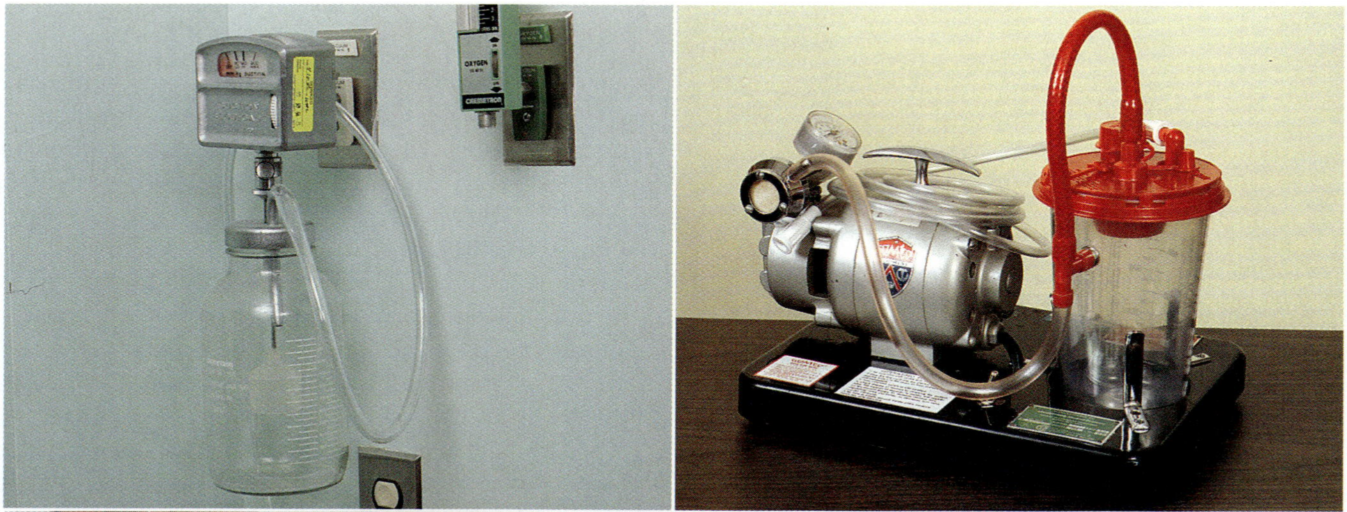

B

C

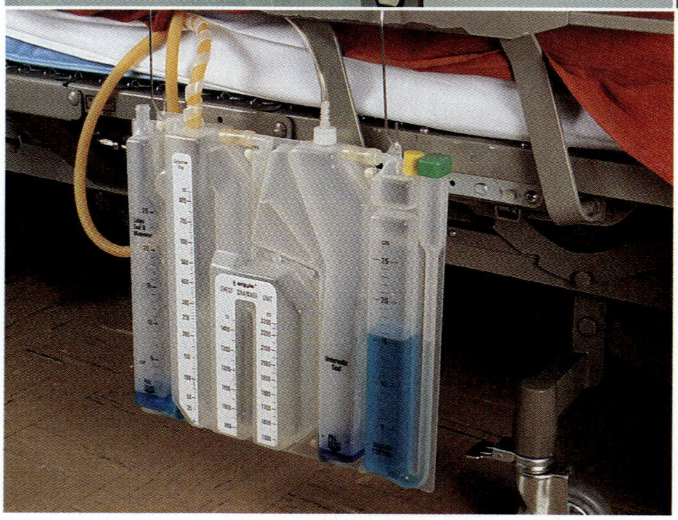

Fig. 24-5 ***A,*** *Wall suction.* ***B,*** *Suction machine.* ***C,*** *Disposable suction apparatus.*

Upper Airway Suctioning

The airway must be clear of secretions for normal breathing. Certain illnesses cause secretions to collect in the upper airway. Usually coughing removes the secretions. If not, the upper airway is suctioned to remove the secretions. A nurse inserts a suction catheter through the mouth or nose into the trachea when suctioning is needed (Fig. 24-6). When suctioning is complete, the catheter is removed. You must be alert for signs and symptoms that signal the need for suctioning. The following are reported to the nurse immediately.

- Tachypnea—rapid breathing; respiratory rate is greater than 24 respirations per minute
- Dyspnea—difficult, labored, or painful breathing
- Moist sounding respirations or gurgling
- Restlessness
- Cyanosis—bluish skin color

Nasogastric Suctioning

A nasogastric tube (NG tube) is used to remove stomach contents and to keep the stomach empty. Gastrointestinal injuries, illnesses, and surgeries often require nasogastric suctioning. A nurse inserts the tube through the person's nose, the esophagus, and into the stomach (see Fig. 17-12, page 420). The tube is connected to the suction source. The NG tube is left in place until the doctor orders its removal.

The NG tube can irritate the nose and mouth. Mouth breathing is common. Usually no oral fluids are allowed. The lips and oral mucous membranes easily dry and crack. A bad taste in the mouth and mouth odor may develop. Therefore oral hygiene is given often. The nose also is kept clean. Pressure and friction from the tube can irritate the nostril. Nasal secretions may harden and form crusts. The tube must not cause pressure on the nose.

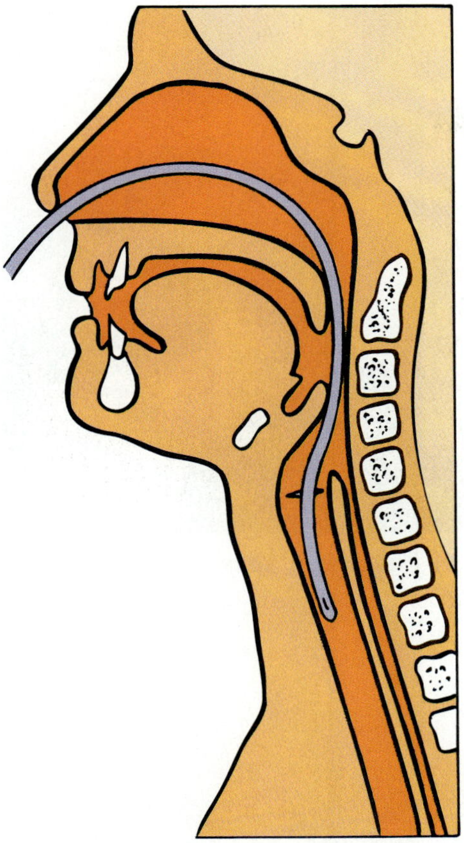

Fig. 24-6 *A suction catheter inserted through the person's nose into the trachea. Tubing connects the catheter to wall suction.*

Wound Suctioning

Surgery or injuries can result in blood and other drainage to collect in a wound. The wound must be suctioned. A drain or catheter is inserted and attached to suction. Often the drain or catheter is inserted during surgery. Chest and abdominal surgeries usually require wound suction.

Safety Rules

The person is protected from harm during suctioning. The suction tubing or catheter and the suction source are handled carefully. You need to practice the safety rules listed in Box 24-3.

OXYGEN THERAPY

Oxygen is a tasteless, odorless, and colorless gas. Oxygen is necessary for survival. Death occurs within 4 minutes if a person stops breathing. Serious health problems develop if a person does not have enough oxygen. During illness, the amount of oxygen in the blood may be less than normal. If so, the doctor orders supplemental oxygen. Surgery, acute illness, respiratory disorders, and heart disease are among the many reasons for supplemental oxygen.

Oxygen is treated as a drug. The doctor orders the amount of oxygen to be given and the device to be used to administer the oxygen. The order also states if oxygen is to be given continuously or intermittently (periodically). *Continuous oxygen therapy* means that the oxygen is never stopped. That is, the administration of oxygen is not interrupted for any reason. *Intermittent oxygen therapy* is for symptom relief. Chest pain and exercise are common reasons for intermittent oxygen. The oxygen helps relieve chest pain. Persons with chronic respiratory diseases may have adequate oxygen at rest. With mild exercise or activities of daily living, they may become short of breath. Oxygen helps to relieve the shortness of breath.

BOX 24-3 Safety Rules when Caring for Persons Needing Suctioning

- Never suction a person.
- Make sure the person is not lying on the catheter or tubing.
- Make sure there are no kinks in the catheter or tubing.
- Never turn off the suction source.
- Do not raise the drainage container above the insertion site.
- Do not empty the drainage container.
- Do not disconnect any part of the suction system.
- Report the appearance of bright red drainage or an increase in the amount of blood to the nurse immediately.
- Observe the amount and appearance of drainage in the container. Report your observations to the nurse at regular intervals. Report unusual observations immediately.
- Make sure there is enough slack in the tubing. There should not be any pull or pressure at the insertion site.

BOX 24-4 Safety Rules for Oxygen Therapy

- Follow the safety precautions for fire and the use of oxygen (see Chapter 8).
- Never remove the device (catheter, mask) used to administer oxygen.
- Never shut off oxygen flow from the wall outlet or tank.
- Give oral hygiene as directed by the nurse.
- Tape or pin the connecting tubing to the person's gown. The tubing must be secured in place.
- Make sure there are no kinks in the tubing.
- Make sure the person is not lying on any part of the tubing.
- Report signs and symptoms of respiratory distress or abnormal breathing patterns to the nurse immediately (see Chapter 18).
- Check the gauge to ensure there is adequate oxygen in the tank (Fig. 24-7). Tell the nurse if the tank is low.
- Check to make sure the oxygen is flowing at the ordered rate. Tell the nurse immediately if there is a problem.

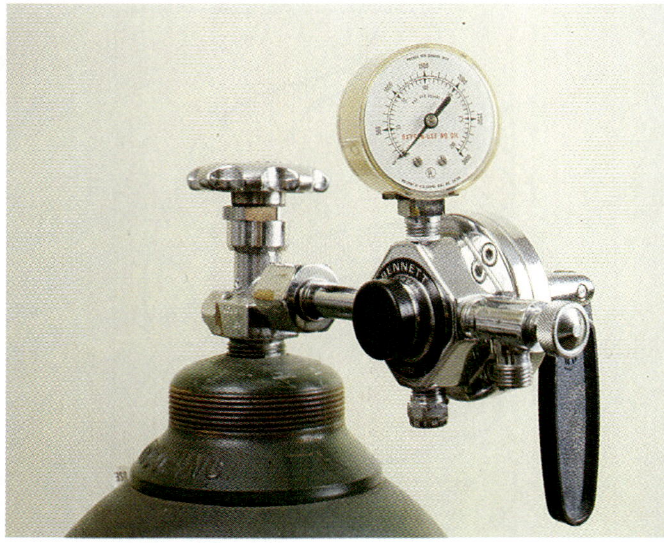

Fig. 24-7 *The oxygen tank gauge shows the amount remaining.*

You are never responsible for administering oxygen. The nurse and respiratory therapist start and maintain oxygen therapy. However, you may care for persons receiving oxygen therapy. Therefore you need to know how to give safe care to these persons. Safety rules for oxygen therapy are listed in Box 24-4.

Devices Used to Administer Oxygen

Oxygen is supplied through wall outlets and from oxygen tanks. Oxygen concentrators are often used in nursing facilities and in private homes.

With the wall outlet (Fig. 24-8), oxygen is piped into each patient or resident unit. Each unit is connected to a centrally located oxygen supply.

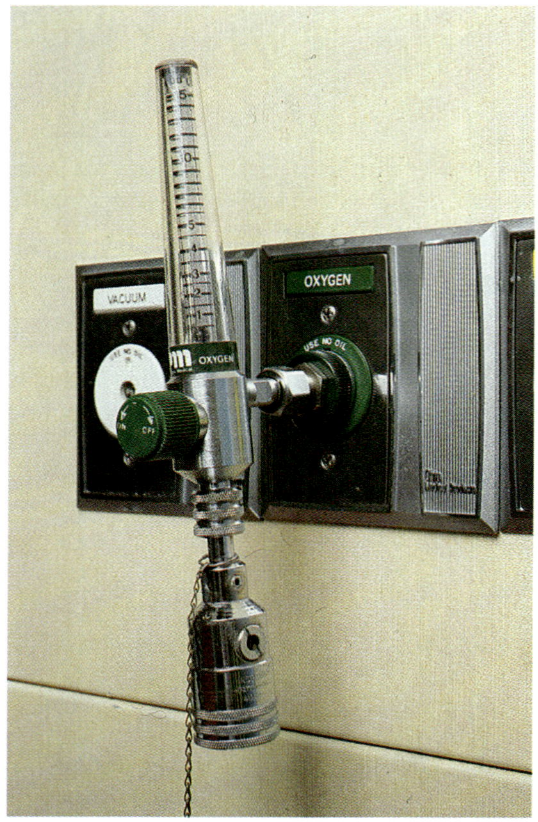

Fig. 24-8 *Wall oxygen outlet.*

The oxygen tank is portable (Fig. 24-9). It is brought to the person's unit when the doctor orders oxygen therapy. Small oxygen tanks are used during emergencies and transfers. Some ambulatory persons need continuous oxygen. Portable oxygen cylinders are used when walking (Fig. 24-10). The large oxygen tank is more common in homes.

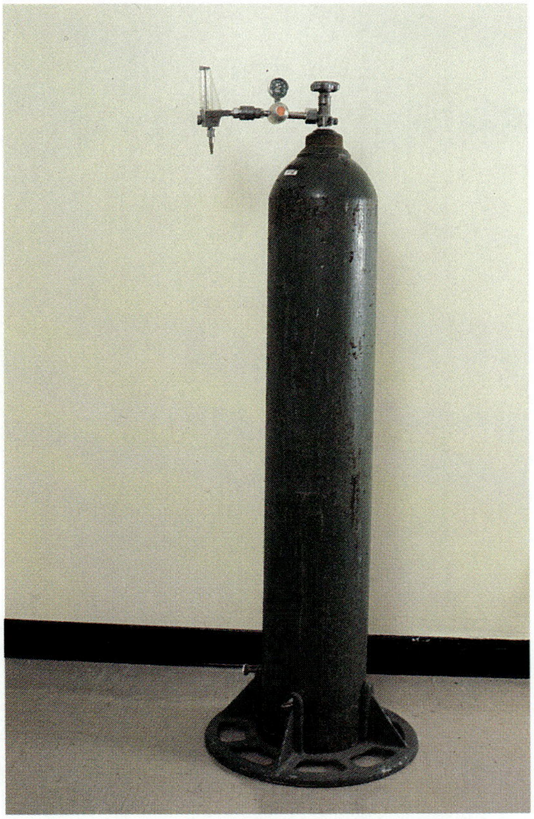

Fig. 24-9 *Oxygen tank.*

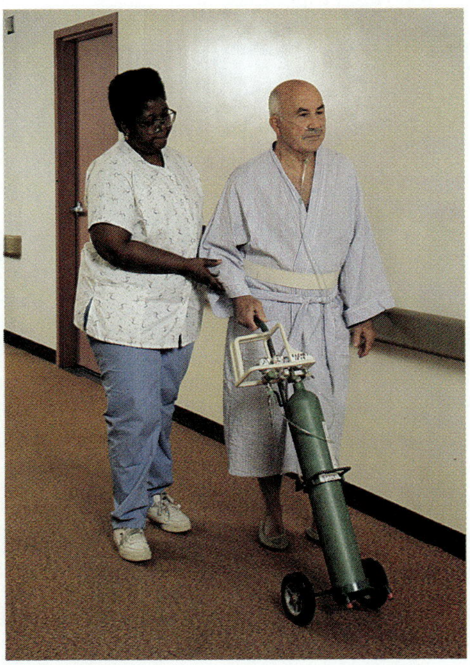

Fig. 24-10 *Portable oxygen cylinder used during ambulation.*

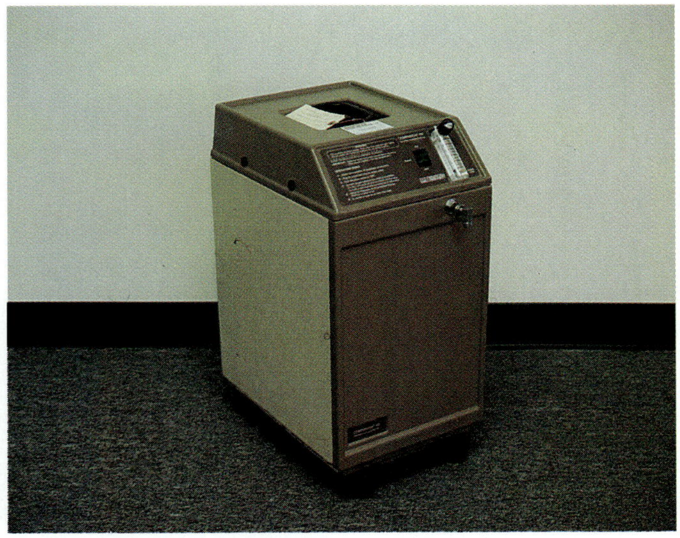

Fig. 24-11 *Oxygen concentrator.*

Oxygen concentrators are often used in home care (Fig. 24-11). They do not require an oxygen source (wall outlet or tank). The concentrator removes oxygen from the air. A power source is required. If the concentrator is not portable, moving about is restricted. The person must be close to the machine. A portable oxygen tank is needed in case of a power failure and for mobility. Higher electric bills are an added expense.

Two devices are commonly used to administer oxygen.

- **Nasal cannula** (Fig. 24-12, A on page 538)—is the most often used. Two prongs project from the tubing. The prongs are inserted a short distance into the nostrils. The elastic headband or tubing is brought behind the ears to keep the cannula in place. The cannula is simple to use. The person can eat and talk with it in place. Nasal irritation occurs if the prongs are too tight. Pressure on the ears can also occur.
- **Face mask** (Fig. 24-12, B on page 538)—covers the nose and mouth. The mask has small holes in the sides of the mask. Carbon dioxide escapes during exhalation. Room air enters during inhalation. The mask is removed for eating and drinking. A nasal cannula is used during meals. Many persons experience fright and feelings of suffocation with face masks. Talking can be difficult. The person's face is kept clean and dry to help prevent irritation from the mask.

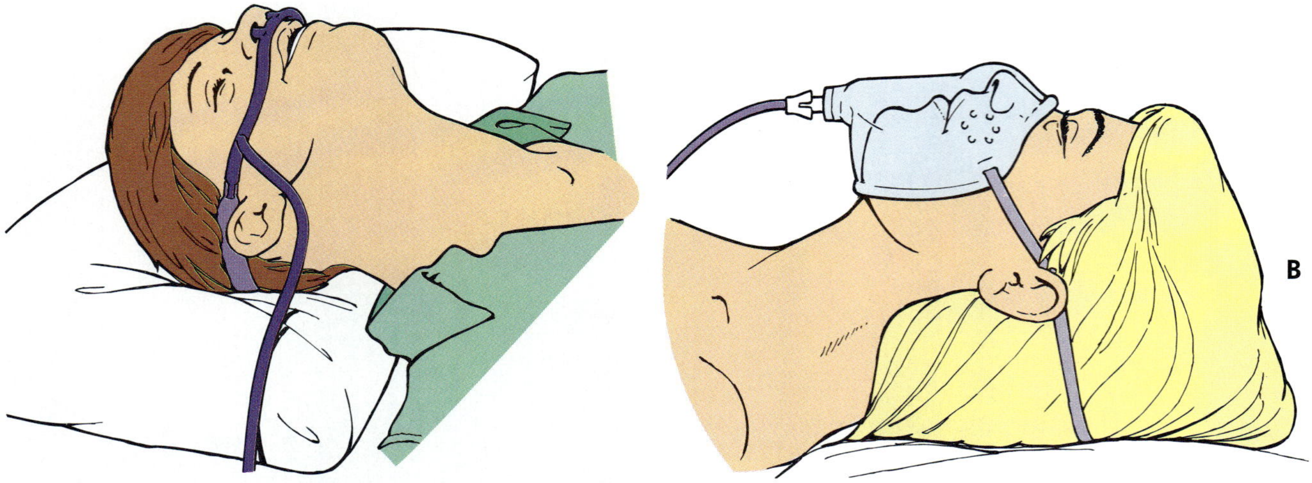

Fig. 24-12 *A, Nasal cannula. B, Oxygen face mask.*

COLLECTING SPUTUM SPECIMENS

Respiratory disorders cause the lungs, bronchi, and trachea to secrete mucus. This mucus is called **sputum** when expectorated (expelled) through the mouth. Sputum is different from saliva. Saliva is a thin, clear liquid produced by the salivary glands in the mouth. Saliva is often called "spit."

Sputum specimens are studied for blood, microorganisms, and abnormal cells. The person coughs up sputum from the bronchi and trachea (Fig. 24-13). Coughing and raising sputum are often painful and difficult. Specimen collection is easier in the early morning. Secretions are usually coughed up upon awakening. The person rinses the mouth with water. Rinsing decreases the amount of saliva and removes food particles. Mouthwash is not used before collecting a sputum specimen. It can destroy some of the microorganisms that may be present.

Collecting a sputum specimen can be embarrassing for the person. Other persons nearby may be upset or nauseated by coughing and expectorating sounds. Also, the appearance of sputum can be disagreeable to the person and others. For these reasons, privacy is protected during the procedure. The specimen container is immediately covered and placed in a bag. Some facilities have covered sputum containers that conceal the contents.

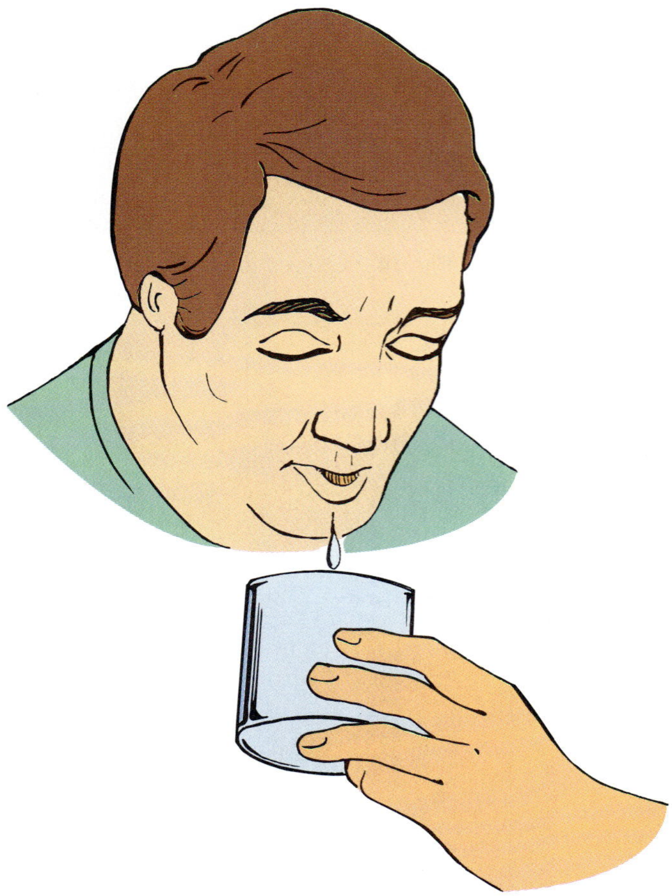

Fig. 24-13 *The person expectorates directly into the center of the specimen container.*

Collecting a Sputum Specimen

Pre-procedure

1 Explain the procedure to the person.
2 Wash your hands.
3 Collect the following:
- Sputum specimen container with cover
- Tissues
- Label
- Laboratory requisition
- Disposable bag
- Disposable gloves

Procedure

4 Label the container.
5 Identify the person. Check the ID bracelet with the requisition.
6 Provide for privacy. If able, the person uses the bathroom to obtain the specimen.
7 Ask the person to rinse the mouth out with clear water.
8 Put on the gloves.
9 Have the person hold the container. Only the outside of the container is touched.
10 Ask the person to cover the mouth and nose with tissues when coughing.
11 Ask him or her to take 2 or 3 deep breaths and cough up the sputum.
12 Have the person expectorate directly into the container (see Fig. 24-13). Sputum should not touch the outside of the container.
13 Collect 1 to 2 tablespoons of sputum unless told to collect more.
14 Put the lid on the container immediately.
15 Place the container in the bag. Attach the requisition to the bag.
16 Remove the gloves.

Post-procedure

17 Make sure the person is comfortable and unscreened.
18 Wash your hands.
19 Take the bag to the laboratory.
20 Wash your hands.
21 Report the following to the nurse:
- The time the specimen was collected and taken to the laboratory
- The amount of sputum collected
- How easily the person raised the sputum
- The consistency and appearance of the sputum (thick, clear, white, green, yellow, or blood-tinged)
- Any other observations

THE VAGINAL IRRIGATION

A **vaginal irrigation (douche)** is the introduction of a fluid into the vagina and the immediate return of the fluid. Doctors order douches to relieve pain and inflammation. They also are ordered to clean the vagina preoperatively or because of discharge. Medications, heat, and cold can be applied by vaginal irrigation. You do not perform the procedure if heat, cold, or a medication is applied. Some facilities and home care agencies do not consider the vaginal irrigation to be a nursing assistant function.

Vaginal irrigations are not done during menstruation. Nor are they done during late pregnancy or during the first 6 to 8 weeks after childbirth. Douching after intercourse is not a birth control method. Normally, douching is not necessary. The vaginal secretions cleanse the vagina naturally and protect it from infection.

A disposable kit has a container, connecting tubing, and nozzle. The nozzle is plastic and is checked for chips and cracks, which could cause vaginal injury. The person is positioned on her back for the procedure. The nozzle is gently inserted backward and upward (Fig. 24-14 on page 542). This follows the angle of the vagina when the person is in the back-lying position.

Vaginal irrigations require touching and exposure of the genital area. The genital area is a sexual area. The person must be protected from sexual abuse. You also must protect yourself from being accused of sexual abuse. Remember, some people do not like being touched. The purpose of the touch can be interpreted the wrong way. Culture, religion, and personal values and beliefs affect the meaning of touch. You must perform the procedure in a competent and professional manner. Be sure to explain the procedure to the person and get the person's consent to proceed. Also protect the right to privacy. Exposure of the person is a form of sexual abuse. How you communicate with the person deserves special attention. You must be careful what you say and do. Some words have different meanings to different people. Your nonverbal communication is important. Follow the principles of communication (see Chapter 4) to protect the person and yourself.

GIVING A VAGINAL IRRIGATION

PRE-PROCEDURE

1 Explain the procedure to the person.
2 Wash your hands.
3 Collect the following:
   - Disposable vaginal irrigation kit
   - 1000 ml of the irrigation solution
   - Bath thermometer
   - Bath blanket
   - Bedpan
   - Toilet tissue
   - Waterproof pad
   - Disposable gloves
   - IV pole
   - Water pitcher
   - Equipment for perineal care
4 Identify the person. Check the ID bracelet with the treatment card.
5 Provide for privacy.
6 Raise the bed to the best level for good body mechanics.

PROCEDURE

7 Offer the bedpan and ask her to void. Her bladder should be empty for the procedure. Provide toilet tissue and ensure privacy.
8 Empty the bedpan. Measure I&O if ordered. Clean and return the bedpan. (Wear gloves for this step.)
9 Wash your hands.
10 Warm the irrigation solution to body temperature or 105° F (40.5° C) as directed by the nurse. If the solution was prepared by central supply, set the container in a basin of hot water. Allow it to warm.
11 Do the following to warm a tap water solution.
   a Fill the pitcher with 1000 ml of warm water.
   b Measure the water temperature.
   c Adjust the water temperature accordingly.

Procedure continued on page 542.

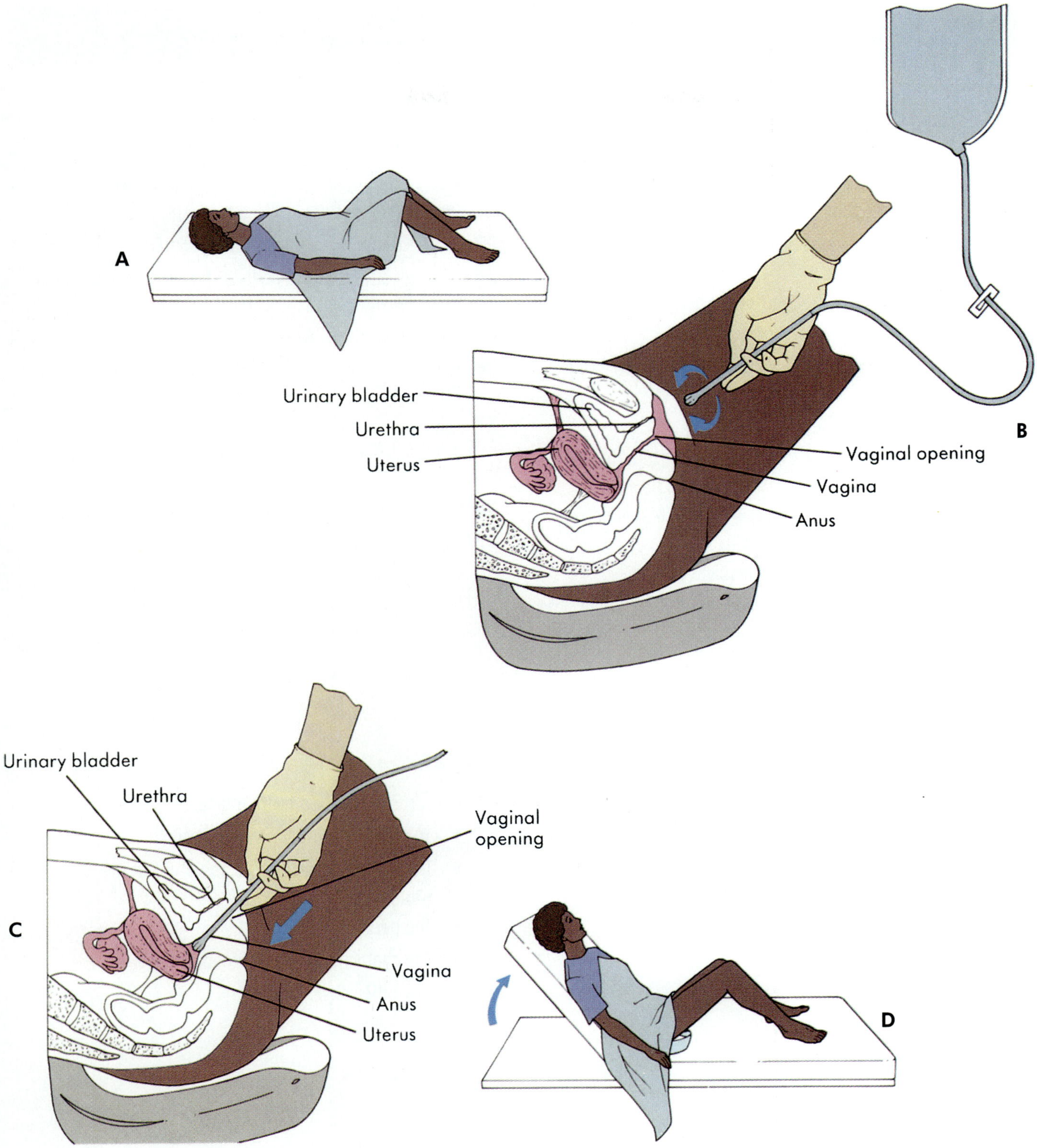

Fig. 24-14 *Vaginal irrigation. A, Position of the person. B, Solution is used to cleanse the vulva. C, Solution flows into the vagina through a nozzle that has been inserted 3 to 4 inches. D, Elevating the head of the bed allows the solution to drain from the vagina.* *(From Dison N: Clinical nursing techniques, ed 4, St Louis, 1979, Mosby–Year Book.)*

GIVING A VAGINAL IRRIGATION—CONT'D

PROCEDURE—CONT'D

12 Cover the person with a bath blanket. Fanfold the top linens to the foot of the bed.

13 Help the person to a back-lying position. Drape her with the bath blanket as for perineal care.

14 Place the waterproof pad under her buttocks.

15 Put on the gloves.

16 Provide perineal care (see *Giving Female Perineal Care,* page 309).

17 Position her on the bedpan.

18 Clamp the irrigation tubing. Pour the solution into the irrigation container.

19 Hang the container from the IV pole. It should be 12 inches above the vagina.

20 Position the nozzle over the vulva. Unclamp the tubing. Let some solution run over the perineal area.

21 Insert the nozzle 3 to 4 inches into the vagina (see Fig. 24-14 on page 542). Rotate the nozzle gently during the procedure.

22 Clamp the tubing when the container is empty. Remove the nozzle.

23 Place the tubing in the irrigation container.

24 Help her sit up on the bedpan. This lets solution drain from the vagina into the bedpan.

25 Help her lie down again.

26 Remove the bedpan. Dry the perineal area with toilet tissue.

27 Take the bedpan into the bathroom. Clean and return it to its proper place. (Make sure side rails are up if ordered.)

28 Remove the waterproof pad.

29 Discard used disposable items.

30 Change damp linen. Remove the gloves.

POST-PROCEDURE

31 Make sure the person is comfortable.

32 Return top linens and remove the bath blanket.

33 Lower the bed to its lowest position. Place the call bell within reach. Unscreen the person.

34 Raise or lower side rails as instructed by the nurse.

35 Wash your hands.

36 Report the following to the nurse:

- The time the irrigation was given
- The amount, type, and temperature of the solution
- The person's response
- The character of the returned solution
- Any other observations

CROSS-TRAINING OPPORTUNITIES

You may be cross-trained for other special procedures. Such procedures are done by phlebotomists, pharmacy clerks, and EKG technicians.

- *Phlebotomist*—draws blood from persons for laboratory study. Blood is taken from a vein. *Phlebotomy* is the process of withdrawing blood from a vein (Fig. 24-15). Phlebotomists work in the laboratory. They are given on-the-job training in phlebotomy or take a course at a community college, technical school, or vocational school.
- *Pharmacy clerk*—works in the pharmacy and is supervised by the pharmacist. The clerk orders and stocks supplies, labels drugs, and cleans equipment and work areas. On-the-job training is given.
- *EKG or ECG technician*—takes electrocardiograms (see Figure 25-2). Training is given on the job.

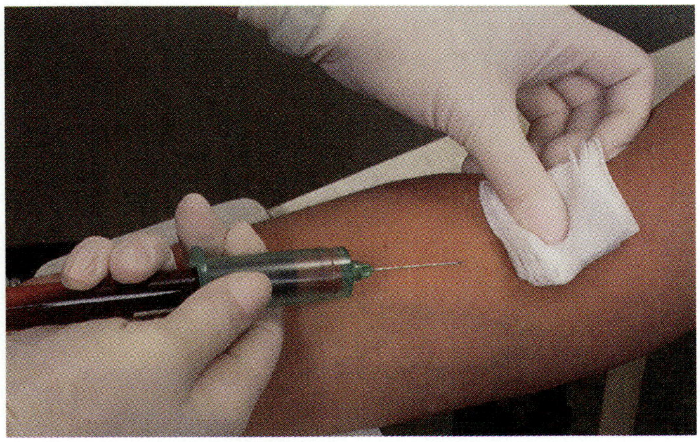

Fig. 24-15 *A phlebotomist draws blood from a person.* (From *Zakus S: Clinical procedures for medical assistants, ed 3, St Louis, 1995, Mosby–Year Book.*)

SUMMARY

You are never responsible for intravenous therapy, suction, and oxygen therapy. However, you may care for persons receiving these therapies. You need to have a sound, basic understanding of their purposes and safety rules. Safety promotes quality of life.

The person's safety is never overlooked. The person is carefully observed. You must promptly report observations and patient or resident complaints. The side effects and complications of some of the treatments and procedures are severe. Every sign, symptom, or complaint is important.

Finally, know your own limits. Do not perform any procedure you do not understand or with which you are unfamiliar. Remember your legal and ethical responsibilities. You have the right to say no. Do not do anything that is beyond your legal scope, preparation, and skill level.

Review Questions

Circle the best *answer.*

1 Cora Jones has an IV infusion. You should
- a Add a new bag if necessary
- b Check the drip chamber to see if fluid is dripping
- c Use the clamp to regulate the flow rate
- d Change the tubing daily

2 Cora Jones sometimes needs her upper airway suctioned. You can
- a Suction her whenever necessary
- b Set up the suction system
- c Observe for signs and symptoms that indicate a need for suction
- d Turn on the suction source

3 Cora Jones has nasogastric suction. You should
- a Give frequent oral hygiene
- b Turn off the suction when transferring her to the chair
- c Irrigate the tube
- d Empty the drainage container

4 These devices are used to administer oxygen. Which allows eating and talking?
- a Wall outlet
- b Nasal cannula
- c Face mask
- d Oxygen tank

5 Cora Jones is receiving supplemental oxygen. You should do the following *except*
- a Follow the safety measures related to fire and the use of oxygen
- b Remove the administration device for meals
- c Give oral hygiene as directed by the nurse
- d Make sure there are no kinks in the tubing

6 You are to collect a sputum specimen. Which is *false?*
- a An early morning specimen is best.
- b Privacy is protected.
- c The person uses mouthwash before raising the sputum.
- d The sputum is expectorated directly into the specimen container.

7 You are to give a vaginal irrigation. You should do the following *except*
- a Have the person void before beginning the procedure
- b Warm the solution to body temperature or to 105° F
- c Check the nozzle for chips or cracks
- d Hang the container 18 to 24 inches above the vagina

Answers to these questions are on page 752.

The Person Having Surgery

25

OBJECTIVES

- Define the key terms listed in this chapter
- Describe the common fears and concerns of surgical patients
- Explain how persons are psychologically prepared for surgery
- Describe how to prepare a room for the postoperative patient
- List the signs and symptoms to immediately report to the nurse during the postoperative period
- Explain why patients must be turned and repositioned after surgery
- Explain why coughing and deep breathing are important
- Explain the purpose of leg exercises and elastic stockings
- Describe binders and bandages and their purposes
- List the complications of wound healing
- Explain why early ambulation is important after surgery
- Describe how to meet the surgical patient's needs for nutrition, fluids, and elimination
- Describe how to provide for personal hygiene after surgery
- Perform the procedures described in this chapter

KEY TERMS

anesthesia The loss of feeling or sensation produced by a drug

atelectasis The collapse of a portion of the lung

dehiscence The separation of the surgical incision

elective surgery Scheduled surgery a person chooses to have at a certain time

embolus A blood clot that travels through the vascular system until it lodges in a distant blood vessel

emergency surgery Unscheduled surgery done immediately to save the person's life or limb

evisceration The separation of the surgical incision along with protrusion of abdominal organs

general anesthesia Unconsciousness and the loss of feeling or sensation produced by a drug

local anesthesia The loss of sensation in a small area

major surgery Complex surgery; the many risks and complications may be life-threatening

minor surgery Simple surgery; there are few risks or complications

pneumonia Infection of the lung

postoperative After the operation or surgery

preoperative Before the operation or surgery

regional anesthesia The loss of sensation or feeling in a part of the body, produced by the injection of a drug; the person does not lose consciousness

thrombus A blood clot

urgent surgery Surgery necessary for the person's health; it must be done soon to prevent further damage or disease

Surgery is done for many reasons. Common reasons include removing a diseased organ or body part, removing a tumor, or repairing injured tissue. Surgery is also done to diagnose a disease, improve appearance, and relieve symptoms. Surgeries are elective, urgent, or emergency.

- **Elective surgery** is done for the person's well-being. It is not lifesaving and may not be necessary for the person's health. The surgery is scheduled anywhere from 1 day to months in advance. Cosmetic surgery—surgery to improve appearance—is usually elective surgery.
- **Urgent surgery** is necessary for the person's health. It must be done soon to prevent further damage or disease. Cancer surgery and coronary artery bypass surgery are examples.
- **Emergency surgery** is done immediately to save a person's life or limb. The need is sudden and unexpected. Accidents, stabbings, and bullet wounds often require emergency surgery.

The person is prepared for what happens before, during, and after surgery. Physical and psychological preparation are necessary. Nurses and doctors prepare the person for the surgical experience.

If you work in a hospital, you may have contact with persons before and after surgery. In nursing facilities, many residents are recovering from surgery. Many postoperative patients need home care. Your role in caring for surgical patients depends on certain factors.

- The employer's policies
- Whether the surgery was major or minor
- The person's condition before surgery
- The person's condition after surgery

PSYCHOLOGICAL CARE

Illness or injury cause persons to have many fears and concerns. The need for surgery increases these fears. The person's deepest and worst fears are often felt. How would you feel if your body was going to be cut open tomorrow? Would you fear cancer or the loss of function of an organ or body part? Would you have fears about pain, nausea and vomiting, or death? Who will care for your children and your home? Who will earn money while you are in the hospital? Imagine you are in an accident. An ambulance takes you to the emergency room. You wake up many hours later. You are told that your right leg was amputated during surgery.

Psychological preparation is important. You must appreciate the person's fears and concerns. The health team must show the person warmth, sensitivity, and caring.

BOX 25-1 COMMON FEARS AND CONCERNS OF SURGICAL PATIENTS

Fears

- The fear of cancer
- The fear of body disfigurement and scarring
- The fear of disability
- The fear of pain during surgery
- The fear of dying during surgery
- The fear of anesthesia and its effects
- The fear of going to sleep or not waking up after surgery
- The fear of exposure
- The fear of severe pain or discomfort after surgery
- The fear of tubes, needles, and other equipment used for care
- The fear of complications
- The fear of prolonged recovery
- The fear that more surgery or treatments will be needed
- The fear of being separated from family and friends

Concerns

- Who will care for children and other family members?
- Are the children being cared for properly?
- Who will take care of pets or plants?
- Who will take care of the house, do the cleaning and laundry, mow the lawn, and tend the garden?
- How will monthly bills, loan payments, mortgages, or rent be paid?
- Will insurance cover hospital and doctor bills?

Fears and Concerns

Feelings are affected by past experiences. Some persons have had surgery before. Others have not. Family and friends usually share their surgical experiences with the person. Their experiences also may affect the person. Most people know about some tragic surgical event—surgery on the wrong person, surgery on the wrong body part, or instruments left inside the body. Some people do not talk about their fears and concerns. Instead there may be quiet and withdrawn behaviors, crying, or constant talking about other things. Some pace, are very cheerful, or show unusual behavior. These behaviors may be due to one or more fears listed in Box 25-1.

What the Person Has Been Told

The doctor explains the need for surgery to the person and family. They are told about the surgical procedure, risks, and possible complications. Probable risks from not having surgery are also explained. Information is given about who will do the surgery, when it is scheduled, and how long it will take. The person and family may want or need more information about the surgery and what to expect. Questions and misunderstandings are cleared up. Instructions about care are also given. All information before surgery is given by the doctor or nurse.

After surgery the doctor tells the patient and the family about the results. The doctor decides what and when to tell them. Often the health team knows before the person does. Patients and families are usually anxious to know the results. They often ask nurses, nursing assistants, and other health workers. Often they ask if reports are back from the laboratory or what the reports say. Knowing what the person has been told is very important. You do not tell of any diagnosis, nor do you give incomplete or inaccurate information. The nurse tells you what and when the person and family have been told.

Nursing Assistant Responsibilities

You can assist in the psychological care of the surgical patient. You can do the following if you are involved in preoperative and postoperative care:

- Listen to the person who voices fears or concerns about surgery
- Refer any questions about the surgery or its results to the nurse
- Explain procedures you will perform to the person and why they are being done
- Follow the rules of communication (see Chapter 3)
- Use verbal and nonverbal communication to relate to the surgical patient (see Chapter 4)
- Provide care and perform procedures in an efficient and competent manner

- Report any verbal and nonverbal indications of patient fear or anxiety to the nurse
- Report a person's request to see a member of the clergy to the nurse

THE PREOPERATIVE PERIOD

The preoperative (before surgery) period may be many days or just a few minutes. If time permits, the person is prepared psychologically and physically for the effects of anesthesia and surgery. Good preoperative preparation prevents postoperative complications.

Preoperative Teaching

The nurse does the preoperative teaching. The person is told about what to expect before and after surgery.

- Preoperative activities are explained—the type and purpose of tests, skin preparation, personal care measures, and the purpose and effects of preoperative medications.
- Deep breathing, coughing, and leg exercises are taught and practiced. After surgery, these activities are done every 1 or 2 hours when the person is awake.
- The importance of turning, repositioning, and early ambulation after surgery is explained.
- The sights and sensations to expect when consciousness is regained are explained.
- The person is told about the recovery room where he or she will wake up (Fig. 25-1).
- It is explained that vital signs are taken frequently until they are stable.
- The person is told about the type and amount of pain to expect. The person is also told that pain medications are given for comfort.
- Certain treatments and equipment may be needed, depending on the type of surgery. The person may be told about an IV infusion, urinary catheter, NG tube, oxygen, or wound suction. Special devices, such as a cast or traction, may also be needed.
- Activity or positioning restrictions are explained.

Special Tests

Before surgery the doctor orders several tests. They are done to evaluate the person's circulatory, respiratory, and urinary systems. These tests include a chest x-ray examination, a complete blood count (CBC), and urinalysis. An electrocardiogram (ECG or EKG) is done to detect any cardiac (heart) problems. The electrocardiogram is a recording of the electrical activity of the heart (Fig. 25-2).

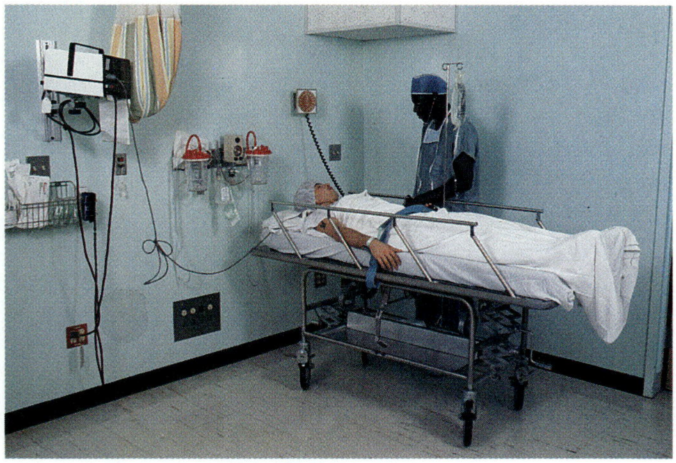

Fig. 25-1 *Recovery room.*

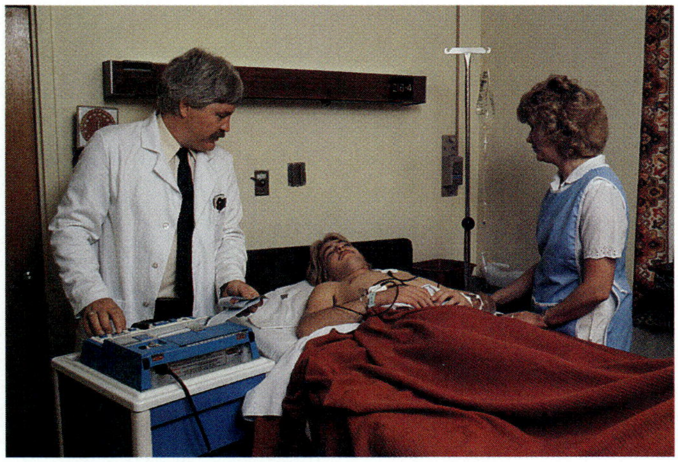

Fig. 25-2 *An electrocardiogram is being taken.*

If blood loss is expected, the person's blood is tested to determine the blood type. The blood is also tested for reactions with blood that may be given. This is called *type and crossmatch.* Other tests are done depending on the person's condition and the surgery. A nurse prepares the person for the tests. The nurse also makes sure the results are on the chart by the time of surgery.

Nutrition and Fluids

The person fasts for 6 to 8 hours before surgery. A light supper is usually allowed the evening before surgery. Then the person is NPO from midnight until otherwise ordered. These measures reduce the risk of vomiting and aspiration during anesthesia and after surgery. Sometimes surgery is scheduled for the afternoon. Then the person has a regular supper and a light breakfast. The NPO restriction begins after breakfast. An NPO sign is placed in the person's room. Remember, the water pitcher and glass are removed when the person is NPO.

Elimination

A suppository or enema may be given the evening before or the morning of surgery. The doctor orders what to give and when. Abdominal surgeries almost always require a preoperative enema. If intestinal surgery is to be done, cleansing enemas are ordered. Cleansing enemas clear the colon of feces. Enemas are also given when straining or a bowel movement could cause postoperative problems. Such problems include pain, severe bleeding (hemorrhage), or stress on the operative area. You may be assigned to give the preoperative enema.

Catheters are ordered for some surgeries. The catheter keeps the bladder empty during surgery. For pelvic and abdominal surgeries, the bladder must be empty. A full bladder is easily injured during surgery.

Personal Care

You may be assigned to assist the person with personal care. Personal care before surgery usually involves the following:

- A complete bed bath, shower, or tub bath the evening before or the morning of surgery. A special soap or cleanser may be ordered. A shampoo is included. The bath and shampoo reduce the number of microbes on the body at the time of surgery.
- Makeup and nail polish are removed before surgery. The person's color and circulation must be observed during and after surgery.
- Long hair is braided. All hairpins, clips, combs, and similar items are removed. Some facilities have both men and women wear surgical caps. A cap keeps hair out of the face and the operative area.
- Oral hygiene is given to promote comfort. Because of being NPO, the person is very thirsty and has a dry mouth. The person must not swallow any water during the procedure.
- Dentures are removed. They are not worn to the operating room. They are removed before preoperative medications are given. They are cleaned and kept moist in a denture cup. They are kept in a safe place. Some persons do not want to be seen without their dentures. If possible, let persons wear their dentures until they must be removed. This helps maintain the person's sense of dignity and esteem.

Valuables

Valuables are removed for safekeeping. These include glasses, contact lenses, hearing aids, and jewelry. These items are easily lost or broken during surgery. They can also be lost or broken during transfers to the operating room, recovery room, and back to the person's room. A note is made on the person's chart about which valuables have been removed and where they are being kept. The person may ask to wear a wedding band or religious medal. The item is secured in place with gauze or tape according to hospital policy.

Skin Preparation

The skin is prepared for surgery by thorough cleansing and hair removal. The skin and hair shafts contain microbes that could enter the body through the surgical incision. A serious infection could result. The skin cannot be sterilized. However, the number of microbes can be reduced by the *skin prep.*

The area to be prepared includes the site where the incision will be made. A large part of the surrounding area is also *prepped.* This helps reduce the possibility of contamination during draping. Hospital policy and the surgeon's preferences determine the area to be prepared for a specific surgery (Fig. 25-3 on pages 552 and 553).

The skin prep is done the evening before or the morning of surgery. The skin prep may be done in the person's room by a nurse or nursing assistant. It may also be done in the operating room area by a member of the surgical team. Hair is removed by applying a depilatory (cream hair remover) or shaving.

For shaving, disposable prep kits are used. A kit has a disposable razor, a sponge filled with soap, a basin, and a disposable drape and towel (Fig. 25-4 on page 554). The skin is lathered with soap. Then the skin is shaved in the direction of hair growth (Fig. 25-5 on page 554). Any break in the skin is a possible site of infection. You may be assigned to do a skin prep. Be very careful not to cut, scratch, or nick the skin during the procedure. Standard Precautions and the Bloodborne Pathogen Standard are followed.

The Surgical Skin Prep

Pre-procedure

1 Explain the procedure to the person.

2 Wash your hands.

3 Collect the following:
- Disposable skin prep kit
- Bath blanket
- Warm water
- Disposable gloves
- Waterproof pad
- Bath towel

4 Identify the person. Check the ID bracelet with the treatment card.

5 Provide for privacy.

Procedure

6 Make sure you have good lighting. There should be no glares or shadows.

7 Raise the bed to the best level for good body mechanics. Lower the side rail.

8 Cover the person with a bath blanket. Fanfold top linens to the foot of the bed.

9 Place the waterproof pad under the area to be shaved.

10 Open the skin prep kit.

11 Position the person for the skin prep. Drape him or her with the disposable drape.

12 Add warm water to the basin. Put on the gloves.

13 Apply soap to the skin with the sponge. Work up a good lather.

14 Hold the skin taut. Shave in the direction of hair growth (see Fig. 25-5).

15 Shave outward from the center using short strokes.

16 Rinse the razor often.

17 Check to see that the entire area is free of hair. Make sure there are no cuts, scratches, or nicks.

18 Rinse the skin thoroughly. Pat dry.

19 Remove the drape and waterproof pad. Remove the gloves.

20 Return top linens. Remove the bath blanket.

Post-procedure

21 Make sure the person is comfortable.

22 Lower the bed to its lowest position. Place the call bell within reach. Unscreen the person.

23 Return equipment to its proper place.

24 Discard used disposable items. Follow facility policy for soiled linen.

25 Wash your hands.

26 Report the following to the nurse:
- The time the procedure was completed
- The area prepared
- Any cuts, nicks, or scratches
- Any other observations

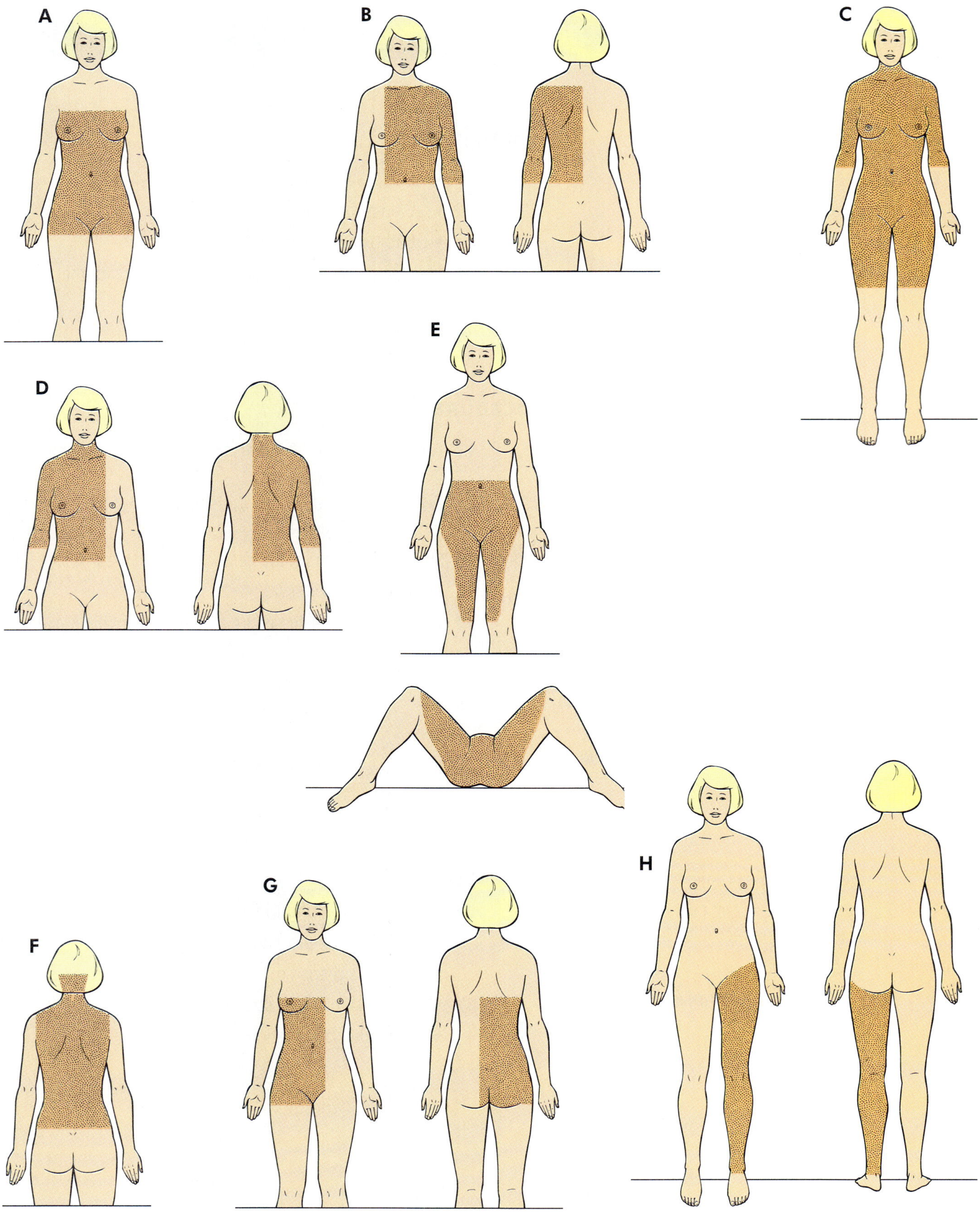

Fig. 25-3 *Skin preparation sites for surgeries on various body areas. The shaded area indicates the area that should be shaved. A, Abdominal surgery. B, Chest or thoracic surgery. C, Open-heart surgery. D, Breast surgery. E, Perineal surgery. F, Cervical spine surgery. G, Kidney surgery. H, Knee surgery.*

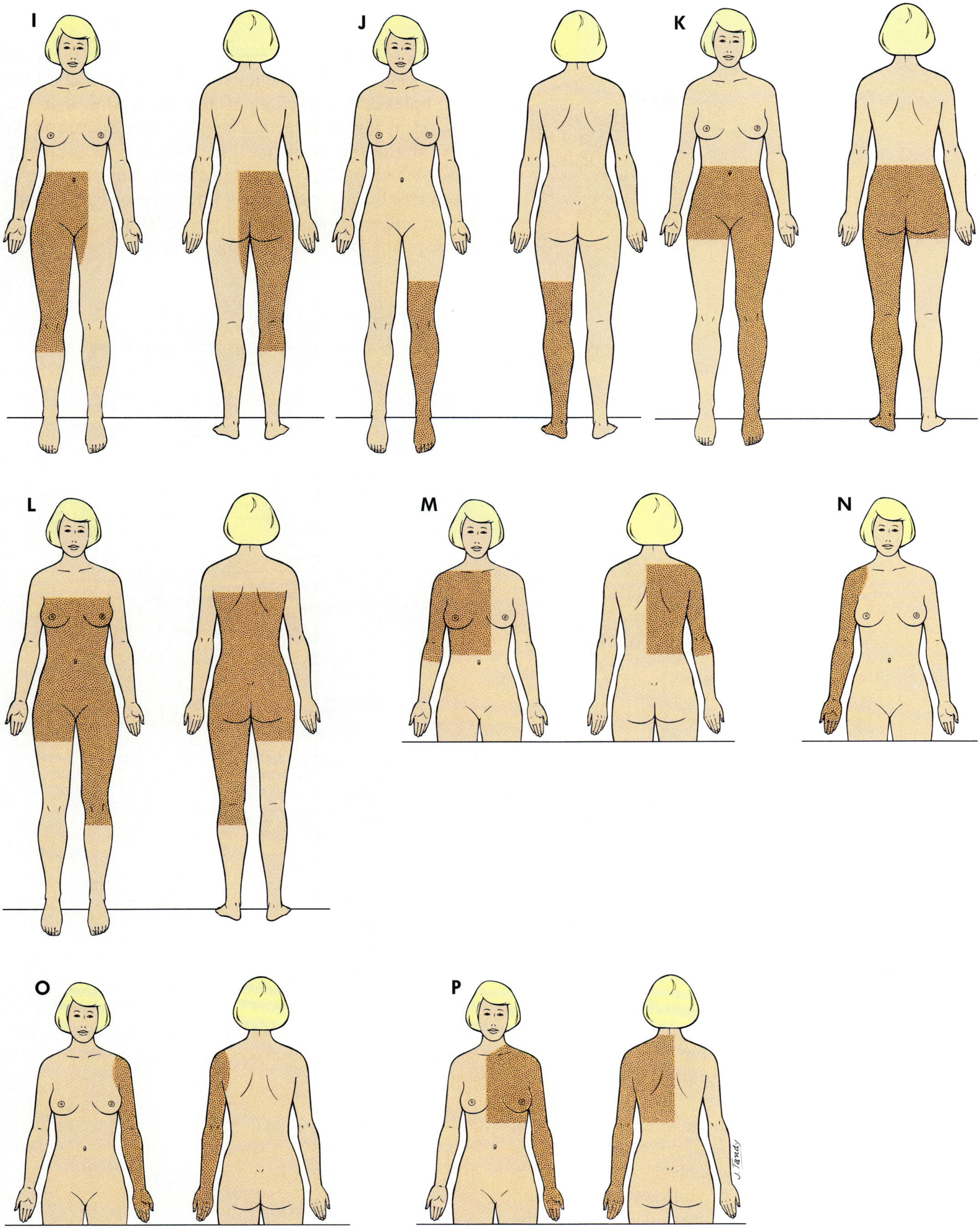

Fig. 25-3—cont'd *I, Hip and thigh surgery. J, Lower leg and foot surgery. K, Complete lower extremity surgery. L, Abdominal and leg surgery. M, Upper arm surgery. N, Lower arm surgery. O, Elbow surgery. P, Upper arm surgery.*

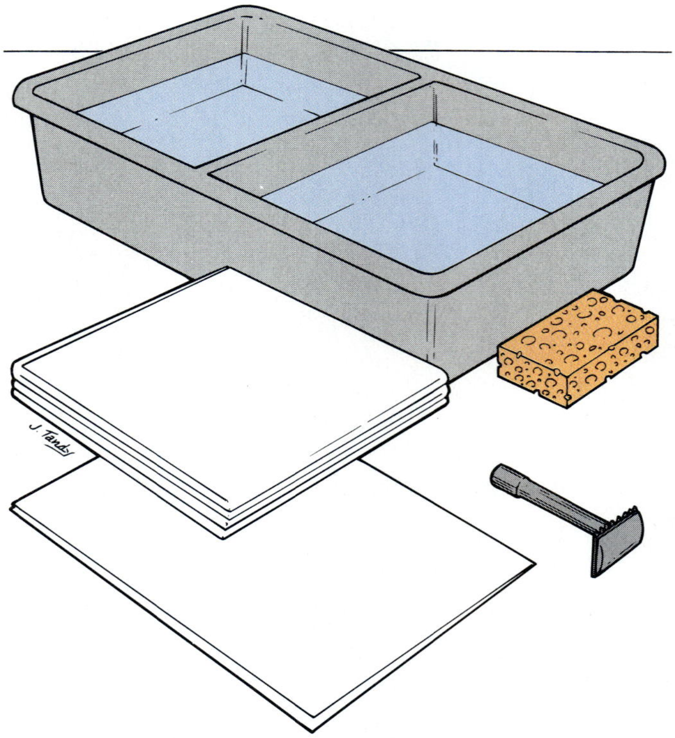

Fig. 25-4 *Skin prep kit.*

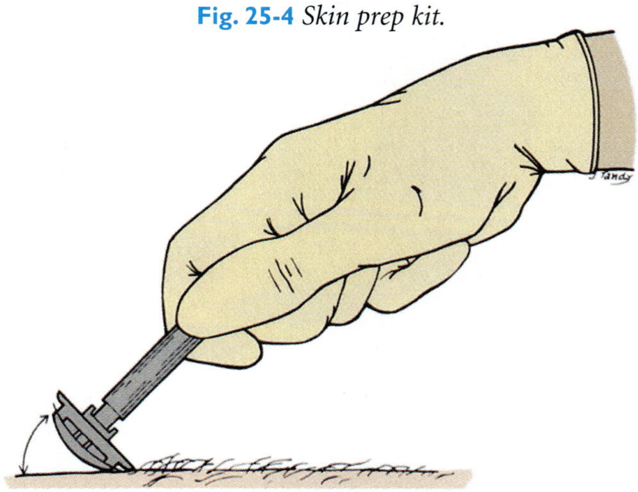

Fig. 25-5 *The skin is held taut. Shaving is done in the direction of hair growth.*

The Consent for Surgery

Before surgery can be done, the person must give permission. The person signs an *operative permit* or *surgical consent.* The consent is signed when the person understands the information given by the doctor. Sometimes the person's spouse or nearest relative is also required to sign the consent. A parent or legal guardian signs the surgical consent of a minor child. The legal guardian signs for a person who is mentally incompetent. The doctor is responsible for securing the person's written consent. However, this responsibility is often delegated to the nurse. *You are never responsible for obtaining the person's written consent for surgery.*

The Preoperative Checklist

A preoperative checklist (Fig. 25-6) is placed on the front of the person's chart. The nurse makes sure the checklist is completed. Completion of the list means that the person is ready for surgery. The nurse may ask you to do some of the things on the list. You need to promptly report when you have completed each activity. Observations are also reported. Except for the preoperative medication and side rails, the entire checklist is completed before preoperative medications are given.

BEND PEEL TAB - FORM #52-1 REVISED 1/77

BARNES HOSPITAL SURGICAL CHECK LIST

NAME: DATE:

ITEM	YES	NO	NURSE SIGNATURE
I.D. band on			
Face sheet in chart			
Name plate in chart			
Operative Permit signed			
History & Physical in chart			
Patient on proper service			
Operative area prepped and checked			
Blood work in chart and within normal limits			
Urinalysis in chart			
Allergies noted as to whether or not present			
Chest X-ray done if ordered EKG			
V.S. taken & charted			
Jewelry removed or secured to patient			
Dentures, eyeglasses, contact lenses, nail polish, hairpins, or prothesis removed			
Patient in hospital pajamas			
Voided or catheterized			
Has patient been NPO			
Pre-op med given TIME______			

Fig. 25-6 *Preoperative checklist. (From Potter PA, Perry AG: Fundamentals of nursing: concepts, process, and practice, ed 3, St Louis, 1993, Mosby–Year Book.)*

Preoperative Medication

Medication is given the night before surgery to help the person sleep. About 45 minutes to 1 hour before surgery, the preoperative medications are given. One medication helps the person relax and feel drowsy. The other dries up respiratory secretions to prevent aspiration. Complaints of drowsiness, lightheadedness, thirst, and dry mouth are normal and expected.

Falls and accidents are prevented after the preoperative medications are given. Side rails are raised and the person is not allowed out of bed. Therefore the person is asked to urinate before the medications are given. Once the medications have been given, the bedpan or urinal is used for voiding. Smoking is not allowed. Dropping a cigarette or falling asleep can occur.

The bed is raised to the highest position at this time. The person is transferred from the bed to a stretcher. Furniture is moved out of the way to make room for the stretcher. The overbed table and bedside stand are cleaned off. This prevents damage to equipment and valuables.

Transporting the Person to the Operating Room

A nurse or attendant from the operating room brings a stretcher to the person's room. The person is transferred onto the stretcher and covered with a bath blanket to provide warmth and prevent exposure. The person is protected from falling. Safety straps are secured, and the side rails are raised. A small pillow may be placed under the person's head for comfort.

Identification checks are made. Then the person's chart is given to the staff member from the operating room.

The nurse responsible for preoperative care may go with the person to the entrance of the operating room area. The family also may be allowed to go this far.

ANESTHESIA

There are three types of anesthetics: general, regional, and local.

- **General anesthesia** produces unconsciousness and the loss of feeling or sensation. A drug is given intravenously or a gas is inhaled (breathed in).
- **Regional anesthesia** produces loss of sensation or feeling in a large area of the body. The person does not lose consciousness. A drug is injected into a body part.
- **Local anesthesia** produces loss of sensation in a small area. A drug is injected at the specific site.

Anesthetics are given by specially educated doctors and nurses. An *anesthesiologist* is a doctor who specializes in the administration of anesthetics. An *anesthetist* is a nurse who has had advanced study in the administration of anesthetics.

THE POSTOPERATIVE PERIOD

After surgery (postoperative) the person is taken to the recovery room (RR) or postanesthesia room (PAR). The recovery room is near the operating room. There the person recovers from the anesthetic. This can take 1 to 2 hours. The person is watched very closely. Vital signs are taken and observations are made often. Certain conditions must be met before the person leaves the recovery room.

- Vital signs must be stable.
- The person must have good respiratory function.
- The person must also be able to respond and call for help when it is needed.

The doctor gives the transfer order when appropriate.

Preparing the Person's Room

The room must be ready for the person's return from the recovery room. A surgical bed is made (see Chapter 12). Equipment and supplies needed for the person's care are brought to the room. The nurse tells you if special preparations and equipment are needed. The room is prepared after the person is taken to the operating room. Preparations include:

- Making a surgical bed
- Placing equipment and supplies in the room
  *Thermometer
  *Stethoscope
  *Sphygmomanometer
  *Kidney basin
  *Tissues
  *Waterproof bed protector
  *Vital signs flow sheet
  *Intake and output record
  *IV pole
  *Other items as directed by the nurse
- Raising the bed to its highest position; the side rails must be down
- Moving furniture out of the way so the stretcher can be brought into the room

Receiving the Person from the Recovery Room

The recovery room nurse calls the nursing unit when the person is ready to be transferred. Sometimes special equipment is needed. If so, the recovery room nurse lists the needed items. The person is transported by the recovery room nurses. The floor nurse receives the person (Fig. 25-7). You may be asked to help transfer the person from the stretcher to the bed. You may also need to help position the person.

Vital signs are taken, and other important observations are made. They are compared with those reported by the recovery room nurse. The nurse checks dressings for bleeding. The placement and functioning of tubes, catheters, and IV infusions are also checked. Side rails are raised, and the call bell is placed within the person's reach. Necessary care and treatments are given. Then the family is allowed to see the person.

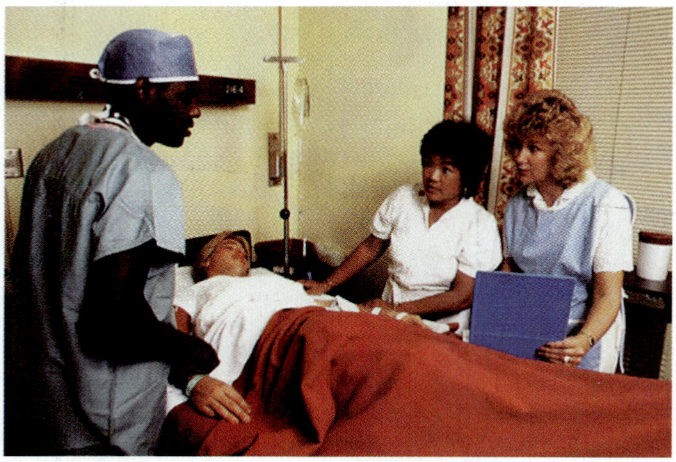

Fig. 25-7 *A patient is brought to the nursing unit from the recovery room. A nurse meets the patient on return to the unit.*

Measurements and Observations

The person's condition and hospital policies affect your role in postoperative care. You may be assigned to measure vital signs and observe the person's condition. The following schedule is common for vital signs and observations:

- Every 15 minutes the first hour
- Every 30 minutes for 1 to 2 hours
- Every hour for 4 hours
- Every 4 hours

The nurse tells you how often to check the person. This is an important responsibility. You must be alert for the signs and symptoms listed in Box 25-2. They are reported to the nurse immediately.

Positioning

Proper positioning promotes comfort and prevents complications. The type of surgery affects positioning. Position restrictions may be ordered. The person is usually positioned for easy and comfortable breathing. Also, stress on the incision is prevented. When supine, the head of the bed is usually raised slightly. The person's head may be turned to the side. These positions prevent aspiration if vomiting occurs.

Repositioning is done every 1 to 2 hours. This helps prevent respiratory and circulatory complications. The person may not want to turn because of pain. Provide support and turn the person with smooth, gentle motions. Pillows and other devices are often used in positioning (see Chapter 10).

The nurse tells you when to reposition the person and what positions are allowed. Usually you assist the nurse. However, you may be responsible for turning and repositioning the person. This may occur when the person's condition is stable and care is simple.

BOX 25-2 Postoperative Observations: What to Report to the Nurse

- Choking
- A drop or rise in blood pressure
- The appearance of bright red blood from the incision, drainage tubes, or suction tubes
- A pulse rate of greater than 100 or less than 60 beats per minute
- A weak or irregular pulse
- A rise or drop in body temperature
- The need for upper airway suctioning (tachypnea, dyspnea, moist sounding respirations or gurgling, restlessness, cyanosis)
- Shallow, slow breathing
- Rapid, gasping, or difficult respirations
- Weak cough
- Complaints of thirst
- Restlessness
- Cold, moist, clammy, or pale skin
- Cyanosis of the lips or nails
- Increased drainage on or under dressings or on bed linens (including draw sheets, bottom sheets, and pillowcases)
- Complaints of pain or nausea
- Vomiting
- Confusion or disorientation
- Additional measurements and observations
  - *The amount, character, and time of the first voiding after surgery
  - *Intake and output
  - *IV flow rate
  - *The appearance of drainage from a urinary catheter, NG tube, or wound suction
  - *Any other observation that can mean a change in the person's condition

Coughing and Deep Breathing

Respiratory complications are prevented. There are two major complications. One is **pneumonia,** an infection in the lung. The other is **atelectasis,** the collapse of a portion of the lung. Atelectasis occurs when mucus collects in the airway. Air cannot get to a part of the lung, and the lung collapses. Coughing and deep breathing exercises help prevent these complications. Mucus is removed by coughing. Deep breathing promotes air movement into most parts of the lungs. These exercises are ordered for persons on bed rest and for those with respiratory disorders.

The person may be afraid to cough and deep breathe. The exercises may be painful, especially after chest and abdominal surgeries. The person may be afraid of breaking open the incision while coughing. However, coughing and deep breathing are necessary to prevent complications.

The frequency of coughing and deep breathing varies. Some doctors order the exercises every 1 or 2 hours while the person is awake. Others want them done 4 times a day. The nurse tells you when coughing and deep breathing need to be done. You are also told how many deep breaths and coughs the person should do. Remember, coughing and deep breathing are done only when directed by the nurse.

Coughing and Deep Breathing Exercises

Pre-procedure

1 Explain the procedure to the person.

2 Identify the person. Check the ID bracelet with the treatment card.

3 Provide for privacy.

Procedure

4 Help the person to a comfortable sitting position: dangling, semi-Fowler's, or Fowler's position.

5 Have the person deep breathe:

- **a** Have the person place the hands over the rib cage (Fig. 25-8).
- **b** Ask the person to exhale. Explain that he or she should exhale until the ribs move as far down as possible.
- **c** Have the person take a deep breath. It should be as deep as possible. Remind him or her to inhale through the nose.
- **d** Ask the person to hold the breath for 3 seconds.
- **e** Ask the person to exhale slowly through pursed lips (Fig. 25-9). He or she should exhale until the ribs move as far down as possible.
- **f** Repeat this step 4 more times.

6 Ask the person to cough:

- **a** Have the person interlace the fingers over the incision (Fig. 25-10, A). The person can also hold a small pillow or folded towel over the incision (Fig. 25-10, B).
- **b** Have the person take in a deep breath as in step 5.
- **c** Ask the person to cough strongly twice with the mouth open.

Post-procedure

7 Assist the person to a comfortable position.

8 Raise or lower side rails as instructed by the nurse.

9 Place the call bell within reach.

10 Unscreen the person.

11 Report your observations to the nurse:

- The number of times the person coughed and deep breathed
- How the person tolerated the procedure

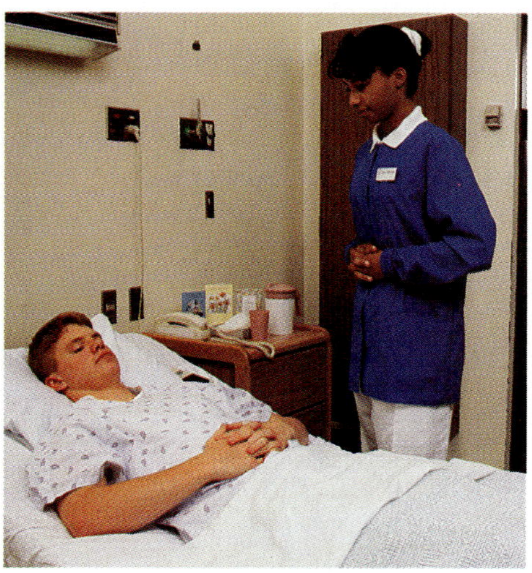

Fig. 25-8 *The hands are placed over the rib cage for deep breathing.*

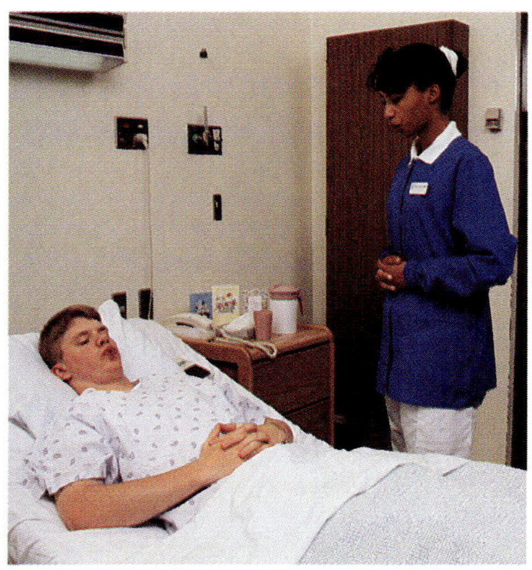

Fig. 25-9 *The patient exhales through pursed lips during the deep breathing exercise.*

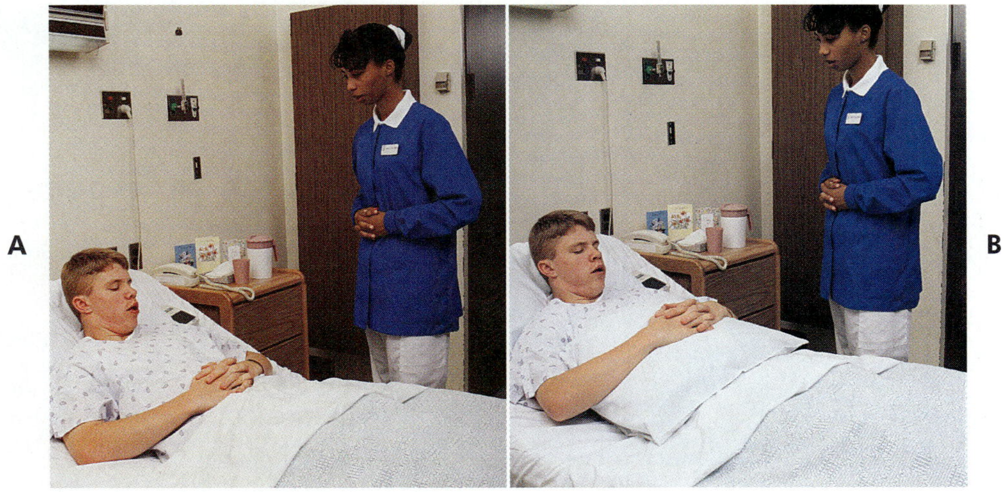

Fig. 25-10 *The incision is supported for the coughing exercise. A, Fingers are interlaced over the incision area. B, A small pillow is held over the incision.*

Leg Exercises

After surgery, circulation must be stimulated. This is especially true for blood flow in the extremities. If blood flow is sluggish, blood clots may form. Blood clots (**thrombi**) can form in the deep leg veins (Fig. 25-11, A). A blood clot (**thrombus**) can break loose and travel through the bloodstream. It then becomes an embolus. An **embolus** is a blood clot that travels through the vascular system until it lodges in a distant vessel (Fig. 25-11, B). An embolus from a vein eventually lodges in the lungs (pulmonary embolus). A pulmonary embolus can cause severe respiratory problems and death.

Leg exercises increase venous blood flow. Therefore they help prevent thrombi. Leg exercises are easy to do. You may have to assist if the person is weak. If the person has had leg surgery, a doctor's order is needed for the exercises. The nurse tells you when to do the exercises. They are done with the person in the supine position. They are done at least every 1 or 2 hours while the person is awake. The following exercises are done 5 times:

- Ask the person to make circles with the toes. This rotates the ankles.
- Have the person dorsiflex and plantar flex the feet (see Chapter 19).
- Have the person flex and extend one knee and then the other (Fig. 25-12 on page 560).
- Ask the person to raise and lower one leg off the bed (Fig. 25-13 on page 560). Repeat this exercise with the other leg.

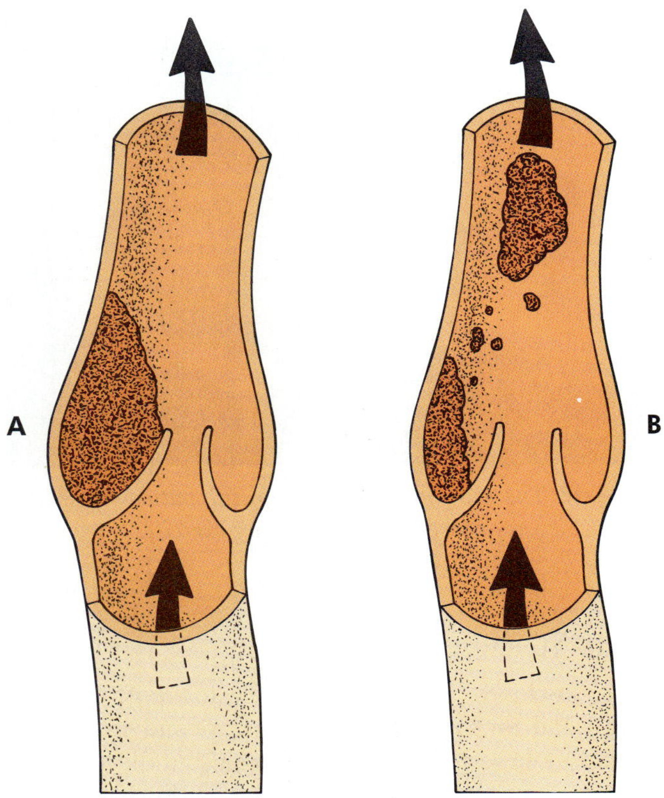

Fig. 25-11 *A, A blood clot is attached to the wall of a vein. The arrows show the direction of blood flow. B, Part of the thrombus has broken off and has become an embolus. The embolus will travel in the bloodstream until it lodges in a distant vessel.*

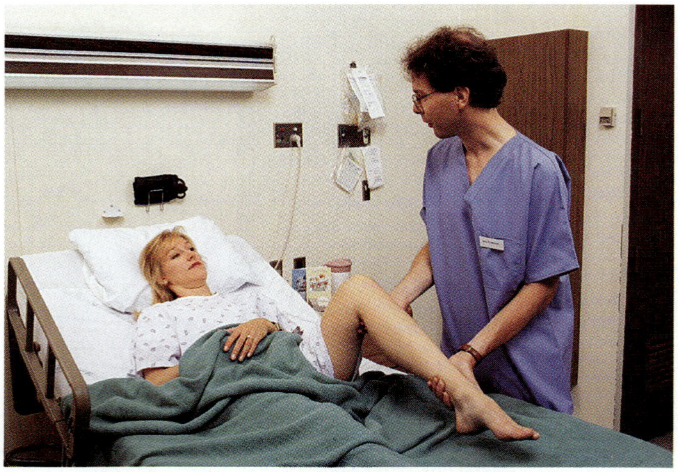

Fig. 25-12 *The knee is flexed and then extended during postoperative leg exercises.*

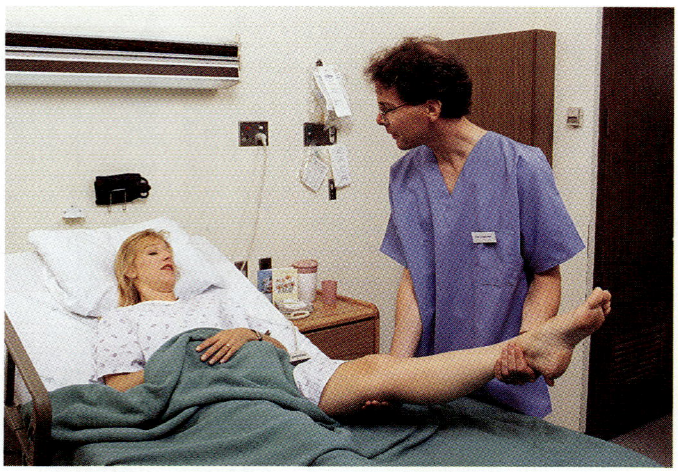

Fig. 25-13 *The nursing assistant helps the patient raise and lower the leg in another postoperative leg exercise.*

Elastic Stockings

Elastic stockings are often ordered for postoperative patients and for those with heart disease and circulatory disorders. Bed rest and pregnancy are also indications for elastic stockings. Affected persons can develop blood clots (thrombi).

Elastic stockings are often called AE hose or antiembolic stockings. They help prevent the development of thrombi. The elastic exerts pressure on the veins, promoting venous blood flow to the heart.

The stockings come in many sizes. Thigh-high or knee-high lengths are available. The nurse measures the person to determine the correct size. The stockings are removed at least twice each day. They are applied before the person gets out of bed.

Applying Elastic Stockings

Pre-procedure

1. Explain the procedure to the person.
2. Wash your hands.
3. Obtain elastic stockings in the correct size.
4. Identify the person. Check the ID bracelet with the treatment card.
5. Provide for privacy.
6. Raise the bed to the best level for good body mechanics.

Procedure

7. Lower the side rail.
8. Position the person supine.
9. Expose the legs. Fanfold top linens back toward the person.
10. Hold the foot and heel of the stocking. Gather the rest of the stocking in your hands.
11. Support the person's foot at the heel.
12. Slip the foot of the stocking over the toes, foot, and heel (Fig. 25-14, A).
13. Pull the stocking up over the leg. It should be even and snug (Fig. 25-14, B).
14. Make sure the stocking is not twisted and has no creases or wrinkles.
15. Repeat steps 10 through 14 for the other leg.
16. Return top linens to their proper position.

Post-procedure

17. Help the person to a comfortable position.
18. Lower the bed to its lowest position. Place the call bell within reach.
19. Raise or lower side rails as instructed by the nurse.
20. Unscreen the person.
21. Wash your hands.
22. Tell the nurse that the stockings have been applied. Report the time of application.

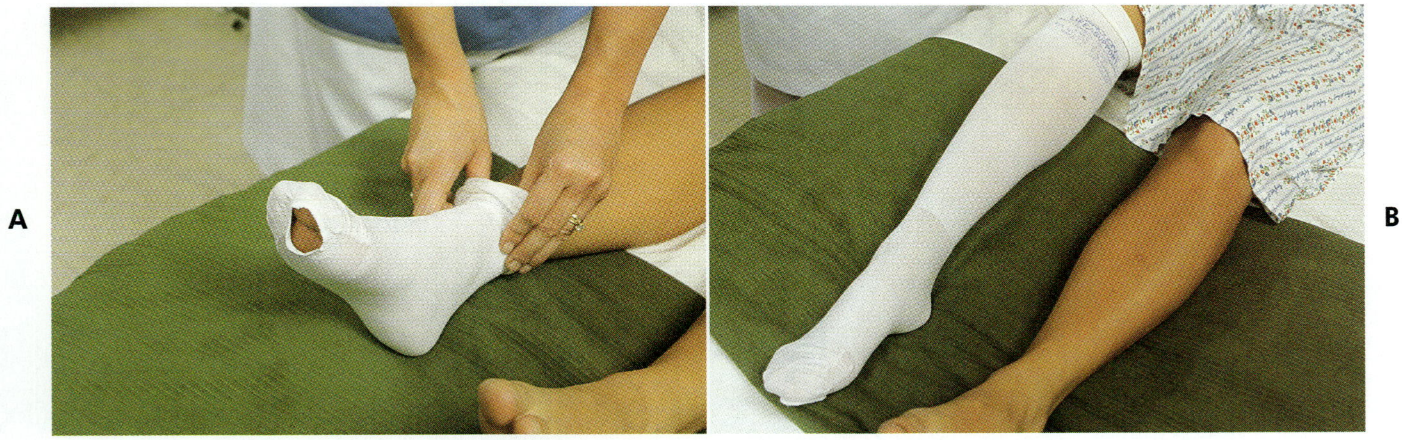

Fig. 25-14 ***A***, *The stocking is slipped over the toes, foot, and heel.* ***B***, *The stocking is pulled up over the leg.*

Bandages and Binders

Bandages are applied to an extremity. Binders are applied to the abdomen, chest, or perineal areas. Bandages and binders are used to:

- Promote comfort
- Promote circulation
- Provide support and pressure
- Promote healing
- Prevent injury
- Hold dressings in place

They must be applied properly. Incorrect application can cause severe discomfort, skin irritation, and circulatory and respiratory complications. The binder's effectiveness and the person's safety depend on correct application. Box 25-3 lists the rules for applying binders.

BOX 25-3 RULES FOR APPLYING BINDERS

- Apply the binder so that firm, even pressure is exerted over the area.
- Apply the binder so it is snug but does not interfere with breathing or circulation.
- Position the person in good alignment when the binder is applied.
- Reapply the binder if it becomes loose, wrinkled, out of position, or causes discomfort.
- Secure pins so they point away from incisional areas.
- Change binders that are moist or soiled to prevent the growth of microorganisms.

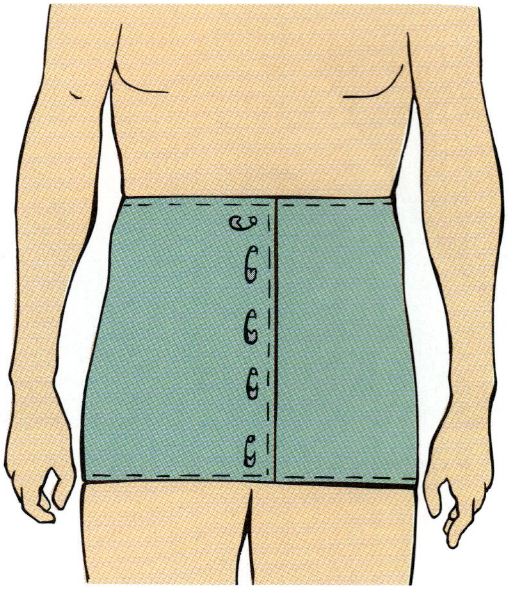

Fig. 25-15 *Straight abdominal binder.*

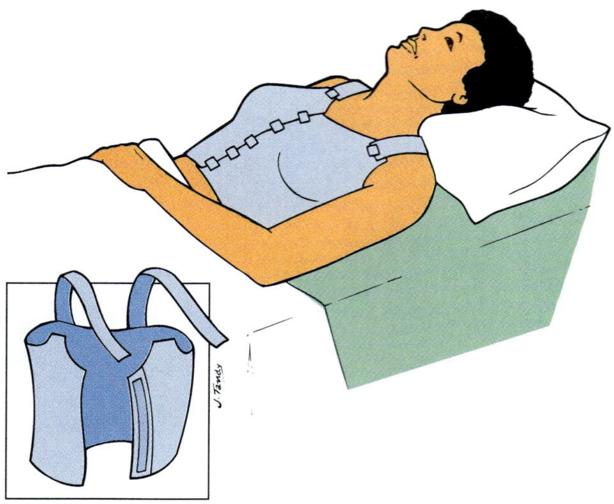

Fig. 25-16 *Breast binder.*

Straight abdominal binders Straight abdominal binders (Fig. 25-15) provide abdominal support and hold dressings in place. The binder is a rectangle. The binder is applied with the person supine. The top part is positioned at the person's waist. The lower part is over the hips. The binder is secured in place with pins, hooks, or Velcro.

Breast binders Breast binders (Fig. 25-16) support the breasts following breast surgery. They also apply pressure to the breasts after childbirth. If the mother does not breast-feed, pressure from the binder helps dry up the milk in the breasts. The binder also promotes comfort and provides support to swollen breasts after childbirth. The woman is supine when the breast binder is applied. The binder is pulled snugly across the chest and secured in place.

T binders T binders are used to secure dressings in place after rectal and perineal surgeries. The single T binder is used for women (Fig. 25-17, A). The double T binder is used for men (Fig. 25-17, B). If perineal dressings are large, women may need double T binders. To apply a T binder, the waist bands are brought around the waist and pinned at the front. The tails are brought between the person's legs and up to the waistband. They are pinned in place at the waistband.

Elastic bandages Elastic bandages are used for the same purposes as elastic stockings. They also provide support and reduce swelling from musculoskeletal injuries. The bandage is applied from the lower (distal) part of the extremity to the top (proximal) part. The nurse gives you directions about the area to be bandaged. The rules for applying bandages are listed in Box 25-4.

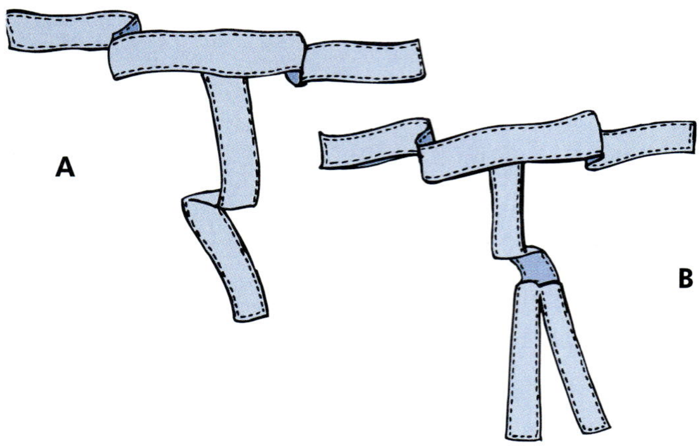

Fig. 25-17 *A, Single T binder. B, Double T binder.*

BOX 25-4 RULES FOR APPLYING BANDAGES

- Use the correct size. The bandage must be the proper length and width to bandage the extremity.
- Position the extremity in good alignment.
- Face the person during the procedure.
- Leave fingers or toes exposed if possible. This allows the circulation to be checked.
- Apply the bandage with firm, even pressure.
- Check the color and temperature of the extremity every hour.
- Reapply a loose or wrinkled bandage.

Applying Elastic Bandages

Pre-procedure

1 Explain the procedure to the person.

2 Wash your hands.

3 Collect the following:
- Elastic bandage as determined by the nurse
- Tape, metal clips, or safety pins

4 Identify the person. Check the ID bracelet with the treatment card.

5 Provide for privacy.

6 Raise the bed to the best level for good body mechanics.

Procedure

7 Help the person to a comfortable position. Expose the part to be bandaged.

8 Make sure the area is clean and dry.

9 Hold the bandage so the roll is up and the loose end is on the bottom (Fig. 25-18, A).

10 Apply the bandage to the smallest part of the wrist, ankle, or knee.

11 Make two circular turns around the part (Fig. 25-18, B).

12 Make overlapping spiral turns in an upward direction. Each turn should overlap about two-thirds of the previous turn (Fig. 25-18, C).

13 Apply the bandage smoothly with firm, even pressure. It should not be tight.

14 Pin, tape, or clip the end of the bandage to hold it in place. The pin or clip must not be under the part.

15 Check the fingers or toes for coldness or cyanosis. Also check for complaints of pain, numbness, or tingling. Remove the bandage if any are noted. Report your observations to the nurse.

Post-procedure

16 Make sure the person is comfortable and the call bell is within reach.

17 Lower the bed.

18 Raise or lower side rails as instructed by the nurse.

19 Unscreen the person.

20 Wash your hands.

21 Report the following to the nurse:
- The time the bandage was applied
- The site of the application
- Any other observations

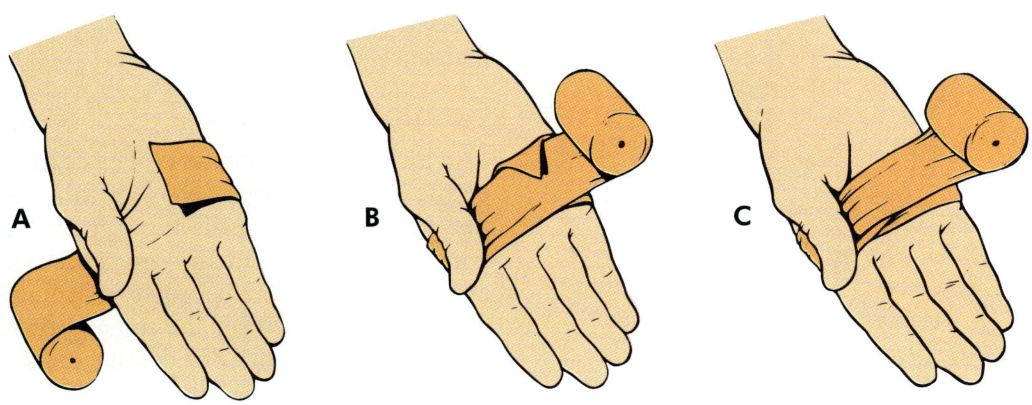

Fig. 25-18 *A, The roll of the elastic bandage is up, and the loose end is on the bottom. B, The bandage is applied to the smallest part with two circular turns. C, The bandage is applied with spiral turns in an upward direction.* (From Parcel GS and Rinear CE: *Basic emergency care of the sick and injured,* ed 4, St Louis, 1989, Mosby–Year Book.)

Wound Healing

The incision must be protected after surgery. Healing must be promoted and infection prevented. Sterile dressing changes are done by the doctor or nurse. Some states allow nursing assistants to do simple dressing changes. All nursing team members take measures to prevent stress on the incision. Coughing, vomiting, and abdominal distention place stress on the incision. Two complications can occur.

- Wound **dehiscence** is the separation of the surgical incision (Fig. 25-19).
- Wound **evisceration** is the separation of the surgical incision along with the protrusion of abdominal organs (Fig. 25-20).

Binders and supporting the incision during coughing and deep breathing help prevent wound dehiscence and evisceration. So does preventing vomiting and abdominal distention.

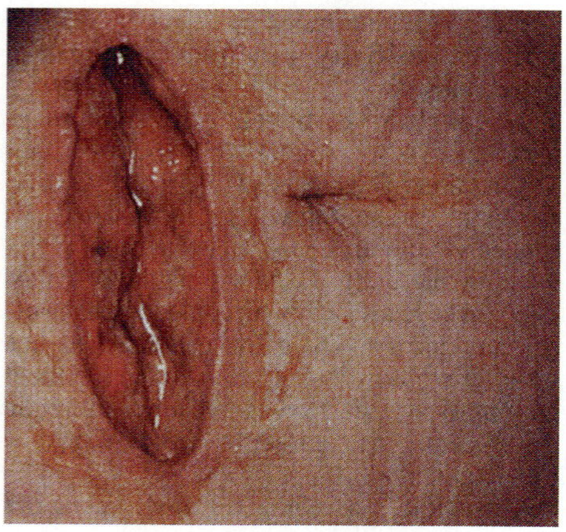

Fig. 25-19 *Wound dehiscence.* *(Courtesy of Morison M: A colour guide to the nursing management of wounds, London, 1992, Wolfe Medical Publishers.)*

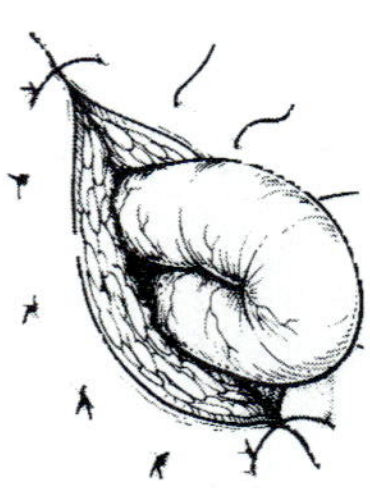

Wound evisceration

Fig. 25-20 *Wound evisceration.* *(From Mosby's medical, nursing & allied health dictionary, ed 4, St Louis, 1994, Mosby–Year Book.)*

Early Ambulation

Early ambulation prevents many postoperative complications. They include thrombi, pneumonia, atelectasis, constipation, and urinary tract infections. The person usually ambulates the evening of surgery or the next day. The person dangles first. Blood pressure and pulse are measured. If they are stable, the person is assisted out of bed. Usually the person does not walk very far, often just a few feet in the room. Distance increases as the person gains strength.

The nurse tells you when to ambulate the person. Usually you assist the nurse the first time.

Nutrition and Fluids

The person has an IV infusion on return from the operating room. The need for continued IV therapy depends on the type of surgery and the person's condition. Anesthesia can cause nausea and vomiting. The person's diet progresses from NPO to clear liquids, to full liquids, to a light diet, to a regular diet. The diet is ordered by the doctor. Frequent oral hygiene is important when the person is NPO.

Elimination

Normal elimination must be established after surgery. Anesthesia, the surgery itself, and being NPO affect normal bowel and urinary elimination. Many pain medications can cause constipation. The measures to promote elimination are practiced as directed by the nurse (see Chapters 15 and 16).

Intake and output are measured postoperatively. The person must urinate within 8 hours after surgery. You must report the person's first voiding. If the person does not void within 8 hours, a catheterization is usually ordered. Some patients have catheters after surgery. See Chapter 15 for care of the person with a catheter.

Fluid intake and return to a regular diet are necessary for bowel elimination. Suppositories or enemas may be ordered for constipation. Rectal tubes may be ordered for flatulence.

Comfort and Rest

Pain is common after surgery. The degree of pain depends on the extent of surgery, the location of the incision, and the presence of drainage tubes, casts, or other devices. Positioning during surgery can cause muscle strains and discomfort. The doctor orders pain medications for the person. The nurse uses the nursing process to promote comfort and rest. Many of the measures listed in Chapter 20 will be part of the person's care plan.

Personal Hygiene

Personal hygiene after surgery is important for the person's physical and mental well-being. Wound drainage and solutions used to prep the skin can irritate the skin and cause discomfort. NPO causes a dry mouth and breath odors. Moist, clammy skin from blood pressure changes or elevated body temperatures is another source of discomfort. Frequent oral hygiene, hair care, and a complete bed bath the day after surgery help refresh and renew the person physically and psychologically. The gown is changed whenever it becomes wet or soiled.

SUMMARY

Surgery is physically and psychologically unpleasant. The more urgent, serious, and complicated the surgery, the greater the effects on the person. The doctor and nurse prepare the person for the surgery. You may assist in certain preoperative activities. Always explain what you are going to do and why. This helps the person psychologically.

After surgery the person recovers from the effects of anesthesia and the operation. Postoperative complications must be prevented. These include bleeding, respiratory distress or infection, thrombi and emboli, and wound infection. Following the rules of safety and medical asepsis helps prevent complications. Turning, repositioning, coughing and deep breathing, and leg exercises also help. You must be alert for signs and symptoms to report to the nurse. Your observations help the nurses and doctors recognize and treat complications.

The nurse tells you what care to give before and after surgery. Remember, the person has many fears and concerns about the surgery and its effects. A kind, caring, and sensitive manner is appreciated by the person.

REVIEW QUESTIONS

Circle the best *answer.*

1 Which is *true* of elective surgery?
- **a** The surgery is done immediately.
- **b** The need for surgery is sudden and unexpected.
- **c** Surgery is scheduled for a later date.
- **d** General anesthesia is always used.

2 Mr. Moore said he was afraid of surgery. He might show his fear by
- **a** Being quiet and withdrawn
- **b** Crying
- **c** Pacing or being unusually cheerful
- **d** All of the above

3 You can assist in Mr. Moore's psychological preparation by explaining
- **a** The reason for the surgery
- **b** Procedures and why they are being done
- **c** The risks and possible complications of surgery
- **d** What to expect during the preoperative and postoperative periods

4 Preoperatively, Mr. Moore is
- **a** NPO
- **b** Allowed only water
- **c** Given a regular breakfast
- **d** Given a tube feeding

5 Cleansing enemas are ordered for Mr. Moore preoperatively. The enemas are given
- **a** To clean the colon of all fecal material
- **b** To prevent postoperative bleeding
- **c** To relieve flatus
- **d** To prevent postoperative pain

6 Mr. Moore's skin prep is done preoperatively to
- **a** Completely bathe the body
- **b** Sterilize the skin
- **c** Reduce the number of microbes on the skin
- **d** Destroy nonpathogens and pathogens

7 When shaving the skin before surgery
- **a** Shave in the direction opposite of hair growth
- **b** Shave toward the center of the specific area
- **c** Be careful not to cut, scratch, or nick the skin
- **d** All of the above

8 Mr. Moore's preoperative medication has been given. He
- **a** Must remain in bed
- **b** Is allowed to smoke with supervision
- **c** Can use the commode for elimination
- **d** Is allowed only sips of water

9 General anesthesia
- **a** Is a specially educated nurse
- **b** Produces unconsciousness and the loss of feeling or sensation
- **c** Is a specially educated doctor
- **d** Produces loss of sensation or feeling in a body part

10 Mr. Moore must cough and deep breathe after surgery to prevent
- **a** Bleeding
- **b** A pulmonary embolus
- **c** Respiratory complications
- **d** Pain and discomfort

11 Leg exercises are ordered for Mr. Moore. Which is *true?*
- **a** Leg exercises are done to stimulate circulation.
- **b** Leg exercises are done to prevent thrombi.
- **c** Leg exercises are done 5 times every 1 or 2 hours.
- **d** All of the above

12 Postoperatively, Mr. Moore's position is changed
- **a** Every 2 hours
- **b** Every 3 hours
- **c** Every 4 hours
- **d** Every shift

Review Questions—Cont'd

13 Mr. Moore wears elastic stockings to

a Prevent blood clots
b Hold dressings in place
c Reduce swelling after musculoskeletal injury
d All of the above

14 Mr. Moore has an abdominal binder. The binder is used to

a Prevent blood clots
b Prevent wound infection
c Provide support and hold dressings in place
d Decrease circulation and swelling

15 When applying an elastic bandage

a The extremity needs to be in good alignment
b The fingers or toes are covered if possible
c It is applied from the largest to smallest part of the extremity
d It is applied from the upper to the lower part of the extremity

Circle T *if the answer is true and* F *if the answer is false.*

16 **T** **F** Hair is usually washed before surgery.

17 **T** **F** Hair is kept out of the face for surgery by using pins, clips, or combs.

18 **T** **F** Nail polish is removed before surgery.

19 **T** **F** Women are allowed to wear makeup to surgery.

20 **T** **F** Pajamas can be worn to the operating room.

21 **T** **F** Valuables are removed preoperatively.

22 **T** **F** A surgical bed is made for the person's return from the recovery room.

23 **T** **F** You are responsible for receiving the person from the recovery room.

24 **T** **F** A drop in a person's blood pressure must be reported to the nurse immediately.

25 **T** **F** Organs protrude with wound dehiscence.

26 **T** **F** The patient never ambulates until the day after surgery

27 **T** **F** After surgery, the person's diet progresses from NPO to full liquids.

28 **T** **F** Intake and output are measured after surgery.

29 **T** **F** A surgical patient should urinate within 8 hours after surgery.

30 **T** **F** Constipation is not a concern after abdominal surgery.

Answers to these questions are on page 752.

Rehabilitation and Restorative Care

26

OBJECTIVES

- Define the key terms listed in this chapter
- Describe how rehabilitation involves the whole person
- Identify the complications that need to be prevented for successful rehabilitation
- Identify ways to help disabled persons perform activities of daily living
- Identify the common psychological reactions of rehabilitation
- Describe how disability affects a person's job status and how rehabilitation can help
- Identify the members of the rehabilitation team
- List the common rehabilitation services and those required by OBRA
- Explain how to promote quality of life during the rehabilitation process
- Describe nursing assistant responsibilities in rehabilitation

KEY TERMS

activities of daily living (ADL) Self-care activities a person performs daily to remain independent and to function in society

prosthesis An artificial replacement for a missing body part

rehabilitation The process of restoring the disabled person to the highest level of physical, psychological, social, and economic functioning possible

Disease, injury, and surgery can result in loss of body function or loss of a body part. Birth injuries and birth defects can also affect functioning. Often more than one function is lost. Everyday activities such as eating, bathing, dressing, and walking may be difficult or seem impossible. The person may be unable to return to a job. The ability to care for children, family, and the home may be seriously affected. The disabled person may be totally or partially dependent on others to meet basic needs. The degree of disability present affects how much function is possible.

Health care is concerned with preventing disability and reducing the degree of disability. Helping the person adjust to the disability is also important. **Rehabilitation** is the process of restoring the disabled person to the highest level of physical, psychological, social, and economic functioning possible. The focus is on improving the person's abilities. For some persons the goal is to return to employment. For others, self-care is the goal. Sometimes improvement is not possible. Then the focus is on maintaining the highest level of functioning possible and preventing further disability.

REHABILITATION AND THE WHOLE PERSON

The rehabilitation process involves the whole person. A physical illness or injury always has some psychological or social effect. A disability has similar effects. How would you feel if a car accident left you paralyzed from the waist down? Would you be angry, afraid, or depressed? Would you deny it happened to you? Could you be involved in your usual social activities? Could you dance, exercise, shop, or go to school? Could you attend church services or visit relatives and friends in their homes? Could you drive a car? Could you return to your present job? Could you find another job with your remaining skills and abilities?

Rehabilitation helps a person adjust to the disability physically, psychologically, socially, and economically. Abilities are emphasized, not the disability. However, complications that can cause further disability must be prevented. Therefore rehabilitation begins when the person first seeks health care.

Physical Considerations

Rehabilitation begins with preventing complications. Complications can occur from bed rest, prolonged illness, or recovery from injury. Contractures, pressure sores, and bowel and bladder problems are prevented. Contractures and pressure sores are prevented with good body alignment, frequent turning and repositioning, range-of-motion exercises, and supportive devices (see Chapters 10 and 19). Good skin care is very important in preventing pressure sores (see Chapter 13).

Bladder training was described in Chapter 15. The method used depends on the person's physical problems, capabilities, and needs. The nurse explains the method planned for the person. The rules to be followed are also explained.

Bowel training was described in Chapter 16. It involves gaining control of bowel movements and developing a regular pattern of elimination. Fecal impaction, constipation, and anal incontinence are prevented (see Chapter 16).

Performing self-care activities is a major goal of rehabilitation. **Activities of daily living** (**ADL**) refer to self-care activities. Activities of daily living are performed daily by the person to remain independent and to function in society. These activities include bathing, oral hygiene, eating, bowel and bladder elimination, and moving about. A person's ability to perform self-care activities and the need for self-help devices are evaluated.

The hands, wrists, and arms may be affected by disease or injury. Self-help devices may be needed for various activities. Equipment can usually be changed or made to meet a person's needs. Special eating utensils may be needed. Glass holders, plate guards, and silverware with curved handles or cuffs (Fig. 26-1) are available. Some

A B C D

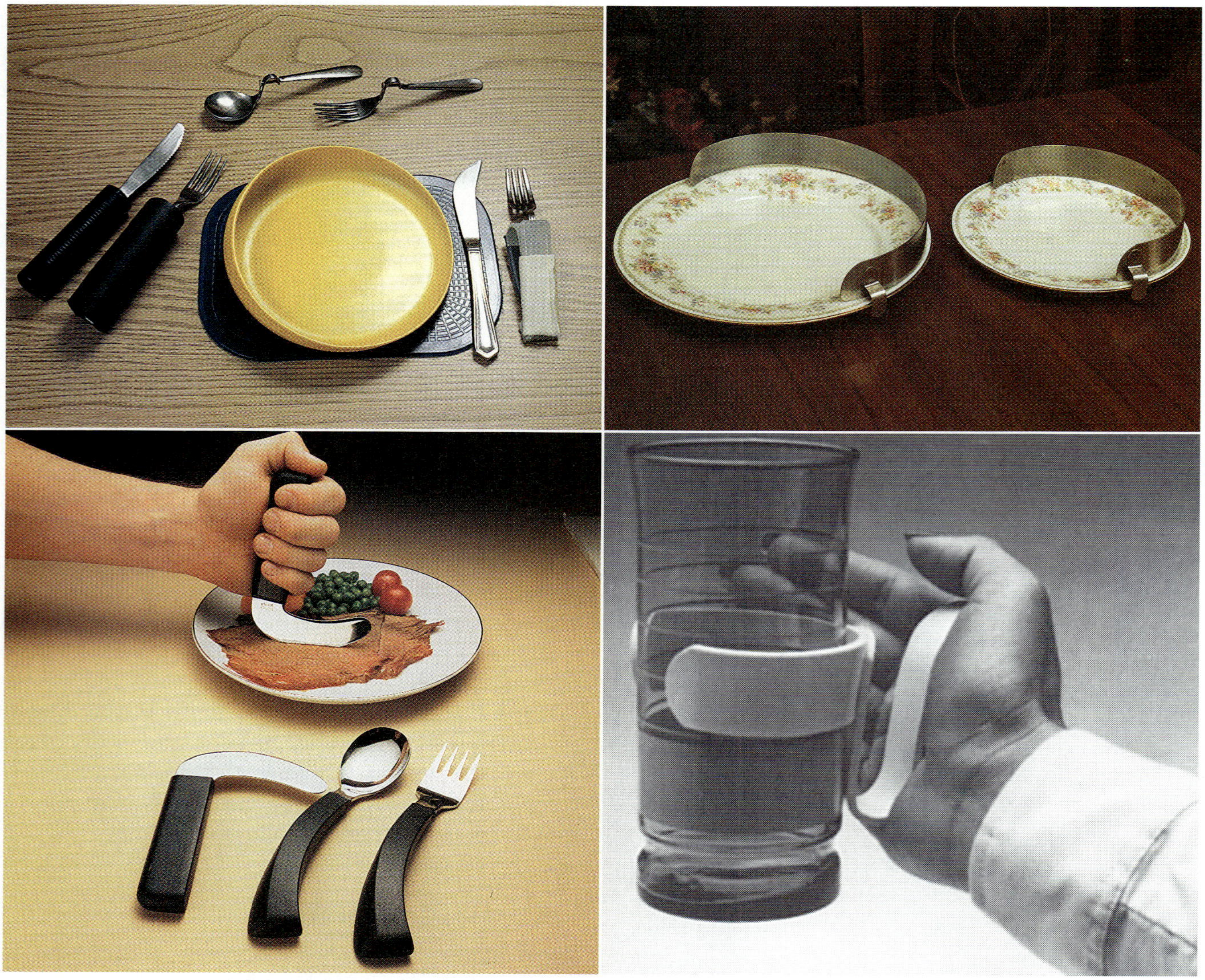

Fig. 26-1 *Eating utensils for persons with special needs. A, Note the cuffed fork, which fits over the hand. The rounded plate helps keep food on the plate. Special grips and swivel handles are helpful for some people. B, Plateguards help keep food on the plate. C, Knives with rounded blades are rocked back and forth to cut food. They eliminate the need to have a fork in one hand and a knife in the other. D, Glass or cup holder.* *(B, C, and D courtesy of BISSELL Healthcare Corp./Fred Sammons, Inc. From Hoeman SP: Rehabilitation/restorative care in the community, St Louis, 1990, Mosby–Year Book.)*

devices are attached to a special splint (Fig. 26-2). Electric toothbrushes are helpful if the person cannot perform the back-and-forth motions necessary for brushing teeth. Longer handles can be attached to combs, brushes, and sponges (Fig. 26-3). There also are self-help devices for preparing meals, using kitchen appliances, dressing, writing, dialing telephones, and for many other activities (Fig. 26-4 on page 572).

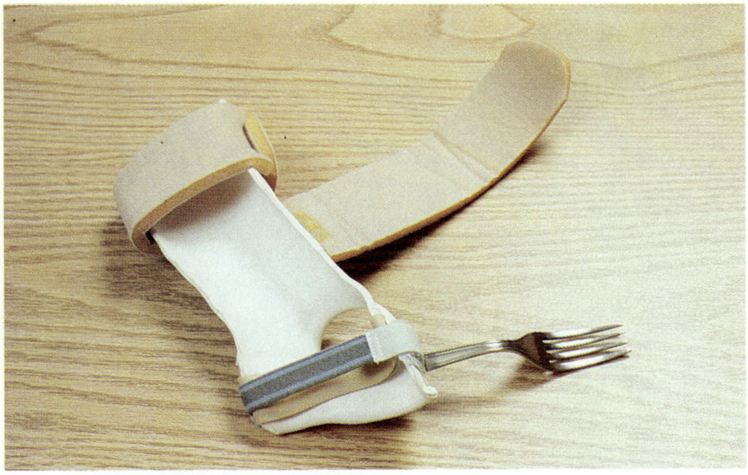

Fig. 26-2 *Self-help devices can be attached to splints.*

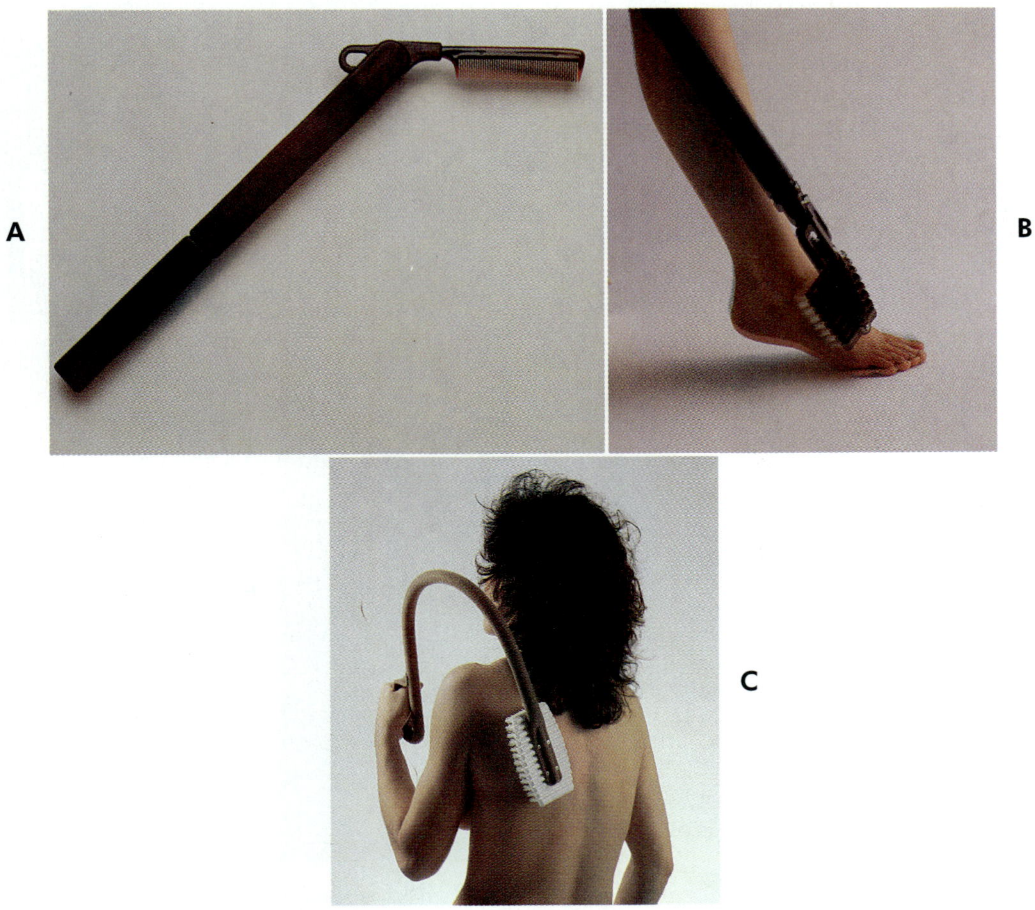

Fig. 26-3 ***A,*** *A long-handled comb for hair care.* ***B,*** *The brush has a long handle for bathing.* ***C,*** *This brush has a curved handle.*
(Courtesy of North Coast Medical, Inc, San Jose, Calif. From Hoeman SP: Rehabilitation/restorative care in the community, St Louis, 1990, Mosby–Year Book.)

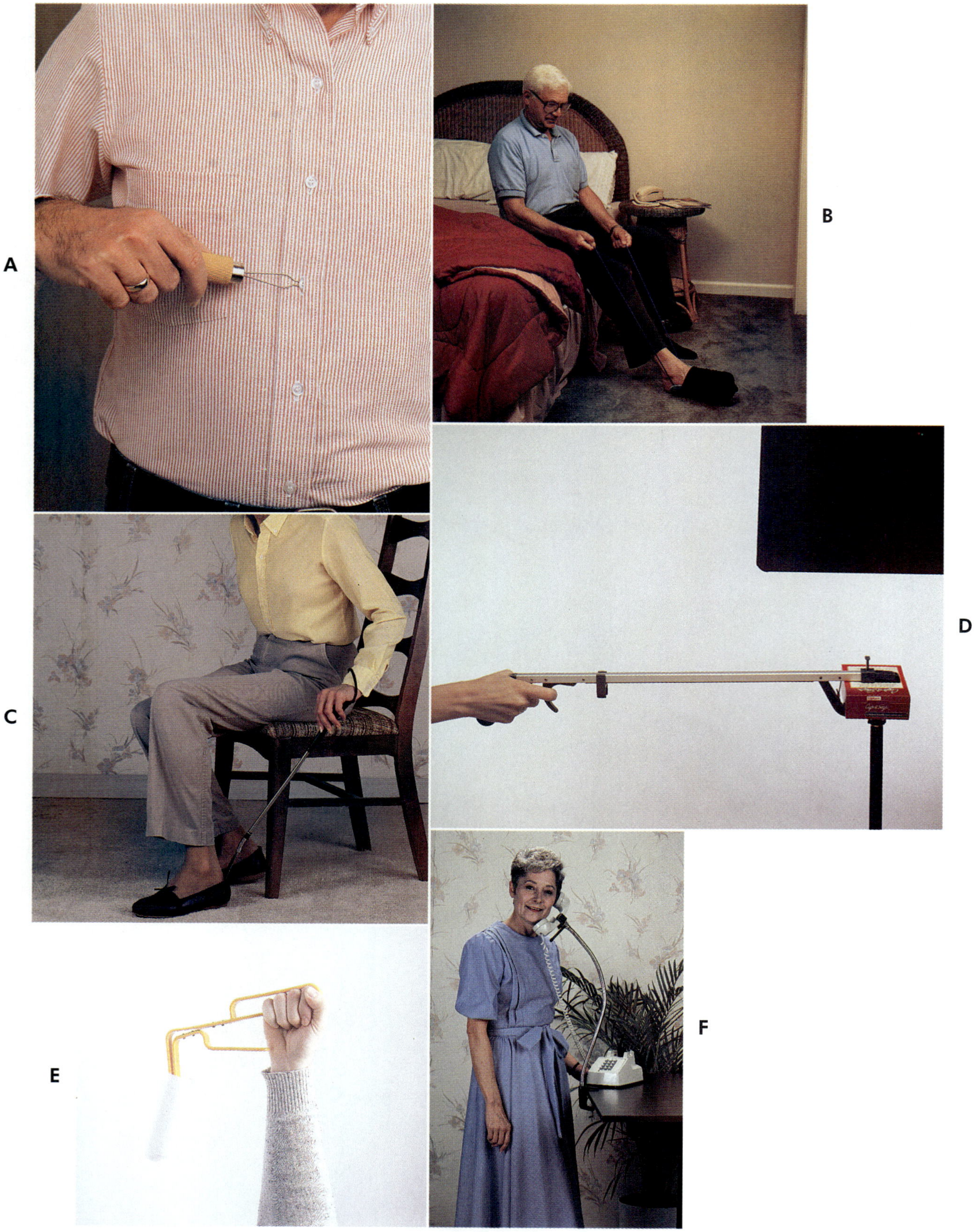

Fig. 26-4 *A, A button hook is used to button and zip clothing. B, A sock puller is used to put on socks and stockings. C, A long-handled shoehorn for putting on shoes. D, Reachers are helpful for those in wheelchairs. E, A toilet paper holder is used for wiping. F, The telephone holder is for those who cannot hold a phone.* (*A, B, D, E courtesy of North Coast Medical Inc, San Jose, Calif. C, F courtesy of BISSELL Healthcare Corp./Fred Sammons, Inc. D from Hoeman SP: Rehabilitation/restorative care in the community, St Louis, 1990, Mosby–Year Book.*)

Some persons have lower-extremity involvement. They may have to learn how to walk with a supportive device or learn to use a wheelchair. If walking is possible, the person is taught to use crutches or a walker, cane, or brace (Fig. 26-5). Both legs may be paralyzed or amputated. If so, a wheelchair is used. Persons paralyzed on one side of the body also need wheelchairs. If possible, the person is taught how to transfer from the bed to the wheelchair without assistance. Other transfers are taught. These include transfers to and from the toilet, bathtub, sofas and chairs, and in and out of cars (Fig. 26-6).

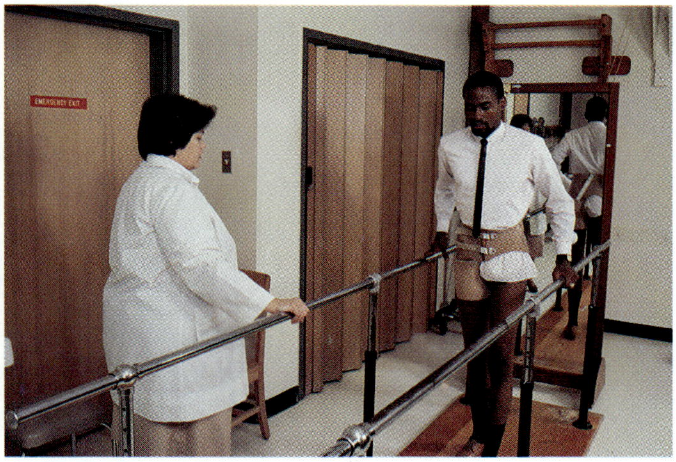

Fig. 26-5 *A person learns how to walk in physical therapy.*

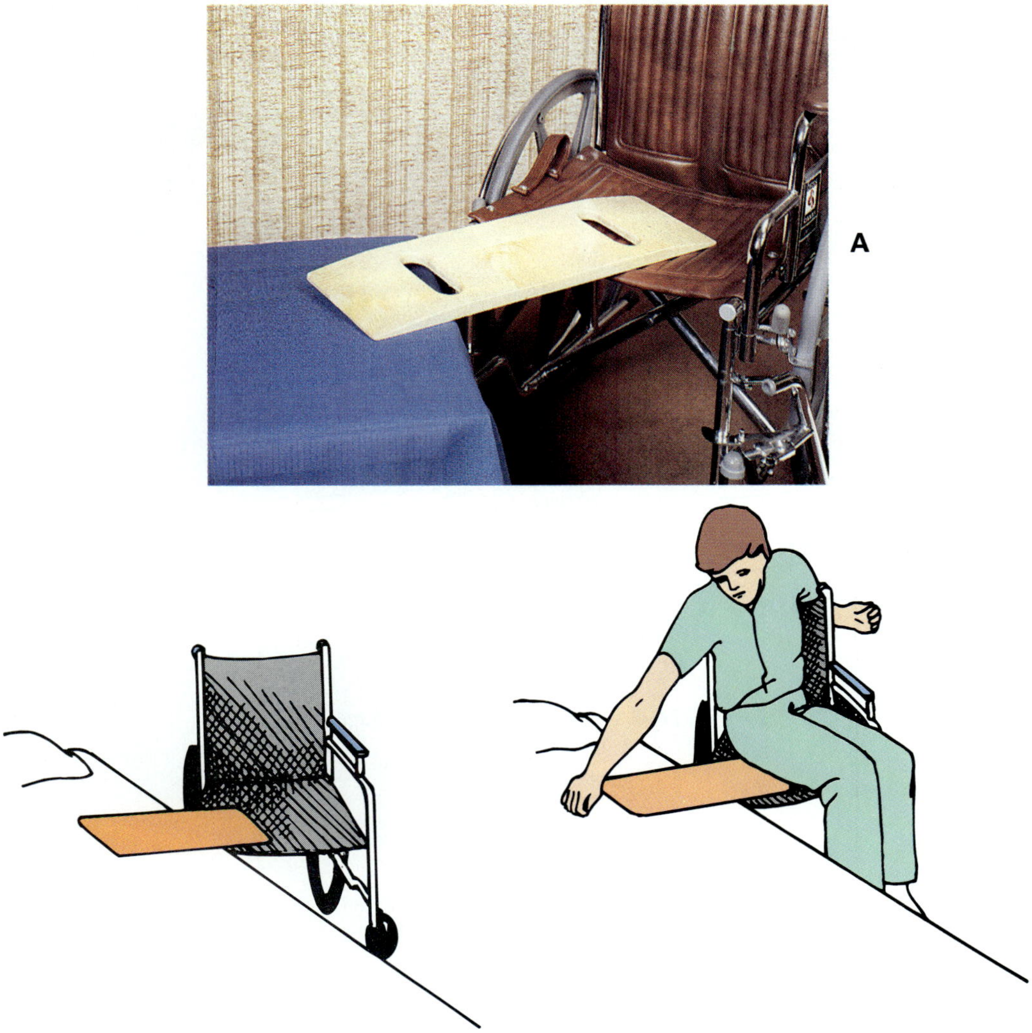

A

B

Fig. 26-6 *A, A transfer board is used to transfer from one seat to another. B, The person transfers from the wheelchair to the bed. C, A transfer from the wheelchair to the bathtub. D, A transfer to the car. The person has left-side paralysis.* *(A courtesy of BISSELL Healthcare Corp./Fred Sammons, Inc. A, B, C, and D from Hoeman SP: Rehabilitation/restorative care in the community, St Louis, 1990, Mosby–Year Book.)*

Continued.

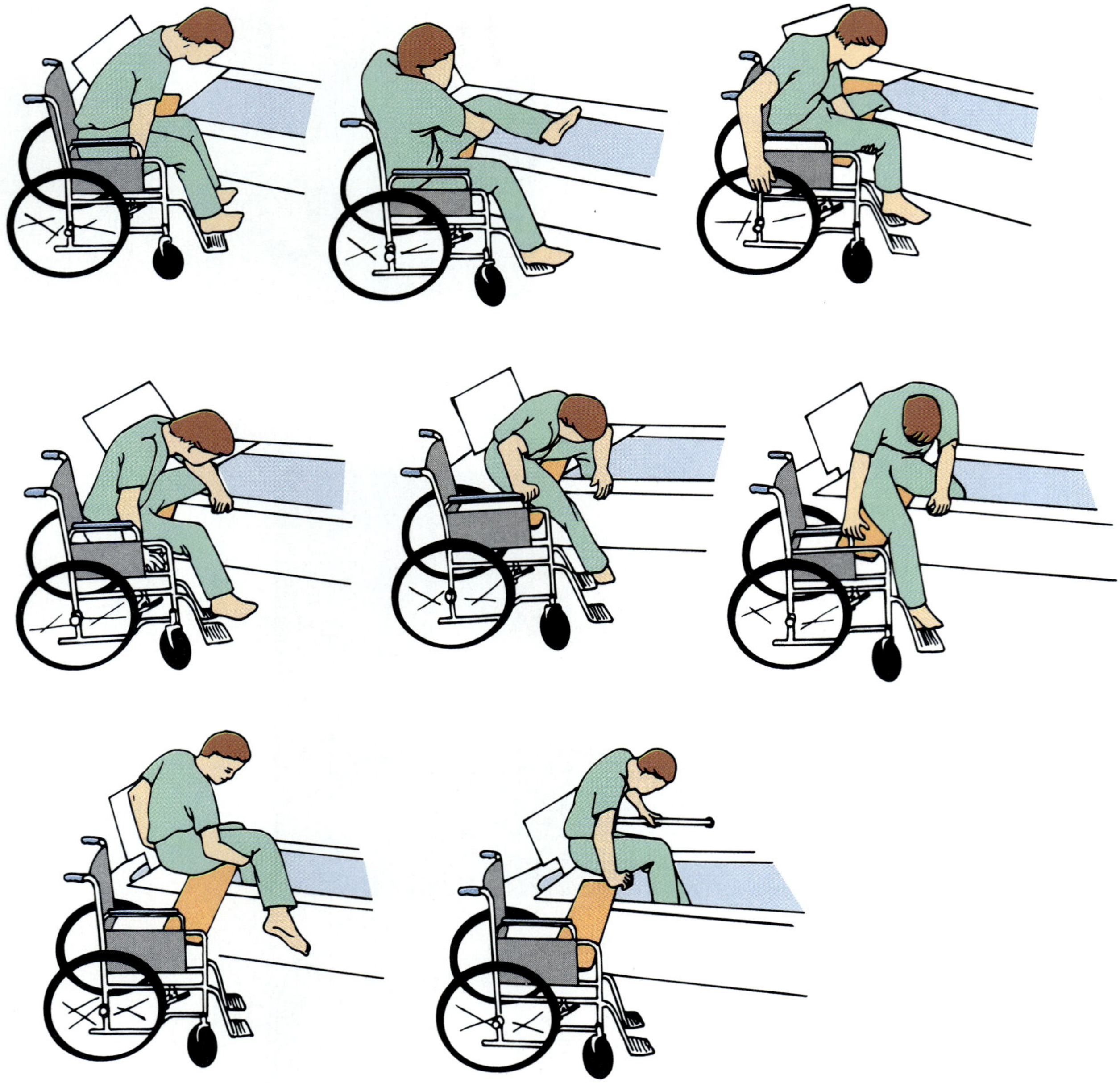

C

Fig. 26-6, cont'd *For legend see page 573.*

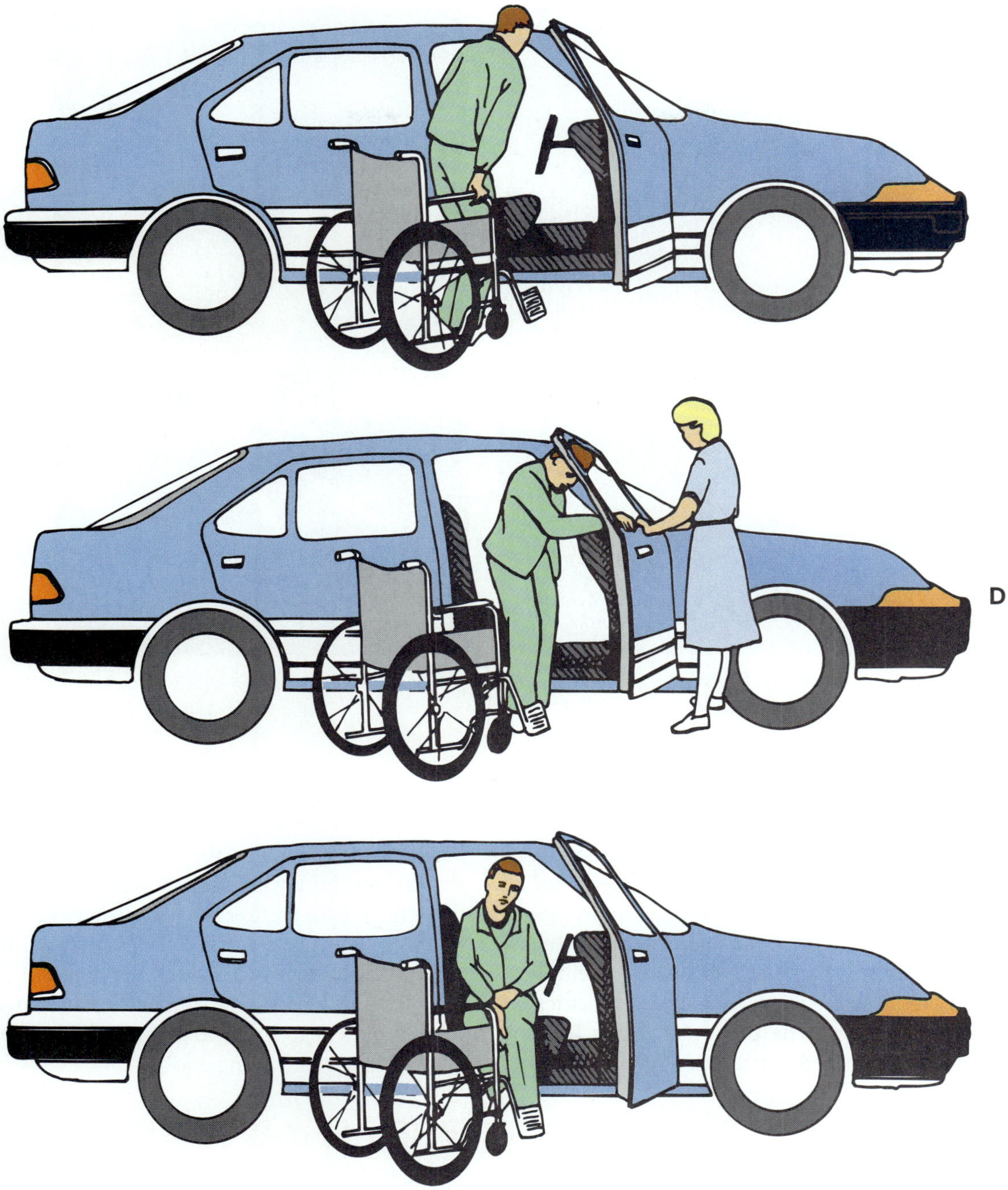

Fig. 26-6, cont'd *For legend see page 573.*

A

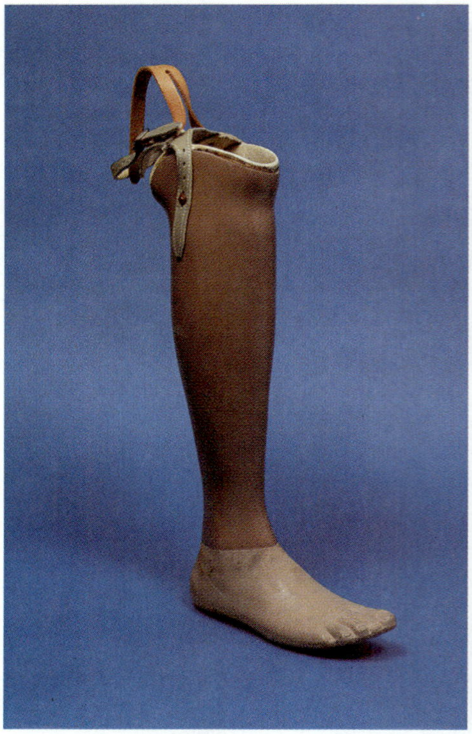

B

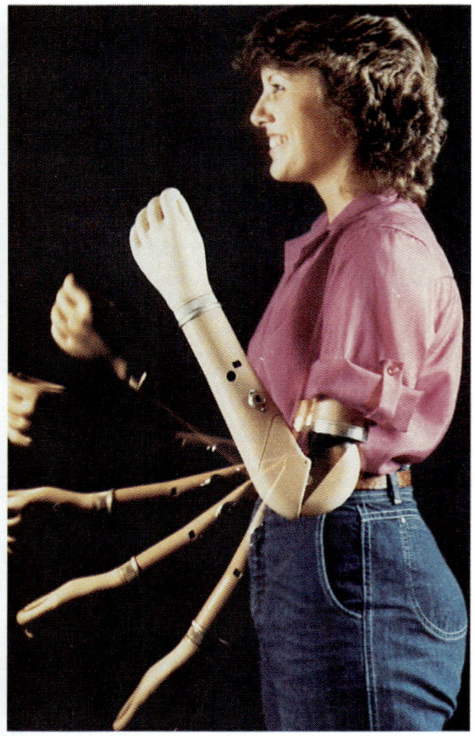

Fig. 26-7 *A, Leg prosthesis. B, Arm prosthesis.* (*B, Courtesy of Motion Control, Division of IOMED Inc., Salt Lake City, Utah.*)

The person with a missing body part may be fitted with a prosthesis. A **prosthesis** is an artificial replacement for a missing body part. A person can usually be fitted with an artificial arm or leg and taught how to use the prosthesis (Fig. 26-7). Artificial eyes are available. There are breast prostheses for women who have had a breast removed. Modern technology will result in more sophisticated prostheses. The goal is for the prosthesis to be like the missing part in function and appearance.

Psychological and Social Considerations

Self-esteem and relationships are often affected by a disability. Changes in appearance and function may cause the person to feel unwhole, unattractive, unclean, or undesirable to others. During the early stages of rehabilitation the person may refuse to acknowledge the disability. The person may be depressed, angry, and hostile.

Successful rehabilitation depends on the person's attitude, acceptance of limitations, and motivation. The person must focus on remaining abilities. Discouragement and frustration are common. Progress may be slow, or efforts unsuccessful. Each new task to be learned is a reminder of the disability. Old fears and emotions may again be experienced. The person needs help accepting the disability and the resulting limitations. Support, reassurance, encouragement, and sensitivity from the health team are necessary.

Economic Considerations

The person may be unable to return to a job held before the disease, injury, or surgery. Rehabilitation services can help the person reenter the work force. The person is evaluated to determine work abilities, past work experiences, interests, and talents. Through the rehabilitation process a job skill may be restored or a new one learned. The goal is for the person to become gainfully employed. Assistance is often given in finding a job.

THE REHABILITATION TEAM

Rehabilitation is a team effort. The team consists of the person, doctor, nursing team, other health professionals and workers, and the family. All assist the disabled person to achieve independence. A physical therapist, occupational therapist, psychiatrist, psychologist, speech therapist, social worker, member of the clergy, dietician, and others may be involved. A vocational counselor evaluates the person's ability to perform a job skill and return to work.

The team meets regularly to discuss and evaluate the person's progress. Goals are set for the person. The person should be involved in the goal setting. Changes in the rehabilitation plan are made as needed. The disabled person and family members are encouraged to attend the meetings.

REHABILITATION SERVICES

Rehabilitation begins at the time of illness or injury. Depending on the person's needs and problems, the process may be continued. The person may require extended hospital care or care in a nursing facility. Some people are transferred to rehabilitation centers, where many specialized services are available. Others can be treated as outpatients. There are centers for the blind, deaf, mentally retarded, physically disabled, those with speech problems, and the mentally ill. Rehabilitation services are available to some people in their homes or in day-care centers. Nursing assistants work in all of these settings.

OBRA Requirements

OBRA requires that nursing facilities provide rehabilitation services. The services may be provided by facility staff. If not, the facility must obtain the service from another source. For example, a facility may not employ a physical therapist. Instead, the facility obtains the service from a local hospital. OBRA rules state that rehabilitation services required by a resident's comprehensive care plan must be provided. If a resident requires physical therapy, it must be provided. If a resident requires occupational therapy, it must be provided. If a resident requires speech therapy, it must be provided. Such rehabilitation services require a doctor's order.

QUALITY OF LIFE

Successful rehabilitation improves the person's quality of life. A hopeful and winning attitude helps motivate the person. However, rehabilitation can be slow and frustrating. You can help the person have the right attitude by taking measures to promote quality of life.

The person's rights must be protected. The right to privacy is important. The person should be able to relearn old or practice new skills in private. The person does not need other patients or residents watching. Others do not need to see mistakes, falls, spills, or clumsiness. Nor do they need to see the person's anger or tears. Providing privacy protects the person's dignity and promotes self-respect.

The right to personal choice gives the person control. Being unable to control body movements or functions is very frustrating. The person is allowed and encouraged to control the other aspects of his or her life to the extent possible. Personal choice is discussed throughout this book. You need to allow personal choice whenever possible. Persons who are sad and depressed may not want to make personal choices. You need to encourage them to do so. Making personal choices helps them feel in control of those things that affect them.

The person is part of the rehabilitation team. The team plans and evaluates the person's rehabilitation program. Being part of the team allows the individual personal choice in planning care.

The person has the right to be free from abuse and mistreatment. Rehabilitation can be a very slow process. Sometimes improvement is not seen for weeks. Learning how to use an assistive device can be painfully slow. Learning to speak again after a stroke can take a long time. So can learning how to dress when there is paralysis on one side. These are just a few examples of the skills that may be part of rehabilitation. What seems so simple to you can be very hard for the person. Repeated explanations and demonstrations may have no or little results. You may become impatient and short with the resident. Or you may see such behavior from other team members or the family. You must protect the person from physical and mental abuse and mistreatment. No one can shout, scream, or yell at the person. Nor can they hit or strike the person. The person cannot be called names. Unkind remarks must not be made. You need to report signs of abuse or mistreatment to the nurse.

You must learn to deal with your own anger and frustration. Remember that the person wants to have function and control of body movements. The person does not choose loss of function. If the process is frustrating to you, just think how the person must feel. Discuss your feelings with the nurse. The nurse can suggest ways to help you control your feelings. Perhaps you can be reassigned to other patients or residents for a while.

Taking part in activities promotes quality of life. The person is encouraged to join in group activities. The person may be concerned about how others view the disability. You need to provide support and reassurance. The person needs to know that others have disabilities. Other patients and residents are likely to be very supportive and understanding because of their own disabilities. Allow personal choice in activities. The person usually chooses those of interest and which are the least threatening.

The person's environment is important for quality of life. It must be safe and meet the person's needs. Adjustments may be needed because of disabilities. Location of the overbed table or the bedside stand may need to be changed. The person may need a special chair. If the call bell cannot be used, another way is needed to communicate with the staff. These and other adjustments are recommended by nurses, occupational and physical therapists, and other team members including nursing assistants. The nurse or therapist explains the need and purpose to the person and family.

NURSING ASSISTANT RESPONSIBILITIES

You are a valuable member of the rehabilitation team. As in other situations, a nurse directs you in performing care activities. Many procedures and care measures already learned will be part of the disabled person's care. Safety, communication, legal, and ethical considerations apply in rehabilitation. The many rules described throughout this book also apply, regardless of the type of disability.

Box 26-1 lists your responsibilities as a member of the rehabilitation team.

CROSS-TRAINING OPPORTUNITIES

Rehabilitation offers cross-training opportunities for nursing assistants. Occupational therapy aides and physical therapy aides are often needed in rehabilitation areas. Both types of aides transport persons to and from therapy, prepare equipment and supplies, and do office work.

BOX 26-1 Nursing Assistant Responsibilities in Rehabilitation

- Follow the instructions and directions given by the nurse very carefully.
- Report early signs and symptoms of complications such as pressure sores, contractures, and bowel and bladder problems.
- Keep the person in good body alignment at all times (see Chapter 10).
- Practice measures to prevent pressure sores (see Chapter 13).
- Turn and reposition the person as directed (see Chapter 10).
- Perform range-of-motion exercises as instructed (see Chapter 19). They must be done as often as indicated by the nurse or the nursing care plan.
- Encourage the person to perform as many activities of daily living as possible and to the extent possible.
- Give genuine praise when even a little progress is made.
- Provide emotional support and reassurance.
- Practice the techniques developed by members of the rehabilitation team when assisting the person. This helps you understand what the person needs to do.
- Know how to apply self-care devices used by the person.
- Try to understand and appreciate the person's situation, feelings, and concerns.
- Do not pity the person or give sympathy.
- Concentrate on the person's abilities, not the disabilities.
- Remember that muscles atrophy if they are not used.
- Practice the task that the person must perform. This helps you guide and direct the person.
- Know how to use and operate special equipment used in the person's rehabilitation program.
- Convey an attitude of hopefulness to the person and family.

Summary

Rehabilitation is challenging and rewarding for the health team. Patience, understanding, and sensitivity are needed when working with disabled persons. Progress may be slow and hard to see. The person may become frustrated and discouraged. You must give support, encouragement, and praise when needed. The disabled person does not need pity or sympathy.

Emphasizing abilities is important. It is necessary to prevent disabling complications. Contractures, pressure sores, and bowel and bladder problems are prevented. Therefore good nursing care is necessary. Besides helping to prevent complications, you need to observe the techniques taught to the disabled person. This helps you guide the person more effectively during care. If the person is expected to perform tasks in different ways, frustration takes the place of progress. Finally, remember that the more the person can do alone, the better the person's quality of life.

Review Questions

Circle the best *answer.*

1 Rehabilitation is concerned with
- **a** Physical disabilities
- **b** Physical capabilities
- **c** The whole person
- **d** Psychological, social, and economic functioning

2 Mrs. Lund's physical rehabilitation begins with the prevention of
- **a** Anger, frustration, and depression
- **b** Contractures and pressure sores
- **c** Illness and injury
- **d** Loss of self-esteem

3 Mrs. Lund has weakness on her right side. ADL should be
- **a** Done by Mrs. Lund to the extent possible
- **b** Done by the nursing assistant
- **c** Postponed until she regains use of her right side
- **d** Supervised by the physical therapist

4 The process of rehabilitation emphasizes Mrs. Lund's
- **a** Disability
- **b** Limitations
- **c** Abilities
- **d** All of the above

5 Which reaction is Mrs. Lund likely to experience?
- **a** Feelings of being undesirable
- **b** Anger and hostility
- **c** Depression
- **d** All of the above

6 Which statement is *false?*
- **a** Disabled people can never work again.
- **b** Disabled people may need to learn a new job skill.
- **c** The disabled person is evaluated to determine the ability to work.
- **d** Disabled people are often given help in finding a job.

7 The rehabilitation team consists of
- **a** The nursing team
- **b** The doctor
- **c** Various members of the health team
- **d** The disabled person and the nurse

8 The nursing assistant
- **a** Plans the rehabilitation program
- **b** Supplies prostheses
- **c** Gives praise when even slight progress is made
- **d** Does as much as possible for the disabled person

REVIEW QUESTIONS—CONT'D

9 Which statement is *false?*

a Sympathy and pity help the person adjust to the disability.

b You should know how to apply self-care devices.

c You should know how to use equipment used in the person's care.

d An attitude of hopefulness must be conveyed to the person.

10 Mrs. Lund requires speech therapy after a stroke. Therapy should be provided in private.

a True

b False

11 Mrs. Lund is in physical therapy to learn how to use a walker. She asks to have music played. You should

a Tell her music is not allowed

b Choose some music

c Ask Mrs. Lund to choose some music

d Ask the person in charge of group activities to choose some music

12 A staff member tells Mrs. Lund that she cannot have dessert until she does her exercises. This is abuse and mistreatment.

a True

b False

13 Mrs. Lund does not want to attend a concert at the facility. This is her right to

a Personal choice

b Privacy

c Be free from abuse and neglect

d All of the above

14 Mrs. Lund's right side is weak. The call bell has been placed on the right side. You move it to the left side of the bed. You have promoted her quality of life by

a Protecting her from abuse and mistreatment

b Allowing personal choice

c Providing a safe environment

d All of the above

Answers to these questions are on page 752

Persons with Hearing and Vision Problems

21

OBJECTIVES

- Define the key terms listed in this chapter
- Explain otitis media and Meniere's disease
- Describe the effects of hearing loss and vision loss
- Describe how to communicate with the hearing impaired person
- Explain how to communicate with the speech impaired person
- Explain the purpose of a hearing aid
- Describe how to care for a hearing aid
- Explain the differences between glaucoma and cataracts
- Care for eyeglasses
- Explain why you should not insert or remove contact lenses
- Describe how to protect an artificial eye from loss or damage
- Explain how to care for a blind person

KEY TERMS

braille A method of writing for the blind; raised dots are arranged to represent each letter of the alphabet; the first ten letters represent the numbers 1 through 9

otitis media Infection *(itis)* of the middle *(media)* ear *(ot)*

tinnitus Ringing in the ears

vertigo Dizziness

Sight and hearing are valuable senses. They allow communication with others, learning, and moving about. They also are important for activities of daily living and countless other activities. Hearing and vision are important for the basic need of being safe and secure. Warning signs of danger need to be heard and seen.

Most people take hearing and vision for granted. However, hearing and vision problems are common among all age groups, especially the elderly. Common causes include birth defects, accidents, infections, diseases, and aging. You will care for many people who have some degree of hearing or vision loss. This chapter describes the measures that will help you communicate with such persons. Their special safety needs are also described.

EAR DISORDERS

The ear is important for hearing and balance (see Chapter 5, pages 103-104). Middle ear infections, Meniere's disease, and hearing loss are presented in this section.

Otitis Media

Otitis media is infection *(itis)* of the middle *(media)* ear *(ot)*. The infection can be acute or chronic. Chronic otitis media can damage the tympanic membrane (eardrum) or the ossicles (see Fig. 5-13). The eardrum and ossicles are needed for hearing. Permanent hearing loss can occur from chronic otitis media.

Fluid buildup occurs in the ear. It causes pain and hearing loss. Other signs and symptoms include fever and ringing in the ears (**tinnitus**). Antibiotics are usually ordered by the doctor.

Meniere's Disease

Meniere's disease involves increased fluid in the inner ear. The increased fluid causes pressure in the middle ear. There are three symptoms. Vertigo is the major symptom. **Vertigo** means dizziness. The person feels whirling and spinning sensations. The person must lie down. Dizziness may be so severe that the person has nausea and vomiting. The two other main symptoms of Meniere's disease are ringing in the ears (tinnitus) and hearing loss.

The doctor can order different medications for the person. Sometimes a low-salt diet is ordered to decrease the amount of fluid in the ear. Safety is important during vertigo. Falls must be prevented. The person must lie down when vertigo is experienced. Side rails are usually ordered. The head should be kept still. The person should avoid turning the head. To talk to the person, stand directly in front of him or her. When movement is necessary, the person should move slowly. Bright or glaring lights are avoided. Assistance is given with ambulation. The person should not walk alone in case vertigo occurs.

Hearing Problems

Hearing losses range from slight hearing impairments to complete deafness. Hearing is needed for many functions. Clear speech, responding to others, safety, and awareness of surroundings all require hearing. Many people deny having difficulty hearing. This is because hearing loss is often associated with aging.

Effects on the person A person may be unaware of gradual hearing loss. Others may see changes in the person's behavior or attitude. However, they may not know that the changes are due to hearing difficulties. Symptoms and effects of hearing loss vary. They are not always obvious to the person or to others.

Infants with hearing impairments often fail to start talking. Lack of attention and failing grades are early signs of poor hearing in children. There are some obvious signs of hearing impairment in children and adults. These include:

- Speaking too loudly
- Leaning forward to hear
- Turning and cupping the better ear toward the speaker
- Answering questions or responding inappropriately
- Asking for words to be repeated

Psychological and social effects are less obvious. People with hearing problems may answer others inappropriately. Therefore they tend to avoid social situations. This is an attempt to avoid embarrassment. However, loneliness, boredom, and feelings of being left out often result. Only parts of conversations may be heard. People with hearing loss may become suspicious. They may think they are being talked about or that others are talking softly on purpose. Some try to control conversations to avoid responding to or answering questions. Straining and working to hear can cause fatigue, frustration, and irritability.

People with hearing loss may have speech problems. You hear yourself as you talk. How you pronounce words and the volume of your voice depend on how you hear yourself. Hearing loss may result in slurred speech and improper word pronunciation. Monotone speech and dropping word endings may also occur.

Communicating with the person Hearing impaired persons may wear hearing aids or read lips. They also watch facial expressions, gestures, and body language to understand what is being said. Sign language may be necessary for the totally deaf (Figs. 27-1 and 27-2 on page 586). Some hearing impaired people have *hearing* dogs. The dog alerts the person to such things as ringing phones, doorbells, sirens, or oncoming cars. Certain measures are needed when communicating with the person. The measures listed in Box 27-1 can help the person hear or speech read (lip read).

The person may have speech problems. Understanding what the person is saying can be hard. Do not assume that you understand what is being said. Do not pretend to understand to avoid embarrassing the person. Serious problems can result if you assume or pretend to understand. The guidelines listed in Box 27-2 on page 587 will help you communicate with the speech impaired person.

BOX 27-1 Communicating with the Hearing Impaired Person

- Gain attention and alert the person to your presence. Raise an arm or hand or lightly touch the person's arm. Do not startle or approach the person from behind.
- Face the person directly when speaking. Do not turn or walk away while you are talking.
- Stand or sit in good light. Shadows and glares affect the person's ability to see your face clearly.
- Speak clearly, distinctly, and slowly.
- Speak in a normal tone of voice. Do not shout.
- Do not cover your mouth, smoke, eat, or chew gum while talking. These things affect mouth movements.
- Stand or sit on the side of the better ear.
- State the topic of conversation first.
- Use short sentences and simple words.
- Write out important names and words.
- Say things in a different way if the person does not seem to understand.
- Keep conversations and discussions short to avoid tiring the person.
- Repeat and rephrase statements as needed.
- Be alert to the messages sent by your facial expressions, gestures, and body language.
- Reduce or eliminate background noises.

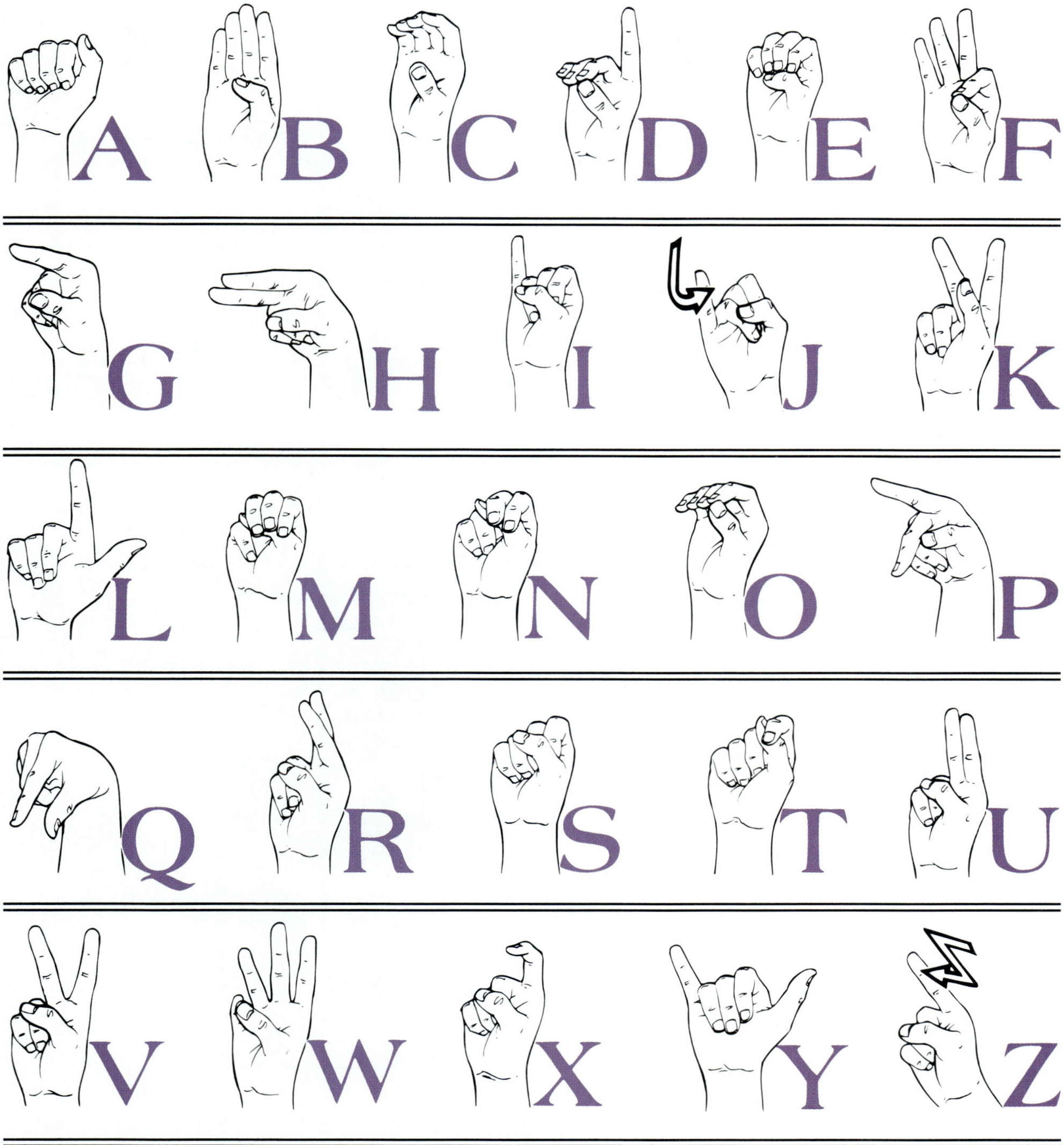

Fig. 27-1 *Manual alphabet.* *(Courtesy of National Association of the Deaf, Silver Springs, Maryland.)*

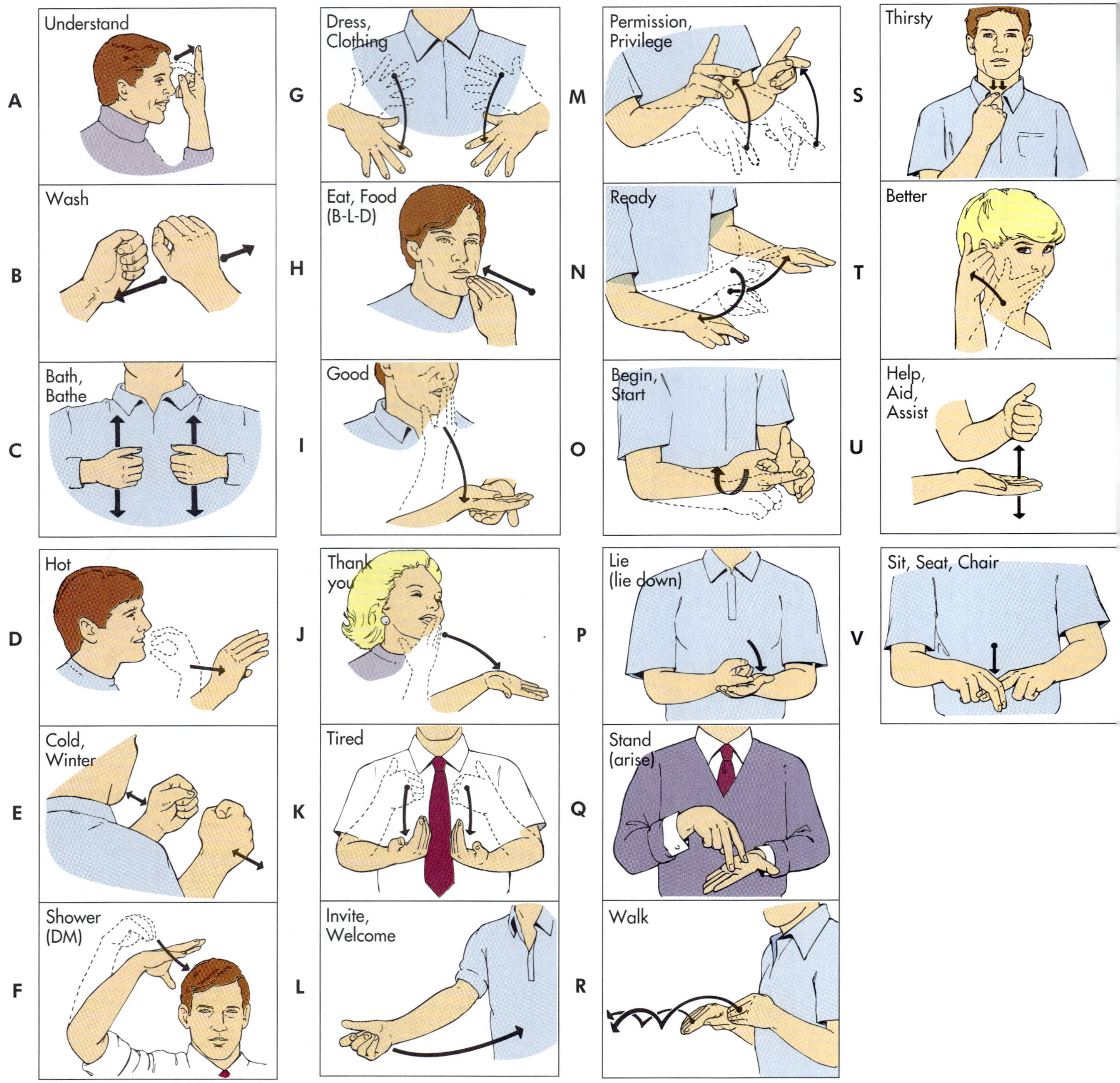

Fig. 27-2 *Sign language.*

BOX 27-2 Communicating with the Speech Impaired Person

- Listen and give the person your full attention.
- Ask the person questions to which you know the answer. This helps you to become familiar with the person's speech.
- Determine the subject being discussed. This helps you to understand main points.
- Ask the person to repeat or rephrase statements if necessary.
- Repeat what the person has said. Ask if you have understood correctly.
- Ask the person to write down key words or the message.
- Watch the person's lip movements.
- Watch facial expressions, gestures, and body language for clues about what is being said.

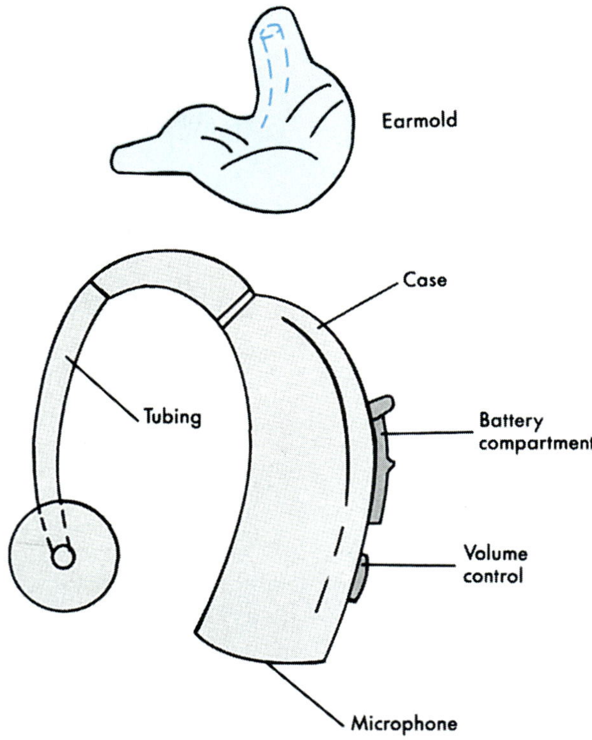

Fig. 27-3 *Parts of a hearing aid.* (*From Long BC, Phipps WJ, and Cassmeyer VL: Medical-surgical nursing: a nursing process approach, ed 3, St Louis, 1993, Mosby—Year Book.*)

Hearing aids A *hearing aid* amplifies sound (Fig. 27-3). It does not correct or cure the hearing problem. The ability to hear is not improved. The person hears better with a hearing aid. This is because the hearing aid makes sounds louder. Both background noise and speech are amplified. Noise must be minimized to help the person adjust to the hearing aid. Remember that the hearing aid does not make speech clearer, only louder. The measures for communicating with hearing impaired persons apply to those with hearing aids.

There are different types of hearing aids (Fig. 27-4 on page 588). Hearing aids operate on batteries. There is an *on* and *off* switch. Sometimes hearing aids do not seem to work properly. Often only simple measures are needed to get them to work.

- Check if the hearing aid is *on.*
- Check the battery position.
- Insert a new battery if needed.
- Clean the earmold if necessary.

Hearing aids are expensive. They must be handled carefully and cared for properly. *Check with the nurse before washing a hearing aid.* Only the earmold is washed. It usually is washed daily with soap and water. Thoroughly dry the earmold before putting it back in place. The battery is removed at night. When not in use, the hearing aid is turned off.

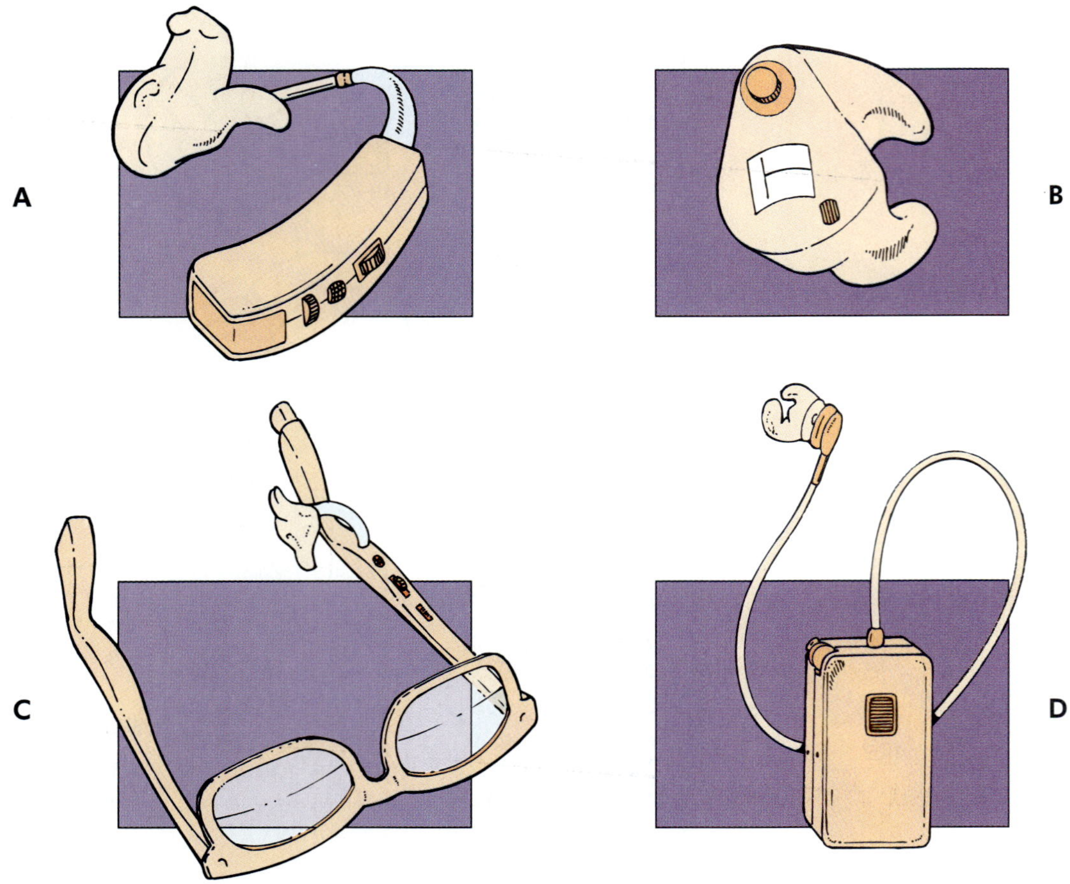

Fig. 27-4 *Types of hearing aids. A, Behind-the-ear hearing aid. B, In-the-ear hearing aid. C, Eyeglass aid. D, Body-worn aid.*

EYE DISORDERS

Vision problems occur at all ages. Problems range from very mild vision loss to complete blindness. Vision loss may be sudden or gradual in onset. One or both eyes may be affected. Surgery, eyeglasses, or contact lenses are often necessary.

Glaucoma

With glaucoma, pressure within the eye is increased. This damages the retina and optic nerve. The result is visual loss with eventual blindness. The disease is gradual or sudden in onset. Signs and symptoms include tunnel vision (Fig. 27-5), blurred vision, and blue-green halos around lights. With sudden onset, there also is severe eye pain, nausea, and vomiting. Glaucoma is a major cause of blindness. Persons over 40 years of age are at risk. The cause is unknown.

Treatment involves drug therapy and possibly surgery. The goal is to prevent further damage to the retina and optic nerve. Damage that has already occurred cannot be reversed.

Cataract

Cataract is an eye disorder in which the lens becomes cloudy (opaque). The cloudiness prevents light from entering the eye (Fig. 27-6). Gradual blurring and dimming of vision occurs. Sight is eventually lost. A cataract can occur in one or both eyes. Aging is the most common cause. Surgery is the only treatment.

The person may have to wear an eye shield or patch for several days after surgery. The shield protects the eye from injury. One or both eyes may be covered. Measures for the blind person are practiced when an eye shield is worn. Even if only one shield is worn, there may be visual loss in the other eye from cataract formation or other causes.

A lens is usually implanted during surgery (Fig. 27-7 on page 590). Vision is returned to near normal. If an implant is not done, the person is fitted with corrective lenses after surgery.

Box 27-3 on page 590 lists the postoperative care required after cataract surgery.

Fig. 27-5 *A, Normal vision. B, Tunnel vision. C, D, E, Visual loss continues, with eventual blindness.*

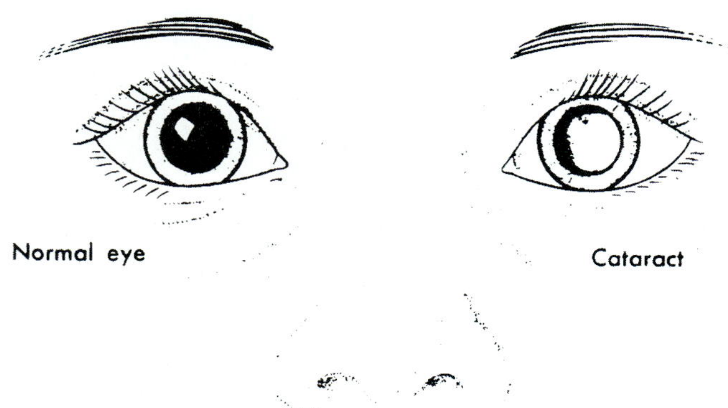

Fig. 27-6 *There is a cataract in the left eye. (From Long BC, Phipps WJ, and Cassmeyer VL: Medical-surgical nursing: a nursing process approach, ed 3, St Louis, 1993, Mosby—Year Book.)*

BOX 27-3 Postoperative Care Following Cataract Surgery

- An eye shield is worn during sleep (including naps) to protect the eye.
- The person sleeps on the unaffected side for 3 to 4 weeks. This prevents pressure on the affected eye.
- The person does not rub the affected eye.
- Showers and shampoos are not allowed until ordered by the doctor.
- The person does not bend at the waist or lift heavy objects. These activities can be resumed in about 1 month.
- Self-help devices (see Chapter 26) may be needed for activities of daily living. When such devices are used, the person does not have to bend at the waist.
- Constipation is prevented. The person must not strain to have a bowel movement.
- Coughing is avoided. Coughing increases pressure within the eye.
- Reading is limited. The back-and-forth movements involved in reading can loosen sutures (stitches) at the operative site.
- Eye drainage or complaints of pain are reported to the nurse immediately.

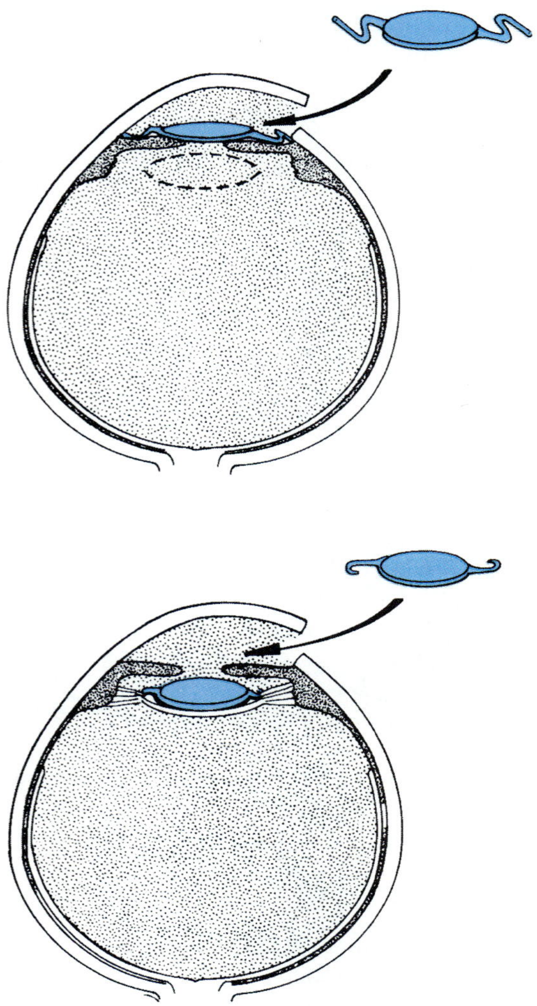

Fig. 27-7 *Lens implant during cataract surgery. (From Long BC, Phipps WJ, and Cassmeyer VL: Medical-surgical nursing: a nursing process approach, ed 3, St Louis, 1993, Mosby–Year Book.)*

Corrective Lenses

Eyeglasses and contact lenses are prescribed to correct vision problems. Sometimes eyeglasses are worn only for certain activities, such as reading or seeing at a distance. Some people wear them all the time while awake. Contact lenses are usually worn continuously while awake.

Eyeglasses People are often upset when glasses are first needed. However, adjustment is usually rapid. Most people know that glasses will be needed sooner or later. Appearance is often a concern. Frames are chosen that fit face shape, personality, and life-style. There are many styles and shapes.

Lenses are made of hardened glass or plastic. They are impact resistant to prevent shattering. Glass lenses are washed with warm water and dried with soft tissue. Plastic lenses are easily scratched. Special cleaning solutions, tissues, and cloths are used to clean and dry them.

Glasses are costly. They are protected from breakage or other damage. When not worn, they are put in their case. The case is put in the drawer of the bedside stand to prevent glasses from being lost or damaged.

Contact lenses Contact lenses fit directly on the eye. There are hard and soft contacts. Many people like contacts because they cannot be seen. They do not break easily and can be worn for sports. However, contacts cost more than eyeglasses and are easily lost. Depending on the type of lens, contacts can be worn for 12 to 24 hours or for 1 week. Contacts are often removed for swimming and sleeping.

Caring for Eyeglasses

Pre-procedure

1 Explain the procedure to the person.
2 Wash your hands.
3 Collect the following:
   - Eyeglass case
   - Cleaning solution or warm water
   - Tissues

Procedure

4 Remove the person's glasses.
   a Hold the frames in front of the ear on both sides (Fig. 27-8, A).
   b Lift the frames from the ears and bring the glasses down away from the face (Fig. 27-8, B).
5 Clean the glass with the cleaning solution or warm water. Dry the lenses with tissues.
6 Open the eyeglass case.
7 Fold the glasses and put them in the case. Do not touch the clean lenses.
8 Place the glass case in the top drawer of the bedside stand. Or put the glasses back on the person as follows:
   a Unfold the glasses.
   b Hold the frame at each side and place them over the ears.
   c Adjust the glasses so the nosepiece rests on the nose.
   d Return the glass case to the drawer in the bedside stand.
9 Wash your hands.

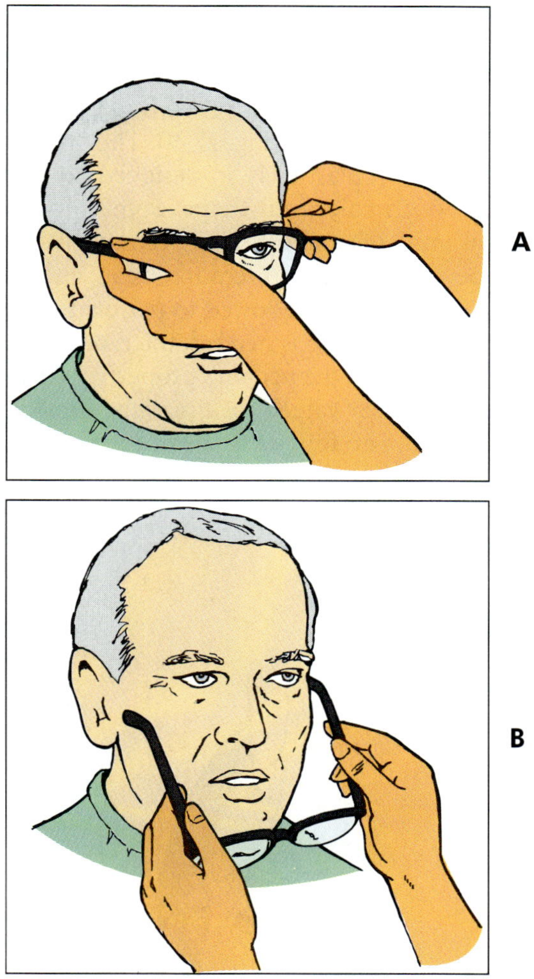

Fig. 27-8 *A, Remove eyeglasses by holding the frames in front of both ears. B, Lift the frames from the ears and bring the glasses down away from the face.*

Persons with contact lenses are taught to insert, remove, and clean them. They should perform these activities personally. However, some persons cannot insert or remove the lenses. A nurse is responsible for helping the person. The eye is easily damaged when inserting or removing contact lenses. Therefore you should not perform these measures.

Artificial Eyes

Removal of an eye is sometimes necessary because of injury or disease. The person is then fitted with an ocular prosthesis or artificial eye (Fig. 27-9). The artificial eye is made of glass or plastic. It is designed to match the remaining eye in color and shape. Some prostheses are permanent implants and others are removable. If removable, the person is taught to remove, clean, and insert the prosthesis. The person is allowed to perform routine care of the prosthesis. If help is needed, the nurse assists.

The artificial eye is the person's property. Like dentures, eyeglasses, and other valuables, it must be protected from loss or damage. The following measures are practiced if the eye is removed and will not be reinserted.

- A container is lined with a soft cloth or 4 × 4 gauze. This prevents the eye from being scratched or damaged.
- The container is filled with water or a saline (salt) solution.
- The eye is placed in the container and the container closed.
- The container is labeled with the person's name and room number.
- The labeled container is placed in the drawer in the bedside stand.

The person is blind on the side of the artificial eye. Vision in the other eye may be normal or impaired.

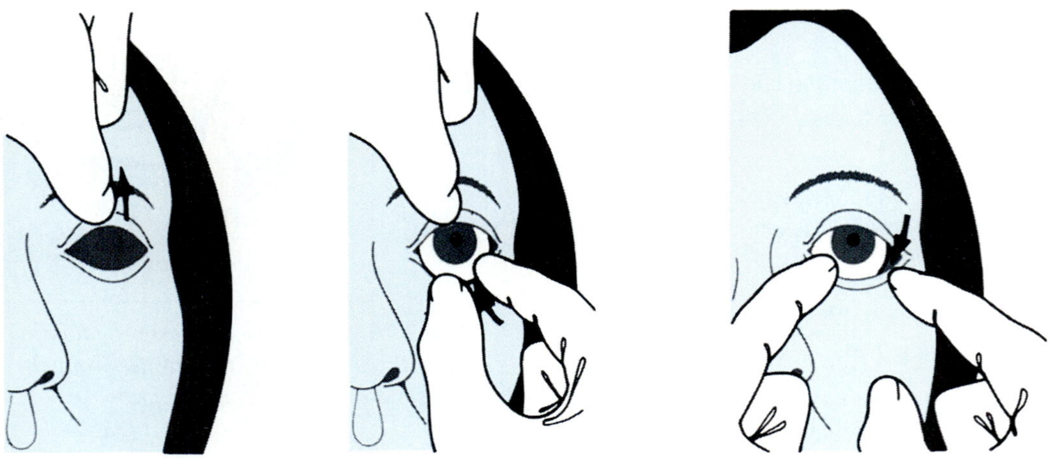

Fig. 27-9 *An artificial eye is inserted. (From Lewis SM and Collier IC: Medical-surgical nursing: assessment and management of clinical problems, ed 3, St Louis, 1992, Mosby—Year Book.)*

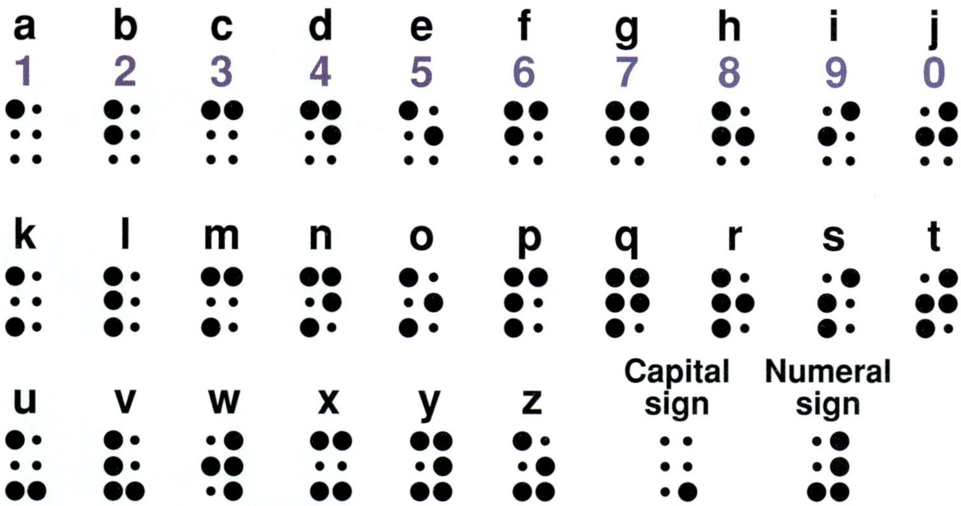

Fig. 27-10 *Braille.*

Special Needs of the Blind Person

Blindness has many causes. Birth defects, accidents, and eye diseases are among the many causes. It can also be a complication of diseases that affect other organs and body systems. Blindness usually occurs later in life. A person's life is seriously affected by the loss of sight. Physical and psychological adjustments are hard and long. Special education and training are needed. Moving about, activities of daily living, reading braille, and using a seeing-eye dog all require training.

Braille is a method of writing for the blind that uses raised dots. Dots are arranged to represent each letter of the alphabet. The first 10 letters also represent the numbers 0 through 9 (Fig. 27-10). The person feels the arrangement of dots with the fingers (Fig. 27-11). Many books, magazines, and newspapers are available in braille. There are also braille typewriters and computer keyboards.

Braille is hard to learn, especially for many elderly people. Entire books and articles are available on compact disks and audiotapes. They can be bought or borrowed from libraries.

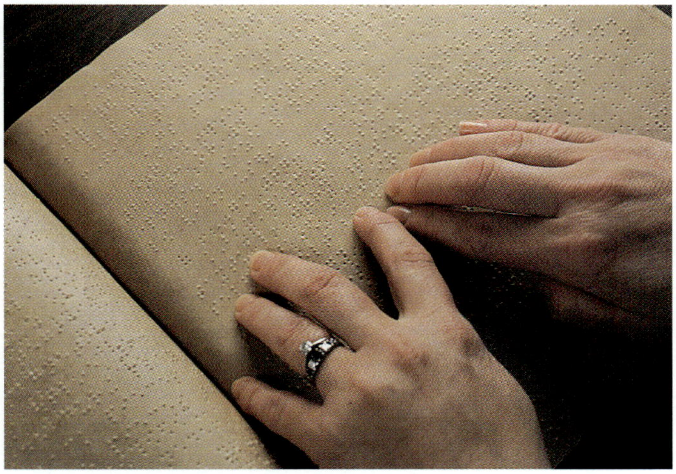

Fig. 27-11 *Braille is "read" with the fingers.*

The blind person can be taught to move about using a white cane with a red tip or a seeing-eye dog or guide dog. Both are recognized worldwide as signs that the person is blind. The dog serves as the eyes of the blind person. The dog recognizes danger and guides the person through traffic.

You must treat the blind person with respect and dignity—not with pity. Most blind people have adjusted well. They lead independent lives. Some have been blind for a long time and others for a short time. Certain practices are necessary when dealing with a blind person. The practices listed in Box 27-4 are necessary no matter how long the person has been blind.

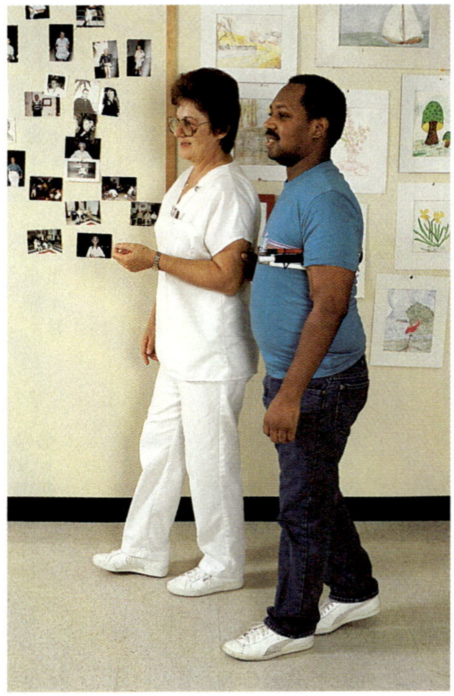

Fig. 27-12 *The blind person walks slightly behind the nursing assistant and touches the assistant's arm lightly.*

BOX 27-4 CARING FOR THE BLIND PERSON

- Identify yourself when you enter the room. Give your name, title, and reason for being there. Do not touch the person until you have indicated your presence in the room.
- Orient the person to the room. Identify the location and purpose of furniture and equipment.
- Let the person move about and touch and locate furniture and equipment if able.
- Do not rearrange furniture and equipment.
- Give step-by-step explanations of procedures as you perform them. Indicate when the procedure is over.
- Tell the person when you are leaving the room.
- Keep doors open or shut, never partially open.
- Assist the person in ambulating by walking slightly ahead of him or her (Fig. 27-12). The person touches your arm lightly. Never push or guide the blind person in front of you.
- Inform the person of steps, doors, turns, furniture, curbs, and other obstructions when assisting with ambulation.
- Assist in food selection by reading the menu to the person.
- Explain the location of food and beverages on the tray. Use the face of a clock (see Fig. 17-5) or guide the person's hand to each item on the tray.
- Cut meat, open containers, butter bread, and perform other similar activities if needed.
- Keep the call bell within the person's reach.
- Provide a radio, compact disks or audiotapes, television, and braille books for entertainment.
- Do not shout or speak in a loud voice. Just because a person is blind does not mean that hearing is impaired.
- Let the person perform self-care if able.

Summary

Hearing and sight allow people to function independently and to recognize dangers. Pleasure, amusement, recreation, entertainment, and communication are also possible because of hearing and vision. Partial or complete loss of one of these senses can seriously affect the person's physical and mental well-being. Safety is also affected.

You must not avoid these persons. Put yourself in the person's situation. How would you feel, react, and want to be treated if you had a vision or hearing problem. You need to appreciate the person's situation. Practicing the guidelines in this chapter will help you communicate and care for persons with hearing and vision problems.

Review Questions

Circle the best *answer.*

1 Mr. Young has Meniere's disease. Which is *true?*
- **a** He has a middle ear infection.
- **b** Vertigo is the major symptom.
- **c** Hearing aids will correct the problem.
- **d** All of the above.

2 Nursing care for Mr. Young includes preventing
- **a** Infection
- **b** Falls
- **c** Constipation
- **d** All of the above

3 Mr. Young is hearing impaired. He may
- **a** Avoid social situations
- **b** Become suspicious
- **c** Control conversations
- **d** All of the above

4 Which is not an obvious effect of hearing loss?
- **a** Loneliness and boredom
- **b** Speaking too loudly
- **c** Asking for things to be repeated
- **d** Answering questions inappropriately

5 You are talking to Mr. Young. You should do the following *except*
- **a** Speak clearly, distinctly, and slowly
- **b** Sit or stand where there is good light
- **c** Shout
- **d** Stand or sit on the side of the better ear

6 You are talking to Mr. Young. You can do the following except
- **a** State the topic of discussion
- **b** Chew gum while talking
- **c** Use short sentences and simple words
- **d** Write out important names and words

7 A person has a speech problem. You should
- **a** Pretend to understand so the person is not embarrassed
- **b** Have the person write out all messages
- **c** Ask the person to repeat or rephrase statements when necessary
- **d** All of the above

8 Mr. Young has a hearing aid. The hearing aid
- **a** Corrects the hearing problem
- **b** Makes sounds louder
- **c** Makes speech clearer
- **d** All of the above

9 Mr. Young's hearing aid does not seem to be working. First, you should
- **a** See if it is turned on
- **b** Wash the entire instrument with soap and water
- **c** Have it repaired
- **d** Remove the batteries

REVIEW QUESTIONS—CONT'D

10 Mr. Young has a cataract. Which is true?
- **a** Surgery is the only treatment.
- **b** There is no cure.
- **c** He will be blind eventually.
- **d** There is pressure in the eye.

11 An eye shield is ordered for Mr. Young. Which is *true?*
- **a** The eye shield protects the eye from injury.
- **b** The eye shield is worn at bedtime and when napping.
- **c** Measures for the blind person are practiced.
- **d** All of the above

12 Mr. Young is not wearing his eyeglasses. They should be
- **a** Soaked in a cleansing solution
- **b** Kept within his reach
- **c** Put in the case and in the top drawer of the bedside stand
- **d** Placed on the overbed table

13 You are allowed to remove and insert contact lenses.
- **a** True
- **b** False

14 Braille involves
- **a** A white cane with a red tip for walking
- **b** Raised dots arranged to represent letters of the alphabet
- **c** An artificial eye
- **d** Books and articles on compact disks or audiotapes

15 Mr. Goldman is blind. You should do the following *except*
- **a** Touch him to get his attention
- **b** Move equipment and furniture to provide variety
- **c** Explain procedures step by step
- **d** Have him walk behind you

16 You can provide for Mr. Goldman's safety by
- **a** Keeping doors partially open
- **b** Informing him of steps and curbs
- **c** Rearranging furniture
- **d** All of the above

Answers to these questions are on page 752.

Common Health Problems

28

OBJECTIVES

- Define the key terms listed in this chapter
- Identify the warning signs of cancer
- List cancer treatments
- Explain how to maintain joint function in persons with arthritis
- Explain how to care for persons in casts, in traction, and with hip pinnings
- Describe osteoporosis and the care required
- Explain why loss of a limb requires psychological adjustment
- Describe cerebrovascular accident, its signs and symptoms, and the care required
- Describe Parkinson's disease and multiple sclerosis
- Identify the causes and effects of head and spinal cord injuries and the care required
- Describe common respiratory disorders and the care required
- Identify the signs, symptoms, and treatment of hypertension
- List the risk factors for coronary artery disease
- Describe angina pectoris, myocardial infarction, heart failure, and the care required
- Describe the care required by persons with disorders of the urinary system
- Identify the signs, symptoms, and complications of diabetes
- Explain how to help the person who is vomiting
- Describe hepatitis and AIDS, their signs and symptoms, and necessary precautions

KEY TERMS

alopecia Loss of hair

amputation The removal of all or part of an extremity

aphasia The inability *(a)* to speak *(phasia)*

arthritis Joint *(arthr)* inflammation *(itis)*

benign tumor A tumor that grows slowly and within a localized area

cancer Malignant tumor

closed fracture The bone is broken but the skin is intact; simple fracture

compound fracture The bone is broken and has come through the skin; open fracture

expressive aphasia Difficulty expressing or sending out thoughts

expressive-receptive aphasia Difficulty expressing or sending out thoughts and difficulty receiving information

fracture A broken bone

gangrene A condition in which there is death of tissue; tissues become black, cold, and shriveled

hemiplegia Paralysis on one side of the body

hyperglycemia High *(hyper)* sugar *(glyc)* in the blood *(emia)*

hypoglycemia Low *(hypo)* sugar *(glyc)* in the blood *(emia)*

malignant tumor A tumor that grows rapidly and invades other tissues; cancer

metastasis The spread of cancer to other parts of the body

paraplegia Paralysis of the legs

quadriplegia Paralysis of the arms, legs, and trunk

receptive aphasia Difficulty receiving information

stomatitis Inflammation *(itis)* of the mouth *(stomat)*

stroke A cerebrovascular accident (CVA); blood supply to a part of the brain is suddenly interrupted

tumor A new growth of cells; tumors can be benign or malignant

This chapter gives basic information about common health problems. People with these disorders need health care. The nurse uses the nursing process to meet the needs of patients and residents with these and other health problems. Knowing something about a disorder makes the required care meaningful. If more information is needed, ask a nurse for additional explanations.

A review of Chapter 5 (Body Structure and Function) will help in studying this chapter.

CANCER

A **tumor** is a new growth of abnormal cells. Tumors can be benign or malignant (Fig. 28-1 on page 600). **Benign** tumors grow slowly and within a localized area. They do not usually cause death. A malignant tumor is cancerous. A **malignant** tumor (**cancer**) grows rapidly and invades healthy tissues (Fig. 28-2 on page 600). Death occurs if the cancer is not treated and controlled. **Metastasis** is the spread of cancer to other parts of the body (Fig. 28-3 on page 600). It occurs if the cancer is not treated and controlled. Cancer can occur in almost any body part. The most common sites are the lungs, colon and rectum, breast, prostate, and uterus. Cancer is the second leading cause of death in the United States.

The exact causes of cancer are unknown. However, certain factors are known to contribute to its development. These include

- A family history of cancer
- Exposure to radiation (including the sun) or certain chemicals
- Smoking
- Alcohol
- High-fat, high-calorie diet
- Food additives
- Viruses
- Hormones

Cancer can be treated and controlled with early detection. The seven warning signs identified by the American Cancer Society are listed in Box 28-1 on page 600.

Treatment depends on the type of tumor, its location, and if it has spread. One treatment or a combination of treatments may be used. The three cancer treatments are surgery, radiotherapy (radiation therapy), and chemotherapy.

Surgery involves removing malignant tissue. Surgery is done to cure cancer or to relieve pain from advanced cancer. Some surgeries are very disfiguring. Surgical patients require the care described in Chapter 25.

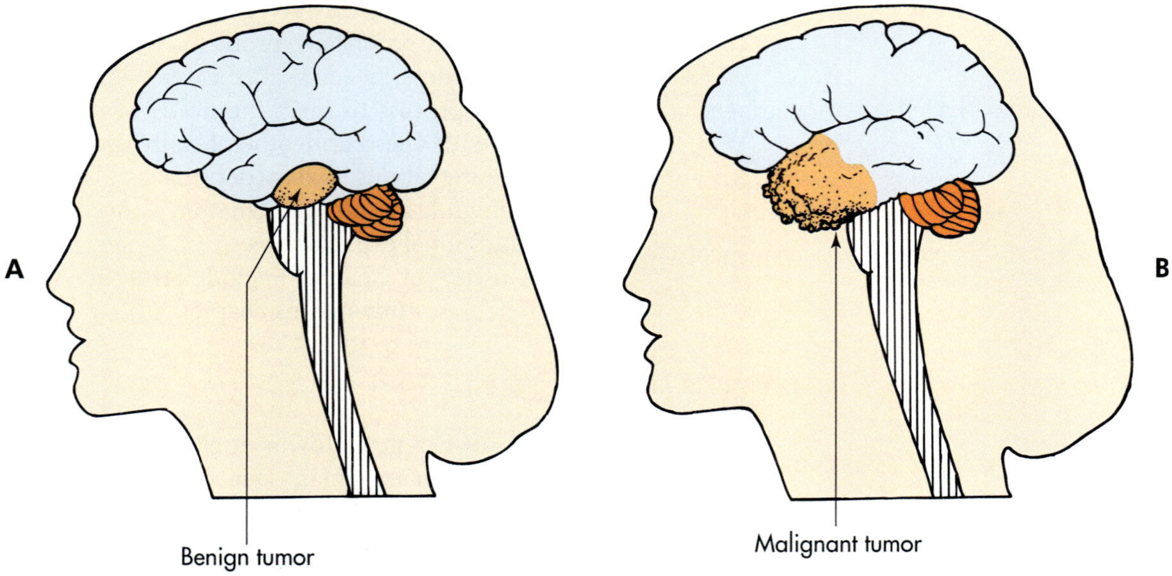

Fig. 28-1 *A, Benign tumors grow within a localized area. B, Malignant tumors invade other tissues.*

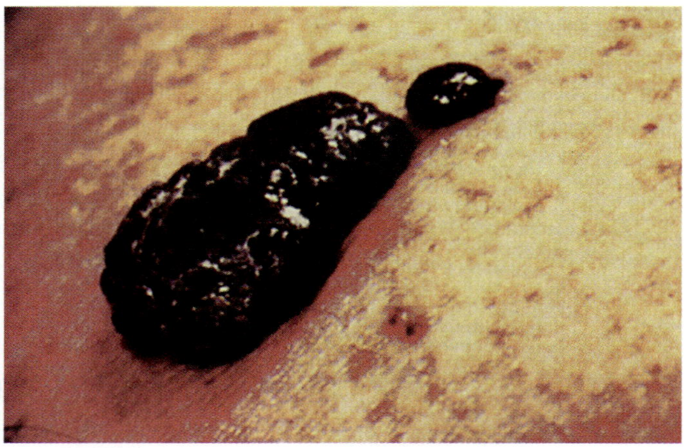

Fig. 28-2 *A malignant tumor on the skin. (From Belcher AE: Cancer nursing, St Louis, 1992, Mosby–Year Book.)*

BOX 28-1 SEVEN WARNING SIGNS OF CANCER

- **C**hange in bowel or bladder habits
- **A** sore that does not heal
- **U**nusual bleeding or discharge from a body opening
- **T**hickening or lump in the breast or elsewhere in the body
- **I**ndigestion or difficulty swallowing
- **O**bvious change in a wart or mole
- **N**agging cough or hoarseness

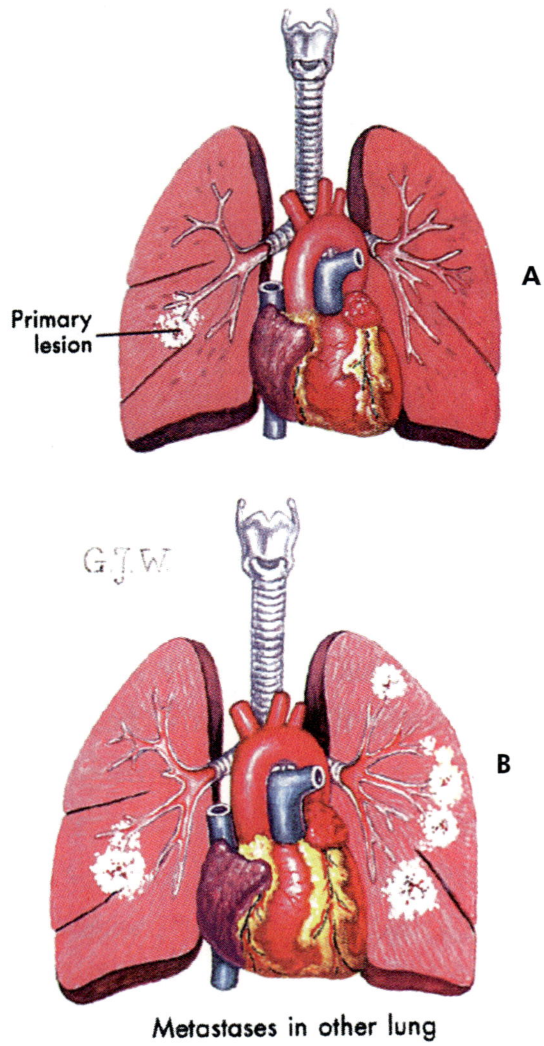

Fig. 28-3 *A, A tumor in the lung. B, The tumor has metastasized to the other lung. (From Belcher AE: Cancer nursing, St Louis, 1992, Mosby–Year Book.)*

Spotlight On...

Anna G of Watsonville, California, *is a nursing assistant working in a hospice program. She went on a home visit to a young female patient who had uterine cancer that had spread throughout her body. The patient had both a urostomy and a colostomy. The husband was the primary caregiver. The urostomy had been leaking constantly, wetting the patient's clothes and bedding. This made it necessary for her to keep a towel over her lap all the time. Because she was young and had visitors it was very embarrassing to her. Anna had just received instruction on ostomy care and knew the urostomy should not be leaking. She remembered that a bonding adhesive would stop the leaking. After bathing the patient and cleaning the urostomy area, Anna applied the adhesive and a new bag. The patient and her husband were relieved and grateful that she could now greet her friends with dignity.*

Radiotherapy destroys living cells. X-rays are directed at the tumor. Cancer cells and normal cells are exposed to radiation. Both are destroyed. Radiotherapy is used to cure certain cancers or to control the growth of cancer cells. Pain can be relieved or prevented by controlling cell growth. Radiotherapy has side effects. Discomfort, nausea, and vomiting are common. Skin breakdown can occur in the exposed area. The doctor may order special skin care procedures.

Chemotherapy involves drugs that kill cells. Like radiotherapy, chemotherapy affects normal cells and cancer cells. It is used to cure cancer or control the growth rate of cancer cells. Side effects can be severe. They are caused by the destruction of normal cells. The gastrointestinal tract is irritated. Nausea, vomiting, and diarrhea result. **Stomatitis,** an inflammation *(itis)* of the mouth *(stomat),* may also develop. Hair loss **(alopecia)** may occur. Decreased production of blood cells occurs. As a result, the person is at risk for bleeding and infection. The heart, lungs, liver, kidneys, and skin may also be affected.

Persons with cancer have many needs. They include:

- Pain control
- Adequate rest and exercise
- Fluids and nutrition
- Prevention of skin breakdown
- Prevention of bowel elimination problems (constipation is a side effect of pain medications; diarrhea occurs from chemotherapy)
- Dealing with the side effects of radiotherapy and chemotherapy
- Psychological and social needs

The person's psychological and social needs are great. The person may be angry, afraid, and depressed. There may be disfigurement from surgery. The person may feel unwhole, unattractive, or unclean. The person and family need much emotional support. The future may be uncertain. The possibility of death may be very real. Put yourself in the person's position. How would you feel and what would you want if you had cancer? Do not be afraid to talk to the person. Avoiding the person because you are uncomfortable is one of the worst things you can do. Use touch to communicate that you care. Listen to the person. Often the person needs to talk and needs someone to listen. Being there when needed is important. You may not have to say anything. Just be there to listen.

MUSCULOSKELETAL DISORDERS

Musculoskeletal disorders are common. They affect the ability to move about. Some are due to injury. Others result from aging. A review of the musculoskeletal system on pages 96-97 in Chapter 5 will be helpful in studying this section.

Arthritis

Arthritis means joint *(arth)* inflammation *(itis).* It is the most common joint disease. Pain and decreased mobility occur in the affected joints. There are two basic types of arthritis.

Osteoarthritis (degenerative joint disease) This type of arthritis occurs with aging. Joint injury and obesity are other causes. The hips and knees are commonly affected. These joints bear the body's weight. Joints in the fingers, thumbs, and spine can also be affected. Symptoms are joint stiffness and pain. Joint stiffness occurs with rest and lack of motion. Pain occurs with weight-bearing and joint motion. Severe pain can interfere with rest and sleep. Cold weather and dampness seem to increase the symptoms. Heberden's nodes (Fig. 28-4 on page 602) are common in the fingers.

Osteoarthritis has no cure. Treatment involves relieving pain and stiffness. Doctors often order aspirin for pain. Local heat or local cold applications may be ordered. For obese persons, weight loss is recommended. A low-fat, low-calorie diet is often ordered. When the condition is advanced, the person may need help walking. A walking aid (cane, walker) may be needed. Assistance with ADL is given as necessary. Joint replacement surgery may be necessary (see page 603).

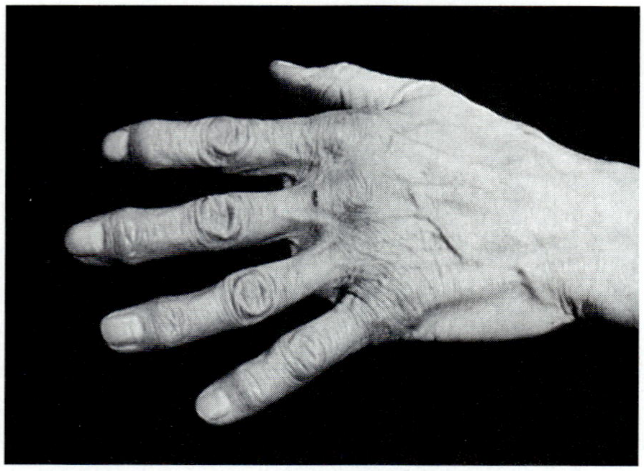

Fig. 28-4 *Heberden's nodes occur in the finger joints.* (*From Lewis SH and Collier IC: Medical-surgical nursing: assessment and management of clinical problems, ed 3, St Louis, 1992, Mosby–Year Book.*)

Rheumatoid arthritis (RA) Rheumatoid arthritis is a chronic disease. It can occur at any age and occurs most often in women. Connective tissue throughout the body is affected. The disease affects the heart, lungs, eyes, kidneys, and skin. However, the joints are mainly affected. Smaller joints in the fingers, hands, and wrists are affected first (Fig. 28-5). Eventually, larger joints are involved. Severe inflammation causes very painful and swollen joints. The person restricts movement with severe pain. As the disease progresses, more and more joints become involved. Changes in other organs eventually occur.

Signs and symptoms of rheumatoid arthritis include:

- Pain, redness, and swelling in the joint area
- Joint stiffness upon awakening and after inactivity
- Limitation of joint motion
- Fever
- Fatigue
- Loss of appetite
- Weight loss
- Muscle aches

The goals in treating rheumatoid arthritis are:

- Maintaining joint motion
- Controlling pain
- Preventing deformities

The person needs a lot of rest. Bed rest may be ordered if several joints are involved and when fever is present. If the person is on bed rest, turning and repositioning are done every 2 hours. Good body alignment is essential. Positioning to prevent contractures and deformities promotes comfort. Bed boards, a bed cradle, trochanter rolls, and pillows are used for body alignment and positioning. Adequate sleep—8 to 10 hours—is needed each night. Morning and afternoon rest periods are also necessary. Rest is balanced with exercise. Range-of-motion exercises are done. Walking aids may be needed. Splints may be applied to the affected body parts. Safety measures to prevent falls are practiced.

Medications are ordered by the doctor for pain. Local heat or local cold applications may be ordered. Back massages are relaxing. Joint replacement surgery may be indicated.

Emotional support and reassurance are needed. The disease is chronic. Death from other organ involvement is always possible. A good attitude is important. Being active is important. The more persons can do for themselves, the better off they are. A person may need someone to talk to. You must be a good listener when the person needs to talk.

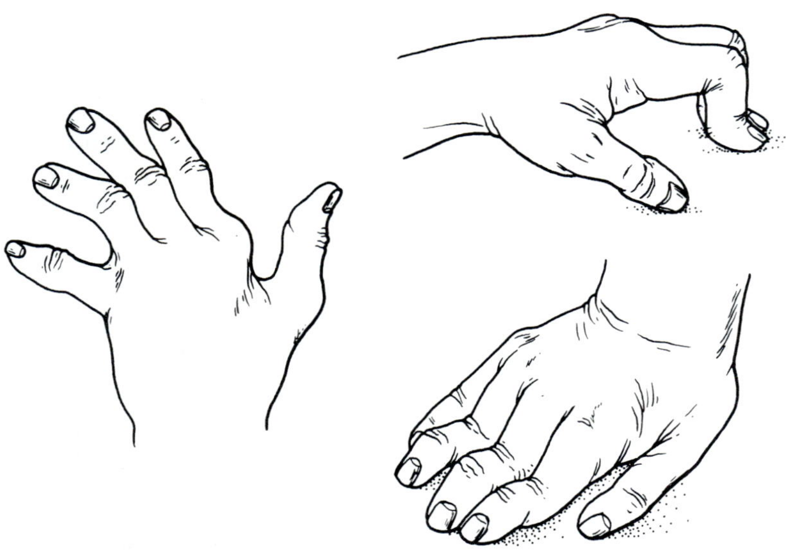

Fig. 28-5 *Finger deformities caused by rheumatoid arthritis.* (*From Lewis SH and Collier IC: Medical-surgical nursing: assessment and management of clinical problems, ed 3, St Louis, 1992, Mosby–Year Book.*)

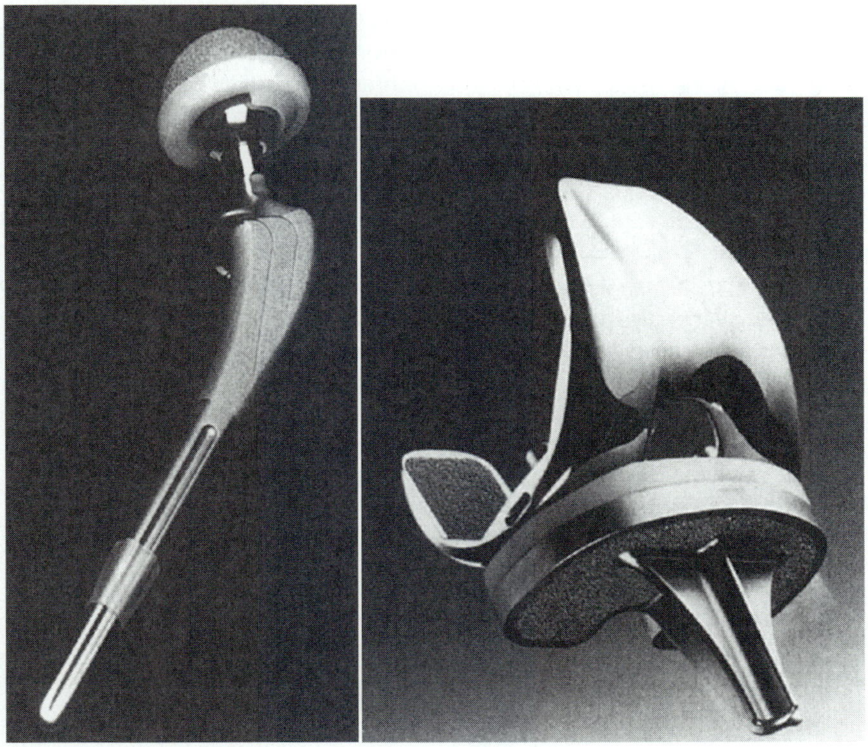

Fig. 28-6 *A, Hip replacement prosthesis. B, Knee replacement prosthesis. (From Thompson JM, McFarland GK, Hirsch JE, Tucker SM: Mosby's clinical nursing, ed 3, St Louis, 1993, Mosby–Year Book.)*

Total joint replacement **Arthroplasty** is the surgical replacement *(plasty)* of a joint *(arthro)*. Ankle, knee, hip, shoulder, wrist, finger, and toe joints can be replaced. The diseased joint is removed and replaced with a prosthesis (Fig. 28-6). The surgery is done to relieve pain and to restore joint motion. You may care for persons who have had joint replacement surgery. The nurse shares the person's care plan with you.

Fractures

A **fracture** is a broken bone. Tissues around the fracture (muscles, blood vessels, nerves, and tendons) are usually injured. Fractures may be open or closed (Fig. 28-7). A **closed fracture (simple fracture)** means the bone is broken but the skin is intact. An **open fracture (compound fracture)** means the broken bone has come through the skin.

Fractures are caused by falls and accidents. Bone tumors, metastatic cancer, and a bone disease called osteoporosis (see page 611) are other causes. Signs and symptoms of a fracture are

- Pain
- Swelling
- Limited movement and loss of function
- Bruising and color changes in the skin at the fracture site
- Bleeding (internal or external)

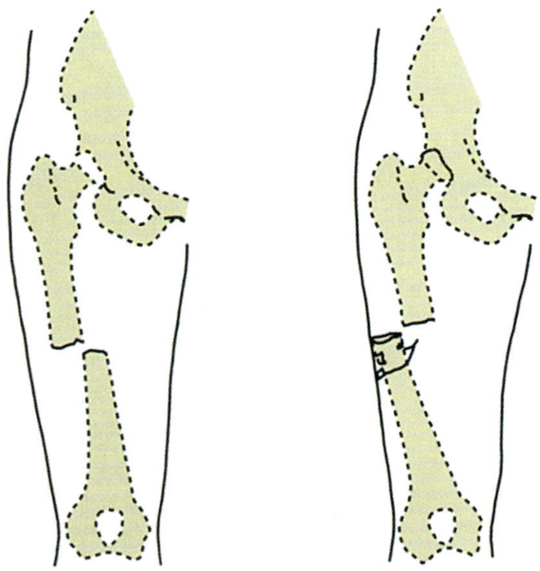

Fig. 28-7 *A, Closed fracture. B, Open fracture. (From Harkness-Hood GH and Dincher JR: Total patient care: foundations and practice of adult health nursing, ed 8, St Louis, 1992, Mosby–Year Book.)*

The bone has to heal. The two bone ends are brought into normal position. This is called reduction. **Closed reduction** involves manipulating the bone back into place. The skin is not opened. **Open reduction** involves surgery. The bone is exposed and brought back into alignment. Nails, rods, pins, screws, metal plates, or wires may

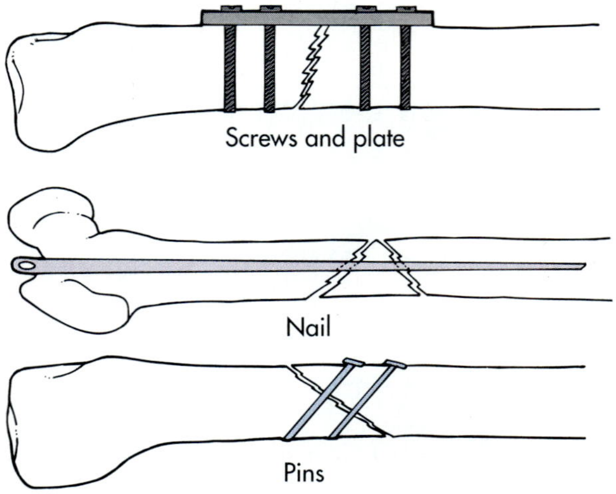

Fig. 28-8 *Devices used to reduce a fracture.* *(From Milliken ME and Campbell G: Essential competencies for patient care, St Louis, 1985, Mosby–Year Book.)*

be used to keep the bone in place (Fig. 28-8). After reduction, the fracture is immobilized. In other words, movement of the two bone ends is prevented. A cast or traction may be used to immobilize the bone.

Cast care Casts are made of plaster of paris, plastic, or fiberglass. The cast covers all or part of an extremity (Fig. 28-9). Before the doctor applies the cast, the extremity is covered with stockinette. This protects the skin. Material for plaster of paris casts, plastic, or fiberglass casts comes in rolls. A roll is moistened and wrapped around the extremity. Several rolls may be used. A plaster of paris cast needs 24 to 48 hours to dry. A dry cast is odorless, white, and shiny. A wet cast is gray, cool, and has a musty smell. Plastic and fiberglass casts dry more quickly. The rules listed in Box 28-2 are for cast care.

BOX 28-2 RULES FOR CAST CARE

- Do not cover the cast with blankets, plastic, or other material. A plaster cast gives off heat as it dries. Covers prevent the heat from escaping. Burns can occur if the heat cannot escape.
- Turn the person as directed by the nurse. All cast surfaces are exposed to the air at one time or another. Even drying is promoted by turning.
- The cast must maintain its shape. Do not place the cast on a hard surface while wet. A hard surface flattens the cast. Pillows are used to support the entire length of the cast (Fig. 28-10 on page 606). When turning and positioning the person, support the cast with your palms (Fig. 28-11 on page 606). Fingers can make dents in the cast. The dents can cause pressure areas that can lead to skin breakdown.
- Protect the person from rough edges of the cast. Cast edges may be covered with tape. This is called petaling (Fig. 28-12 on page 607). If stockinette is used, the doctor pulls it up over the cast. The stockinette is then secured in place with a roll of cast material.
- Keep a plaster cast dry. A wet plaster cast loses its shape. It must be protected from moisture from the perineal area. The nurse may apply a waterproof material around the perineal area once the cast is dry.
- Do not let the person insert anything into the cast. Itching often occurs under the cast and causes an intense desire to scratch. Skin can be broken by items used for scratching (pencils, coat hangers, knitting needles, back scratchers). The open area under the cast can become infected. Items used for scratching can also wrinkle the stockinette. The object can be lost into the cast. Both can cause pressure, which leads to skin breakdown.
- A casted extremity is elevated on pillows. Elevation of an arm or leg reduces swelling.
- Have enough help when turning and repositioning the person. Plaster casts are heavy and awkward. Balance can be lost easily.
- Lying on the injured side is usually not allowed. The nurse tells you what positions are allowed.
- Report these signs and symptoms immediately:
  - *Pain—a warning sign of a pressure sore, poor circulation, or nerve damage
  - *Swelling and a tight cast—blood flow to the part may be affected
  - *Pale skin—reduced blood flow to the part
  - *Cyanosis—reduced blood flow to the part
  - *Odor—an infection may be present
  - *Inability to move the fingers or toes—the cast may be causing pressure on a nerve
  - *Numbness—the cast may be causing pressure on a nerve; there may be reduced blood flow to the part
  - *Temperature changes—cool skin means poor circulation; hot skin means inflammation
  - *Drainage on or under the cast—there may be an infection under the cast
  - *Chills, fever, nausea, and vomiting—there may be an infection under the cast

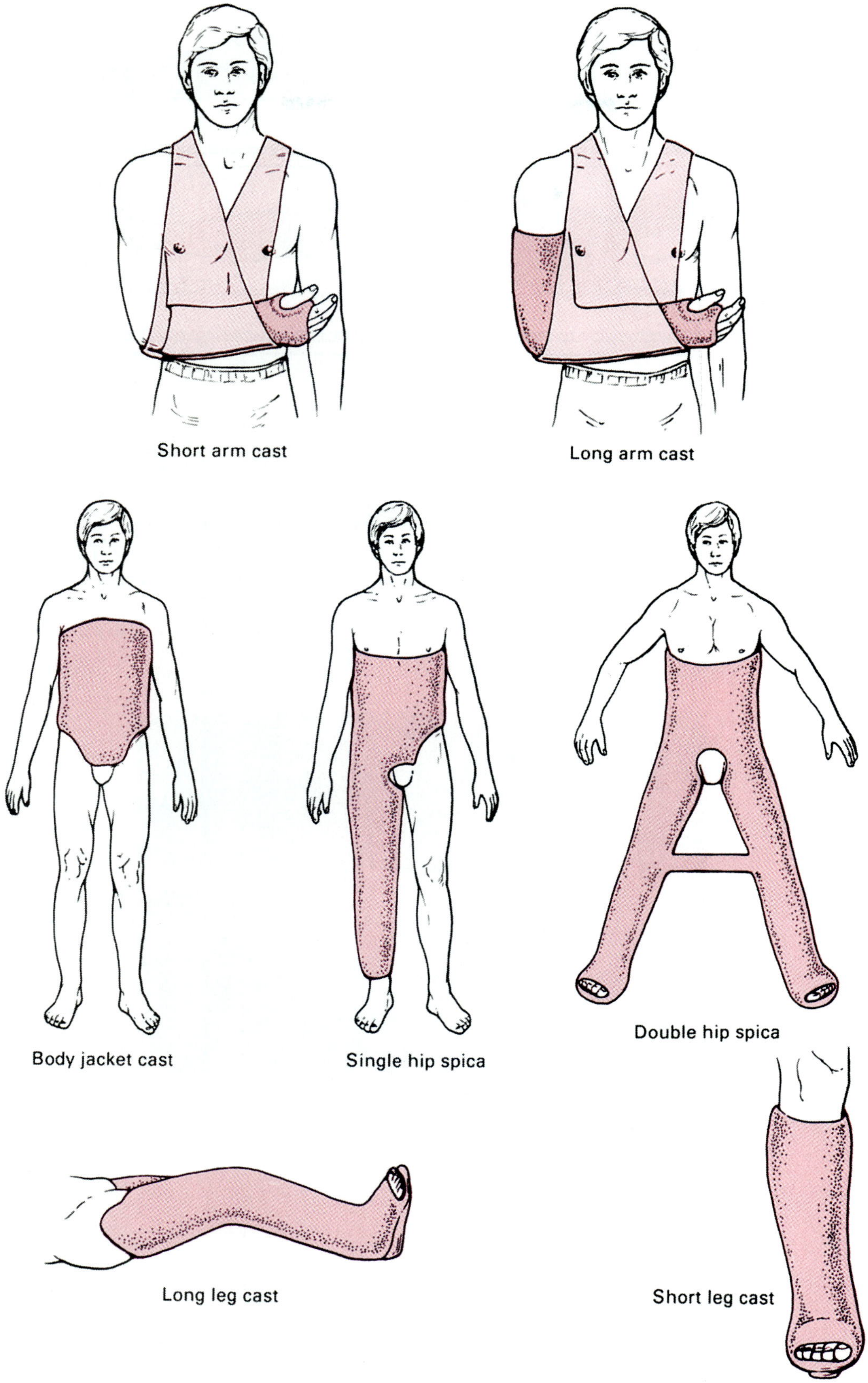

Fig. 28-9 *Common casts. (From Lewis SH and Collier IC: Medical-surgical nursing: assessment and management of clinical problems, ed 3, St Louis, 1992, Mosby–Year Book.)*

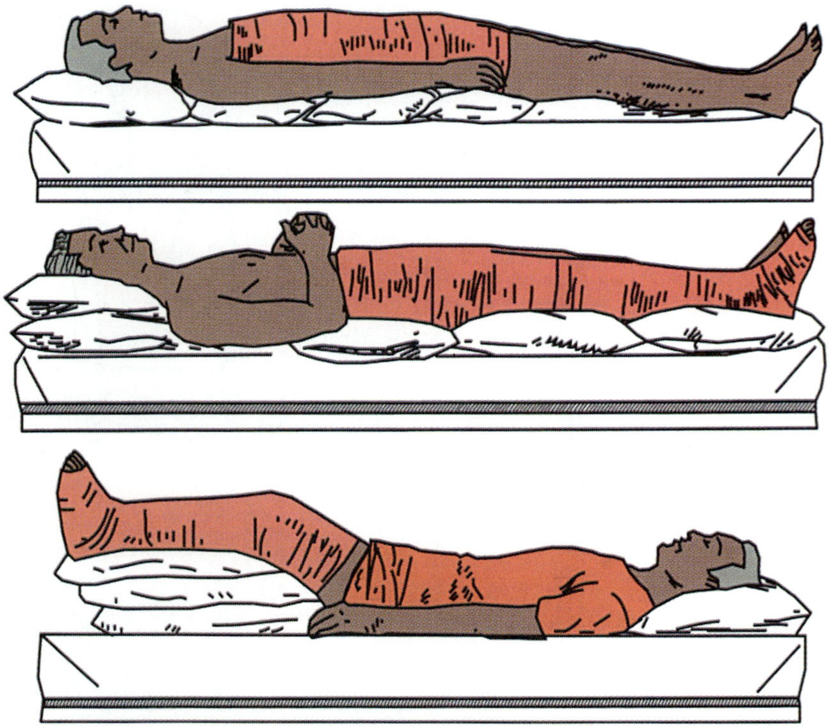

Fig. 28-10 *Pillows support the entire length of the wet cast.* *(From Harkness-Hood GH and Dincher JR: Total patient care: foundations and practice for adult health nursing, ed 8, St Louis, 1992, Mosby-Year Book.)*

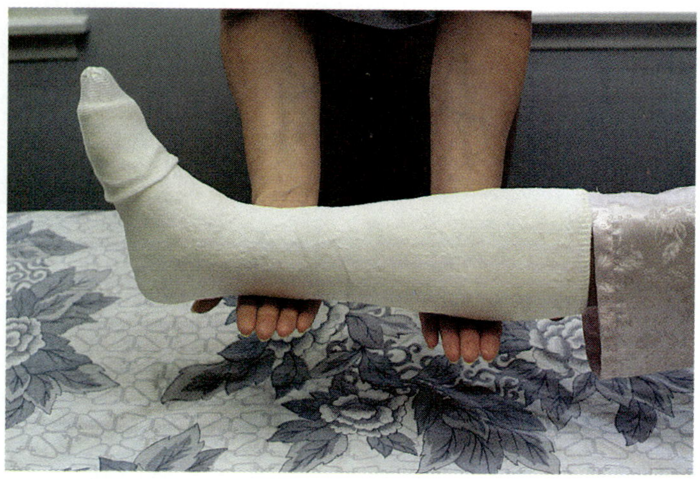

Fig. 28-11 *The cast is supported with the palms during lifting.*

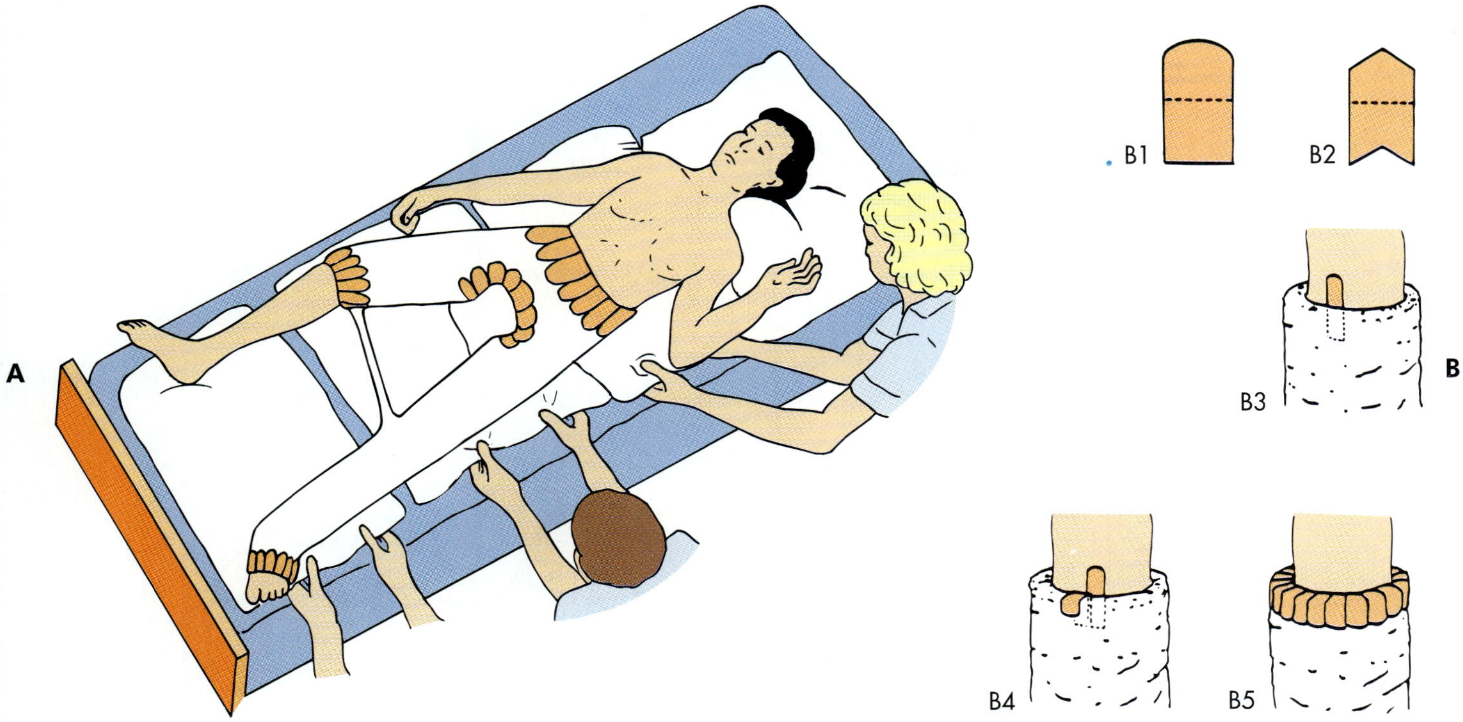

Fig. 28-12 *A, The edges of the cast are petaled. B, Pieces of tape are used to make petals. The petal is placed inside the cast and then brought over the edge.* *(From Billings DM and Stokes LG: Medical-surgical nursing: common health problems of adults and children across the life span, ed 2, St Louis, 1987, Mosby–Year Book.)*

Traction Traction is used to reduce and immobilize fractures. A steady pull from two directions keeps the fractured bone in place. Traction is also used for muscle spasms, to correct or prevent deformities, and for other musculoskeletal injuries. Weights, ropes, and pulleys are used (Fig. 28-13 on page 608). Traction can be applied to the neck, arms, legs, or pelvis.

Traction is applied by the doctor to the skin or to the bone. *Skin traction* involves applying bandages and strips of material to the skin. Weights are attached to the material or bandage (see Fig. 28-13). Traction applied directly to the bone is called *skeletal traction.* It is used for some arm and leg fractures. A pin is inserted through the bone (Fig. 28-14 on page 608). For traction to the cervical spine, tongs are applied to the skull (Fig. 28-15 on page 608). Weights are attached to the pin or tongs.

The rules listed in Box 28-3 apply when caring for a person in traction.

BOX 28-3 Caring for Persons in Traction

- Keep the person in good body alignment and pulled up in bed. This is necessary to maintain the proper pull of the traction.
- Do not remove the traction.
- Keep weights off the floor. Weights must hang freely from the traction setup (see Fig. 28-13).
- Do not remove weights from the traction setup.
- Do not add weights to the traction setup.
- Perform range-of-motion exercises for the uninvolved body parts as directed by the nurse.
- Check with the nurse about turning and positioning. Usually only the back-lying position is allowed.
- Provide the fracture pan for elimination.
- Give skin care often.
- Put bottom linens on the bed from the top down. The person uses the trapeze to raise the body off the bed (Fig. 28-16 on page 609).
- Check the insertion site of pins or tongs for redness, drainage, or odors. Report any observations to the nurse immediately.
- Observe for the signs and symptoms listed under cast care. Report these observations to the nurse immediately.

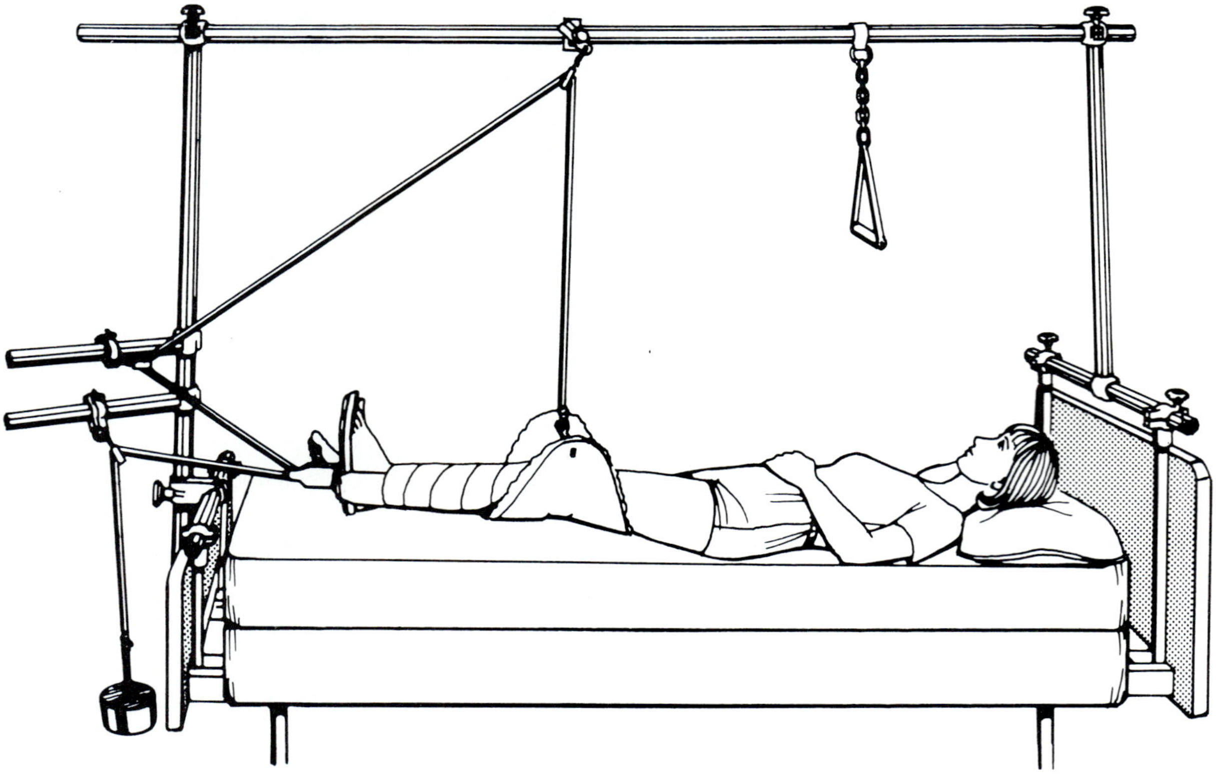

Fig. 28-13 *Traction setup. Note the weights, pulleys, and ropes. (From Long BC, Phipps WJ, and Cassmeyer VL: Medical-surgical nursing: a nursing process approach, ed 3, St Louis, 1993, Mosby–Year Book.)*

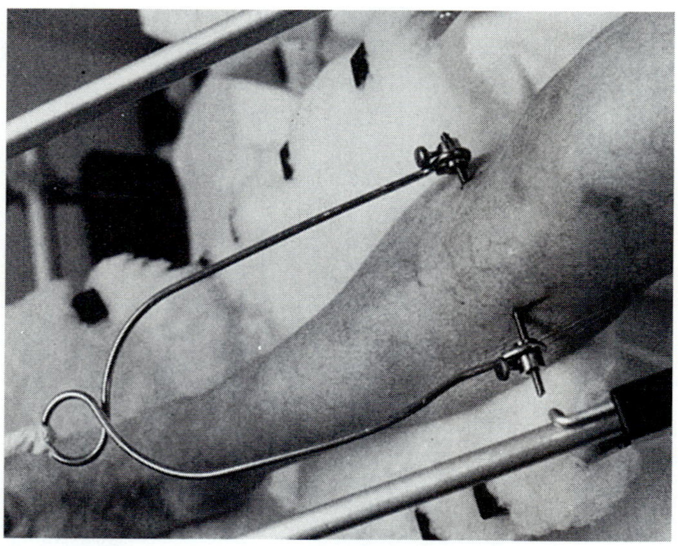

Fig. 28-14 *Skeletal traction is attached to the bone. (From Long BC, Phipps WJ, and Cassmeyer VL: Medical-surgical nursing: a nursing process approach, ed 3, St Louis, 1993, Mosby–Year Book.)*

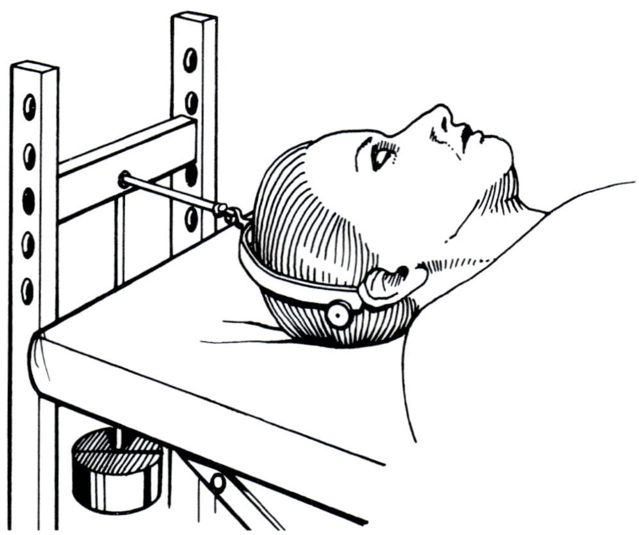

Fig. 28-15 *Tongs are inserted into the skull for traction to the cervical spine. (From Long BC, Phipps WJ, and Cassmeyer VL: Medical-surgical nursing: a nursing process approach, ed 3, St Louis, 1993, Mosby–Year Book.)*

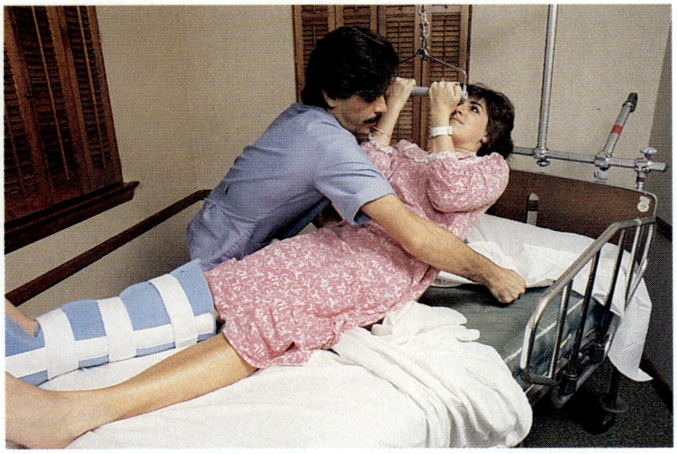

Fig. 28-16 *A bed is made from the top down for the person in traction. The person uses the trapeze to lift the buttocks off the bed. Then the linens are pulled down over the bed.*

Hip fractures Fractured hips are common in the elderly (Fig. 28-17). They are especially serious because healing is slower in older people. The person may have other disorders. These disorders and slow healing may complicate the person's condition and care. The person is also at great risk for postoperative complications. These include pneumonia and atelectasis, pressure sores, constipation, thrombi in the leg veins, and confusion.

Open reduction is usually required. The fracture is fixed in position with a pin, nail, plate, screw, or prosthesis (Fig. 28-18). The person needs preoperative and postoperative care as described in Chapter 25. A cast or traction is sometimes used. Therefore care of the person in a cast or in traction may also be required. The person also requires the care described in Box 28-4 on page 610.

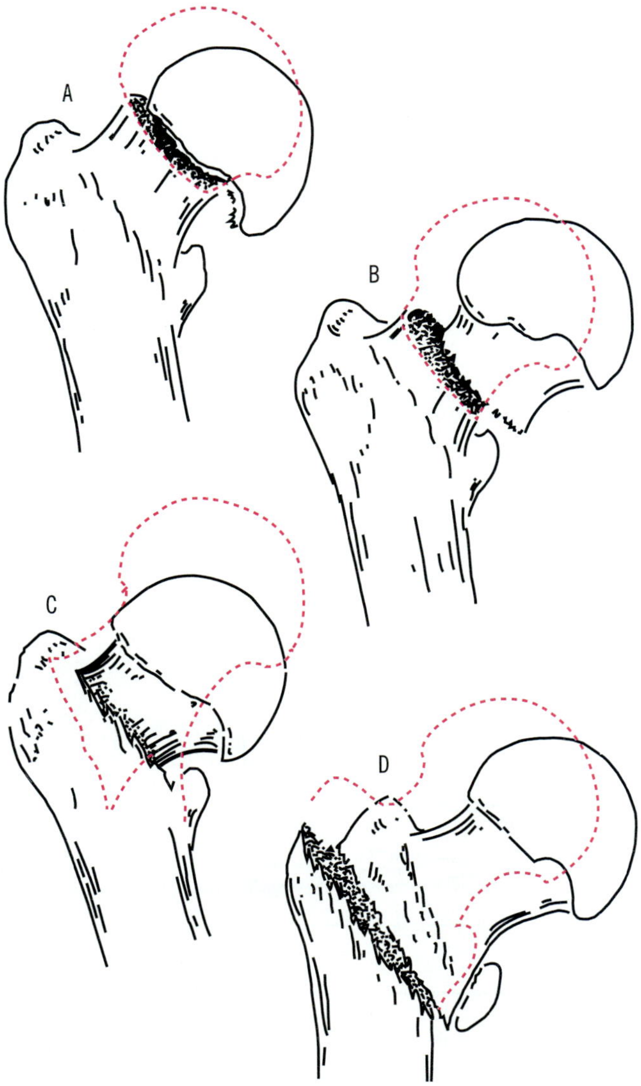

Fig. 28-17 *Hip fractures.* *(From Long BC, Phipps WJ, and Cassmeyer VL: Medical-surgical nursing: a nursing process approach, ed 3, St Louis, 1993, Mosby–Year Book.)*

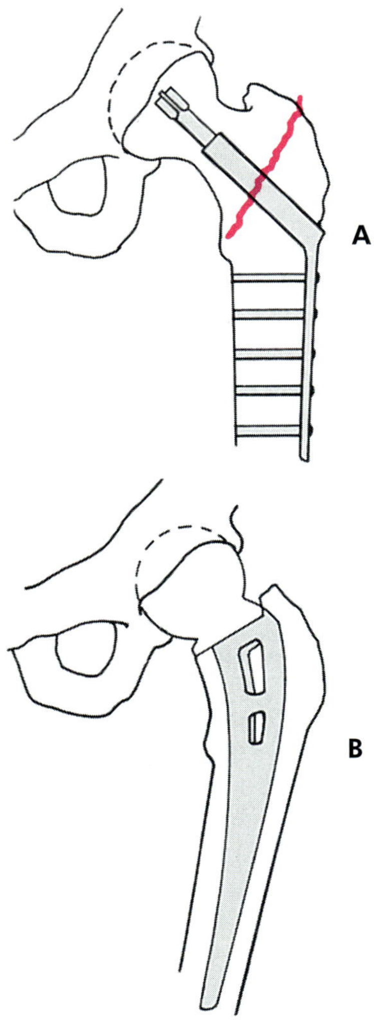

Fig. 28-18 *A, Nail used to repair a hip fracture. B, Prosthesis used to repair a hip fracture.* *(From Long BC, Phipps WJ, and Cassmeyer VL: Medical-surgical nursing: a nursing process approach, ed 3, St Louis, 1993, Mosby–Year Book.)*

BOX 28-4 Care of the Person with a Hip Fracture

- Give good skin care. Skin breakdown can occur rapidly.
- Turn and reposition the person as directed by the nurse. The doctor's orders for turning and positioning depend on the type of fracture and the surgery performed.
- Keep the operated leg abducted at all times. The leg is abducted when the person is supine, being turned, or in a side-lying position (Fig. 28-19, A). Pillows or abductor splints can be used as directed (Fig. 28-19, B).
- Prevent external rotation of the hip (Fig. 28-20). Use trochanter rolls or abduction splints as directed.
- Perform range-of-motion exercises as directed. Do not exercise the affected leg.
- Provide a straight-backed chair with armrests when the person is to be up. A low, soft chair is not used.
- Place the chair on the unaffected side.
- Assist the nurse in transferring the person from the bed to the chair as directed.
- Do not let the person stand on the operated leg unless allowed by the doctor.
- Support and elevate the leg as directed when the person is in the chair.

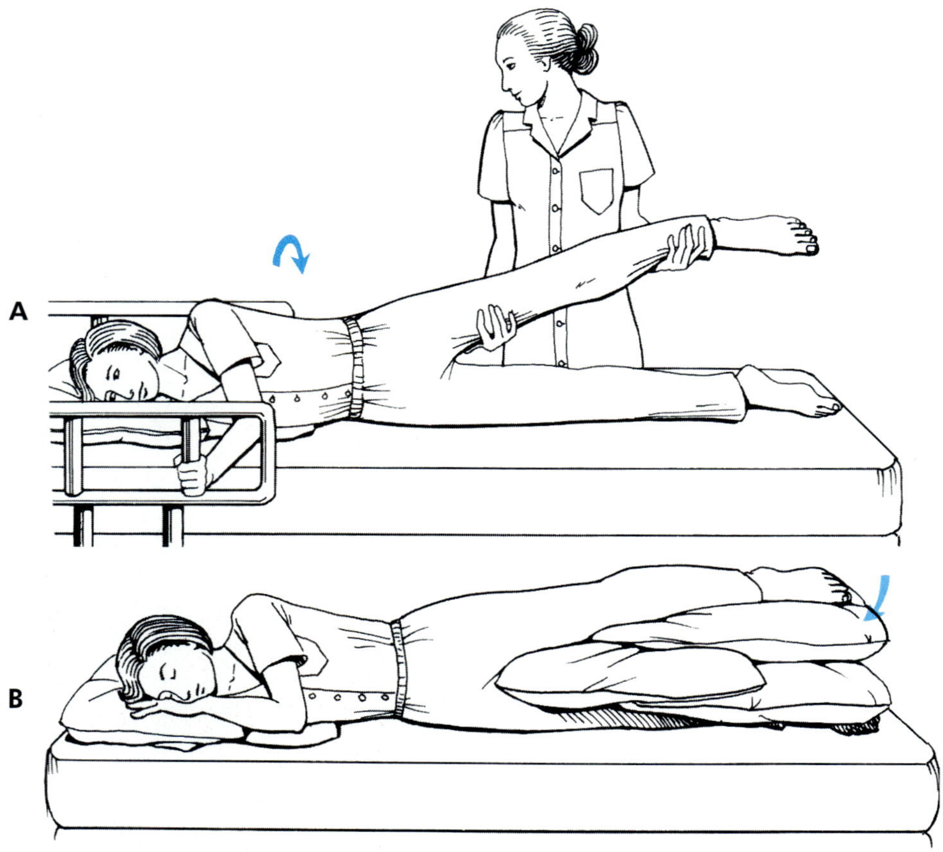

Fig. 28-19 *A, The hip is abducted when the person is turned. B, Pillows are used to maintain the hip in abduction.* *(From Long BC, Phipps WJ, and Cassmeyer VL: Medical-surgical nursing: a nursing process approach, ed 3, St Louis, 1993, Mosby–Year Book.)*

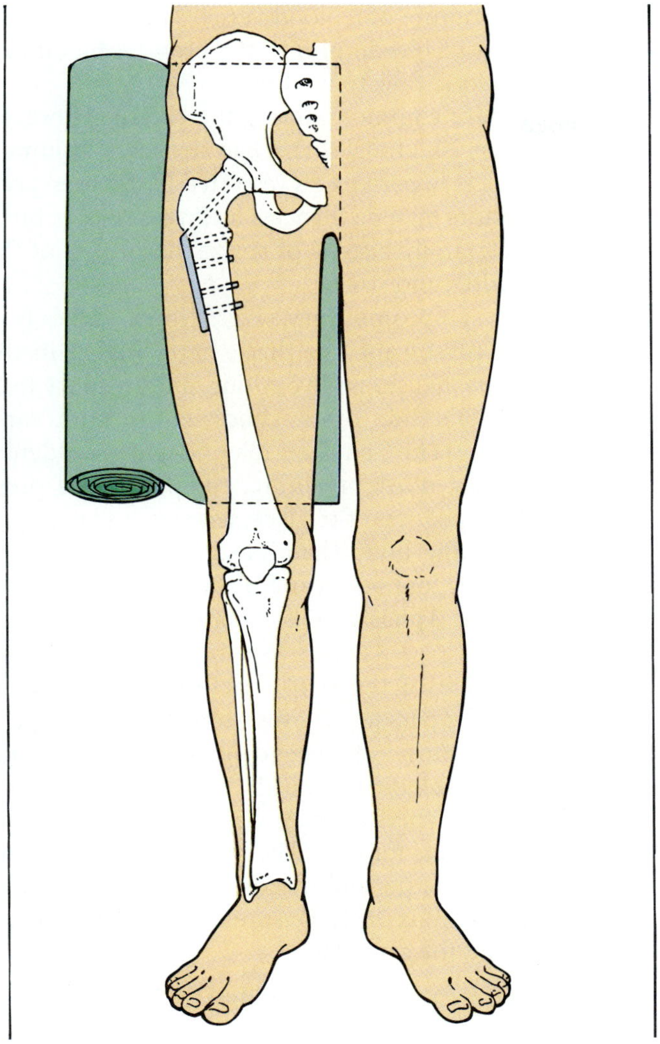

Fig. 28-20 *A trochanter roll is used to prevent external rotation after a hip pinning.*

Osteoporosis

Osteoporosis is a bone *(osteo)* disorder in which the bone becomes porous and brittle *(porosis)*. Bones of the spine, hips, and wrists are affected most often. It is common in the elderly and in women after menopause. The ovaries do not produce the hormone estrogen after menopause. The lack of estrogen results in bone changes. Lack of dietary calcium is also a major cause of osteoporosis. Bed rest and immobility are other causes because they do not allow for proper bone use. For bone to form properly, it must be used to bear weight. If it is not, calcium is absorbed and the bone becomes porous and brittle.

Signs and symptoms of osteoporosis include low back pain, gradual loss of height, and stooped posture. Fractures are a major threat. Sometimes bones are so brittle that the slightest stress can cause a fracture. Turning in bed or getting up from a chair can cause a fracture. Fractures are a great risk if the person falls or has an accident.

Osteoporosis is treated with calcium and vitamin supplements. Estrogen may be given to women. Exercise, good posture, and a back brace or corset are also important. Walking aids may be needed. Bed rest is avoided. Caution is used when turning and positioning the person. The person must be protected from falls and accidents (see Chapter 8).

Loss of a Limb

An **amputation** is the removal of all or part of an extremity. Usually the part is removed surgically. Traumatic amputations can occur from vehicle accidents. Severe injuries, bone tumors, severe infections, and circulatory disorders may require amputations.

Gangrene is a condition in which there is death of tissue. Infection, injuries, and circulatory disorders may result in gangrene. These conditions interfere with blood supply to the tissues. The tissues do not receive enough oxygen and nutrients. Poisonous substances and waste products build up in the affected tissues. Tissue death results. The tissue becomes black, cold, and shriveled (Fig. 28-21) and eventually falls off. If untreated, gangrene spreads through the body and causes death.

All or part of an extremity may be amputated. Fingers, the hand, forearm, or entire arm may be removed. Toes, the foot, lower leg, upper leg, or entire leg may be amputated. A below-the-knee amputation is called a BK (below the knee) or BKA (below knee amputation). An above-the-knee amputation is called an AK (above the knee) or AKA (above knee amputation).

Much support is needed. A major psychological adjustment is necessary. The person's life is affected by the amputation. Appearance, activities of daily living, moving about, and the job are just a few areas affected. Put yourself in the person's position. How would you feel if you lost an arm or leg?

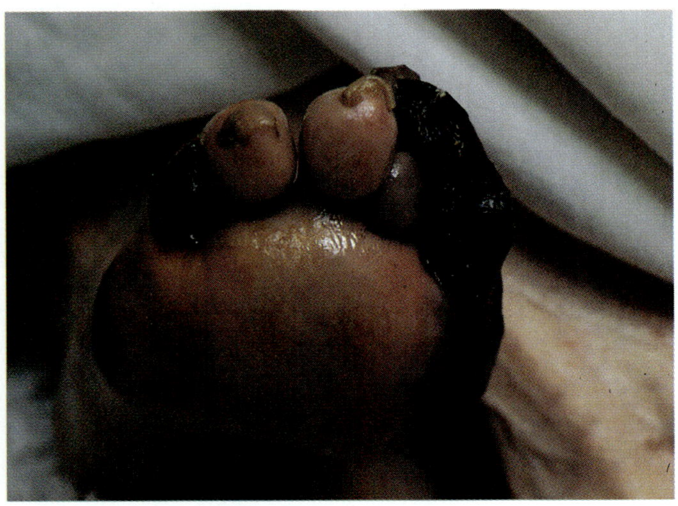

Fig. 28-21 *Gangrene.*

Nurses are responsible for the person's preoperative and postoperative care. At some point most persons are fitted with a prosthesis (see Fig. 26-7, page 558). The stump is conditioned so the prosthesis fits. Stump conditioning involves shrinking and shaping the stump into a cone shape. Bandaging is used to shrink and shape the stump (Fig. 28-22). Exercises are ordered to strengthen the other limbs. Physical therapists help the person use the prosthesis (Fig. 28-23). Occupational therapy is necessary if the stump or prosthesis is used for activities of daily living.

The person may feel that the limb is still there or may complain of pain in the amputated part. This is called *phantom limb pain.* The exact cause is unknown. However, it is a normal reaction. The sensation may occur only for a short time after surgery. However, some persons have phantom limb pain for many years.

NERVOUS SYSTEM DISORDERS

Nervous system disorders can affect mental and physical functions. The ability to speak, understand, feel, see, hear, touch, think, control bowels and bladder, or move may be affected. There are many causes and types of nervous system disorders. The common ones are described here.

Cerebrovascular Accident

A cerebrovascular accident (CVA) is commonly called a **stroke.** Blood supply to a part of the brain is suddenly interrupted. Brain damage occurs. The interruption can be due to the rupture of a blood vessel. This causes hemorrhage (excessive bleeding) into the brain. A blood clot can obstruct blood flow to the brain.

Stroke is more common among the elderly. However, persons in their 20s and 30s have had strokes. A common cause of stroke is hypertension (elevated blood pressure). Other risk factors include diabetes mellitus, obesity, birth control pills, a family history of stroke, hardening of the arteries, smoking, and stress.

Signs and symptoms vary. Sometimes there is a warning. The person may be dizzy, have ringing in the ears, a headache, nausea and vomiting, and memory loss. Weakness on one side of the body is often an early warning sign. The stroke may occur suddenly. Unconsciousness, noisy breathing, elevated blood pressure, slow pulse, redness of the face, seizures, and paralysis on one side of the body (**hemiplegia**) may occur. The stroke victim may lose bowel and bladder control and the ability to speak. **Aphasia** is the inability *(a)* to speak *(phasia).*

Emergency care of the stroke victim is described in Chapter 33. If the person survives, some brain damage is likely. The functions lost depend on the area of brain damage (Fig. 28-24 on page 614). Rehabilitation starts immediately. The person may be partially or totally dependent on others for care. The nurse uses the nursing process to meet the person's needs. Common care measures are listed in Box 28-5. Be sure to follow the nurse's instructions and the care plan.

BOX 28-5 CARE OF THE PERSON WITH A CEREBROVASCULAR ACCIDENT (CVA, STROKE)

- The lateral position is used to prevent aspiration.
- Coughing and deep breathing are encouraged.
- The bed is kept in semi-Fowler's position.
- Side rails are kept up except when giving care.
- Turning and repositioning are done at least every 2 hours.
- Elastic stockings are usually ordered to prevent thrombi (blood clots) in the legs.
- Range-of-motion exercises are performed to prevent contractures.
- A catheter may be inserted or a bladder training program started.
- A bowel training program may be necessary.
- Safety precautions are practiced.
- Assistance is given for self-care activities. The person is encouraged to do as much as possible.
- Communication methods are established. Magic slates, pencil and paper, a picture board, or other methods may be used.
- Good skin care is given to prevent pressure sores.
- Speech therapy, physical therapy, and occupational therapy may be ordered.
- Emotional support and encouragement are given. Praise is given for even the slightest accomplishment.

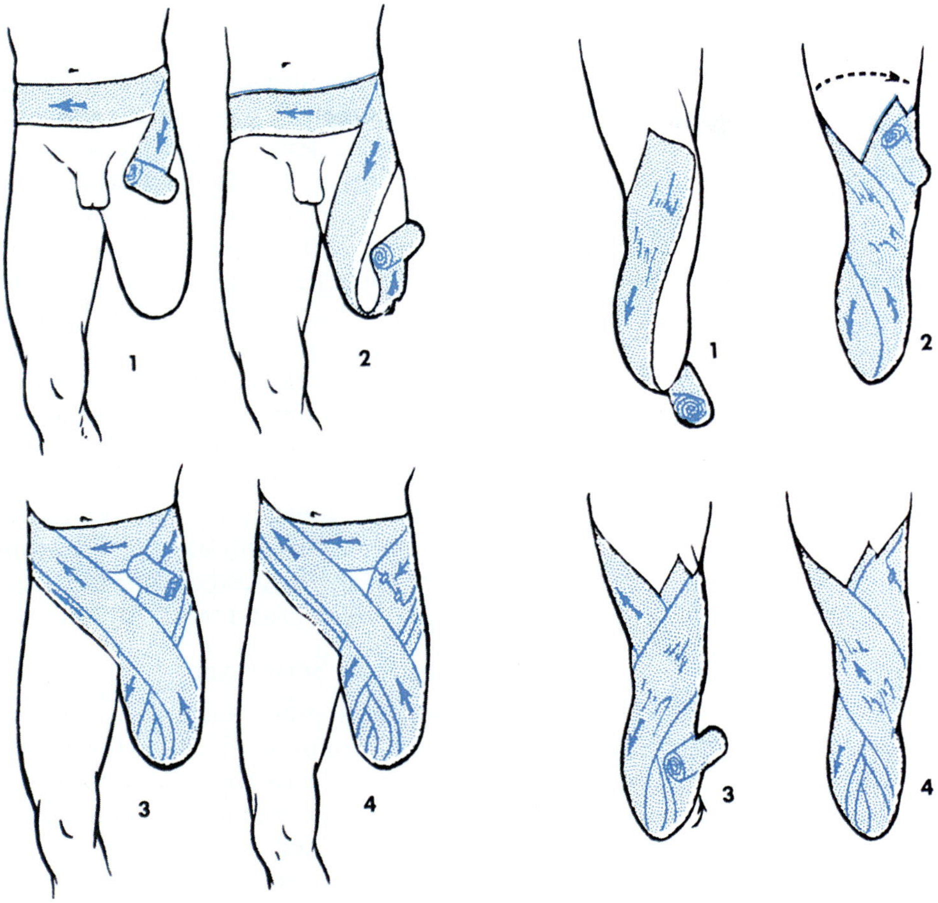

Fig. 28-22 *An above-the-knee amputation is bandaged to shrink and shape the stump. (From Long BC, Phipps WJ, and Cassmeyer VL: Medical-surgical nursing: a nursing process approach, ed 3, St Louis, 1993, Mosby–Year Book.)*

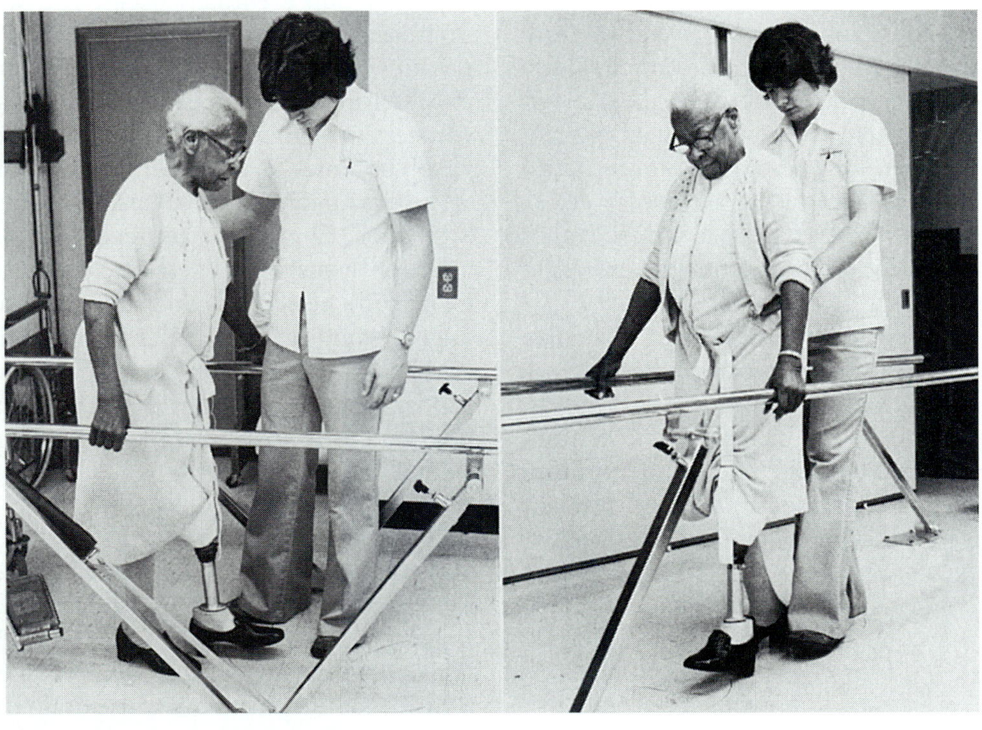

Fig. 28-23 *Use of the prosthesis is learned in physical therapy. (From Long BC, Phipps WJ, Cassmeyer VL: Medical-surgical nursing, ed 3, St Louis, 1993, Mosby–Year Book.)*

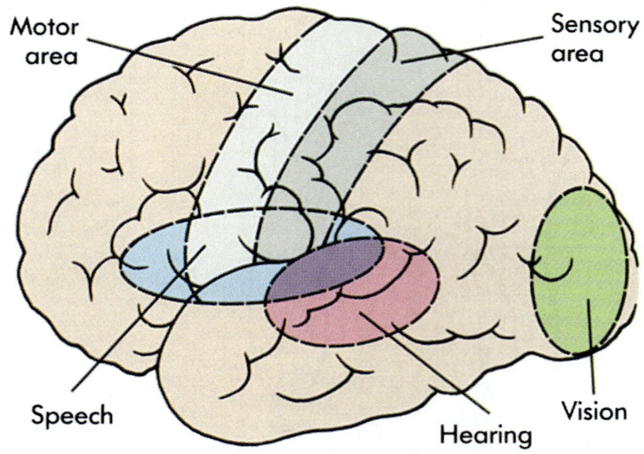

Fig. 28-24 *Functions lost from a stroke depend on the area of brain damage.* (*From Milliken ME and Campbell G: Essential competencies for patient care, St Louis, 1985, Mosby–Year Book.*)

Aphasia Speech is controlled by the left side of the brain. Persons with right-sided hemiplegia may also have aphasia. There are two basic types of aphasia. **Expressive aphasia** relates to difficulty expressing or sending out thoughts. There are problems with speaking, spelling, counting, gesturing, or writing. The person thinks one thing but says another. For example, the person thinks about food but asks for a newspaper. People are called the wrong names even when correct names are known. Or the person thinks clearly but cannot speak. Some only produce sounds and no words. The person may cry or swear for no apparent reason.

Receptive aphasia relates to receiving information. The person has trouble understanding what is said or read. Everyday objects are not recognized. The person may have no idea what to do with a fork, toilet, water glass, television, telephone, or other items. The person may not recognize people. Remember, for communication to occur, the message sent must be received and correctly interpreted. The person with *receptive* aphasia simply cannot interpret the message received. The person with *expressive* aphasia cannot send messages.

Some people have both expressive and receptive aphasia. This is called **expressive-receptive aphasia.**

Persons with aphasia have many emotional needs. Frustration, depression, and anger are common. Communication is important for independent functioning and for relationships. Remember, the resident wants to communicate but cannot. You need to be patient and kind.

Parkinson's Disease

Parkinson's disease is a slow, progressive disorder. Degeneration of a part of the brain occurs. There is no cure. The disease is usually seen in the elderly. Signs and symptoms are a masklike facial expression, tremors, pill-rolling movements of the fingers, a shuffling gait, stooped posture, stiff muscles, slow movements, slurred or monotone speech, and drooling. Mental function is usually not affected at first. As the disease progresses, confusion and forgetfulness may develop.

Drugs specifically for Parkinson's disease are ordered by the doctor. Physical therapy may be ordered. The person may need help with eating and other self-care activities. Measures to promote normal bowel elimination are practiced. Constipation is a risk because of decreased activity and poor nutrition. Safety practices are followed to prevent injury. Remember, mental function may not be affected. Talk to and treat the person as an adult.

Multiple Sclerosis

Multiple sclerosis (MS) is a progressive disease. The myelin sheath (which covers the nerves), the spinal cord, and the white matter in the brain are destroyed. Therefore nerve impulses cannot be sent to and from the brain in a normal manner.

Symptoms begin in young adulthood. The onset is gradual. There is blurred or double vision. Difficulty with balance and walking occur. Tremors, numbness and tingling, weakness, dizziness, urinary incontinence, anal incontinence or constipation, behavior changes, and incoordination eventually occur. The person's condition progressively worsens over many years. Blindness, contractures, paralysis of all extremities (quadriplegia), loss of bowel and bladder control, and respiratory muscle weakness are among the person's many problems. The person becomes totally dependent on others for care.

There is no known cure. Persons are kept active as long as possible. They are encouraged and allowed to do as much for themselves as possible. Nursing care depends on the person's needs and condition. Skin care, hygiene, and range-of-motion exercises are important. Measures are taken to prevent injury and to promote bowel and bladder elimination. Turning, positioning, coughing, and deep breathing are also important. Complications from bed rest are prevented.

Head Injuries

The scalp, skull, and brain tissue can be injured. Some injuries are minor. There may be only temporary loss of consciousness. Others are more serious. Permanent brain damage or death may result. Brain tissue can be bruised or torn. Skull fractures can cause brain damage. Bleeding from head injuries can occur in the brain or surrounding structures.

Head injuries are caused by falls, vehicle accidents, industrial accidents, and sports injuries. Other body parts also may be injured. Spinal cord injuries are likely. Birth injuries are another major cause of head trauma. If the person survives a severe head injury, some permanent damage is likely. Paralysis, mental retardation, personality changes, speech problems, breathing difficulties, and loss of bowel and bladder control may be permanent. Rehabilitation is required. Nursing care depends on the person's needs and remaining abilities.

Spinal Cord Injuries

Spinal cord injuries can permanently damage the nervous system. These injuries usually occur from stab or bullet wounds, vehicle accidents, industrial accidents, falls, or sports injuries. Cervical traction (a form of skeletal traction) is often necessary (see Fig. 28-15). The person in cervical traction is placed on a Stryker frame.

The type of damage depends on the level of the injury. The higher the level of injury, the greater the loss of function (Fig. 28-25). If the injury is in the lumbar area, muscle function in the legs is lost. Injuries at the thoracic level cause loss of muscle function below the chest. Persons with injuries at the lumbar or thoracic levels are paraplegics. **Paraplegia** is paralysis of the legs. Cervical injuries may result in loss of function to the arms, chest, and all muscles below the chest. Persons with these injuries are quadriplegics. **Quadriplegia** is paralysis of the arms, legs, and trunk.

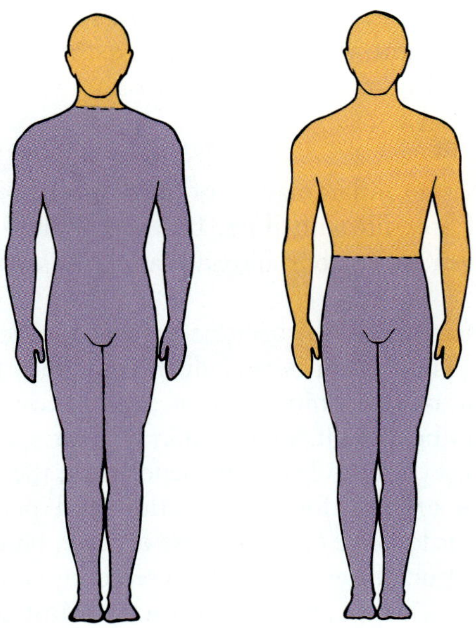

Fig. 28-25 *The shaded areas indicate the areas of paralysis. (From Milliken ME, Campbell G: Essential competencies for patient care, St Louis, 1985, Mosby–Year Book.)*

If the person survives, rehabilitation is necessary. The person's needs and the rehabilitation program depend on the functions lost and remaining abilities. Emotional needs cannot be overlooked. These persons have severe emotional reactions to paralysis and the loss of function. Paralyzed persons generally need the care listed in Box 28-6.

BOX 28-6 Care of Persons with Paralysis

- Protect the person from falls. Keep side rails up, the bed in low position, and the call bell within reach.
- Protect the person from burns. Bath water, heat applications, and food must be at the proper temperature.
- Turn and reposition the person at least every 2 hours.
- Give skin care and other measures to prevent pressure sores.
- Maintain good body alignment at all times. Use pillows, trochanter rolls, foot boards, and other devices as needed.
- Carry out bowel and bladder training programs.
- Perform range-of-motion exercises to maintain muscle function and prevent contractures. Other exercises may be ordered.
- Assist with food and fluids as needed. The person may have to be fed. Self-help devices may be needed.
- Give emotional and psychological support. Psychiatrists or psychologists may be involved in the person's care.
- Physical therapy, occupational therapy, and vocational rehabilitation may be ordered. They help the person regain independent functioning to the extent possible.

RESPIRATORY DISORDERS

Persons with respiratory disorders are often seen in hospital and nursing facilities. Some need home care. The respiratory system brings oxygen into the lungs and removes carbon dioxide from the body. Respiratory disorders interfere with this function and threaten life. A review of the respiratory system on page 106 in Chapter 5 will help in studying this section.

Chronic Obstructive Pulmonary Disease (COPD)

Three disorders are grouped under chronic obstructive pulmonary disease (COPD). They are chronic bronchitis, asthma, and emphysema. These disorders interfere with the normal exchange of oxygen and carbon dioxide in the lungs. They obstruct air flow.

Chronic bronchitis Chronic bronchitis occurs after repeated episodes of bronchitis (inflammation of the bronchi). Cigarette smoking is the major cause. Air pollution is another cause. *Smoker's cough* in the morning is usually the first symptom. At first the cough is dry. Eventually the person coughs up mucus, which may contain pus and blood. The cough becomes more frequent as the disease progresses. The person has difficulty breathing and may tire easily. The mucus and inflamed breathing passages *obstruct* airflow into the lungs. Therefore the body cannot get normal amounts of oxygen.

The person must stop smoking. Oxygen therapy and breathing exercises are often ordered. Respiratory tract infections must be prevented. Should a respiratory infection occur, prompt treatment is essential.

Emphysema In emphysema, the alveoli become enlarged. Walls of the alveoli are less elastic. They do not expand and shrink normally with inspiration and expiration. As a result, some air is trapped in the alveoli during expiration. Trapped air is not exhaled. As the disease progresses, more alveoli are involved. Therefore more air is trapped. The normal exchange of oxygen and carbon dioxide cannot occur in affected alveoli. Chronic bronchitis and emphysema often occur together.

Cigarette smoking is the most common cause. Signs and symptoms include shortness of breath and smoker's cough. At first, shortness of breath occurs with exertion. As the disease progresses, it may occur at rest. Sputum may contain pus. As more air is trapped in the lungs, the person develops a *barrel chest* (Fig. 28-26). Persons usually prefer to sit upright and slightly forward. Breathing is easier in this position.

The person must stop smoking. Respiratory therapy, breathing exercises, oxygen, and drug therapy are ordered.

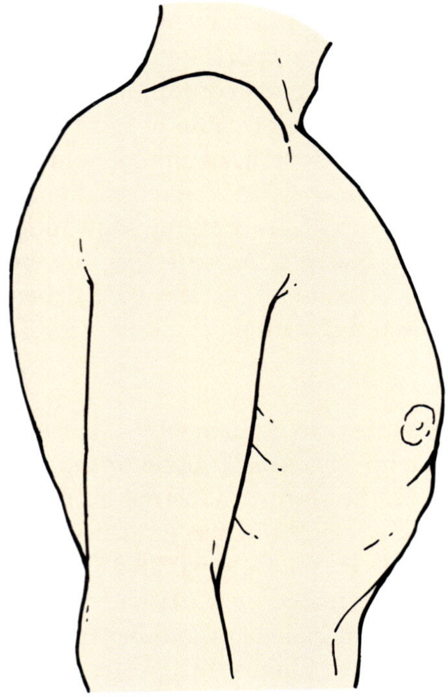

Fig. 28-26 *Barrel chest from emphysema.*

Asthma Air passages narrow with asthma. Difficulty in breathing results. Allergies and emotional stress are common causes. Episodes occur suddenly and are called *asthma attacks.* Besides dyspnea, there is shortness of breath, wheezing, coughing, rapid pulse, perspiration, and cyanosis. The person is very frightened during the attack. Fear causes the attack to become worse.

Drugs are used to treat asthma. Emergency room treatment may be necessary for severe attacks. The person and family are taught how to prevent asthma attacks. Repeated attacks can damage the respiratory system.

Pneumonia

Pneumonia is an inflammation of lung tissue. Alveoli in the affected area fill with fluid. Because of fluid in the alveoli, oxygen and carbon dioxide cannot be exchanged normally.

Pneumonia is caused by bacteria, viruses, aspiration, or immobility. The person is very ill. Fever, chills, painful cough, pain on breathing, and a rapid pulse occur. Cyanosis may be present. Sputum may be clear, green, yellowish, or rust colored. The color depends on the cause.

Drugs are ordered for the infection and pain. The doctor may order *force fluids* because of fever. Fluids also help to thin mucous secretions. Thin secretions are easier to cough up. Oxygen may be necessary. Most persons prefer semi-Fowler's position for breathing. Standard Precautions are followed. Other isolation precautions may be necessary, depending on the cause. Mouth care is important. Frequent linen changes are needed because of fever.

Tuberculosis (TB)

Tuberculosis (TB) is a bacterial infection. The lungs are affected. However, TB can also occur in the kidney and bones. TB was a major cause of death in the early 1900s. Drug therapy specific for TB was introduced in the 1940s and 1950s. This resulted in a dramatic decline in the number of TB cases each year. However, TB still occurs and is a major health problem. In the late 1980s the number of cases began to increase. There has been a steady increase in TB since then.

The bacteria causing TB are spread by airborne droplets (see Chapter 9). Bacteria are spread when the person coughs, sneezes, speaks, or sings. Others in the environment can inhale the bacteria. Generally many bacteria must be inhaled for the infection to develop. Persons who have close, frequent contact with an infected person are at risk. TB is more likely to occur in close, crowded environments such as inner-city neighborhoods. Persons with HIV infection (pages 627-628) are also at risk.

An infection develops in the lung. Sometimes the bacteria do not produce an infection until many years later. The person may not have symptoms at first. The disease may be found when routine chest x-rays are done or when a TB skin test is required for a job. Early signs and symptoms are tiredness, loss of appetite, weight loss, fever in the late afternoon, and night sweats. Coughing occurs. The cough is more frequent as the disease progresses. Sputum production also increases. Chest pain occurs.

Treatment involves drug therapy specific for TB. Hospital care usually is not necessary. Persons with TB need to cover their noses and mouths with tissues when coughing or sneezing. Tissues are flushed down the toilet or placed in a paper bag and burned. Handwashing after contact with sputum is essential. If hospital care is needed, the person wears a mask. Standard Precautions and Airborne Precautions are practiced.

CARDIOVASCULAR DISORDERS

Cardiovascular disorders are the leading causes of death in the United States. Problems occur in the heart or in the blood vessels.

Hypertension

Hypertension *(high blood pressure)* is a condition in which the blood pressure is abnormally high. The systolic pressure is 140 mm Hg or higher. Or the diastolic pressure is 90 mm Hg or higher. Elevated measurements must occur on two different occasions. Risk factors for hypertension are listed in Box 28-7. Narrowed blood vessels are a common cause. When vessels are narrow, the heart must pump with more force to move blood through the vessels. Kidney disorders, head injuries, some complications of pregnancy, and tumors of the adrenal gland can also cause hypertension.

BOX 28-7 Risk Factors for Hypertension

- Age—the risk increases with aging beginning at about age 35
- Sex—men are at greater risk than women
- Race—blacks are at greater risk than whites
- Family history—tends to run in families
- Obesity—related to lack of exercise and atherosclerosis
- Stress—increased sympathetic nervous system activity
- Cigarette smoking—nicotine causes narrowing of blood vessels
- High-salt diet—sodium causes fluid retention; increased fluid raises the blood volume
- Alcohol—increases chemical substances in the body that increase blood pressure
- Lack of exercise—leads to obesity
- Atherosclerosis—arteries narrow because of fatty buildup in the vessels

Hypertension can damage other body organs. The heart may enlarge so it can pump with more force. Blood vessels in the brain may burst and cause a stroke. Blood vessels in the eyes and kidneys may be damaged.

At first, hypertension may not cause signs or symptoms. Usually it is discovered when blood pressure is measured. Signs and symptoms develop as the disorder progresses. Headache, blurred vision, and dizziness may be reported. Complications of hypertension include stroke, heart attack, kidney (renal) failure, and blindness.

There are many medications for lowering blood pressure. The person is advised to quit smoking, exercise regularly, and get enough rest. A sodium-restricted diet may also be ordered. If the person is overweight, a low-calorie diet is ordered.

Coronary Artery Disease (CAD)

The coronary arteries are in the heart. They provide the heart with its own blood supply. In coronary artery disease, the coronary arteries become narrowed. One or all of the arteries may be affected. Because of narrowed vessels, blood supply to the heart muscle is reduced. The most common cause is atherosclerosis. In atherosclerosis, fatty material collects on the arterial walls (Fig. 28-27). The arteries narrow and obstruct blood flow. Blood flow through an artery may be totally blocked. Permanent damage occurs in the part of the heart receiving its blood supply from that artery.

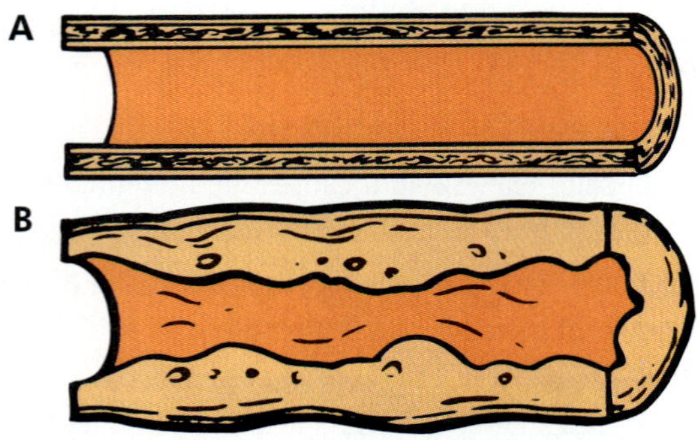

Fig. 28-27 *A, Normal artery. B, Fatty deposits collect on the walls of arteries in atherosclerosis.*

Risk factors for CAD have been identified. They include:

- Obesity
- Cigarette smoking
- Lack of exercise
- A diet high in fat and cholesterol
- Hypertension

CAD is more common in men and older people. The type A personality is also a risk factor. This personality type is aggressive, competitive, and hard working. The person has difficulty relaxing, has a sense of urgency, and does things at a rapid pace.

The two major complications of coronary artery disease are angina pectoris and myocardial infarction (heart attack).

Angina pectoris Angina *(pain)* pectoris *(chest)* means chest pain. The chest pain is due to reduced blood flow to a part of the heart muscle (myocardium). Angina pectoris occurs when the heart needs more oxygen. Normally, blood flow to the heart increases when the heart's need for oxygen increases. Physical exertion, a heavy meal, emotional stress, and excitement increase the heart's need for oxygen. In CAD, the narrowed vessels prevent increased blood flow.

Signs and symptoms of angina include chest pain. The pain may be described as a tightness or discomfort in the left side of the chest. Pain may radiate to other sites (Fig. 28-28). Pain in the left jaw and down the inner aspect of

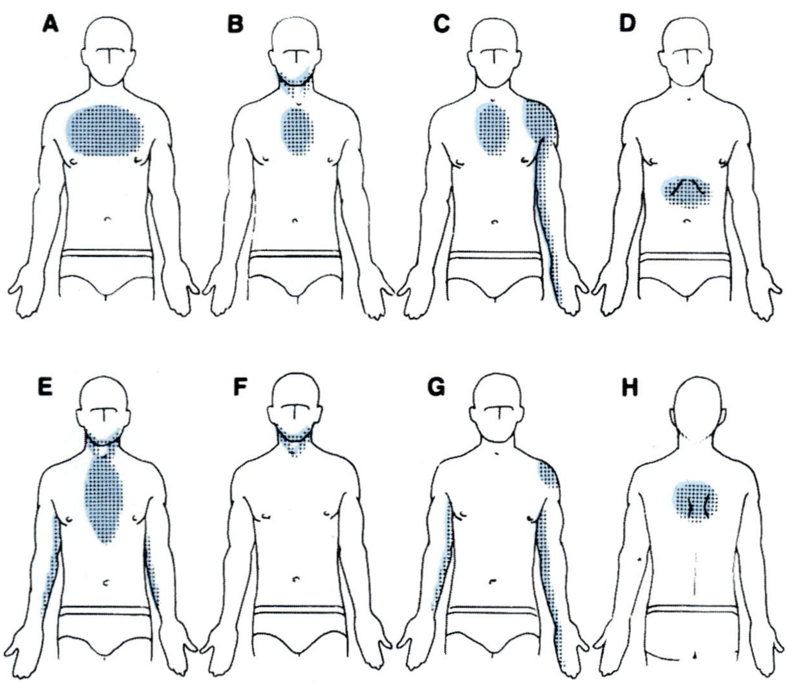

Fig. 28-28 *Shaded areas show where the pain of angina pectoris is located.* *(From Long BC, Phipps WJ, and Cassmeyer VL: Medical-surgical nursing: a nursing process approach, ed 3, St Louis, 1993, Mosby–Year Book.)*

the left arm is common. The person may be pale, feel faint, and perspire. Dyspnea may be present. These signs and symptoms cause the person to stop activity and rest. Rest often relieves the symptoms in 3 to 15 minutes. Rest reduces the heart's need for oxygen. Therefore normal blood flow is achieved and heart damage is prevented.

Besides rest, a medication called *nitroglycerin* is taken to relieve angina. A nitroglycerin tablet is taken when an angina attack occurs. The nitroglycerin is put under the tongue. It dissolves under the tongue and is rapidly absorbed into the bloodstream. Most doctors want the nitroglycerin kept at the bedside. The person takes a tablet when one is needed and then tells the nurse. The person does not have to wait for a nurse to answer the call bell and then go get the tablet. The person should have nitroglycerin tablets nearby at all times. This includes when the person goes to physical therapy, occupational therapy, the x-ray department, the dining room, lounge, or other parts of the facility. Persons at home should keep the tablets close by.

Persons are taught to avoid situations that are likely to cause angina pectoris. These include overexertion, heavy meals and overeating, and emotional situations. They are advised to stay indoors during cold weather or during hot, humid weather. Exercise programs supervised by doctors may be developed.

Some people need coronary artery bypass surgery. The surgery bypasses the diseased part of the artery (Fig. 28-29) and increases blood flow to the heart. Many persons with angina pectoris eventually have heart attacks. Chest pain that is not relieved by rest and nitroglycerin may have a more serious cause.

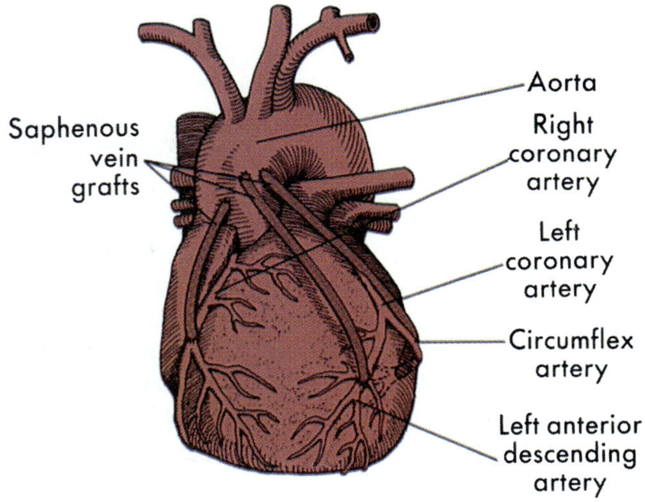

Fig. 28-29 *Coronary artery bypass surgery. The diseased part of the area is bypassed with a vein graft.* (*Modified from Long BC and Woods NF: Medical-surgical nursing: concepts and clinical practice, ed 3, St Louis, 1987, Mosby–Year Book.*)

Myocardial infarction (MI) A myocardial infarction is due to lack of blood supply to the heart muscle (myocardium). Tissue death occurs (infarction). Common terms for MI are *heart attack, coronary, coronary thrombosis,* and *coronary occlusion.* Blood flow to the myocardium is suddenly interrupted. Usually a thrombus (blood clot) obstructs blood flow through an artery. The area of damage may be small or large. Sudden cardiac death *(cardiac arrest)* can occur (see Chapter 33).

The person may have one or more signs and symptoms listed in Box 28-8. Myocardial infarction is an emergency.

BOX 28-8 Signs and Symptoms of Myocardial Infarction

- Sudden, severe chest pain
- Pain is usually on the left side
- Pain is described as crushing, stabbing, or squeezing; some describe pain in terms of someone sitting on the chest
- Pain may radiate to the neck and jaw, and down the arm or to other sites
- Pain is more severe and lasts longer than angina pectoris
- Pain is not relieved by rest and nitroglycerin
- Indigestion
- Dyspnea
- Nausea
- Dizziness
- Perspiration
- Pallor
- Cyanosis
- Cold and clammy skin
- Low blood pressure
- Weak and irregular pulse
- Fear and apprehension
- A feeling of doom

Efforts are directed at relieving pain, stabilizing vital signs, giving oxygen, and calming the person. Many drugs are given. The person is treated in a coronary care unit (CCU). The unit has emergency equipment and drugs needed during cardiac arrest. Measures are taken to prevent life-threatening complications.

The person is in the CCU for at least 3 days. When stable, the person is transferred. Activity is increased gradually. Drug therapy and measures to prevent complications are continued. A cardiac rehabilitation program is planned for the person. This includes an exercise program, teaching about medications, and dietary changes. Changes in life-style and sexual activity may be necessary. The goal of cardiac rehabilitation is to prevent another heart attack.

Heart Failure

Heart failure occurs when the heart cannot pump blood normally. Blood backs up and causes congestion of tissues. Left-sided heart failure, right-sided heart failure, or both, can occur.

When the left side of the heart fails to pump efficiently, blood backs up into the lungs. Signs and symptoms of respiratory congestion occur. These include dyspnea, increased sputum production, cough, and gurgling sounds in the lungs. In addition, blood is not pumped out of the heart to the rest of the body in adequate amounts. Organs do not receive enough blood. Signs and symptoms occur because of effects on the organs. For example, poor blood flow to the brain causes confusion, dizziness, and fainting. Poor blood flow to the kidneys causes reduced kidney function and decreased urinary output. The skin becomes pale or cyanotic. Blood pressure falls. A very severe form of left-sided failure is *pulmonary edema* (fluid in the lungs). Pulmonary edema is an emergency. Death can occur.

The right side of the heart may fail. Blood backs up into the venae cavae and into the venous system. Feet and ankles swell. Neck veins bulge. Congestion occurs in the liver; liver function decreases. The abdomen becomes congested with fluid. The right side of the heart cannot pump blood to the lungs efficiently. Therefore normal blood flow does not occur from the lungs to the left side of the heart. Less blood than normal is pumped from the left side of the heart to the rest of the body. As with left-sided heart failure, the body's organs have a reduced blood supply. The signs and symptoms described in the previous paragraph eventually occur.

Heart failure is usually caused by a weakened heart. Myocardial infarction and hypertension are common causes. Damaged heart valves are another cause.

Heart failure can be treated and controlled. Drugs are given to strengthen the heart and to reduce the amount of fluid in the body. A sodium-restricted diet is ordered. Oxygen is given. Most persons prefer semi-Fowler's or Fowler's position for breathing. Many elderly people suffer from heart failure. They may need home care or care in a nursing facility. You may be involved in these aspects of the person's care:

- Maintaining bed rest or a limited activity program
- Measuring intake and output
- Measuring weight daily
- Restricting fluids as ordered by the doctor
- Giving good skin care to prevent skin breakdown
- Performing range-of-motion exercises
- Assisting with transfers or ambulation
- Assisting with self-care activities
- Maintaining good body alignment
- Applying elastic stockings

DISORDERS OF THE URINARY SYSTEM

The kidneys, ureters, bladder, and urethra are the major structures of the urinary system. Disorders can occur in one or more of these structures.

Urinary Tract Infections (UTI)

Urinary tract infections (UTI) are common. They can occur in the bladder or in a kidney. Infection in one area can lead to infection of the entire system. Normally the urinary system is sterile. There are no pathogens or nonpathogens. Microbes can enter the urinary system through the urethra. Catheterization, urological examinations, sexual intercourse, and poor perineal hygiene are common causes. Urinary tract infection is a common nosocomial infection (see Chapter 9).

Women are at greater risk for UTIs than men. Women have a shorter urethra which microbes can easily enter. Also, fluid secreted by the prostate gland in men offers protection from UTIs. Older men and young girls are also at risk.

Cystitis Cystitis is inflammation *(itis)* of the bladder *(cyst)*. It is caused by bacteria. Often there are no signs or symptoms. Or the person may have one or more of the following:

- Urinary frequency
- Urgency
- Dysuria—difficult or painful *(dys)* urination *(uria)*
- Pain
- Foul-smelling urine
- Hematuria—blood *(hemat)* in the urine *(uria)*
- Pyuria—pus *(py)* in the urine *(uria)*

Antibiotics are the treatment of choice.

Pyelonephritis Pyelonephritis is inflammation *(itis)* of the pelvis *(pyelo)* kidney *(nephr)*. Infection is the most common cause. Chills and fever occur along with the signs and symptoms of cystitis. Treatment consists of antibiotics and fluids.

Renal Calculi

Renal calculi are kidney *(renal)* stones *(calculi)*. White men between the ages of 20 and 55 have the greatest risk. Bed rest and immobility also are risk factors. Stones vary in size. Signs and symptoms include:

- Severe pain in the flank, back, abdomen, thigh, and urethra
- Fever and chills
- Dysuria—difficult or painful *(dys)* urination *(uria)*
- Nausea and vomiting
- Urinary frequency and urgency
- Oliguria—scant *(olig)* urine *(uria)*
- Hematuria—blood *(hemat)* in the urine *(uria)*

Treatment involves pain relief and forcing fluids. The person needs to drink about 4000 ml of fluid a day. Forcing fluids helps promote passage of the stone through the urine. All urine is strained (see Chapter 15). Surgical removal of the stone may be necessary.

Renal Failure

In renal failure (kidney failure) the kidneys do not function or are severely impaired. Waste products cannot be removed from the blood. Fluids are retained in the body. Heart failure and hypertension easily result. Renal failure may be acute or chronic. The person is very ill.

Acute renal failure Acute renal failure occurs suddenly. Severe decreased blood flow to the kidneys is a common cause. The many causes of decreased blood flow to the kidneys includes postoperative bleeding, bleeding from trauma, myocardial infarction (heart attack), severe congestive heart failure, burns, and severe allergic reactions.

There are three phases.

- **Oliguric phase**—oliguria (scant amount of urine) occurs at first. Urine output is less than 400 ml in 24 hours. Oliguria is followed by anuria (absence of urine). This phase may last from a few days to 2 weeks.
- **Diuretic phase**—diuresis occurs. Diuresis means the process *(esis)* of passing *(di)* the urine *(ur)*. Large amounts of urine are produced. Urine output can range from 1000 to 5000 ml a day.
- **Recovery phase**—kidney function improves and returns to normal. This phase can take anywhere from 1 month to 1 year. Some persons develop chronic renal failure.

Every body system is affected by the buildup of waste products in the blood. Death can occur. It may be due to renal failure, infection, gastrointestinal bleeding, or the cause of the renal failure.

The doctor orders drug therapy, restricted fluids, and diet therapy. The person's diet is low in protein, high in carbohydrates, and low in potassium. The nurse plans for the person's physical and psychological needs. The person's care plan is likely to include:

- Measuring and recording urine output every hour; an output of less than 30 ml per hour is reported to the nurse immediately
- Measuring and recording intake and output
- Restricting fluid intake
- Daily weight measurements with the same scale
- Turning and repositioning at least every 2 hours
- Measures to prevent pressure sores
- Frequent oral hygiene
- Measures to prevent infection
- Coughing and deep breathing exercises
- Measures to meet the person's emotional needs

BOX 28-9 Signs and Symptoms of Chronic Renal Failure

- Yellow, tan, or dusky skin
- Dry, itchy skin
- Thin, brittle skin
- Bruises
- Bad breath (halitosis)
- Stomatitis (inflammation of the mouth)
- Nausea and vomiting
- Loss of appetite
- Diarrhea or constipation
- Bleeding tendencies
- Susceptibility to infection
- Hypertension
- Congestive heart failure
- Ulcers in the gastrointestinal tract
- Irregular pulse
- Abnormal breathing patterns
- Burning sensation in the legs and feet
- Muscle twitching
- Leg cramps at night
- Convulsions
- Confusion
- Coma

Chronic renal failure In chronic renal failure the kidneys can no longer meet the needs of the body. Nephrons of the kidney are slowly destroyed over many years. Infections, obstructions of the urinary tract, hypertension, tumors, and diabetes are among the many causes. Some children are born with abnormalities that lead to renal failure.

Signs and symptoms appear when 80 to 90 percent of kidney function is lost. Every body system is affected by the buildup of waste products in the blood. Box 28-9 lists some of the signs and symptoms that occur.

Treatment includes fluid restriction, diet therapy, drugs, and dialysis. **Dialysis** is the process of removing waste products from the blood. It is a complex process. Specially trained nurses perform the procedure. Some persons have kidney transplants.

Nursing measures for the person in chronic renal failure are listed in Box 28-10.

BOX 28-10 Care of the Person in Chronic Renal Failure

- A diet low in protein, potassium, and sodium
- Fluid restriction
- Measuring blood pressure in the supine, sitting, and standing positions
- Measuring weight daily (with the same scale)
- Measuring and recording intake and output
- Turning and repositioning
- Measures to prevent pressure sores
- Range-of-motion exercises
- Measures to prevent itching (bath oils, lotions, and creams)
- Measures to prevent injury and bleeding
- Frequent oral hygiene
- Measures to prevent infection
- Measures to prevent diarrhea or constipation
- Measures to meet the person's emotional needs

THE ENDOCRINE SYSTEM

The endocrine system is made of glands. The endocrine glands secrete hormones that affect other organs and glands. A review of the endocrine system on pages 112-113 in Chapter 5 will help you in studying this section. The most common endocrine disorder is diabetes mellitus.

Diabetes Mellitus

In this disorder the body cannot use sugar properly. Insulin is needed for the proper use of sugar. Insulin is secreted by the pancreas. In diabetes mellitus, the pancreas does not secrete enough insulin. Sugar builds up in the blood. Cells do not have enough sugar for energy. Therefore cells cannot perform their specific functions.

Diabetes mellitus occurs in children and adults. Risk factors include a family history of diabetes and obesity. The risk increases after age 40.

There are two main types of diabetes mellitus.

- *Insulin-dependent (type I) diabetes*—occurs most often in children and young adults. The pancreas does not secrete insulin. The person must have daily insulin injections.
- *Non-insulin-dependent (type II) diabetes*—occurs in adults. The pancreas secretes some insulin. The amount secreted is not enough to meet the body's needs.

Signs and symptoms include increased urine production, increased thirst, hunger, and weight loss. Blood tests show increased sugar levels. Urine test shows sugar in the urine (see Chapter 15). If diabetes is not controlled, complications occur. These include changes in the retina that can lead to blindness, kidney damage, nerve damage, and circulatory disorders. Kidney damage can lead to renal failure. Circulatory disorders can lead to a stroke, heart attack, and slow wound healing. Foot and leg wounds are very serious. Infection and gangrene can occur and require amputation of the part.

Insulin-dependent (type I) diabetes is treated with daily insulin therapy, diet, and exercise (see Chapter 17). The amount of sugar in the diet is limited. Meals are served on time to balance insulin needs. Remember, food raises the blood sugar and insulin lowers blood sugar. The person needs to eat all foods served.

Non-insulin-dependent (type II) diabetes is treated with diet and exercise. The number of calories and sugar in the diet are restricted. If the person is overweight, weight loss needs to occur. Oral medications may be ordered. Some persons with type II diabetes need insulin.

Blood tests or urine tests for sugar are done daily or before meals. Good foot care is very important.

Hypoglycemia (insulin shock) occurs with too much insulin. **Hypoglycemia** means low *(hypo)* sugar *(glyc)* in the blood *(emia)*. Hyperglycemia (diabetic coma) develops if a person does not get enough insulin. **Hyperglycemia** means high *(hyper)* sugar *(glyc)* in the blood *(emia)*. Table 28-1 on page 624 summarizes the causes, signs, and symptoms of hypoglycemia and hyperglycemia. Both can lead to death if not corrected.

TABLE 28-1

HYPOGLYCEMIA AND HYPERGLYCEMIA

	Causes	Signs and Symptoms
Hypoglycemia (Insulin Shock)	Too much insulin Omitting a meal Eating too little food Increased exercise Vomiting	Hunger Weakness Trembling Perspiration Headache Dizziness Rapid pulse Low blood pressure Confusion Cold, clammy skin Convulsions Unconsciousness
Hyperglycemia (Diabetic Coma)	Undiagnosed diabetes Not enough insulin Eating too much food Too little exercise Stress from surgery, illness, emotional upset, and so on	Weakness Drowsiness Thirst Hunger Frequent urination Flushed face Sweet breath odor Slow, deep, and labored respirations Rapid, weak pulse Low blood pressure Dry skin Headache Nausea and vomiting Coma

DIGESTIVE DISORDERS

The digestive system breaks down food so it can be absorbed by the body. Another function is the elimination of solid wastes. Some digestive disorders have already been discussed in Chapter 16: diarrhea, constipation, flatulence, anal incontinence, and care of persons with colostomies and ileostomies.

Vomiting

Vomiting is the act of expelling stomach contents through the mouth. It is a sign of illness or injury. It can be life-threatening. The vomitus (material vomited) can be aspirated and obstruct the airway. Shock can also occur if large amounts of blood are vomited. The following measures are practiced.

- Use Standard Precautions and follow the Bloodborne Pathogen Standard. Wear gloves if possible.
- Turn the person's head well to one side. This prevents aspiration.
- Place an emesis basin under the person's chin.
- Remove the vomitus from the person's immediate environment.
- Let the person use mouthwash and perform oral hygiene. This helps eliminate the taste of vomitus.
- Eliminate odors.
- Change linens as necessary.
- Observe vomitus for color, odor, and undigested food. Vomitus that looks like coffee grounds contains digested blood. This indicates bleeding.

- Measure the amount of vomitus. The amount is reported to the nurse and recorded on the I&O record.
- Save a specimen for laboratory study.
- Do not discard vomitus until it has been observed by the nurse.

COMMUNICABLE DISEASES

Communicable diseases (contagious or infectious diseases) can be transmitted from one person to another. They can be transmitted in the following ways:

- Direct—from the infected person
- Indirect—from dressings, linens, or surfaces
- Airborne—from the person through sneezing or coughing
- Vehicle—through ingestion of contaminated food, water, drugs, blood, or fluids
- Vector—from animals, fleas, and ticks

This section discusses hepatitis and AIDS. Table 28-2 and Table 28-3 on page 626 outline common childhood and adult communicable diseases. A review of Chapter 9 may be helpful in studying this section.

TABLE 28-2

COMMON COMMUNICABLE CHILDHOOD DISEASES

Disease	Signs and Symptoms	Mode of Transmission	Infective Material
Bacterial meningitis	Fever, severe headache, stiff neck, sore throat	Direct contact	Oral, nasal secretions
Chicken pox (varicella)	Fever, rash, cutaneous vesicles	Airborne, direct contact with drainage	Respiratory secretions, drainage from vesicles
German measles (rubella)	Fever, rash	Airborne, direct contact with oral secretions	Oral secretions
Hepatitis A	Fever, loss of appetite, jaundice, fatigue	Direct contact, oral ingestion of virus	Urine, stool
Measles (rubeola)	Fever, rash, bronchitis	Airborne, direct contact with secretions	Oral secretions
Mumps	Fever, swelling of salivary glands (parotid)	Airborne, direct contact	Saliva
Whooping cough (pertussis)	Violent cough at night, whooping sound when cough subsides	Airborne, direct contact	Oral secretions
Scarlet fever	Fever, headache, nausea, vomiting	Airborne, direct contact	Oral secretions

Reprinted and adapted with permission from Heckman JD: Emergency care and the transportation of the sick and injured, ed 4, Park Ridge, Ill, 1987, American Academy of Orthopaedic Surgeons, pp 361-362.

TABLE 28-3

COMMON ADULT COMMUNICABLE DISEASES

Disease	Signs and Symptoms	Mode of Transmission	Infective Material
AIDS	Fever, night sweats, weight loss, cough	Sexual contact, blood, needles	Blood, semen, possibly saliva
Gonorrhea	Discharge from the urethra or vagina, lower abdominal pain, fever	Sexual contact	Genitourinary secretions
Hepatitis B	Fever, fatigue, loss of appetite, nausea, headache	Blood, oral secretions, sexual contact	Blood, saliva, semen
Hepatitis C	Fever, headache, fatigue, jaundice	Blood	Blood
Malaria	Cyclic fever, chills, fever	Blood-mosquito vector	Blood
Mononucleosis	Fever, sore throat, fatigue	Mouth-to-mouth contact	Oral secretions
Pneumonia	Fever, cough	Airborne	Sputum
Syphilis	Genital and cutaneous lesions, nerve degeneration (late)	Sexual contact, blood	Drainage from genital lesions, blood
Tuberculosis	Fever, night sweats, weight loss, cough	Airborne	Sputum

Reprinted and adapted with permission from Heckman JD: Emergency care and the transportation of the sick and injured, ed 4, Park Ridge, Ill, 1987, American Academy of Orthopaedic Surgeons, pp 361-362.

Hepatitis

Hepatitis is an inflammatory disease of the liver. There are different types of hepatitis.

Type A (infectious hepatitis) is usually spread by the fecal-oral route. Food, water, or drinking or eating vessels can be contaminated with feces. The virus is ingested when the person eats or drinks contaminated food or water. It can also be ingested when a person eats or drinks from a vessel contaminated with the virus. Causes include poor sanitation, crowded living conditions, poor nutrition, and poor hygiene practices. The disease is more common in children. You must be careful when handling bedpans, feces, and rectal thermometers. Good handwashing is essential for you and the person. Standard Precautions are followed.

Type B (serum hepatitis) is usually transmitted by blood and sexual contact. The type B virus is present in blood, saliva, semen, and urine of infected persons. The virus is spread by contaminated blood or blood products and by sharing needles and syringes among IV drug users. There is a vaccine to prevent hepatitis B. See Chapter 9 for a review of the Occupational Safety and Health Administration (OSHA) standard for occupational exposure to bloodborne pathogens.

Hepatitis can be mild or can cause death. The signs and symptoms of hepatitis include:

- Loss of appetite
- Weakness, fatigue, exhaustion
- Nausea
- Vomiting
- Fever
- Skin rash
- Dark urine
- Jaundice (yellowish skin color)
- Light-colored stools
- Headache
- Chills
- Abdominal pain

You must protect yourself and others from the hepatitis virus. Standard Precautions and OSHA's Bloodborne Pathogen Standard are necessary to prevent the spread of hepatitis. Transmission-Based Precautions may be ordered (see Chapter 9, page 204).

Acquired Immunodeficiency Syndrome (AIDS)

Acquired immunodeficiency syndrome (AIDS) is caused by a virus. The virus is called the human immunodeficiency virus (HIV). The virus attacks the body's immune system. It affects the person's ability to fight other diseases. There is presently no cure for AIDS and no vaccine to prevent the disease. AIDS eventually causes death.

The virus is carried in blood, semen, vaginal secretions, and breastmilk of infected persons. HIV is not spread by insects or casual contact. AIDS is transmitted mainly by

- Sexual contact (oral, anal, or vaginal) with an infected person
- Needle-sharing among intravenous drug users
- Transfusions of infected blood
- HIV-infected mothers before, during, or shortly after childbirth

The virus enters the bloodstream through the rectum, vagina, penis, or mouth. Small breaks in the mucous membrane of the vagina or rectum may occur when the penis, finger, or other objects are inserted. Gum disease can cause breaks in the mucous membrane of the gums. The breaks in the mucous membrane of the mouth, vagina, or rectum provide a route for the virus to enter the bloodstream.

Intravenous drug users transmit AIDS through the use of contaminated needles and syringes. The virus is carried in the contaminated blood left in needles or syringes. When needles and syringes are used by others, contaminated blood enters their bloodstreams.

Infection can also occur when infected body fluids come in contact with open areas on the skin. Babies can become infected during pregnancy or shortly after birth.

Persons at risk for AIDS are:

- Homosexual or bisexual men
- Intravenous drug users
- Sex partners of those who are homosexual, bisexual, and intravenous drug users
- Infants born to infected mothers
- Persons who received contaminated blood or blood products

Signs and symptoms of AIDS are listed in Box 28-11. Some persons infected with HIV do not develop AIDS for

BOX 28-11 Signs and Symptoms of Acquired Immunodeficiency Syndrome (AIDS)

- Loss of appetite
- Weight loss greater than 10 pounds without reason
- Fever
- Night sweats
- Diarrhea
- Tiredness, extreme or constant
- Skin rashes
- Swollen glands in the neck, underarms, and groin
- Dry cough
- White spots in the mouth or on the tongue
- Purple blotches or bumps on the skin that look like bruises but do not disappear
- Dementia (see Chapter 30)

as long as 10 to 12 years. They may not show signs or symptoms of the disease. However, they are carriers of the virus. They can spread the disease to others.

Persons with AIDS develop other diseases. Their bodies do not have the ability to fight disease. Their immune system, which fights diseases, is damaged. The person is at risk for pneumonia, Kaposi's sarcoma (a type of cancer), and central nervous system damage. The person with central nervous system damage may show memory loss, loss of coordination, paralysis, and mental disorders.

You may care for persons with AIDS or HIV carriers (Box 28-12). You may have contact with the person's blood, body fluids, secretions, and excretions. Mouth-to-mouth contact is possible during CPR. Certain precautions are necessary to protect yourself and others from the AIDS virus. Standard Precautions and the Bloodborne Pathogen Standard are followed (see Chapter 9, pages 204-208). *These precautions apply when caring for all persons.* Remember, you may care for a person who has the HIV virus but shows no symptoms. You may also care for a person who has not yet been diagnosed as having AIDS.

BOX 28-12 Caring for the Person with AIDS

- Practice Standard Precautions (see Chapter 9).
- Follow the Bloodborne Pathogen Standard (see Chapter 9).
- Provide daily hygiene; avoid harsh soaps that irritate the skin.
- Provide oral hygiene before meals and at bedtime. Make sure the person uses a toothbrush with soft bristles.
- Provide oral fluids as ordered.
- Measure and record intake and output.
- Measure weight daily.
- Have the person perform deep breathing and coughing exercises as ordered.
- Practice measures to prevent pressure sores.
- Assist with range-of-motion exercises and ambulation as ordered.
- Encourage the person to perform self-care as able. Assistive devices may be needed (walkers, commode, eating devices).
- Encourage the person to be as active as possible.
- Change linens, gowns, or pajamas as often as needed when fever is present.
- Be a good listener and provide emotional support.

SUMMARY

A person may have one or more disorders. For example, Martha Powers has arthritis, diabetes, heart disease, and osteoporosis. Problems increase if a fracture occurs. She is then at risk for infection, pneumonia, and complications from bed rest. The care required depends on the nature and number of health problems.

Quality of life is important for persons with health problems. The care you give them has been presented in previous chapters. Safety, good alignment, turning and repositioning, preventing infection, skin care, urinary and bowel elimination, and nutrition are some examples.

The right to privacy and confidentiality is very important. Remember, only discuss the person's problems with the nurse and health team members involved in the person's care. You are not responsible for giving information to families and visitors. You must not discuss patients or residents outside the facility. Your own family and friends should not hear about patients and residents.

The right to personal choice must be protected. Be sure to explain what you are going to do. The person's consent is necessary. Also involve the person in deciding when to begin care or procedures.

Be sure to protect the person from abuse, mistreatment, and neglect. This is very important for persons with communicable diseases. Health team members may tend to avoid the person out of fear of getting the disease. Standard Precautions and the Bloodborne Pathogen Standard serve to protect others from contamination and infection.

Only very basic information was given about each disorder. Entire textbooks have been written on many of these disorders. You are not expected to have an in-depth understanding of every health problem. However, the information in this chapter gives you a better understanding of the physical, psychological, and social needs of patients and residents.

REVIEW QUESTIONS

Circle the best *answer.*

1 The spread of cancer to other body parts is
- **a** A malignant tumor
- **b** Metastasis
- **c** Gangrene
- **d** A benign tumor

2 Which is *not* a warning sign of cancer?
- **a** Painful, swollen joints
- **b** A sore that does not heal
- **c** Unusual bleeding or discharge from a body opening
- **d** Nagging cough or hoarseness

3 Martha Powers has arthritis. Care does *not* include
- **a** Measures to prevent contractures
- **b** Range-of-motion exercises
- **c** A cast or traction
- **d** Assistance with activities of daily living

4 A cast needs to dry. Which is *false?*
- **a** The cast is covered with blankets or plastic.
- **b** The person is turned as directed so the cast dries evenly.
- **c** The entire length of the cast is supported with pillows.
- **d** The cast is supported by the palms when lifted.

5 A person has a cast. Which are reported immediately?
- **a** Pain, numbness, or inability to move the fingers or toes
- **b** Chills, fever, or nausea and vomiting
- **c** Odor, cyanosis, or temperature changes of the skin
- **d** All of the above

6 A person is in traction. You should do the following *except*
- **a** Perform range-of-motion exercises as directed
- **b** Keep the weights off the floor
- **c** Remove the weights if the person is uncomfortable
- **d** Give skin care at frequent intervals

7 A person has had a hip pinning. The operated leg is
- **a** Abducted at all times
- **b** Adducted at all times
- **c** Externally rotated at all times
- **d** Flexed at all times

8 Martha Powers has osteoporosis. She is at risk for
- **a** Fractures
- **b** An amputation
- **c** Phantom limb pain
- **d** All of the above

9 A person has had an amputation. Why will the person have a psychological adjustment?
- **a** Activities of daily living are affected.
- **b** Appearance is affected.
- **c** The person's job may be affected.
- **d** All of the above.

10 A person has had a CVA. Which is *false?*
- **a** Blood supply to part of the brain was interrupted.
- **b** Hemiplegia may occur.
- **c** Aphasia may occur.
- **d** Changes in brain tissue are progressive.

11 A person has had a stroke. The nurse tells you to do the following. Which should you question?
- **a** Elevate the head of the bed to a semi-Fowler's position.
- **b** Do range-of-motion exercises every 2 hours.
- **c** Turn, reposition, and give skin care every 2 hours.
- **d** Keep the bed in the highest horizontal position.

12 A person has receptive aphasia. This means that the person
- **a** Cannot talk
- **b** Cannot write
- **c** Has trouble understanding messages
- **d** All of the above

REVIEW QUESTIONS—CONT'D

13 A person has Parkinson's disease. Which is *false?*

- **a** Parkinson's disease affects part of the brain.
- **b** The person's mental function is affected first.
- **c** Signs and symptoms include stiff muscles, slow movements, and a shuffling gait.
- **d** The person is protected from injury.

14 A person has multiple sclerosis. Which is *false?*

- **a** Nerve impulses are sent to and from the brain in a normal manner.
- **b** Symptoms begin in young adulthood.
- **c** There is no cure.
- **d** The person is eventually paralyzed and totally dependent on others for care.

15 Persons with head or spinal cord injuries require

- **a** Rehabilitation
- **b** Speech therapy
- **c** Care in a nursing facility
- **d** Psychiatric care

16 A quadriplegic has paralysis

- **a** Of the legs, arms, and trunk
- **b** On one side of the body
- **c** Of the legs
- **d** Of the legs and trunk

17 A person has emphysema. Which is *false?*

- **a** The person has dyspnea only with activity.
- **b** Cigarette smoking is the most common cause.
- **c** The person will probably breathe easier sitting upright and slightly forward.
- **d** Sputum may contain pus.

18 A person has pneumonia. Standard Precautions are required.

- **a** True
- **b** False

19 A person has hypertension. Which complication can occur?

- **a** Stroke
- **b** Heart attack
- **c** Renal failure
- **d** All of the above

20 A person has hypertension. Treatment will probably include the following *except*

- **a** No smoking and regular exercise
- **b** A high-sodium diet
- **c** A low-calorie diet if the person is obese
- **d** Medications to lower the blood pressure

21 A person has angina pectoris. Which is *true?*

- **a** Damage to the heart muscle occurs.
- **b** The pain is described as crushing, stabbing, or squeezing.
- **c** The pain is relieved with rest and nitroglycerin.
- **d** All of the above.

22 A person is having a myocardial infarction. You know that

- **a** The person is having a heart attack
- **b** This is an emergency situation
- **c** The person may have a cardiac arrest
- **d** All of the above

23 A person has heart failure. The following measures have been ordered. Which should you question?

- **a** Force fluids
- **b** Measure intake and output
- **c** Measure weight daily
- **d** Perform range-of-motion exercises

24 A person has cystitis. This is

- **a** A kidney infection
- **b** Kidney stones
- **c** A urinary tract infection
- **d** An inflammation of the bladder

25 A person has acute renal failure. Recovery is likely.

- **a** True
- **b** False

26 A person has chronic renal failure. Care will include all of the following *except*

- **a** A diet low in protein, potassium, and sodium
- **b** Measuring urinary output every hour
- **c** Measures to prevent pressure sores
- **d** Measuring weight daily

REVIEW QUESTIONS—CONT'D

27 Which is not a sign of diabetes mellitus?
- **a** Increased urine production
- **b** Weight gain
- **c** Hunger
- **d** Increased thirst

28 Martha Powers has diabetes. She needs all of the following *except*
- **a** Her meals served on time
- **b** Good foot care
- **c** Oral insulin
- **d** Diet therapy

29 Vomiting is dangerous because of
- **a** Aspiration
- **b** Cardiac arrest
- **c** Fluid loss
- **d** Stroke

30 AIDS and hepatitis require
- **a** Airborne Precautions
- **b** Contact Precautions
- **c** Standard Precautions
- **d** Droplet Precautions

31 AIDS is usually spread by contact with infected
- **a** Blood
- **b** Urine
- **c** Tears
- **d** Saliva

32 These statements are about HIV and AIDS. Which is *false?*
- **a** Standard Precautions are practiced and the Blood Pathogen Standard is followed.
- **b** There may be signs and symptoms of central nervous system damage.
- **c** The person is at risk for infection.
- **d** The person always shows some signs and symptoms.

Answers to these questions are on page 752.

Mental Health Problems

29

OBJECTIVES

- Define the key terms listed in this chapter
- Explain the difference between mental health and mental illness
- List the causes of mental illness
- Explain how an individual's personality develops
- Describe three levels of awareness
- Describe anxiety
- Understand the defense mechanisms used to relieve anxiety
- Explain three anxiety disorders
- Describe common phobias
- Explain schizophrenia
- Describe bipolar disorder and depression
- Describe three types of personality disorders
- Describe substance abuse, anorexia nervosa, and bulimia
- Describe the care required by a person with a mental health disorder

KEY TERMS

affect Feelings and emotions

anxiety A vague, uneasy feeling that occurs in response to stress

compulsion The uncontrolled performance of an act

conscious Awareness of the environment and experiences; the person knows what is happening and can control thoughts and behaviors

defense mechanism An unconscious reaction that blocks unpleasant or threatening feelings

delusion A false belief

delusion of grandeur An exaggerated belief about one's own importance, wealth, power, or talents

delusion of persecution A false belief that one is being mistreated, abused, or harassed

ego The part of the personality dealing with reality; deals with thoughts, feelings, good sense, and problem solving

emotional illness Mental illness, mental disorder, psychiatric disorder

hallucination Seeing, hearing, or feeling something that is not real

id The part of the personality at the unconscious level; concerned with pleasure

mental Relating to the mind; something that exists in the mind or is performed by the mind

mental disorder Mental illness; emotional disorder, psychiatric disorder

mental health A state of mind in which the person copes with and adjusts to the stresses of everyday living in ways acceptable to society

mental illness A disturbance in the person's ability to cope or adjust to stress; behavior and functioning are impaired; mental disorder, emotional illness, psychiatric disorder

obsession A persistent thought or idea

panic An intense and sudden feeling of fear, anxiety, terror, or dread

paranoia A disorder *(para)* of the mind *(noia);* false beliefs (delusions) and suspicion about a person or situation

personality The set of attitudes, values, behaviors, and characteristics of a particular person

phobia Fear, panic, or dread

psychiatric disorder Mental illness, mental disorder, emotional disorder

psychosis A serious mental disorder; the person does not view or interpret reality correctly

stress The response or change in the body caused by any emotional, physical, social, or economic factor

stressor Any emotional, physical, social, or economic factor that causes stress

subconscious Memory, past experiences, and thoughts of which the person is not aware; they can be easily recalled

superego The part of the personality concerned with what is right and wrong

unconscious Experiences and feelings that cannot be remembered

The whole person has physical, social, psychological, and spiritual parts. As explained in Chapter 4, these parts cannot be separated. Each part affects the other. A physical problem affects the person socially, mentally, and spiritually. Likewise, mental health problems affect the person physically, socially, and spiritually. A social problem can have physical, mental health, and spiritual effects.

You will care for patients and residents who have physical problems. In turn, emotional or mental health problems may develop. Or a person with a mental health problem may need hospital care because of physical illness. You may also work in a mental health setting. The setting may be a mental health hospital, a mental health unit in a hospital, or a community health agency. Persons with mental health problems are also seen in home settings. Mentally ill persons often have physical problems resulting from mental health problems.

BASIC CONCEPTS

Mental health and mental illness are opposites (Fig. 29-1). However, just like physical health and physical illness, there are levels of seriousness. At one extreme is the person with the common cold. The person has chills, fever, and respiratory congestion. At the other extreme is a person with a life-threatening illness. Mental health has the same extremes.

Mental Health

Mental relates to the mind. It is something that exists in the mind or is performed by the mind. Therefore mental health involves the mind. There are many definitions of mental health and mental illness. Different textbooks have different definitions. So do various cultures. Most definitions include the concept of stress. For purposes of this textbook, the following definitions are used.

- **Stress** is the response or change in the body caused by any emotional, physical, social, or economic factor.
- **Mental health** is a state of mind in which the person copes with and adjusts to the stresses of everyday living in ways acceptable to society.
- **Mental illness** is a disturbance in the person's ability to cope or adjust to stress. The person's behavior and functioning are impaired. **Mental disorder, emotional illness,** and **psychiatric disorder** also mean mental illness.

Mental health disorders have many causes. Some result when the person cannot cope or adjust to stress. Others are caused by chemical imbalances in the body. Some are genetic in origin. Genes are found in chromosomes. Characteristics from parents are passed onto children through genes contained in the chromosomes. Other causes include drug or substance abuse. Social and cultural factors can also lead to mental illness.

Personality

Personality is the set of attitudes, values, behaviors, and characteristics of a particular person. Personality development starts at birth. Genes, culture, environment, parenting, and social experiences are among the many factors that affect and influence personality development.

Maslow's theory of basic needs (see Chapter 4) affects personality development. Lower level needs must be met before higher level needs. Safety and security, love and belonging, esteem, and self-actualization needs cannot be met unless the physical needs are met. A child who grows up hungry, neglected, cold, or abused will not feel safe and secure. Higher level needs cannot be met. Unmet needs at any age affect personality development.

The growth and development tasks presented in Chapter 6 also affect personality development. Remember, there is a sequence, order, and pattern to growth and development. Certain developmental tasks must be accomplished at each stage. Each stage lays the foundation for the next stage.

Sigmund Freud's theory of personality development involves the id, ego, and superego. To understand his theory, you need to understand three levels of awareness:

- **Conscious**—awareness of the environment and experiences; the person knows what is happening and can control thoughts and behavior.
- **Subconscious**—the memory, past experiences, and thoughts of which the person is not aware. Such thoughts, experiences, and memory are easily recalled.
- **Unconscious**—experiences and feelings that cannot be remembered.

The **id** part of the personality is at the unconscious level. The id is concerned with pleasure. The need for pleasure must be satisfied almost immediately. The id deals with hunger, comfort, sex, and warmth. The person is not aware that he or she behaves and acts in ways to satisfy the id.

The **ego** deals with reality, with what is happening in the person's world. Thoughts, feelings, reasoning, good sense, and problem-solving occur in the ego. The ego decides what to do and when.

The **superego** is concerned with what is right and wrong. Morals and values are in the superego. The superego judges what the ego thinks and does. It is like a parent helping a child look at behaviors.

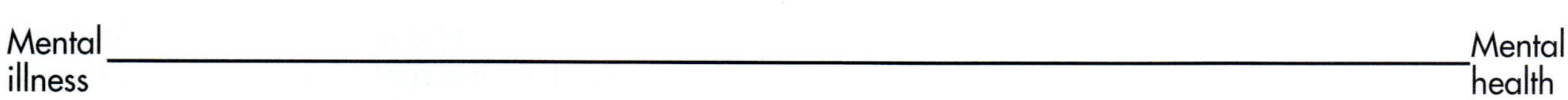

Fig 29-1 *Mental health and mental illness are at two extremes. There are various levels of seriousness in between the extremes.*

Anxiety

Anxiety is a vague, uneasy feeling. It is a response to stress. The person may not know the source or cause of the uneasy feeling. The person has a sense of danger or harm. Danger or harm may be real or imagined. Anxiety is usually a normal emotion. The person acts to relieve the unpleasant feeling. Anxiety generally occurs when the person's needs are not met. Anxiety is seen in all mental health disorders.

There are many signs and symptoms of anxiety (Box 29-1). They depend on the degree of anxiety. Persons with mental health disorders have higher levels of anxiety.

The level of anxiety depends on the stressor. A **stressor** is any emotional, physical, social, or economic factor that causes stress. Past experiences with the same or a similar stressor affect how a person reacts. The number of stressors also affects the person's reaction. A stressor at one time in a person's life may produce only mild anxiety. The same stressor may produce a higher level of anxiety at another time.

BOX 29-1 Signs and Symptoms of Anxiety

- A "lump" in the throat
- "Butterflies" in the stomach
- Rapid pulse
- Rapid respirations
- Increased blood pressure
- Rapid speech
- Voice changes
- Dry mouth
- Perspiration
- Nausea
- Diarrhea
- Urinary frequency
- Urinary urgency
- Poor attention span
- Difficulty following directions
- Difficulty sleeping
- Loss of appetite

Coping and defense mechanisms are used to relieve anxiety. Common coping mechanisms include eating, drinking, smoking, exercising, talking about the problem, and fighting. Some people play music, go for a walk, take a hot bath, or want to be alone. Some coping mechanisms are healthier than others.

Defense mechanisms are unconscious reactions that block unpleasant or threatening feelings. Defense mechanisms protect the ego. They are used by everyone. Some use of defense mechanisms is normal. They relieve anxiety. Persons with mental health disorders use defense mechanisms inappropriately. Box 29-2 on page 638 describes the common defense mechanisms.

MENTAL HEALTH DISORDERS

There are many types of mental health disorders. Some affect thinking, others affect mood. There are anxiety disorders and personality disorders. Substance abuse and eating disorders also are mental health problems. Changes in the brain are another cause. Dementia can occur (see Chapter 30).

Anxiety Disorders

Persons with anxiety disorders have high degrees of anxiety. Signs and symptoms depend on the anxiety level.

Panic disorder Panic is the highest level of anxiety. **Panic** is an intense and sudden feeling of fear, anxiety, terror, or dread that occurs suddenly with no obvious reason. The person cannot function and has severe signs and symptoms of anxiety. *Panic attacks* can last for a few minutes or for hours. They can occur several times a week.

BOX 29-2 Defense Mechanisms

Compensation—compensate means to make up for, replace, or substitute. Compensation means to make up for or substitute a strength for a weakness.
Example: Joe Williams is not good in sports. But he learns to play the guitar well.

Conversion—to convert means to change. Conversion is when an emotion is expressed or changed into a physical symptom.
Example: Danny Monroe knows that he will have to read out loud in school today. He does not want to go to school. He complains of a stomach ache.

Denial—to deny means to refuse to accept or believe something that is true or correct. Denial is when the person refuses to face or accept something that is unpleasant or threatening.
Example: Greg Adams had a heart attack. He is told to quit smoking and to eat a low fat diet. He continues to smoke and eat fatty foods.

Displacement—to displace means to move or take the place of. Displacement is when an individual moves his or her behavior or emotions from one person, place, or thing to another person, place, or thing. The behavior or emotion is directed at a safe person, place, or thing.
Example: You are angry with your supervisor. Instead of yelling at your supervisor, you yell at your husband when you get home.

Identification—to identify means to relate or recognize. Identification is when a person assumes the ideas, behaviors, and traits of another person.
Example: A little girl admires her neighbor who is a high school cheerleader. The little girl practices cheerleading in her back yard.

Projection—project means to blame or assign responsibility to another. Projection is blaming another person or object for one's own unacceptable behavior, emotions, ideas, or wishes.
Example: Molly and June are in the same class. Molly fails a test and blames June for not helping her study.

Rationalization—rational means sensible, reasonable, or logical. To rationalize means to give some acceptable reason or excuse for one's behavior or actions. The real reason is not given.
Example: Jane Doe does not study for a test and gets a poor grade. Jane says that the teacher is too hard and doesn't like her.

Reaction formation is when a person acts in a way that is opposite to what he or she truly feels.
Example: Peter Smith does not like his boss. Peter buys the boss an expensive gift for Christmas.

Regression—to regress means to move back or to retreat. Regression means to retreat or move back to an earlier time or condition.
Example: A 3-year-old wants to drink from a baby bottle when a new baby comes into the family.

Repression—to repress means to hold down or keep back. Repression is keeping unpleasant or painful thoughts or experiences from the conscious mind. Such thoughts and experiences are in the unconscious mind and cannot be recalled or remembered.
Example: When she was 8 years old, Terry Taft was sexually abused by her father. She is now 33 years old and has no memory of the event.

Phobic disorders **Phobia** means fear, panic, or dread. The person with a phobia has an intense fear of an object or situation. Common phobias are described in Box 29-3.

BOX 29-3 Common Phobias

Agoraphobia—*agora* means marketplace; *phobia* means fear
Fear of being in an open, crowded, or public place

Algophobia—*algo* means pain; *phobia* means fear
Fear of being in pain or seeing others in pain

Aquaphobia—*aqua* means water; *phobia* means fear
Fear of water

Claustrophobia—*claustro* means closing, *phobia* means fear
Fear of being in or being trapped in an enclosed or narrow space

Gynephobia—*gyne* means woman; *phobia* means fear
Fear of women

Laliophobia—*lalio* means to talk or babble; *phobia* means fear
Fear of talking because of the fear of stuttering

Mysophobia—*myso* means anything that is disgusting; *phobia* means fear
Fear of the slightest uncleanliness; fear of dirt or contamination

Nyctophobia—*nycto* means night or darkness; *phobia* means fear
Fear of night or darkness

Photophobia—*photo* pertains to light; *phobia* means fear
Fear of light with the need to avoid light places

Pyrophobia—*pyro* means fire; *phobia* means fear
Fear of fire

Xenophobia—*xeno* means strange; *phobia* means fear
Fear of strangers

Obsessive-compulsive disorder An **obsession** is a persistent thought or idea. The thought or idea may be violent. **Compulsion** is the uncontrolled performance of an act. The person knows the act is wrong but has much anxiety if the act is not done. Some eating disorders are obsessive-compulsive. The person is obsessed with thoughts of food and eats constantly. Constant handwashing because of mysophobia (fear of dirt or contamination) is another. Some obsessive-compulsive disorders involve violent acts.

Schizophrenia

Schizophrenia means split *(schizo)* mind *(phrenia)*. The following terms are important to understand schizophrenia:

- **Psychosis** means a serious mental disorder. The person does not view or interpret reality correctly.
- **Delusion** is a false belief. A person believes he or she is God, a movie star, or some other person.
- **Hallucination** is seeing, hearing, or feeling something that is not real. A person may see animals, insects, or people that are not present.
- **Paranoia** means a disorder *(para)* of the mind *(noia)*. The person has false beliefs (delusions) and is suspicious about a person or situation. For example, a woman believes she is being stalked or person believes his food and drinks are poisoned.
- **Delusion of grandeur** is an exaggerated belief about one's own importance, wealth, power, or talents. For example, a person believes he is Superman or a woman believes she is the Queen of England.
- **Delusion of persecution** is the false belief that one is being mistreated, abused, or harassed. For example, a person believes that a person or group is "out to get" him or her.

The person with schizophrenia has a disorder of the mind (psychosis). Thinking and behavior are disturbed. The person has delusions (false beliefs) and hallucinations (seeing, hearing, or feeling things that are not real). The person has difficulty relating to others and may be paranoid (suspicion about a person or situation). The person's responses are inappropriate. Communication is disturbed. The person may ramble or repeat what another says. Sometimes speech cannot be understood. The person may withdraw from others and the world. That is, the person lacks interest in others and is not involved with people or society. The person may sit for hours alone without moving, speaking, or responding. Some persons *regress*. To regress means to retreat or move back to an earlier time or condition. For example, it is normal for a 5-year-old to regress back to bedwetting when there is a new baby in the family. It is not normal for an adult to have the behaviors of an infant or child. However, that is often seen in schizophrenia.

Affective Disorders

Affect relates to feelings and emotions. Affective disorders involve feelings, emotions, and moods. There are two major affective disorders.

Bipolar disorder *Bipolar* means two *(bi)* poles or ends *(polar)*. The person with bipolar disorder has extreme mood swings. Depression is at one extreme. Mania (elation) is at the other extreme. The person may:

- Be more depressed than manic
- Be more manic than depressed
- Alternate between depression and mania

When depressed, the person is very sad and feels lonely, worthless, empty, and hopeless. Self-esteem is low. The person may think about suicide.

In the manic phase, the person is excited, has much energy, is very busy, cannot sleep, and does not take time to eat or tend to self-care needs. Delusions of grandeur are common.

Major depression The person is very unhappy, lacks motivation, and feels unwanted. These feelings are extreme. There also are problems with concentration. Body functions are depressed. Sleeping problems and inactivity are common. Constipation can occur.

Personality Disorders

The individual with a personality disorder has rigid, inflexible, and maladaptive behaviors. To *adapt* means to change or adjust. *Mal* means bad, wrong, or ill. Maladaptive means to change or adjust in the wrong way. Because of their behaviors, individuals with personality disorders cannot function well in society. Personality disorders include:

- **Abusive personality**—the person copes with anxiety by abusing others. The person's behavior may be violent.
- **Paranoid personality**—the person is very suspicious. There is distrust of others.
- **Antisocial personality**—the person has poor judgment, lacks responsibility, is hostile, and has no loyalty to any person or group. Morals and ethics are lacking. The person blames others for actions and behaviors. The rights of others are not considered. The person has no guilt and does not learn from past experiences or punishment. The person is often in trouble with law enforcement authorities.

Substance Abuse

Substance abuse occurs when a person physically or psychologically depends on drugs or alcohol. Alcohol is abused more than any other drug or substance. Both legal and illegal drugs are abused. Legal drugs are those approved for use in the United States. They are prescribed by doctors. Illegal drugs have not been approved for use. They are obtained through illegal means. Commonly abused drugs are listed in Box 29-4. Abused substances affect the central nervous system. Some have a depressing effect. Others stimulate the nervous system. All affect the mind and thinking.

BOX 29-4 Commonly Abused Substances

NARCOTICS

- Opium
- Morphine
- Codeine
- Heroin
- Meperidine (Demerol)
- Methadone

DEPRESSANTS

- Chloral Hydrate (Noctec)
- Barbiturates (Nembutal, Phenobarbital, Secobarbital, Tuinal)
- Benzodiazepines (Dalmane, Diazepam, Halcion, Librium, Tranxene, Valium, Xanax)

STIMULANTS

- Cocaine (Coke, Flake, Snow)
- Amphetamines (Uppers)

HALLUCINOGENS

- LSD (Acid)
- Mescaline and Peyote (Mesc, Buttons, Cactus)
- Phencyclidine (PCP, Angel dust, Hog)

CANNABIS

- Marijuana (Pot, Acapulco Gold, Grass, Reefer, Sinsemilla, Thai Sticks)
- Hashish (Hash)
- Hashish Oil (Hash)

Modified from Rawlins RP, Williams SR, and Beck CK: Mental health-psychiatric nursing: a holistic life-cycle approach, ed 3, St Louis, 1993, Mosby—Year Book.

Eating Disorders

There are two common eating disorders: anorexia nervosa and bulimia.

Anorexia nervosa Anorexia nervosa occurs when a person has an abnormal fear of weight gain and obesity. The disorder is seen in adolescent girls. The person believes she is fat despite body weight and appearance. She has a poor self-image. Sleep disturbances, depression, and amenorrhea occur. *Amenorrhea* means lack of *(a)* monthly *(meno)* flow *(rrhea)*. In other words, she stops having monthly menstrual periods. There also may be suicidal thoughts. The person with anorexia nervosa is severely emaciated (Fig. 29-2). *Emaciation* means extreme leanness from disease or poor nutrition.

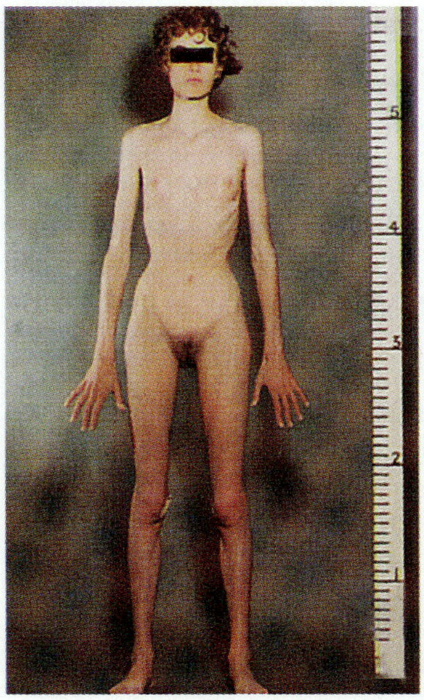

Fig. 29-2 *Emaciation from anorexia nervosa.* *(From Color atlas and text of clinical medicine, second edition by Forbes & Jackson, 1996. Mosby-Wolfe Limited, London, UK.)*

Bulimia *Bulimia* comes from the Greek words that mean ox *(bous)* and hunger *(limos)*. The person with bulimia craves food. There is often constant eating or binge eating. After eating, the person induces vomiting. That is, the body is purged (rid) of the food eaten. Some take diuretics. Diuretics cause the kidneys to produce large amounts of urine. Extra fluid in the body is lost. This results in weight loss. Laxative abuse may occur. Laxatives are drugs that rid the intestines of feces through defecation.

CARE OF PERSONS WITH MENTAL HEALTH DISORDERS

Treatment of mental health disorders involves having the person explore his or her thoughts and feelings. Psychotherapy, group therapy, occupational therapy, art therapy, and family therapy allow and encourage feelings to be expressed. Often medications are ordered. Drugs may be ordered for anxiety or depression.

The nurse uses the nursing process to meet the person's needs. The needs of the total person must be met. This includes the person's physical, safety and security, and emotional needs. The nurse shares the person's care plan with you. You also may be involved in sessions to plan the person's care.

Communication is important in caring for persons with mental health disorders. You need to review pages 45-46 in Chapter 3 and pages 81-87 in Chapter 4. You must be alert to nonverbal communication. This includes the person's nonverbal communication and your own.

SUMMARY

Mental health disorders occur in persons of all ages. There are many causes. Mentally ill people are seen in all health care settings. The person may need treatment for a physical problem or for the mental health problem. Whatever the reason for care, the person is treated as a physical, psychological, social, and spiritual being. The person's basic needs must be met. The person's rights must also be protected.

The nurse explains the person's care to you. Often strict limits are placed on the person's behavior. If you do not understand the purpose of a certain care measure, be sure to ask the nurse.

Communication is very important. Be sure to review Chapters 3 and 4. You must observe the person's body language. Be sure to report what the person says and does to the nurse. Also be careful of your own body language. Mentally ill persons are often very alert to the body language of others.

Review Questions

Circle the best *answer.*

1 Patty Walls has a mental health problem. The doctor says that she is under stress. Stress is
- **a** The way she copes with and adjusts to everyday living
- **b** A response or change in the body caused by some factor
- **c** A mental or emotional disorder
- **d** A thought or idea

2 The doctor asks Patty's parents about her personality development. Personality is
- **a** The id and the ego
- **b** A person's attitudes, values, behaviors, and characteristics
- **c** The coping and defense mechanisms used by a person
- **d** All of the above

3 The doctor says that Patty has many unpleasant experiences in her subconscious. You know that Patty
- **a** Can remember those experiences
- **b** Cannot remember those experiences
- **c** Is aware of those experiences
- **d** Is projecting those experiences to others

4 Which part of Patty's personality is concerned with right and wrong?
- **a** The id
- **b** The ego
- **c** The superego
- **d** The conscious

5 Patty uses defense mechanisms. Defense mechanisms are used to
- **a** Blame others
- **b** Make excuses for behavior
- **c** Return to an earlier time
- **d** Block unpleasant feelings

6 These statements are about defense mechanisms. Which is *false?*
- **a** Mentally healthy persons do not use defense mechanisms.
- **b** Defense mechanisms protect the ego.
- **c** Defense mechanisms relieve anxiety.
- **d** All of the above.

7 Patty also has phobias. A phobia is
- **a** A serious mental disorder
- **b** A false belief
- **c** An intense fear of an object or situation
- **d** Feelings and emotions

8 Patty believes she is married to a rock singer. She is constantly trying to telephone him. This behavior is a
- **a** Delusion
- **b** Hallucination
- **c** Compulsion
- **d** Obsession

9 Patty's belief that she is married to a rock singer is called a
- **a** Fantasy
- **b** Delusion of grandeur
- **c** Delusion of persecution
- **d** Hallucination

10 Patty believes that her parents are against her and her marriage. This belief is called
- **a** Fantasy
- **b** Delusion of grandeur
- **c** Delusion of persecution
- **d** Hallucination

REVIEW QUESTIONS—CONT'D

11 Patty's roommate has bipolar disorder. This means that the person

- **a** Is very suspicious
- **b** Has poor judgment, lacks responsibility, and is hostile
- **c** Is very unhappy and feels unwanted
- **d** Has severe mood swings

12 A person has an abusive personality. You know that the person

- **a** Abuses drugs or alcohol
- **b** Has an eating disorder
- **c** Has bulimia
- **d** May have violent behavior

Answers to these questions are on page 753.

Confusion and Dementia

30

OBJECTIVES

- Define the key terms listed in this chapter
- Describe confusion and its causes
- List the measures that help confused persons
- Describe Alzheimer's disease
- Describe the signs, symptoms, and behaviors associated with Alzheimer's disease
- Explain the care required by persons with Alzheimer's disease
- Describe the effects of Alzheimer's disease on the family

Key Terms

delusion A false belief

dementia The term used to describe mental disorders caused by changes in the brain

hallucination Seeing, hearing, or feeling something that is not real

pseudodementia False *(pseudo)* disorder of the mind *(dementia)*

sundowning Increased signs, symptoms, and behaviors of Alzheimer's disease during hours of darkness

Some changes in the brain and nervous system occur normally with aging (Box 30-1 on page 646). Certain diseases can also cause changes in the brain. No matter the cause, changes in the brain can affect the person's cognitive function. (Cognitive relates to knowledge.) Cognitive functioning relates to memory, thinking, reasoning, ability to understand, judgment, and behavior.

CONFUSION

Confusion has many causes. Diseases, infections, losses of hearing and sight, and reactions to medications are some major causes. Brain injury and physical changes from aging are other causes. With aging, there is reduced blood supply to the brain and progressive loss of brain cells. Sometimes personality and mental changes result. Memory and the ability to make judgments are lost. The person may not know people, the time, or the place. There also may be gradual loss in the ability to perform activities of daily living. Behavior changes are common. Anger, restlessness, depression, and irritability may occur.

Acute confusion (delirium) occurs suddenly. Acute confusion is usually caused by infection, illness, injury, or medications. It can occur postoperatively. Treatment is aimed at the cause of the confusion. Usually acute confusion is temporary.

Confusion caused by physical changes cannot be cured. Some measures help to improve the person's functioning (Box 30-2 on page 646). The person's physical and safety needs must be met.

DEMENTIA

Dementia is the term used to describe mental disorders that are caused by changes in the brain. The prefix *de* means opposite, away, off of, to remove, down, or from. *Mentia* comes from the Latin word for mind. Dementias are chronic. There is no cure, and they become progressively worse.

Pseudodementia means false *(pseudo)* dementia. The person has the signs and symptoms of dementia. However, changes in the brain do not occur. This can occur with depression (see Chapter 29).

There are many causes and types of dementia. Brain injury, vascular problems, stroke, tumors, and infection are some causes. Dementia occurs with AIDS and Parkinson's disease. Changes in the brain from aging is another cause. To determine the cause and type of problem, the doctor orders many tests. Treatment depends on the cause and problem. Most dementias are due to the Alzheimer's type.

BOX 30-1 Changes in the Nervous System from Aging

- Brain cells are lost
- Nerve conduction slows
- Response and reaction times are slower
- Reflexes are slower
- Vision and hearing decrease
- Decreased senses of taste and smell
- Reduced sense of touch and sensitivity to pain
- Reduced blood flow to the brain
- Changes in sleep patterns
- Shorter memory
- Forgetfulness
- Confusion
- Dizziness

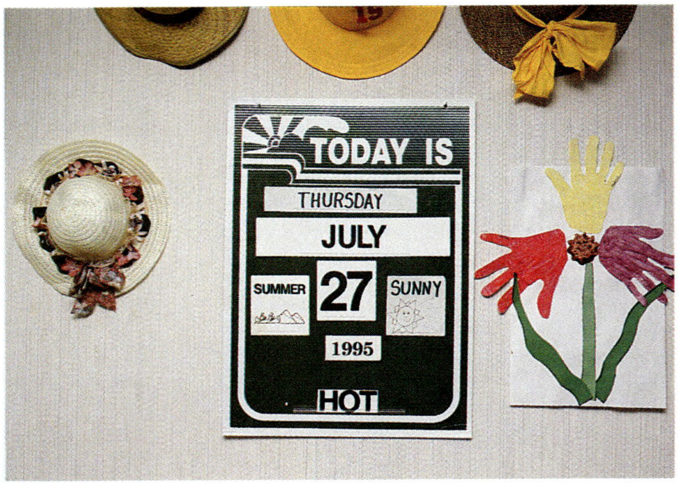

Fig. 30-1 *A large calendar is within the person's view.*

BOX 30-2 Caring for the Confused Person

- Follow the person's care plan to meet basic needs.
- Provide for the person's safety.
- Face the person and speak clearly and slowly.
- Call the person by name every time you are in contact with him or her.
- State your name and show your name tag.
- Tell the person the date and time each morning. Repeat the information as often as necessary during the day or evening.
- Explain what you are going to do and why.
- Give clear and simple answers to questions.
- Ask clear and simple questions. Allow enough time for the person to respond.
- Give short, simple instructions.
- Keep calendars and clocks with large numbers in the person's room and in nursing areas (Fig. 30-1).
- Encourage the person to wear glasses and a hearing aid if needed.
- Use touch to communicate (see Chapter 4).
- Allow the person to place familiar objects and pictures within view.
- Provide newspapers and magazines. Read to the person if appropriate.
- Discuss current events with the person.
- Provide access to television and radios.
- Maintain the day-night cycle. Open curtains, shades, and drapes during the day and close them at night. Use a night-light at night. Encourage the person to wear regular clothes during the day rather than gowns or pajamas.
- Maintain a calm, relaxed, and peaceful atmosphere. Prevent loud noises, rushing, and congested hallways and dining rooms.
- Maintain the person's routine. Meals, bathing, exercise, television programs, and other activities are on a schedule. This promotes a sense of order and anticipation of what to expect.
- Do not rearrange furniture or the person's belongings.
- Encourage the person to participate in self-care activities.
- Be consistent.
- Remind the person of holidays, birthdays, and other special events.

ALZHEIMER'S DISEASE

Alzheimer's disease is a brain disease. Brain cells that control intellectual function are damaged. The disease is progressive. That is, it gets worse and worse. It occurs in both men and women. Though more common in the elderly, it also occurs in younger people. Some people in their 40s and 50s have Alzheimer's disease. The cause is unknown.

Stages of Alzheimer's Disease

There are three stages of Alzheimer's disease (Box 30-3). Signs and symptoms become more severe with each stage. The disease ends in death.

Wandering, sundowning, hallucinations, delusions, and catastrophic reactions occur. Agitation, restlessness, aggression, and combative behaviors are other problems.

Wandering Persons with Alzheimer's disease are disoriented to person, time, and place. They may wander from home or the facility and not find their way back. They may be with caregivers one moment and gone the next. Judgment is poor and they cannot tell what is safe or dangerous. They are in danger of accidents. A person may walk into traffic or into a nearby river or lake. If not properly dressed, exposure is a risk in cold climates.

Sundowning **Sundowning** occurs in the late afternoon and evening hours. As daylight ends and darkness occurs, confusion, restlessness, and other symptoms increase. The person's behavior is worse after the sun goes down. Sundowning may relate to being tired or hungry. Inadequate light may cause the person to see things that are not there. Persons with Alzheimer's disease may be afraid of the dark.

Hallucinations A **hallucination** is seeing, hearing, or feeling something that is not really there. Senses are dulled. Affected persons see animals, insects, or people

BOX 30-3 STAGES OF ALZHEIMER'S DISEASE

Stage 1
- Memory loss—forgetfulness; forgets recent events
- Poor judgment; bad decisions
- Disoriented to time
- Lack of spontaneity—less outgoing or interested in things
- Blames others for mistakes, forgetfulness, and other problems
- Moodiness

Stage 2
- Restlessness; increases during the evening hours
- Sleep disturbances
- Memory loss increases—may not recognize family and friends
- Dulled senses—cannot tell the difference between hot and cold; cannot recognize dangers
- Bowel and bladder incontinence
- Needs assistance with activities of daily living—problems with bathing, feeding, and dressing self; afraid of bathing; will not change clothes
- Loses impulse control—may use foul language, have poor table manners, be sexually aggressive, or be rude
- Movement and gait disturbances—walks slowly, has a shuffling gait
- Communication problems—cannot follow directions; has problems with reading, writing, and math; speaks in short sentences or single words; statements may not make sense
- Repeats motions and statements—may move things back and forth constantly; may say the same thing over and over again
- Agitation—behavior may become violent

Stage 3
- Seizures (Chapter 33)
- Cannot communicate—may groan, grunt, or scream
- Does not recognize self or family members
- Depends totally on others for all activities of daily living
- Disoriented to person, time, and place
- Totally incontinent of urine and feces
- Cannot swallow—choking and aspiration are risks
- Sleep disturbances increase
- Becomes bed bound—cannot sit or walk
- Coma
- Death

that are not present. Some hear voices. They may feel bugs crawling on their bodies or feel that they are being touched.

Delusions **Delusions** are false beliefs. People with Alzheimer's disease may think they are God, movie stars, or some other person. Some believe they are in jail, are going to be murdered, or are being attacked. A person may believe that the caregiver is actually someone else. Many other false beliefs can occur.

Catastrophic reactions Catastrophic reactions are extreme responses. The person reacts as if a disaster or tragedy has occurred. The person may scream, cry, or be agitated or combative. These reactions often occur when the person has too much stimuli at one time. Eating, music or television playing, and being asked questions all at one time can overwhelm the person.

Agitation and restlessness The person who is agitated and restless may pace, hit, or yell. Such behaviors may be due to pain or discomfort, anxiety, lack of sleep, sensory overload or sensory deprivation (see Chapter 20), hunger, or the need to eliminate. A calm, quiet environment and meeting basic needs helps calm the person.

Sometimes agitation and restlessness are caused by caregivers. A caregiver may rush the person or be impatient. Or a caregiver's communication may be giving mixed verbal and nonverbal messages. Caregivers always need to look at how their behaviors affect other persons.

Aggression and combativeness Aggressive and combative behaviors occur in some persons. They may result from agitation and restlessness. Examples include hitting, pinching, grabbing, biting, or swearing. Such behaviors are frightening to caregivers, to others in the home, or to patients and residents. Sometimes aggressive and combative behaviors are part of the person's personality.

Care of the Person with Alzheimer's Disease

Alzheimer's disease is frustrating to the person, family, and caregivers. Usually the person is cared for at home until symptoms become severe. Adult day care may help. Care in a nursing facility is often required. The person may develop other illnesses and need hospital care. Thus you may care for a person with Alzheimer's disease in an adult day care setting or in a hospital, nursing facility, or private home. The person needs your support and understanding. So does the family.

Remember, people with Alzheimer's disease do not choose to be forgetful, incontinent, agitated, or rude. Nor do they choose to have all of the other behaviors, signs, and symptoms of the disease. They have no control over what is happening to them. The disease causes the behaviors. Thus when the person does something that a healthy individual would not do, remember that the disease is responsible, not the person.

Care of persons with Alzheimer's disease is described in Box 30-4. The nurse uses the nursing process to plan measures to meet the person's specific needs. The person's safety, personal hygiene, nutrition and fluids, elimination, and activity needs must be met. So must the need for comfort and sleep. Many of the measures listed in Box 30-4 will be part of the person's care plan.

Your observations are important. The person can develop other health problems or be injured. However, the person may not know there is pain, fever, constipation, incontinence, or other signs and symptoms. You need to carefully observe the person. Any change in the person's usual behavior must be reported to the nurse.

Infection is a major risk in persons with Alzheimer's disease. Remember, the person's ability to give full attention to activities of daily living is greatly reduced. Infection can occur from poor hygiene. This includes skin care, oral hygiene, and perineal care after bowel and bladder elimination. Inactivity and immobility can lead to pneumonia and pressure sores.

Besides the measures listed in Box 30-4, other activities and therapies are ordered. These are intended to make the person feel useful, worthwhile, and active. They help the person's self-esteem. The therapist may work with one person, a small group, or a large group. Therapies and activities focus on the person's strengths and past successes. For example:

- A person used to cook. The person is given the task of cleaning vegetables.
- Another person was a good dancer. Activities are planned so the person can dance.

Crafts, exercise, meal preparation, and household chores are among the activities planned for the person. All activities are supervised. Sing-alongs, reminiscing, and board games are other activities.

> ### *Spotlight On…*
>
> ***Janice P of Milwaukee, Wisconsin,*** *a nursing assistant in a nursing home, called upon several of her personal talents when she was assigned to give a tub bath to a resident suffering from Alzheimer's disease. While in the tub the resident became combative and difficult to control. In a soothing manner, Janice began stroking the resident with her soapy hands while softly singing a gospel hymn. The resident became calm, allowing Janice to safely complete the bath.*

BOX 30-4 Care of the Person with Alzheimer's Disease

Environment

- Follow established routines.
- Avoid changing rooms or roommates.
- Place picture signs on rooms, bathrooms, dining rooms, and other areas (Fig. 30-2 on page 650).
- Keep personal items where the person can see them.
- Stay within the person's sight to the extent possible.
- Place memory aids (large clocks and calendars) where the person can see them.
- Keep noise levels low.
- Play music and show movies from the person's past.
- Keep tasks and activities simple.

Communication

- Approach the person in a calm, quiet manner.
- Follow the rules of communication described in Chapter 4.
- Practice measures to promote communication (see Chapter 4).
- Provide simple explanations of all procedures and activities.
- Give consistent responses.

Safety

- Remove harmful, sharp, and breakable objects from the environment. This includes knives, scissors, glass, dishes, razors, and tools.
- Provide plastic eating and drinking utensils. This helps prevent breakage and cuts.
- Place safety plugs in electrical outlets.
- Keep cords and electrical equipment out of reach.
- Childproof caps should be on medicine containers and household cleaners.
- Store household cleaners and medicines in locked storage areas.
- Practice safety measures to prevent falls (see Chapter 8, page 155).
- Practice safety measures to prevent fires (see Chapter 8, page 175).
- Practice safety measures to prevent burns (see Chapter 8, page 156).
- Practice safety measures to prevent poisoning (see Chapter 8, page 157).

Wandering

- Make sure doors and windows are securely locked. Locks are often placed at the top and bottom of doors (Fig. 30-3 on page 650). The person is not likely to look for a lock at the top or bottom of the door.
- Make sure door alarms are turned on. The alarm goes off when the door is opened. These are common in nursing facilities.
- Make sure the person wears an ID bracelet at all times.
- Exercise the person as ordered. Adequate exercise often reduces wandering.
- Do not restrain the person. Restraints require a doctor's order. They also tend to increase confusion and disorientation.
- Do not argue with the person who wants to leave. Remember, the person does not understand what you are saying.
- Go with the person who insists on going outside. Make sure he or she is properly dressed. Guide the person inside after a few minutes (Fig. 30-4 on page 651).
- Let the person wander in enclosed areas if provided. Many nursing facilities have enclosed areas where residents can walk about (Fig. 30-5 on page 651). These areas provide a safe place for the person to wander.

Sundowning

- Provide a calm, quiet environment late in the day. Treatments and activities should be done early in the day.
- Do not restrain the person.
- Encourage exercise and activity early in the day.
- Make sure the person has eaten. Hunger can increase the person's restlessness.
- Promote urinary and bowel elimination. A full bladder or constipation can increase restlessness.
- Do not try to reason with the person. Remember, he or she cannot understand what you are saying.
- Do not ask the person to tell you what is bothering him or her. The person's ability to communicate is impaired. He or she does not understand what you are asking. The person cannot think or speak clearly.

Continued.

BOX 30-4 Care of the Person with Alzheimer's Disease—cont'd

Hallucinations and delusions

- Do not argue with the person. He or she does not understand what you are saying.
- Reassure the person. Tell him or her that you will provide protection from harm.
- Distract the person with some item or activity.
- Use touch to calm and reassure the person (Fig. 30-6).

Basic needs

- Provide for the person's food and fluid needs (see Chapter 17).
- Provide good skin care (see Chapter 13). Make sure the person's skin is free of urine and feces.
- Promote urinary and bowel elimination (see Chapters 15 and 16).
- Promote exercise and activity during the day (see Chapter 19). This helps reduce wandering and sundowning behaviors. The person may also sleep better.
- Reduce the person's intake of coffee, tea, and cola drinks. These contain caffeine. Caffeine is a stimulant. The person's restlessness, confusion, and agitation can increase because of caffeine.
- Provide a quiet, restful environment (see Chapter 20). Soft music is better in the evening than loud television programs.
- Promote personal hygiene (see Chapter 13). Do not force the person into a shower or tub. People with Alzheimer's disease are often afraid of bathing. Try bathing the person when he or she is calm.
- Provide oral hygiene (see Chapter 13).
- Have equipment ready for any procedure ahead of time. This reduces the amount of time the person has to be involved in care measures.
- Observe for signs and symptoms of other disorders or diseases (see Chapter 3).
- Protect the person from infection (see Chapter 9).

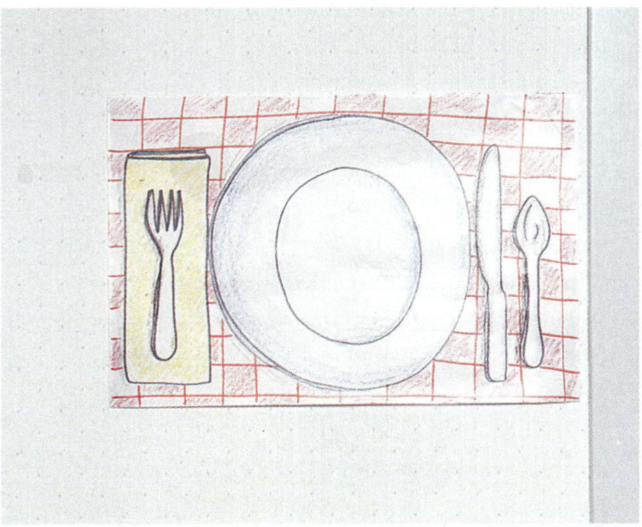

Fig. 30-2 *Signs provide cues to the person with dementia.*

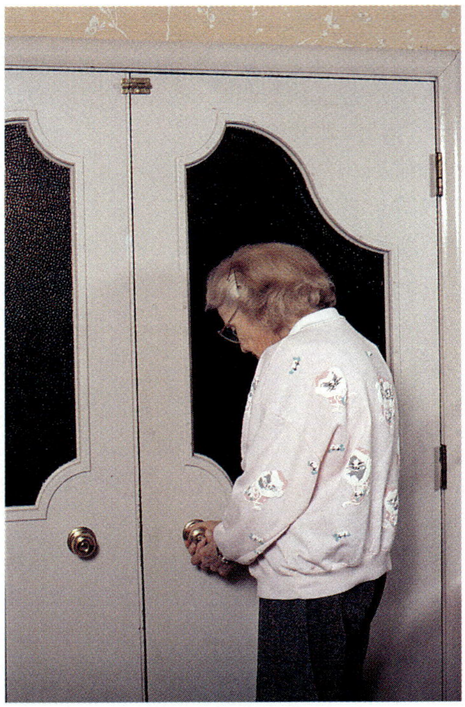

Fig. 30-3 *A slide lock is at the top of the door. The person tries to open the lock on the knob.*

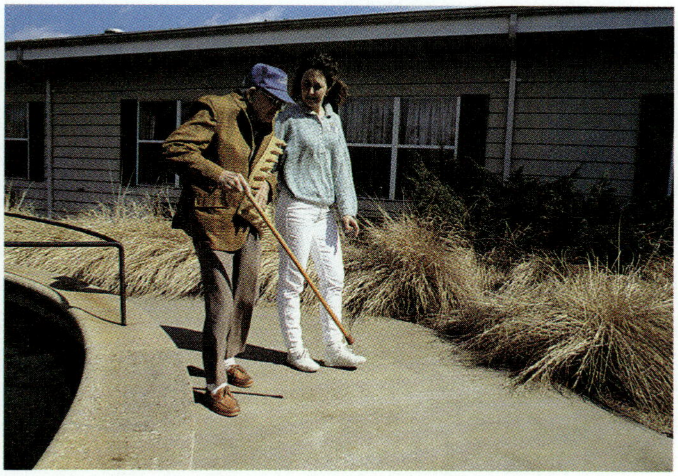

Fig. 30-4 *The nursing assistant walks outside with the person who wanders. He is guided back into the facility.*

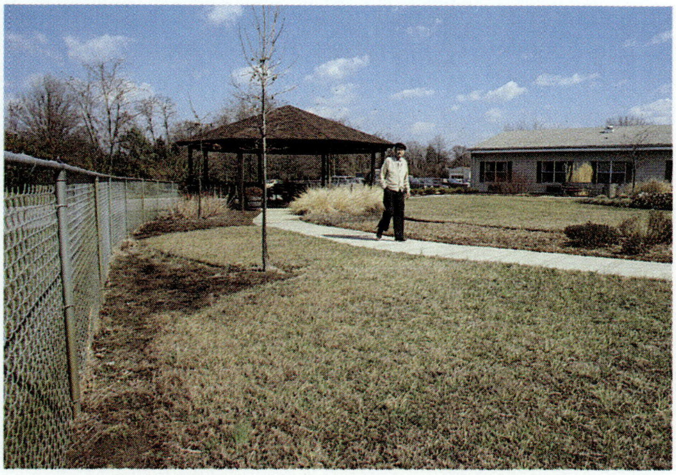

Fig. 30-5 *An enclosed garden allows persons with Alzheimer's disease to wander in a safe environment.*

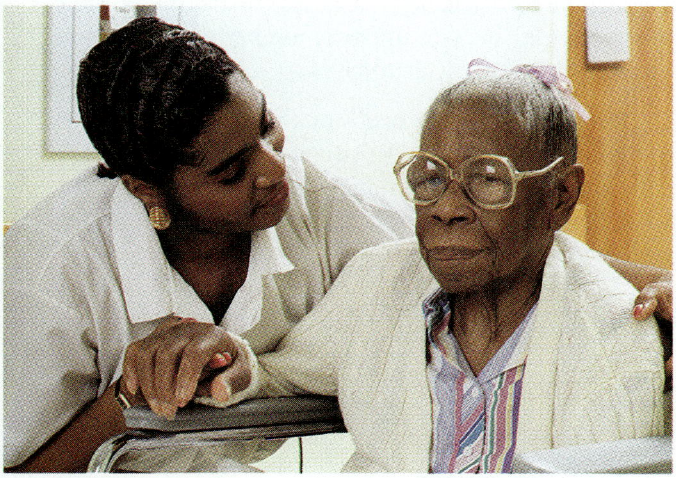

Fig. 30-6 *The nursing assistant uses touch to calm a person with Alzheimer's disease.*

The Family

Persons with Alzheimer's disease may live at home or with children or other family members. Care is given by family members in the household. Or arrangements are made for a family member or someone else to stay with the person. Help is sought from health professionals when family members can no longer deal with the situation or meet the person's needs. Home health care may help for awhile. Adult day care is another option (see Chapter 7). The decision for long-term care is usually made when:

- Family members can no longer meet the person's needs
- The person with Alzheimer's disease no longer knows the caregiver
- Family members have health problems
- Financial problems occur
- The person has behaviors that are dangerous to self or others

Medical care is very expensive. Diagnostic tests, doctor's visits, medicines, and home care are costly. Long-term care is even more expensive. The person's medical care can drain family finances.

The family has special needs. Care of the person at home or in a nursing facility is stressful. There are physical, emotional, social, and financial stresses. Children find themselves in the *sandwich generation.* They are in the middle between their own children who need to be taken care of and an ill parent who needs care. The stress of caring for two families is great. Often caregiving children have jobs too.

Caring for loved ones can be exhausting. Caregivers need much support and encouragement. Many join Alzheimer's disease support groups. These groups are sponsored by hospitals, nursing facilities, and the Alzheimer's Association. The Alzheimer's Association has chapters in cities and towns across the country. Support groups offer encouragement, advice, and ideas about care. People in similar situations share their feelings, anger, frustration, guilt, and other emotions.

The family often feels helpless. No matter what is done for the loved one, the person only gets worse. Much time, money, energy, and emotion are required to care for the person. Anger and resentment may result. The family may then feel guilty because of their anger and resentment. They know that the person did not choose to develop the disease. The family also knows that the person does not choose to have the signs, symptoms, and behaviors of the disease. They may be frustrated and angry that the loved one can no longer show love or affection. How would you feel if your mother, father, husband, or wife did not recognize you? Sometimes the person's behavior is embarrassing.

The family has to learn some of the same care measures and procedures that you learn. They need to learn how to bathe, feed, dress, and give oral hygiene to the person. They also need to learn how to provide a safe environment. The nurse and support group will help them learn to give necessary care.

QUALITY OF LIFE

Quality of life is important for all persons with confusion and dementia. Those in nursing facilities have the same rights under OBRA as other residents. Confused and demented residents may not know or be able to exercise their rights. However, the family is aware of the resident's rights. They need to know that their loved one's rights are being protected. The family also needs to know that the loved one is being treated with respect and dignity.

Confused and demented residents have the right to privacy and confidentiality. You must protect the person from exposure. Only those involved in the person's care are present for care and procedures. The resident is allowed to visit with others in private. When family and friends visit, they are given a space where they can visit privately. Confidentiality is also important. The resident's care and condition are not shared with others.

Even confused and demented residents have the right to personal choice. Some can still make simple choices. For example, a person may be able to choose between wearing a dress or slacks. Choosing to watch or not watch television may be a simple choice. Others cannot make choices themselves. The family may do so. Bath times, menus, clothing, activities, and other aspects of care may be chosen by the family.

The resident has the right to keep and use personal possessions. Some items comfort the resident. A pillow, blanket, afghan, or sweater may be important to the person. The resident may not be able to tell you why or even recognize the item. Still, it is important. Personal items kept by the resident need to be safe. You must also protect the person's property from loss or damage.

Confused and demented residents must be kept free from abuse, mistreatment, and neglect. Caring for these people can be very frustrating. The person's behaviors may be difficult to deal with. Family and staff can become short-tempered and angry. The resident must be protected from abuse (see Chapter 7, page 143). Be sure to report any signs of abuse to the nurse right away. You need to be patient and calm when caring for these residents. Talk with the nurse if you find yourself becoming frustrated. Sometimes an assignment change is needed for a while.

All residents have the right to be free from restraints. Remember, restraints require a doctor's order. They must be used only when it is the best method of protecting the resident. They are not used for staff convenience. Restraints can make confusion and demented behaviors worse. The nurse tells you when restraints are to be used.

Activity and a safe environment promote quality of life. Box 30-4 identifies safety measures for confused and demented residents. These residents also need activities that are safe, calm, and quiet. The recreation therapist and other health team members will find activities that are best for each confused or demented resident. These will be part of the person's care plan.

SUMMARY

Confusion and dementia affect a person's ability to think, reason, and understand. Memory, judgment, and behavior are also affected. Therefore dementia affects the ability to meet basic needs. Physical, safety, love and belonging, esteem, and self-actualization needs are all affected.

Persons with dementia do not choose to be forgetful, to wander, or to have poor manners. The disease is responsible for their behaviors. As frustrating as their behaviors may be, you must remember that they have no control over their actions.

The person and family need much encouragement and emotional support. Required care can be physically, emotionally, and financially draining. There are no cures. However, a kind, caring nursing assistant can be comforting.

REVIEW QUESTIONS

Circle the best *answer.*

1 A patient is confused after surgery. The confusion is likely to be

- **a** Permanent
- **b** Temporary
- **c** Due to an infection
- **d** Due to brain injury

2 The confused person must be protected from

- **a** Danger
- **b** Infection
- **c** Incontinence
- **d** Constipation

3 Joe Dunn has dementia. Dementia describes

- **a** A false belief
- **b** Mental disorders caused by changes in the brain
- **c** Seeing, hearing, or feeling something that is not real
- **d** Alzheimer's disease

4 Joe Dunn was diagnosed with Alzheimer's disease. Which is *true?*

- **a** Alzheimer's disease occurs only in the elderly.
- **b** Diet and medications can control the disease.
- **c** Alzheimer's disease and confusion are the same.
- **d** Alzheimer's disease ends in death.

5 Joe Dunn and other persons with Alzheimer's disease

- **a** Have memory loss, poor judgment, and sleep disturbances
- **b** Lose impulse control and the ability to communicate
- **c** May wander or have delusions and hallucinations
- **d** All of the above

6 Sundowning means that

- **a** The person becomes sleepy when the sun sets
- **b** Behaviors become worse in the late afternoon and evening hours
- **c** Behavior improves at night
- **d** The person is in the third stage of the disease

7 Alzheimer's disease support groups do the following *except*

- **a** Provide care
- **b** Offer encouragement and care ideas
- **c** Provide support for the family
- **d** Promote the sharing of feelings and frustrations

8 Joe Dunn tends to wander. You should

- **a** Make sure doors and windows are locked
- **b** Make sure he wears an ID bracelet
- **c** Help him with exercise as ordered
- **d** All of the above

9 Safety is important for Joe Dunn. Which is *false?*

- **a** Safety plugs are placed in electrical outlets.
- **b** Cleaners and medications should be out of his reach.
- **c** He can keep smoking materials.
- **d** Sharp and breakable objects are removed from his environment.

10 You have been assigned to care for Joe Dunn. Which is *false?*

- **a** It is possible to reason with him.
- **b** Touch can calm and reassure him.
- **c** A calm, quiet environment is important.
- **d** Assistance is needed with ADL.

Answers to these questions are on page 753.

Sexuality

31

OBJECTIVES

- Define the key terms listed in this chapter
- Describe the differences between sex and sexuality
- Explain the importance of sexuality throughout life
- Describe five types of sexual relationships
- Explain how injury and illness can affect sexuality
- Identify the illnesses, injuries, and surgeries that often affect sexuality
- Explain how aging affects sexuality in the elderly
- Explain how the nursing team can promote a person's sexuality
- List the reasons persons may become sexually aggressive
- Describe how to deal with sexually aggressive persons
- Explain how sexually transmitted diseases are spread
- Describe the common sexually transmitted diseases

KEY TERMS

bisexual A person who is attracted to people of both sexes

heterosexual A person who is attracted to members of the opposite sex

homosexual A person who has a strong attraction to members of the same sex

impotence The inability of the male to have an erection

menopause The time when menstruation stops; it marks the end of the woman's reproductive years

sex The physical activities involving the organs of reproduction; the activities are done for pleasure or to produce children

sexuality That which relates to one's sex; those physical, psychological, social, cultural, and spiritual factors that affect a person's feelings and attitudes about his or her sex

transsexual A person who believes that he or she is really a member of the opposite sex

transvestite A person who becomes sexually excited by dressing in the clothes of the opposite sex

Patients and residents must be viewed as total persons. They do not have just physical needs or problems. Attention must be given to the psychological and social effects of a disorder. The needs of love and belonging, esteem, and self-actualization cannot be overlooked. The person's physical, psychological, social, and spiritual needs must be met.

There is another part of the person that involves the physical, psychological, social, and the spiritual. That part is sexuality. Illness and injury can affect a person's sexuality. This chapter describes the effects of illness, injury, and aging on sexuality. Box 31-1 on page 656 contains a review of the structure and functions of the male and female reproductive systems. A review of growth and development in Chapter 6 also will help you to study this chapter.

SEX AND SEXUALITY

Sex and sexuality are different. **Sex** is the physical activities involving the reproductive organs. The activities are done for pleasure or to produce children. **Sexuality** involves the whole personality and the body. A person's attitudes and feelings are involved. Besides physical and psychological factors, sexuality is influenced by social, cultural, and spiritual factors. How a person behaves, thinks, dresses, and responds to others is related to his or her sexuality.

Sexuality is present from birth. A boy or girl name is given when the baby's sex is known. The color blue is used for boys, and pink for girls. Toys reflect sexuality. Dolls are traditionally for girls. Trains are for boys. By the age of 2, children know their own sex. A 3-year-old knows the sex of other children. Children learn male and female roles from their parents (Fig. 31-1). Children learn early that there are certain behaviors for boys and certain ones for girls.

As children grow older, their interest about the human body and how it works increases. Body changes during adolescence bring more interest and curiosity about sex and the body. Their bodies respond to stimulation. Adolescents engage in various sexual behaviors. These may range from kissing, embracing, or petting to sexual intercourse. Pregnancy and sexually transmitted diseases (page 662) are great risks for sexually active teenagers.

Sex has more meaning as young adults mature. Attitudes and feelings are important. Decisions about sexuality become more important. Sexual partners are selected. Sex before marriage and birth control are other decisions.

Sexuality continues to be important into adulthood and old age. Attitudes and the need for sex change as a person grows older. Life circumstances change. Changes may include divorce, death of a spouse, injury, and illness.

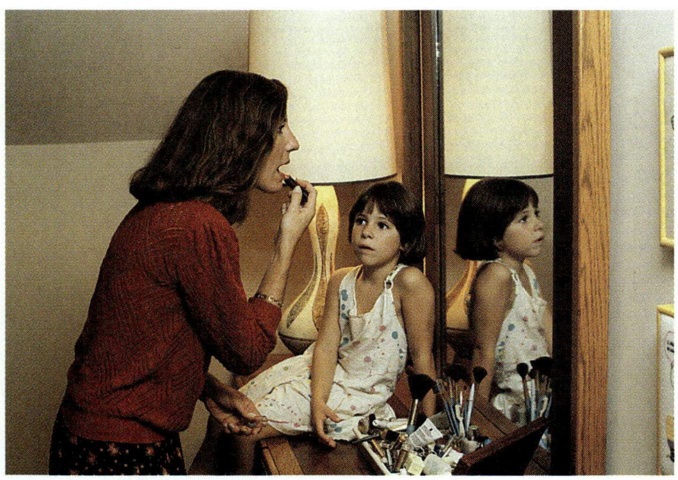

Fig. 31-1 *This little girl is learning female roles from her mother.*

BOX 31-1 Review of the Structure and Function of the Reproductive System

The Male Reproductive System

The structures of the male reproductive system are shown in Figure 31-2. The *testes (testicles)* are the male sex glands *(gonads).* Male sex cells *(sperm cells)* are produced in the testes. So is *testosterone,* the male hormone. This hormone is needed for reproductive organ function and for the development of male secondary sex characteristics (see Chapter 6). The testes are suspended between the thighs in a sac called the *scrotum.*

Sperm travel from the testis to the *epididymis.* The epididymis is a coiled tube on top and to the side of the testis. From the epididymis, sperm travel through a tube called the *vas deferens.* Eventually each vas deferens joins a *seminal vesicle.* The two seminal vesicles store sperm and produce *semen.* Semen is a fluid that carries sperm from the male reproductive tract. The ducts of the seminal vesicles join to form the *ejaculatory duct.* The ejaculatory duct passes through the prostate gland.

The *prostate gland,* shaped like a doughnut, lies just below the bladder. The gland secretes fluid into the semen. As the ejaculatory ducts leave the prostate they join the *urethra,* which also runs through the prostate. The urethra is the outlet for urine and semen. The penis contains the urethra.

The *penis* is outside the body and has *erectile* tissue. When the man is sexually aroused, blood fills the erectile tissue. The penis becomes enlarged, hard, and erect. The erect penis can enter the vagina of the female reproductive tract. The semen, which contains sperm, is released into the vagina.

The Female Reproductive System

The structures of the female reproductive system are shown in Figure 31-3. The female gonads are two almond-shaped glands called *ovaries.* There is an ovary on each side of the uterus in the abdominal cavity. The ovaries contain *ova* (eggs). Ova are female sex cells. One ovum (egg) is released monthly during the woman's reproductive years. Release of an ovum from an ovary is called *ovulation.* The ovaries also secrete the female hormones *estrogen* and *progesterone.* These hormones are needed for reproductive system function and the development of female secondary sex characteristics (see Chapter 6).

When an ovum is released from an ovary, it travels through a *fallopian tube.* There are two fallopian tubes, one on each side. The tubes are attached at one end to the uterus. The ovum travels through a fallopian tube to the *uterus.* The uterus is a hollow, muscular organ shaped like a pear. The uterus is in the center of the pelvic cavity behind the bladder and in front of the rectum. The main part of the uterus is the *fundus.* The neck or narrow section of the uterus is the *cervix.* Tissue lining the uterus is called the *endometrium.* The endometrium has many blood vessels. If sex cells from the male and female unite into one cell, that cell implants into the endometrium. There it grows into a baby. The uterus serves as a place for the unborn baby to grow and receive nourishment.

The cervix projects into a muscular canal called the *vagina.* The vagina opens to the outside of the body and is located just behind the urethra. The vagina receives the penis during sexual intercourse and is part of the birth canal. Glands in the vaginal wall keep it moistened with secretions.

The external genitalia of the female are called the *vulva* (Fig. 31-4). The *mons pubis* is covered with hair in the adult female. The *labia majora* and *labia minora* are two folds of tissue on each side of the vaginal opening. The *clitoris* is a small organ composed of erectile tissue. The clitoris becomes enlarged and hard when sexually stimulated.

Menstruation

The endometrium is rich in blood to nourish the cell that grows into an unborn baby *(fetus).* If pregnancy does not occur, the endometrium breaks up and is discharged through the vagina to the outside of the body. This process is called *menstruation.* Menstruation occurs about every 28 days. Therefore it is also called the *menstrual cycle.*

The first day of the cycle starts with menstruation. Blood flows from the uterus through the vaginal opening. Menstrual flow lasts 3 to 7 days. Ovulation occurs during the next phase. An ovum is released from the ovary. Ovulation usually occurs on or about day 14 of the cycle. Meanwhile, the ovaries secrete estrogen and progesterone (female hormones). These hormones cause the endometrium to thicken for possible pregnancy. If pregnancy does not occur, the hormones decrease in amount. Blood supply to the endometrium decreases because of the decrease in hormones. The endometrium breaks up and is discharged through the vagina. Another menstrual cycle begins.

Fertilization

For reproduction to occur, a male sex cell (sperm) must unite with a female sex cell (ovum). The uniting of the sperm and ovum into one cell is called *fertilization.* A sperm and an ovum each have 23 chromosomes. When the two cells unite, the fertilized cell has 46 chromosomes.

During intercourse, millions of sperm are deposited in the vagina. Sperm travel up the cervix, through the uterus, and into the fallopian tubes. If a sperm and an ovum unite in a fallopian tube, fertilization occurs and pregnancy results. The fertilized cell travels down the fallopian tube to the uterus. After a short time, the fertilized cell implants in the thick endometrium and grows during pregnancy.

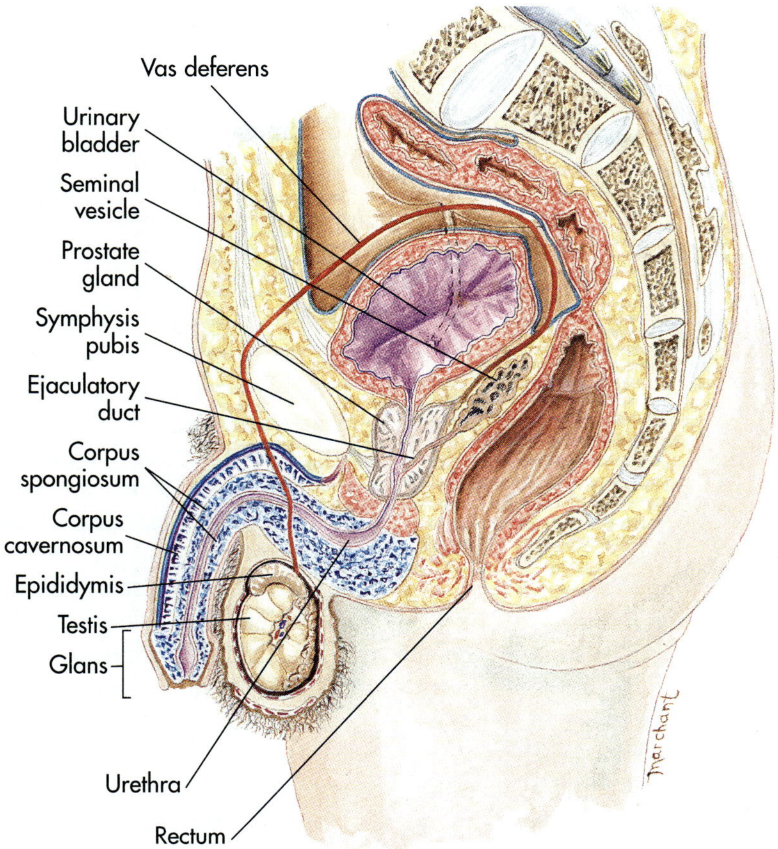

Fig. 31-2 *Male reproductive system.*

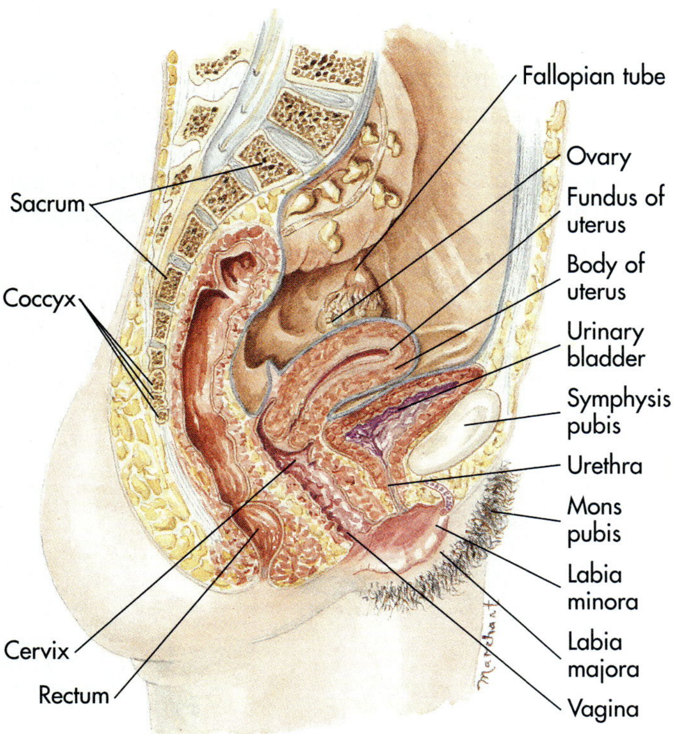

Fig. 31-3 *Female reproductive system.*

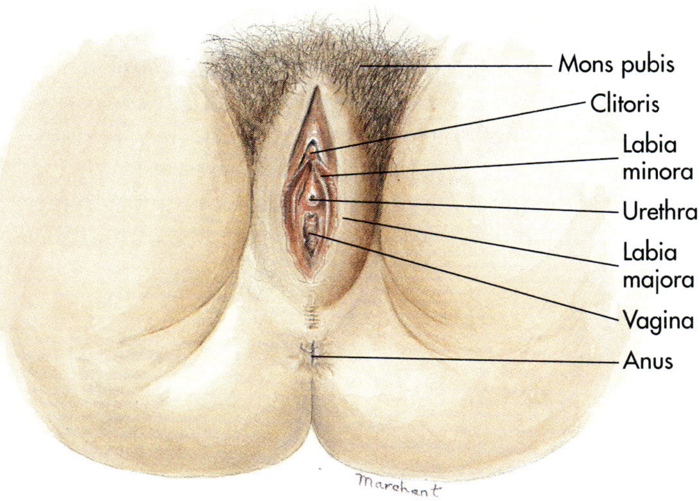

Fig. 31-4 *External female genitalia.*

SEXUAL RELATIONSHIPS

Sex and sexuality usually involve a partner. Most people are heterosexual. A **heterosexual** is a person who is attracted to people of the other sex. Men are attracted to women, and women are attracted to men. Sexual activities involve someone from the opposite sex. However, you may care for people who are not heterosexual.

A **homosexual** is attracted to members of the same sex. The person has sexual relationships and is aroused by a member of the same sex. Men are attracted to men, and women are attracted to women. *Gay* is often used in referring to homosexuals. A female homosexual is called a *lesbian.*

Homosexuality has existed for centuries. Since the 1960s and 1970s it has become more apparent in society. Before, it was hidden. Now many homosexuals are more open about their sexual preference and relationships.

Bisexuals are attracted to both sexes. They are aroused and excited by men or women. Some alternate between homosexual and heterosexual relationships. Bisexuals are often married and have children. They may seek a homosexual relationship or experience outside of marriage.

Some people believe that they are really members of the opposite sex. These people are **transsexuals.** A male believes he is really a woman in a man's body. A woman believes she is really a man in a woman's body. Transsexuals often describe feelings of being "trapped" in the wrong body. Most transsexuals have had these feelings for as long as they can remember. As children they usually show tendencies and interests of the opposite sex. Many transsexuals undergo psychiatric treatment. Some have sex-change operations. Psychiatric treatment and sex-change operations are not always effective in helping these people.

Transvestites become sexually excited by dressing in clothes appropriate to the opposite sex. Most are male. They are usually married and heterosexual. They dress normally as men most of the time. Dressing as a woman is usually done in private. Some dress completely as women. Others focus on bras and panties. The sex partner may not know about the practice. Some women know that their husbands or partners are transvestites. If they agree, women may be included in transvestite activities. Some transvestites have same-sex friends with similar interests.

INJURY AND ILLNESS

Sexuality and sex involve the mind and body. Injury and illness affect how the body works. The mind can also be affected. A person may feel unclean, unwhole, unattractive, or mutilated after disfiguring surgery. Attitudes about sex may change. The person may feel unattractive or incapable of being loved. These feelings affect the person's ability to be close and loving. Therefore the person may develop sexual problems that are psychological. Time, understanding, and a caring partner are very helpful. Counseling or psychiatric help may be needed.

Many illnesses, injuries, and surgeries affect the nervous, circulatory, and reproductive systems. If one or more of these systems are affected, the person's sexual ability may change. Most chronic illnesses affect sexual functioning.

Impotence may occur. Impotence is the inability of the male to have an erection. Diabetes mellitus, spinal cord injuries, multiple sclerosis, and alcoholism are common causes. Circulatory disorders and medications can affect the ability to achieve an erection. Impotence is a side effect of some medications to control high blood pressure.

Heart disease, stroke, chronic obstructive pulmonary disease, and nervous system disorders can affect the ability to have sex. Some reproductive system surgeries have physical and psychological effects. Removal of the prostate or the testes affects erections. Removal of the uterus, ovaries, or a breast may affect a woman psychologically. A colostomy or ileostomy may psychologically affect both men and women.

You will care for persons with disorders that can affect sexual functioning. Changes in sexual functioning greatly impact the person. Fear, anger, worry, and depression often occur. These are seen in the person's behavior and comments. The person's feelings are very normal and are expected.

SEXUALITY AND THE ELDERLY

Sexual relationships are psychologically and physically important to the elderly (Fig. 31-5). They fall in love, hold hands, embrace, and have sex. They need sex, love, and affection. Many are capable of sexual intercourse.

Love, affection, and intimacy are needed throughout life. As other losses occur, feeling close to another person becomes more important. Children leave home. Friends and relatives die. Jobs are lost because of retirement. Health problems may develop. These losses may be compounded by decreasing strength and a changing appearance.

Reproductive organs change during the aging process. However, the changes do not remove sexual needs or abilities. In men, the hormone testosterone decreases. The hormone affects strength, sperm production, and reproductive tissues. These changes affect sexual activity. It takes longer for an erection to occur. The phase between erection and orgasm is also longer. Orgasm is less forceful than in the younger years. After orgasm, the erection is lost quickly. The time between erections is also longer. Older men may need the penis stimulated for sexual arousal. Younger men can become sexually excited just by thinking about sex or a sexual partner.

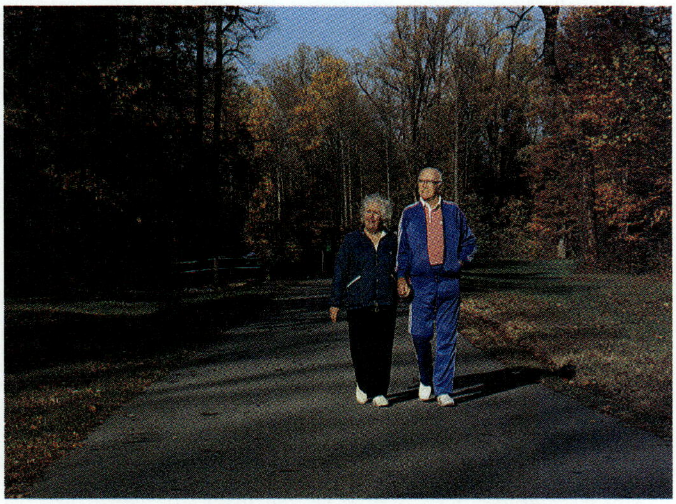

Fig. 31-5 *Love and affection are important to the elderly.*

The frequency of sexual activity usually decreases in elderly men. That is because of the physical changes just described. Mental and physical fatigue, overeating, and excessive drinking affect erections. Some men fear not being able to perform. Therefore sexual activity may be avoided. Pain and reduced mobility from illness and aging can affect frequency. One or both partners may have a chronic illness. The illness may result in decreased frequency or the complete absence of sexual activity.

Physical changes occur in women. **Menopause** occurs around 50 years of age. Menopause is when a woman stops menstruating. Her reproductive years end. A related change is the decreased secretion of the female hormones (estrogen and progesterone). Reduced hormone levels affect reproductive tissues. The uterus, vagina, and external genitalia atrophy. The vagina can still receive the penis during intercourse. However, intercourse may be uncomfortable or painful. This is because the vaginal walls thin and there is vaginal dryness. Like elderly men, older women have changes in sexual excitement. Sexual arousal takes longer. The time between excitement and orgasm is longer. Orgasm is less intense. The woman returns to a pre-excitement state more quickly.

Frequency of sexual activity decreases for many women. Reasons relate to weakness, mental and physical fatigue, pain, and reduced mobility. These may be due to the normal aging process or chronic illness.

Some elderly people do not have sexual intercourse. This does not mean loss of sexual needs or desires. Their needs may be expressed in other ways. Hand holding, touching, caressing, and embracing are ways of expressing closeness and intimacy.

Having a sexual partner is also important. Death and divorce result in loss of a sexual partner. The partner may also be in a hospital or nursing facility. These situations are seen in adults of all ages.

MEETING THE PERSON'S SEXUAL NEEDS

Sexuality is part of the total person. Some people are so ill that sexual activity is impossible. Others want and are able to have sexual activity with their partners. Sexual activity does not always mean intercourse. It may be expressed in other ways. Nursing personnel used to discourage any form of sexual expression, especially among the elderly. Hand holding was okay. But two people were not to get any closer! More attention is now given to sexuality in health and illness. The nursing team has an important role in allowing patients and residents to meet their sexual needs. The measures in Box 31-2 are appreciated by patients and residents. They are carried out in cooperation with the nurse supervising your work.

BOX 31-2 PROMOTING SEXUALITY

- Let the person practice grooming routines. This includes applying makeup, nail polish, and body lotion, and wearing cologne. Hair care and shaving are also important. Women may want to shave their legs and underarms and pluck their eyebrows. Men may wish to use after-shave lotion. Help may be needed with these activities.
- Let the person choose clothing. Hospital gowns embarrass both men and women. Street clothes are worn if the person's condition permits.
- Protect the right to privacy. Avoid exposing the person. The person must be draped and screened appropriately.
- Accept the person's sexual relationships. The person may not share your sexual attitudes, values, or practices. Do not expect the person to act according to your standards. The person may have a homosexual, premarital, or extramarital relationship. There may be more than one sexual partner. Do not make judgments or gossip about relationships.
- Allow privacy. You can usually tell when two people want to be alone. If the person has a private room, close the door for privacy. Some facilities have *Do Not Disturb* signs for doors. Let the person and partner know how much time they can expect to have alone. For example, remind them when to expect a meal tray, medications, or a treatment. This gives them an idea of when to expect someone. Knocking before you enter any room is a common courtesy. It shows respect for privacy. Other staff members should be told that the person wants some time alone. Other measures are necessary if there is a roommate. Consideration must be given to the roommate. The privacy curtain provides little privacy. Privacy can be arranged when the roommate is out of the room. Sometimes roommates volunteer to leave for a while when they sense that couples need time alone. If the roommate cannot leave, other areas on the nursing unit can be found for privacy.
- Allow privacy for masturbation. Remember, it is a normal form of sexual expression and release. Pull the privacy curtain and close the door. Knocking before you enter any room can save you and the person embarrassment. Sometimes persons with dementia masturbate in public areas. You need to lead the person to a private area or engage his or her interest in some other activity.
- Allow elderly persons their right to be sexual. The measures described previously apply to the elderly and other age groups.
- Allow couples in nursing facilities to share the same room. This is now an OBRA requirement. The couple should not be separated. They may have lived together for years. Being in a nursing facility is no reason to separate them in male and female rooms. They are allowed to share the same bed if their conditions permit. A double, queen-, or king-size bed may be provided by the facility or by the couple.
- Allow single elderly people to develop new relationships. Sexual partners are lost through death and divorce. A single resident may develop a relationship with another single resident. Instead of trying to keep them separated, measures should be taken to allow them time together (Fig. 31-6).

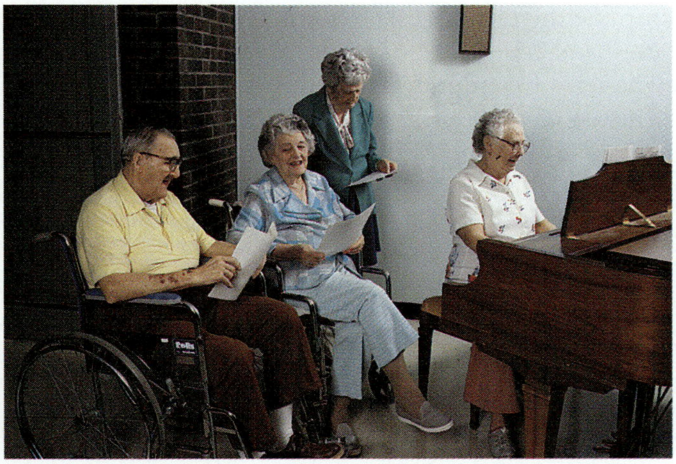

Fig. 31-6 *Intimate relationships occur in nursing facilities.*

THE SEXUALLY AGGRESSIVE PERSON

Some persons try to have their sexual needs met by health workers. They may flirt, make sexual advances or comments, expose themselves, masturbate, or touch workers. Health workers are usually angry or embarrassed when this happens. These reactions are normal. Often there are reasons for the person's behavior. Understanding this may help you to deal with the situation.

Illness, injury, surgery, or aging may threaten the male's sense of manhood. He may try to reassure or prove to himself that he is still attractive and able to perform sexually. He may do so by behaving sexually toward health workers.

Some sexually aggressive behaviors are due to confusion or disorientation. Nervous system disorders, medications, fever, dementia, and poor vision are common causes of confusion and disorientation. The person may confuse a worker with his or her sexual partner. Or the person cannot control behavior because of changes in mental function. Normally the person would be able to control urges toward a worker. However, changes in the brain can make control difficult. Sexual behavior in these situations is usually innocent on the person's part.

Some persons do touch workers inappropriately. Their purpose is sexual. However, sometimes touch is the only way the person can get the worker's attention. For example, Mr. Green had a stroke. His right side is paralyzed and he cannot speak. Your back is to him and you are bending over. Your buttocks are the closest part of your body to him. To get your attention, he touches your buttocks. You should not consider his behavior to be sexual in this situation.

Sexual advances may be intentional. You need to deal with the situation in a professional manner. However, there is no ideal way to deal with the advances. The following suggestions may be helpful.

- Discuss the situation with the nurse. The nurse can help you deal with or understand the person's behavior.
- Ask the person not to touch you in places where you were touched.
- Explain to the person that you have no intention of doing what he or she suggests.
- Explain to the person that his or her behavior makes you uncomfortable. Then politely ask the person not to act in that way.
- Allow privacy if the person is becoming sexually aroused. Provide for safety (raise side rails if they are used by the person, place the call bell within reach, and so on) and tell the person when you will return.

SEXUALLY TRANSMITTED DISEASES

Some diseases are spread by sexual contact. They are grouped under the heading of sexually transmitted diseases (STDs) (Table 31-1). Some people are not aware of being infected. Others know but do not seek treatment. Embarrassment is a common reason for not seeking treatment.

The genital area is usually associated with STDs. However, other body areas may be involved. These areas include the rectum, ears, mouth, nipples, throat, tongue, eyes, and nose. Most STDs are spread by sexual contact. The use of condoms helps prevent the spread of STDs. The use of condoms is very important for preventing the spread of HIV and AIDS (see Chapter 28, pages 627-628). Some STDs are also spread through a break in the skin, by contact with infected body fluids (blood, sperm, saliva), or by contaminated blood or needles.

Standard Precautions are necessary. Handwashing before and after giving care is essential. The Bloodborne Pathogen Standard is also followed.

TABLE 31-1

SEXUALLY TRANSMITTED DISEASES

Disease	Signs and Symptoms	Treatment
Genital herpes	Painful, fluid-filled sores on or near the genitalia (Fig. 31-7) The sores may have a watery discharge Itching, burning, and tingling in the genital area Fever Swollen glands	No known cure Medications can be given to control discomfort
Venereal warts	Male—Warts appear on the penis, anus, or genitalia Female—Warts appear near the vagina, cervix, and labia	Application of special ointment that causes the warts to dry up and fall off Surgical removal may be necessary if the ointment is not effective
AIDS (Acquired immunodeficiency syndrome)	See Chapter 28, pages 627-628	No known treatment at this time
Gonorrhea	Burning on urination Urinary frequency and urgency Vaginal discharge in the female Urethral discharge in the male	Antibiotic medications
Syphilis	*Stage 1*—10 to 90 days after exposure Painless chancre on the penis, in the vagina, or on genitalia (Fig. 31-8); the chancre may also be on the lips or inside of the mouth, or anywhere else on the body *Stage 2*—About 2 months after the chancre General fatigue, loss of appetite, nausea, fever, headache, rash, sore throat, bone and joint pain, hair loss, lesions on the lips and genitalia *Stage 3*—3 to 15 years after infection Damage to the cardiovascular system and central nervous system, blindness	Antibiotic medications

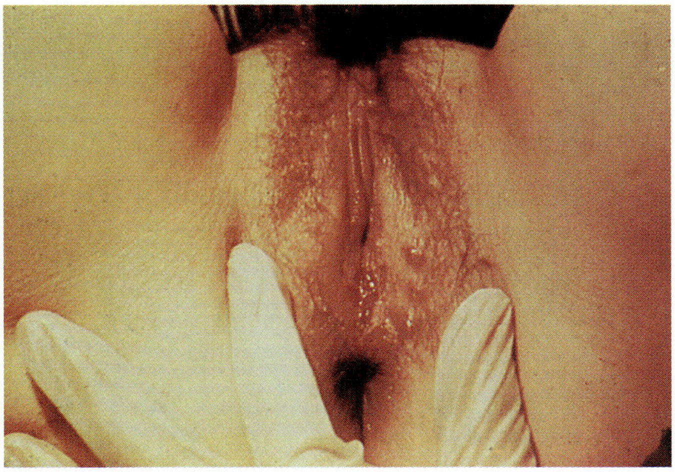

Fig. 31-7 *Genital herpes sore.*

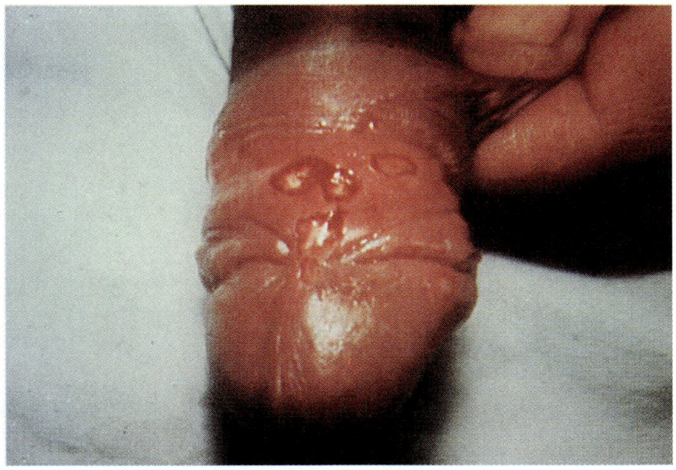

Fig. 31-8 *Chancre caused by syphilis.*

SUMMARY

Sexuality is part of the total person. Ill or injured persons still need love, affection, and closeness with other people. Health workers should promote, not discourage, a person's sexual expression. This is especially true for the elderly.

Illness, injury, and surgery may affect a person's sexuality. The problem may be temporary or permanent. Reproductive organs, the circulatory system, or the nervous system may be affected. As a result, the person may have problems in sexual performance. Some injuries and surgeries are disfiguring. Persons may feel unclean and unattractive to others. Their sexuality and sexual performance may be affected psychologically. Persons who have physical or psychological changes in sexuality need understanding and caring. You must try to understand the person's situation.

REVIEW QUESTIONS

Circle the best *answer.*

1 Sex involves
- **a** The organs of reproduction
- **b** Attitudes and feelings
- **c** Cultural and spiritual factors
- **d** All of the above

2 Sexuality is important to
- **a** Small children
- **b** Teenagers and young adults
- **c** Middle-aged adults
- **d** Persons of all ages

3 Mr. and Mrs. Green are most likely
- **a** Heterosexuals
- **b** Homosexuals
- **c** Bisexuals
- **d** Transsexuals

4 Either illness or injury can result in impotence. Impotence is
- **a** When menstruation stops
- **b** A psychological reaction to disfigurement
- **c** The inability of the male to achieve an erection
- **d** The complete absence of sexual activity

5 Mr. and Mrs. Green's reproductive organs have changed with aging. These changes make sexual activity difficult or impossible.
- **a** True
- **b** False

6 Mr. and Mrs. Green live in the same nursing facility. Which will *not* promote their sexuality?
- **a** Allowing their normal grooming routines
- **b** Having them wear hospital gowns
- **c** Allowing them privacy
- **d** Accepting their relationship

7 An elderly lady and an elderly gentleman live in the same nursing facility as Mr. and Mrs. Green. They seem to be developing a relationship. Nursing staff should keep them separated.
- **a** True
- **b** False

8 Mr. Green requests time alone with his wife. The nurse tells you this is okay. You should
- **a** Close the door to the room
- **b** Put a *Do Not Distur*b sign on the door
- **c** Tell other staff that Mr. and Mrs. Green want some time alone
- **d** All of the above

9 Mr. and Mrs. Green should be assigned to separate rooms.
- **a** True
- **b** False

10 A male patient is being sexually aggressive. The behavior may be
- **a** An attempt to prove he is still attractive and able to perform sexually
- **b** Due to confusion or disorientation
- **c** Done on purpose
- **d** All of the above

11 A patient has made sexual advances to you. You should do the following *except*
- **a** Discuss the situation with the nurse
- **b** Do what the person asks
- **c** Explain to the person that the behavior makes you uncomfortable
- **d** Ask the person not to touch you in places where you were touched

12 Which statement is *false?*
- **a** STDs are usually spread by sexual contact.
- **b** STDs can affect the genital area and other parts of the body.
- **c** Signs and symptoms of STDs are always obvious.
- **d** Some STDs result in death.

Answers to these questions are on page 753.

Caring for Mothers and Newborns

32

OBJECTIVES

- Describe how to meet an infant's safety and security needs
- Identify the signs and symptoms of illness in infants
- Explain how to help mothers with breast-feeding
- Describe three forms of baby formulas
- Explain how to bottle-feed babies
- Explain how to burp a baby
- Describe how to give cord care
- Describe the purposes of circumcision, the necessary observations, and the required care
- Identify planning, safety, temperature, and other factors related to bathing infants
- Explain why infants are weighed
- Perform the procedures described in this chapter

KEY TERMS

circumcision The surgical removal of foreskin

rooting reflex The baby turns his or her head when the cheek or mouth is stroked; the head is turned toward the direction of the stimulus and the baby starts to suck

umbilical cord The structure that carries blood, oxygen, and nutrients from the mother to the fetus

You may care for new mothers, infants, and children. New mothers and newborns are cared for in hospital maternity departments. These departments are called family birth centers or similar names in some hospitals. Pediatric units are for infants and children. A mother or newborn may need home care.

There are many reasons for home care. A mother may have complications before or after childbirth. There may be other young children. A new baby and other children can be overwhelming. Multiple births (twins, triplets, and so on) are another reason. Sometimes mothers simply need help with home maintenance.

A review of growth and development will help you care for babies and children (see Chapter 6). Babies are helpless. They depend on others for their basic needs. Besides physical needs, babies have safety and security and love and belonging needs. You can help meet the baby's basic needs.

INFANT SAFETY AND SECURITY

Babies cannot protect themselves. Like people of all ages, babies need to feel safe and secure. They feel secure when warm and when wrapped and held snugly. Babies cry to communicate. They cry when wet, hungry, uncomfortable, or in pain. Responding to their cries and feeding them when hungry promote safety and security. Infant safety is discussed in Chapter 8. The measures listed in Box 32-1 on page 668 are also important for hospital or home care.

SIGNS AND SYMPTOMS OF ILLNESS

Your observations are important for the infant's safety and well-being. Babies can become ill quickly. Signs and symptoms may be sudden. Therefore you must be very alert. Box 32-2 on page 669 lists the signs and symptoms that must be reported to the nurse immediately.

Tell the nurse when a sign or symptom began. You may need to take an infant's or child's temperature, pulse, and respirations (see Chapter 18). Tympanic, rectal, or axillary temperatures are taken on children younger than 5 years of age. The nurse tells you which method to use for the child. Apical pulses are taken on infants and young children.

BOX 32-1 Infant Safety

- Follow the safety measures listed in Chapter 8 (see page 152).
- Keep the baby warm. Check windows for drafts. Close windows securely.
- Keep your fingernails short. Do not wear rings or bracelets. Long nails and jewelry can scratch the baby.
- Use both hands to lift a newborn.
- Hold the baby securely. Use the cradle hold, football hold, or shoulder hold (Fig. 32-1).
- Support the baby's head and neck when lifting or holding the baby (see Fig. 32-1). Neck support is necessary for the first 3 months after birth.
- Handle the baby with gentle, smooth movements. Avoid sudden or jerking movements. Do not startle the baby.
- Hold and cuddle infants. This is comforting and helps them learn to feel love and security.
- Talk, sing, or play with the baby often. Be sure to talk to the baby during the bath, dressing, and diapering.
- Respond to the baby's crying. Babies cry when they are hungry, uncomfortable, wet, frightened, or when they want attention. This is their way of communicating. Responding to their cries helps them feel safe and secure.
- Do not leave a baby unattended on a table, bed, sofa, or other high surface. Keep one hand on the baby if you must look away (see Fig. 8-1, page 152).
- Use safety straps for babies in infant seats or high chairs.
- Make sure the crib is within hearing distance of the caregivers.
- Keep crib rails up at all times.
- Do not put a pillow in the crib. Pillows can cause suffocation.
- Change the baby's position often. Do not always put the baby in the same position. Alternate between side-lying positions. Support the baby in the side-lying position with a rolled towel or small blanket (Fig. 32-2).
- Do not lay babies on their stomachs for sleep. This can interfere with chest expansion and breathing.
- Keep pins and small objects out of the baby's reach.

A B C

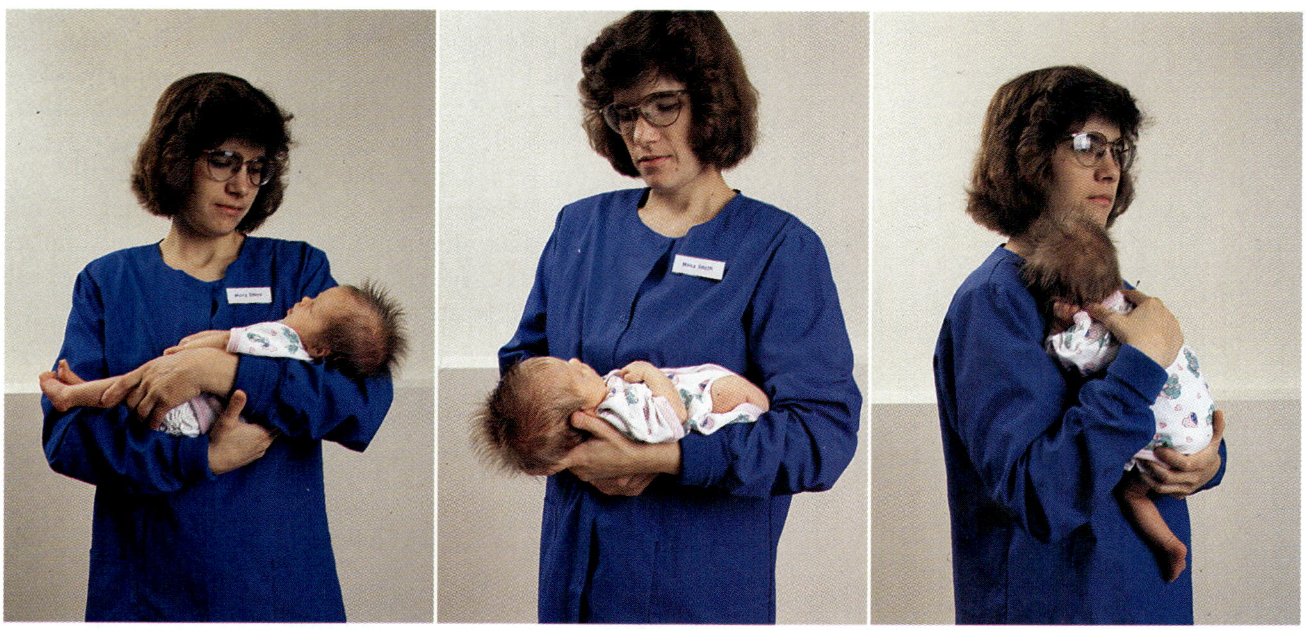

Fig. 32-1 *A, The cradle hold. B, The football hold. C, The shoulder hold.*

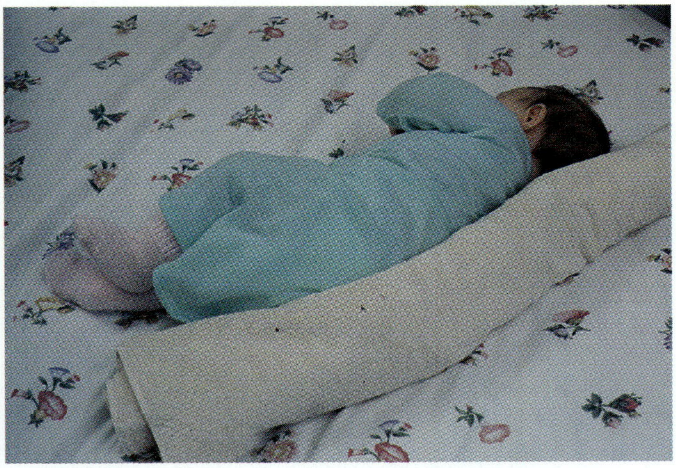

Fig. 32-2 *The baby is supported in the side-lying position with a rolled towel.*

BOX 32-2 Signs and Symptoms of Illness in Babies

- The baby looks sick.
- The baby is limp and slow to respond.
- The baby cries all the time or does not stop crying.
- The baby is flushed, pale, or perspiring.
- The baby has noisy, rapid, difficult, or slow respirations.
- The baby is coughing or sneezing.
- The baby has reddened or irritated eyes.
- The baby turns his or her head to one side or puts a hand to one ear (signs of an earache).
- The baby screams for a long time.
- The baby has skipped feedings.
- The baby has vomited most of the feeding or vomits between feedings.
- The baby has hard, formed stools or watery stools.
- The baby has a rash.

HELPING MOTHERS BREAST-FEED

Many mothers breast-feed their babies. Breast-fed babies usually nurse every 2 or 3 hours. They are fed on demand. In other words, they are fed when hungry, not on a schedule. At first, babies nurse for a short time (5 minutes at each breast). Eventually, nursing time takes up to 30 minutes.

Nurses help new mothers learn to breast-feed. They also teach breast care. Mothers and babies learn how to nurse in a very short time. If the mother or baby is having problems breast-feeding, you must call the nurse.

Mothers may need help getting ready to breast-feed. They may need help with positioning. You may be responsible for bringing babies to mothers. You must help as needed. When you leave the room, make sure the call bell is within reach. The mother and baby need privacy during breast-feeding. In home care settings, you need to stay within hearing distance in case the mother needs help. Box 32-3 on page 670 describes how you can help with breast-feeding.

The nursing mother needs good nutrition. If you are providing home care, you may need to plan meals and grocery shop (Chapter 35). Remember the following when planning meals or grocery shopping.

- Calorie intake may be increased. Your supervisor tells you how much to increase the mother's calorie intake.
- The mother should drink 6 or more cups of milk a day. She can drink whole, 2 percent, or skim milk.
- Include foods high in calcium in the diet.
- The mother should avoid spicy and gas-forming foods. They can cause cramping and diarrhea in the infant. She should avoid onions, garlic, spices, cabbage, brussel sprouts, asparagus, and beans. Chocolate, cola beverages, and coffee can also cause cramping and diarrhea.

Box 32-3 Helping with Breast-Feeding

- Help the mother wash her hands. Handwashing is necessary before she handles her breasts.
- Help the mother to a comfortable position. She may want to nurse sitting up in bed, in a chair, or in the side-lying position (Fig. 32-3).
- Change the baby's diaper if necessary. Bring the baby to the mother.
- Make sure the mother holds the baby close to her breast.
- Have the mother stroke the baby's cheek closest to the breast (Fig. 32-4). This stimulates the **rooting reflex.** The baby turns his or her head when the cheek or mouth is stroked. The head is turned toward the direction of the stimulus and the baby starts to suck. If the right cheek is stroked, the baby turns the head to the right.
- Have the mother keep breast tissue away from the baby's nose with her thumb (Fig. 32-5).
- Give her a baby blanket to cover the baby and her breast. This promotes privacy during the feeding.
- Encourage nursing from both breasts at each feeding. If the baby finished the last feeding at the right breast, the baby starts the next feeding at the left breast.
- Remind her how to remove the baby from the breast. She needs to break the seal or suction between the baby and the breast. She can press a finger down on her breast close to the baby's mouth. Or she can insert a finger into a corner of the baby's mouth (Fig. 32-6).
- Help the mother burp the baby if necessary (page 674). The baby is burped after nursing at each breast.
- Have the mother put a diaper pin on the bra strap of the breast last used. This reminds her which breast to use at the next feeding.
- Change the baby's diaper after the feeding. Lay the baby in the crib if he or she has fallen asleep.
- Encourage the mother to wear a nursing bra day and night. The bra supports the breasts and promotes comfort.
- Encourage the mother to place cotton pads in the bra. The pads absorb leaking milk.
- Have the mother apply cream (if prescribed) to her nipples after each feeding. The cream prevents nipples from drying and cracking.
- Help the mother straighten clothing after the feeding if necessary.

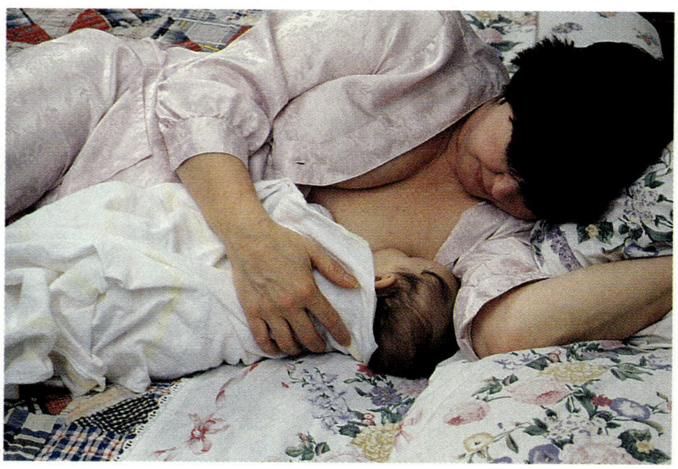

Fig. 32-3 *A mother nursing in the side-lying position.*

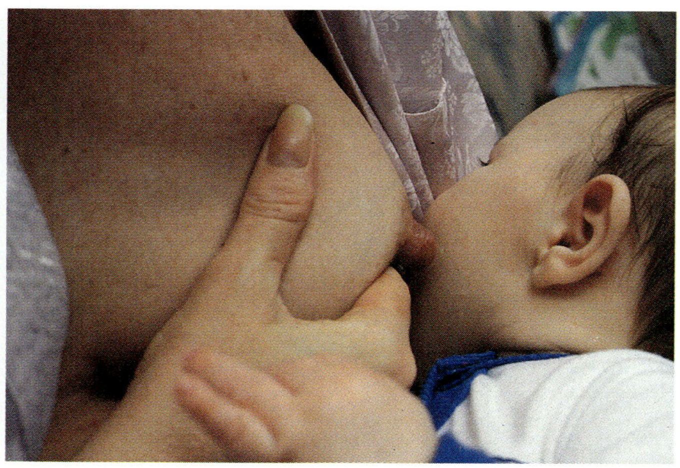

Fig. 32-4 *The mother strokes the baby's cheek with her breast. This stimulates the rooting reflex.*

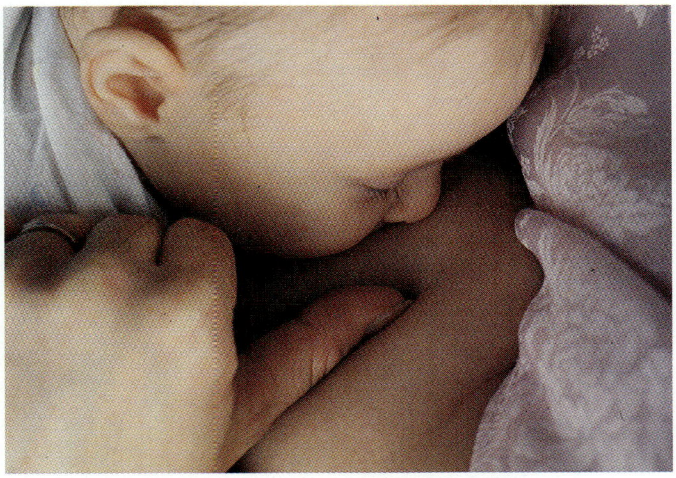

Fig. 32-5 *The thumb is used to keep breast tissue away from the baby's nose.*

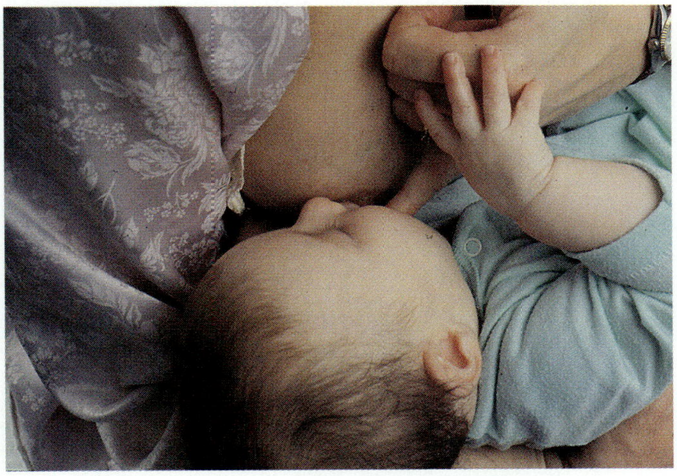

Fig. 32-6 *The mother inserts a finger in the baby's mouth to remove the baby from the breast.*

BOTTLE-FEEDING BABIES

Formula is given to babies who are not breast-fed. The doctor prescribes the formula. It provides the essential nutrients needed by the infant.

Formula comes in three forms. The *ready-to-feed* form is ready to use. It is poured directly from the can into the baby bottle (Fig. 32-7). Water is added to *powdered* and *concentrated* formula. Container directions tell how much formula to use and how much water to add. Bottles are prepared one at a time, or in batches for the whole day. Extra bottles are capped (Fig. 32-8) and stored in the refrigerator. These bottles are used within 24 hours.

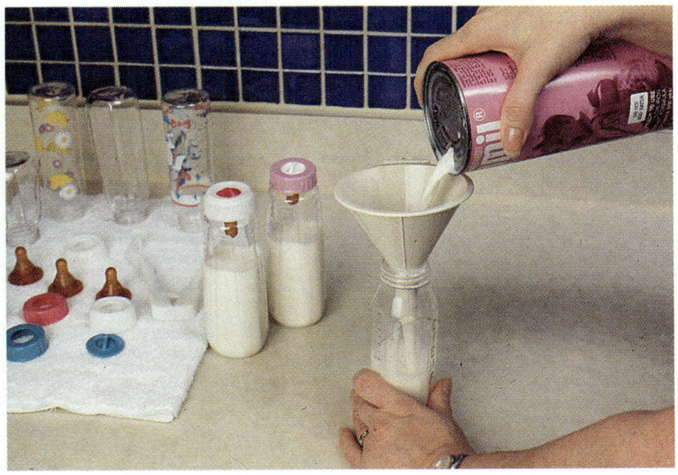

Fig. 32-7 *Ready-to-feed formula is poured from the can into the bottle. A funnel is used to prevent spilling.*

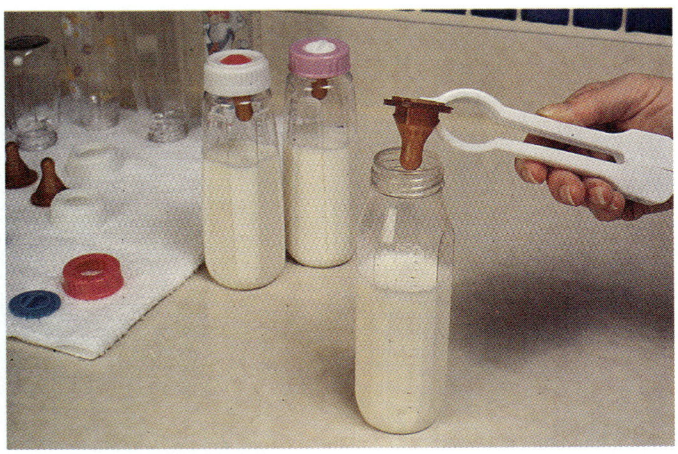

Fig. 32-8 *Bottles are capped for storage in the refrigerator.*

Babies must be protected from infection. Therefore baby bottles, caps, and nipples must be as clean as possible. Disposable equipment is used in hospitals. Reusable equipment may be used in homes. Reusable bottle-feeding equipment is carefully washed in hot, soapy water or in a dishwasher. Complete rinsing is needed to remove all soap. Some mothers use plastic nursers (Fig. 32-9). They require plastic liners that are used once and then discarded.

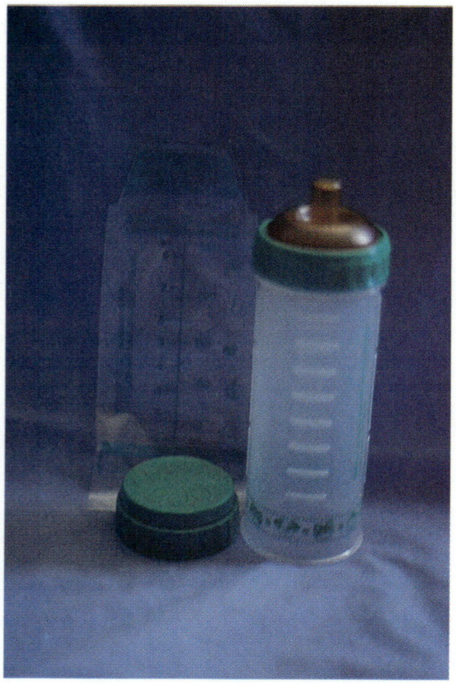

Fig. 32-9 *Plastic nursers have disposable liners.*

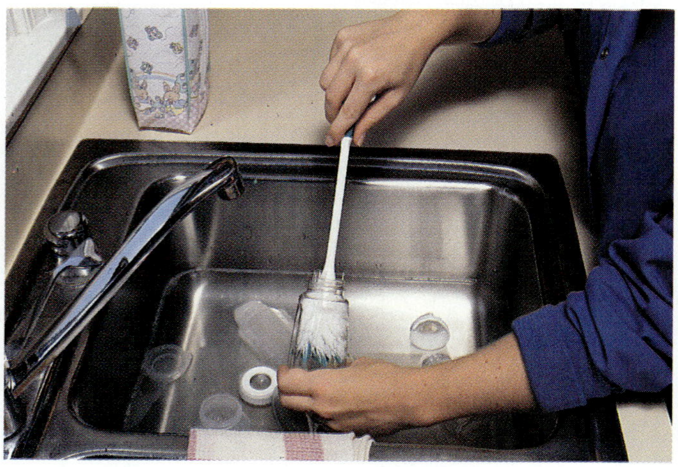

Fig. 32-10 *A bottle brush is used to clean the inside of the bottle.*

Cleaning Baby Bottles

Pre-procedure

1. Wash your hands.
2. Collect the following:
   - Bottles, nipples, and caps
   - Funnel
   - Can opener
   - Bottle brush
   - Dishwashing soap
   - Other items used to prepare formula
   - Towel

Procedure

3. Wash bottles, nipples, caps, funnel, and the can opener in hot, soapy water. Wash other items used to prepare formula.
4. Clean inside baby bottles with the bottle brush (Fig. 32-10).
5. Squeeze hot, soapy water through the nipples (Fig. 32-11). This removes formula from them.
6. Rinse all items thoroughly in hot water. Squeeze hot water through the nipples to remove soap.
7. Lay a clean towel on the countertop.
8. Stand the bottles upside down to drain. Place the nipples, caps, and other items on the towel. Let the items dry.

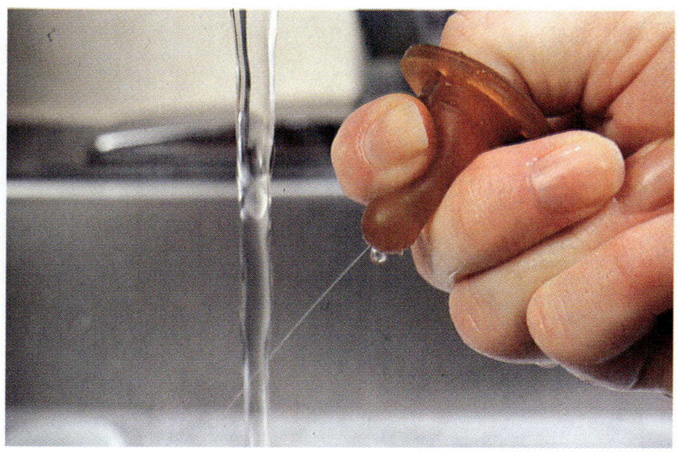

Fig. 32-11 *Water is squeezed through the nipples during cleaning.*

Feeding the Baby

Babies want to be fed every 3 to 4 hours. The amount of formula taken increases as they grow older. The nurse or the mother tells you how much formula a baby needs at each feeding. Babies usually take as much formula as they need. The baby stops sucking and turns away from the bottle when satisfied.

Babies are not given cold formula out of the refrigerator. A bottle is warmed before the feeding. You can warm the bottle in a pan of water. The formula should feel warm. Test the temperature by sprinkling a few drops on your wrist (Fig. 32-12). Do not set the bottle out to warm at room temperature. This takes too long and allows the growth of microorganisms. Do not heat formula in microwave ovens. The formula can heat unevenly and burn the baby's mouth.

The guidelines in Box 32-4 will help you bottle-feed babies.

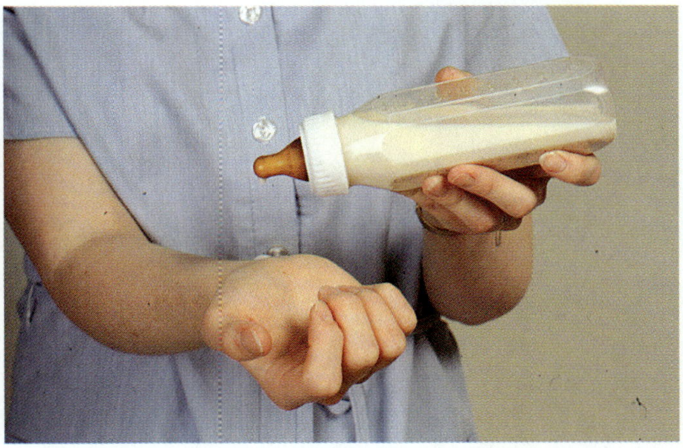

Fig. 32-12 *A home health aide tests formula temperature. Formula should feel warm on her wrist.*

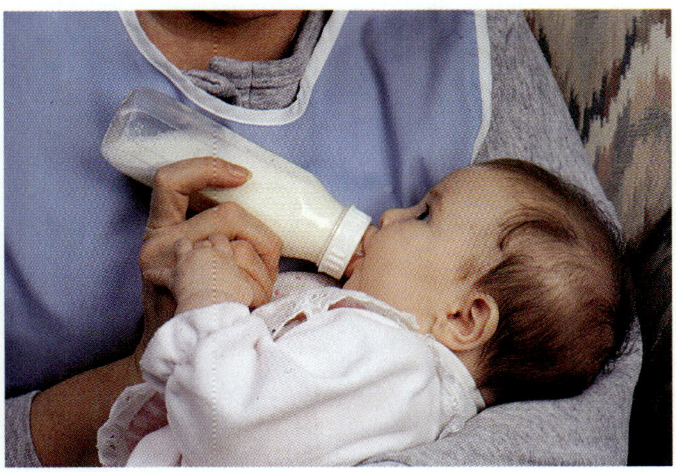

Fig. 32-13 *The bottle is tilted so that formula fills the bottle neck and nipple.*

BOX 32-4 BOTTLE-FEEDING BABIES

- Warm the bottle so the formula feels warm to your wrist.
- Assume a comfortable position for the feeding.
- Hold the baby close to you. Relax and snuggle the baby.
- Tilt the bottle so that the neck of the bottle and the nipple are always filled (Fig. 32-13). Otherwise there will be some air in the neck or nipple. The baby sucks air into the stomach. The air causes cramping and discomfort.
- Do not prop the bottle and lay the baby down for the feeding (Fig. 32-14).
- Burp the baby when he or she has taken half the formula (page 674). Also burp the baby at the end of the feeding.
- Do not leave the baby alone with a bottle.
- Discard remaining formula.
- Wash the bottle, cap, and nipple after the feeding (see *Cleaning Baby Bottles,* page 672).

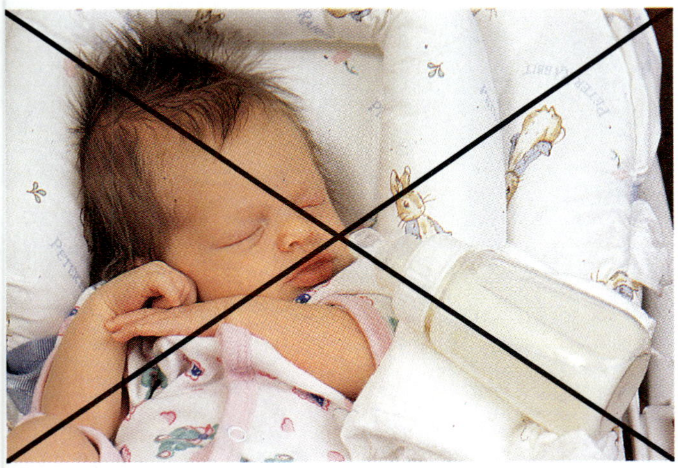

Fig. 32-14 *Do not prop the bottle to feed the baby.*

Burping the Baby

Babies take in air when they nurse. Bottle-fed babies take in more air than breast-fed babies. Air in the stomach and intestines causes cramping and discomfort. This can lead to vomiting. Burping helps to get rid of the air. Burping a baby is sometimes called *bubbling*.

There are two ways to position the baby for burping (Fig. 32-15). One way is to hold the infant over your shoulder. First place a clean diaper or towel over your shoulder. This protects your clothing if the baby "spits up." You can also support the baby in a sitting position on your lap. The towel or diaper is held in front of the baby. To burp the baby, gently pat or rub the baby's back with circular motions.

DIAPERING

Babies urinate several times a day. Breast-fed babies usually have bowel movements after feedings. Bottle-fed babies may have 3 bowel movements a day. Stools are usually soft and unformed. Hard, formed stools mean the baby is constipated. This is reported to the nurse immediately. Watery stools mean diarrhea. Diarrhea is very serious in infants. Their water balance can be upset quickly (see Chapter 17, page 412). Tell the nurse immediately if you suspect a baby has diarrhea.

A

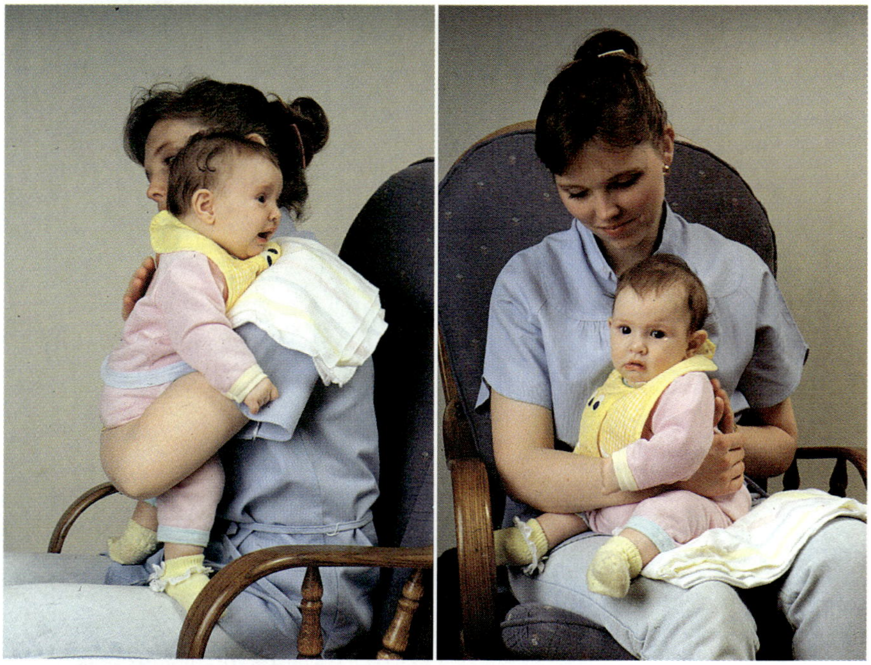

B

Fig. 32-15 *A, The baby is held over the aide's shoulder for burping. B, The baby is supported in the sitting position for burping.*

Diapers are changed when wet. Changing the diaper after a feeding is usually a good idea. Cloth and disposable diapers are available. Cloth diapers are washed, dried, and folded for reuse. They are washed daily or every 2 days with a laundry detergent made especially for use in washing baby clothes. Putting them through the wash cycle a second time without detergent helps remove all soap. If possible, you should hang diapers outside to dry. This gives them a fresh, clean smell.

Disposable diapers are placed in the trash. They are not flushed down the toilet. The use of disposable diapers is more costly.

DIAPERING A BABY

PRE-PROCEDURE

1. Wash your hands.
2. Collect the following:
   - Disposable gloves
   - Clean diaper
   - Waterproof changing pad
   - Washcloth
   - Disposable wipes or cotton balls
   - Basin of warm water
   - Baby soap
   - Baby lotion or cream
3. Place the changing pad under the baby.

PROCEDURE

4. Put on the gloves.
5. Unfasten the dirty diaper. Place diaper pins out of the baby's reach.
6. Wipe the genital area with the front of the diaper (Fig. 32-16 on page 676). Wipe from the front to the back.
7. Fold the diaper so urine and feces are well inside. Set the diaper aside.
8. Clean the genital area from front to back. Use a wet washcloth, disposable wipes, or cotton balls. Wash with mild soap and water if there is a lot of feces or if the baby has a rash. Rinse thoroughly and pat the area dry.
9. Give cord care and clean the circumcision at this time (pages 677-678).
10. Apply cream or lotion to the genital area and buttocks. Do not use too much, because caking can occur.
11. Raise the baby's legs. Slide a clean diaper under the buttocks.
12. Fold a cloth diaper so that there is an extra thickness in front for a boy (Fig. 32-17, A on page 676). For girls, fold the diaper so the extra thickness is at the back (Fig. 32-17, B).
13. Bring the diaper between the baby's legs.
14. Make sure the diaper is snug around the hips and abdomen. It should be loose near the penis if the circumcision has not healed. The diaper should be below the umbilicus if the cord stump has not healed.
15. Secure the diaper in place. Use the plastic tabs on disposable diapers (Fig. 32-18, A on page 677). Make sure the tabs stick in place. Use baby pins for cloth diapers. Pins should point away from the abdomen (Fig. 32-18, B on page 677).
16. Apply plastic pants if cloth diapers are worn. Do not use plastic pants with disposable diapers. They already have waterproof protection.
17. Put the baby in the crib, infant seat, or other safe location.

POST-PROCEDURE

18. Rinse feces from the cloth diaper in the toilet.
19. Store used cloth diapers in a covered pail or plastic bag. Take the disposable diaper to the trash.
20. Remove the gloves and wash your hands.
21. Note and report your observations.

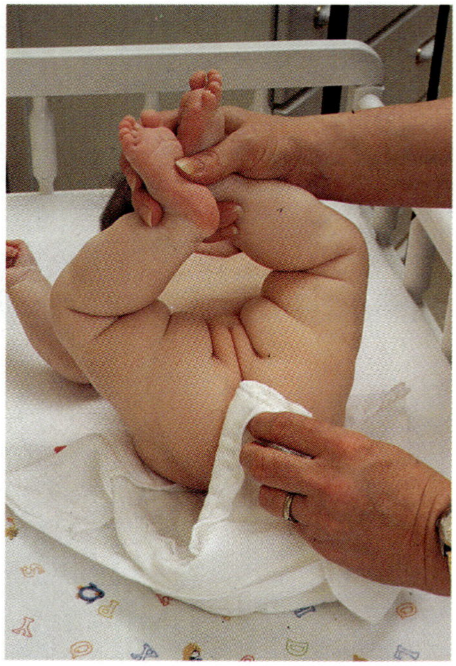

Fig. 32-16 *The front of the diaper is used to clean the genital area.*

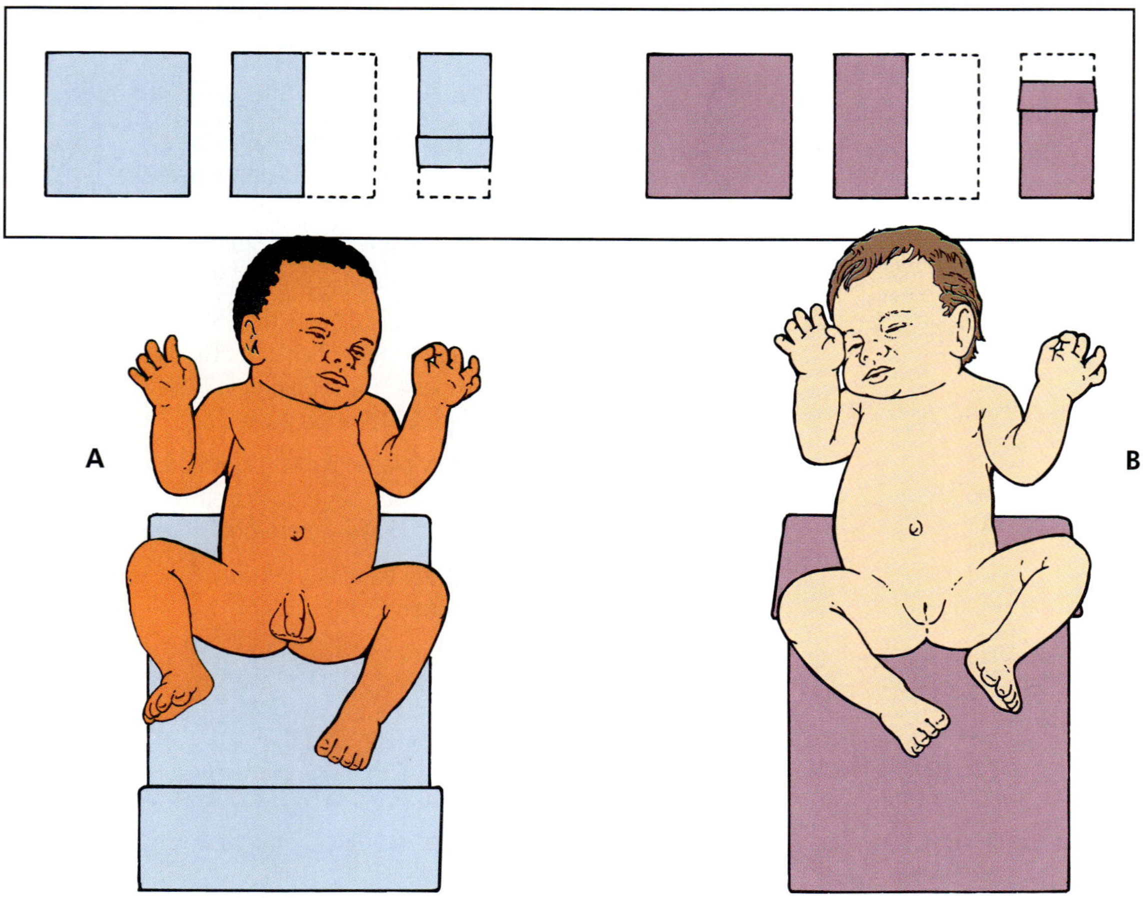

Fig. 32-17 *A, A cloth diaper is folded in front for boys. B, The diaper has a fold in the back for girls.*

A

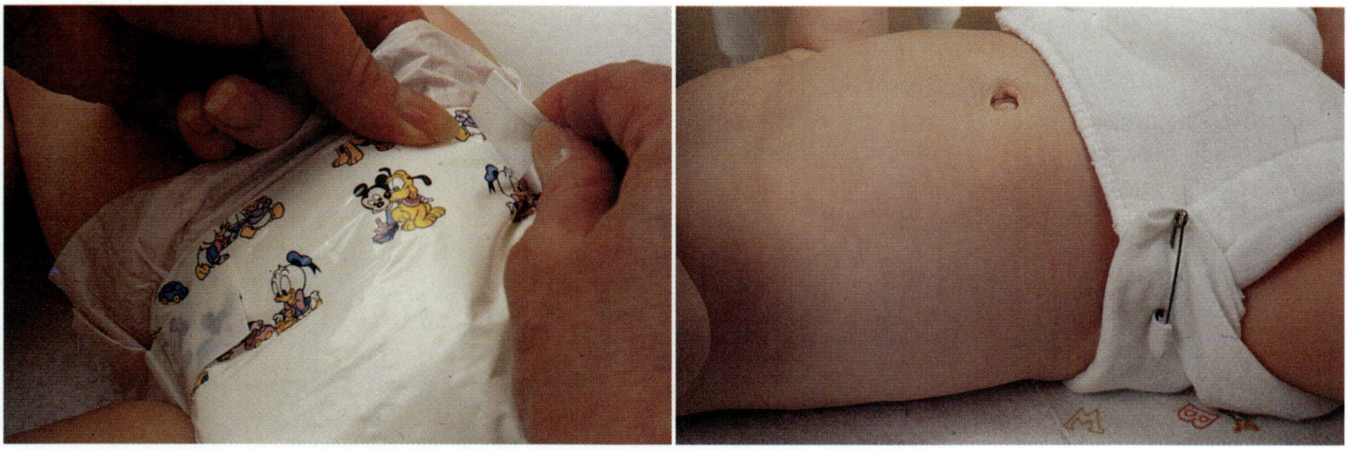

B

Fig. 32-18 *A, A disposable diaper is secured in place with plastic tabs.* ***B,*** *Pins are used to secure cloth diapers. Pins point away from the abdomen.*

CARE OF THE UMBILICAL CORD

The **umbilical cord** connects the mother and the fetus (unborn baby). It carries blood, oxygen, and nutrients from the mother to the fetus (Fig. 32-19). The umbilical cord is not needed after birth. Shortly after delivery, the doctor clamps and cuts the cord. A stump of cord is left on the baby. The stump dries up and falls off in 7 to 10 days. There may be a small amount of blood when the cord comes off.

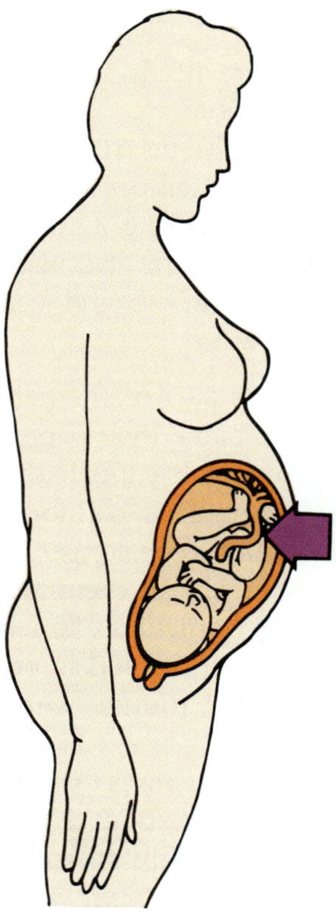

Fig. 32-19 *The umbilical cord connects the mother and fetus. (From Wernig J and Sorrentino SA: The homemaker/home health aide, St Louis, 1989, Mosby–Year Book.)*

The cord provides an area for the growth of microorganisms. Therefore it must be kept clean and dry. Cord care is done at each diaper change. Cord care is continued for 1 or 2 days after the cord comes off. It consists of the following:

- Keep the stump dry. Do not get the stump wet.
- Wipe the base of the stump with alcohol (Fig. 32-20). Use an alcohol wipe or a cotton ball moistened with alcohol. The alcohol promotes drying.
- Keep the diaper below the cord as in Figure 32-18. This prevents the diaper from irritating the stump. It also keeps the cord from becoming wet from urine.
- Report any signs of infection. These include redness or odor or drainage from the stump.
- Give sponge baths until the cord falls off. Then the baby can have a tub bath.

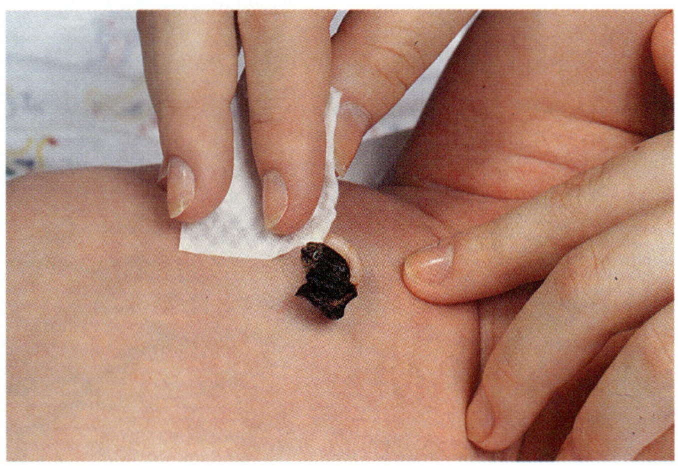

Fig. 32-20 *The cord stump is wiped at the base with alcohol.*

CIRCUMCISION

Boys are born with foreskin on the penis. The surgical removal of foreskin is called a **circumcision** (see Fig. 15-12, page 354). The procedure allows good hygiene and is thought to prevent cancer of the penis. If a circumcision is done, it is usually performed in the hospital before the baby goes home. For those of the Jewish faith, circumcision is a religious ceremony.

The penis will look red, swollen, and sore. However, the circumcision should not interfere with urination. You must carefully check for signs of bleeding and infection. There should be no odor or drainage. You should check the diaper for bleeding. The area should completely heal in 10 to 14 days.

The penis is thoroughly cleaned at each diaper change. Cleaning is especially important if the baby has had a bowel movement. Mild soap and water or commercial wipes are used. The diaper is loosely applied. This prevents the diaper from irritating the penis. Some doctors advise applying petrolatum jelly to the penis. This protects the penis from urine and feces. It also prevents the penis from sticking to the diaper. A cotton swab is used to apply the petrolatum jelly (Fig. 32-21). The nurse tells you if other measures are needed.

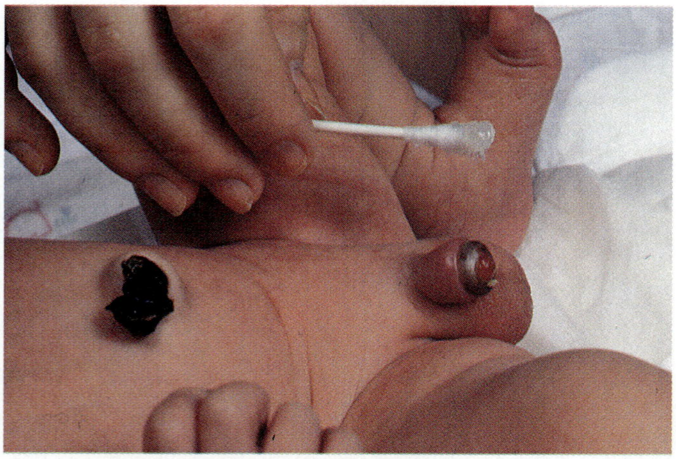

Fig. 32-21 *Petrolatum jelly is applied to the circumcised penis.*

BATHING AN INFANT

A bath is important for cleanliness. Though babies do not get very dirty, they need good skin care. Baths comfort and relax babies. They also provide a wonderful time to hold, touch, and talk to babies. Stimulation is important for development. Being touched and held helps babies learn safety, security, and love and belonging.

Planning is an important part of the bath. You cannot leave the baby alone if you forget something. Therefore you need to gather equipment, supplies, and the baby's clothes before you start the bath. Everything you need must be within your reach.

Safety measures are also very important.

- Never leave the baby alone on a table or in the bath tub.
- Always keep one hand on the baby if you must look away for a moment.
- Hold the baby securely throughout the bath. Babies are very slippery when they are wet. A wet, squirming baby can be very hard to hold.
- Room temperature should be 75° to 80° F for the bath. You may need to turn up the thermostat and close windows and doors about 20 minutes before the bath. The room temperature may be uncomfortable for you. You may want to remove a sweater or lab coat or roll up your sleeves before starting the bath.
- Water temperature needs special attention. Babies have delicate skin and are easily burned. Bath water temperature should be 100° to 105° F (38° to 40.5° C). Bath water temperature is measured with a bath thermometer. If one is not available, test the water temperature with the inside of your wrist (Fig. 32-22). The water should feel warm and comfortable to your wrist.

Bath time should be part of the baby's daily routine. Some mothers like to bathe their babies in the morning. Others prefer the evening. Evening baths have two important advantages. The bath is comforting and relaxing. This helps some babies sleep longer at night. Working fathers are usually home in the evening. The evening bath lets them be involved. Sometimes fathers bathe babies to give mothers time to rest or tend to other children. You must follow the family's routine when working in the home.

There are two bath procedures for babies. Sponge baths are given until the baby is about 2 weeks old. They are given until the cord stump falls off and the umbilicus and circumcision heal. *The cord must not get wet.* The tub bath is given after the cord site and circumcision heal (Fig. 32-23).

Text continued on page 682.

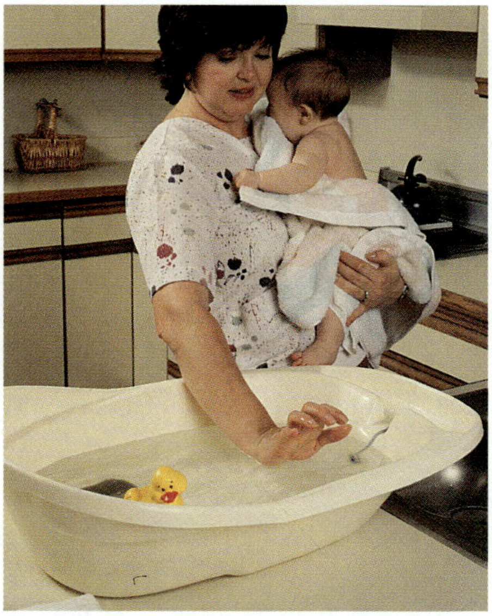

Fig. 32-22 *The wrist is used to test the temperature of the bath water.*

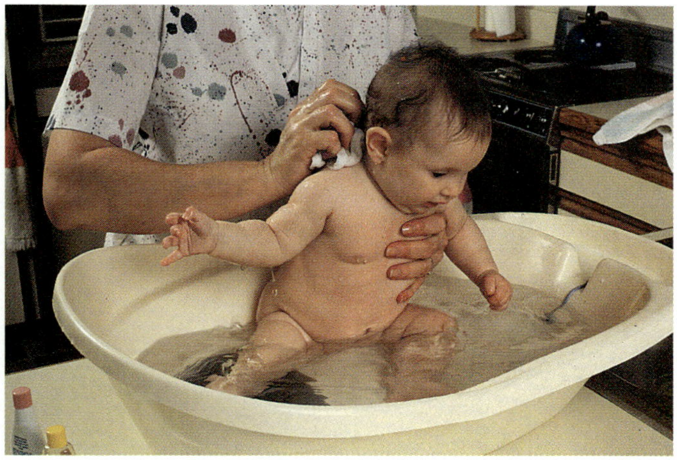

Fig. 32-23 *The baby is given a tub bath.*

Giving a Baby a Sponge Bath

Pre-procedure

1 Wash your hands.
2 Place the following items in your work area:
- Bath basin
- Bath thermometer
- Bath towel
- Two hand towels
- Receiving blanket
- Washcloth
- Clean diaper
- Clean clothing for the baby
- Cotton balls
- Baby soap
- Baby shampoo
- Baby lotion
- Disposable gloves

Procedure

3 Fill the bath basin with warm water. Water temperature should be 100° to 105° F (38° to 40.5° C). Measure water temperature with the bath thermometer or use the inside of your wrist. The water should feel warm and comfortable on your wrist.
4 Provide for privacy.
5 Identify the baby. Check the ID bracelet.
6 Undress the baby. Leave the diaper on.
7 Wash the baby's eyes (Fig. 32-24 on page 680):
   a Dip a cotton ball into the water.
   b Squeeze out excess water.
   c Wash one eye from the inner part to the outer part.
   d Repeat this step for the other eye with a new cotton ball.
8 Moisten the washcloth. Clean the outside of the ear and then behind the ear. Repeat this step for the other ear. Be gentle.
9 Rinse and squeeze out the washcloth. Make a mitt with the washcloth (see Fig. 13-10, page 299).

Continued.

PROCEDURE—CONT'D

10 Wash the baby's face (Fig. 32-25). Clean inside the nostrils with the washcloth. *Do not use cotton swabs to clean inside the ears.* Pat the face dry.

11 Pick up the baby. Hold the baby over the bath basin using the football hold. Support the baby's head and neck with your wrist and hand.

12 Wash the baby's head (Fig. 32-26):

- **a** Squeeze a small amount of water from the washcloth onto the baby's head.
- **b** Apply a small amount of baby shampoo to the head.
- **c** Wash the head with circular motions.
- **d** Rinse the head by squeezing water from a washcloth over the baby's head. Be sure to rinse thoroughly. Avoid getting soap in the baby's eyes.
- **e** Use a small hand towel to dry the head.

13 Lay the baby on the table.

14 Put on the gloves.

15 Remove the diaper.

16 Wash the front of the body. Use a soapy washcloth. You may also apply soap to your hands and wash the baby with your hands (Fig. 32-27). Do not get the cord wet. Rinse thoroughly. Pat dry. Be sure to dry all creases.

17 Turn the baby to the prone position. Repeat step 16 for the back and buttocks.

18 Give cord care and clean the circumcision.

19 Apply baby lotion to the baby's body as directed by the nurse.

20 Put a clean diaper and clean clothes on the baby.

21 Remove the gloves.

22 Wrap the baby in the receiving blanket. Put the baby in the crib or other safe location.

POST-PROCEDURE

23 Clean and return equipment and supplies to the proper place. Do this step when the baby is settled.

24 Wash your hands.

25 Note and report your observations.

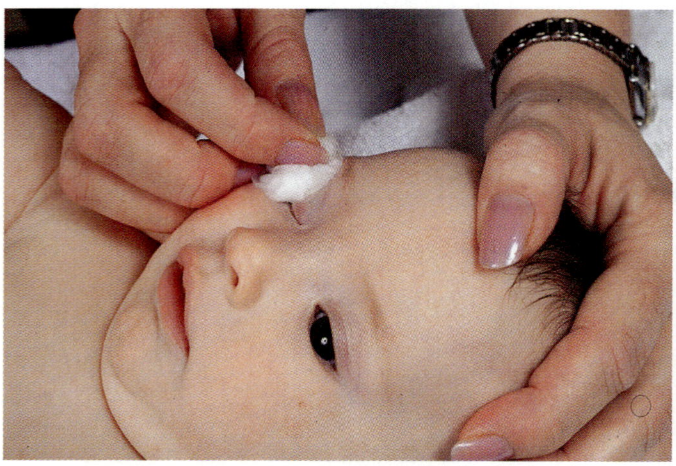

Fig. 32-24 *The baby's eyes are washed with cotton balls. The eye is cleaned from the inner to the outer part.*

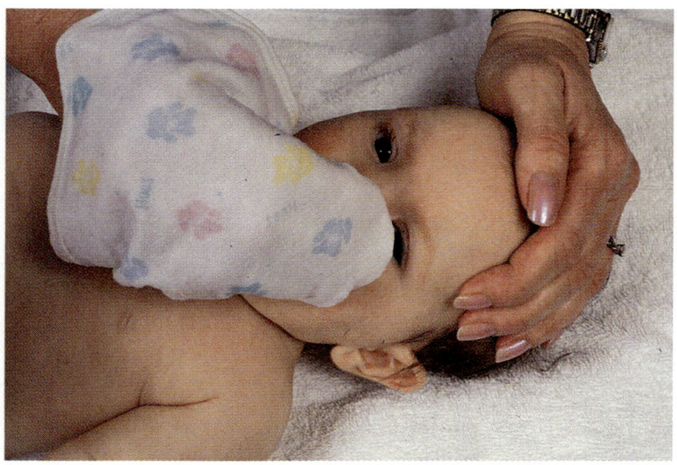

Fig. 32-25 *The baby's face is washed with a mitted washcloth.*

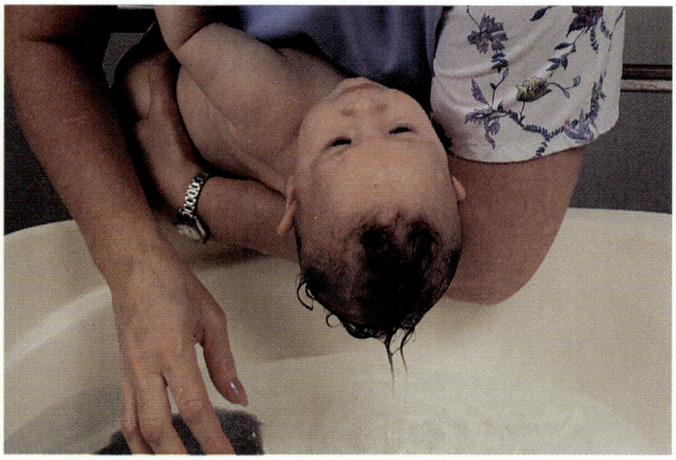

Fig. 32-26 *The baby's head is washed over the basin.*

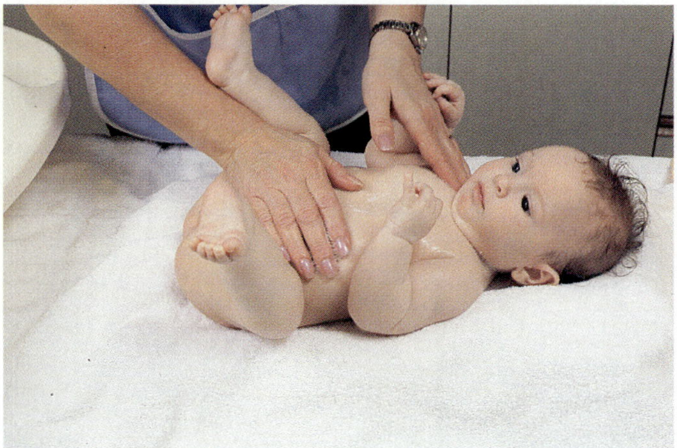

Fig. 32-27 *The hands are used to wash the baby.*

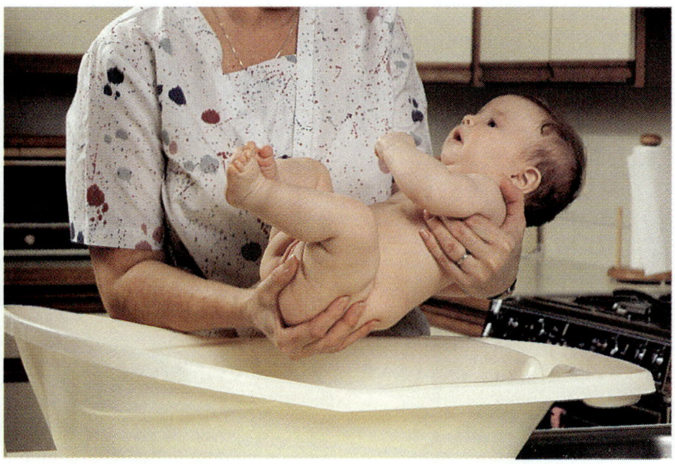

Fig. 32-28 *The baby is held for the tub bath.*

Giving a Baby a Tub Bath

Procedure

1. Follow steps 1 through 15 in the sponge bath procedure (see pages 679-680).
2. Hold the baby as in Figure 32-28:
   - **a** Place your right hand under the baby's shoulders. Your thumb should be over the baby's right shoulder. Your fingers should be under the right arm.
   - **b** Use your left hand to support the baby's buttocks. Slide your left hand under the thighs. Hold the right thigh with your left hand.
3. Lower the baby into the water feet first.
4. Wash the front of the baby's body. Be sure to wash all folds and creases. Rinse thoroughly.
5. Reverse your hold. Use your left hand to hold the baby.
6. Wash the baby's back as in Figure 32-23. Rinse thoroughly.
7. Reverse your hold again. Use your right hand to hold the baby.
8. Wash the genital area.
9. Lift the baby out of the water and onto a towel.
10. Wrap the baby in the towel. Also cover the baby's head.
11. Pat the baby dry. Be sure to dry all folds and creases.
12. Follow steps 21-25 of the sponge bath (pages 679-680).

WEIGHING INFANTS

Infants are weighed at birth. The birth weight serves as the baseline for measuring the infant's growth. The nurse uses weight measurements as part of the assessment step of the nursing process. It is also used to evaluate how much breast milk was taken during breast-feeding. The baby is weighed before and after breast-feeding. The difference in the weights is the amount of milk taken in during breast-feeding. The nurse uses this information to determine if the baby is getting enough milk.

The nurse tells you when to weigh the baby. The baby's safety needs must be met. The baby is protected from chills. The room must be warm and free of drafts. The baby is also protected from falling. Always keep a hand over the baby when taking the weight measurement. Remember to keep one hand on the baby if you need to look away. Breast-fed babies wear the same diaper, clothes, and blanket for each weight measurement.

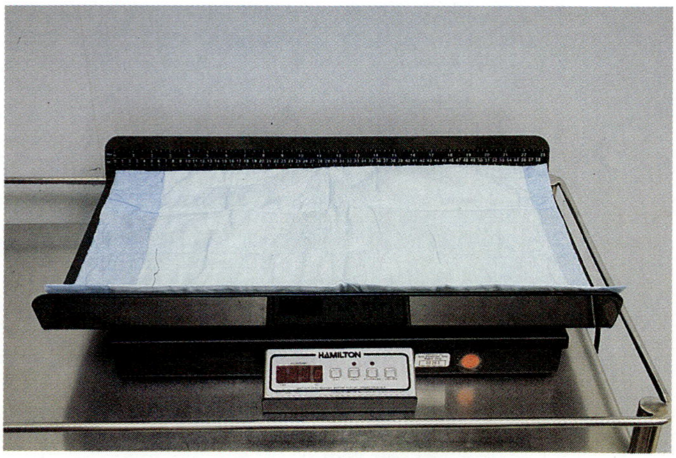

Fig. 32-29 *Digital infant scale.*

WEIGHING AN INFANT

PRE-PROCEDURE

1. Wash your hands.
2. Collect the following:
   - Baby scale
   - Paper for the scale
   - Items for diaper changing (see *Diapering a Baby,* page 675)

PROCEDURE

3. Identify the baby.
4. Place the paper on the scale. Adjust the scale to zero (0).
5. Put on the gloves.
6. Undress the baby and remove the diaper. Clean the genital area.
7. Lay the baby on the scale. Keep one hand over the baby to prevent falling.
8. Read the digital display (Fig. 32-29) or move the pointer until the scale is balanced.
9. Diaper and dress the baby. Lay the baby in the crib.
10. Remove and discard the gloves.

POST-PROCEDURE

11. Return the scale to its proper place.
12. Wash your hands.
13. Report your observations to the nurse.
14. Record the weight according to facility policy.

SUMMARY

Caring for new mothers and infants can be a wonderful experience. Infant safety is very important. Babies cannot protect themselves. They depend on others for their needs. Their physical needs must be met. Babies must also feel safe, secure, and loved. Be sure to talk, sing, and play with babies while you meet their basic needs.

Review Questions

Circle the best *answer.*

1 Andrew is a newborn. His head must be supported for the first
- **a** 7 to 10 days
- **b** Month
- **c** 3 months
- **d** 6 months

2 When holding Andrew, you should
- **a** Hold him securely
- **b** Cuddle him
- **c** Sing and talk to him
- **d** All of the above

3 Which is *false?*
- **a** Andrew's crib should be within hearing distance of caregivers.
- **b** Andrew should have a pillow for sleep.
- **c** Andrew's position should be changed often.
- **d** Crib rails should be up at all times.

4 Report the following to your supervisor *except*
- **a** Andrew looks flushed and is perspiring
- **b** Andrew has watery stools
- **c** Andrew's eyes are red and irritated
- **d** Andrew spits up a small amount when burped

5 Andrew will be breast-fed. The mother should
- **a** Wash her hands
- **b** Hold Andrew close to her breast
- **c** Stimulate the rooting reflex
- **d** All of the above

6 A breast-fed baby should be burped
- **a** Every 5 minutes
- **b** After nursing from one breast
- **c** After nursing from both breasts
- **d** After the feeding

7 Andrew is being switched to bottle-feedings. You do the grocery shopping. Which formula should you buy?
- **a** The one that is on sale
- **b** The ready-to-feed type
- **c** The one ordered by the doctor
- **d** The powdered form

8 You are to warm Andrew's bottle. Which is *true?*
- **a** The bottle is warmed for 5 minutes in the microwave.
- **b** The formula should warm at room temperature.
- **c** The formula should feel warm on your wrist.
- **d** The formula is warmed in a pan for 5 minutes.

9 When bottle-feeding Andrew, you should
- **a** Burp him every 5 minutes
- **b** Save remaining formula for the next feeding
- **c** Tilt the bottle so that formula fills the neck of the bottle and the nipple
- **d** All of the above

10 Andrew's diapers are changed whenever he is wet.
- **a** True
- **b** False

11 Andrew's cord has not yet healed. His diaper should be
- **a** Loose over the cord
- **b** Snug over the cord
- **c** Below the cord
- **d** Disposable

12 Andrew's cord stump is cleaned with
- **a** Soap and water
- **b** Baby shampoo
- **c** Plain water
- **d** Alcohol

Review Questions—Cont'd

13 Andrew's cord and the circumcision are cleaned

- **a** Once a day
- **b** When he has a bowel movement
- **c** Three times a day
- **d** At every diaper change

14 Andrew's cord and circumcision have not healed. He should have a sponge bath.

- **a** True
- **b** False

15 Bath water for Andrew should be

- **a** 85° to 90° F
- **b** 90° to 95° F
- **c** 95° to 100° F
- **d** 100° to 105° F

16 Which should you use to wash Andrew's eyes?

- **a** A mitted washcloth
- **b** Alcohol wipes
- **c** A cotton swab
- **d** Cotton balls

17 Cotton swabs are used to clean inside Andrew's ears.

- **a** True
- **b** False

18 Andrew is being breast-fed. He is weighed with his diaper on.

- **a** True
- **b** False

Answers to these questions are on page 753.

Basic Emergency Care

33

OBJECTIVES

- Define the key terms listed in this chapter
- Describe the general rules of emergency care
- Identify the signs of cardiac arrest and the signs of an obstructed airway
- Describe basic life support and basic life support procedures
- Explain the difference between internal and external hemorrhage
- Explain the difference between arterial and venous bleeding
- Explain how to control hemorrhage
- Identify the signs of, and emergency care for, shock
- Describe two types of seizures and how to care for a person during a seizure
- Describe burns, their causes, and emergency care
- Identify the common causes of, and emergency care for, fainting
- Describe the signs of, and emergency care for, stroke

Key Terms

cardiac arrest The heart and breathing stop suddenly and without warning

convulsion Violent and sudden contractions or tremors of muscles; seizure

first aid Emergency care given to an ill or injured person before medical help arrives

hemorrhage The excessive loss of blood in a short period of time

respiratory arrest Breathing stops but the heart still pumps blood for several minutes

seizure A convulsion

shock A condition that results when there is not enough blood supply to organs and tissues

Emergencies can occur anywhere. They happen in health care facilities, homes, public places, or on highways. Knowing what to do can mean the difference between life and death. This chapter describes some common emergencies and the basic care that is given. You are encouraged to take a first aid course from the National Safety Council or the American Red Cross. A basic life support course given by the American Heart Association, National Safety Council, or the American Red Cross is also recommended. These courses prepare you to give care in emergency situations.

GENERAL RULES OF EMERGENCY CARE

First aid is the emergency care given to an ill or injured person before medical help arrives. The goals of first aid are to:

- Prevent death
- Prevent injuries from becoming worse

When an emergency occurs, the local Emergency Medical Services (EMS) system must be activated. The system involves emergency personnel (paramedics, emergency medical technicians) who have been trained and educated in emergency care. They know how to treat, stabilize, and transport persons with life-threatening conditions. Their emergency vehicles have the equipment, supplies, and drugs used in emergencies. Emergency personnel communicate by telephone or two-way radio with doctors based in hospital emergency rooms. The doctors tell them what to do. In many areas the EMS system is activated by dialing 911. Calling the local fire or police department or the telephone operator can also activate the system.

Each emergency is different. However, the rules in Box 33-1 on page 688 apply to any emergency.

BASIC LIFE SUPPORT (BLS)

When the heart and breathing stop, the person is clinically dead. Blood and oxygen are not circulated through the body. Permanent brain damage and other organ damage occur within 4 to 6 minutes. Death may be expected. Death is expected in persons suffering from illnesses for which there is no hope of recovery. However, the heart and breathing can stop suddenly and without warning. This is a state of **cardiac arrest.**

Cardiac arrest is a sudden, unexpected, and dramatic event. Cardiac arrest can occur while driving, shoveling snow, playing golf or tennis, watching television, eating, and sleeping. It can occur anywhere and at any time. Common causes include heart disease, drowning,

BOX 33-1 General Rules of Emergency Care

- Know your limits. Do not do more than you are able. Do not perform an unfamiliar procedure. Do what you can under the circumstances.
- Stay calm. This helps the victim feel more secure.
- Practice Standard Precautions and follow the Bloodborne Pathogen Standard to the extent possible.
- Check for signs of life-threatening problems. Check for breathing, a pulse, and bleeding.
- Keep the victim lying down or in the position in which he or she was found. Moving the victim could make an injury worse.
- Perform necessary emergency measures.
- Call for help or tell someone to activate the EMS system. An operator will send emergency vehicles and personnel to the scene. *Do not hang up until the operator has hung up.* Give the operator the following information:
  *Your location—street address and city or town you are in. Give names of cross streets or roads and landmarks if possible.
  *Telephone number you are calling from
  *What has happened (heart attack, accident, and so on)—police, fire equipment, and ambulances may be needed
  *How many people need help
  *Condition of victims, any obvious injuries, and any life-threatening situations
  *What aid is being given
- Do not remove the victim's clothing unless you have to. If clothing must be removed, tear or cut garments along the seams.
- Keep the victim warm. Cover the victim with a blanket. Or use coats and sweaters.
- Reassure the conscious victim. Explain what is happening and that help has been called.
- Do not give the victim any food or fluids.
- Do not move the victim. Emergency personnel have been trained to do so.
- Keep bystanders away from the victim. Bystanders tend to stare, give advice, and comment about the victim's condition. The victim may think the situation is worse than it really is. Also, the victim's privacy is invaded by onlookers.

electrical shock, severe injury, airway obstruction, and drug overdose. The victim suffers permanent brain damage unless breathing and circulation are restored.

Respiratory arrest is when breathing stops but the heart still pumps blood for several minutes. Causes of respiratory arrest include drowning, stroke, obstructed airway, drug overdose, electrocution, lightning strike, smoke inhalation, suffocation, heart attack (myocardial infarction), coma, and other injuries. If breathing is not restored, cardiac arrest occurs. If the person still has a pulse, rescue breathing (page 689) can often prevent cardiac arrest.

Basic life support involves preventing or promptly recognizing cardiac arrest or respiratory arrest. BLS procedures support breathing and circulation. These life-saving measures require speed, skill, and efficiency. Prompt activation of the EMS system is also part of basic life support.

Cardiopulmonary Resuscitation

There are three major signs of cardiac arrest—no pulse, no breathing, and unconsciousness. The person's skin is cool, pale, and gray. The person has no blood pressure.

Cardiopulmonary resuscitation (CPR) must be started as soon as cardiac arrest occurs. CPR provides oxygen to the brain, heart, kidneys, and other organs until more advanced emergency care can be given. CPR has three basic parts (the ABCs of CPR):

- Airway
- Breathing
- Circulation

The person must be supine on a hard, flat surface. The arms are positioned at the sides. If turning is necessary, use the logrolling procedure. There may be other injuries. Therefore the person must be turned as a unit to prevent twisting of the spinal cord.

Airway The respiratory passages (airway) must be open to restore breathing. The airway is often blocked or obstructed during cardiac arrest. The victim's tongue falls toward the back of the throat and blocks the airway. The

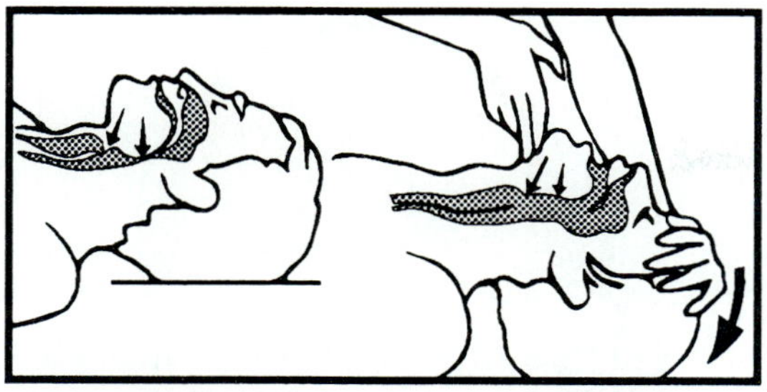

Fig. 33-1 *The head-tilt/chin-lift maneuver is used to open the airway. One hand is on the victim's forehead, and pressure is applied to tilt the head back. The fingers of the other hand are placed under the chin. The chin is lifted forward with the fingers.*

head-tilt/chin-lift maneuver is used to open the airway (Fig. 33-1):

- Place one hand on the victim's forehead.
- Apply pressure on the forehead with the palm to tilt the head back.
- Place the fingers of the other hand under the bony part of the chin.
- Lift the chin forward as the head is tilted backward with the other hand.

When the airway is open, check for vomitus, loose dentures, or other foreign bodies. These can obstruct the airway during rescue breathing. Vomitus is wiped away with your index and middle fingers. Wear disposable gloves or cover your fingers with a cloth. Dentures are removed. Though time must not be wasted, try to protect the dentures from loss or damage.

Breathing Air is not inhaled when breathing stops. The victim must get oxygen. Otherwise, permanent brain and organ damage occur. Breathing is done for the victim. This is called rescue breathing.

Before rescue breathing is started, breathlessness is determined (Fig. 33-2). It should take 3 to 5 seconds to do the following:

- Maintain an open airway.
- Place your ear over the person's mouth and nose.
- Observe the person's chest.
- *Look* to see if the chest rises and falls.
- *Listen* for the escape of air.
- *Feel* for the flow of air.

Mouth-to-mouth resuscitation (Fig. 33-3) is the most common method of rescue breathing. The airway is kept open to give mouth-to-mouth resuscitation. The victim's nostrils are pinched shut with the thumb and index finger

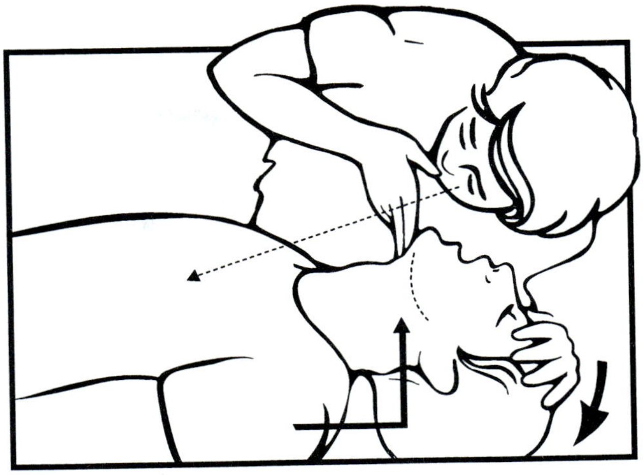

Fig. 33-2 *Breathlessness is determined by* looking *to see if the chest rises and falls,* listening *for the escape of air, and* feeling *for the flow of air.*

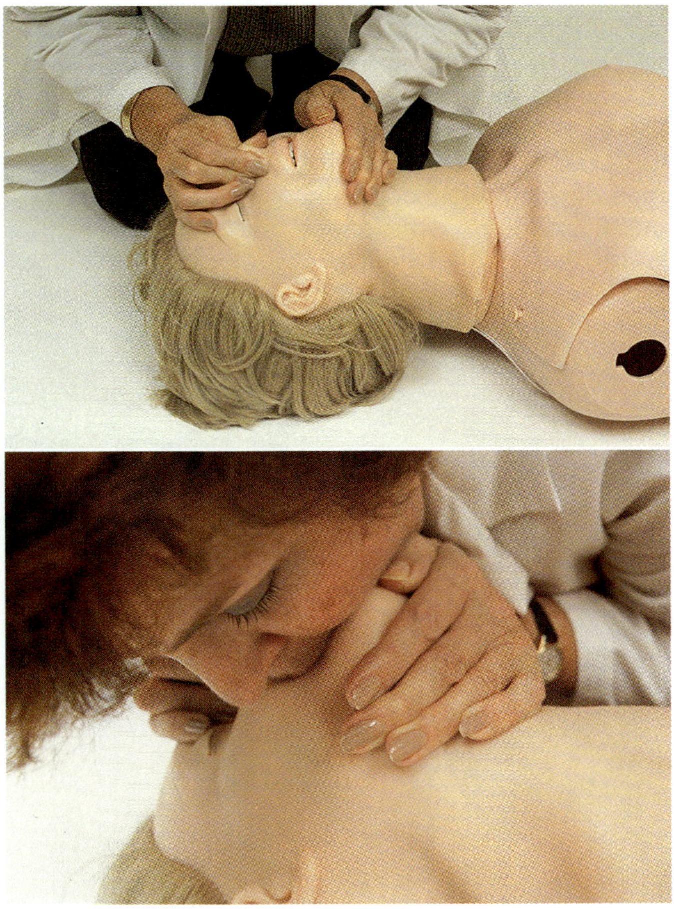

A

B

Fig. 33-3 *Mouth-to-mouth resuscitation. A, The victim's airway is opened, and the nostrils are pinched shut. B, The victim's mouth is sealed by the rescuer's mouth.*

of the hand on the forehead. Shutting the nostrils prevents the escape of air from the nose. After taking a deep breath, place your mouth tightly over the victim's mouth. Slowly blow air into the victim's mouth. You should see the victim's chest rise as the lungs fill with air. You should also hear the escape of air when the person exhales. After giving a ventilation, remove your mouth from the victim's mouth. Then take in a quick, deep breath.

Mouth-to-mouth resuscitation is not always indicated or possible. The *mouth-to-nose* technique may be necessary. The mouth-to-nose technique is used when:

- You cannot ventilate the victim's mouth
- You cannot open the mouth
- You cannot make a tight seal for mouth-to-mouth resuscitation
- The mouth is severely injured

The mouth is closed for mouth-to-nose resuscitation. The head-tilt/chin-lift method is used to open the airway. Pressure is placed on the chin to close the mouth. To give the ventilation, place your mouth over the victim's nose and blow air into the nose (Fig. 33-4). After the ventilation, remove your mouth from the person's nose.

Some people breathe through openings *(stomas)* in their necks (Fig. 33-5). They need *mouth-to-stoma* ventilation during cardiac or respiratory arrest. You will seal your mouth around the stoma and blow air into the stoma (Fig. 33-6). Before giving mouth-to-mouth or mouth-to-nose resuscitation, always check to see if a

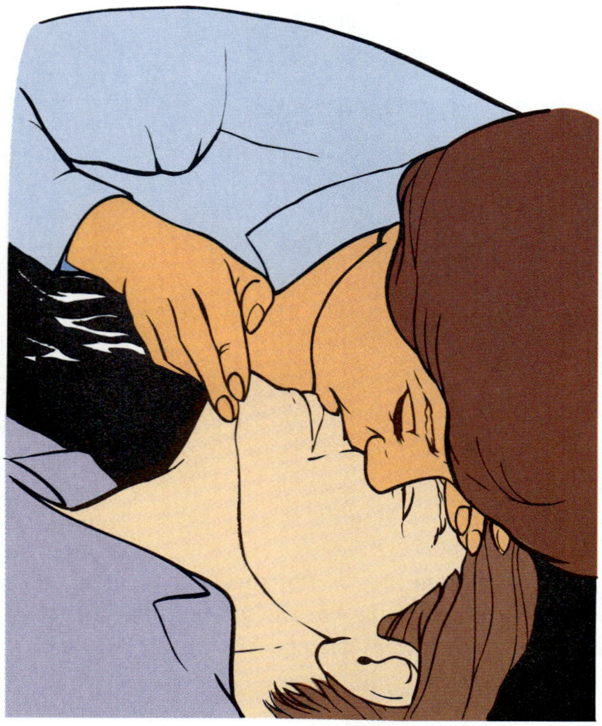

Fig. 33-4 *Mouth-to-nose resuscitation.*

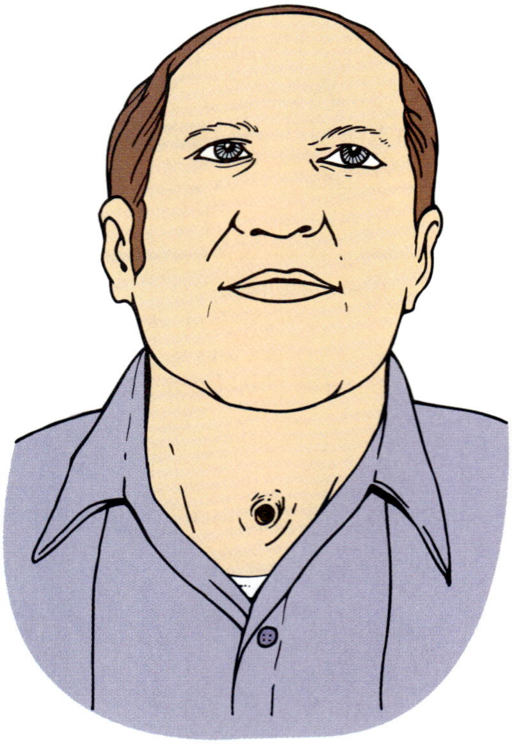

Fig. 33-5 *A stoma in the neck. The person breathes air in and out of the stoma.*

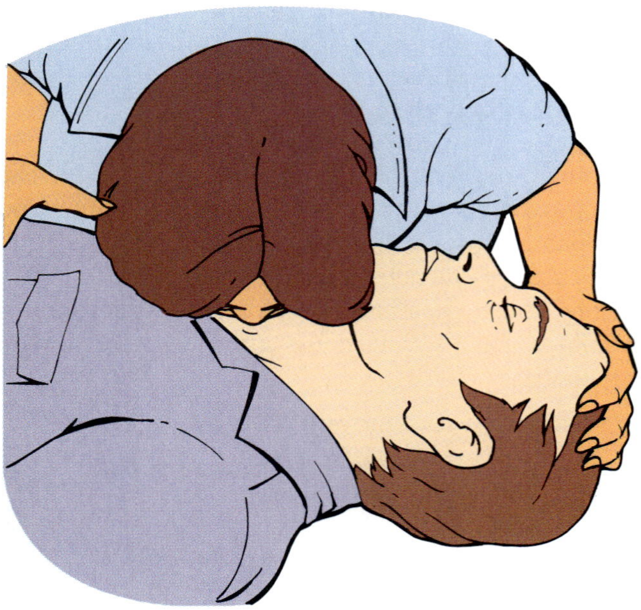

Fig. 33-6 *Mouth-to-stoma resuscitation.*

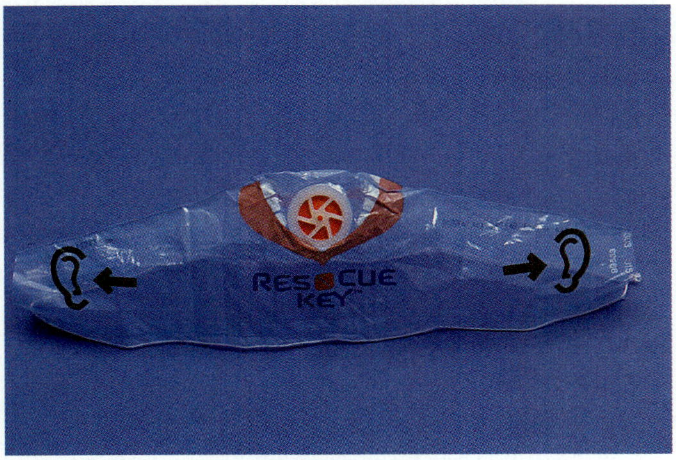

Fig. 33-7 *Mask device.*

person has a stoma. Other methods of rescue breathing are not effective if the person has a stoma.

You will have contact with the victim's body fluids or body substances during rescue breathing. Barrier devices prevent contact with the victim's mouth and body fluids or body substances. Mask devices are available (Fig. 33-7). *Mouth-to-barrier device* is another method of rescue breathing. The barrier device is placed over the person's mouth and nose. There must be a tight seal. You breathe into the barrier device.

When CPR is started, two breaths are given at first. Exhalation is allowed after each breath. Then breaths are given at a rate of 10 to 12 breaths per minute. During one-rescuer CPR, 2 breaths are given after every 15 chest compressions. During two-rescuer CPR, a breath is given after every 5 chest compressions.

Circulation Blood flow to the brain and other organs must be maintained. Otherwise, permanent damage results. The heart has stopped beating in cardiac arrest. Therefore blood must be pumped through the body in some other way. Artificial circulation is accomplished by chest compression. Each chest compression forces blood through the circulatory system.

Before chest compressions are started, pulselessness must be determined. The carotid artery on the side near you is used to check for pulselessness. To find the carotid pulse, place the tips of your index and middle fingers on the victim's trachea (windpipe). Then slide your fingertips down off the trachea to the groove of the neck (Fig. 33-8).

The heart lies between the sternum (breastbone) and the spinal column. When pressure is applied to the sternum, the sternum is depressed. This compresses the heart between the sternum and spinal column (Fig. 33-9). For effective chest compressions, the victim must be supine and on a hard, flat surface.

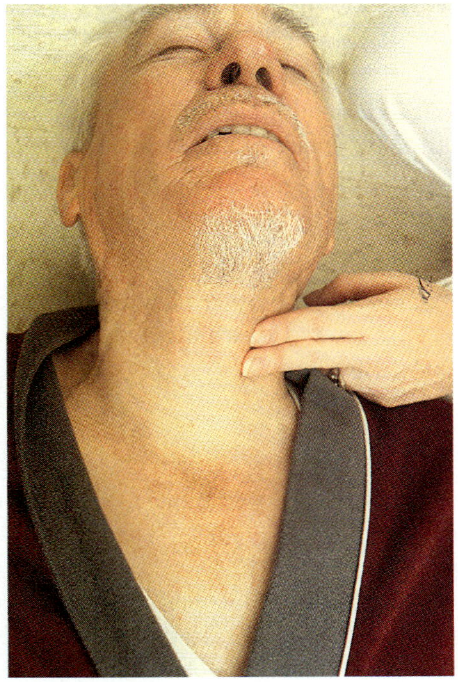

Fig. 33-8 *Locating the carotid pulse. Index and middle fingers are placed on the trachea. The fingers are moved down into the groove of the neck where the carotid pulse is located.*

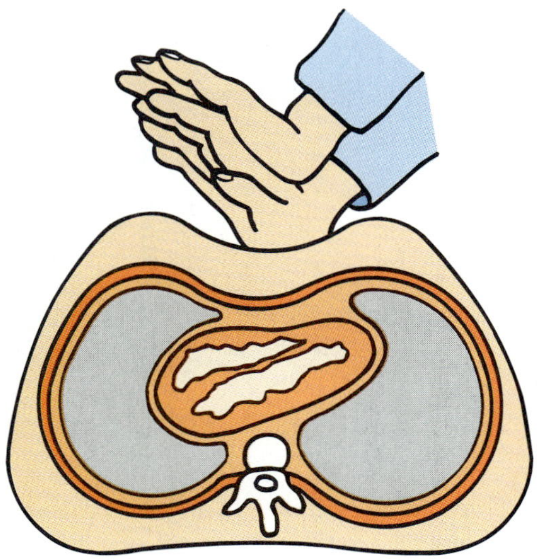

Fig. 33-9 *The heart lies between the sternum and spinal cord. The heart is compressed when pressure is applied to the sternum.* (From Rosen P, et al.: Emergency medicine: concepts and clinical practice, ed 3, St Louis, 1992, Mosby—Year Book.)

Proper hand position is important for chest compressions. The process for locating hand position for adults is shown in Figure 33-10.

- Use your index and middle fingers to locate the lower part of the victim's rib cage on the side near you.
- Then run your fingers up along the rib cage to the notch at the center of the chest. The notch is where the ribs and sternum meet.
- Place the heel of your other hand on the lower half of the sternum next to your index finger.
- Remove your index and middle fingers from the notch.
- Place that hand on the hand already on the sternum.
- Extend or interlace your fingers. Keep your fingers off the chest.

You must be positioned properly for chest compressions. Your elbows are straight. Your shoulders are directly over the victim's chest (Fig. 33-11). Firm downward pressure is exerted to depress the sternum about 1½ to 2 inches in the adult. Then pressure is released without removing your hands from the chest. Compressions are given in a regular rhythm.

Performing CPR CPR is done only for cardiac arrest. You must determine if cardiac arrest or fainting has occurred. CPR is done when there is unresponsiveness, breathlessness, and pulselessness. That is, the person does not respond, is not breathing, and has no pulse. Basic life support involves the following sequence:

1. Determine unresponsiveness. Tap or gently shake the victim and shout "Are you OK?" If there is no response, the victim is unconscious.
2. *Activate the EMS system immediately if the person is unresponsive.*
3. Determine breathlessness. *Look* at the victim's chest to see if it rises and falls. *Listen* for the escape of air during expiration. *Feel* for the flow of air.
4. Open the airway and give two breaths if the person is not breathing.
5. Determine pulselessness.
6. Start chest compressions if the person has no pulse.

Cardiopulmonary resuscitation can be done alone or with another person. CPR is *never* practiced on another person. Serious damage can be done. Mannequins are used to learn CPR.

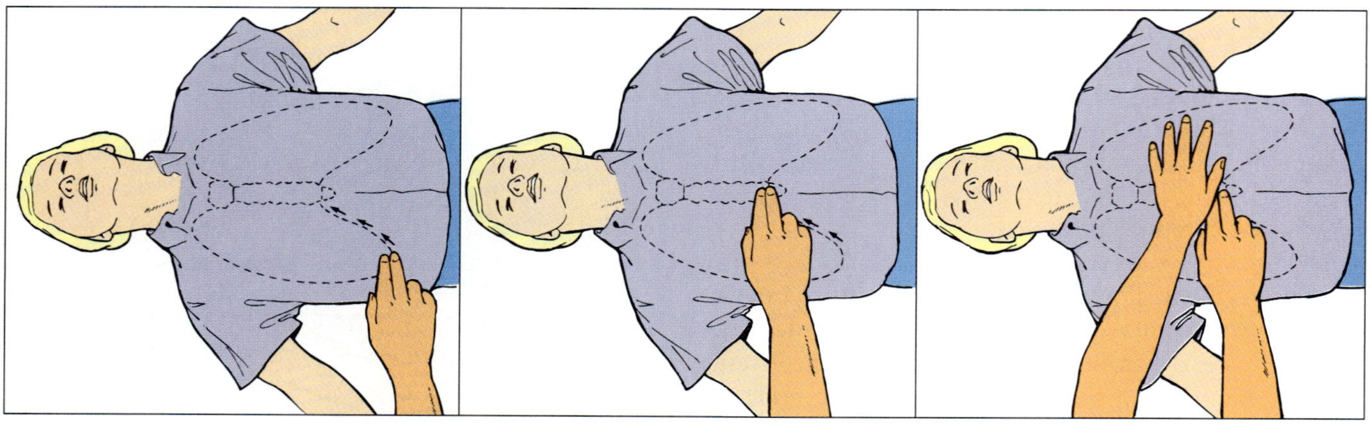

A B C

Fig. 33-10 *Proper hand position for CPR. A, Locate the rib cage. B, Run the fingers along the rib cage to the notch. C, The heel of the hand is placed next to the index finger.*

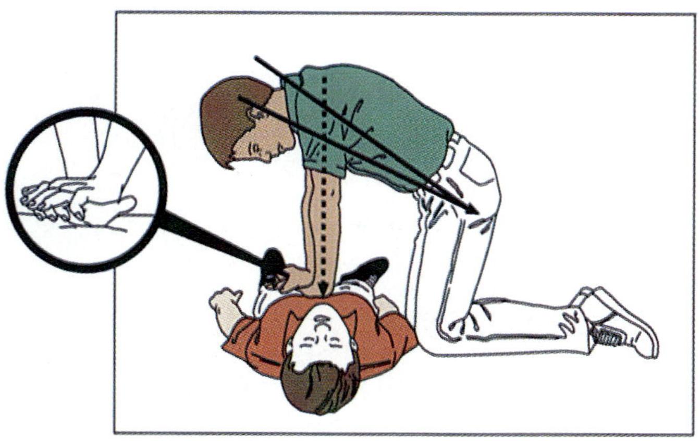

Fig. 33-11 *Position of the shoulders for CPR.*

Adult CPR—One Rescuer

Procedure

1 Check for unresponsiveness.

2 Activate the EMS system.

3 Position the victim supine. Logroll the victim so there is no twisting of the spine. The victim must be on a hard, flat surface. Place the victim's arms alongside the body.

4 Open the airway. Use the head-tilt/chin-lift maneuver.

5 Check for breathlessness.

6 Give 2 breaths. Each should be 1½ seconds long. Let the victim's chest deflate between breaths.

7 Check for pulselessness. Check the pulse for 5 to 10 seconds. Use your other hand to keep the airway open with the head-tilt maneuver.

8 Give chest compressions at a rate of 80 to 100 per minute. Give 15 compressions and then 2 breaths.

   a Establish a rhythm and count out loud (try: "1 and, 2 and, 3 and, 4 and, 5 and, 6 and, 7 and, 8 and, 9 and, 10 and, 11 and, 12 and, 13 and, 14 and, 15").

   b Open the airway and give 2 breaths.

   c Repeat this step until 4 cycles of 15 compressions and 2 breaths have been given.

9 Check for a carotid pulse (5 seconds).

10 Give 2 breaths if pulselessness continues.

11 Repeat step 8. Check for a pulse every few minutes. Do not interrupt CPR for more than 5 seconds.

Adult CPR—Two Rescuers

Procedure

1 Perform one-person CPR until a helper arrives.

2 Continue chest compressions. The helper says, "I know CPR. Can I help?"

3 Indicate that you want help. Ask that the EMS system be activated, if not already done.

4 Do not stop chest compressions. The helper kneels on the other side of the victim. The two-rescuer procedure starts after you complete a cycle of 15 compressions and 2 breaths.

5 Stop compressions for 5 seconds. The helper checks for a carotid pulse. The helper states "No pulse."

6 Perform two-person CPR (Fig. 33-12 on page 694) as follows:

   a The helper gives 2 breaths.

   b Give chest compressions at a rate of 80 to 100 per minute. Count out loud in a rhythm (try: "1 and, 2 and, 3 and, 4 and, 5").

   c The helper gives a breath immediately after the fifth compression. Pause for 1 to 1½ seconds for the breath. Continue chest compressions after the breath.

   d A breath is given after every fifth compression. Your helper checks for a pulse during the compressions.

7 Stop compressions after 1 minute. Your helper checks for breathing and a pulse. After the first minute, compressions are stopped every few minutes to check for breathing and circulation. Compressions are stopped for only 5 seconds.

8 Call for a switch in positions when you are tired.

9 Change positions quickly.

   a Helper gives a breath after you give the fifth compression.

   b Helper moves down to kneel at the victim's shoulder and finds the proper hand position.

   c You move to the victim's head after giving the fifth compression.

   d Check for a pulse (5 seconds).

   e Say "No pulse."

   f Give 1 breath before your helper starts chest compressions.

10 Give 1 breath after every fifth compression.

11 Switch positions when the person giving the compressions is tired. Check for a pulse and breathing at every position change.

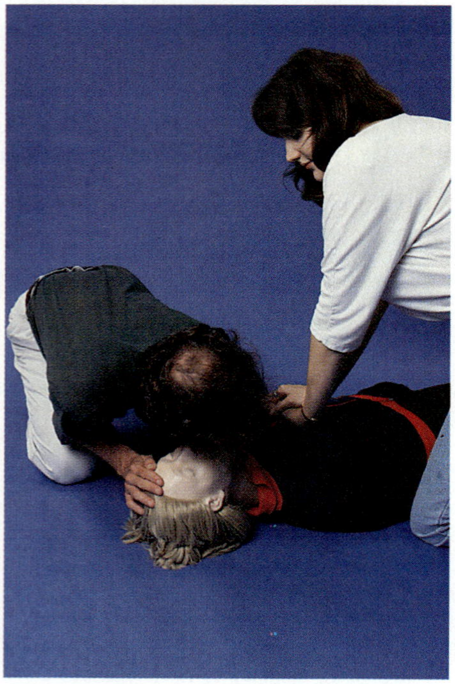

Fig. 33-12 *Two people performing CPR.*

Basic Life Support for Infants and Children

Cardiac arrest due to heart disease is rare in children. More common causes involve diseases and injuries that lead to respiratory arrest or circulatory failure. Sudden infant death syndrome (SIDS), respiratory diseases, airway obstruction, drowning, infection, and nervous system diseases are the most common causes in children under one year of age. Injuries are the most common cause in children older than one year. They include motor vehicle injuries, street injuries, bicycle injuries, drowning, burns, and firearm injuries.

Sequence of BLS for infants and children

Like for adults, basic life support for infants and young children involves determining unresponsiveness, activating the EMS system, and determining breathlessness and pulselessness. However, there are some important differences.

- Injuries are a likely cause of respiratory or cardiac arrest. Head, neck, and spinal cord injury are possible. Therefore the victim is not moved or shaken to determine unresponsiveness. Unresponsiveness is determined by tapping or shouting to get a response.
- Shout for help or send a second rescuer to activate the EMS system.
- If you are alone, provide basic life support for 1 minute before activating the EMS system. This can prevent respiratory arrest from advancing to cardiac arrest.
- If there are no injuries and if the victim is small, carry the victim to the telephone. This makes calling the EMS system easier.
- Move any victim from a dangerous location. Also move the victim if CPR cannot be performed where the victim is lying.
- If the victim must be moved, make sure the head does not roll, twist, or tilt. The head and body must be held straight without twisting. Use the logrolling procedure for turning the victim.
- The head-tilt/chin-lift maneuver also is used for infants and children. The head is not hyperextended as in the adult. Rather the head is tilted to a normal (neutral) or *sniffing* position (Fig. 33-13).
- If neck injury is suspected, the jaw-thrust maneuver is used. To perform the *jaw-thrust maneuver* (Fig. 33-14):
  1. Place 2 or 3 fingers under each side of the lower jaw at the angle of the jaw.
  2. Use your other finger to lift the jaw upward and outward.
  3. Rest your elbows on the surface on which the infant or child is lying.
- The airway is kept open throughout CPR. Only one hand is used for chest compressions. The other is kept on the forehead to maintain the head tilt. For children, both hands are used for the head-tilt/chin-lift maneuver when giving breaths.
- CPR involves 20 breaths and 100 chest compressions per minute.

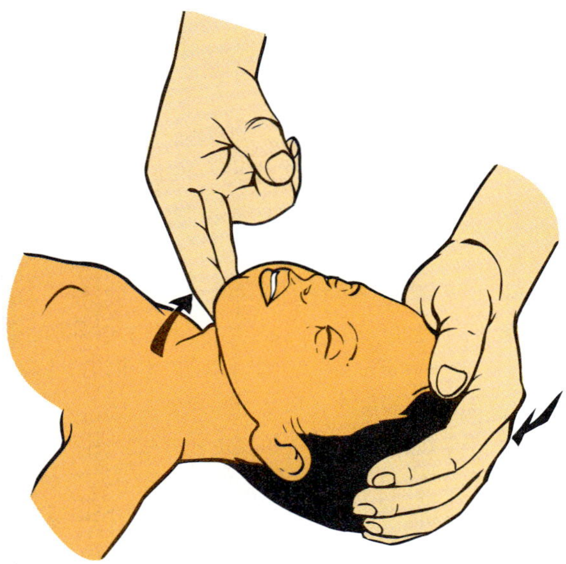

Fig. 33-13 *The head-tilt/chin-lift maneuver is used for infants. The infant's head is not tilted as far back as that of the adult. The infant's head is in a neutral or "sniffing" position.*

PROCEDURE

1 Check for unresponsiveness.

2 Activate the EMS system.

3 Logroll the victim onto his or her back. Support the head and neck when turning the victim. Position the infant or child supine on a hard, flat surface.

4 Open the airway. Use the head-tilt/chin-lift maneuver. Do not hyperextend the head. Extension of the head usually opens an infant's or child's airway (see Fig. 33-13).

5 Check for breathlessness.

6 Give 2 slow breaths. Use enough force to make the chest rise. Each breath should take 1 to 1½ seconds. Cover an infant's nose and mouth with your mouth when giving a breath (Fig. 33-15). Let the chest deflate between breaths.

7 Check for pulselessness. Use the brachial artery for infants and the carotid artery for children. Keep the airway open.

8 Give chest compressions to an *infant:*

- **a** Locate hand position (Fig. 33-16 on page 696).
  - **1** Draw an imaginary line between the nipples.
  - **2** Place your index finger just under the imaginary line.
  - **3** Place your middle and ring fingers next to your index finger. The area for chest compression is below your middle and ring fingers.
- **b** Give compressions using your middle and ring fingers. The sternum is compressed ½ to 1 inch at least 100 times per minute. Release pressure after each compression. Do not remove your fingers from the chest.
- **c** Count out loud in a rhythm (try: "1, 2, 3, 4, 5").
- **d** Give 1 breath after every fifth compression.
- **e** Check for a pulse after 20 cycles of 5 compressions and 1 breath (about 1 minute).
- **f** Continue chest compressions and ventilation if there is no pulse.
- **g** Check for a pulse every few minutes.

9 Give chest compressions to a *child* (use the adult method if the child is large or older than age 8):

- **a** Locate proper hand position (Fig. 33-17 on page 696).
  - **1** Run your middle finger up along the rib cage to the notch at the center of the chest.
  - **2** Mark the notch with your middle finger.
  - **3** Place your index finger next to your middle finger.
  - **4** Place the heel of the same hand next to where the index finger was located.
- **b** Depress the sternum 1 to 1½ inches with the heel of your hand. Keep your fingers off the chest. Keep the airway open with your other hand.
- **c** Give 80 to 100 compressions per minute. Count out loud in a rhythm (try: "1 and 2 and 3 and 4 and 5").
- **d** Give a breath after every fifth compression.
- **e** Check for a pulse after 20 cycles of 5 compressions and 1 breath.
- **f** Continue chest compressions and breaths if there is no pulse.
- **g** Check for a pulse every few minutes.

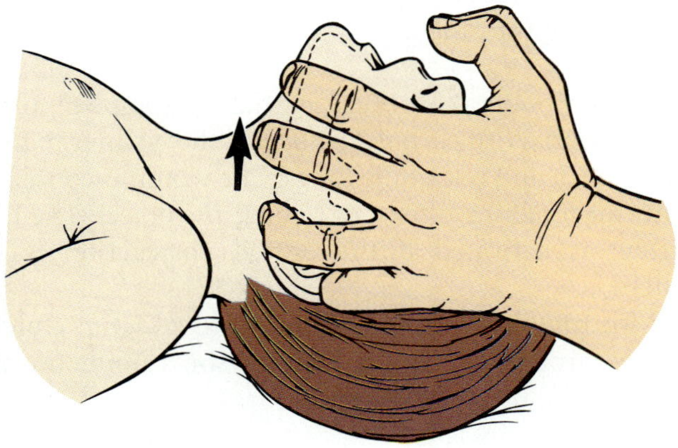

Fig. 33-14 *The jaw-thrust maneuver. Two or 3 fingers are placed on the lower jaw. The other fingers are used to lift the jaw upward and outward.*

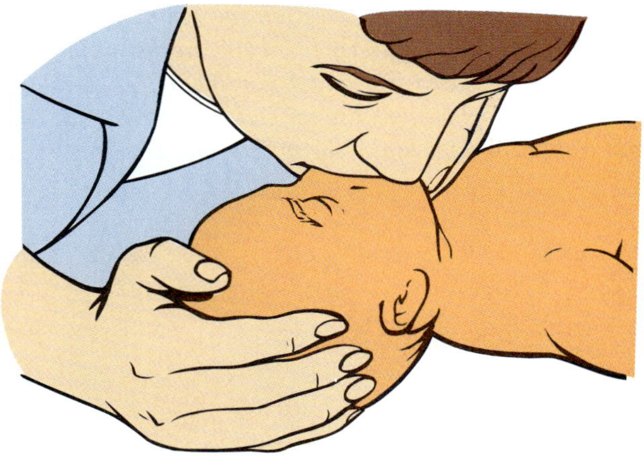

Fig. 33-15 *The infant's mouth and nose are covered during mouth-to-mouth resuscitation.*

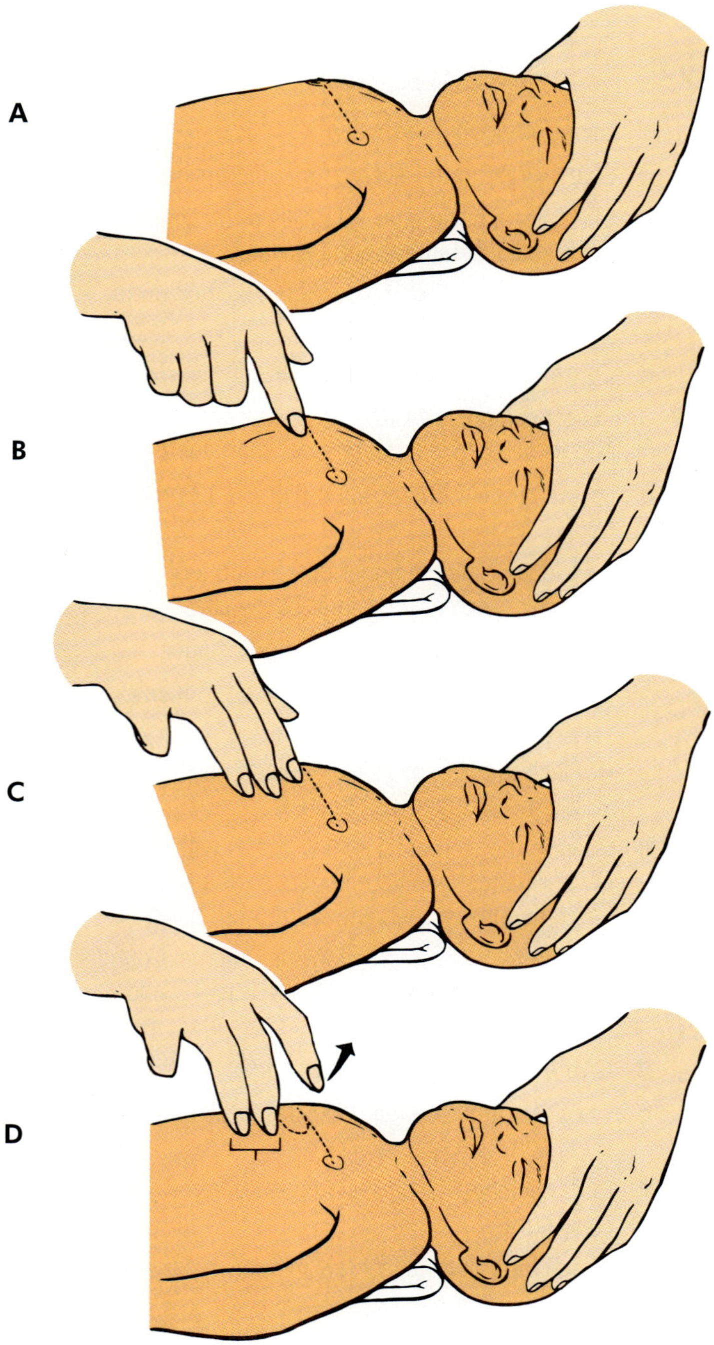

Fig. 33-16 *Locating hand position for infant chest compressions. A, Draw an imaginary line between the nipples. B, The index finger is placed just under the line. C, The middle and ring fingers are placed next to the index finger. D, The area for chest compressions is under the middle and ring fingers.*

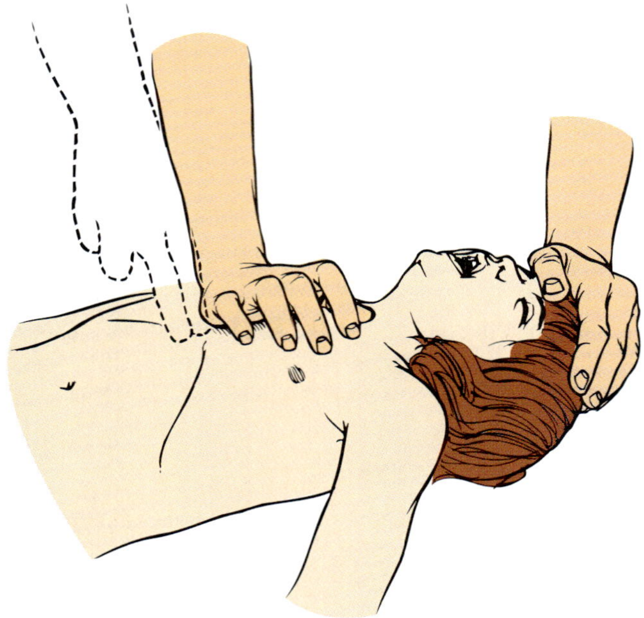

Fig. 33-17 *The heel of one hand is used for CPR on a child. The heel is placed over the lower end of the sternum as for an adult.*

Obstructed Airway

Airway obstruction (choking) can lead to cardiac arrest. Air cannot pass through the air passages to the lungs. The body does not get oxygen.

Foreign bodies can cause airway obstruction. This often occurs during eating. Meat is the most common food causing airway obstruction. Choking often occurs on large, poorly chewed pieces of meat. Laughing and talking while eating can also cause choking. Adults can choke on dentures. Excessive alcohol intake is another cause. Children have choked on small objects such as pieces of hot dogs, marbles, hard candy, coins, and beads. Peanuts, peanut butter, and popcorn can cause choking if not chewed well. They should not be given to young children.

Airway obstruction can occur in unconscious persons. Common causes are aspiration of vomitus and the tongue falling back into the airway. These occur during cardiac arrest.

Foreign bodies can cause partial or complete airway obstruction. With *partial obstruction,* the victim can move some air in and out of the lungs. The victim is conscious. Forceful coughing often can remove the object. The EMS system is activated if the partial obstruction is not relieved.

With *complete airway obstruction,* the victim clutches at the throat (Fig. 33-18). The person cannot breathe,

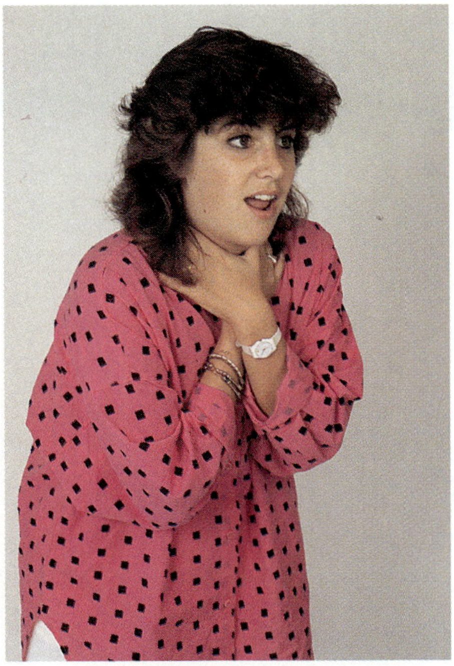

Fig. 33-18 *A choking person will usually clutch the throat.*

speak, or cough. The victim is pale and cyanotic. Air does not move in and out of the lungs. If conscious, the victim is very apprehensive. The obstruction must be removed immediately before cardiac arrest occurs. Obstructed airway is an emergency. The EMS system must be activated.

The *Heimlich maneuver* is used to relieve an obstructed airway caused by a foreign body. It involves abdominal thrusts. The maneuver is performed with the victim standing, sitting, or lying down. The *finger sweep* is used with the Heimlich maneuver when an adult victim is unconscious.

The Heimlich maneuver is not effective in extremely obese persons and in pregnant women. Chest thrusts are used for them. Chest thrusts are described in Box 33-2.

BOX 33-2 Obstructed Airway: Chest Thrusts for Obese or Pregnant Persons

The victim is sitting or standing:

a Stand behind the victim.

b Place your arms under the victim's underarms. Wrap your arms around the victim's chest.

c Make a fist. Place the thumb side of the fist on the middle of the sternum (breastbone).

d Grasp the fist with your other hand.

e Give backward chest thrusts until the object is expelled or the victim becomes unconscious.

The victim is lying down or unconscious:

a Position the victim supine.

b Kneel next to the victim's body.

c Position your hands as for external chest compression.

d Give chest thrusts until the object is expelled or the victim becomes unconscious.

Clearing the Obstructed Airway—The Victim is Standing or Sitting

Procedure

1. Ask the victim if he or she is choking.
2. Determine if the victim can cough or speak.
3. Perform the Heimlich maneuver if the person is choking (Fig. 33-19).
   a. Stand behind the victim.
   b. Wrap your arms around the victim's waist.
   c. Make a fist with one hand.
   d. Place the thumb side of the fist against the abdomen. The fist is in the middle above the navel and below the end of the sternum (breastbone).
   e. Grasp your fist with your other hand.
   f. Press your fist and hand into the victim's abdomen with a quick, upward thrust.
   g. Repeat the abdominal thrust until the object has been expelled or the victim loses consciousness.

Clearing the Obstructed Airway—The Victim is Lying Down

Procedure

1. Ask the victim if he or she is choking.
2. Determine if the victim can cough or speak.
3. Perform the Heimlich maneuver if the person is choking (Fig. 33-20).
   a. Position the victim supine.
   b. Kneel next to the victim's thighs.
   c. Place the heel of one hand against the abdomen. It should be in the middle above the navel and below the end of the sternum (breastbone).
   d. Place your second hand on top of your first hand.
   e. Press into the abdomen with a quick, upward thrust.
   f. Repeat abdominal thrusts until the object has been expelled or the victim loses consciousness.

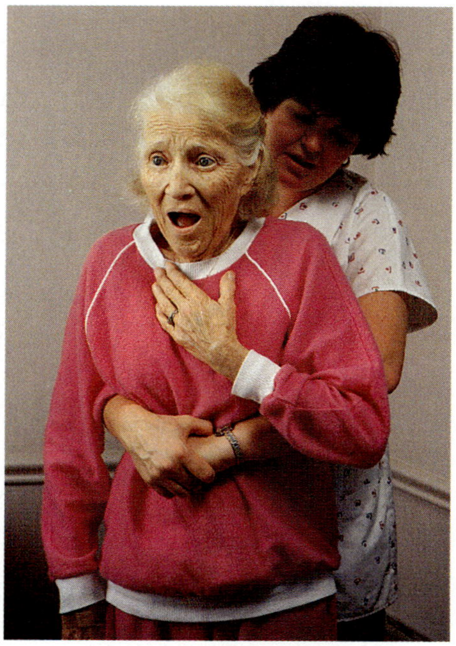

Fig. 33-19 *Abdominal thrusts with the victim standing.*

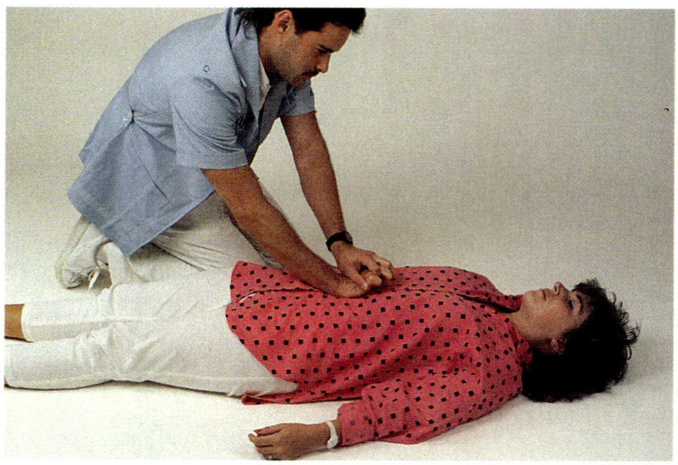

Fig. 33-20 *Abdominal thrusts with the victim lying down.*

Clearing the Obstructed Airway—The Unconscious Adult

Procedure

1 Check for unresponsiveness.

2 Logroll the victim to the supine position with his or her face up. The victim's arms should be at the sides.

3 Open the airway. Use the head-tilt/chin-lift maneuver.

4 Check for breathlessness.

5 Give 1 breath. Reposition the victim's head and open the airway if you could not ventilate. Give 1 breath.

6 Do the Heimlich maneuver if you could not ventilate the victim.

- a Kneel by the victim's thighs.
- b Place the heel of one hand against the victim's abdomen. It should be in the middle of the abdomen between the lower end of the sternum and the navel.
- c Place your other hand on top of the hand on the victim's abdomen (see Fig. 33-20).
- d Give an abdominal thrust. Press inward and upward.
- e Give no more than 5 abdominal thrusts.

7 Do the finger sweep maneuver to check for a foreign object (Fig. 33-21).

- a Open the victim's mouth. Use the tongue-jaw lift maneuver (see Fig. 33-21, A).
    - 1 Grasp the tongue and lower jaw with your thumb and fingers.
    - 2 Lift the lower jaw upward.
- b Insert your other index finger into the mouth along the side of the cheek and deep into the throat (Fig. 33-21, B). Your finger should be at the base of the tongue.
- c Form a hook with your index finger.
- d Try to dislodge and remove the object. Do not push it deeper into the throat.
- e Grasp and remove the object if it is within reach.

8 Open the airway with the head-tilt/chin-lift method.

9 Give 1 breath.

10 Repeat steps 6 through 9 for as long as necessary.

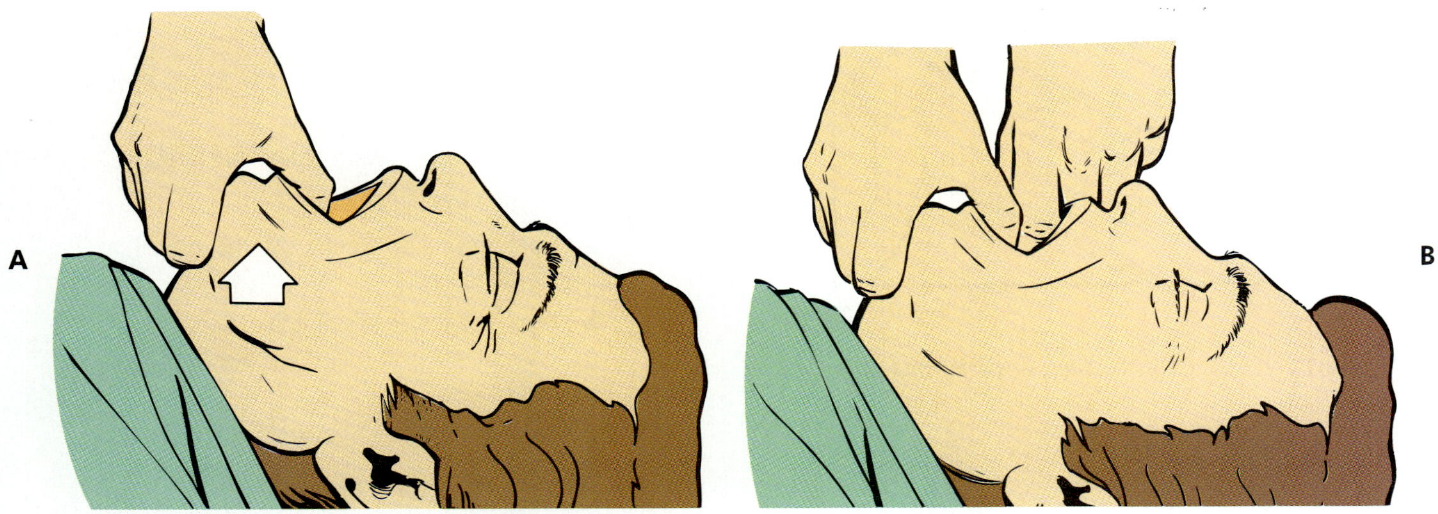

Fig. 33-21 *Tongue-jaw lift maneuver. A, The victim's tongue is grasped, and the jaw is lifted forward with one hand. B, The index finger of the other hand is used to check for a foreign object.*

Clearing an Obstructed Airway—the Conscious Child

Procedure

1. Stand behind the child.
2. Wrap your arms under the child's underarms and around the chest.
3. Make a fist with one hand. Place the thumb side of the fist against the child's abdomen. The fist should be in the middle, above the navel and below the end of the sternum (breastbone).
4. Grab the fist with the other hand.
5. Give a quick inward and upward thrust.
6. Repeat the abdominal thrusts until the object is expelled or the child loses consciousness.
7. Lay the child down if he or she loses consciousness. (See *Clearing an Obstructed Airway—the Unconscious Child.*)

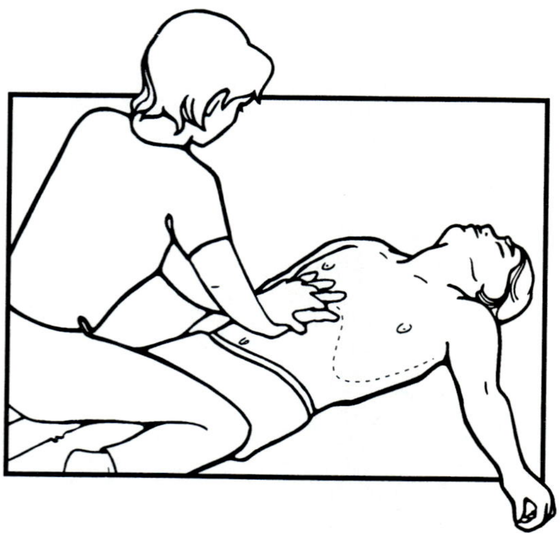

Fig. 33-22 *The Heimlich maneuver performed on an unconscious child.*

Clearing an Obstructed Airway—the Unconscious Child

Procedure

1. Logroll the child if he or she is face down. Support the head and neck. Position the child supine.
2. Do the following if you saw the child lose consciousness or if you suspect a foreign body obstruction.
   - **a** Use the tongue-jaw lift maneuver to lift the chin.
   - **b** Look for a foreign object.
   - **c** Remove the foreign object with the finger sweep maneuver.
3. Open the airway. Use the head-tilt/chin-lift maneuver.
4. Give 1 breath. Reposition the child's head if you could not ventilate the child. Give 1 more breath.
5. Do the Heimlich maneuver if you could not ventilate the child (Fig. 33-22).
   - **a** Kneel beside the child or straddle the hips if he or she is on the floor.
   - **b** Place the heel of one hand against the child's abdomen. The hand is in the middle and slightly above the navel and below the end of the sternum (breastbone).
   - **c** Place your other hand directly on top of your fist.
   - **d** Give 5 quick, upward abdominal thrusts.
6. Check for a foreign object.
   - **a** Open the child's mouth. Use the tongue-jaw lift maneuver.
   - **b** Look into the child's mouth. Do the finger sweep maneuver *only* if you see a foreign object.
   - **c** Remove the foreign object if it is seen.
7. Open the airway. Use the head-tilt/chin-lift maneuver.
8. Give 1 breath.
9. Repeat steps 5 through 8 as often as necessary.

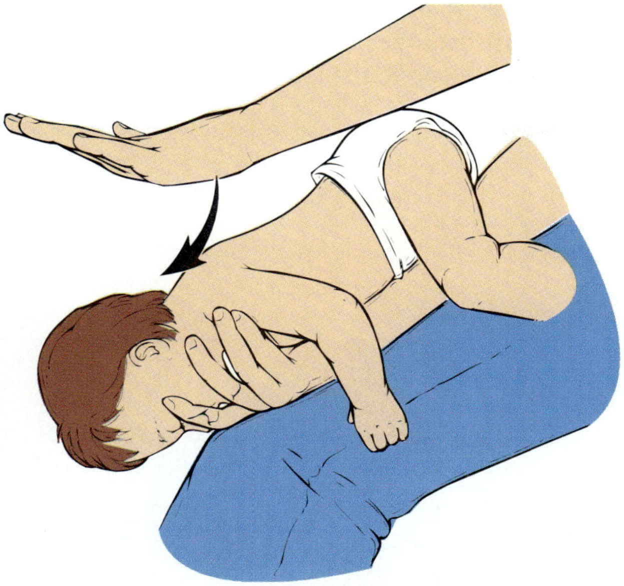

Fig. 33-23 *The infant is held face down and supported with one hand. The rescuer supports her arm on her thigh. Back blows are given with the heel of one hand. The blows are given between the infant's shoulder blades.*

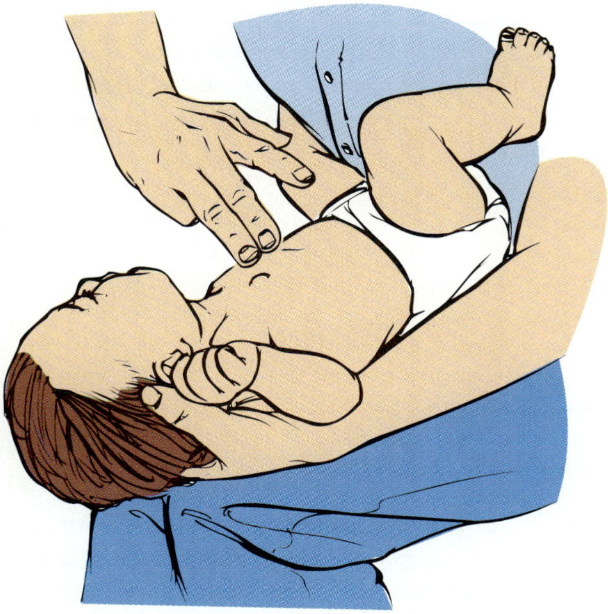

Fig. 33-24 *The infant is positioned on the rescuer's thigh for chest thrusts. Hand position for chest thrusts in the infant is the same as for chest compressions.*

Clearing an Obstructed Airway—the Conscious Infant

Procedure

1. Determine if the infant has an airway obstruction.
2. Hold the infant face down over your forearm or thigh with one hand. The infant's head should be lower than the trunk. Hold the infant's jaw to support the head.
3. Give up to 5 back blows with the heel of one hand. The blows are given between the infant's shoulder blades (Fig. 33-23).
4. Support the infant's back with your free hand. Your other hand supports the neck, jaw, and chest. Turn the infant.
5. Place the infant over your thigh. The baby's head is lower than the trunk.
6. Give chest thrusts (Fig. 33-24 on page 702):
   - **a** Locate hand position as for chest compressions.
   - **b** Give up to 5 downward chest thrusts (chest compressions).
7. Remove the foreign body if it is seen:
   - **a** Use the tongue-jaw lift maneuver to lift the chin.
   - **b** Look for a foreign object.
   - **c** Remove the foreign object with the finger sweep maneuver.
8. Open the airway. Use the head-tilt/chin-lift maneuver.
9. Repeat back blows, chest thrusts, and rescue breathing until the object is expelled. Continue basic life support until the infant is breathing.

Self-Administered Heimlich Maneuver

You may choke yourself. You can perform the Heimlich maneuver to relieve the obstructed airway. To do so:

- Make a fist with one hand.
- Place the thumb side of the fist under your navel and below the lower end of the sternum.
- Grasp your fist with your other hand.
- Press inward and upward quickly.
- Press the upper abdomen against a hard surface if the thrust did not relieve the obstruction. Use the back of a chair, a table, or a railing.
- Use as many thrusts as needed.

HEMORRHAGE

Life and body functions require an adequate blood supply. Blood must circulate through the body. If a blood vessel is torn or cut, bleeding and blood loss occur. The larger the blood vessel, the greater the bleeding and blood loss. **Hemorrhage** is the excessive loss of blood in a short period of time. If the bleeding is not stopped, death results.

Hemorrhage may be internal or external. Internal hemorrhage cannot be seen. Bleeding occurs inside the body into tissues and body cavities. Pain, shock, vomiting blood, coughing up blood, and loss of consciousness are signs of internal hemorrhage. There is little you can do for internal bleeding. Keep the person warm, flat, and quiet until medical help arrives. Fluids are not given.

External bleeding is usually seen. However, it may be hidden by clothing. Hemorrhage may be from an injured artery or vein. Bleeding from an artery is bright red and occurs in spurts. There is a steady flow of blood from a vein. External bleeding must be stopped. You can do the following to control external hemorrhage.

- Activate the EMS system.
- Practice Standard Precautions and follow the Bloodborne Pathogen Standard. Wear gloves if possible.
- Place a sterile dressing directly over the wound. Use any clean material (handkerchief, towel, cloth, or sanitary napkin) if there is no sterile dressing.
- Apply pressure with your hand directly over the bleeding site (Fig. 33-25). Do not release the pressure until the bleeding is controlled.
- If direct pressure does not control bleeding, apply pressure over the artery above the bleeding site (Fig. 33-26). Use your first three fingers. For example, if bleeding is from the lower arm, apply pressure over the brachial artery. The brachial artery supplies blood to the lower arm.

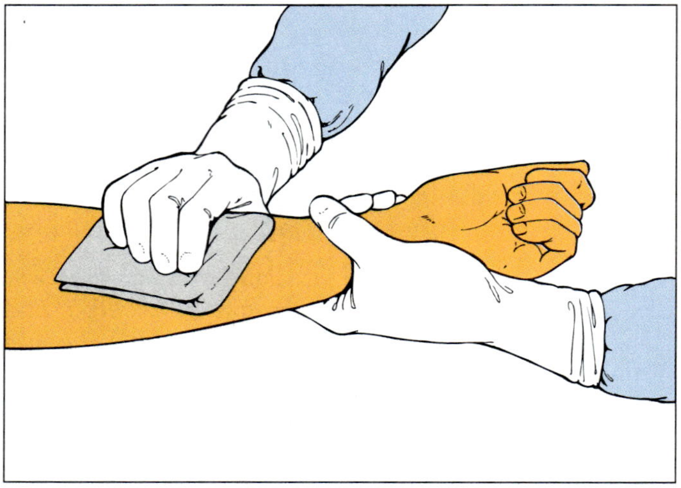

Fig. 33-25 *Direct pressure is applied to the wound to stop bleeding. The hand is placed over the wound.* (*From Parcel GS and Rinear CE: Basic emergency care of the sick and injured, ed 4, St Louis, 1990, Mosby—Year Book.*)

Spotlight On…

Shelly S of Canton, Illinois, *a nursing assistant working in a nursing home, was asked to help a resident with a nosebleed. When Shelly entered the resident's room, she found the frail woman lying in a pool of blood. Shelly knew this amount of bleeding was abnormal for a nosebleed. She calmly asked another nursing assistant to get the nurse. She then covered the resident with blankets, but left the blood because she knew the paramedics would need to know how much blood loss had occurred to determine if a transfusion was needed. Shelly remained with the resident and comforted her until the paramedics arrived.*

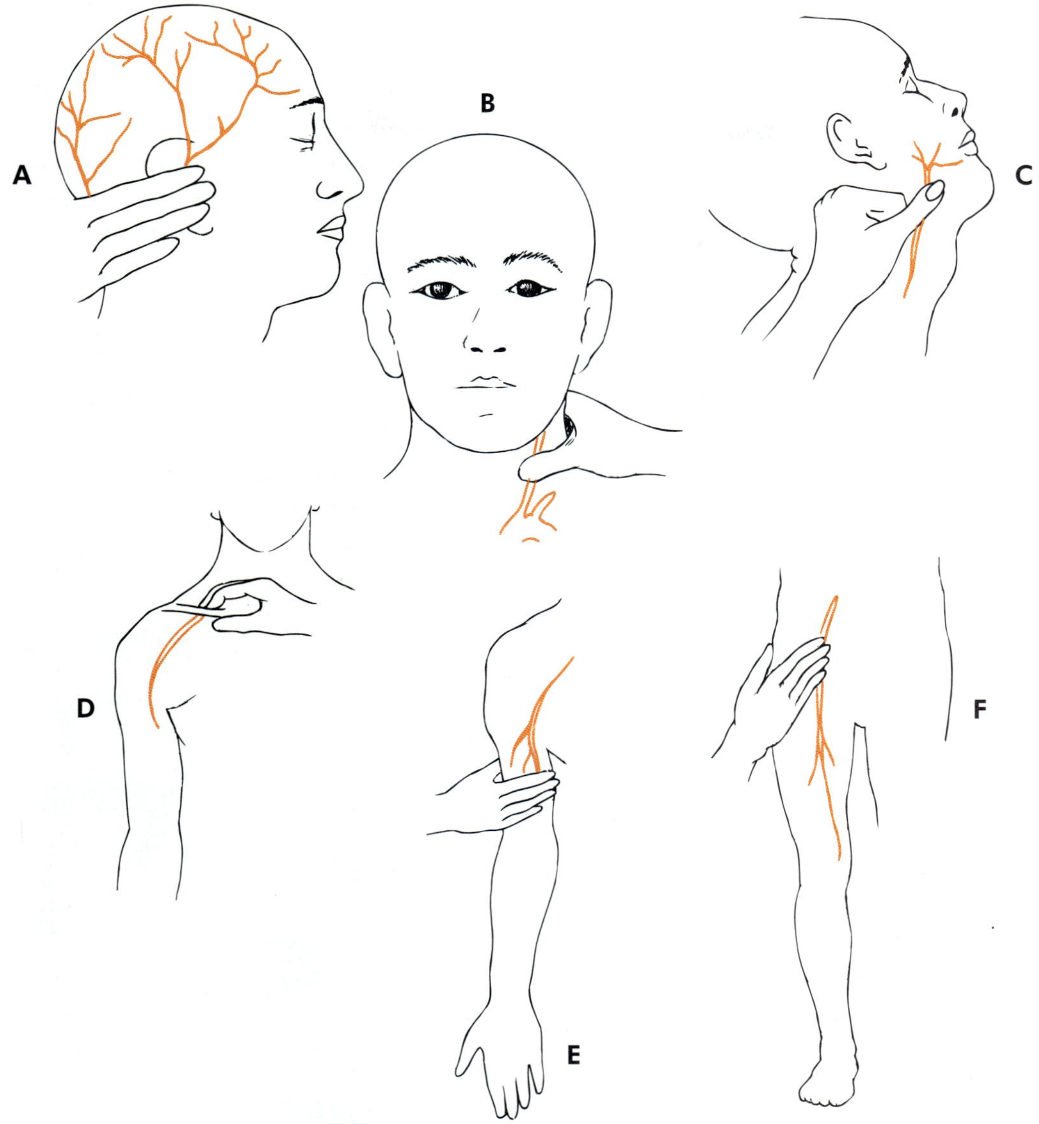

Fig. 33-26 *Pressure points to control bleeding. A, Temporal artery. B, Carotid artery. C, External maxillary artery. D, Subclavian artery. E, Brachial artery. F, Femoral artery. (From Billings DM and Stokes LG: Medical-surgical nursing: common health problems of adults and children across the lifespan, St Louis, 1982, Mosby—Year Book.)*

SHOCK

Shock results when there is not enough blood supply to organs and tissues. Blood loss, heart attack (myocardial infarction), burns, and severe infection can cause shock. Signs and symptoms include:

- Low or falling blood pressure
- Rapid and weak pulse
- Rapid respirations
- Cold, moist, and pale skin
- Thirst
- Restlessness
- Confusion and loss of consciousness as shock worsens

Shock is possible in any person who is acutely ill or injured. Do the following to prevent and treat shock:

- Keep the victim lying down.
- Control hemorrhage.
- Keep the victim warm. Place a blanket over and under the victim if possible.
- Reassure the victim.
- Activate the EMS system.

SEIZURES

Seizures (convulsions) are violent and sudden contractions of muscles. Muscle contractions are involuntary. Seizures are caused by an abnormality in the brain. The abnormality may be caused by head injury during birth or from trauma, high fever, brain tumors, poisoning, and central nervous system infections. Head trauma and lack of blood flow to the brain can also cause seizures.

The terms "attack" and "fits" have been used by non-health care workers in referring to seizures. Do not use these terms. They have unpleasant and disturbing meanings.

There are many types of seizures. You need to be aware of two types. The *tonic-clonic seizure (grand mal seizure, generalized seizure)* has two phases. The tonic phase is first. The person loses consciousness. If standing or sitting, the person falls to the floor. The body is rigid because all muscles contract at once. The clonic phase is next. Muscle groups contract and relax. This causes jerking and twitching movements of the body. Urinary and anal incontinence may occur. After the seizure, the person usually falls into a deep sleep. There may be confusion and headache on awakening.

The *generalized absence (petit mal)* seizure usually lasts a few seconds. There is loss of consciousness, twitching of the eyelids, and staring. These seizures are more common in children and adolescents. However, they can occur in persons of all ages.

The person must be protected from injury during a seizure. The following measures are performed:

- Call for help.
- Lower the person to the floor.
- Place a folded bath blanket or towel under the person's head. You may cradle the person's head in your lap or on a pillow (Fig. 33-27). This prevents the person's head from striking the hard surface of the floor.
- Turn the head to one side.
- Loosen tight clothing around the person's neck. This includes ties, scarves, or collars.
- Move furniture and equipment away from the person. The person may strike these objects during the uncontrolled body movements.
- Do not try to restrain body movements during the seizure.
- Position the person on one side if possible.
- Summon medical help. Do not leave the person during the seizure.
- Do not put your fingers between the person's teeth. The person can bite down on your fingers during the seizure.

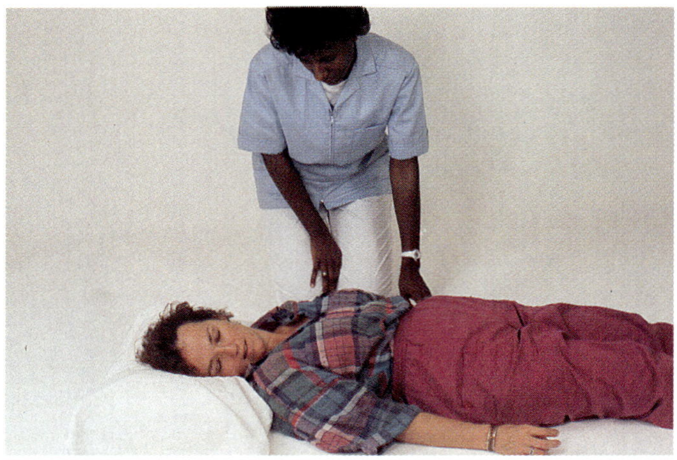

Fig. 33-27 *The head is protected during a seizure.*

BURNS

Burns can severely disable a person (Fig. 33-28). They can also cause death. Most burn injuries occur in the home. Infants and children are the usual victims. The elderly are also at great risk. Common causes of burns and fires are:

- Scalds from hot liquids
- Playing with matches and lighters
- Electrical injuries (Fig. 33-29)
- Cooking accidents (barbecues, microwaves, stoves, ovens)
- Falling asleep while smoking
- Fireplaces
- Space heaters
- No smoke detectors or nonfunctioning smoke detectors
- Sunburn
- Chemicals

The skin has two layers: the dermis and epidermis. Burns are described as partial thickness or full thickness. *Partial-thickness burns* involve the dermis and part of the epidermis. These burns are very painful. Nerve endings are exposed. *Full-thickness burns* involve the dermis and the entire epidermis. The fat layer, muscle, and bone may be injured or destroyed. Full-thickness burns are not painful. Nerve endings are destroyed.

Burns vary in seriousness. Burn size and depth, the body part involved, and the victim's age affect the severity of the burn. Burns to the face, eyes, ears, hands, and feet are more serious than burns to an arm or leg. Infants, young children, and the elderly have a greater risk of dying than do persons of other ages.

The EMS system must be activated as soon as possible. Emergency care of burns includes the following:

- Do not touch the victim if he or she is in contact with an electrical source. Have the power source turned off or remove the electrical source first. Use an object that does not conduct electricity (rope or wood) to remove the electrical source.
- Remove the victim from the fire or burn source.
- Stop the burning process. Extinguish flames with water or roll the person in a blanket. A coat, sheet, or towel can be used.
- Remove hot clothing that is not sticking to the skin. Also remove jewelry and any tight clothing. If hot clothing cannot be removed, cool the clothing with water.
- Provide basic life support as needed. This includes activating the EMS system.

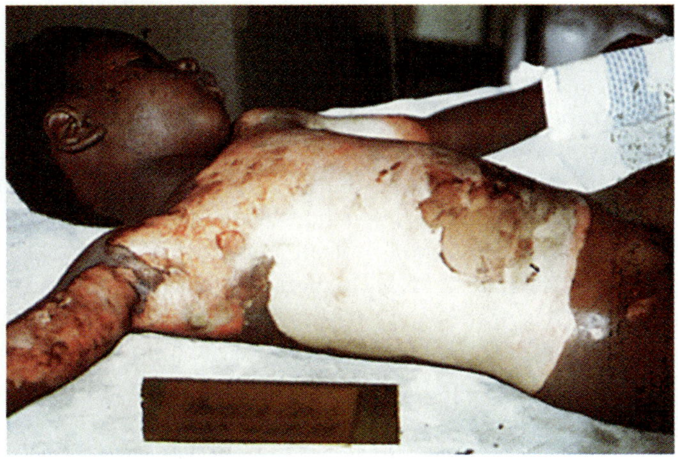

Fig. 33-28 *Full-thickness burn from flames.* (From Sanders M: *Mosby's paramedic text,* St Louis, 1994, Mosby–Year Book.)

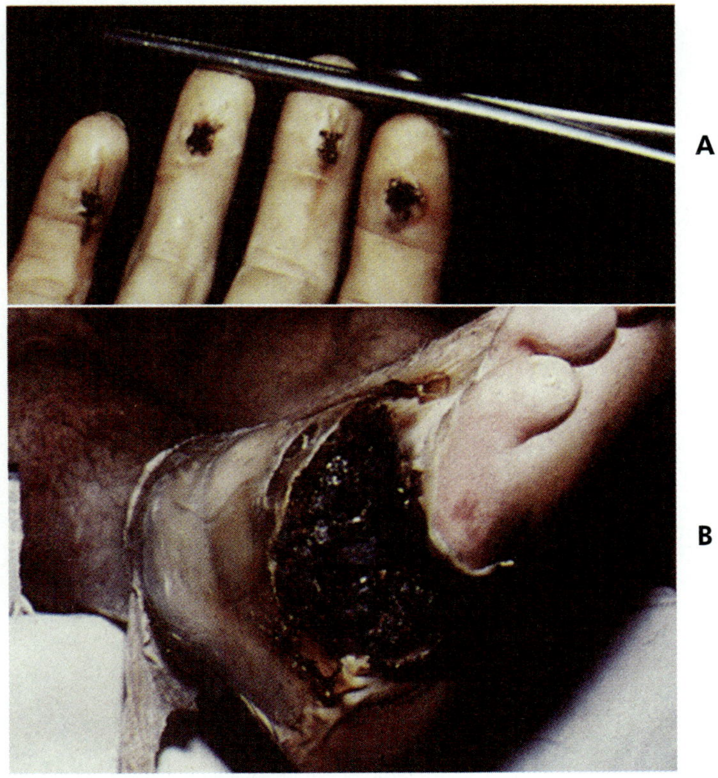

Fig. 33-29 *An electrical burn.* ***A,*** *The electrical current enters through the hand.* ***B,*** *The electrical current exits through the foot.* (From Sanders M: *Mosby's paramedic text,* St Louis, 1994, Mosby—Year Book.)

- Cover the burn wounds with a clean, moist covering. You can use towels, sheets, or any other clean cloth. Keep the covering wet.
- Do not put oil, butter, salve, or ointments on the burns.
- Cover the victim with a blanket or coat to prevent heat loss.

FAINTING

Fainting is the sudden loss of consciousness from an inadequate blood supply to the brain. Hunger, fatigue, fear, and pain are common causes. Some people faint at the sight of blood or injury. Standing in one position for a long time or being in a warm, crowded room can lead to fainting. Dizziness, perspiration, and blackness before the eyes are warning signals. The person looks pale. The pulse is weak. Respirations are shallow if consciousness is lost. Emergency care for fainting includes the following:

- Have the person sit or lie down before fainting occurs.

  *If sitting, the person bends forward and places his or her head between the knees (Fig. 33-30).

  *If the victim is lying down, the legs are elevated.
- Loosen tight clothing.
- Keep the person lying down if fainting has occurred.
- Do not let the person get up until symptoms have subsided for about 5 minutes.
- Help the person to a sitting position after recovery from fainting. Observe for symptoms of fainting.

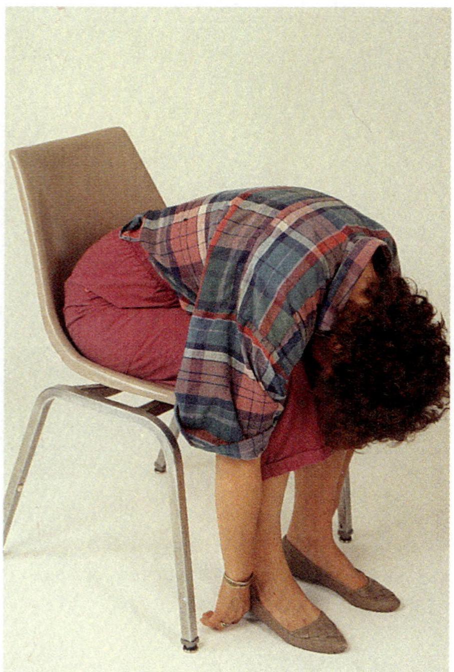

Fig. 33-30 *The person bends forward and places the head between the knees to prevent fainting.*

STROKE

Stroke (cerebrovascular accident) was described in Chapter 28. A stroke occurs when the brain is suddenly deprived of its blood supply. Usually only part of the brain is affected. A stroke may be caused by a thrombus, an embolus, or cerebral hemorrhage. Cerebral hemorrhage is due to the rupture of a blood vessel in the brain.

The signs of stroke vary. They depend on the size and location of brain injury. Loss of consciousness or semiconsciousness, rapid pulse, labored respirations, elevated blood pressure, vomiting, and hemiplegia are signs of stroke. The person may have aphasia (the inability to speak). Convulsions may occur.

Emergency care includes the following:

- Turn the person onto the affected side. The affected side is limp and the cheek appears puffy.
- Elevate the head without flexing the neck.
- Loosen tight clothing.
- Keep the person quiet and warm.
- Reassure the person.
- Activate the EMS system.

SUMMARY

Emergencies are sudden and unexpected. They are frightening for the victim and others nearby. Quick action may be needed to save the victim's life and to prevent injuries from becoming worse. Emergencies can occur anywhere. You may be with the victim when an emergency happens. Staying calm, knowing what to do, and calling for help are important for the victim's physical and mental well-being.

Cardiac arrest and airway obstruction are deadly and frightening emergencies. They may occur anywhere and at any time. A basic life support course will prepare you for these emergencies. You may be able to save a person's life with basic life support procedures.

A first aid course is also helpful. A first aid course prepares you to handle many injuries. Examples include insect stings, fractures, frostbite, poisoning, and eye injuries. The general rules of emergency care apply to any emergency. You may not know how to care for the specific injury. However, you can help the victim by following the general rules of emergency care.

Quality of life must be protected during emergencies. The victim is a person. He or she must be treated with dignity and respect.

The right to privacy and confidentiality are protected. Do not expose the person unnecessarily. You may be in a place where you cannot close doors, shades, and curtains. The victim may be in a lounge, dining area, or public place. Do what you can to protect the person's privacy.

Onlookers are major threats to privacy and confidentiality. If you are giving emergency care, your main concern is the victim's illness or injuries. It is hard to give care and manage onlookers at the same time. Ask someone else to deal with the onlookers. If another person is giving care, you can help by keeping onlookers away from the victim.

People are naturally curious. They want to know what happened, the extent of injuries or illness, and if the person will be okay. You must be careful not to discuss the situation. Remember, information about the person's care, treatment, and condition are confidential. Also remember that only doctors can make diagnoses. You can make observations about signs and symptoms. Only the doctor can determine what is wrong with the person.

The right to personal choice must be protected. It is often hard to give choices in emergencies. They are given when possible. Hospital care may be required. The person has the right to choose which hospital to be taken to.

Personal possessions must be protected from loss and damage. Dentures and eyeglasses are often lost or broken in emergencies. Watches and other jewelry are easily lost. Clothing may be torn or cut. You must be very careful to protect the person's property. In public places, personal items are given to family members, police, or EMS personnel.

Physical and psychological safety are important. The person is protected from further injury. For example, a stroke victim is protected from falls. The person having a seizure is protected from head injuries. All emergency victims need to feel safe and secure. Reassurance, explanations about care, and a calm approach are important. They help the person feel safe and secure.

Review Questions

Circle the best *answer.*

1 The goals of first aid are to

a Call for help and keep the victim warm

b Prevent death and prevent injuries from becoming worse

c Stay calm and perform emergency measures

d Reassure the victim and keep bystanders away

2 When giving first aid, you should

a Be aware of your own limitations

b Move the victim

c Give the victim fluids

d Perform any necessary emergency measures

3 The person is in cardiac arrest. Cardiac arrest is

a The same as stroke

b The sudden stopping of heart action and breathing

c The sudden loss of consciousness

d The condition that results when there is inadequate blood supply to the organs and tissues of the body

4 Which is *not* a sign of cardiac arrest?

a No pulse

b No breathing

c A sudden drop in blood pressure

d Unconsciousness

5 You are to give mouth-to-mouth rescue breathing. You should do the following *except*

a Pinch the victim's nostrils shut

b Place your mouth tightly over the victim's mouth

c Blow air into the victim's mouth as you exhale

d Cover the victim's nose with your mouth

6 External chest compressions are performed. The chest is compressed

a ½ to 1 inch with the index and middle fingers

b 1 to 1½ inches with the heel of one hand

c 1½ to 2 inches with two hands

d With one hand in the middle of the sternum

7 Which does not determine breathlessness?

a Looking to see if the chest rises and falls

b Counting respirations for 30 seconds

c Listening for the escape of air

d Feeling for the flow of air

8 Which is used to feel for a pulse during adult CPR?

a The apical pulse

b The brachial pulse

c The carotid pulse

d The dorsalis pedis pulse

9 How many breaths are given at the beginning of CPR?

a 1

b 2

c 3

d 4

10 You are performing adult CPR alone. Which is *false?*

a Give 2 breaths after every 15 compressions

b Check for a pulse after 1 minute

c Give 1 breath after every fifth compression

d Count out loud

11 Adult CPR is being given by two people. Breaths are given

a After every fifth compression

b After every fifteenth compression

c After every compression

d Only when the positions are changed

12 External cardiac compressions are given to an infant at a rate of

a 60 per minute

b 75 per minute

c 80 per minute

d 100 per minute

13 The most common cause of obstructed airway in adults is

a A loose denture

b Meat

c Marbles

d Candy

REVIEW QUESTIONS—CONT'D

14 If airway obstruction occurs, the victim usually
- **a** Clutches at the throat
- **b** Can speak, cough, and breathe
- **c** Is calm
- **d** Has a seizure

15 The Heimlich maneuver is used to relieve an obstructed airway. Which is *false?*
- **a** The victim can be standing, sitting, or lying down.
- **b** A fist is made with one hand.
- **c** The thrusts are given inward and upward at the lower end of the sternum.
- **d** The hands are positioned in the middle between the waist and lower end of the sternum.

16 A victim has an obstructed airway. Poking motions are used with the finger-sweep maneuver.
- **a** True
- **b** False

17 Arterial bleeding is suspected. Arterial bleeding
- **a** Cannot be seen
- **b** Occurs in spurts
- **c** Is dark red
- **d** Oozes from the wound

18 A person is hemorrhaging from the left forearm. The first action is to
- **a** Lower the body part
- **b** Apply pressure to the brachial artery
- **c** Apply direct pressure to the wound
- **d** Cover the victim

19 A person is in shock. The signs of shock are
- **a** Rising blood pressure, rapid pulse, and slow respirations
- **b** Rapid pulse, rapid respirations, and warm skin
- **c** Falling blood pressure; rapid pulse and respirations; and skin that is cold, moist, and pale
- **d** Falling blood pressure; slow pulse and respirations; thirst; restlessness; and warm, flushed skin

20 A person in shock needs
- **a** Mouth-to-mouth resuscitation
- **b** To be kept lying down
- **c** Clothes removed
- **d** To be placed in Trendelenburg's position

21 These statements relate to tonic-clonic seizures. Which is *false?*
- **a** There is contraction of all muscles at once
- **b** The person may stop breathing
- **c** The seizure usually lasts about 10 to 20 seconds
- **d** There is loss of consciousness during the seizure

22 A person has been burned. There are no complaints or signs of pain. You know that
- **a** The burn is minor
- **b** The burn is partial thickness
- **c** The burn is full thickness
- **d** The dermis has been destroyed

23 Burns should be covered with
- **a** A clean, moist cloth or dressing
- **b** Butter, oil, or salve
- **c** Water
- **d** Nothing

24 A person is about to faint. Which is *false?*
- **a** Take the person outside for some fresh air.
- **b** Have the person sit or lie down.
- **c** Loosen tight clothing.
- **d** Elevate the legs if the person is lying down.

25 Emergency care of the stroke victim includes the following *except*
- **a** Positioning the person on the affected side
- **b** Giving the person sips of water
- **c** Loosening tight clothing
- **d** Keeping the person quiet and warm

Answers to these questions are on page 753.

The Dying Person

34

OBJECTIVES

- Define the key terms listed in this chapter
- Describe terminal illness
- Identify the psychological forces that influence living and dying
- Explain how culture and religion influence attitudes about death
- Describe how different age groups view death
- Describe the five stages of dying
- Explain how to meet the dying person's psychological, social, and spiritual needs
- Explain how you can help meet the physical needs of the dying person
- Describe the needs of the family during the dying process
- Describe hospice care
- Explain the importance of the Patient Self-Determination Act
- Explain what is meant by a *do not resuscitate* order
- Explain how to promote quality of life for the dying person
- Identify the signs of approaching death and the signs of death
- Assist in giving postmortem care

Key Terms

advance directive A written document stating a person's wishes about health care when that person is no longer able to make his or her own decisions

postmortem After *(post)* death *(mortem)*

reincarnation The belief that the spirit or soul is reborn in another human body or in another form of life

rigor mortis The stiffness or rigidity *(rigor)* of skeletal muscles that occurs after death *(mortis)*

terminal illness An illness or injury for which there is no reasonable expectation of recovery

Dying people are cared for in hospitals, nursing facilities, or at home. Many are in hospice programs (see Chapter 1). Death may be sudden and without warning. Often it is expected.

Health workers see death often. Many are unsure of their feelings about death. They are uncomfortable with dying persons and the subject of death. Dying persons represent helplessness and failure to cure. They also remind us of our own eventual death.

You must examine your feelings about death. Your attitudes about death and dying affect the care you give. You will help meet the person's physical, psychological, social, and spiritual needs. Therefore you need to understand the dying process. Then you can approach the dying person with care, kindness, and respect.

TERMINAL ILLNESS

Many illnesses and diseases can be cured or controlled. Others have no cure. Many injuries can be repaired. Others are so serious that the body cannot function. Recovery is not expected. The disease or injury ends in death. An illness or injury for which there is no reasonable expectation of recovery is a **terminal illness.**

Doctors cannot predict the exact time of death. A person may have days, months, weeks, or years to live. Predictions have been wrong. People expected to live for only a short time have lived for years. Others have been expected to live for a longer time. They have died sooner than expected.

Modern medicine has found cures or has prolonged life in many cases. Future research will bring new cures. However, two very powerful psychological forces influence living and dying. They are hope and the will to live. People have died sooner than expected or for no apparent reason when they have lost hope or the will to live.

ATTITUDES ABOUT DEATH

Experiences, culture, religion, and age influence a person's attitude about death. Many people fear death. Others do not believe they will die. Some look forward to and accept death. Attitudes and beliefs about death often change as a person grows older. They are also affected by changing circumstances.

Dying people are usually cared for in health facilities or at home. The family is often involved in the person's care. Family members usually gather at the bedside to comfort the person and to say their last farewells. The family also comforts each other. When death occurs, the funeral director is called. The funeral director takes the body from the facility and prepares it for funeral practices.

Many adults and children have never had contact with a dying person. Nor have they been present when death occurred. Some have never attended a visitation or funeral. They have not seen the process of dying and death. Therefore it is frightening, morbid, and a mystery.

Culture and Religion

American practices and attitudes are different from those of other cultures (Table 34-1). In some cultures, dying people are cared for at home by the family. Some families care for the body after death and prepare it for burial.

Attitudes about death are closely related to culture and religion. Some believe that life after death is free of suffering and hardship. They also believe there will be reunion with family and loved ones. Many believe there is punishment and suffering in the afterlife for sins and misdeeds. Others do not believe in the afterlife. They believe death is the end of life. There are also religious beliefs about the form of the human body after death. Some believe the body keeps its physical form. Others believe that only the spirit or soul is present in the afterlife. **Reincarnation** is the belief that the spirit or soul is reborn into another human body or into another form of life. Many people strengthen their religious beliefs when dying. Religion also provides comfort for the dying person and the family.

Age and Beliefs About Death

Ideas about death change as people grow older. Infants and toddlers have no concept of death. Children between the ages of 3 and 5 start to be curious and have ideas about death. They recognize the death of family members or pets and notice dead birds or bugs. They think death is temporary. Children often blame themselves when someone or something dies. They see the death as punishment for being bad. When children ask questions about death, adults often give answers that cause fear and confusion. Children who are told, "He is sleeping," may be afraid to go to sleep.

Children between the ages of 5 and 7 years know death is final. They do not think that they will die. Death happens to other people. They also think death can be avoided. Children associate death with punishment and body mutilation. It is also associated with witches, ghosts, goblins, and monsters. These ideas come from fairy tales, cartoons, movies, video games, and television.

Adults have more fears about death than children. They fear pain and suffering, dying alone, and the invasion of privacy. They also fear loneliness and separation from family and loved ones. They worry about who will care for and support those left behind. Adults often resent death. This is particularly true when it interferes with plans, hopes, dreams, and ambitions.

Elderly people usually have fewer fears than younger adults. They accept that death will occur. They have had more experiences with dying and death. Many have lost family members and friends. Some welcome death as freedom from pain, suffering, and disability. Death also means reunion with those who have died first. Like younger adults, elderly persons often fear dying alone.

THE STAGES OF DYING

Dr. Elisabeth Kübler-Ross has described five stages of dying. They are denial, anger, bargaining, depression, and acceptance.

- *Denial* is the first stage. Persons refuse to believe they are dying. "No, not me" is a common response. The person believes a mistake has been made. Information about the illness or injury is not heard. The person cannot deal with any problem or decision about the illness or injury. This stage can last for a few hours, days, or much longer. Some people are still in denial when they die.
- *Anger* is the second stage of dying. The person thinks "Why me?" People in this stage feel anger and rage. They envy and resent those who have life and health. Family, friends, and the health team are usually targets of anger. They blame others. Fault is found with those who are loved and needed the most. The health team and family may have a hard time dealing with persons during this stage. Remember that anger is a normal, healthy reaction. Do not take the person's anger personally. You must control any urge to attack back or avoid the person.
- *Bargaining* is the third stage. Anger has passed. The person now says "Yes, me, but. . . ." Often there is bargaining with God for more time. Promises are made in exchange for more time. The person may want to see a child marry, see a grandchild, have one more Christmas, or live for some important event. Usually more promises are made as the person makes "just one more" request. This stage may not be obvious to you. Bargaining is usually done privately and on a spiritual level.
- *Depression* is the fourth stage. The person thinks "Yes, me" and is very sad. There is mourning over things that have been lost and the future loss of life. The person may cry or say little. Sometimes the person talks about people and things that will be left behind.
- *Acceptance* of death is the fifth and final stage of dying. The person is calm and at peace. The person has said what needs to be said. Unfinished business is completed. The person is ready to accept death. A person may be in this stage for many months or years. Reaching the acceptance stage does not mean death is near.

TABLE 34-1

TOP TEN COUNTRIES OF ORIGIN OF IMMIGRANTS TO THE UNITED STATES*: DEATH RITES

Country	Death Rites
Mexico	Small children may not be part of dying and death rituals. Family members take turns staying around the clock with the dying person in the hospital. Grief can be expressive; for example, *el ataque* consists of hyperkinetic (increased muscle movement) or seizure-type behavior patterns. These behavior patterns serve to release emotions.
Vietnam	Quality of life is more important than length of life because of beliefs in reincarnation. There is also the expectation of less suffering in the next life. Therefore the dying are helped to recall their past good deeds and to achieve a fitting mental state. Autopsies are allowed. Cremation is preferred. Death at home is preferred over death in the hospital. Upon death the body is washed and wrapped in clean white sheets. In some areas a coin or jewels (a wealthier family) and rice (a poorer family) are put in the dead person's mouth. This is from the belief that they will help the soul go through the encounters with gods and devils, and the soul will be born rich in the next life. Relatives sew small pillows to place under the neck, feet, and wrists of the body. The body is placed in a coffin, and burial is in the ground.
Philippines	The person is protected from knowing about a poor prognosis because it will only add to his or her suffering. After death, emotional grief responses may occur.
Former Soviet Union	The family is told first of a serious prognosis. They decide if the person should be informed.
Dominican Republic	No information
Mainland China	The Chinese have an aversion to death and to anything concerning death. Autopsy and disposal of the body are individual preferences and are not prescribed by religion. Euthanasia is allowed. Donation of body parts is encouraged. The eldest son is responsible for all arrangements for the deceased. The deceased is initially buried in a coffin. After 7 years the body is exhumed and cremated. The urn is reburied in the tomb. White clothing is worn for mourning.
India	Hindu persons may make indirect references to their own deaths, often accepting God's will. The person's desire to be clearheaded as death approaches must be assessed in planning medical treatment. Providing a time and place for prayer is essential for the family and the person. Prayer helps them deal with anxiety and conflict. The Hindu priest or anyone present may read from the Holy Sanskrit books. Some priests tie strings (signifying a blessing) around the neck or wrist. After death the priest pours water into the mouth of the deceased. Families may prefer that only Hindus touch the body and may wash the body themselves. Blood transfusions, organ transplants, and autopsies are allowed. Cremation is preferred. Reincarnation is a Hindu belief.
El Salvador	No information
Poland	The body is not embalmed. It is placed in the home for the wake. Church services and ground burial follow. Feelings of grief may be verbally expressive.
United Kingdom	No information

*Information obtained from U.S. Dept. of Immigration and Naturalization Services.
From Geissler EM: Pocket guide to cultural assessment, St Louis, 1994, Mosby–Year Book.

> *Spotlight On...*
>
> ***Denneatta L of Elkins, West Virginia,*** *was caring for a nursing home resident as the resident began expressing her fear of dying. The woman was worried about her family and children and how they would get along without her. Denneatta spent a long time talking to the resident and reassuring her, and the woman seemed very relieved. Two days later as Denneatta was working with her, the resident said, "This is the first time in months I haven't been afraid of dying." That evening the woman passed away.*

Dying persons do not always pass through all five stages. A person may never get beyond a certain stage. Some people move back and forth between stages. For example, a person who has reached acceptance may move back to bargaining. Then the person may move forward to acceptance. Some people are in one stage until death.

PSYCHOLOGICAL, SOCIAL, AND SPIRITUAL NEEDS

Dying people continue to have psychological, social, and spiritual needs. They may want family and friends present. They may want to talk about the fears, worries, and anxieties of dying. Some want to be alone. Often they want to talk to a nursing team member. Persons often need to talk during the night. Things are quiet, there are few distractions, and there is more time to think.

There are two very important aspects of communication when dealing with the dying person. These are listening and touch.

- *Listening.* The dying person is the one who needs to talk, express feelings, and share worries and concerns. Just being there and listening helps to meet the person's psychological and social needs. Do not worry about saying the wrong thing. Nor should you worry about finding the right words to comfort and cheer the person. Nothing really must be said. Being there for the person is what counts.
- *Touch.* Touch can convey caring and concern when words cannot. Sometimes a person does not want to talk but needs you nearby. Do not feel that you need to talk. Silence, along with touch, is a powerful and meaningful way to communicate.

Spiritual needs are important. The person may wish to see a priest, rabbi, minister, or other clergy. The person may also want to participate in religious practices. Privacy is provided during prayer and spiritual moments. Courtesy is given to the clergy. The person is allowed to have religious objects nearby (medals, pictures, statues, Bibles, the Koran, the Torah, or other religious writings). You must handle these items like other valuables.

PHYSICAL NEEDS

Dying may take a few minutes, hours, days, or weeks. There is general slowing of body processes, weakness, and changes in levels of consciousness. The person is allowed to be as independent as possible. As the person's condition weakens, the nursing team helps meet basic needs. The person may totally depend on others for basic needs and activities of daily living. Every effort is made to promote the person's physical and psychological comfort. The person is allowed to die in peace and with dignity.

Vision, Hearing, and Speech

Vision becomes blurred and gradually fails. The person naturally turns toward light. A darkened room may frighten the person. The eyes may be half open. Secretions often collect in the corners of the eyes. Because of failing vision, you need to explain what is being done to the person or in the room. The room should be well lit. However, bright lights and glares are avoided. Good eye care is essential (see Chapter 13). If the eyes stay open, a nurse may apply a protective ointment. Then the eyes are covered with moistened pads to prevent injury.

Hearing is one of the last functions to be lost. Many people hear until the moment of death. Even if unconscious, the person may hear. Always assume that the dying person, or any unconscious person, can hear. Speak in a normal voice, provide reassurance and explanations about care, and offer words of comfort. Avoid topics that could upset the person.

Speech becomes difficult. It may be hard to understand the person. Sometimes the person cannot speak. The nursing team needs to anticipate the person's needs. The person is not asked questions that have long answers. "Yes" or "no" questions are asked. These are kept to a minimum. Though speech may be hard or impossible, you must still talk to the person.

Mouth, Nose, and Skin

Oral hygiene is essential for comfort. Routine mouth care is given if the person can eat and drink. Frequent oral hygiene is given as death approaches and when there is difficulty taking oral fluids. Oral hygiene is also important if mucus collects in the mouth and the person cannot swallow.

Crusting and irritation of the nostrils can occur. Common causes are increased nasal secretions, an oxygen cannula, or an NG tube. The nose is carefully cleaned. The nurse may have you apply a lubricant to the nostrils.

Circulation fails and body temperature rises as death approaches. Though body temperature rises, the skin is cool, pale, and mottled (blotchy). Perspiration increases. Good skin care, bathing, and the prevention of pressure sores are necessary. Linens and gowns are changed whenever needed because of perspiration. Although the skin feels cool, only light bed coverings are needed. Blankets may make the person feel warm and cause restlessness.

Elimination

Dying persons may have urinary and anal incontinence. Waterproof bed protectors are used. Perineal care is given as necessary. Some persons are constipated and have urinary retention. Doctors may order enemas and Foley catheters.

Comfort and Positioning

Measures are taken to promote comfort. Good skin care, personal hygiene, back massages, and oral hygiene help to increase comfort. Some persons have severe pain. The nurse gives pain medications ordered by the doctor. Frequent position changes promote comfort. So does good body alignment using supportive devices. Care is taken when turning the person. You may need help to turn the person slowly and gently. Persons with breathing difficulties usually prefer semi-Fowler's position.

The Person's Room

The person's room should be as pleasant as possible. It should be well lit and well ventilated. Unnecessary equipment is removed. Some equipment is upsetting to look at (suction machines, drainage containers). If possible, these items are kept out of the person's sight. The room should be near the nurse's station. The person can be watched more carefully.

Mementos, pictures, cards, flowers, religious objects, and other significant items comfort and reassure the person. Arranging them within the person's view is appreciated. The person and family are allowed to arrange the room as they wish. This helps meet the needs of love, belonging, and esteem. The room should be comfortable, pleasant, and reflect the person's choices. This promotes physical and mental comfort.

THE FAMILY

The family is going through a hard time. It may be very hard to find the right words to comfort them. You can show your feelings to the family by being available, courteous, and considerate. Also use touch to show your concern.

The family usually spends a lot of time with their loved one. Normal visiting hours do not apply if the person is dying. You must respect the person's and family's right to privacy. They need as much time together as possible. However, the person's care cannot be neglected just because the family is present. Most facilities let family members help give care. If they do not want to help, you can suggest that they take a break for a beverage or meal.

The family may be very tired, sad, and tearful. They need support and understanding. Watching a loved one die is very painful. So is dealing with the eventual loss of that person. The family is given every possible courtesy and respect. They may find comfort in a visit from a member of the clergy. You need to communicate this request to the nurse immediately.

HOSPICE CARE

Hospice care is an option for the terminally ill (see Chapter 1). Hospices are concerned with the physical, emotional, social, and spiritual needs of dying persons and their families. Care does not focus on cures or with life-saving procedures. Rather, pain relief and comfort measures are stressed. The goal of hospice care is to improve the dying person's quality of life.

A hospice may be part of a health facility or a separate facility. Many hospices offer home care. Follow-up care and support groups for survivors are other hospice services.

LEGAL ISSUES AND QUALITY OF LIFE

Much attention has been given to the right to die. Many people do not want to be kept alive by machines or other measures. Consent must be given for any treatment. Patients and residents make their own decisions when they are able. Some make their wishes known about prolonging death before the time comes.

The Patient Self-Determination Act

The Patient Self-Determination Act gives persons the right to accept or refuse medical treatment. They also have the right to make advance directives. An **advance directive** is a written document stating a person's wishes about health care when that person is no longer able to make his or her own decisions. Advance directives usually prohibit certain types of care if there is no hope of recovery. Living wills and durable power of attorney are common advance directives.

All health care facilities must inform all persons of the right to advance directives on admission. This information must be in writing. The person's medical record must document whether the person has made advance directives. The law also protects the person's quality of care. Quality of care cannot be less because the person has made advance directives.

Living wills A living will is a person's written statement about the use of life-sustaining measures. Life-sustaining measures are those that support or maintain life. Tube feedings, artificial respirators, and cardiopulmonary resuscitation are some examples. These measures and other machines keep the person alive when death is likely. A living will instructs doctors

- Not to start measures that prolong dying
- To remove measures that prolong dying

Durable power of attorney Durable power of attorney for health care is another type of advance directive. The power to make decisions about health care is given to another person. Usually this is a family member or friend. Sometimes it is a lawyer. A person may no longer be able to make decisions about his or her own health care. Then the person with durable power of attorney has the legal authority to do so.

"Do Not Resuscitate" Orders

When death is sudden and unexpected, every effort is made to save the person's life. CPR is started (see Chapter 33) and an emergency *code* is called. Nurses, doctors, and emergency staff rush to the person's bedside. They bring emergency and life-saving equipment with them. CPR and other life-support measures are continued until the person is resuscitated or until the doctor declares the person dead.

Doctors often write *do not resuscitate (DNR)* or *no code* orders for terminally ill persons. This means that no attempts will be made to resuscitate the person. The person will be allowed to die in peace and with dignity. The orders are often written after the person or family has been consulted. Some persons have advance directives that address resuscitation.

Quality of Life

Quality of life is important to patients, residents, and their families. A person has the right to die in peace and with dignity. Box 34-1 contains the dying person's bill of rights. The dying person also has rights under OBRA.

You must protect the person's right to privacy and confidentiality. Remember the person must not be exposed unnecessarily. The person has the right not to have his or her body seen by others. Proper draping and screening procedures are important.

The person and family or other visitors have the right to visit in private. The dying person is likely to be too weak to leave the bed or room. Therefore the roommate may have to leave the room. The nurse will try to work out an arrangement that is satisfactory to both roommates. The dying resident may be moved to a private room. This gives the resident and family privacy. The family can also stay as long as they like. Plus, a roommate's right to privacy is protected.

The right to confidentiality is important. This right is protected before and after death. The person's condition and diagnoses are shared only with those involved with

BOX 33-1 The Dying Person's Bill of Rights

- I have the right to be treated as a living human being until I die.
- I have the right to maintain a sense of hopefulness, however changing its focus may be.
- I have the right to be cared for by those who can maintain a sense of hopefulness, however changing this might be.
- I have the right to express my feelings and emotions about my approaching death, in my own way.
- I have the right to participate in decisions concerning my care.
- I have the right to expect continuing medical and nursing attention even though "cure" goals must be changed to "comfort" goals.
- I have the right not to die alone.
- I have the right to be free from pain.
- I have the right to have my questions answered honestly.
- I have the right not to be deceived.
- I have the right to have help from and for my family accepting my death.
- I have the right to die in peace and dignity.
- I have the right to retain my individuality and not be judged for my decisions, which may be contrary to the beliefs of others.
- I have the right to discuss and enlarge my religious and/or spiritual experiences, regardless of what they may mean to others.
- I have the right to expect that the sanctity of the human body will be respected after death.
- I have the right to be cared for by caring, sensitive, knowledgeable people who will attempt to understand my needs and will be able to gain some satisfaction in helping me face my death.

Modified From Barbus AJ: Am J Nurs 75(1):99, 1975

the person's care. The person's final moments and cause of death are also kept confidential. So are statements, conversations, and family reactions.

The dying person has the right to be free from abuse, mistreatment, and neglect. Some health workers avoid the dying person. They are uncomfortable with death and dying. Others have superstitions or religious beliefs about being near dying people. Abuse and mistreatment may occur. Family members or health workers may be the sources of such actions. The person may be too weak to report the abuse or mistreatment. Or the person may feel that punishment is deserved for needing so much care. The person has the right to receive kind and respectful care before and after death. Be sure to report signs of abuse, mistreatment, or neglect to the nurse.

Freedom of restraint applies to the dying person. Restraints are used only if ordered by the doctor. Dying persons are often too weak to be dangerous to themselves or others.

You must protect the individual's personal possessions. The person may want certain photos and religious items nearby. Religious items may include medals, a rosary, a Bible, a crucifix, candles, and so on. Such items should be provided if possible. The person's property must be protected from loss or damage before and after death. They may be passed on as family treasures or mementos.

Nursing facility residents have the right to a safe and homelike environment. They usually depend on others for safety. All health workers must keep the environment safe and homelike. Remember, the facility is the person's home. Try to keep equipment and supplies out of view. The room should also be free of unpleasant odors and noises. Do your best to keep the room neat and clean.

The right to personal choice is especially important. Remember, the person has the right to be involved in treatment and care. The dying person may refuse treatment. The person may also have a living will. The person may not be mentally able to be involved in treatment decisions. The family or legal representative will act on the person's behalf. The decision may be to allow the person to die with peace and dignity. Choices to refuse treatment or not prolong life need to be respected by the health team.

SIGNS OF DEATH

There are signs of approaching death. They may occur rapidly or slowly.

- Movement, muscle tone, and sensation are lost. This usually starts in the feet and legs. It eventually spreads to the rest of the body. When the mouth muscles relax, the jaw drops. The mouth may stay open. There is often a peaceful facial expression.
- Peristalsis and other gastrointestinal functions slow down. There may be abdominal distention, anal incontinence, impaction, nausea, and vomiting.
- Circulation fails and body temperature rises. The person feels cool or cold, looks pale, and perspires heavily. The pulse is fast, weak, and irregular. Blood pressure starts to fall.
- The respiratory system fails. Cheyne-Stokes, slow, or rapid and shallow respirations are observed. Mucus collects in the respiratory tract. This causes the *death rattle* that is heard.
- Pain decreases as the person loses consciousness. However, some people are conscious until the moment of death.

The signs of death include no pulse, respirations, or blood pressure. The pupils are fixed and dilated. A doctor determines that death has occurred and pronounces the person dead.

CARE OF THE BODY AFTER DEATH

Care of the body after *(post)* death *(mortem)* is called **postmortem** care. A nurse gives postmortem care. You may be asked to assist. The care begins as soon as the doctor pronounces the person dead. Standard Precautions and the Bloodborne Pathogen Standard are followed. You may have contact with infected blood, body fluids, secretions, or excretions.

Postmortem care is done to maintain the body's appearance. Discoloration and skin damage are prevented. Postmortem care also includes gathering valuables and personal items for the family. The right to privacy and the right to be treated with dignity and respect apply after death.

Within 2 to 4 hours after death, rigor mortis develops. **Rigor mortis** is the stiffness or rigidity *(rigor)* of skeletal muscles. It occurs after death *(mortis)*. Postmortem care involves positioning the body in normal alignment before rigor mortis sets in. The family may want to see the body before it is taken to the morgue or funeral home. The body should appear in a comfortable and natural position for this viewing.

In some facilities the body is prepared only for viewing. Postmortem care is completed later by the funeral director.

Repositioning of the body is often required during postmortem care. The repositioning is done to bathe soiled areas and to put the body in good alignment. Movement of the body can cause remaining air in the lungs, stomach, and intestines to be expelled. When air is expelled, the body produces sounds. Do not be alarmed or frightened by these sounds. They are normal and to be expected.

ASSISTING WITH POSTMORTEM CARE

PRE-PROCEDURE

1. Wash your hands.
2. Collect the following:
   - Postmortem kit if used in your facility (shroud, gown, two tags, gauze squares, and safety pins)
   - Valuables list
   - Waterproof bed protectors
   - Wash basin
   - Bath towels
   - Washcloth
   - Tape
   - Dressings
   - Disposable gloves
   - Cotton balls
3. Provide for privacy.
4. Raise the bed to its highest level.

PROCEDURE

5. Make sure the bed is flat.
6. Put on the gloves.
7. Position the body supine. Arms and legs are straight. Place a pillow under the head and shoulders (Fig. 34-1).
8. Close the eyes. Gently pull the eyelids over the eyes. Apply a moistened cotton ball gently over the eyelids if the eyes will not stay closed.
9. Insert dentures if it is facility policy. If not, put them in a labeled denture container.
10. Close the mouth. Place a rolled towel under the chin to support the mouth in the closed position if necessary.
11. Follow facility policy about jewelry. Remove all jewelry except for wedding rings if this is facility policy. List the jewelry that was removed. Place the jewelry and the list in an envelope for the family.
12. Place a cotton ball over the wedding ring. Secure it in place with tape.
13. Remove drainage bottles, bags, and containers. Leave tubes and catheters in place if an autopsy is to be performed. Ask the nurse about removal of tubes.
14. Bathe soiled areas with plain water. Dry thoroughly.
15. Place a bed protector under the buttocks.
16. Remove soiled dressings and replace them with clean ones.
17. Put a clean gown on the body. Make sure the body is positioned as in step 7.
18. Brush and comb the hair if necessary.
19. Fill out the ID tags. Tie one to an ankle or to the right big toe.
20. Cover the body to the shoulders with a sheet if the family will view the body.
21. Gather all of the person's belongings. Put them in a bag labeled with the person's name.
22. Remove all used supplies, equipment, and linens except the shroud and the other ID tag. Make sure the room is neat. Adjust lighting so it is soft.
23. Remove the gloves and wash your hands.
24. Let the family view the body. Provide for privacy. Give the person's belongings to the family.
25. Get a stretcher if the body will be taken to the morgue.
26. Put on another pair of gloves.
27. Place the body on the shroud or cover the body with a sheet after the family has left the room. Apply the shroud as in Figure 34-2.
    a. Bring the top down over the head.
    b. Fold the bottom up over the feet.
    c. Fold the sides over the body.
28. Secure the shroud in place with safety pins or tape.

PROCEDURE—CONT'D

29 Attach the second ID tag to the shroud.

30 Take the body to the morgue:

- **a** Move the body onto the stretcher with the help of co-workers.
- **b** Have the doors to other rooms along the hallway closed.
- **c** Transport the body to the morgue. Leave the denture cup with the body.
- **d** Return the stretcher to its proper place.

31 Leave the body on the bed if it will be taken directly to the funeral home. Leave the denture cup with the body. Close the door or pull privacy curtain around the bed.

POST-PROCEDURE

32 Remove the gloves and wash your hands.

33 Strip the person's unit when the body has been removed. Wear gloves for this step.

34 Wash your hands.

35 Report the following to the nurse:

- The time the body was taken by the funeral director
- What was done with jewelry and personal items
- What was done with dentures

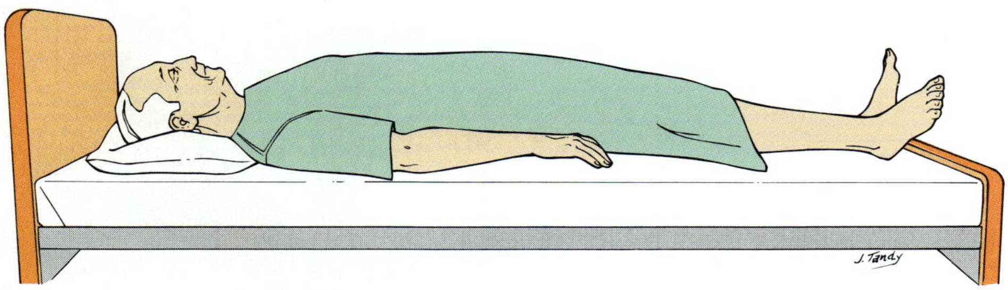

Fig. 34-1 *The body is in the dorsal recumbent position. Arms are straight at the sides. There is a pillow under the head and shoulders.*

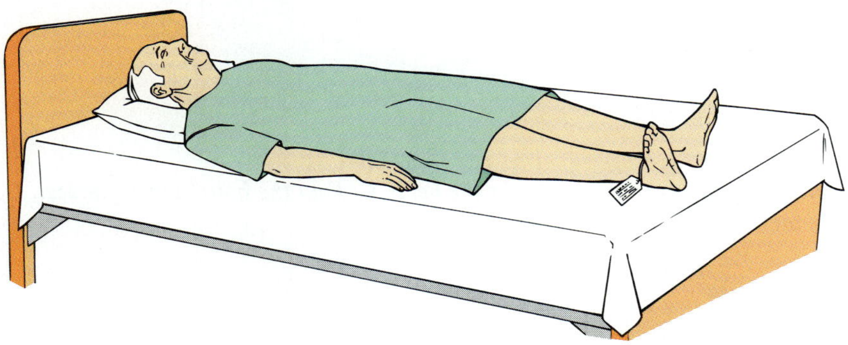

Fig. 34-2 *Applying a shroud. A, Place the body on the shroud.*

Continued.

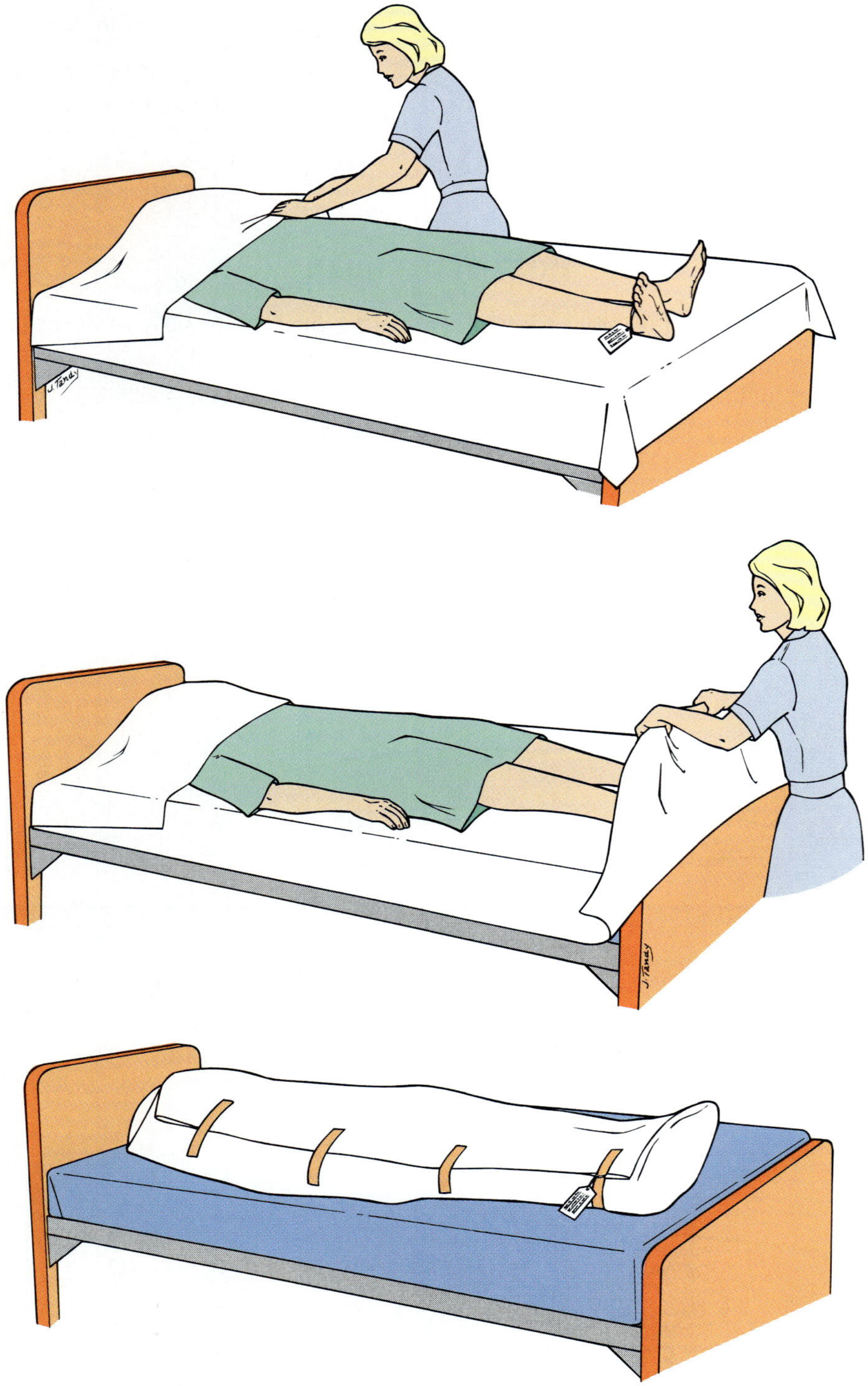

Fig. 34-2—cont'd *B, Bring the top of the shroud down over the head. C, Fold the bottom over the feet. D, Fold the sides over the body, tape or pin the sides together, and attach the ID tag.*

SUMMARY

American society values youth, beauty, and life. The topic of death is usually avoided. Many people die in health facilities. Therefore health workers see death often.

You may be uncomfortable with the subject of death. If so, you will be uncomfortable with the dying person. Some people believe that medicine should keep people alive. These people may be angry and frustrated with the dying person. Certain behaviors are seen when health workers do not feel comfortable with death and dying. They include avoiding the person, nervous talking, hurried care, rough handling, and minimizing the person's needs. You may need to discuss your feelings about death with a nurse, other health workers, or a member of the clergy. This will help you develop a more positive attitude about death.

The nurse uses the nursing process to meet the person's needs. The terminally ill person should be allowed to die with peace and dignity. The person is encouraged to be independent for as long as possible. As the person's condition weakens, the nursing team is needed more and more for care and comfort. Even though the person is dying, basic needs continue.

The health team also is concerned with the dying person's psychological, social, and spiritual comfort. Visits from the clergy are often appreciated. The dying person may like to have family and staff members visit often, sit quietly at the bedside, and use touch. Remember that silence and touch are very effective ways to communicate with the person and family. The person's right to privacy also needs your attention. The right to privacy is protected before and after death.

Postmortem care is given after death. Each facility has its own policies and procedures about care of the body after death. Postmortem care always includes treating the body with dignity and respect, and respecting the right to privacy.

REVIEW QUESTIONS

Circle the best *answer.*

1 Which is *true?*

- **a** Death from terminal illness is sudden and unexpected.
- **b** Doctors know when death will occur.
- **c** An illness is terminal when there is no reasonable hope of recovery.
- **d** All severe injuries result in death.

2 Which psychological forces influence living and dying?

- **a** Hope and the will to live
- **b** Reincarnation and belief in the afterlife
- **c** Denial and anger
- **d** Bargaining and depression

3 These statements relate to attitudes about death. Which is *false?*

- **a** Dying people are often cared for in health facilities.
- **b** Attitudes about death are influenced by religion.
- **c** Infants and toddlers understand death.
- **d** Young children often blame themselves when someone dies.

4 Reincarnation is the belief that

- **a** There is no afterlife
- **b** The spirit or soul is reborn into another human body or another form of life
- **c** The body keeps its physical form in the afterlife
- **d** Only the spirit or soul is present in the afterlife

REVIEW QUESTIONS—CONT'D

5 Children between the ages of 5 and 7 view death as
- **a** Temporary
- **b** Final
- **c** Adults do
- **d** Going to sleep

6 Adults and the elderly usually fear
- **a** Dying alone
- **b** Reincarnation
- **c** The five stages of dying
- **d** All of the above

7 Persons in the stage of denial
- **a** Are angry
- **b** Make "deals" with God
- **c** Are sad and quiet
- **d** Refuse to believe they are dying

8 Jenny Parker is dying. At one point she tried to gain more time. She was in the stage of
- **a** Anger
- **b** Bargaining
- **c** Depression
- **d** Acceptance

9 When caring for Jenny Parker, you should
- **a** Use touch and listening
- **b** Do most of the talking
- **c** Keep the room darkened
- **d** Speak in a loud voice

10 As death nears, the last sense to be lost is
- **a** Sight
- **b** Taste
- **c** Smell
- **d** Hearing

11 Jenny Parker's care includes the following *except*
- **a** Eye care
- **b** Mouth care
- **c** Active range-of-motion exercises
- **d** Position changes

12 Jenny Parker is positioned in
- **a** The supine position
- **b** The Fowler's position
- **c** Good body alignment
- **d** The dorsal recumbent position

13 A "do not resuscitate" order has been written for Jenny Parker. This means that
- **a** CPR will not be done
- **b** She has a living will
- **c** Life-prolonging measures will be carried out
- **d** She will be kept alive as long as possible

14 Which are *not* signs of approaching death?
- **a** Rapid pulse and slowing of gastrointestinal functions
- **b** Loss of movement and muscle tone
- **c** Increased pain and blood pressure
- **d** Cheyne-Stokes respirations and the death rattle

15 The signs of death are
- **a** Convulsions and incontinence
- **b** No pulse, respirations, or blood pressure
- **c** Loss of consciousness and convulsions
- **d** The eyes stay open, there are no muscle movements, and the body is rigid

16 Postmortem care is done
- **a** After rigor mortis sets in
- **b** After the doctor pronounces the person dead
- **c** When the funeral director arrives for the body
- **d** After the family has viewed the body

Answers to these questions are on page 753.

The Home Health Care Assistant

35

OBJECTIVES

- Describe home health care and agencies that employ home health care assistants
- Describe the responsibilities, qualities, and characteristics of the home health care assistant
- List the emergency phone numbers to be kept by the phone
- Identify aspects of the home environment and family relationships that need consideration
- Describe how to save time when doing housekeeping
- Identify infection control measures to be practiced in the home
- Explain how to keep the kitchen and bathroom clean
- Describe your responsibilities in preparing meals and shopping
- Explain how to read and use food labels
- Explain how laundry should be done
- Identify what to record and report to the nurse
- Explain how to provide for your own safety

KEY TERMS

Daily Reference Values (DRVs) The maximum daily intake values for total fat, saturated fat, cholesterol, sodium, carbohydrate, and dietary fiber

Daily Value (DV) How a serving fits into the daily diet; it is expressed in a percentage based on a daily diet of 2,000 calories

Many chronically ill and disabled people are cared for at home. Home care is often preferred for many reasons. Hospital and nursing facility costs are high. Some people do not want to be in a nursing facility. There is a more important reason for home care. Most people are happier and more secure in their own homes.

Home health care aide, home health aide, and *home health care assistant* are some of the titles referring to nursing assistants who give home care.

HOME HEALTH CARE

The person needing home care is assisted with meeting basic needs. Other services may include housekeeping, laundry, shopping, and meal preparation. Visiting Nurse Associations, public health departments, some hospitals, and social service agencies provide home care. Other home health agencies are owned by corporations or private companies. You may work for one of these groups or for the family.

You must always work under the supervision of RNs or doctors. The same ethical and legal guidelines must be followed when working in a hospital, nursing facility, or private home (see Chapter 2). The procedures and rules presented in this book can be practiced in the home. They are performed as directed by the RN or doctor.

You may be needed in the home for many reasons. The family may need help giving care. They may need help to turn, reposition, transfer, or ambulate the person. Some families cannot give care. A job and small children may take the family's time. The spouse or family members may also have physical limits. You may tend to all of the individual's personal care needs. Some assignments include providing a safe, clean living area.

You may care for the same person in one home every day. Or you may be assigned to 2 or 3 people in different homes. Assignments depend on the care and housekeeping required.

Persons needing home care vary in age. Infants, young children, teenagers, adults, and elderly persons need home care (Fig. 35-1). Their diseases, disabilities, and conditions also vary. Problems may be acute or chronic. Home care may be needed for a short or long time.

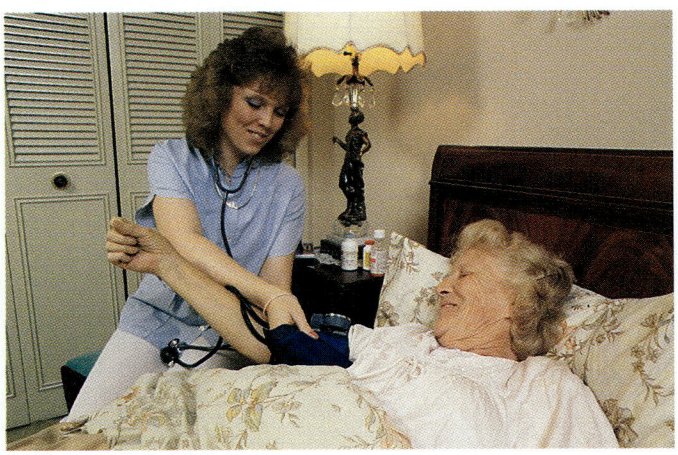

Fig. 35-1 *A home health care assistant caring for a person in the home.*

THE HOME HEALTH CARE ASSISTANT

Home health care assistants provide personal care and home services. Home services depend on the needs of the person and family.

Responsibilities

Your roles, responsibilities, and related legal and ethical guidelines are described in Chapter 2. Besides personal care, you may be assigned to:

- Perform light housekeeping so rooms are clean and neat.
- Do laundry. Clothing and linens are washed, ironed, and mended as needed. Family laundry may also be done.
- Shop for groceries and household items as needed and directed.
- Prepare and serve nutritious meals. This includes planning menus, following special diets, and feeding the person if necessary.
- Clean and use home appliances for personal care and housekeeping duties.

There are limits to the services provided by home health care assistants. Heavy housekeeping is not done. This includes moving heavy furniture, waxing floors, shampooing carpets, washing windows, cleaning rugs or drapes, and carrying firewood, coal, or ash containers. The person may have a doctor's or other appointments. The supervisor's permission is needed before taking the person anywhere outside of the home. It is also needed for providing transportation or running errands for the person or family.

Qualities and Characteristics

Home health care assistants must have the qualities and characteristics described in Chapter 2. Home settings are different from health care facilities. You work alone in the home. An RN can be reached by phone. The RN makes some home visits. However, an RN is not immediately available to give bedside help or to handle emergencies.

You must understand the person's needs. Personal care and other procedures must be performed skillfully and safely. You must be able to work alone without supervision. Self-discipline is essential. You must arrive at homes on time. Organize activities so personal care needs and housekeeping tasks are fulfilled. Avoid temptations. This includes watching television, talking on the telephone, and stopping for an extra cup of coffee. Time is spent on assignments, not visiting with the person or family. Efficient use of time is necessary.

Home health care presents certain situations not found in health facilities. You may be asked to shop. You must be honest and thrifty with the person's money. Items purchased, cost with receipts, total amount spent, and amount of money returned are accurately reported to the person or family. Nursing assistants handle valuables and personal property in health facilities. However, access to the person's property is greater in the home. Home furnishings, appliances, linens, and household items are used for personal care and housekeeping. Personal and family property must be treated with respect. Damage must be prevented. Read the manufacturer's instructions before using any appliance. Clean the appliance after use.

Home care assignments, like any other assignment, must be completed. You must never leave in the middle of an assignment. Nor should you leave before someone from the next shift arrives. Unfortunately, conflicts or problems may occur. Make every effort to finish the assignment. Explain the problem to your supervisor. The supervisor will try to make any needed changes. You must not walk out on the person. That would leave the person in an unsafe situation. Walking out is a most unethical behavior.

Emergency Situations

Emergencies may occur. You must be calm. Good judgment is required. Basic first aid or emergency care may be necessary (see Chapter 33). The appropriate people must be notified. Sometimes your supervisor is called first. At other times, the emergency medical services (EMS) system is activated first. Then the supervisor is called. These telephone numbers are kept by the phone:

- Fire department
- Police department
- Ambulance
- Supervisor
- Doctor
- Hospital
- Responsible family member (home and work numbers)
- Poison control center

The urgency and nature of the situation determine who is notified first. Some situations require simple first aid. Others threaten the life of the person and those in the home. You need to learn the differences between simple and life-threatening emergencies.

Safety hazards in the home must be identified. The supervisor and appropriate family members are informed of safety hazards. You must be ready to act if there is a fire. Identify exits from the home when you start an assignment. Also know how to move the person out of the home. Chapter 8 describes fire safety and accident prevention in the home.

THE HOME ENVIRONMENT

Homes vary in size, cleanliness, and furnishings. Equipment for care and housekeeping also varies. Some homes are luxurious. Others reflect poverty. Whether rich or poor, each person and family is treated with respect, kindness, and dignity. Do not make judgments about the person's life-style, habits, religion, or culture. Such practices are included in the nursing process. They are reflected in meal planning and preparation (see Chapter 17).

You must always respect and protect the person's and family's property. All items, even a scrap of paper, are treated as valuable. An item may not seem important to you. However, it can have great meaning and significance to the person or family.

Family Relationships

Family personalities and attitudes affect the mood in the home. Many family relationships are happy and supportive. However, poor relationships exist. Mental illness, alcoholism, drug addiction, unemployment, delinquency, and physical illness may affect the family. Some families have difficulty adjusting to or accepting the person's illness or disability.

Your supervisor explains the nature of any family problems to you. Do not get involved in family problems. Always maintain a professional manner. Have empathy and be understanding. However, do not give advice, take sides, or make judgments about family conflicts.

The Person's Room

The person may have one room or a section of the home. The person may move about with assistive devices. Sometimes home adjustments are needed. A person may be unable to climb stairs in a two-story home. Then the person's bedroom is moved downstairs. If needed, a hospital bed, commode, overbed table, and other hospital furnishings are bought or rented. A nurse, social worker, physical therapist, and occupational therapist can advise and assist the family in making changes and in obtaining equipment.

Homes do not always have health care equipment and conveniences. Substitutes may be needed for plastic drawsheets, bath basins, supportive devices, trays, and other items. The nurse gives advice about getting substitutes. Imagination and creativity can produce many items for personal care and other procedures (Fig. 35-2).

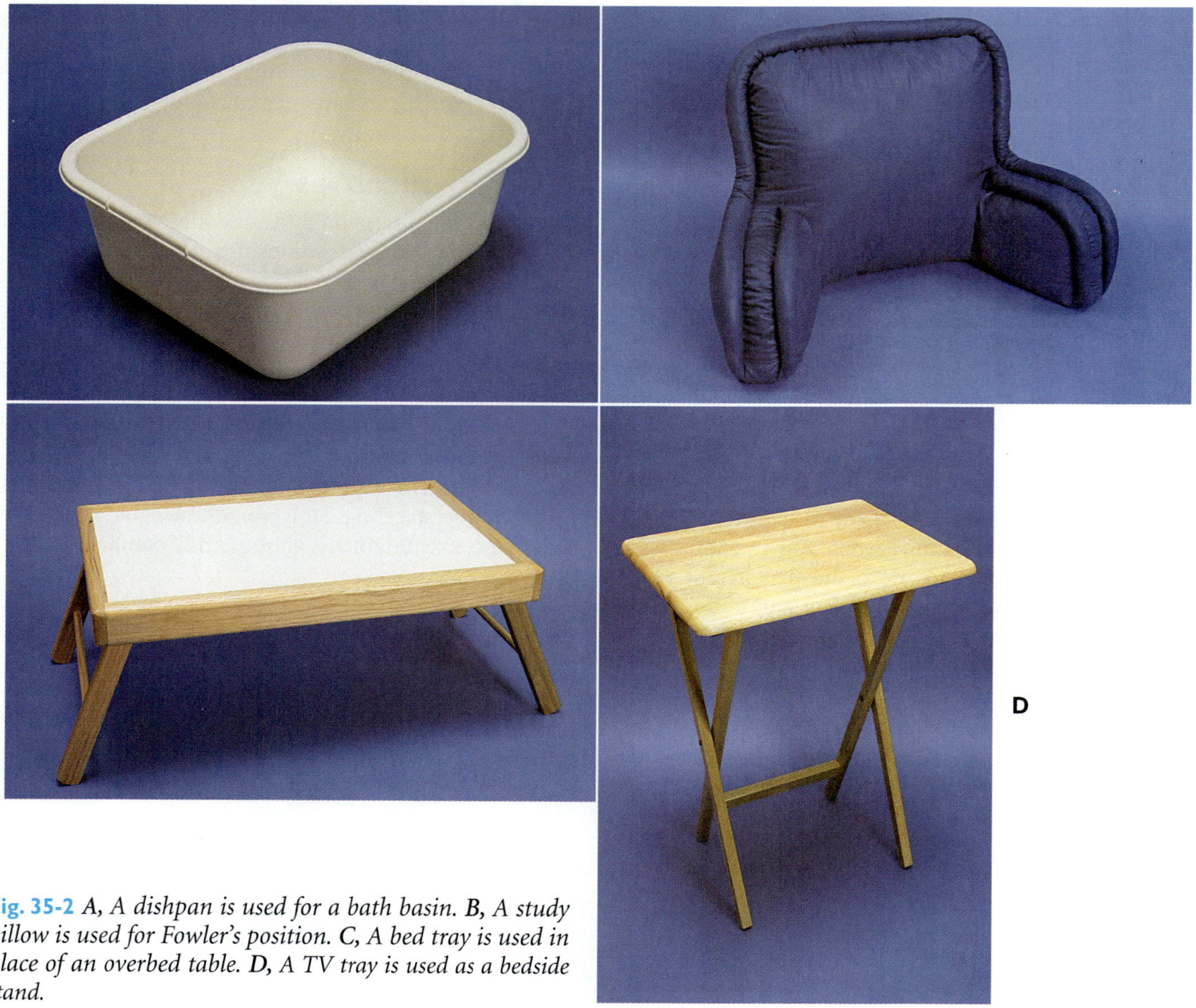

Fig. 35-2 *A, A dishpan is used for a bath basin. B, A study pillow is used for Fowler's position. C, A bed tray is used in place of an overbed table. D, A TV tray is used as a bedside stand.*

HOUSEKEEPING SERVICES

Organizing the person's care and housekeeping assignments is important. The person's care is your first concern. However, you cannot neglect assigned housekeeping duties. Plan carefully. List all the personal care activities and tasks to be done each day. Do housekeeping tasks while the person is sleeping, visiting with family or friends, or watching television.

Cleaning the Home

Housekeeping functions include cleaning the person's room, the kitchen, bathroom, and other rooms. Some tasks are done weekly: vacuuming, washing floors, polishing furniture, and changing bed linens (Fig. 35-3). Others are done daily or many times a day so the home is neat and orderly. Newspapers, toys, and magazines are picked up as needed. Ashtrays and wastebaskets are emptied often. Beds are made and furniture is dusted daily. Daily cleaning usually takes about an hour. Cleaning time depends on the size of the home. Cleaning can be done after personal care. It can also be done when the person is sleeping or doing other things.

Helpful Hints

Home health care may include cleaning, shopping, and preparing meals. Do the following to save time and work efficiently.

- Collect all supplies and items needed for personal care or for a housekeeping task.
- Use a pail, tray, shopping bag, or laundry basket to carry needed supplies and items from room to room (Fig. 35-4).
- Keep paper and pencil in your pocket. Jot down items to buy or replace.
- Secure a shopping list to a bulletin board, refrigerator door, or other handy place. Note food, cleaning supplies, paper products, and other items that must be bought. Ask the family to use the list.
- Wipe up spills and crumbs right away. Hardened spills and foods are difficult to remove.
- Plan major tasks for certain days. Try not to shop, do laundry, vacuum, and wash floors all on the same day.
- Use time well. Personal care can be given, a meal made, or the kitchen cleaned while clothes are in the washer or dryer.

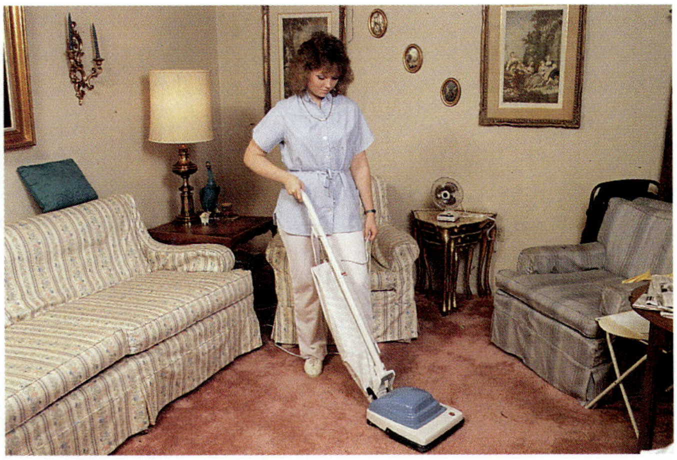

Fig. 35-3 *Some housecleaning tasks are done weekly.*

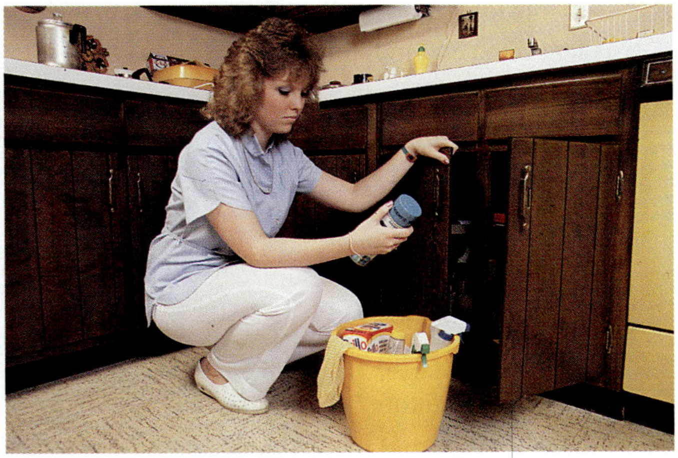

Fig. 35-4 *A pail is used to carry cleaning supplies from one room to another.*

Spotlight On…

Jorge C of Albuquerque, New Mexico, *was working as a student in a home health care clinical rotation when he was asked to help bridge a communication gap with a family that was being followed. The nurses following this family did not speak the mother's native language, so they were unsure if they were correctly picking up signs of infant abuse or neglect going on in the home. To get a clearer picture of the family's situation, the RNs in charge asked Jorge to go along with the home health aide on a family visit and speak to the mother in her native language. After visiting and speaking with the mother, Jorge reported to the RNs that he had not seen or heard any signs of abuse going on in the home.*

Infection Control

You must prevent the spread of microorganisms in the home. The person must also be protected from microbes brought into the home. If the person has an infection, measures are taken to prevent its spread (see Chapter 9). Handwashing is very important. Hands are washed before and after each contact with the person and at other appropriate times. Standard Precautions prevent contact with the person's blood, body fluids, secretions, and excretions. The Bloodborne Pathogen Standard is followed as needed. Other infection control measures include:

- Washing dishes and other eating and cooking utensils
- Cleaning kitchen appliances, counters, tables, and other surfaces
- Dusting furniture
- Vacuuming and mopping floors
- Washing clothes and linens
- Cleaning bathroom fixtures
- Disposing of garbage, leftover food, and other soiled supplies
- Washing fruits and vegetables before storing and eating them
- Handling meat and poultry safely as instructed on safe-handling labels (Fig. 35-5) required by the U.S. Dept. of Agriculture
- Cooking meats and poultry adequately
- Cleaning baby bottles

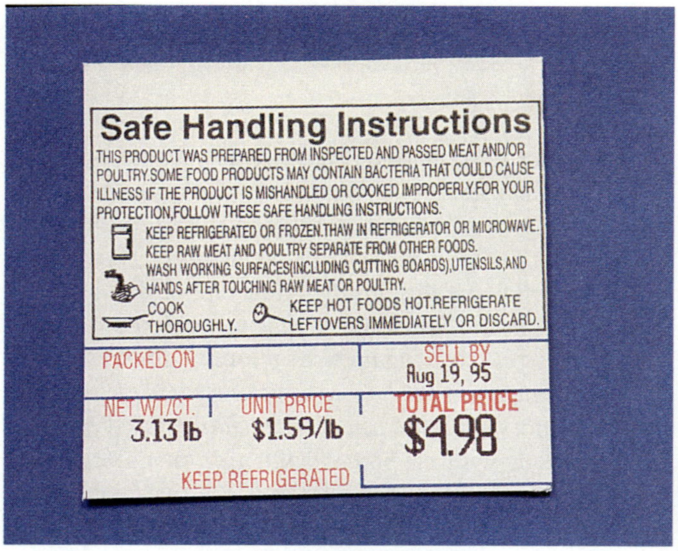

Fig. 35-5 *Safe-handling instructions for meat and poultry required by the U.S. Dept. Agriculture.*

The Kitchen

The kitchen is cleaned more often than any other room. It is cleaned up after each meal. Cleaning the kitchen is not left until the end of the day. Housekeeping tasks include disposing of garbage, storing leftovers, washing dishes, and wiping surfaces. Cleaning floors, cabinets, and drawers is also included.

Garbage consisting of paper, boxes, and cans is placed in either a paper or plastic bag or in recycle bins. Garbage of food or wet articles is placed in a container lined with a plastic bag. If available, use a garbage disposal for food and liquid garbage. Do not put bones in the garbage disposal. Garbage is emptied at least once a day. Some homes have trash compactors. They save storage space by crushing garbage. Trash compactors help keep kitchens fresh and clean and keep garbage hidden from view. Some states and communities recycle paper, glass, plastic, and other substances. Recycling procedures are followed as required.

Leftover food is placed in small containers. The containers are covered with lids, foil, or plastic wrap. Then they are dated. The containers are refrigerated as soon as possible and used within the next 2 to 3 days.

Dishwashing is a method of infection control. If there is no dishwasher, dishes are washed by hand with liquid detergent and hot water. Glasses and cups are washed first. They are followed by silverware, plates, bowls, and then pots and pans. All are rinsed well with hot water and placed in a drainer to dry. Air drying handwashed items is more aseptic than towel drying. If using a dishwasher, rinse dishes before loading them into the dishwasher (Fig. 35-6). Special dishwasher detergent is used. You should wait until there is a full load before turning on the wash cycle. This saves water and electricity. Pots and pans and cast iron, wood, and most plastic items are not washed in a dishwasher. Dishes are put away after they have dried.

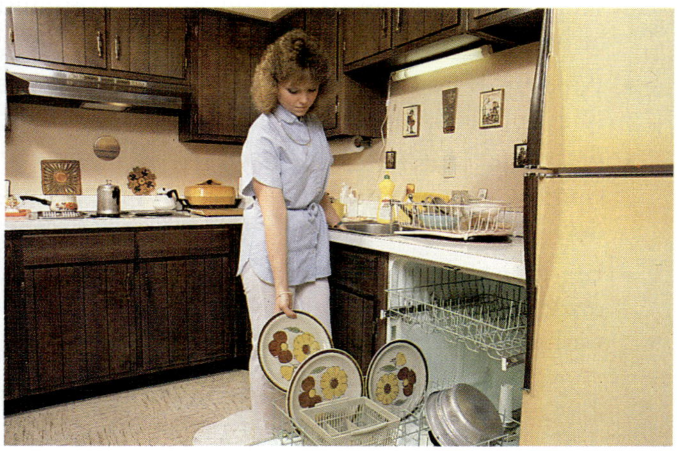

Fig. 35-6 *Dishes are rinsed and then stacked in the dishwasher.*

Countertops, tables, the stove, and the refrigerator are wiped clean. A sponge or dishcloth moistened with warm water and a detergent is used. Grease, spills, and splashes from cooking are thoroughly removed. Some people use liquid surface cleaners after surfaces are wiped. The sink is cleaned with a scouring powder.

Uncarpeted floors are damp-mopped at least weekly. Spills are wiped up right away. A dust mop or broom is used for routine sweeping. A dustpan is used to collect dust and crumbs. Sweeping is done daily or more often if needed.

Kitchen drawers and cabinets and the items in them are cleaned 3 or 4 times a year. Drawers and cabinets are kept orderly by storing and putting items away neatly. Outside surfaces of cabinets and drawers are wiped clean weekly.

The Bathroom

Microorganisms easily grow and spread in bathrooms. Therefore you must maintain a clean bathroom.

Every family member has a role in keeping the bathroom clean. Aseptic measures must be practiced whenever the bathroom is used. These include:

- Flushing the toilet after each use
- Rinsing the sink after washing, shaving, or oral hygiene
- Wiping out the tub or shower after each use
- Removing and disposing of hair from the sink, tub, or shower
- Hanging towels out to dry or placing them in a hamper
- Wiping up water spills

The bathroom is cleaned every day. All surfaces are cleaned (Fig. 35-7). A disinfectant or a solution of water and detergent is used. The surfaces to be cleaned include:

- The toilet bowl, seat, and outside areas
- The floor
- The sides, walls, and curtain or door of the shower or tub
- Towel racks
- Toilet tissue, toothbrush, and soap holders
- The mirror
- The sink
- Windowsills

A vinyl or linoleum floor is mopped. A carpeted floor is vacuumed. The wastebasket is emptied. Clean towels and washcloths are placed on the towel racks. Bathroom windows may be opened for a short time, and air freshener may be used. These help eliminate odors and give a fresh smell to the bathroom. Bath mats, the wastebasket, and the laundry hamper or basket are washed weekly. Finally, toilet and facial tissue are replaced whenever needed.

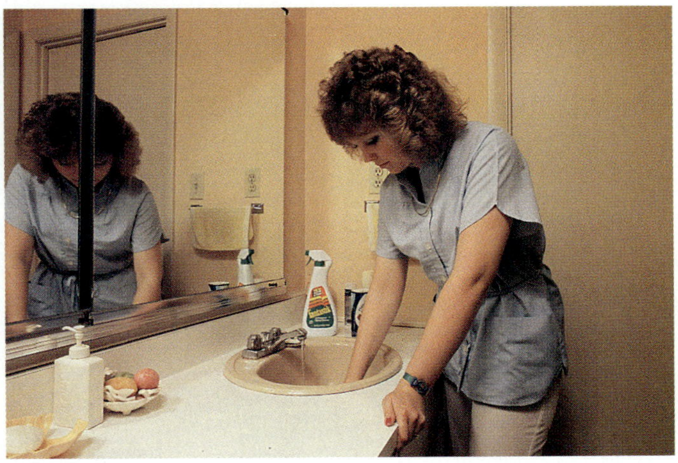

Fig. 35-7 *Bathroom surfaces are cleaned daily to control the spread of microorganisms.*

Preparing Meals and Shopping

You may be asked to plan menus and shop for groceries. You must consider the person's diet, food preferences, and finances. Menus are planned for a full week. Recipes are checked to make sure all ingredients are on hand or are on the shopping list. Money can be saved by checking newspapers for sales and using coupons. All grocery receipts are saved for the person or family member.

Foods must be properly stored when you return from the store. Dairy products and most fresh fruits and vegetables are refrigerated right away. Meats, poultry, fish, and frozen foods are put in the freezer if not for immediate use. Dried, packaged, canned, and bottled foods keep well in cabinets.

Meal planning and preparation requires knowledge of the Food Guide Pyramid, basic nutrition, and cooking methods. A review of Chapter 17 is advised. Also review what foods are allowed on the person's diet. Special eating and digestive problems due to illness, injury, or aging are considered when preparing and serving meals (Fig. 35-8). A good cookbook is a helpful guide for planning and preparing meals.

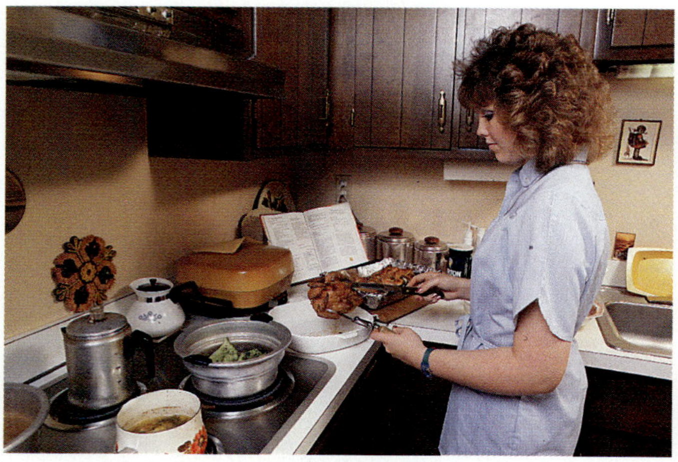

Fig. 35-8 *The person's special needs are considered when preparing meals.*

Food labels The Nutrition Labeling and Education Act of 1990 (NLEA) requires food labeling for almost all foods (Fig. 35-9). Food labels for raw fruits, vegetables, meat, fish, and poultry are found at the point of purchase. That is, the food label is at the fruit, vegetable, or meat counter in the store. Food labels are useful for planning a healthy diet and for following special diets ordered by the doctor. Food labels allow informed, healthy food choices.

The food label (Fig. 35-10) has information about:

- Serving size and how the serving fits into the daily diet
- Total number of calories per serving and the number of calories from fat
- The total amount of fat and the amount of saturated fat
- Amount of cholesterol
- Sodium content
- Total amount of carbohydrates and the amount of dietary fiber and sugars
- Protein
- Vitamins A and C
- Calcium
- Iron

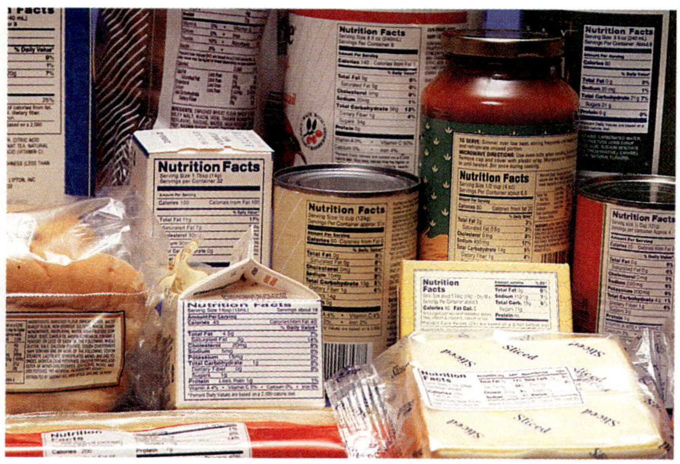

Fig. 35-9 *Food labels are required on most foods.*

How a serving fits into the daily diet is called the **Daily Value (DV).** This helps you understand how a food fits into the daily diet. The Daily Value is expressed in a percent. The percent is based on a daily diet of 2,000 calories. Some food labels show the maximum daily intake values for total fat, saturated fat, cholesterol, sodium, carbohydrate, and dietary fiber. These are **Daily Reference Values (DRVs).** The DV and DRVs are used as follows:

- For a healthy diet, no more than 30 percent of the calories in the daily diet should come from fat.
- Based on a 2,000-calorie diet, there should be no more than 65 grams of fat in the diet.
- The food label in Figure 35-10 shows that one serving has 13 grams of fat or 20 percent of the Daily Value.
- The person can have 52 more grams of fat (80 percent) that day.

Nutrition Facts
Serving Size 1 cup (228g)
Servings Per Container 2

Amount Per Serving

Calories 260 Calories from Fat 120

	% Daily Value*
Total Fat 13g	**20%**
Saturated Fat 5g	**25%**
Cholesterol 30mg	**10%**
Sodium 660mg	**28%**
Total Carbohydrate 31g	**10%**
Dietary Fiber 0g	**0%**
Sugars 5g	
Protein 5g	

Vitamin A 4% • Vitamin C 2%
Calcium 15% • Iron 4%

* Percent Daily Values are based on a 2,000 calorie diet. Your daily values may be higher or lower depending on your calorie needs:

	Calories:	2,000	2,500
Total Fat	Less than	65g	80g
Sat Fat	Less than	20g	25g
Cholesterol	Less than	300mg	300mg
Sodium	Less than	2,400mg	2,400mg
Total Carbohydrate		300g	375g
Dietary Fiber		25g	30g

Calories per gram:
Fat 9 • Carbohydrate 4 • Protein 4

Fig. 35-10 *Information contained on a food label. (From U.S. Food and Drug Administration: FDA consumer: an FDA consumer special report, May 1993.)*

Labels are not required for all foods. Food labels are voluntary for raw fruits, vegetables, meats, fish, and poultry. Labels are not required for:

- Coffee and tea
- Some spices and flavorings
- Ready-to-eat foods prepared on site (deli, bakery, and restaurant food)
- Food produced by small business
- Foods in small packages (the size of Life Savers)

Laundry

Laundry must be protected from damage or discoloration. The person and family are asked about the detergents, bleaches, and fabric softeners to use. Clothing labels are checked for washing instructions (Fig. 35-11). Labels also indicate the need for dry cleaning or hand washing.

Clothes are sorted before washing. White clothes, blends, and dark clothes are separated. Towels and sheets are usually washed separately. Items are checked for spots or stains. Pockets are checked for money, pens, pencils, tissues, and other items. Clothes are buttoned or zipped. Belts and adornments are removed if possible to prevent loss or damage.

Clothing to be ironed is folded neatly to prevent wrinkling and creasing. Permanent press items are promptly removed from the dryer and are folded or put on hangers. Clothing is mended when needed. Freshly laundered and ironed clothing and linens are promptly and neatly returned to drawers and closets.

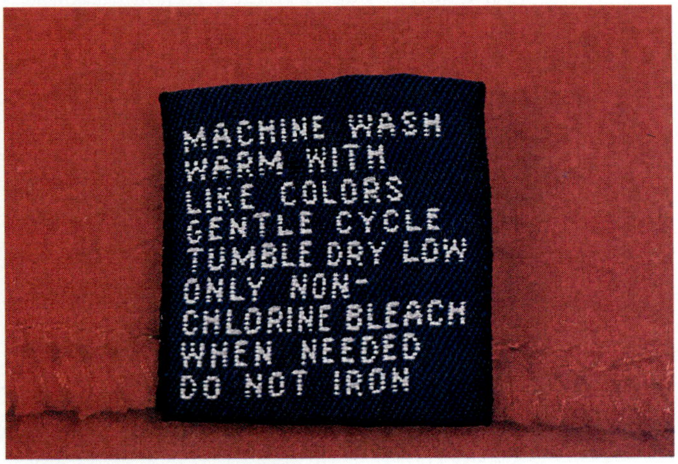

Fig. 35-11 *Clothing labels contain washing instructions.*

REPORTING AND RECORDING

Accurate observations must be made. Observations are reported to the nurse and recorded in the person's records (see Chapter 3). Observations include vital signs, treatments, intake and output, bowel movements, appetite, and skin condition.

You need to keep a record of your activities. The nurse explains what records to keep and how to complete the forms. Some agencies require mileage records. They are needed if agency cars are used or if you are reimbursed for mileage. Records are also kept of the following:

- The time of your arrival at the person's home
- The time a personal care activity or housekeeping task was started and finished
- The time you left the person's home
- The time it took to travel to the next home

YOUR PERSONAL SAFETY

Your personal safety is important. Sometimes you have to go into unsafe areas. You may have to work at night. Box 35-1 contains some common-sense safety tips. Safety should be practiced all the time, not just when you are working.

BOX 35-1 PERSONAL SAFETY PRACTICES

- Know the area you will be visiting. Ask your supervisor about the area.
- Make a "dry run" of the area. Know the route in advance. The shortest route is not always the safest.
- Make sure you have plenty of gas and that the car is in good working order.
- Keep a flashlight with working batteries, flares, a fire extinguisher, and a first aid kit in your car.
- Raise the hood and use the flares if the car breaks down. Stay in the car and call the police if you have a cellular phone. If someone stops by to help, ask that person to call the police.
- Check for places to park. Choose a well-lit area. If using a parking garage, park near entrances, exits, and on the lower level. Try to get close to the attendant if possible. Remember, the closest space near the home is not always the safest for parking.
- Park your car so that you can leave quickly and easily. Park at corners so no one can park in front of you. In parking lots, back in. You can see more from your front windshield than from the back window.
- Lock your car. However, there are times you may consider leaving your car unlocked. If you need to get in the car fast, you do not want to fumble with keys. Use your judgment. Do not leave anything in the car if you leave it unlocked.
- Have your car key ready when you leave the home. You do not want to be fumbling for keys on the way to or at the car. You want to get into the car quickly.
- Check the back seat before getting into the car. Make sure there is no one in the car. Leave immediately if there is someone in the car.
- Lock car doors when you get in the car and keep windows rolled up.
- Keep purses and other valuables under the seat or near your side. Do not leave them on the seat. They are an easy target for smash-and-grab robberies.
- Use well-lit and busy streets if you have to walk. Avoid vacant lots, alleys, wooded areas, and construction sites. Again, the shortest way is not always the safest.
- Note the location of phone booths or carry a cellular phone. Know your location and keep phone calls simple.
- Go to a police or fire station or a store if you think you are being followed.
- Carry money for phone calls and for bus, train, or taxi fairs. Have money in your pocket so you do not have to fumble with a purse or wallet.
- Stand with others and near the ticket booth if using public transportation. Sit near the driver or conductor.
- Do not hitchhike or pick up hitchhikers.
- Try not to go alone. If policy permits, take another staff member with you.
- Let someone know where you are at all times. Let someone know when you are leaving a home and when you arrive at the next assignment. If you do not call in when expected, someone will know that something is wrong.

BOX 35-1 Personal Safety Practices—cont'd

- Make it known that you do not carry drugs, needles, or syringes.
- Do not carry valuables with you. Leave them at home, at the agency, or in the trunk of the car. If someone wants what you have with you, give it. The only thing of value is *you.*
- Carry wallets and purses safely. A wallet should be in an inside coat or pants pocket. Never carry a wallet in the rear pocket. Keep a firm grip on a purse and keep it close to your body (Fig. 35-12).
- Do not wear headphones when walking. They keep you from hearing cars and people around you.
- Carry a whistle or shriek alarm.
- Scream as loud and as long as you can. Keep screaming. Both men and women should scream.
- Use your car keys as a weapon. Carry them in your strong hand and have one key extended (Fig. 35-13). Hold the key firmly. If you are attacked, go for the person's face. Use the key to slash the person's face. Do not use poking motions. Also, do not try for a specific target because you might miss. Do not be shy because your attacker will not be.
- Remember, you have two arms, two hands, two feet, and two knees. This means that you can attack from four directions at once. Do not be shy—your attacker will not be. Push, pull, yank, and so on. You can attack the genital area of either a man or woman.
- Use your thumbs as weapons. Go for the eyes and push hard.
- Carry a travel size of aerosol hair spray. Go for the face.

Modified from McLean County Sheriff's Department, Bloomington, IL, and the Illinois Criminal Justice Information Authority.

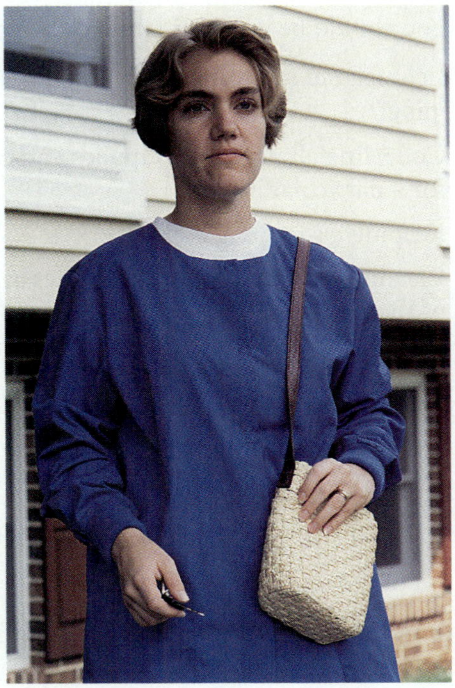

Fig. 35-12 *The nursing assistant has a firm grip on her purse and holds it close to her body.*

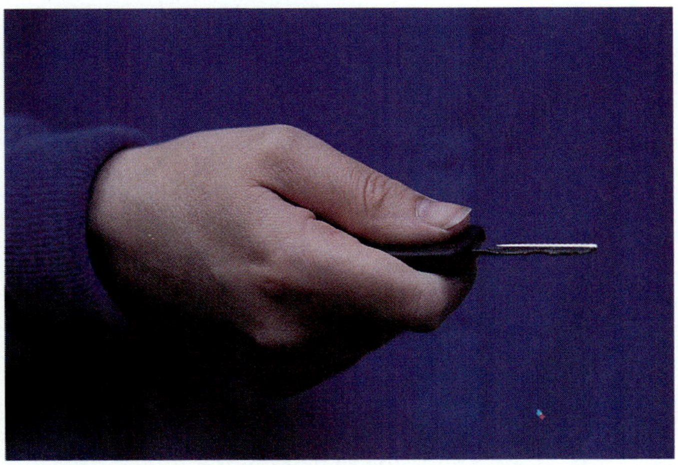

Fig. 35-13 *Car keys are held so that a key can be used as a weapon.*

Summary

Home health care offers many challenges. An RN directs and supervises your work. However, the RN is not in the home for immediate guidance and assistance. You must be able to work alone. Personal care procedures are performed the same way in the home as in health facilities. However, you may not have health care equipment to use. Be creative and use what is available.

Personal care is your first priority. Housekeeping may be part of your assignment. Activities are organized to allow enough time for personal care and housekeeping tasks. A safe, clean living environment is maintained for the person. The person's home and property are treated with care and respect. The home is not reorganized and rearranged to meet your likes and needs.

The person's family also deserves consideration. Family relationships can be loving and healthy. Sometimes there are conflicts among family members. You need to be aware of any family problems. However, you should not get personally involved with the family or their problems.

Review Questions

Circle the best *answer.*

1 Home health care involves
- a Personal care and housekeeping tasks
- b Emergency medical care and rehabilitation
- c Housekeeping and laundry services
- d Personal care and baby-sitting services

2 You are caring for 38-year-old Kathy Kane. A car accident left her a quadriplegic. When caring for Kathy, you can do all of the following *except*
- a Do light housekeeping
- b Give medications
- c Do the laundry
- d Prepare meals

3 Kathy Kane's parents ask for help with the following. Which can you do?
- a Heavy housework
- b Family errands
- c Provide family members with transportation
- d Shop for groceries

4 As a home health care assistant, you must be
- a Able to solve family quarrels
- b Honest and able to work alone
- c Able to meet all of the needs of the person and family
- d Able to give advice about family matters

5 Which is *false?*
- a Each person and family member is treated with respect, kindness, and dignity.
- b Cultural and religious practices are respected.
- c You should get involved with family problems.
- d You should be aware of family problems.

6 Which will *not* save time when doing housekeeping?
- a Collecting all necessary supplies and equipment for a particular activity
- b Keeping a shopping list
- c Cleaning spills, surfaces, and dishes at the end of the day
- d Planning major tasks for certain days

7 Infection control measures include
- a Handwashing and washing dishes
- b Dusting and vacuuming
- c Doing the laundry and cleaning the bathroom
- d All of the above

8 The best way to dispose of food and liquid garbage is to
- a Put it in a trash compactor
- b Put it in a garbage disposal
- c Put it in a paper bag
- d Flush it down the toilet

Review Questions—cont'd

9 Which is *true?*

a Leftovers are kept warm on the stove.

b Dishes are washed in cold water.

c Any detergent can be used in a dishwasher.

d Kitchen surfaces are wiped clean as often as necessary.

10 Daily bathroom cleaning does *not* include

a Cleaning all bathroom surfaces

b Cleaning the bath mat, wastebasket, and laundry hamper

c Damp-mopping the floor

d Replacing soiled towels

11 When shopping for groceries, consider

a The person's diet

b Food preferences

c The amount of money for food

d All of the above

12 These statements are about food labels. Which is *true?*

a They are required on all foods.

b They are only used for special diets.

c Information is given about the amount of calories and the amount of fat.

d They include safe-handling instructions.

13 When doing laundry

a Wash light and dark clothes together

b Always use bleach

c Always check labels for washing instructions

d All of the above

14 These statements are about personal safety. Which practice is unsafe?

a Take the shortest route to the person's home.

b Walk in well-lit areas and on busy streets.

c Have your car keys ready when you leave the home.

d Use your car key as a weapon.

15 When parking your car, you should do the following *except*

a Back in if possible

b Park at a corner

c Park near the entrance in a parking garage

d Park as close to the home as possible

Answers to these questions are on page 754.

Medical Terminology

36

OBJECTIVES

- Define the key terms listed in this chapter
- Identify three word elements used in medical terms
- Translate Greek and Latin prefixes and suffixes into English
- Combine word elements into medical terms
- Translate medical terms into English
- Identify the four abdominal regions
- Define the directional terms that describe the positions of the body in relation to other body parts
- Identify the abbreviations used in health care and their meanings

KEY TERMS

abbreviation A shortened form of a word or phrase

combining vowel A vowel added between two roots or a root and a suffix to make pronunciation easier

prefix A word element placed at the beginning of a word to change the meaning of the word

root A word element containing the basic meaning of the word

suffix A word element placed at the end of a root to change the meaning of the word

word element A part of a word

Many people find medical language mysterious and secretive—the private language of doctors and nurses. Yet people use medical terms every day. You probably know the terms *flu, diarrhea, cancer, appendectomy, cardiac,* and *pneumonia.* Health and medicine get a lot of attention on television and in newspapers and magazines. Because of such great news coverage, many medical terms are commonly understood.

Learning medical terminology is important for nursing assistants. As you gain more knowledge and experience, you will understand and use medical terms often and with ease. Learning medical terms for illnesses, diseases, and common things like bruises, baldness, and a "runny nose" can be fun and educational. This chapter introduces medical terminology and the common abbreviations used in health care.

THE WORD ELEMENTS OF MEDICAL TERMS

Like all words, medical terms are made up of parts or **word elements.** These elements are combined in various ways to form medical terms. A term is translated by separating the word into its elements. Important word elements are prefixes, roots, and suffixes.

Prefixes

A **prefix** is a word element placed at the beginning of a word. A prefix changes the meaning of the word. The prefix *olig* (scant, small amount) can be placed before the word *uria* (urine) to make *oliguria.* It means a scant amount of urine. Prefixes are always combined with other word elements. They are never used alone. Most prefixes are Greek or Latin. You need to learn the following prefixes to begin understanding medical terminology.

Prefix	Meaning
a-, an-	without, not, lack of
ab-	away from
ad-	to, toward, near
ante-	before, forward, in front of
anti-	against
auto-	self
bi-	double, two, twice
brady-	slow
circum-	around
contra-	against, opposite
de-	down, from
dia-	across, through, apart
dis-	apart, free from
dys-	bad, difficult, abnormal
ecto-	outer, outside
en-	in, into, within
endo-	inner, inside
epi-	over, on, upon
eryth-	red
eu-	normal, good, well, healthy
ex-	out, out of, from, away from
hemi-	half
hyper-	excessive, too much, high
hypo-	under, decreased, less than normal
in-	in, into, within, not
infra-	within
inter-	between
intro-	into, within
leuk-	white
macro-	large
mal-	bad, illness, disease
meg-	large
micro-	small
mono-	one, single
neo-	new
non-	not
olig-	small, scant
para-	beside, beyond, after
pre-	by, through
peri-	around
poly-	many, much
post-	after, behind
per-	before, in front of, prior to
pro-	before, in front of
re-	again, backward
retro-	backward, behind
semi-	half
sub-	under, beneath
super-	above, over, excess
supra-	above, over
tach-	fast, rapid
trans-	across
uni-	one

Roots

The **root** contains the basic meaning of the word. It is combined with another root, with prefixes, and with suffixes in various combinations to form a medical term. Like prefixes, roots are mainly from the Greek and Latin languages.

A vowel may be added when two roots are combined or when a suffix is added to a root. The vowel is called a **combining vowel** and is usually an *o*. An *i* is sometimes used. An *i* is used when there is no vowel between the two combined roots or between the root and the suffix. A combining vowel makes pronunciation easier.

The most common roots and their combining vowels are listed here.

Root (combining vowel)	Meaning
abdomin (o)	abdomen
aden (o)	gland
adren (o)	adrenal gland
angi (o)	vessel
arterio	artery
arthr (o)	joint
broncho	bronchus, bronchi
card, cardi (o)	heart
cephal (o)	head
chole, chol(o)	bile
chondr (o)	cartilage
colo	colon, large intestine
cost (o)	rib

Root (combining vowel)	Meaning
crani (o)	skull
cyan (o)	blue
cyst (o)	bladder, cyst
cyt (o)	cell
dent (o)	tooth
derma	skin
duoden (o)	duodenum
encephal (o)	brain
enter (o)	intestines
fibr (o)	fiber, fibrous
gastr (o)	stomach
gloss (o)	tongue
gluc (o)	sweetness, glucose
glyc (o)	sugar
gyn, gyne, gyneco	woman
hem, hema, hemo, hemat (o)	blood
hepat (o)	liver
hydr (o)	water
hyster (o)	uterus
ile (o), ili (o)	ileum
laparo	abdomen, loin, or flank
laryng (o)	larynx
lith (o)	stone
mamm (o)	breast, mammary gland
mast (o)	mammary gland, breast
meno	menstruation
my (o)	muscle
myel (o)	spinal cord, bone marrow
necro	death
nephr (o)	kidney
neur (o)	nerve
ocul (o)	eye
oophor (o)	ovary
ophthalm (o)	eye
orth (o)	straight, normal, correct
oste (o)	bone
ot (o)	ear
ped (o)	child, foot
pharyng (o)	pharynx
phleb (o)	vein
pnea	breathing, respiration
pneum (o)	lung, air, gas
proct (o)	rectum
psych (o)	mind
pulmo	lung
py (o)	pus
rect (o)	rectum
rhin (o)	nose
salping (o)	eustachian tube, uterine tube
splen (o)	spleen
sten (o)	narrow, constriction
stern (o)	sternum
stomat (o)	mouth
therm (o)	heat
thoraco	chest
thromb (o)	clot, thrombus
thyr (o)	thyroid
toxic (o)	poison, poisonous
toxo	poison
trache (o)	trachea
urethr (o)	urethra
urin (o)	urine
uro	urine, urinary tract, urination
uter (o)	uterus
vas (o)	blood vessel, vas deferens
ven (o)	vein
vertebr (o)	spine, vertebrae

Suffixes

A **suffix** is placed at the end of a root to change the meaning of the word. Suffixes cannot be used alone. Like prefixes and roots, they are from Greek and Latin. When translating medical terms, begin with the suffix.

A combining vowel is needed if the root ends with a consonant. If the root ends with a vowel and the suffix begins with a vowel, the vowel at the end of the root is dropped. For example, the term *nephritis* means inflammation of the kidney. It was formed by combining *nephro* (kidney) and *itis* (inflammation). The *o* in *nephro* was dropped because the suffix began with a vowel.

You need to learn the suffixes listed in this chapter.

Suffix	Meaning
-algia	pain
-asis	condition, usually abnormal
-cele	hernia, herniation, pouching
-centesis	puncture and aspiration of
-cyte	cell
-ectasis	dilation, stretching
-ectomy	excision, removal of
-emia	blood condition
-genesis	development, production, creation
-genic	producing, causing
-gram	record
-graph	a diagram, a recording instrument
-graphy	making a recording
-iasis	condition of
-ism	a condition
-itis	inflammation
-logy	the study of
-lysis	destruction of, decomposition
-megaly	enlargement
-meter	measuring instrument
-metry	measurement
-oma	tumor
-osis	condition
-pathy	disease
-penia	lack, deficiency

Suffix	Meaning
-phasia	speaking
-phobia	an exaggerated fear
-plasty	surgical repair or reshaping
-plegia	paralysis
-ptosis	falling, sagging, dropping, down
-rrhage, -rrhagia	excessive flow
-rrhaphy	stitching, suturing
-rrhea	profuse flow, discharge
-scope	examination instrument
-scopy	examination using a scope
-stasis	maintenance, maintaining a constant level
-stomy, -ostomy	creation of an opening
-tomy, -otomy	incision, cutting into
-uria	condition of the urine

Combining Word Elements

Medical terms are formed by combining word elements. A root can be combined with prefixes, roots, or suffixes. The prefix *dys* (difficult) can be combined with the root *pnea* (breathing). This forms the term *dyspnea*, meaning difficulty in breathing.

Roots can be combined with suffixes. The root *mast* (breast) combined with the suffix *ectomy* (excision or removal) forms the term *mastectomy*. It means the removal of a breast.

Combining a prefix, root, and suffix is another way to form medical terms. *Endocarditis* consists of the prefix *endo* (inner), the root *card* (heart), and the suffix *itis* (inflammation). *Endocarditis* means inflammation of the inner part of the heart.

There are more complex combinations of prefixes, roots, and suffixes.

- Two prefixes, a root, and a suffix
- A prefix, two roots, and a suffix
- Two roots and a suffix

The important things to remember are that prefixes always come before roots and suffixes always come after roots. You can practice forming medical terms by combining the word elements listed in this chapter.

ABDOMINAL REGIONS

The abdomen is divided into regions in order to help describe the location of body structures, pain, or discomfort. The four regions (quadrants) are shown in Figure 36-1. The regions are the

- Right upper quadrant (RUQ)
- Left upper quadrant (LUQ)
- Right lower quadrant (RLQ)
- Left lower quadrant (LLQ)

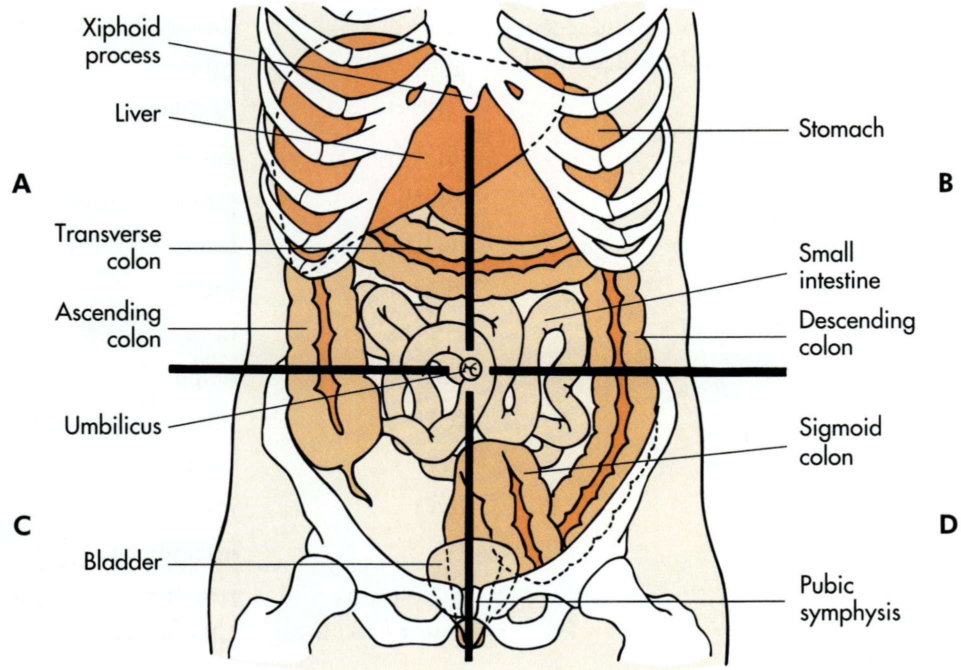

Fig. 36-1 *The four regions of the abdomen.* ***A,*** *Right upper quadrant.* ***B,*** *Left upper quadrant.* ***C,*** *Right lower quadrant.* ***D,*** *Left lower quadrant.*

DIRECTIONAL TERMS

Certain terms are often used to describe the position of one body part in relation to another. These terms give the direction of the body part when a person is standing and facing forward. The following directional terms are derived from some of the prefixes listed in this chapter:

- *Anterior (ventral)*—located at or toward the front of the body or body part
- *Distal*—the part farthest from the center or from the point of attachment
- *Lateral*—relating to or located at the side of the body or body part
- *Medial*—relating to or located at or near the middle or midline of the body or body part
- *Posterior (dorsal)*—located at or toward the back of the body or body part
- *Proximal*—the part nearest to the center or to the point of origin

ABBREVIATIONS

Abbreviations are shortened forms of words or phrases. They are often used in written communication to save time and space. Some facilities use abbreviations other than the ones listed here. Most facilities have a list of the abbreviations they accept. You should get the list when you are hired and use only the abbreviations accepted by that facility. If you are unsure if an abbreviation is acceptable, write the term out in full to communicate accurately.

Abbreviation	Meaning
abd	abdomen
ac	before meals
ADL	activities of daily living
ad lib	as desired
Adm (adm)	admitted or admission
AM (am)	morning
amb	ambulatory
amt	amount
ap	apical
approx	approximately
bid	twice a day
BM (bm)	bowel movement
BP	blood pressure
BRP	bathroom privileges
$\bar{c}$	with
C	centigrade
Ca	cancer, calcium
CA	cancer
Cath	catheter
CBC	complete blood count
CBR	complete bed rest
cc	cubic centimeter
CCU	coronary care unit
CNA	certified nursing assistant
c/o	complains of
CPR	cardiopulmonary resuscitation
dc (d/c)	discontinue
DOA	dead on arrival
DON	director of nursing
drsg	dressing
Dx	diagnosis
ECG (EKG)	electrocardiogram
EEG	electroencephalogram
ER	emergency room
F	Fahrenheit
FBS	fasting blood sugar
FF	force fluids
fl (fld)	fluid
ft	foot or feet
gal	gallon
GB	gallbladder
GI	gastrointestinal
GSW	gunshot wound
h (hr)	hour
H_2O	water
HS (hs)	hour of sleep
ht	height
ICU	intensive care unit
in	inch
I&O	intake and output
IV	intravenous
L	left, liter
Lab	laboratory
lb	pound
liq	liquid
LLQ	left lower quadrant
LMP	last menstrual period
LPN	licensed practical nurse
lt	left
LVN	licensed vocational nurse
LUQ	left upper quadrant
meds	medications
mid noc	midnight
min	minute
ml	milliliter
NA	nursing assistant
neg	negative
nil	none
no	number
noc	night
NPO (npo)	nothing by mouth
O_2	oxygen
OB	obstetrics
OJ	orange juice

Abbreviation	Meaning
OOB	out of bed
OR	operating room
OT	occupational therapy
oz (Oz)	ounce
PAR	postanesthesia room
pc	after meals
Peds	pediatrics
per	by, through
PM (pm)	after noon
po (per os)	by mouth
postop (post op)	postoperative
preop (pre op)	preoperative
prep	preparation
prn	when necessary
Pt (pt)	patient
PT	physical therapy
q	every
qd	every day
qh	every hour
q2h, q3h, etc.	every 2 hours, every 3 hours, and so on
qhs	every night at bedtime
qid	four times a day
qod	every other day
R	rectal temperature; respiration, right
RBC	red blood cell; red blood count
RLQ	right lower quadrant
RN	registered nurse
ROM	range of motion

Abbreviation	Meaning
RR	recovery room
RUQ	right upper quadrant
s	without
SOB	shortness of breath
Spec (spec)	specimen
SSE	soapsuds enema
stat	at once, immediately
Surg	surgery
tbsp	tablespoon
tid	three times a day
TLC	tender loving care
TPR	temperature, pulse, and respirations
tsp	teaspoon
U/a (U/A, u/a)	urinalysis
VS (vs)	vital signs
WBC	white blood cell; white blood count
w/c	wheelchair
wt	weight

Spotlight On…

Gloria T of Rhinelander, Wisconsin, *is a nursing assistant working as a home health aide for a hospital-based home health agency. During a home visit, Gloria noticed that her patient was having radiating chest pain and shortness of breath. Gloria immediately called to report the symptoms to the primary RN. This resulted in the patient being admitted to the hospital ICU with a pneumothorax. The patient was treated and released back to home care after a 3-day hospital stay.*

SUMMARY

Medical terminology involves word elements derived mainly from Greek and Latin. Word elements are prefixes, roots, and suffixes. They are combined in various ways to form medical words. Prefixes go before roots, and suffixes go after roots. They are never used alone. You can practice forming and translating medical words by learning the word elements listed in this chapter. Use a nursing dictionary to check your accuracy.

Knowing commonly accepted abbreviations will also help you communicate with other health workers. Abbreviations save time and space when you make notes about assignments and patient or resident observations. If you are allowed to chart in medical records, use abbreviations accepted by your facility whenever possible.

Review Questions

Fill in the blanks.

1 Word elements used in medical terminology are
  a ____________________
  b ____________________
  c ____________________

2 A ____ is placed at the beginning of a word to change the meaning of the word.

3 A ____ is placed at the end of a word to change the meaning of the word.

4 The four regions of the abdomen are
  a ____________________
  b ____________________
  c ____________________
  d ____________________

Match the item in column A with the item in column B.

Column A	Column B
5 Distal	**a** The part nearest to the center or point of origin
6 Proximal	**b** Relating to or located at the side of the body or body part
7 Anterior (ventral)	**c** Located at or toward the front part of the body or body part
8 Medial	**d** The part farthest from the center or point of attachment
9 Posterior (dorsal)	**e** Located at or toward the back of the body or body part
10 Lateral	**f** Relating to or located at or near the middle or the midline of the body or body part

Write the definition of the following prefixes.

11 a- ____________________
12 dys- ____________________
13 bi- ____________________
14 ab- ____________________
15 trans- ____________________
16 post- ____________________
17 olig- ____________________
18 hyper- ____________________
19 per- ____________________
20 hemi- ____________________
21 hypo- ____________________
22 ad- ____________________

Write the definition of the following suffixes.

23 -algia ____________________
24 -itis ____________________
25 -ostomy ____________________
26 -ectomy ____________________
27 -emia ____________________
28 -osis ____________________
29 -rrhage ____________________
30 -penia ____________________
31 -pathy ____________________
32 -otomy ____________________
33 -rrhea ____________________
34 -plasty ____________________

Write the definition of the following roots.

35 cranio ____________________
36 cardio ____________________
37 mammo ____________________
38 veno ____________________
39 urino ____________________
40 pnea ____________________
41 cyano ____________________
42 arterio ____________________
43 colo ____________________
44 arthro ____________________
45 litho ____________________

REVIEW QUESTIONS—CONT'D

46 gastro ____________________

47 encephalo ____________________

48 gluco ____________________

49 hemo ____________________

50 hystero ____________________

51 hepato ____________________

52 myo ____________________

53 nephro ____________________

54 phlebo ____________________

55 oculo ____________________

56 osteo ____________________

57 neuro ____________________

58 pneumo ____________________

59 toxico ____________________

60 psycho ____________________

61 thoraco ____________________

Match the item in column A with the item in column B.

Column A	Column B
62 Intravenous	**a** Inflammation of a joint
63 Apnea	**b** Blood in the urine
64 Hemiplegia	**c** Excessive flow of blood
65 Thoracotomy	**d** Paralysis on one side
66 Arthritis	**e** Surgical removal of the uterus
67 Bronchitis	**f** No breathing
68 Anuria	**g** Inflammation of the bronchi
69 Hematuria	**h** Incision into the chest
70 Hysterectomy	**i** No urine
71 Hemorrhage	**j** Within a vein

Write the abbreviation for the following terms.

72 Bathroom privileges ____________________

73 As desired ____________________

74 Complains of ____________________

75 Twice a day ____________________

76 Hour of sleep ____________________

77 Intake and output ____________________

78 Nothing by mouth ____________________

79 When necessary ____________________

80 Postoperative ____________________

81 Every ____________________

82 Wheelchair ____________________

83 At once, immediately ____________________

Answers to these questions are on page 754.

ANSWERS TO REVIEW QUESTIONS

CHAPTER 1: *INTRODUCTION TO HEALTH CARE FACILITIES*

1 c
2 c
3 a
4 b
5 a
6 c
7 False
8 True
9 False
10 True
11 True
12 True
13 False
14 True

CHAPTER 2: *THE NURSING ASSISTANT*

1 c
2 b
3 d
4 a
5 c
6 d
7 d
8 a
9 b
10 b
11 d
12 b
13 a
14 b
15 d
16 a
17 a
18 d
19 c
20 a
21 b
22 a
23 b
24 d
25 c
26 b
27 c
28 d
29 b
30 a
31 b
32 a
33 b
34 a

CHAPTER 3: *COMMUNICATING IN THE HEALTH CARE FACILITY*

1 True
2 False
3 False
4 False
5 True
6 False
7 False
8 False
9 True
10 a
11 d
12 b
13 b
14 a
15 c
16 c
17 b
18 c
19 d
20 d
21 c
22 d

CHAPTER 4: *UNDERSTANDING THE PERSONS YOU CARE FOR*

1 c
2 d
3 c
4 b
5 a
6 c
7 a
8 a
9 d
10 a
11 b
12 d
13 c
14 a
15 c
16 a
17 d
18 d

CHAPTER 5: *BODY STRUCTURE AND FUNCTION*

1 a
2 b
3 b
4 d
5 c
6 c
7 d
8 c
9 b
10 a
11 b
12 c
13 d
14 d
15 b

16 a
17 d
18 b
19 b
20 b
21 c
22 d
23 a
24 d
25 a
26 b

CHAPTER 6: *GROWTH AND DEVELOPMENT*

1 b
2 c
3 d
4 b
5 d
6 a
7 b
8 a
9 c
10 b
11 c
12 c
13 c
14 d
15 c
16 a
17 b
18 c
19 a
20 d
21 c

CHAPTER 7: *CARE OF THE ELDERLY*

1 a
2 d
3 c
4 d
5 c
6 a
7 b
8 d
9 c
10 c
11 d
12 c
13 a
14 c
15 a
16 c
17 a
18 b
19 a
20 c

CHAPTER 8: *SAFETY*

1 a
2 d
3 d
4 b
5 c
6 b
7 a
8 a
9 a
10 d
11 d
12 c
13 a
14 b
15 c
16 d
17 a
18 b
19 c
20 b
21 b
22 c
23 a
24 a
25 a
26 b
27 a
28 c
29 d
30 d
31 b
32 a

CHAPTER 9: *PREVENTING INFECTION*

1 True
2 True
3 True
4 True
5 True
6 False
7 False
8 False
9 True
10 True
11 True
12 False
13 True
14 False
15 d
16 a
17 d
18 d
19 b
20 d
21 a
22 b
23 d
24 c
25 c
26 c
27 a
28 d
29 d
30 d
31 a
32 c
33 a
34 d
35 c

CHAPTER 9—continued

36 c
37 a
38 d

CHAPTER 10: *BODY MECHANICS*

1 False
2 True
3 True
4 False
5 True
6 True
7 True
8 True
9 True
10 True
11 True
12 False
13 True
14 True
15 False
16 False
17 False
18 True
19 False
20 True
21 c
22 a
23 a
24 d
25 c

CHAPTER 11: *THE PATIENT/RESIDENT UNIT*

1 b
2 d
3 a
4 d
5 a
6 c
7 True
8 False
9 True
10 False
11 True
12 True

CHAPTER 12: *BEDMAKING*

1 True
2 False
3 False
4 False
5 True
6 False
7 False
8 True
9 True
10 False
11 True
12 False
13 True
14 True
15 True
16 False
17 True
18 True
19 False
20 False

CHAPTER 13: *CLEANLINESS AND SKIN CARE*

1 True
2 False
3 False
4 False
5 False
6 False
7 False
8 True
9 False
10 False
11 False
12 False
13 True
14 True
15 True
16 True
17 True
18 d
19 d
20 b
21 b
22 c
23 c
24 d
25 c

CHAPTER 14: *PERSONAL CARE AND GROOMING*

1 d
2 b
3 c
4 a
5 d
6 c
7 b
8 b
9 d
10 b
11 b
12 a
13 a
14 a

CHAPTER 15: *URINARY ELIMINATION*

1 c
2 b
3 d
4 a
5 b
6 b
7 a
8 a

9 d
10 c
11 d
12 b
13 a
14 c
15 d
16 b

CHAPTER 16: *BOWEL ELIMINATION*

1 a
2 d
3 b
4 d
5 d
6 c
7 d
8 b
9 c
10 a
11 d
12 a

CHAPTER 17: *FOODS AND FLUIDS*

1 b
2 d
3 a
4 a
5 d
6 d
7 c
8 a
9 c
10 d
11 a
12 b
13 c
14 b
15 d
16 a
17 c
18 c
19 b
20 b
21 d
22 d

CHAPTER 18: *MEASUREMENT OF VITAL SIGNS*

1 c
2 b
3 a
4 d
5 c
6 a
7 a
8 c
9 d
10 d
11 b
12 c
13 a
14 b

CHAPTER 19: *EXERCISE AND ACTIVITY*

1 a
2 b
3 c
4 d
5 b
6 c
7 a
8 b
9 c
10 b
11 False
12 False
13 True
14 False
15 True
16 False

CHAPTER 20: *COMFORT, REST, AND SLEEP*

1 a
2 c
3 d
4 d
5 d
6 a
7 c
8 a
9 b
10 d
11 b
12 a
13 b
14 c
15 d
16 b
17 d
18 a
19 c
20 d
21 c
22 d
23 a
24 b
25 d
26 b
27 b
28 a
29 d
30 a

CHAPTER 21: *ADMISSIONS, TRANSFERS, AND DISCHARGES*

1 False
2 True
3 True

CHAPTER 21—continued

4 True
5 False
6 True
7 False
8 False
9 True
10 True
11 True
12 False

CHAPTER 22: *ASSISTING WITH THE PHYSICAL EXAMINATION*

1 b
2 d
3 c
4 b
5 c
6 d

CHAPTER 23: *HEAT AND COLD APPLICATIONS*

1 d
2 b
3 d
4 b
5 d
6 c
7 c
8 a
9 d
10 a
11 d
12 a
13 c
14 a
15 d
16 b

CHAPTER 24: *SPECIAL PROCEDURES AND TREATMENTS*

1 b
2 c
3 a
4 b
5 b
6 c
7 d

CHAPTER 25: *THE PERSON HAVING SURGERY*

1 c
2 d
3 b
4 a
5 a
6 c
7 c
8 a
9 b
10 c
11 d
12 a
13 a
14 c
15 a
16 True
17 False
18 True
19 False
20 False
21 True
22 True
23 False
24 True
25 False
26 False
27 False
28 True
29 True
30 False

CHAPTER 26: *REHABILITATION AND RESTORATIVE CARE*

1 c
2 b
3 a
4 c
5 d
6 a
7 c
8 c
9 a
10 a
11 c
12 a
13 a
14 c

CHAPTER 27: *PERSONS WITH HEARING AND VISION PROBLEMS*

1 b
2 b
3 d
4 a
5 c
6 b
7 c
8 b
9 a
10 a
11 d
12 c
13 b
14 b
15 b
16 b

CHAPTER 28: *COMMON HEALTH PROBLEMS*

1 b
2 a
3 c
4 a
5 d
6 c
7 a
8 a
9 d

10 d
11 d
12 c
13 b
14 a
15 a
16 a
17 a
18 a
19 d
20 b
21 c
22 d
23 a
24 d
25 a
26 b
27 b
28 c
29 a
30 c
31 a
32 d

CHAPTER 29: *MENTAL HEALTH PROBLEMS*

1 b
2 b
3 a
4 c
5 d
6 a
7 c
8 c
9 b
10 c
11 d
12 d

CHAPTER 30: *CONFUSION AND DEMENTIA*

1 b
2 a
3 b
4 d
5 d
6 b
7 a
8 d
9 c
10 a

CHAPTER 31: *SEXUALITY*

1 a
2 d
3 a
4 c
5 b
6 b
7 b
8 d
9 b
10 d
11 b
12 c

CHAPTER 32: *CARING FOR MOTHERS AND NEWBORNS*

1 c
2 d
3 b
4 d
5 d
6 b
7 c
8 c
9 c
10 a
11 c
12 d
13 d
14 a
15 d
16 d
17 b
18 a

CHAPTER 33: *BASIC EMERGENCY CARE*

1 b
2 a
3 b
4 c
5 d
6 c
7 b
8 c
9 b
10 c
11 a
12 d
13 b
14 a
15 c
16 b
17 b
18 c
19 c
20 b
21 c
22 c
23 a
24 a
25 b

CHAPTER 34: *THE DYING PERSON*

1 c
2 a
3 c
4 b
5 b
6 a
7 d
8 b
9 a
10 d
11 c
12 c
13 a
14 c

CHAPTER 34—continued

15 b

16 b

CHAPTER 35: *THE HOME HEALTH CARE ASSISTANT*

1 a

2 b

3 d

4 b

5 c

6 c

7 d

8 b

9 d

10 b

11 d

12 c

13 c

14 a

15 d

CHAPTER 36: *MEDICAL TERMINOLOGY*

1 a Prefix
b Root
c Suffix

2 Prefix

3 Suffix

4 a Right upper quadrant
b Left upper quadrant
c Right lower quadrant
d Left lower quadrant

5 d

6 a

7 c

8 f

9 e

10 b

11 Without or not

12 Bad, difficult, abnormal

13 Double, two, twice

14 Away from

15 Across, over

16 After, behind

17 Scant, small

18 Excessive, too much

19 Before, prior to

20 Half

21 Decreased, less than normal

22 Toward

23 Pain

24 Inflammation

25 Creation of an opening

26 Removal of, excision

27 Blood condition

28 Condition

29 Excessive flow

30 Lack, deficiency

31 Disease

32 Incision, cutting into

33 Profuse flow, discharge

34 Surgical repair or reshaping

35 Skull

36 Heart

37 Breast

38 Vein

39 Urine

40 Breathing, respiration

41 Blue

42 Artery

43 Colon, large intestine

44 Joint

45 Stone

46 Stomach

47 Brain

48 Glucose, sweetness

49 Blood

50 Uterus

51 Liver

52 Muscle

53 Kidney

54 Vein

55 Eye

56 Bone

57 Nerve

58 Lung

59 Poison

60 Mind

61 Chest

62 j

63 f

64 d

65 h

66 a

67 g

68 i

69 b

70 e

71 c

72 BRP

73 ad lib

74 c/o

75 bid

76 HS (hs)

77 I&O

78 NPO (npo)

79 prn

80 postop (post op)

81 q

82 w/c

83 stat

GLOSSARY

abduction Moving a body part away from the body

abbreviation A shortened form of a word or phrase

acetone Ketone bodies that appear in the urine because of the rapid breakdown of fat for energy

active physical restraint A restraint attached to the person's body and to a stationary (nonmovable) object; movement and access to one's body are restricted

activities of daily living (ADL) Self-care activities a person performs daily to remain independent and to function in society

acute illness A sudden illness from which a person is expected to recover

acute pain Pain that is felt suddenly from injury, disease, trauma, or surgery; it generally lasts less than 6 months

adduction Moving a body part toward the body

admission Official entry of a person into a facility or nursing unit

advance directive A written document stating a person's wishes about health care when that person is no longer able to make his or her own decisions

affect Feelings and emotions

alopecia Loss of hair

AM care Routine care performed before breakfast; early morning care

amputation The removal of all or part of an extremity

anal incontinence The inability to control the passage of feces and gas through the anus

anesthesia The loss of feeling or sensation produced by a drug

anorexia Loss of appetite

antiperspirant A skin care product that reduces the amount of perspiration

anxiety A vague, uneasy feeling that occurs in response to stress

aphasia The inability *(a)* to speak *(phasia)*

apical-radial pulse Taking the apical and radial pulses at the same time

apnea The lack or absence of *(a)* breathing *(pnea)*

artery A blood vessel that carries blood away from the heart

arthritis Joint *(arthr)* inflammation *(itis)*

asepsis Being free of disease-producing microorganisms

aspiration Breathing fluid or an object into the lungs

assault Intentionally attempting or threatening to touch a person's body without the person's consent

atelectasis The collapse of a portion of the lung

atrophy A decrease in size or a wasting away of tissue

autoclave A pressurized steam sterilizer

base of support The area on which an object rests

battery Unauthorized touching of a person's body without the person's consent

bedsore A decubitus ulcer; a pressure sore; a pressure ulcer

benign tumor A tumor that grows slowly and within a localized area

biohazardous waste Items contaminated with blood, body fluids, or body substances and that may be harmful to others; bio means life and hazardous means dangerous or harmful

bisexual A person who is attracted to people of both sexes

blood pressure The amount of force exerted against the walls of an artery by the blood

body alignment The way in which body parts are aligned with one another; posture

body language Facial expressions, gestures, posture, and body movements that send messages to others

body mechanics Using the body in an efficient and careful way

body temperature The amount of heat in the body that is a balance between the amount of heat produced and the amount lost by the body

bradycardia A slow *(brady)* heart rate *(cardia);* the rate is less than 60 beats per minute

bradypnea Slow *(brady)* breathing *(pnea);* the respiratory rate is less than 10 respirations per minute

braille A method of writing for the blind; raised dots are arranged to represent each letter of the alphabet; the first 10 letters represent the numbers 1 through 9

calorie The amount of energy produced from the burning of food by the body

cancer Malignant tumor

capillary A tiny blood vessel; food, oxygen, and other substances pass from the capillaries to the cells

cardiac arrest The heart and breathing stop suddenly and without warning

carrier A human being or animal that is a reservoir for microorganisms but does not have signs and symptoms of infection

case management A nursing care pattern; a case manager (an RN) coordinates a person's care from admission through discharge and into the home setting

caster A small wheel made of rubber or plastic

catheter A tube used to drain or inject fluid through a body opening

catheterization The process of inserting a catheter

cell The basic unit of body structure

chart Another term for the medical record

Cheyne-Stokes A pattern of breathing in which respirations gradually increase in rate and depth and then become shallow and slow; breathing may stop for 10 to 20 seconds

chronic illness An illness, slow or gradual in onset, for which there is no known cure; the illness can be controlled, and complications can be prevented

chronic pain Pain lasting longer than 6 months; it may be constant or occur off and on

chyme Partially digested food and fluid that pass from the stomach into the small intestine

circumcision The surgical removal of foreskin

civil law Laws concerned with relationships between people; private law

clean technique Medical asepsis

closed fracture The bone is broken but the skin is intact; simple fracture

closed wound A wound in which the skin is intact; tissues below the skin are injured

colostomy An artificial opening between the colon and abdominal wall

coma A state of being unaware of one's surroundings and being unable to react or respond to people, places, or things

combining vowel A vowel added between two roots or a root and a suffix to make pronunciation easier

comfort A state of well-being; the person has no physical or emotional pain and is calm and at peace

communicable disease A disease caused by pathogens that are easily spread; a contagious disease

communication The exchange of information; a message sent is received and interpreted by the intended person

compound fracture The bone is broken and has come through the skin; open fracture

compulsion The uncontrolled performance of an act

conscious Awareness of the environment and experiences; the person knows what is happening and can control thoughts and behaviors

constipation The passage of a hard, dry stool

constrict To narrow

contagious disease Communicable disease

contamination The process by which an object or area becomes unclean

contracture The abnormal shortening of a muscle

convulsion Violent and sudden contractions or tremors of muscles; seizure

crime An act that is a violation of a criminal law

criminal law Laws concerned with offenses against the public and society in general; public law

culture The values, beliefs, habits, likes, dislikes, customs, and characteristics of a group that are passed from one generation to the next

cyanosis Bluish discoloration of the skin

Daily Reference Values (DRVs) The maximum daily intake values for total fat, saturated fat, cholesterol, sodium, carbohydrate, and dietary fiber

Daily Value (DV) How a serving fits into the daily diet; it is expressed in a percentage based on a daily diet of 2,000 calories

dandruff The excessive amount of dry, white flakes from the scalp

decubitus ulcer A bedsore, pressure sore, or pressure ulcer

defamation Injuring a person's name and reputation by making false statements to a third person

defecation The process of excreting feces from the rectum through the anus; a bowel movement

defense mechanism An unconscious reaction that blocks unpleasant or threatening feelings

dehiscence The separation of the surgical incision

dehydration A decrease in the amount of water in body tissues

delusion A false belief

delusion of grandeur An exaggerated belief about one's own importance, wealth, power, or talents

delusion of persecution A false belief that one is being mistreated, abused, or harassed

dementia The term used to describe mental disorders caused by changes in the brain

deodorant A skin preparation that masks and controls body odors

development Changes in a person's psychological and social functioning

developmental task That which the person must complete during a stage of development

diabetes mellitus A chronic disease in which the pancreas fails to secrete enough insulin; the body is prevented from using sugar for energy

diarrhea The frequent passage of liquid stools

diastole The period of heart muscle relaxation

diastolic pressure The pressure in the arteries when the heart is at rest

digestion The process of physically and chemically breaking down food so that it can be absorbed for use by the cells

dilate To expand or open wider

disaster A sudden catastrophic event in which many people are injured and killed, and property is destroyed

discharge Official departure of a person from a facility or nursing unit

discomfort To ache, hurt, or be sore; pain

disinfection The process by which pathogens are destroyed

distraction To change the person's center of attention

dorsal recumbent position The supine or backlying examination position; the legs are together

dorsiflexion Bending backward

douche Vaginal irrigation

drawsheet A small sheet placed over the middle of the bottom sheet; it helps keep the mattress and bottom linens clean and dry and can be used to turn and move the person in bed; the cotton drawsheet

dysphagia Difficulty or discomfort *(dys)* in swallowing *(phagia)*

dyspnea Difficult, labored, or painful *(dys)* breathing *(pnea)*

dysuria Painful or difficult *(dys)* urination *(uria)*

edema The swelling of body tissues with water

ego The part of the personality dealing with reality; deals with thoughts, feelings, good sense, and problem solving

elective surgery Scheduled surgery a person chooses to have at a certain time

embolus A blood clot that travels through the vascular system until it lodges in a distant blood vessel

emergency surgery Unscheduled surgery done immediately to save the person's life or limb

emotional illness Mental illness, mental disorder, psychiatric disorder

empathy The ability to see things from another person's point of view

enema The introduction of fluid into the rectum and lower colon

enuresis Urinary incontinence in bed at night

esteem The worth, value, or opinion one has of a person

ethics Knowledge of what is right and wrong conduct

evening care HS care or PM care

evisceration The separation of the surgical incision along with protrusion of abdominal organs

expressive aphasia Difficulty expressing or sending out thoughts

expressive-receptive aphasia Difficulty expressing or sending out thoughts and difficulty receiving information

extension Straightening of a body part

external rotation Turning the joint outward

face mask A device used to administer oxygen; it covers the nose and mouth

false imprisonment Unlawful restraint or restriction of a person's movement

fecal impaction The prolonged retention and accumulation of feces in the rectum

feces The semisolid mass of waste products in the colon

first aid Emergency care given to an ill or injured person before medical help arrives

flatulence The excessive formation of gas in the stomach and intestines

flatus Gas or air in the stomach or intestines

flexion Bending a body part

Foley catheter A catheter that is left in the urinary bladder so urine drains continuously into a collection bag; an indwelling or retention catheter

footdrop Plantar flexion

Fowler's position A semisitting position; the head of the bed is elevated 45° to 60°

fracture A broken bone

fraud Saying or doing something to trick, fool, or deceive another person

friction The rubbing of one surface against another

functional incontinence The involuntary, unpredicted passage of urine from the bladder; the person does not have nervous system or urinary system diseases or injuries

functional nursing A nursing care pattern; nursing personnel are given specific tasks to do for all assigned patients or residents

gait belt A transfer belt

gangrene A condition in which there is death of tissue; tissues become black, cold, and shriveled

gastrostomy A surgically created opening *(stomy)* in the stomach *(gastro)* that allows feeding

gavage Tube feeding

general anesthesia Unconsciousness and the loss of feeling or sensation produced by a drug

geriatrics The branch of medicine concerned with the problems and diseases of old age and the elderly; the care of aging people

germicide A disinfectant applied to skin, tissues, or inanimate objects

gerontology The study of the aging process

glucosuria Sugar *(glucos)* in the urine *(uria);* glycosuria

glycosuria Sugar *(glycos)* in the urine *(uria);* glucosuria

goal That which is desired in or by the person as a result of nursing care

graduate A calibrated container used to measure fluid

ground That which carries leaking electricity to the earth and away from the electrical appliance

growth The physical changes that can be measured and that occur in a steady, orderly manner

guided imagery Creating and focusing on an image

hallucination Seeing, hearing, or feeling something that is not real

health care system Health care agencies that have joined together as one provider of care; include one or more hospitals, nursing facilities, home care agencies, hospice settings, and doctors

health team A group of workers who work together to provide health care for patients and residents

hematuria Blood *(hemat)* in the urine *(uria)*

hemiplegia Paralysis on one side of the body

hemoglobin The substance in red blood cells that carries oxygen and gives blood its color

hemorrhage The excessive loss of blood in a short period of time

heterosexual A person who is attracted to members of the opposite sex

hirsutism Excessive body hair in women and children

home care agency An agency that provides nursing care and assistance to persons in their homes

homosexual A person who has a strong attraction to members of the same sex

horizontal recumbent position The dorsal recumbent position

hormone A chemical substance secreted by the glands into the bloodstream

hospice A health care facility or program for persons dying of terminal illness

host The environment in which microorganisms live and grow; reservoir

hyperextension Excessive straightening of a body part

hyperglycemia High *(hyper)* sugar *(glyc)* in the blood *(emia)*

hypertension Persistent blood pressure measurements above the normal systolic (140 mm Hg) or diastolic (90 mm Hg) pressures

hyperventilation Respirations that are rapid and deeper than normal

hypoglycemia Low *(hypo)* sugar *(glyc)* in the blood *(emia)*

hypotension A condition in which the systolic blood pressure is below 90 mm Hg and the diastolic pressure is below 60 mm Hg

hypoventilation Respirations that are slow, shallow, and sometimes irregular

hs or HS care Care given in the evening at bedtime; evening care or PM care

id The part of the personality at the unconscious level; concerned with pleasure

ileostomy An artificial opening between the ileum (small intestine) and the abdominal wall

immunity Protection against a specific disease

impotence The inability of the male to have an erection

indwelling catheter A retention or Foley catheter

insomnia A chronic condition in which the person cannot sleep or stay asleep throughout the night

intake The amount of fluid taken in by the body

internal rotation Turning the joint inward

intravenous therapy Fluid administered through a needle within a vein; IV, IV therapy, and IV infusion

invasion of privacy A violation of a person's right not to have his or her name, photograph, or private affairs exposed or made public without giving consent

Kardex A type of card file that summarizes information found in the medical record; includes medications, treatments, diagnosis, routine care measures, and special equipment used by the patient or resident

ketone body Acetone

knee-chest position The person kneels and rests the body on the knees and chest; the head is turned to one side, the arms are above the head or flexed at the elbows, the back is straight, and the body is flexed about 90 degrees at the hips

laryngeal mirror An instrument used to examine the mouth, teeth, and throat

lateral position The sidelying position

law A rule of conduct made by a government body

legal That which pertains to a law

libel Defamation through written statements

licensed practical nurse (LPN) An individual who has completed a 1-year nursing program and has passed the licensing examination for practical nurses

lithotomy position The person is in a backlying position, the hips are brought down to the edge of the examination table, the knees are flexed, the hips are externally rotated, and the feet are supported in stirrups

local anesthesia The loss of sensation in a small area

logrolling Turning the person as a unit in alignment with one motion

long-term care facility A health care facility in which persons live and are given nursing care; nursing facility or nursing home

major surgery Complex surgery; the many risks and complications may be life-threatening

malignant tumor A tumor that grows rapidly and invades other tissues; cancer

malpractice Negligence by a professional person

medical asepsis The practices used to remove or destroy pathogens and to prevent their spread from one person or place to another person or place; clean technique

medical diagnosis The identification of a disease or condition by a doctor

medical record A written account of a person's illness and response to the treatment and care given by the health team; chart

menarche The time when menstruation first begins

menopause The time when menstruation stops; it marks the end of the woman's reproductive years

menstruation The process in which the lining of the uterus breaks up and is discharged from the body through the vagina

mental Relating to the mind; something that exists in the mind or is performed by the mind

mental disorder Mental illness; emotional disorder, psychiatric disorder

mental health A state of mind in which the person copes with and adjusts to the stresses of everyday living in ways acceptable to society

mental illness A disturbance in the person's ability to cope or adjust to stress; behavior and functioning are impaired; mental disorder, emotional illness, psychiatric disorder

metabolism The burning of food for heat and energy by the cells

metastasis The spread of cancer to other parts of the body

microbe A microorganism

microorganism A small *(micro)* living plant or animal *(organism)* that cannot be seen without the aid of a microscope; a microbe

micturition The process of emptying the bladder; urination or voiding

minimum data set (MDS) A form used by nurses in nursing facilities to assess a resident's mental, physical, and psychosocial functioning

minor surgery Simple surgery; there are few risks or complications

mitered corner A way of tucking linens under the mattress to help keep them straight and smooth

morning care Care given after breakfast; cleanliness and skin care measures are more thorough at this time

nasal cannula A two-pronged device used to administer oxygen; the prongs are inserted into the nostrils

nasal speculum An instrument used to examine the inside of the nose

need That which is necessary or desirable for maintaining life and mental well-being

negligence An unintentional wrong in which a person fails to act in a reasonable and careful manner and causes harm to a person or to the person's property

nocturia Frequent urination *(uria)* at night *(noct)*

nonpathogen A microorganism that does not usually cause an infection

nonverbal communication Communication that does not involve words

normal flora Microorganisms that usually live and grow in a certain location

nosocomial infection An infection acquired after admission to a health care facility

NREM sleep The stage of sleep when there is no rapid eye movement; nonREM sleep

nursing assistant An individual who gives basic nursing care under the supervision of a registered nurse or an LPN; other titles include nurse's aide, nursing attendant, patient care assistant, health care assistant, and patient care technician

nursing care plan A written guide that gives direction about the nursing care a patient or resident should receive

nursing diagnosis A statement describing a health problem that can be treated by nursing measures

nursing facility A long-term care facility or nursing home

nursing intervention An action or measure taken by a nursing team member to help the person reach a goal

nursing process The method used by nurses to plan and deliver nursing care; it has five steps: assessment, nursing diagnosis, planning, implementation, and evaluation

nursing team Individuals who provide nursing care—registered nurses, LPNs, and nursing assistants

nutrient A substance that is ingested, digested, absorbed, and used by the body

nutrition The many processes involved in the ingestion, digestion, absorption, and use of foods and fluids by the body

objective data Information that can be seen, heard, felt, or smelled by another person; signs

observation Using the senses of sight, hearing, touch, and smell to collect information about a person

obsession A persistent thought or idea

obstetrics The branch of medicine concerned with the care of women during pregnancy, labor, and childbirth, and for the 6 to 8 weeks after birth

oliguria Scant amount *(olig)* of urine *(uria);* usually less than 500 ml in 24 hours

open wound A wound in which the skin is broken

ophthalmoscope A lighted instrument used to examine the internal structures of the eye

oral hygiene Measures performed to keep the mouth and teeth clean; mouth care

organ Groups of tissues with the same function

ostomy The surgical creation of an artificial opening

otitis media Infection *(itis)* of the middle *(media)* ear *(ot)*

otoscope A lighted instrument used to examine the external ear and the eardrum (tympanic membrane)

output The amount of fluid lost by the body

pain Discomfort

panic An intense and sudden feeling of fear, anxiety, terror, or dread

paranoia A disorder *(para)* of the mind *(noia);* false beliefs *(delusions)* and suspicion about a person or situation

paraphrasing Restating the person's message in your own words

paraplegia Paralysis from the waist down; paralysis of the legs

passive physical restraint A restraint near but not directly attached to the person's body; it does not totally restrict freedom of movement and allows access to certain body parts

pathogen A microorganism that is harmful and capable of causing an infection

patient-focused care (PFC) A delivery strategy that uses cross-trained staff and moves services from departments to the bedside

patient/resident pack Personal care equipment provided by the health care facility (wash basin, emesis or kidney basin, bedpan, urinal, water pitcher and glass, soap, and soap dish)

patient/resident unit The furniture and equipment provided for the person by the health care facility

pediatrics The branch of medicine concerned with the growth, development, and care of children ranging in age from the newborn to the adolescent

pediculosis (lice) The infestation with lice

pediculosis capitis The infestation of the scalp *(capitis)* with lice

pediculosis corporis The infestation of the body *(corporis)* with lice

pediculosis pubis The infestation of the pubic *(pubis)* hair with lice

percussion hammer An instrument used to tap body parts to test reflexes

pericare Perineal care

perineal care Cleansing the genital and anal areas

peristalsis Involuntary muscle contractions in the digestive system that move food through the alimentary canal; the alternating contraction and relaxation of intestinal muscles

personal protective equipment Specialized clothing or equipment (gloves, gown, mask, goggles, face shield) worn for protection against a hazard

personality The set of attitudes, values, behaviors, and characteristics of a particular person

phantom pain Pain felt in a body part that is no longer there

phobia Fear, panic, or dread

plantar flexion The foot is bent; footdrop

plaque A thin film that sticks to the teeth; it contains saliva, microorganisms, and other substances

plastic drawsheet A drawsheet made of plastic; it is placed between the bottom sheet and the cotton drawsheet to keep the mattress and bottom linens clean and dry

PM care HS care or evening care

pneumonia Infection of the lung

polyuria The production of abnormally large amounts *(poly)* of urine *(uria)*

postmortem After *(post)* death *(mortem)*

postoperative After the operation or surgery

posture The way in which body parts are aligned with one another; body alignment

prefix A word element placed at the beginning of a word to change the meaning of the word

preoperative Before the operation or surgery

pressure sore An area where the skin and underlying tissues are eroded because of a lack of blood flow; a decubitus ulcer; a bed sore; a pressure ulcer

pressure ulcer A bed sore; a decubitus ulcer; a pressure sore

primary caregiver The person in the child's environment who is mainly responsible for providing or assisting with the child's basic needs

primary nursing A nursing care pattern; a registered nurse is responsible for the total care of persons on a 24-hour basis

pronation Turning downward

prosthesis An artificial replacement for a missing body part

pseudodementia False *(pseudo)* disorder of the mind *(dementia)*

psychiatric disorder Mental illness, mental disorder, emotional disorder

psychiatry The branch of medicine concerned with the diagnosis and treatment of people with mental health problems

psychosis A serious mental disorder; the person does not view or interpret reality correctly

puberty The period when the reproductive organs begin to function and secondary sex characteristics appear

pulse The beat of the heart felt at an artery as a wave of blood passes through the artery

pulse deficit The difference between the apical and radial pulse rates

pulse rate The number of heartbeats or pulses felt in 1 minute

quadriplegia Paralysis from the neck down; paralysis of the arms, legs, and trunk

radiating pain Pain felt at the site of tissue damage and in nearby areas

range of motion The movement of a joint to the extent possible without causing pain

receptive aphasia Difficulty receiving information

recording Writing or charting patient or resident care and observations

reflex An involuntary movement

regional anesthesia The loss of sensation or feeling in a part of the body produced by the injection of a drug; the person does not lose consciousness

registered nurse (RN) An individual who has studied nursing for 2, 3, or 4 years and has passed a licensing examination

rehabilitation The process of restoring the disabled person to the highest level of physical, psychological, social, and economic functioning possible

reincarnation The belief that the spirit or soul is reborn in another human body or in another form of life

relaxation To be free from mental or physical stress

religion Spiritual beliefs, needs, and practices

REM sleep The stage of sleep when there is rapid eye movement

reporting A verbal account of patient or resident care and observations

reservoir The environment in which microorganisms live and grow; the host

resident assessment protocol (RAP) Triggers and guidelines used in developing the comprehensive care plan

respiration The process of supplying the cells with oxygen and removing carbon dioxide from them; the act of breathing air into (inhalation) and out of (exhalation) the lungs

respiratory arrest Breathing stops but the heart still pumps blood for several minutes

rest To be calm, at ease, and relaxed; to be free of anxiety and stress

restraint Any item, object, device, garment, material, or chemical that restricts a person's freedom of movement or access to one's body

retention catheter A Foley or indwelling catheter

reverse Trendelenburg's position The head of the bed is raised, and the foot of the bed is lowered

rigor mortis The stiffness or rigidity *(rigor)* of skeletal muscles that occurs after death *(mortis)*

root A word element containing the basic meaning of the word

rooting reflex The baby turns his or her head when the cheek or mouth is stroked; the head is turned toward the direction of the stimulus and the baby starts to suck

seizure A convulsion

self-actualization Experiencing one's potential

semi-Fowler's position The head of the bed is raised 45°, and the knee portion is raised 15°; or the head of the bed is raised 30°

sex The physical activities involving the organs of reproduction; the activities are done for pleasure or to produce children

sexuality That which relates to one's sex; those physical, psychological, social, cultural, and spiritual factors that affect a person's feelings and attitudes about his or her sex

shearing When skin sticks to a surface and the muscles slide in the direction the body is moving

shock A condition that results when there is not enough blood supply to organs and tissues

sidelying position The lateral position

signs Objective data

Sims' position A sidelying position in which the upper leg is sharply flexed so that it is not on the lower leg and the lower arm is behind the person

slander Defamation through oral statements

sleep A state of unconsciousness, reduced voluntary muscle activity, and lowered metabolism

sphygmomanometer The instrument used to measure blood pressure

spore A bacterium protected by a hard shell that forms around the microorganism

sputum Mucus secreted by the lungs, bronchi, and trachea during respiratory illnesses or disorders

sterile The absence of all microorganisms

sterile technique Surgical asepsis

sterilization The process by which all microorganisms are destroyed

stethoscope An instrument used to listen to the sounds produced by the heart, lungs, and other body organs

stoma An opening; see colostomy and ileostomy

stomatitis Inflammation *(itis)* of the mouth *(stomat)*

stool Feces that have been excreted

stress The response or change in the body caused by any emotional, physical, social, or economic factor

stress incontinence The leakage of small amounts of urine (less than 50 ml)

stressor Any emotional, physical, social, or economic factor that causes stress

stroke A cerebrovascular accident (CVA); blood supply to a part of the brain is suddenly interrupted

subconscious Memory, past experiences, and thoughts of which the person is not aware; they can be easily recalled

subjective data That which is reported by a person and cannot be observed by using the senses; symptoms

suction The process of withdrawing or sucking up fluids

suffix A word element placed at the end of a root to change the meaning of the word

suffocation Termination of breathing that results from lack of oxygen

sundowning Increased signs, symptoms, and behaviors of Alzheimer's disease during hours of darkness

superego The part of the personality concerned with what is right and wrong

supination Turning upward

supine position The backlying or dorsal recumbent position

suppository A cone-shaped solid medication that is inserted into a body opening; it melts at body temperature

surgical asepsis The practices that keep equipment and supplies free of all microorganisms; sterile technique

symptoms Subjective data

system Organs that work together to perform special functions

systole The period of heart muscle contraction

systolic pressure The amount of force it takes to pump blood out of the heart into the arterial circulation

tachycardia A rapid *(tachy)* heart rate *(cardia);* the heart rate is over 100 beats per minute

tachypnea Rapid *(tachy)* breathing *(pnea);* the respiratory rate is usually greater than 24 respirations per minute

tartar Hardened plaque on teeth

team nursing A nursing care pattern; an RN serves as a team leader; RNs, LPNs, and nursing assistants are assigned to care for certain persons

terminal illness An illness or injury for which there is no reasonable expectation of recovery

thrombus A blood clot

tissue A group of cells with the same function

total incontinence The continuous loss of urine from the bladder; the passage of urine cannot be predicted

tort A wrong committed against a person or the person's property

transfer Moving a person from one room, nursing unit, or facility to another

transfer belt A belt used to hold onto a person during a transfer or when walking with the person; a gait belt

transsexual A person who believes that he or she is really a member of the opposite sex

transvestite A person who becomes sexually excited by dressing in the clothes of the opposite sex

Trendelenburg's position The head of the bed is lowered, and the foot of the bed is raised

triggers Clues that direct the caregiver to the appropriate resident assessment protocol (RAP)

tumor A new growth of cells; tumors can be benign or malignant

tuning fork An instrument used to test hearing

umbilical cord The structure that carries blood, oxygen, and nutrients from the mother to the fetus

unconscious Experiences and feelings that cannot be remembered

urge incontinence The involuntary passage of urine after feeling a strong need to void

urgent surgery Surgery necessary for the person's health; it must be done soon to prevent further damage or disease

urinary frequency Voiding at frequent intervals

urinary incontinence The inability to control the passage of urine from the bladder

urinary urgency The need to void immediately

urination The process of emptying the bladder; micturition or voiding

vaccination The administration of a vaccine to produce immunity

vaccine A preparation containing weakened or dead microorganisms

vaginal irrigation The introduction of a fluid into the vagina and the immediate return of the fluid; douche

vaginal speculum An instrument used to open the vagina so that it and the cervix can be examined

vein A blood vessel that carries blood back to the heart

verbal communication Communication that uses the written or spoken word

vertigo Dizziness

vital signs Temperature, pulse, respirations, and blood pressure

voiding Urination or micturition

will A legal statement of how a person's property is to be distributed after the person's death

word element A part of a word

wound An injury to tissue

INDEX

Note that page numbers followed by "f" designate figures and those followed by "t" designate tables.